Contemporary Issues In
BIOETHICS
SECOND EDITION

Contemporary Issues In
BIOETHICS
SECOND EDITION

Edited by

Tom L. Beauchamp and LeRoy Walters
Kennedy Institute of Ethics and Department of Philosophy
Georgetown University

Wadsworth Publishing Company
Belmont, California
A Division of Wadsworth, Inc.

Philosophy Editor: Kenneth King
Production: Del Mar Associates
Cover Design: Neiheisel • Slick

Printed in the United States of America

1 2 3 4 5 6 7 8 9 10 — 86 85 84 83 82

Library of Congress Cataloging in Publication Data

Main entry under title:

Contemporary issues in bioethics.

   Bibliography: p.
   1. Bioethics. I. Beauchamp, Tom L.
II. Walters, LeRoy. [DNLM: 1. Bioethics—Collected
works. 2. Ethics, Medical—Collected works. W 50
C761]
QH332.C66 1982   174′.2   81-22015
ISBN 0-534-01102-0   AACR2

Preface

Recent developments in the biomedical fields have led to considerable moral perplexity about the rights and duties of health professionals and researchers, patients and research subjects. Since about 1970 members of a number of academic disciplines—including biology, medicine, philosophy, religious studies, and law—have become involved in an ongoing discussion of the complex ethical issues raised by these developments. This anthology provides a systematic overview of that discussion: It presents an introduction to ethical theory and a set of carefully selected readings on some of the most important contemporary issues in bioethics.

The essays in this book have been choosen on the basis of their clarity of conceptual and ethical reflection, their teachability, and their significance for current controversies in bioethics. Whenever possible, the essays have been arranged in a debate-like format: Divergent viewpoints have been juxtaposed, so that the reader may explore the strengths and weaknesses of alternative positions on an issue. Each chapter of readings is preceded by an editor's introduction, which sets the essays in context and surveys the major arguments on the chapter topic. At the end of each chapter we have recommended readings and have listed bibliographical resources that contain numerous additional citations.

Although this second edition retains the general structure of the first, the book has been thoroughly revised. Chapter 1 is a completely new introduction to ethical theory written by one of the editors to provide students with a background for understanding the readings and for applying moral philosophy to biomedical issues. In addition, this edition contains new chapters on personhood (Chapter 3), the disclosure of information (Chapter 5), health policy (Chapter 10), and scientific freedom and its limits (Chapter 12).

We owe a great debt of gratitude to several friends who assisted us in the preparation of this edition. Ray Moseley made many suggestions regarding selections, prepared the author identifications, and contributed substantially to the animal research section of Chapter 12. Our assistants, Elizabeth Holmes and Mary Ellen Timbol, typed the introductions and bibliographies and were responsible for preparing the manuscript copy of the entire work. Ms. Holmes and Ms. Timbol, ably assisted by Ellen Aho, Timothy Hodges, Michael Miyazaki, and Kyle Ward, also proofread the pages of the volume. Without the dedicated efforts of these conscientious people, our book quite simply could not have been brought to completion. Our appreciation also goes to the individuals who reviewed this book: Martin Benjamin, Michigan State University; Norman Daniels, Tufts University; Robert G. Friedman, University of Virginia; Jon R. Hendrix, Ball State University; Robert Lipkin, Northwestern University; and Ronald J. Wilburn, University of Pennsylvania.

We also wish to thank Nancy Sjoberg of Del Mar Associates for expertly overseeing the production of this work, and Kenneth King and Sandra Craig of Wadsworth Publishing Company for their helpful editorial advice on a variety of questions. Our research colleagues at the Kennedy Institute of Ethics contributed many suggestions for improving the first edition, and our library and information colleagues kept us abreast of the most recent literature in bioethics. Finally, we acknowledge with gratitude the sustained support provided to the Kennedy Institute by the Joseph P. Kennedy, Jr., Foundation and the personal interest that Sargent and Eunice Kennedy Shriver have devoted to our research and publication efforts.

Washington, D. C.
November 1981

T. L. B.
L. W.

Contents

PART II The Patient-Professional Relationship 117

PART III Life and Death 215

PART IV Allocation and Health Policy   381

PART V Biomedical Research   503

Part I

MORAL AND CONCEPTUAL FOUNDATIONS

1.
Ethical Theory and Bioethics

The moral problems discussed in this book have emerged from professional practice in the fields of clinical medicine, biomedical research, nursing, and in some cases the social and behavioral sciences. The goal of this first chapter is to provide a basis in moral philosophy sufficient for reading and criticizing the essays in the ensuing eleven chapters. Many of these essays are not written by philosophers, of course, and thus an acquaintance with legal theories, psychiatric theories, and the like can often play a role in the understanding of an author's orientation and purposes. Nonetheless, the unifying theme in the volume is that of critical moral reflection, and ethical theory is the field that engages in such reflection.

FUNDAMENTAL PROBLEMS

THE STUDY OF MORALITY

The term "ethical theory" refers to the study of the nature and justification of general ethical principles that can be applied to special areas where moral problems arise. The term "morality," however, is different. It is used to refer to traditions of belief about right and wrong human conduct. Many aspects of morality naturally lead us to classify it as a social institution with a history and a code of learnable rules. Like political constitutions and languages, morality exists before we are instructed in its relevant rules, and we learn its requirements as we grow up. We learn moral rules alongside other important social rules, and this is one reason why it later becomes difficult to distinguish the two. For example, we are constantly reminded in our early years that we must observe such social rules as saying "Please" when we want something and "Thank you" when we receive it. We are also taught that certain things ought or ought not to be done because they affect the interests of other people: "It is better to give than to receive." "Respect the rights of others." These are elementary instructions in morality; they express what society expects of us in terms of taking the interests of other people into account. We thus learn about moral instructions and expectations.

Morality can be studied and developed by a variety of methods. Not all of these methods can correctly be called "ethical theory," but at least some can. In particular four ways of either studying moral beliefs or doing moral philosophy have dominated the literature of ethics. Two of these approaches presumably describe and analyze morality without taking moral positions, and these approaches are therefore called "nonnormative." Two other approaches do involve taking moral positions, and are therefore called "normative." These four approaches, each of which is characterized briefly below, can be summarized as follows:

        A. Nonnormative approaches
          1. Descriptive ethics
          2. Metaethics
        B. Normative approaches
          3. General normative ethics
          4. Applied ethics

It would be a mistake to regard these categories as expressing rigid and always clearly distinguishable differences of approach. They are often undertaken jointly. Nonetheless, when understood as broad polar contrasts exemplifying models of inquiry, these distinctions are important.

First among the two nonnormative fields of inquiry into morality is *descriptive ethics,* or the factual description and explanation of moral behavior and beliefs. Anthropologists, sociologists, and historians who study moral behavior employ this approach when they explore how moral attitudes, codes, and beliefs differ from person to person and from society to society. We often find such descriptions in novels about foreign lands in foreign times. These works dwell in great detail on the sexual practices, codes of honor, and rules governing permissible killing in a society. A more commonplace example is the sociological study of biomedical research involving human subjects and the standards of informed consent used in performing the research (see Chapter 11). Descriptive ethics thus investigates a wide variety of moral beliefs and behavior. Although philosophers do not generally range into descriptive ethics in their work, some have combined descriptive ethics with philosophical ethics, for example, by analyzing the ethical practices of American Indian tribes.

A second nonnormative field, *metaethics,* involves (presumably nonevaluative) analysis of the meanings of central terms in ethics, such as "right," "obligation," "good," "virtue," and "responsibility." The proper analysis of the term "morality" and the distinction between the moral and the nonmoral is a typical example of a metaethical problem. In addition to the analysis of central terms, the structure or logic of moral reasoning is examined in metaethics, including the nature of moral justifications and inferences. (Descriptive ethics and metaethics may, of course, not be the only forms of nonnormative inquiry. In recent years there has been considerable discussion of the biological bases of moral behavior and the ways in which humans do and do not differ from animals. This form of inquiry is obviously different from the study of attitudes, codes, or beliefs.)

General normative ethics attempts to formulate and defend basic principles and virtues governing the moral life. Ideally, any such ethical theory will provide a whole system of moral principles or virtues and reasons for adopting them, and will defend claims about the range of their applicability. In the course of this chapter the most prominent of these theories will be examined in detail, as will the principles of autonomy, justice, and beneficence—three principles that have often played a major role in these theories.

The principles found in general normative ethics are commonly applied to specific moral problems, such as abortion, widespread hunger, racial and sexual discrimination, and research involving human subjects, and this use of ethical theory is referred to as *applied ethics.* Philosophical treatments of medical ethics, engineering ethics, journalistic ethics, jurisprudence, and business ethics all involve an application of general ethical principles to moral problems that arise in these professions. Substantially the same general ethical principles apply to problems across these professional fields and in areas beyond professional ethics as well. One might appeal to principles of justice, for example, in order to illuminate and resolve issues of taxation, health care distribution, criminal punishment, and reverse discrimination (see Chapter 9). Similarly, principles of veracity (truthfulness) apply to debates about secrecy and deception in international politics, misleading advertisements in business ethics, balanced reporting in journalistic ethics, and the disclosure of the nature and extent of an illness to a patient in medical ethics (see Chapter 5).

Applied ethics is the main type of moral philosophy found in the readings in this volume. It has frequently been employed in recent years in contexts of public policy and professional ethics, where an interdisciplinary approach is required. Members of the profession bring experience and technical information to the discussion, while moral philosophers bring familiarity with traditions of ethical reflection, insights into various distinctions and categories that can illuminate moral issues, and skill in probing the presuppositions and implications of positions.

MORAL DILEMMAS AND DISAGREEMENTS

In the teaching of ethics in professional schools, moral problems are often examined through case studies, since these cases can involve dilemmas that require students to identify the moral principles at issue. Several articles in this collection also employ analyses of cases in order to reach their conclusions, and we shall now use the same method to look at moral dilemmas and disagreements.

Moral Dilemmas. In a case presented in Chapter 5, two judges became entangled in apparent moral disagreement when confronted with a murder trial. A woman named Tarasoff had been killed by a man who previously had confided to a psychiatrist his intention to kill her as soon as she returned home from a summer vacation. Owing to obligations of confidentiality between patient and physician, a psychologist and a consulting psychiatrist did not report the threat to the woman or to her family, though they did make one unsuccessful attempt to commit the man to a mental hospital. One judge held that the therapist could not escape liability, saying that, "When a therapist determines, or pursuant to the standards of his profession should determine, that his patient presents a serious danger of violence to another, he incurs an obligation to use reasonable care to protect the intended victim against such danger." Notification of police and direct warnings to the family were mentioned as possible instances of due care. The judge argued that although medical confidentiality must generally be observed by physicians, it was overridden in this particular case by a duty to the possible victim and to the "public interest in safety from violent assault." In the minority opinion, a second judge stated his firm disagreement. He argued that a patient's rights are violated when rules of confidentiality are not observed, that psychiatric treatment would be frustrated by nonobservance, and that patients would subsequently lose confidence in psychiatrists and would fail to provide full disclosures. He also suggested that violent assaults would actually increase because mentally ill persons would be discouraged from seeking psychiatric aid.[1]

The Tarasoff case is an instance of a moral dilemma, for strong moral reasons support the quite opposite conclusions of the two judges. The most difficult and recalcitrant moral controversies that we shall encounter in this volume are almost always similarly dilemmatic. They involve what Guido Calabresi has called "tragic choices." Everyone who has been faced with a difficult decision—such as whether to have an abortion, to have a pet "put to sleep," or to commit a member of one's family to a mental institution—knows through deep anguish what is meant by a personal dilemma. Such dilemmas occur whenever good reasons for mutually exclusive alternatives can be cited; if any one set of reasons is acted upon, outcomes desirable in some respects but undesirable in others will result.

It is important to note that parties on both sides of dilemmatic disagreements can *correctly* marshal moral principles in support of their substantially different conclusions. Most moral dilemmas present a need to balance competing ideal claims in untidy circumstances. The reasons on each side of many moral problems are weighty, and none is obviously the right set of reasons. Indeed, there is a sense in which all the reasons ought to be acted on, for each, considered by itself, is a good reason. Situations involving dilemmas that lead to disagreements can be analyzed as taking one of two forms: (1) Some evidence indicates that an act is morally right, and some evidence indicates that the act is morally wrong, but the evidence on both sides is inconclusive. Abortion, for example, is sometimes said to be a terrible dilemma for women who see the evidence in this way (see Chapter 6). (2) It is clear to the agent that on moral grounds he or she both ought and ought not to perform an act. The question of whether one ought to assist the suicide of a helpless, pain-ridden patient already near death seems to take this form (see Chapter 8).

One possible response to the problem of moral dilemmas and disputes is that we do not have and are not likely ever to have a single ethical theory or a single method for resolving disagreements. In any pluralistic culture there may be many sources of moral value and consequently a pluralism of moral points of view on many issues: bluffing in business deals, providing national health insurance to all citizens, involuntarily committing the mentally disturbed, civil disobedience, etc. If this response is correct, it is obvious why there seem to be intractable moral controversies both inside and outside professional philosophy. On the other hand, there may be ways out of at least some dilemmas and disputes, as we shall now see.

The Resolution of Moral Disagreements. Can we hope—in light of complex dilemmas and other sources of dispute—to resolve moral disagreements? If so, on what principles and procedures should we rely? Probably no single set of considerations will prove consistently reliable as a means of ending disagreement and controversy (and resolutions of cross-cultural conflicts will always be especially elusive). Nonetheless, several methods for dealing constructively with moral disagreements have been employed in the past, and each deserves recognition as a method of easing and perhaps even settling controversies. A number of these methods are exemplified in the readings in this volume.

First, many moral disagreements can be at least partially resolved by obtaining factual information concerning points of moral controversy. It has often been uncritically assumed that moral disputes are (by definition) produced solely by differences over moral principles or their application, and not by a lack of information. This assumption is overly simplistic, however, because disputes over what morally ought or ought not to be done often have nonmoral elements as central ingredients. For example, debates about the allocation of health dollars to preventive and educational measures (see Chapter 9) have often bogged down over factual issues of whether such measures actually function to prevent illness and promote health.

In some cases new information has made possible a move toward negotiation and even resolution of disagreements. New scientific information about the alleged dangers involved in certain kinds of scientific research, for instance, have turned public controversies regarding the risks of science and the rights of scientific researchers in unanticipated directions. In one recent controversy over so-called recombinant DNA research (see Chapter 12), it had been feared that the research might create an organism of pathogenic capability that known antibodies would be unable to combat and that could produce widespread contagion. Accusations of unjustifiable and immoral research were heard in the corridors of certain universities and even congressional hearing rooms, although the researchers contended that the risks were minimal. New scientific information from risk-assessment studies indicating that the research was less dangerous than had been feared had a dramatic effect on the moral and political controversy about the justifiability of the risks to society presented by this scientific research.

Controversies about saccharin, toxic substances in the workplace, IQ research, fluori-dation, and the swine-flu vaccine, among others, have been similarly laced with issues of both values and facts. The arguments used by disagreeing parties may turn on some dispute about liberty or justice and therefore may be primarily moral, but they may also rest on factual disagreements over, for example, the efficacy of a product or treatment. New information may have only a limited bearing on the resolution of some of these controversies, whereas in others it may have a direct and almost overpowering influence. The problem is that rarely, if ever, is all the information obtained that would be sufficient to settle even these factual matters.

Second, controversies have been settled by reaching conceptual or definitional agree-ment over the language used by disputing parties. In some cases stipulation of a definition or a clear explanation of what is meant by a term may prove sufficient, but in other cases agreement cannot be so conveniently achieved. Controversies over the morality of euthanasia, for example, are often needlessly entangled because disputing parties use different senses of the term yet have much invested in their particular definitions. For example, it often happens that one party equates euthanasia with mercy killing and another party equates it with voluntarily elected natural death. Obviously the resulting moral ''controversy'' over ''euthanasia'' is hopelessly embedded in terminological problems (see Chapter 8). There is no common point of contention in such cases, for the parties will be addressing entirely separate issues through their conceptual assumptions. Although conceptual agreement provides no guarantee that a dispute will be settled, it should at least facilitate discussion of the issues. For this reason, many essays in this volume dwell at some length on issues of conceptual analysis. This is especially true of Chapters 2 and 3, where the difficult concepts of person, health, and disease are treated.

Third, resolution of moral problems can be facilitated if disputing parties can come to agreement on a common set of moral principles. If this method requires a complete shift from one starkly different moral point of view to another, agreement will rarely if ever be achieved. Differences that divide persons at the level of their most cherished principles are deep divisions, and conversions are infrequent. Various forms of discussion and negotia-tion can, however, lead to the adoption of a new or changed moral framework that can serve as a common basis for discussion.

For example, Chapter 11 contains a discussion of some of the work of a recent U.S. National Commission appointed to study ethical issues in research involving human subjects. This Commission began its deliberations by unanimously adopting a common framework of moral principles, which provided the general background for deliberations about particular problems. Commissioners developed a framework of three moral princi-ples: respect for persons, beneficence, and justice. These principles were analyzed in detail in the light of contemporary philosophical ethics and were then applied to a wide range of moral problems that confronted the Commission.[2] There is ample evidence in the transcripts of this body's deliberations to indicate that the common framework of moral principles facilitated discussion of the controversies they addressed and led to many agreements that might otherwise have been impossible.

Fourth, resolution of moral controversies can be aided by a method of example and opposed counterexample. Cases or examples favorable to one point of view are brought forward, and counterexamples to these cases are thrown up by a second person against the examples and claims of the first. Such use of example and counterexample serves as a format for weighing the strength of conflicting considerations. This form of debate occurred, for example, when the National Commission mentioned in the preceding paragraph came to consider the level of risk that can justifiably be permitted in scientific research involving children as subjects where no therapuetic benefit is offered to the child (see Chapter 11). On the basis of principles of acceptable risk used in their own previous deliberations, Commissioners were at first inclined to accept the view that only very low risk or "minimal risk" procedures could be justified in the case of children (where "minimal risk" refers analogically to the level of risk present in standard medical examinations of patients). However, examples from the history of medicine were cited that revealed how certain significant diagnostic, therapeutic, and preventive advances in medicine would have been unlikely, or at least retarded, unless procedures that posed a higher level of risk had been employed. Counterexamples of overzealous researchers who placed children at too much risk were then thrown up against these examples, and the debate continued for several months. Eventually a majority of Commissioners abandoned their original view that nontherapeutic research involving more than minimal risk was unjustified. Instead, they accepted the position that a higher level of risk can be justified by the benefits provided to other children, as when a group of terminally ill children become subjects of research in the hope that something will be learned about their disease that can be applied to other children. Once a consensus on this particular issue crystallized, resolution was quickly achieved on the entire moral controversy about the involvement of children as research subjects (although a small minority of Commissioners never agreed).

Fifth and finally, one of the most important methods of philosophical inquiry, that of exposing the inadequacies and unexpected consequences of an argument, can also be brought to bear on moral disagreements. If an argument is inconsistent, then pointing out the inconsistency will change the argument and shift the focus of discussion. There are, in addition, many more subtle ways of attacking an argument than pointing to straightforward inconsistencies. For example, in Chapters 3, 6, and 7 a number of writers have discussed the nature of "persons" when dealing with problems of abortion, fetal rights, and the definition of death. Some of these writers have not appreciated that their arguments about persons—used, for example, to discuss fetuses and those who are irreversibly comatose—were so broad that they carried important but unnoticed implications for both infants and animals. Their arguments implicitly provided reasons they had not noticed for denying rights to infants that adults have, or for granting (or denying) the same rights to fetuses that infants have, and in some cases for granting (or denying) the same rights to animals that infants have. It may, of course, be correct to hold that infants have fewer rights than adults, or that fetuses and animals should be granted the same rights as infants (see Chapter 12 on "Research Involving Animals"). The point is that if a moral argument leads to conclusions that a proponent is not prepared to defend and did not previously anticipate, then part of the argument will have to be changed, and this process may reduce the distance between those who disagree. This style of argument is often supplemented by one or more of the other four ways of reducing moral disagreement. Much of the work published in philosophical journals takes precisely these forms of attacking arguments, using counterexamples, and proposing alternative frameworks of principles.

Much moral disagreement may not be resolvable by any of the five means discussed. Philosophy need not contend that moral disagreements can always be resolved, or even that every rational person must accept the same method for approaching such problems. There is always a possibility of ultimate disagreement. However, *if* something is to be done about problems of justification in contexts of disagreement, a resolution is most likely to occur if the methods outlined in this section are used. These strategies will often be found in the articles included in this anthology.

RELATIVISM

The fact of moral disagreement raises questions about appropriate criteria for *correct* or *objective* moral judgments. People's awareness of cultural differences relative to moral judgment, and of moral disagreements among friends over issues like abortion, has led many to doubt the possibility that there are correct and objective positions in morals. This doubt is fed by popular aphorisms which assert that morality is more properly a matter of taste than reason, that it is ultimately arbitrary what one believes, and that there is no neutral standpoint from which to view disagreements. Accordingly, many individuals may be inclined to think that moral views are simply based on feelings or on how a society accommodates the desires of its citizens, not on some deeper set of objectively justifiable principles. These same individuals, however, tend to view morality as more than a matter of individual taste when they themselves feel strongly about a particular moral position. When they are firmly convinced that another person or nation is acting unjustly, they do not regard their convictions as *mere* matters of feeling or taste.

Tension between the belief that morality is purely subjective and the belief that it has an objective grounding leads to issues of relativism in morals. One basic issue is whether an objective morality is possible and whether reason has any substantial role to play in ethics. Proponents of relativism believe that all moral beliefs and principles relate only to individual cultures or individual persons: One person's or one culture's values do not govern the conduct of others. Relativists defend this position by appeal to anthropological data indicating that moral rightness and wrongness vary from place to place and that there are no absolute or universal moral standards that could apply to all persons at all times. They add that rightness is contingent on individual or cultural beliefs and that the concepts of rightness and wrongness are therefore meaningless apart from the specific contexts in which they arise.

Moral relativism is no newcomer to the scene of moral philosophy. Ancient thinkers were as perplexed by cultural and individual differences as moderns, as is evidenced by Plato's famous battle with a relativism popular in his day. Nevertheless, it was easier in former times to ignore cultural differences than it is today, because there was once greater uniformity within cultures, as well as less commerce between them. The contrast between ancient Athens and modern Manhattan is evident, and any contemporary pluralistic culture is saturated with individuality of belief and lifestyle. Almost every day, the news media point up the differences between Anglo-American culture and, say, the customs prevalent in Iran, China, and India. The differences are sometimes so staggering that we can scarcely believe we live in the same world, or at least the same world of morals. At the same time, we tend to reject the claim that this diversity compels us to tolerate racism, social caste systems, sexism, genocide, and a wide variety of inequalities of treatment that we deeply believe morally wrong but find sanctioned either in our own culture or in others.

Problems of apparent moral diversity offer a serious challenge to moral philosophy. If rightness and wrongness are completely determined or exhausted by particular contexts, a universal ethical system seems a hopeless ideal. Although it has at times been a fashionable view in the social sciences that relativism is a correct and highly significant doctrine, moral philosophers have generally tended to reject relativism. They find relativistic views unconvincing, both because they seem irrelevant to the main task of moral philosophy and because the counterarguments seem at least as good as the arguments defending relativism. Furthermore, there are so many different notions subsumed under the theme of relativism that arguments often seem undirected and confused. In an effort to clarify these notions of relativism, the two main forms it has taken are discussed.

Cultural Relativism. Anthropologists have often asserted that patterns of culture can only be understood as unique wholes. Moral beliefs about normal behavior are thus closely connected in a culture to other cultural characteristics, such as language and fundamental political institutions. Studies show, they maintain, that what is deemed worthy of moral approval or disapproval in one society varies, both in detail and as a whole pattern, from moral standards in other societies. So far as universality is concerned, these anthropologists believe that their data show at most that in all societies persons possess a moral conscience, that is, a general sense of right and wrong. Their reasoning is that although in every culture some actions and intentions are approved as right or good and others are disapproved, the *particular* actions, motives, and rules that are praised and blamed vary greatly from culture to culture—practices of abortion, euthanasia, patient consent, and research involving human subjects being but a few among thousands of possible examples.

From the perspective taken by these anthropologists, a moral standard is simply a historical product sanctioned by custom—nothing more, nothing less. Psychological and historical versions of this same thesis hold that the moral beliefs of individuals vary according to historical, environmental, and familial differences. It is now a generally accepted psychological premise that most moral beliefs, including our sense of conscience, must somehow be learned in a social context. Moreover, the evolution and transformation over time of these beliefs either in cultures or in individuals can often be reconstructed by historians. The weight of anthropological, psychological, and historical evidence thus conspires to suggest, according to relativists, that moral beliefs are relative to groups or individuals and that there are no universal norms, let alone universally *valid* ones.

This form of relativism has plagued moral philosophy, and many philosophical arguments have been advanced against it. Among the best known are arguments that there is a universal *structure* of human nature or at least a universal set of human needs which leads to the adoption of similar or even identical principles in all cultures. This line of argument rests at least partially on empirical claims about what actually is believed across different cultures. More important than this empirical thesis, however, is the claim that even though cultural or individual beliefs vary, it does not follow that people ultimately or fundamentally disagree about moral standards. That is, two cultures may agree about an ultimate *principle of morality,* yet disagree about the ''ethics'' of a particular situation or practice. If a moral conflict were truly fundamental, then the conflict could not be removed even if there were perfect agreement about the facts of a case, about the analysis of concepts involved, and about background beliefs. Much anthropological evidence suggests that conflicts between moral beliefs across cultures are not basic or fundamental, because disagreements over critical *facts* or *concepts* are the underlying source of ''moral'' diversity. For example, in many cultures it is thought that people are reborn just as they die; individuals who die in a senile and broken-hearted state will be reborn in the same state. To avoid this condition in the afterlife, people in these cultures execute their parents at what is considered an age immediately prior to senility. Although this practice is vastly different from that sanctioned in nations most familiar to the readers of this volume, the difference in moral judgment at a fundamental level is not as great as it appears at first, because both cultures appeal to a similar ultimate moral principle to justify their treatment of the aged. That is, they both appeal to beneficent concern for the ultimate welfare of their parents.

Mere disagreements or differences in practice do not alone defeat belief in moral objectivity. When two parties argue for or against some moral view—the morality of research involving children as subjects, killing animals, abortion, or withholding information from patients—most people tend to think that at least one party is mistaken or that some genuinely fair compromise can be reached, or perhaps they remain uncertain while on the lookout for a best argument to emerge. But they do not infer from the mere fact of a conflict between beliefs that there is no way to establish one view as correct, or at least as better argued than the other. The more absurd the position advanced by one party, the more convinced they become that some views being defended are mistaken or require supplementation. They are seldom tempted to conclude that there could not be any correct moral theory that might resolve such a dispute among reasonable persons. In fact, the existence of diverse and culturally bound customs is perfectly compatible with each of the nonrelativist ethical theories discussed in a later section of this chapter—utilitarianism and deontology, in particular.

Normative Relativism.   Cultural relativists might reasonably be said to hold that "What is right at one place or time may be wrong at another." This statement is ambiguous, however, and can easily be interpreted as a second form of relativism. Some relativists interpret "What is right at one place or time may be wrong at another" to mean that it *is right* in one context to act in a way that it *is wrong* to act in another. This thesis is normative, because it discloses standards, or norms, of right and wrong behavior. One form of this normative relativism asserts that one ought to do what one's *society* determines to be right (a group or social form of normative relativism), and a second form holds that one ought to do what one *personally* believes (an individual form of normative relativism).

This normative position has sometimes crudely been translated as "anything is right or wrong whenever some individual or some group sincerely thinks it is right or wrong." However, less crude formulations of the position can be given, and more or less plausible examples can be adduced. One can hold the slightly more sophisticated view, for example, that in order to be right something must be conscientiously and not merely customarily believed. Alternatively, it might be formulated as the view that whatever is believed is right if it is part of a well-formed traditional moral code of rules in a society.

Support is sometimes claimed for these relativist contentions by appeal to the belief that it is inappropriate to criticize one culture from the perspective of another. Thus, normative relativism has been said to include the following thesis: Because moral norms are valid only when accepted by a group or an individual, it is morally illegitimate to apply any norm to another culture or individual. The claim is that the validity of moral norms is limited in scope and that the norms themselves are binding only in a specific domain, much as principles of etiquette and custom are binding only in certain locations.

The apparent inconsistency of this form of relativism with many cherished moral beliefs is one major source of objections directed at normative relativism by both philosophers and nonphilosophers. For example, most of us believe that better and worse moral beliefs can sometimes be identified, and that moral progress or moral retrogression can occur in cultures and individuals. Moreover, no theory of normative relativism is likely to convince us that we must tolerate all acts of others. At least some moral views seem relatively enlightened, no matter how great the variability of beliefs; the idea that practices such as slavery cannot be evaluated across cultures by some common standards seems patently unacceptable to many. It is one thing to suggest that such practices might be excused, and quite another to suggest that they are right.

Another objection to normative relativism derives from its claim to provide a *standard* for right belief. Suppose a kidney patient is dying and comes to believe in assisted suicide, even though it is strictly prohibited in his society. What is he bound to do? If he has conscientious convictions that conflict with the generally accepted rules in his culture, where do his obligations lie? Besides the problem of individual versus social-group norms, the concept of a social group is itself difficult to interpret. Americans, for example, do not share a uniform set of convictions, nor do members of seemingly more homogeneous groups, such as Episcopalians or business executives. Significant moral disagreement can emerge within all such groups, and it is sometimes even unclear whether individual persons are members of a social group. These matters need clarification before normative relativism becomes a plausible and attractive thesis.

A final objection is the following: If we interpret normative relativism as requiring tolerance of other views, the theory is imperiled by inconsistency. The proposition that we ought to tolerate the views of others, or that it is right not to interfere with others, is not permitted by the theory itself, for such a proposition bears the marks of a *nonrelative* account of moral rightness—one based on, but not reducible to, the cross-cultural findings of anthropologists. If there can be relativity of belief in the case of every other ethical issue, then there can be relativity over whether the practices of another society or person are to be tolerated. If the relativist holds that a principle of tolerance is demanded by ''morality itself,'' then other fundamental normative propositions cannot be excluded from similar standing in the purportedly relativist theory. Indeed, it looks as though a (universal) principle of respect for persons underlies and gives moral force to the normative relativists' appeal for tolerance and respect. But if this moral principle is recognized as valid, it can of course be employed as an instrument for criticizing such cultural practices as the denial of human rights to minorities and beliefs such as that of racial superiority. A moral principle requiring tolerance of other practices and beliefs thus leads inexorably to the abandonment of normative relativism.

MORAL JUSTIFICATION

One general and important question implicit in every section of this introduction thus far is, ''Can answers about what is morally good and right be justified?'' This question arises repeatedly even in popular discussions of morality. Questions of justification are matters of immediate practical significance, and at the same time they are related to the most theoretical dimensions of philosophy. A good case can be made that philosophy in general, in all of its fields, is primarily concerned with the criticism and justification of positions or points of view—whether the subject matter under discussion is religion, science, law, education, mathematics, or some other field. Similarly, a good case can be made that the central questions in ethics are those of justification. But what is required in order to justify some moral point of view?

Moral judgments are justified by giving reasons for them. Not all reasons, however, are *good* reasons, and not all good reasons are *sufficient* for justification. For example, as discussed in Chapter 4, a good reason for involuntarily committing certain mentally ill persons to institutions is that they present a clear and present danger to other persons. Many believe that this reason is also sufficient to justify various practices of involuntary commitment. By contrast, a reason for commitment that is sometimes *offered* as a good reason, but which many people (such as Thomas Szasz in an essay in this volume) consider a *bad* reason (because it involves a deprivation of liberty), is that some mentally ill persons are dangerous to themselves. If someone holds that commitment on grounds of danger to self is a good reason and is solely sufficient to justify commitment, that person should be able to give some further account of *why* this reason is good and sufficient. That is, the person should be able to give further justifying reasons for the belief that the reason offered is good and sufficient. The person might refer, for example, to the dire consequences for the mentally ill that will occur if someone fails to intervene. The person might also invoke certain principles about the importance of caring for the needs of the mentally ill, etc. In short, the person is expected to give a set of reasons that amounts to an argued defense of his or her perspective on the issues.

Moral Arguments. Every belief we hold is subject to challenge and therefore to justification by reasoned argument. No matter what we believe about the justifiability of intervening to protect the mentally ill, our views are subject to criticism and require defense. However, because not all reasons that are offered in support of a belief are sufficient reasons, many reasons that are advanced in an argument fail to support the conclusion reached. Logic is that branch of philosophy concerned with the relationship between reasons and conclusions drawn from the reasons. More precisely, logic describes the relationship between premises and conclusions that are correctly drawn from the premises. Logic is thus concerned to explain why arguments succeed and fail. But what is an argument—in particular a moral argument—and what role do arguments play in the attempt at justification?

An argument is a group of related statements where one statement in the group, the conclusion, is claimed to be either the consequence of the others or to be justified by the others, which are called variously evidence, reasons, grounds, and premises. In general, every argument can be put into the following form: *X* is correct; therefore, *Y* is correct. Arguments are rarely presented in this simplified form, however. More often they are submerged in complex patterns of discourse; they are disguised by rhetoric, irrelevancies, redundancies, and subtle connections with other arguments.

Moreover, an argument in which conclusions correctly follow from premises does not necessarily constitute a *proof*. The term "proof" refers to a *sound* argument, that is, one that establishes the correctness of its conclusion. Just as there are good and bad reasons, so there are good and bad arguments, and a person may argue adeptly for some conclusion and still not prove anything. In general, logic is not concerned with soundness or proofs because (with one minor exception) logic alone cannot determine whether the premises in an argument are correct or incorrect. Thus, in ethics some form of evidence or reflection must determine whether the premises used are acceptable in order to know whether an argument proves anything. It is the business of *logic* to tell us whether conclusions *follow* from premises; it is the business of some substantive inquiry such as *ethics* to tell us whether the premises should be *accepted* in the first place. Only ethics, not logic, can tell us if it is ever morally permissible to deceive those who are sick or dying (a subject discussed in Chapter 5). But only logic can tell us whether we have made a mistake in the way we formally argue about this topic. For example, it can tell us if we have made mistaken inferences, are guilty of inconsistencies, have a sufficient number of premises, etc.

Levels of Justification in Moral Argument. Different kinds of discourse are involved in moral reasoning and argument. A moral *judgment,* for example, expresses a decision, verdict, or conclusion about a particular action or character trait. Moral *rules* are general guides governing actions of a certain kind; they assert what ought (or ought not) to be done in a range of particular cases. Moral *principles* are more general and more fundamental than such rules, and serve (at least in some systems of ethics) as the justifying reasons for accepting rules. A simple example of a moral rule is, "It is wrong to deceive patients," but the principle of autonomy (as discussed below) may be the basis of several moral rules of the deception-is-wrong variety. Finally, ethical *theories* are bodies of principles and rules that are more or less systematically related.

The different kinds of moral discourse can also be developed as a theory of *levels* of justification.[3] Judgments about what ought to be done can be viewed as justified (i.e., good and sufficient independent reasons for the judgments given) by rules, which in turn are justified by principles, which then are justified by ethical theories (which are discussed in the following section). This thought can be diagrammed as follows (where the arrow indicates the direction of *justification,* the particular or less general moral assertion being justified by appeal to the more general):

Theory
↑
Principle
↑
Rule
↑
Judgment

Many justifications found in this volume either conform to or can be reconstructed to conform to this diagram. Consider again, for example, the Tarasoff case. One argument and justification used by the psychiatrist (the defendant) and indeed by one of the judges can be diagrammed as follows:

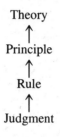

Consequential theory (perhaps utilitarianism)
↑
Principle of autonomy
↑
Rule of confidentiality of a physician's information
↑
Judgment that the psychiatrist's confidential information
should remain confidential (undisclosed to others)

The particular judgment made by the psychiatrist (and one judge) that confidential information should remain undisclosed in this case is shown in this diagram to be justified in terms of a rule of confidentiality, which in turn is justified in terms of a more general principle of autonomy, which is then justified by a more general theory that recognizes the importance of consequentialist appeals. (Of course, more than one rule or principle may be invoked at these levels in the attempt to justify a judgment.)

This discussion of justification and argument implicitly raises the question of the best justifying reasons and theories—and thus of the best premises to use in moral arguments.

CLASSICAL ETHICAL THEORIES

A structured normative ethical theory is a system of principles by which to determine what ought and ought not to be done. Modern ethical theory has come to be classified in terms of deontological and utilitarian approaches. Because in almost every chapter in this volume at least one author defends some utilitarian-based conclusion, this general ethical theory requires examination.

UTILITARIAN THEORIES

Utilitarianism is rooted in the thesis that an action or practice is right (when compared to any alternative action or practice) if it leads to the greatest possible balance of good consequences or to the least possible balance of bad consequences in the world as a whole. In taking this perspective, utilitarians invite us to consider the whole point or function of morality as a social institution, where "morality" is understood to include our shared rules of justice and other principles of the moral life. The point of the institution of morality, they insist, is to promote human welfare by minimizing harms and maximizing benefits: There would be no point at all in having moral codes and understandings unless they served this purpose. Utilitarians thus see moral rules as the means to the fulfillment of individual needs as well as to the achievement of broad social goals. A good example of this way of thinking is found in Chapter 11, devoted to ethical issues of research involving human subjects. At least two authors in that chapter (Chalmers and Eisenberg) see both the purpose of biomedical research and the purpose of rules that constrain the involvement of humans in such research as the minimization of harm (in the form of injury and disease) and the maximization of benefits (health benefits, in particular).

Mill's Utilitarianism. The major exposition of utilitarianism has generally been regarded as that of John Stuart Mill in his work *Utilitarianism* (1863). In this work Mill discusses two foundations of utilitarianism: (1) a *normative* foundation in the principle of utility, and (2) a *psychological* foundation in human nature. The principle of utility, or the Greatest Happiness Principle, he proposes as the foundation of morals: "Actions are right in proportion as they tend to promote happiness, wrong as they tend to produce the reverse of happiness, i.e., pleasure or absence of pain." Pleasure and freedom from pain, Mill argues, are alone desirable as ends; all desirable things (which are numerous) are therefore desirable either for the pleasure inherent in them, or as means to the promotion of pleasure and the prevention of pain.

Mill's second foundation of utilitarianism derives from his belief that most and perhaps all persons have a basic desire for unity and harmony with their fellow human beings. Whereas Mill's utilitarian predecessor, Jeremy Bentham, had tried to justify the principle of utility by claiming that it is in our own self-interest to promote everyone's interest, Mill appeals to social feelings of mankind for his justification. Just as we feel horror at crimes, he says, so we have a basic moral sensitivity to the needs of others. In the end his view seems to be that the purpose of morality is at once to tap natural human sympathies so as to benefit others, while at the same time controlling unsympathetic attitudes that cause harm to others. The principle of utility is conceived as the best means to these basic human goals.

For Mill and many other utilitarians, moral theory is grounded in a theory of the general goals of life, which they conceive as the pursuit of pleasure and the avoidance of pain. The production of pleasure and pain assumes moral and not merely personal significance when the consequences of our actions affect the pleasurable or painful states of others. Moral rules and moral and legal institutions, as they see it, must be grounded in a general theory of value, and morally good actions are alone determined by these final values. Utilitarians, as we shall now see, have not always agreed on these goals and values, but one main task for any utilitarian is to provide an acceptable theory that explains which things are intrinsically good and why they are so. Additionally, there is a question of *whose* goals are to count in a utilitarian calculation. For example, when discussing the morality of biomedical research, are the pains of animals to count (a topic taken up in Chapter 12); and in considering euthanasia for defective newborns, are the interests of fetuses and newborns to count, and if so, by what utilitarian criteria (a topic considered in Chapter 7)?

The Theory of Value. Within utilitarian theories of value, a major distinction is drawn between *hedonistic* and *pluralistic* utilitarians. Bentham and Mill are hedonistic, because they conceive utility entirely in terms of pleasure. In effect, they argue that the good life is constituted by happiness, which is equivalent to pleasure (though they did not argue that the word "good" *means* happiness or pleasure in ordinary language). All good things are valuable only as means to the production of pleasure or the avoidance of pain. Hedonistic utilitarianism, then, holds that acts or practices which maximize pleasure are right actions. Pluralistic utilitarian philosophers, by contrast, believe that no single goal or state constitutes *the* good and that many values besides happiness possess intrinsic worth—for example, the values of friendship, knowledge, love, devotion, health, beauty, and perhaps even certain moral qualities such as fairness. Those who subscribe to this pluralistic approach prefer to interpret the principle of utility as demanding that the rightness or wrongness of an action be assessed in terms of the total range of intrinsic values ultimately produced by the action, not in terms of pleasure alone. The greatest aggregate good, then, must be determined by considering multiple intrinsic goods. Several essays in this volume appear to interpret health as such an intrinsic good and suggest utilitarian schemes for the public distribution of this good. The debate over health-care allocation and the right to health care in Chapter 9, for example, is indicative of the ongoing significance of this utilitarian argument, as is the argument over genetic policy found in Chapter 10.

Although not as part of the dispute between hedonists and pluralists, Mill went to considerable lengths to clarify his use of the term "happiness." He insisted that happiness does not refer merely to "pleasurable excitement" but rather encompasses a realistic appraisal of the pleasurable moments afforded in life, whether they take the form of tranquillity or passion. Mill and Bentham both believed that pleasure and the freedom from pain could at least in rough ways be measured and compared, and Bentham argued that pleasure and pain can be measured by using a hedonic calculus. To determine the moral value of an action, he said, one must add up the total happiness to be produced, subtract the pains involved, and then determine the balance, which expresses the moral value of the act. Thus, a person literally is able, in Bentham's scheme, to calculate what ought morally to be done.

Many philosophers have objected to such quantification, arguing that it either is impossible or would take too long to be practical for determining what we ought to do in daily life. Whatever the merits of this objection, which is taken up below, Mill and Bentham realized that it is unrealistic in our daily practical affairs to pause and rationally calculate in detail on every occasion where choices must be made. They maintained that we must rely heavily on our common sense, our habits, and our past experience, as do contemporary utilitarians. For example, most people know that too frequent use of x-ray examinations is dangerous and that utility is maximized by prudent utilization of such tests. But our knowledge of the consequences of x-rays over time is quite limited, and predictions are risky when those involved try to formulate hospital policies and legislation to protect against such dangers. Mill and Bentham were agreed that we can only ask reasonable predictability and choice in such cases—not perfect predictability and error-free calculations.

Both the hedonistic and the pluralistic approaches have nonetheless seemed to some recent philosophers relatively useless for purposes of objectively aggregating widely different interests in order to determine where maximal value, and therefore right action, lies. Many utilitarians thus interpret the good as that which is subjectively desired or wanted; the *satisfaction* of desires or wants is seen as the goal of our moral actions. This third approach is based on individual *preferences,* and utility is analyzed in terms of an individual's actual preferences, not in terms of intrinsically valuable experiences or states of affairs. To maximize an individual's utility is to maximize what he or she has chosen or would choose from the available alternatives. To maximize the utility of those persons affected by an action or policy is to maximize the utility of the aggregate group. This theory, too, plays a role in some articles in this anthology—especially those centered on health policy (Chapter 10) and the allocation of resources (Chapter 9).

This preference-based utilitarian approach to value has been viewed by many as superior to its predecessors, but it is not trouble free as a general theory of morals. A major theoretical problem arises when individuals have morally unacceptable preferences. For example, a person's strong sexual preference may be to rape young children, but such a preference is morally intolerable. We reject such preferences. Utilitarianism based purely on subjective preferences is satisfactory, then, only if a range of *acceptable* preferences can be formulated. This task has proved difficult in theory, and an attempt to limit or discount actual preferences may even be inconsistent with a pure preference approach. Nonetheless, some plausible replies to this objection are open to utilitarians. First, since most people are not perverse and do have morally acceptable (albeit some-times odd) values, utilitarians believe they are justified in proceeding under the assumption that the preference approach is not fatally marred by a speculative problem. As Mill noted, any moral theory whatever may lead to unsatisfactory outcomes if one assumes universal idiocy. Second, because ''perverse'' desires have been determined on the basis of past experience to cut against the objectives of utilitarianism by creating conditions productive of unhappiness, the desires (preferences) could never even be permitted to count. We discount preferences to rape children not only because they obstruct the preferences of children but because, more generally, such preferences eventuate in a great deal of unhappiness to society. Preferences that serve merely to frustrate the preferences of others are thus ruled out by the goal of utilitarianism. As Mill himself argued, the cultivation of certain kinds of desires is built into the ''ideal'' of utilitarianism.

Still, even if most persons are not perverse and if the ideals of utilitarianism are well entrenched in society, some rational agents may have preferences that are immoral or unjust, and a major problem for utilitarian theory is that it may stand in need of a supplementary criterion of value in addition to mere preference. (Many critics have suggested that at least a principle of justice must supplement the principle of utility.)

Act and Rule Utilitarianism. A significant dispute has arisen among utilitarians over whether the principle of utility is to be applied to particular *acts* in particular cir-cumstances or to *rules* of conduct that determine which acts are right and wrong. For the *rule* utilitarian, actions are justified by appeal to such rules as ''Don't deceive'' and ''Don't break promises.'' These rules, in turn, are justified by appeal to the principle of utility. An *act* utilitarian simply justifies actions directly by appeal to the principle of utility.

Act utilitarianism is often characterized as a "direct" or "extreme" theory because the act utilitarian directly asks, "What good and evil consequences will result directly from *this action in this circumstance?*"—not "What good and evil consequences will result generally from this *sort* of action?" In this formulation, the right act is the one that has the greatest utility *in the circumstances*. This approach seems natural because utilitarianism aims at maximizing value, and the most direct means to this goal would seem to be that of maximizing value on every single occasion. This position does not demand, however, that every single time we act we must determine what should be done without any reference to general guidelines. We clearly learn from past experience, and the act utilitarian does permit summary rules of thumb. The act utilitarian thus regards rules such as "You ought to tell the truth to patients" as useful but not as valid for all circumstances. An act utilitarian would not hesitate to break such rules if a violation would actually lead to the greatest good for the greatest number in a particular case.

Consider the following case, which recently occurred in the state of Kansas and which anticipates some issues about euthanasia encountered in Chapter 8: An elderly woman lay ill and dying. Her suffering came to be too much for either her or her faithful husband of 54 years to endure, so she requested that he kill her. Stricken with grief and unable to bring himself to perform the act, the husband hired another man to kill his wife. An act utilitarian might reason that in this case hiring another to kill the woman was justified, even though in general we would not permit physicians, for example, to engage in such a practice. After all, only this woman and her husband were directly affected, and relief of her pain was the main issue. It would be unfortunate, the act utilitarian might reason, if our "rules" against killing failed to allow for selective killings of this sort, for it is extremely difficult to generalize from case to case. The jury, as it turned out, convicted the husband of murder in this case, and he was sentenced to 25 years in prison. An act utilitarian might maintain that the application of rules of criminal justice inevitably leads to injustices and that rule utilitarianism cannot escape this consequence of a rule-based position.

Many philosophers object vigorously to act utilitarianism, charging its exponents with basing morality on mere expediency. On act-utilitarian grounds, they say, it is desirable for a physician to kill babies with many kinds of birth defects, since the death of the child would relieve the family and society of a great burden and inconvenience and thus in some respects would lead to the greatest good for the greatest number. Many opponents of act utilitarianism have thus argued that strict rules, which cannot be set aside for the sake of convenience, must be maintained. Many of these apparently desirable rules can be justified by the principle of utility, so utilitarianism need not be abandoned even if act utilitarianism is judged unworthy.

Rule utilitarians hold that rules have a central position in morality and cannot be compromised by the demands of particular situations. Such compromise would threaten the very effectiveness of the rules; effectiveness is judged by determining that the observance of a given rule would, in theory, maximize social utility better than would any possible substitute rule (or no rule). The rule utilitarian believes that this position is capable of escaping such counterexamples and objections to act utilitarianism as the one about defective newborns mentioned above, because rules are not subject to change by the demands of individual circumstances. Utilitarian rules are, in theory, firm and protective of all classes of individuals, independent of factors of social convenience and momentary need.

Still, it is necessary to ask whether rule-utilitarian theories can escape the very criticisms they acknowledge as tarnishing act utilitarianism. Dilemmas often arise that involve conflicts among moral rules—for example, rules of confidentiality conflict with rules protecting individual welfare, as in the Tarasoff case. Many believe a pregnant woman's rights can conflict with the rights of a fetus, as discussed in relation to abortion in Chapter 6. If the moral life were so ordered that we always knew which rules and rights should receive priority, there would be no serious problem for moral theory. Yet such a ranking of rules seems clearly impossible, and in a pluralistic society there are many rules that some persons accept and others reject. Even if everyone agreed on the same rules and on their interpretation, in one situation it might be better to break a confidence in order to protect someone, and in another circumstance it might be better to keep the information confidential.

Mill briefly considered this problem. He held that the principle of utility should itself decide in any given circumstance which rule is to take priority. However, if this solution is accepted by *rule* utilitarians, then their theory must rely directly on some occasions on the principle of utility to decide *in particular situations* which *action* is preferable to which alternative action in the absence of a governing rule. If whole sets of utility-based rules or statements of rights cannot determine whether a woman who has become pregnant because of rape is justified in seeking an abortion, how is rule utilitarianism to be distinguished from act utilitarianism? And do all the same criticisms and counterexamples that rule utilitarians (and others) bring against act utilitarians apply to rule utilitarianism itself?

The rule utilitarian can reply to this criticism by asserting that a sense of relative weight and importance should be built directly into moral rules, at least insofar as possible. For example, the rule utilitarian might argue that rules prohibiting the active killing of newborn babies are of such vital social significance (i.e., have such paramount social utility) that they can never be overridden by appeal to rules that allow parents the freedom to make fundamental choices for their children. Rule utilitarians may acknowledge that weights cannot be so *definitely* formulated and built into principles that irresolvable conflicts among rules will *never* arise. What they need not concede is that this problem is unique to rule utilitarianism. Every moral theory, after all, has certain practical limitations in cases of conflict. This is a general problem with the moral life itself, the rule utilitarian will argue, and thus not unique to a particular theory. It will nonetheless be possible to distinguish theories that require strict observance of rules from those, such as act utilitarianism, that do not. This form of rule utilitarian argument emerges in Chapter 8, where the adequacy of present rules governing killing (and the basis of such rules in utility) is discussed. (See the first four essays in that chapter in particular.)

Criticisms of Utilitarianism. Two criticisms of utilitarianism are of major importance for our purposes in this volume. The first centers on the suggestion that goods can be measured and comparatively weighed. Because utility is to be maximized, one who makes a utilitarian choice must be in a position to compare the different possible utilities of an action. But can units of happiness or some other utilitarian value be measured and compared so as to determine the best among alternatives? In deciding how to allocate resources, for example, how is a state legislature to compare the value of a good screening program for genetic disease with the value of regular medical examinations at publicly funded clinics for checkups—or either with public health education? It is difficult for individuals to rank their *own* preferences, and still more difficult to compare one person's preferences with the preferences of others. Yet at least a rough comparison is required if the utility of everyone affected by the actions is to be maximized.

The utilitarian reply to these criticisms is that we make crude, rough and ready comparisons of values every day. For example, we decide to go on a picnic rather than have an office party because we think one activity will be more pleasurable or will satisfy more members of a group than the other. Physicians commonly recommend courses of treatment or nontreatment to families based on judgments of pain avoidance and family welfare. It is easy to overestimate the demands of utilitarianism and the precision with which its exponents have thought it could be employed. Accurate measurements of others' goods or preferences can seldom be provided because of limited knowledge and time. In everyday affairs—such as medical practice, hospital administration, or legislative decision-making—prior knowledge about the consequences of our actions is severely limited. What is important, morally speaking, is that a person conscientiously attempt to determine the most favorable action, and then with equal seriousness attempt to perform that action.

A second criticism is that utilitarianism can easily lead to injustices, especially to unjust social distributions. The argument may be expressed as follows: The action that produces the greatest balance of value for the *greatest number* of people may bring about unjustified harm or disvalue to a minority. An ethical theory requiring that the rights of individuals be surrendered in the interests of the majority seems plainly deficient; if a fair opportunity is denied the minority or the sick, the theory supporting such a recommendation is clearly unjust. Moreover, many political philosophers and legal theorists have argued that documents such as the Bill of Rights in the United States Constitution or the Patients' Bill of Rights studied in Chapter 4 of this text contain a set of rules based on nonutilitarian principles, for such rights rigidly protect citizens from invasions in the name of the public good. Several writers in Chapter 9 also accuse utilitarianism of leading to unfair treatments when appealed to in the allocation of scarce health resources and when used to determine whether people have a right to health care.

Consider a real-life example of this problem, one explored in Chapters 9 and 10. Utilitarian reasoning is closely connected to so-called cost/benefit analysis, which is widely used in contemporary business, government, and health policy. According to cost/benefit models, an evaluation of all benefits and costs of a potential program or action must be made in order to determine which among alternative programs or actions is to be recommended. These costs and benefits can include both economic and noneconomic factors. Opponents of utilitarianism and cost/benefit analysis argue as follows: At least some cost/benefit analyses will reveal that a particular government program or new technology will prove highly beneficial to some members of society at a "justifiable" financial cost, yet the costs of providing this benefit might function to deny basic medical or welfare services to the most disadvantaged members of society. These critics suggest that the disadvantaged ought to be subsidized as a matter of justice, either in terms of health services or financial awards—no matter what cost/benefit analyses reveal. Planning efforts employing cost/benefit analysis that cut out minority interests are morally mistaken, they say, because they fail to account for considerations of distributive justice.

A utilitarian reply to these objections might begin by agreeing that it would not always be permissible to follow the dictates of *single, short-range* cost/benefit calculations. For example, suppose that a new diagnostic device significantly increased health benefits for the wealthy, who alone could afford it, but exposed operators of the equipment to near fatal doses of radiation. A rule utilitarian would agree that it would be immoral to use this equipment, even if statistical calculations indicated a highly favorable overall cost/benefit equation: many lives saved and only a few technicians lost. The rule utilitarian bases this reply on a framework of moral rules that follows from the general program of moral philosophy governing rule-utilitarian thinking. The point here is that considerations of social utility and the basic rules of justice determined by those considerations set a limit on the risk of harm that can be permitted, under utilitarian theory, on the basis of short-range cost/benefit calculations.

This utilitarian reply rests on two strategies of argument. First, utilitarians insist that all the entailed costs and benefits must be considered. In the case of the sick and dying, for example, costs include protests from advocates of the poor and minorities, impairment to social ideals, further alienation of the poor from the government and public officials, and the like. Second, rule utilitarian analyses emphatically deny that single cost/benefit determinations ought to be accepted. Such utilitarian analyses propose that general rules of justice (justified by broad considerations of utility) ought to constrain particular actions or uses of cost/benefit analysis in all cases. They also claim that the criticisms regarding possible denial of services to the disadvantaged as a result of cost/benefit analyses are short-sighted, for they focus on injustices that might be done through a too superficial or short-term application of the principle of utility. If one takes a long-range view, utilitarians argue, one will see that utility never eventuates in overall unjust outcomes. This problem recurs later in the chapter, when the subject of justice is discussed.

Utilitarianism, then, conceives the moral life in terms of intrinsic value and the means to produce such value. Deontologists, by contrast, argue that moral standards exist independently of utilitarian ends and that the moral life is wrongly conceived in terms of means and ends. (The Greek word *deon,* or binding duty, is the source of the term "deontology.") An act or rule is right, in their view, insofar as it satisfies the demands of some overriding principle(s) of duty.

DEONTOLOGICAL THEORIES

Deontologists urge us to consider that actions are morally wrong not because of their consequences but because the action type—the class of which the actions are instances—involves a moral violation. A radical deontologist will even argue that consequences are irrelevant to moral evaluations: An act is right if and only if it conforms to an overriding moral duty and wrong if and only if it violates the overriding moral duty or principle. Many deontological theories are not so radical, however, holding that moral rightness is only in part independent of utilitarian conceptions of goodness.

Deontologists believe that our duties to others are manifold and diverse, some springing from special relationships that utilitarians unjustifiably ignore. These relationships include, for example, those of parent and child, physician and patient, and employer and employee. Physicians have obligations to their patients that they do not have to other individuals, no matter the utilitarian outcome of treating their patients and not treating others. Children incur special obligations to their parents, and vice-versa; parents have a moral obligation to oversee and support the health and welfare needs of their children that they do not have in regard to other children in their neighborhood. (Paul Ramsey expresses precisely such a view in discussing the use of children in research in Chapter 11.)

Deontologists also believe that utilitarians give too little consideration to the performance of acts in the past that create obligations in the present. If a person has promised something or has entered into a contract, he or she is bound to the terms of the agreement, no matter what the consequences of keeping it. If one person harms another, the person who inflicted the injury is bound to compensate the injured one, whether the compensation serves utilitarian goals or not.

Since deontologists believe that moral standards are independent of utilitarian ends, what is the source of these standards and how is moral duty based on these standards?

Throughout the history of philosophy deontologists have identified starkly different ultimate principles of duty as the final moral standards. Although these many different views cannot be surveyed here, it is possible to briefly distinguish several different grounds to which they have appealed. Perhaps the best known deontological account is the Divine Command theory. The will of God is the ultimate standard in this account, and an action or action type is right or wrong if and only if commanded or forbidden by God. Other deontologists hold that some actions or action types are naturally right or wrong, good or evil, requiring no reason having to do with religion, politics, or social organization. In Chapters 6 and 8, for example, principles concerning the preservation of human life are discussed. Many deontologists believe these principles right as a fundamental matter. (Some claim that the moral value of principles—and therefore actions—can be known through reason, whereas others hold that their value can only be known through intuition.)

Finally, some deontologists appeal to a social contract reached under conditions of absolute fairness as the source of moral duty. The ultimate principle of duty is action in accordance with moral rules fairly derived from a situation of mutual agreement. Many writers in this volume appeal to the recent work of John Rawls on the topic of justice, and Rawls is one representative of the social contract point of view. His work is discussed at length later in this chapter. (Norman Daniels appeals to the Rawlsian position in his contribution to Chapter 9, where he discusses the appropriate distribution of health care goods and services.)

Types of Deontological Theory. Just as there are act and rule utilitarians, there are also act and rule deontologists. Act deontologists hold that the individual in any given situation must grasp immediately what ought to be done without relying on rules. Because each situation is potentially unique, and so not subsumable under general rules, they emphasize the particular and changing features of moral experience. However, these theories have not made a strong appeal in contemporary ethics.

Rule deontology, on the other hand, continues to hold great appeal. According to this theory, types of acts are right or wrong because of their conformity or nonconformity to one or more principles or rules. Such guides are more significant than mere rules of thumb based on past experience, and they are valid independently of their general tendency to promote good consequences. Such a rule-deontological theory may envisage only one supreme principle—a *monistic* theory—or many principles—a *pluralistic* theory. Monistic deontological theories generally maintain that one fundamental principle provides the source from which other more specific moral rules can be derived. A simple theory of this description is that all moral rules and duties ultimately derive from the golden rule, which states that you should treat others as you would wish to be treated yourself. Pluralistic deontologists, by contrast, affirm two or more irreducible moral principles.

Rule deontology seems to have made a greater appeal than act deontology for several reasons. First, rules facilitate decision making. We often have no opportunity or time to think through the steps from basic principles to conclusions. Second, act theories present problems for cooperation and trust. Lawyers, physicians, teachers, and even our friends would not be bound by any firm moral obligations, and a recognition of this fact would stand to diminish our trust that they will live up to their normal obligations. Third, act deontologists reduce moral rules—e.g., "Do not deceive"—to mere rules of thumb approximating the (nonmoral) rule "Have a medical checkup once a year." Such rules obviously allow individual discretion. Rule deontologists find this view unsatisfactory as an account of *moral* rules, which they see as more binding than optional rules of thumb. Rules that prohibit murder, rape, torture, and cruelty, for example, cannot simply be set aside on any given occasion in the way ''Wash your hair once a day'' or ''Have a medical checkup once a year'' can be set aside. For example, codes of medical and nursing ethics set limits on the way human subjects may be involved in biomedical research. These limits are not optional ones that can be set aside by individual discretion. (See, for example, the introduction to Chapter 11, which discusses such rules as *necessary conditions* of morally justified research.)

Kant's Ethical Theory. The single most widely studied deontological theory is the rule-oriented theory developed by Immanuel Kant, whose influential views will provide much of the framework for the remaining discussion of deontological theories. Kant tries to establish the ultimate basis for the validity of moral rules in pure (practical) reason, not in intuition, conscience, or the production of utility. Morality, he contends, provides a rational framework of principles and rules that constrain and guide everyone, without regard to their own personal goals and interests. Moral rules apply universally, and any rule qualifies as universally acceptable only if it cannot be rationally rejected. The ultimate basis of morality, then, rests on principles of reason that all rational agents possess.

Kant thought all considerations of utility and self-interest secondary, because the moral worth of an agent's action depends exclusively on the moral acceptability of the rule on the basis of which the person is acting—or, as Kant prefers to say, moral acceptability depends on the rule that determines the agent's *will*. An action, therefore, has moral worth only when performed by an agent who possesses what Kant calls a good will, and a person has a good will only if moral duty based on a universally valid rule is the sole motive for the action.

Kant lays great emphasis on performing one's duty for the sake of duty and not for any other reason, and this emphasis is one indicator that he espouses a pure form of deontology. All persons, he insists, must act not only *in accordance with duty* but *for the sake of duty*. That is, the person's motive for acting must rest in a *recognition* of an act as required by duty. It is not good enough, in Kant's view, that one merely perform the morally correct action, for one could perform one's duty for self-interested reasons having nothing to do with morality. If one does what is morally right simply because one is scared, because one derives pleasure from doing that kind of act, because one is selfish, or because the action is in one's own interest, then there is nothing morally praiseworthy about the action. For example—to take up a subject found in Chapter 5—if a physician tells the truth to a patient only because the physician fears a malpractice suit if he or she tells a lie and not because of a belief in the importance of patient autonomy and truth telling, then such a person acts rightly but deserves no moral credit.

When a person behaves according to binding moral rules valid for everyone, Kant considers that person to have an *autonomous* will. Kant compares autonomy with what he calls heteronomy—the determination of the will by persons or conditions other than oneself. Autonomy of the will is present when one knowingly governs oneself in accordance with universally valid moral principles. His concept of autonomy, however, does not simply imply personal liberty of action in accordance with a plan chosen by oneself. (For contrasting views, see the discussion of the principle of autonomy later in this chapter.) Under ''heteronomy'' Kant includes many kinds of coercive determinations of human conduct.

The difference between governance of oneself by moral obligation and governance by coercive force is critical to Kant's moral theory. Coerced acts such as being raped at knifepoint are obviously heteronomously produced, but Kant also holds that actions done from desire, impulse, or personal inclination are heteronomous actions. For example, refraining from theft merely out of fear of being caught is clearly an instance of heteronomy. Actions that are autonomous and morally right, by contrast, are based on moral principles that we accept (but have the freedom to reject). It is, however, easy to misunderstand this argument. To say that an agent "accepts" a moral principle does not mean either that the principle is merely subjective or that each individual must wholly create (author or originate) his or her own moral principles. Kant holds only that each individual must *will the acceptance* of the moral principles to be acted upon. A person's autonomy consists in the ability to govern himself or herself according to these moral principles. Moreover, Kant urges, moral relationships between persons are contingent on mutual respect for autonomy by all the parties involved. Kant develops this notion into a fundamental moral demand that persons be treated as ends in themselves and never solely as means to the ends of others. This Kantian principle, which will be discussed in detail in following paragraphs, is invoked repeatedly by many authors in this volume.

Kant's supreme principle, also called "the moral law," is actually expressed in several ways in his writings. In what appears to be his favored formulation, the principle is stated as follows: "I ought never to act except in such a way that I can also will *that my maxim should become a universal law*." This Kantian principle has often been compared to the Golden Rule, but Kant calls it the "categorical imperative." He gives several examples of moral maxims that are made imperative by this fundamental principle: "Help others in distress"; "Do not commit suicide"; and "Work to develop your abilities." The categorical imperative is *categorical*, he argues, because it admits of no exceptions and is absolutely binding. It is *imperative* because it gives instruction about how one must act.

Kant clarifies this basic moral law—the very condition of morality, in his view—by drawing a distinction between a categorical imperative and a *hypothetical* imperative. A hypothetical imperative takes the form *"If* I want to achieve such and such an end, then I must do so and so." These prescriptions—so reminiscent of utilitarian thinking—tell us what we must do provided that we already have certain desires, interests, or goals. An example would be, "If you want to regain your health, then you must take this medication," or "If you want to improve infant mortality rates, then you must improve your hospital facilities." Such imperatives are obviously not commanded for their own sake; they are commanded only as *means* to an end that has already been willed or accepted. Hypothetical imperatives are not *moral* imperatives because moral imperatives tell us what must be done independently of our goals or desires.

Kant's imperative is an unusual ultimate principle because it mentions nothing about the *content* of moral rules. For this reason, it is often said to be a purely formal principle. It does not, for instance, dictate anything so substantive as "An action is right if and only if it produces the greatest good." The categorical imperative offers only the *form* any rule must have in order to be an acceptable rule of morality.[4] As noted earlier, Kant states his categorical imperative in a distinctly different formulation (which many interpreters take to be a wholly different principle). This form is probably more widely quoted and endorsed in contemporary philosophy than the first form, and certainly it is more frequently invoked in biomedical ethics. Kant's later formulation stipulates that "One must act to treat every person as an end and never as a means only." This imperative insists that one must treat persons as having their own autonomously established goals and that one must never treat them solely as the means to one's own personal goals.

It has been widely stated in contemporary textbooks that Kant is arguing categorically that we can never treat another as a means to our ends. This interpretation, however, seems to misrepresent his views. He argues only that we must not treat another *exclusively* as a means to our own ends. When adult human research subjects are asked to volunteer to test new drugs, for example, they are treated as a means to someone else's ends (perhaps society's ends), but they are not exclusively used for others' purposes, because they do not become mere servants or objects. (This assertion is somewhat controversial, however, as the readings in Chapter 11 reveal.) Kant does not prohibit this use of persons categorically and without qualification. His imperative demands only that persons in such situations be treated with the respect and moral dignity to which every person is entitled at all times, including the times when they are used as means to the ends of others. To treat persons merely as means, strictly speaking, is to disregard their personhood by exploiting or otherwise using them without regard to their own thoughts, interests, and needs.

As appealing as his ethical theory may be, Kant has often been criticized on grounds that he leaves unresolved how duty is to be determined when two or more different duties are in conflict. This criticism is similar to the one directed at rule utilitarians. For example, if one rule demands truth telling to patients while another rule demands the protection of patients from unnecessary harm, what ought to be done in a situation where the disclosure of a piece of information the patient has requested will bring him or her great harm—perhaps a heart attack or the end of a treasured marriage? The categorical imperative seems to give no advice in this regard; it seems, in fact, to demand that both relevant duties be fulfilled. As mentioned above, it may be that no ethical theory can resolve this problem. But Kant's philosophy not only seems unable to help; it apparently *obliges* moral agents to perform two or more actions when only one can be performed.

W. D. Ross, a prominent twentieth-century British philosopher, developed a *pluralistic* rule-deontological theory intended to assist in resolving this problem of a conflict of duties. Ross's views are based on an account of what he calls prima facie duties, which he contrasts with *actual* duties. A *prima facie* duty is a duty that is always to be acted upon unless it conflicts on a particular occasion with an equal or stronger duty. A prima facie duty, then, is always right and binding, all other things being equal; it is "conditional on not being overridden or outweighed by competing moral demands." One's *actual* duty, by contrast, is determined by an examination of the respective weights of competing prima facie duties. Prima facie duties are thus not absolute, since they can in principle be overridden, but at the same time they have far greater moral significance than mere rules of thumb.

As Ross admits, neither he nor any other deontologist has ever been able to present a system of moral rules free of conflicts and exceptions. Ross argues that this is no more of a problem for him than for anyone else, Kant included, because the complexity of the moral life simply makes an exception-free hierarchy of rules and principles impossible.

Rawls's Theory. In recent years a book in the Kantian tradition has had great currency in deontological ethics. John Rawls's *A Theory of Justice* (1971) presents a deontological theory as a direct challenge to utilitarianism on grounds of social justice. Rawls's basic objection to utilitarianism is that social distributions produced by maximizing utility could entail violations of basic individual liberties and rights that ought to be guaranteed by social justice. Utilitarianism, which is concerned with the *total* satisfaction in a society, is indifferent as to the *distribution* of satisfactions among individuals. This indifference would, in Rawls's view, permit the infringement of some people's rights and liberties if the infringement genuinely promised to produce a proportionately greater utility for others.

Rawls therefore sets as his task the development of an alternative ethical theory that is capable of grounding satisfactory principles of justice. Rawls turns for this purpose to a hypothetical social contract procedure that is strongly indebted to what he calls the

"Kantian conception of equality." According to this social contract account, valid principles of justice are those to which we would all agree if we could freely and impartially consider the social situation from a standpoint (the "original position") outside any actual society. Impartiality is guaranteed in this situation by a conceptual device Rawls calls the "veil of ignorance." This notion stipulates that in the original position, each person is (at least momentarily) ignorant of all his or her particular fortuitous characteristics. For example, the person's sex, race, IQ, family background, and special talents or handicaps are unrevealed in this hypothetical circumstance.

The veil of ignorance prevents people from promoting principles of justice biased toward their own combinations of talents and characteristics. Rawls argues that under these conditions, people would unanimously agree on two fundamental principles of justice. The first requires that each person be permitted the maximum amount of equal basic liberty compatible with a similar liberty for others. The second stipulates that once this equal basic liberty is assured, inequalities in social primary goods (e.g., income, rights, and opportunities) are to be allowed only if they benefit everyone and only if everyone has fair equality of opportunity. Rawls considers social institutions to be just if and only if they are in conformity with these two basic principles.

Rawls's theory makes equality a basic characteristic of the original position from which the social contract is forged. Equality is built into that hypothetical position in the form of a free and equal bargain among all parties, where there is equal ignorance of all individual characteristics and advantages that persons have or will have in their daily lives. Furthermore, people behind this veil of ignorance would choose to make the equal possession of basic liberties the first commitment of their social institutions. Nevertheless, Rawls rejects radical egalitarianism, arguing that equal distribution cannot be justified as the sole moral principle. If inequalities were to be introduced that rendered everyone better off by comparison to initial equality, these inequalities would be desirable—as long as they were consistent with equal liberty and fair opportunity. More particularly, if these inequalities work to enhance the position of the most disadvantaged persons in society, then it would be self-defeating for the least advantaged or anyone else to seek to prohibit the inequalities. Rawls thus rejects radical egalitarianism in favor of his second principle of justice.

The first part of his second principle is called the "difference principle." This principle permits inequalities of distribution as long as they are consistent with equal liberty and fair opportunity. Rawls formulates this principle more precisely so that such inequalities would be justifiable only if they most enhance the position of the *"representative* least advantaged" person—that is, a hypothetical individual particularly unfortunate in the distribution of fortuitous characteristics or social advantages. Formulated in this way, the difference principle could allow, for instance, extraordinary economic rewards to entrepreneurs if the resulting economic stimulation were to produce improved job opportunities and working conditions for the least advantaged members of society. A strong egalitarian flavor is retained, however, in that such inequalities would be permissible only if it could be demonstrated that they worked to the greatest advantage of those who were worst off.

The difference principle rests on the view that because inequalities of birth, historical circumstance, and natural endowment are undeserved, society should correct them by improving the unequal situation of naturally disadvantaged members. This is a deontologically based demand that Rawls believes fundamental to moral life in society.

Criticisms of Deontological Theories. Although some arguments against deontological theories have been woven into the preceding discussion, there are two additional criticisms expressed in contemporary philosophy that require examination, together with responses that deontologists might offer to these criticisms.

Deontological theories vary in the consideration they give to the consequences of actions. Kant, as we have seen, asserts that actions are determined to be right or wrong independent of particular consequences, whereas Ross admits that consequences are relevant, even though not the only consideration. An important utilitarian criticism is that deontologists *covertly* appeal to consequences in order to demonstrate the rightness of actions. John Stuart Mill, for example, argues that even Kant's theory does not avoid appeal to the consequences of an action in determining whether it is right or wrong. According to Mill's interpretation of Kant, the categorical imperative demands that an action be morally prohibited if "the *consequences* of (its) universal adoption would be such as no one would choose to incur." Kant fails "almost grotesquely," as Mill puts it, to show that any form of formal contradiction or certification of a moral rule appears when we universalize rules of conduct. Mill argues that Kant's theory relies on a covert appeal to the utilitarian principle that if the consequences of the universal performance of a certain type of action can be shown to be undesirable overall, then that sort of action is wrong.

One possible defense of Kant against such charges is the following: It is not entirely accurate to say that Kant urges us to disregard consequences, or even that he believes an action is morally right (or wrong) without regard to its consequences. Kant holds only that the features of an action making it right are not dependent upon any particular outcome; he never advises that we disregard consequences entirely. The consequences of an action often cannot be separated from the nature of the action itself, and so they too must be considered when an agent universalizes the action in order to determine whether it is permissible. Kant occasionally overstates his views by too strongly condemning consequential reasoning, but his writings indicate that he was more than willing to consider the consequences as an integral part of the universalization process.

A second criticism is centered on *pluralistic* deontological theories. The contention is that pluralistic theories lack unity, coherence, and systematic organization. Critics suggest that whereas the principle of utility tells us what makes right actions right on all occasions, thinkers such as Ross merely provide a disconnected list of diverse right-making considerations. If one takes the basic task of philosophical ethics to be that of providing ultimate good and sufficient reasons for our moral judgments, then pluralistic deontological theories fail. They tend to retreat into an intuitionist theory, where we either intuit on given occasions which duty is the stronger or else must remain uncertain as to where duty lies.

Those who propose this criticism naturally believe that a unified theory is superior to any pluralistic deontological account. Ross was himself concerned about this problem and acknowledged that his catalogue of duties is unsystematic and probably incomplete. His response to those who criticize deontologists for this alleged shortcoming follows the lines of his general criticisms of Kant's appeal to a single categorical imperative. He argues that critics are forcing an "architectonic" of "hastily reached simplicity" on ethics. Although his critics maintain that his views lack systematic unity, he sees disunity as an integral feature of the moral life. Untidiness and complexity may be unfortunate features of morality, but if they are nonetheless true characterizations, his theory of morality can hardly be faulted for taking account of them. Indeed, it is the obligation of a moral philosopher, from Ross's perspective, to point out a lack of systematic unity if it is inescapable.

It is also open to deontologists to argue that their theories are no worse off than utilitarian theories in this regard. Rule utilitarians have an extremely general principle of duty based on certain views about goodness, from which a number of competing rules of duty are derived. These rules are not given systematic unity in utilitarian theories (beyond their derivation from the principle of utility itself). Deontologists could point out that the general demand to act on the most stringent *prima facie* duty is a rule that provides all the cohesion and unity that can reasonably be expected. They might conclude that this principle overrides all other principles on every occasion, and that this measure of systematic unity is all that one needs or could hope to find.

MAJOR ETHICAL PRINCIPLES

How are we to determine, in light of the preceding theories and account of justification, the moral acceptability of a particular act? Understandably, this question is complex, and there is no way to answer it with confident finality. But this much, at least, seems reasonable to assume: If a particular act is wrong, then it will have certain similarities, certain shared features, with other wrong actions; conversely, if a particular act is morally required, it will share similar features with other actions that are morally required. Philosophers who have tried to develop a general normative theory of right and wrong have, of course, tried to discover what these shared features are.

Theories of the two general sorts just discussed have also been used by moral philosophers to support a great many derivative moral principles (and rules—such as the one stating that it is right to keep our promises and wrong to break them). Not all such principles are needed for or even applicable to a discussion of any given moral problem—for example, the morality of suicide. But in order to take a reasoned approach to these problems, we need principles that permit us to take a consistent position on specific and related issues. Three moral principles have proved to be directly relevant to discussions of the issues found in this book: autonomy, beneficence, and justice.

One important qualification is that the three principles identified and explicated here should not be construed as jointly forming a complete moral system. Certainly other moral principles may turn out to be relevant to the problems discussed in this volume. Nonetheless, these three principles are the ones most widely employed in discussions of the moral problems to be encountered, and they are sufficiently comprehensive to provide an analytical framework by means of which moral problems of biomedical ethics can be evaluated. Moreover, most types of general ethical theories would recognize these three principles as valid, although theories differ over their derivation, scope, and relative significance. But let us see what these principles are before discussing questions of derivation and priority.

AUTONOMY

The first principle deserving mention is one commonly referred to as the Principle of Respect for Persons, by which is usually meant something like the following: Because humans act morally and have a capacity for rational choice, they possess value independently of any special circumstances conferring value, and because all human beings and only human beings have such unconditional value, it is always inappropriate to treat them as if they had merely the conditional value possessed by natural objects and (so some believe) by animals. Human beings, as it is sometimes put, have an incalculable worth or moral dignity not possessed by other things or creatures, which are valuable *only under certain conditions*. To respect persons is to see them as unconditionally worthy agents, and so to recognize that they should not be treated as conditionally valued things that serve our own purposes. By contrast, to treat persons as mere means to our own ends is to treat them as if they were not moral agents.

From this perspective, to exhibit a lack of respect for persons is either to reject a person's considered judgments or to deny the person the liberty to act on those judgments. This notion of respect for persons demands that we allow persons the freedom to form their own judgments and perform whatever actions they choose (within other moral limits, of course). Such respect is demanded for no other reason than that those who possess moral dignity are rightfully the determiners of their own destinies. For purposes of this discussion, the import is that individuals should be allowed to be self-determining agents, making their own evaluations and choices when their own interests are at stake. This narrowed version of ''respect for persons'' will be referred to here as respect for the autonomy of persons—or, more briefly, as the Principle of Autonomy. What is entailed by this principle?

There is an almost uniform agreement in the history of philosophy that a person who lacks critical internal capacities for self-rule in some organized fashion—and not mere freedom from external constraint—lacks something integral to freedom and control. Thus, in order to be autonomous, the person must be both *free of external control* and *in control of his or her own affairs*. One is autonomous in this sense only if one's ruling part is in control, if one is subject to no other governing conditions except those to whose control one has consented, and if one is capable of controlled deliberation and action.

To *respect* the autonomy of such self-determining agents is to recognize them as entitled to determine their own destiny, with due regard to their considered evaluations and view of the world, even if it is strongly believed that their evaluation or their outlook is wrong and even potentially harmful to them. They must be accorded the moral right to have their own opinions and to act upon them, as long as those actions produce no serious harm to other persons. Thus, in evaluating the self-regarding actions of others, we are obligated to respect them as persons with the same right to their judgments as we possess to our own, and they in turn are obligated to treat us in the same way.

The *principle of autonomy* can be formulated as follows: Insofar as an autonomous agent's actions do not infringe on the autonomous actions of others, that person should be free to perform whatever action he or she wishes (presumably even if it involves considerable risk to himself or herself and even if others consider the action to be foolish). Some philosophers have believed that autonomy is the primary moral principle and takes precedence over all other moral considerations. However, others consider it merely *one* important principle among others. (Some possible qualifications of this principle are discussed later, in the section on law, authority, and liberty.)

The controversial problems with such a noble-sounding principle, as with all moral principles, arise when we must determine precise limits on its application and how to handle situations when it conflicts with such other moral principles as beneficence and justice. The best known problems of conflict involve overriding refusals of treatment by patients—as in Jehovah's Witnesses' refusals of blood transfusions. Even though the handling of these cases is controversial, the principle of autonomy must not be interpreted as applying to all persons—despite the historical link to ''respect for persons.'' Some persons cannot act autonomously because they are immature, incapacitated, ignorant, or coerced. A person of diminished autonomy is highly dependent on others, less than self-reliant, and in at least some respect incapable of choosing a plan on the basis of controlled deliberations. For example, children and institutionalized populations such as the mentally retarded may have diminished autonomy in this sense. For such persons the principle is inapplicable, except perhaps through some principle of proxy consent or substituted judgment, as discussed in Chapter 11.

The obligation to obtain informed consent in research and clinical contexts, generally said to be grounded in a principle of autonomy, raises many issues about the proper limits of the principle. Whether the principle is the fundamental one or even a primary one justifying consent requirements is a controversial matter, but more important issues concern the exact demands the principle makes in the consent context. These controversies involve questions about the conditions under which a person's right to autonomous expression demand disclosures of information. For example, some writers have argued that where risks of harm are extremely low or nonexistent, disclosures need not be made at all, and consent need not be obtained. This claim has been made about studies of abandoned human tissue, observational and interviewing methods in social research, and routine medical examinations. Others have argued that risk should play no role in the obligation to obtain consent—just as when a psychiatrist assures us that confidentiality will be respected, we do not interpret that assurance to mean that confidentiality will be kept solely under conditions where risk is involved. (These issues are considered primarily in Chapters 5 and 11.)

Among the most important demands made by the principle of autonomy is that of telling the truth. Principles of veracity, as they are called, can easily be treated in moral theory as derivative exclusively from the principle of autonomy. The philosopher Henry Sidgwick, however, observed that it has never been clearly agreed whether these principles state *independent* duties or are special applications of some higher principle such as autonomy. Although it must be admitted that Sidgwick is right, principles of veracity can be treated as derivative from autonomy, as can several other moral principles—such as those of confidentiality and privacy. Certainly autonomy has often been treated in moral theory as such an umbrella concept.

BENEFICENCE

Among the most quoted principles in the history of codes of medical ethics is the maxim *primum non nocere*—"above all, do no harm." Other duties in medicine, nursing, public health, and research are expressed in terms of a more positive obligation to come to the assistance of those in need of treatment or in danger of injury. In the International Code of Nursing Ethics, for example, it is said that "[T]he nurse shares with other citizens the responsibility for initiating and supporting action to meet the health and social needs of the public."[5] Section 10 of the 1977 Principles of Medical Ethics of the American Medical Association expresses a virtually identical point of view.[6] The range of duties requiring abstention from harm and positive assistance may be conveniently clustered under the single heading of the Principle of Beneficence.

The term "beneficence" has broad usage in English; its meanings include the doing of good and the active promotion of good, kindness, and charity. But in the present context the duty of beneficence has a narrower meaning. In its most general form, the principle of beneficence requires us to abstain from injuring others and to help others further their important and legitimate interests, largely by preventing or removing possible harms.[7] Presumably such acts are required when they can be performed with minimal risk to the actors—not under all circumstances of risk. According to William Frankena, this principle can be expressed as including the following four elements: (1) One ought *not to inflict* evil or harm (a principle of nonmaleficence). (2) One ought to *prevent* evil or harm. (3) One ought to *remove* evil or harm. (4) One ought to *do or promote good*.[8] Frankena suggests that the fourth element may not be a duty at all (being an act of benevolence that is over and above duty) and contends that these elements appear in a hierarchical arrangement so that the first takes precedence over the second, the second over the third, and the third over the fourth.

There are philosophical reasons for separating passive nonmaleficence (as expressed in 1) and active beneficence (as expressed in 2–4), and even ordinary moral discourse expresses the view that certain duties not to injure others are more compelling than duties to benefit them. For example, many people see the duty not to injure a patient by abandonment as stronger than the duty to prevent injury to a patient who has been abandoned by another, even though both may be moral duties. Nonetheless, the duty expressed in (1) may not always be stronger than those expressed in (2–4), and demands to benefit others and not to injure them can be unified under a single principle of beneficence—taking care to distinguish, as appropriate, between strong and weak requirements of this principle corresponding roughly to the ordering from 1 to 4.

Firmly established in the history of ethics, in practices of international relations, and in public policy formulation in most countries is the conviction that the failure to increase the good of others when one is knowingly in a position to do so is morally wrong. Preventive medicine and active public health interventions exemplify this conviction. Once methods of treating yellow fever and smallpox were discovered, for example, it was universally agreed that governments ought to take positive steps to establish programs to protect public health. Many welfare programs presumably have a similar moral justification. The existence of both health and welfare programs is one reason why there is now so much discussion of the right to health care and various welfare rights of the sort discussed in Chapters 9 and 10.

Still, there are problems with appeals to beneficence, some of which were implicitly encountered in discussing utilitarianism. Because beneficence potentially demands extreme generosity in the moral life, some philosophers have argued that it is commonly *virtuous,* but not a *duty,* to act beneficently. From this perspective the positive benefiting of others by providing health and welfare services, for example, is based on personal or social ideals beyond the call of duty, and thus is supererogatory rather than obligatory. In what respects and within what limits, then, is beneficence a duty, if it is a duty at all? And how does it apply to such problems as health care allocation and public funding of biomedical research?

Public support of biomedical and behavioral research has often been taken as indicative that some beneficent social actions are morally appropriate and perhaps even morally demanded. This research is undertaken to benefit members of society, including future generations, in highly significant ways, and the benefits produced are generally cited as the primary justification of all publicly funded research. Many similar examples of actions justified through the principle of beneficence could be cited. Still, it is one thing to maintain that actions or programs are morally *justified* and another to maintain that they are morally *required.* It remains controversial which, if any, beneficent actions are actually demanded by duties—a problem that recurs in many readings in this text. (Contrast, for example, the essays by Leon Eisenberg and Hans Jonas in Chapter 11 on the subject of the moral justification of biomedical research.)

Several moral philosophers have offered proposals to resolve this problem by showing that beneficence does, in fact, generate duties. These attempts are too diverse and complex to be considered here,[9] but despite this unresolved problem, it seems reasonable to assume that *some* forms of beneficence are morally required. That we are morally obligated on at least some occasions to assist others or to abstain from harming them is, after all, hardly a matter of moral controversy (even if the exact basis of the obligation is in dispute). For example, we are often morally obligated to benefit someone because of a role we have voluntarily assumed. Beneficent acts are built into our very understanding of the relationship between patients and health care professionals. Through the Hippocratic Oath, the physician pledges to "come for the benefit of the sick" and to "apply dietetic measures for the benefit of the sick according to [his or her] ability and judgment" (see Chapter 4). The physician on duty in an emergency room is obligated to attend to an injured, delirious, uncooperative patient, sometimes at considerable risk both to himself and to the patient. Those engaged in medical practice and research also know that risks of harm presented by medical interventions must constantly be weighed against possible benefits for patients, subjects, or the public interest. This is recognized in the Nuremberg Code, for example, which states that "The degree of risk to be taken should never exceed that determined by the humanitarian importance of the problem to be solved by the experiment" (see Chapter 11).

The responsibilities of physicians, nurses, and public health officials commonly require a balancing of risks and benefits. This balancing can lead to situations where health care professionals view their obligations to a patient differently from the patient's own assessment. The patient may refuse to follow a prescribed regimen, for example, and forcing the patient to accept it would involve a refusal to respect autonomy. Even patients who are competent can exert poor judgment when they are ill or injured, and a crisis arises if they will not consent to a proposed treatment. Some health care professionals are inclined to accept the patient's refusal as valid, whereas others are inclined to ignore the lack of consent and to "benefit" the patient by a medical intervention. This problem of whether to override the decisions of patients in order to benefit them is one dimension of the problem of paternalism, which is treated in detail later in this introduction in the section on Law, Authority, and Liberty. It is shown there how the problem of paternalism is generated by a conflict between principles of autonomy and beneficence, each of which can be and has been conceived by different parties as the overriding principle in cases of conflict. Conflict between the demands of beneficence and autonomy underlies a broad range of controversies in this volume (see especially Chapters 4, 5, 8, and 10).

JUSTICE

Some moral philosophers have held that principles of justice have a moral priority over other moral principles, or at least that certain controversial moral issues can only be grounded within the broad framework of a theory of distributive justice. What, then, is justice, and what makes it unique?

Basic notions of both individual and social justice have been explicated in terms of fairness and "what is deserved." A person has been treated justly when he has been given what he or she is due or owed, what he or she deserves or can legitimately claim. What is deserved may be either a benefit or a burden. If a patient is morally entitled to confidentiality of information, for example, justice has been done when that information is kept confidential, even if discharging the duty of nondisclosure is inconvenient and difficult. Naturally, any denial of something to which a person has a right or entitlement is an injustice. It is also an injustice to place an undue burden on the exercise of a right—for example, to make a deserved piece of information unreasonably difficult to obtain (see Chapter 5).

The more restricted expression "distributive justice" refers to the proper distribution of social benefits and burdens. Usually it refers to the distribution of what Rawls calls "primary social goods," such as economic goods and fundamental political rights. But social burdens must also be considered. Paying taxes and being drafted into the armed services to fight a war are distributed burdens; Medicare checks and grants to do research are distributed benefits. Recent literature on distributive justice has tended to focus on considerations of fair *economic* distribution, especially unjust distributions in the form of inequalities of income between different classes of persons and unfair tax burdens on certain classes. But there are many problems of distributive justice besides strictly economic ones, including the issues raised in prominent contemporary debates over health care distribution, as discussed in Chapter 9.

The notion of justice has been analyzed in different ways in rival theories. But common to all theories of justice is this minimal principle: Like cases should be treated alike—or, to use the language of equality, equals ought to be treated equally and unequals unequally. This elementary principle is referred to as the formal principle of justice, or sometimes as the formal principle of equality—*formal* because it states no particular respects in which people ought to be treated. It merely asserts that whatever respects are under consideration, *if* persons are equal in those respects, they should be treated alike. Thus, the formal principle of justice does not tell us how to *determine* equality or proportion in these matters, and it therefore lacks substance as a specific guide to conduct. In any group of persons there will be many respects in which they are both similar and different, and therefore this account of equality must be understood as "equality in relevant respects."

Because this formal principle leaves space for differences in the interpretation of how justice applies to particular situations, philosophers have developed diverse theories of justice. Again, however, one theme common to many theories is that programs or services designed to assist people of a certain class must, as a matter of justice, be made available to *all* members of that class. To provide some with access to such programs while denying access to others who are equally qualified (and so entitled) is declared unfair. The principle of justice thus understood is particularly applicable to problems of health care allocation and health policy—issues intrinsically related to innovations in public policy (see Chapters 9 and 10).

Theories of justice attempt to be more specific than the formal principle by systematically and precisely elaborating the notions of equality or proportion in distribution; they specify in detail what counts as a relevant respect in terms of which people are to be compared and what it means to give people their due. Philosophers achieve this specificity by developing *material* principles of justice, so called because they put material content into a theory of justice. Each material principle of justice identifies a relevant property that serves as a basis for distributing burdens and benefits. The following is a sample list of major candidates for the position of valid principles of distributive justice (though longer lists have been proposed): 1. To each person an equal share. 2. To each person according to individual need. 3. To each person according to that person's rights. 4. To each person according to individual effort. 5. To each person according to societal contribution. 6. To each person according to merit. There is no obvious barrier to acceptance of more than one of these principles, and some theories of justice accept all six as valid. Most societies use several in the belief that different rules are appropriate to different situations. The role of these principles is taken up again in Chapter 9, where distributions of health care goods and services are discussed.

Egalitarian theories of justice emphasize equal access to primary goods; *Marxist* theories emphasize need; *libertarian* theories emphasize rights to social and economic liberty; and *utilitarian* theories emphasize a mixed use of such criteria so that public and private utility are maximized. (These differences are illustrated at various points in the text.) The acceptability of any such theory of justice is determined by the quality of its moral argument that some one or more selected material principles ought to be given priority (or perhaps even exclusive consideration) over the others.

Claims of injustice and propositions about the demands of justice have frequently appeared in the literature on biomedical ethics, especially when it is believed that someone's legal or moral rights have been violated. These concerns are not usually as broad and far-reaching as the kinds of concerns expressed in general theories of justice. For example, in the literature on research involving some risk to human subjects where there is withholding of information as well, the research is often denounced as an unjust denial of information to which subjects are entitled. Another complaint is that physicians have been unjustly accorded greater control over patients' lives and decisions than they deserve.

These complaints of injustice can easily be linked to violations of the principle of autonomy. However, not all accusations of injustice can be accounted for by appeal to this moral principle—or to other principles. For example, as discussed in Chapter 11, there have been complaints that research on children is immoral *not* because it involves a violation of autonomy but rather because subjects of research are unjustly used as means to the ends of others. Whether or not this Kantian allegation of injustice is correct, the complaint is not easily reduced to some argument that there has been a violation of autonomy, because in this case the concerns center on nonautonomous persons. Moreover, the contention is not reducible to the argument that subjects have been harmed and that therefore there has been a violation of beneficence, because the same Kantian argument about the use of persons as means can be applied to risk-free research as well (e.g., deception research on child learning or observational research on parent-child bonding in hospitals).

These practical concerns about justice and injustice, as earlier noted, seem rather distant from very general theories of justice such as Rawls's (or libertarian and utilitarian theories for that matter). There is, perhaps, a reason for this apparent distance. There seem to be severe limits to philosophy's capacity to resolve public-policy issues through theories of distributive justice; many believe these theories are simply unsuited for public-policy formulation. A widely shared view is that there is no single consistent set of principles of justice that can reliably be invoked to handle practical problems of justice. These critics believe both that there are many such principles and that different contexts compel different uses of such principles. They thus hold that it is too idealistic to suppose that a theory of justice can order these principles *a priori* in determining which must take precedence in particular political or moral contexts.

It would be wrong to argue the extreme thesis that philosophers cannot provide any form of analytical framework that helps policy makers and professionals with their moral problems. But such analytical frameworks must have some measure of immediate practical bearing or philosophy will seem embarrassingly remote as an "applied" field, as these debates about distributive justice well illustrate. The final section of this chapter looks at possible ways in which moral reasoning can assist in the formulation of public policy.

ETHICS, LAW, AND PUBLIC POLICY

ETHICS AND PUBLIC AFFAIRS

There are at least two ways in which applied ethics often overlaps with, and even provides foundations for, law and public policy. First, there are conceptual problems that require careful explication in order that people communicate clearly and efficiently. What is meant in various contexts when crucial terms are used, such as "liberty," "fair distribution,'' ''competence,'' ''rights,'' ''paternalism,'' ''responsibility,'' and ''coercion by law''? At stake is not whether and how justice or liberty should be ensured or what rights and responsibilities should be granted to what persons. The point of conceptual analysis of these fundamental terms is to be as clear and precise as possible without begging any substantive moral issue. The importance of such conceptual clarification became obvious in the discussion of moral disagreement.

Second, normative problems require equally careful attention, in order that we determine what ought to be done in law and social policy. Here, philosophers must abandon the neutrality about issues involved in conceptual clarification, for they are engaged in that controversial world of human affairs where there are conflicting interests, goals, and ideals. Their objective should be to formulate and apply general principles that can be fairly used to guide social policy. For example, a theory of human rights might be developed that determines which rights all persons have and a theory of justice that explains how goods should be distributed in society without regard to the special interest of any person or class of persons. (Chapter 9, on the allocation of scarce medical resources, deals with precisely these questions.)

Many articles in this volume are concerned with concepts and principles in ethical theory that can be applied to public affairs. Joel Feinberg has made a suggestive comment about how the problems raised in these essays might ideally be viewed:

It is convenient to think of these problems as questions for some hypothetical and abstract political body. An answer to the question of when liberty should be limited or how wealth ideally should be distributed, for example, could be used to guide not only moralists, but also legislators and judges toward reasonable decisions in particular cases where interests, rules, or the liberties of different parties appear to conflict. . . . We must think of an ideal legislator as somewhat abstracted from the full legislative context, in that he is free to appeal directly to the public interest unencumbered by the need to please voters, to make ''deals'' with colleagues, or any other merely ''political'' considerations. . . . The principles of the ideal legislator . . . are still of the first practical importance, since they provide a target for our aspirations and a standard for judging our successes and failures.[10]

An example to illustrate this possible deployment of moral philosophy arises from current concern in social scientific, medical, nursing, public health, legal, and government sectors about adequate guidelines for and practices of obtaining informed consent—a concern found in a number of current federal regulations or proposed regulations. (The subject of informed consent is of current interest in public health as well as clinical and research contexts, and those interests are manifested in Chapters 4, 5, 11, and 12.) Hospitals and all levels of health-care professionals and health policy makers, as well as individual physicians and patients, constantly confront problems of informed consent. Lawyers and social scientists have found themselves confused by past court cases and by operative federal regulations, yet are frustrated by having no developed alternatives. For example, issues of consent arise regarding the right to refuse treatment, the competence of patients to understand, the nature and limits of the physician's privilege (''therapeutic privilege'') not to disclose material information under certain conditions, the effects of disclosed information, research involving deception, research involving randomized clinical trials, and so-called proxy consent. Other similarly important issues could be added to this sample list.

Many of these issues have immediate practical implications for patients, subjects, government officials, and lawyers; and many are overtly and traditionally philosophical—for example, issues about the nature of voluntariness, the concept of autonomy, the moral problem of paternalism, and the validity of refusals of treatment. The lack of viable standards of informed consent, as well as the lack of information regarding the quality and value of current practices in obtaining consent, is now impeding both health-care delivery and health-policy development and can retard research, as well. Even large-scale public-health efforts, such as the swine-flu inoculation program and federally funded sterilization and mass genetic screening programs, have been delayed and subjected to criticism because of uncertainty about appropriate standards for the consent of participants. A large sector of the public is therefore interested in this moral problem: research investigators, medical practitioners, policy makers, members of review boards for research, and scholars in the field of biomedical, behavioral, and social ethics.

Another example of ethics at work in the formulation of public policy is found in the work of the National Commission for the Protection of Human Subjects of Biomedical and Behavioral Research, which was established in 1974 by a federal law. Its mandate was to develop ethical guidelines for the conduct of research involving human subjects and to make recommendations to the Department of Health and Human Services (DHHS). To discharge its duties, the Commission studied the nature and extent of various forms of research, its purposes, the ethical issues surrounding the research, present federal regulations, and the views of representatives of professional societies and federal agencies. The Commission engaged in extensive deliberations on these subjects in public, a process in which persons from various fields of ethics were as intimately involved as the representatives of any other discipline. Subsequent government regulations regarding research (issued by DHHS) show the imprint of the Commission in virtually every clause. These regulations cannot be regarded as exclusively ethical in orientation, but much distinctive philosophical material is found in the Commission documents, and ethical analysis provided the framework for its deliberations and recommendations. The Commission also issued one exclusively philosophical volume, which sets forth the moral framework that underlies the various policy recommendations it made.[11] It is perhaps the best example to date both of the use of moral frameworks for policy development and of a philosophical publication issued through a government body.

A recognition that public policy can be buttressed by moral argument must not, of course, be taken as a denial that this relationship sometimes proves controversial. Governments are notoriously prone to invoke "ethical" justifications in defense of laws and policies whose actual foundations rest on narrow grounds of special interests, or at least of narrow interests. As discussed in Chapter 8, laws prohibiting or discouraging such "victimless crimes" as voluntary euthanasia and suicide provide contemporary examples where the legitimacy and propriety of legal appeals to "ethical" considerations have been heavily criticized. Many issues about government regulation of biomedical research, as discussed in Chapters 11 and 12, have been similarly criticized. One central question, for example, concerns the scope of the government's freedom to restrict or place conditions on the use of government-funded research.

However one views these controversies, it is worth noting that the arguments on all sides often appeal to the *rights* of patients, subjects, citizens, and health professionals. Such appeals to rights are now commonplace, and when rights are violated we often become appropriately indignant.

LEGAL AND MORAL RIGHTS

Only recently has Western society emphasized the importance of human rights, and only recently have they come to play an important role in public policy discussions. Until the seventeenth and eighteenth centuries, even problems of political philosophy were rarely discussed in terms of rights, perhaps because duties to lord, king, state, church, and

God (as well as duties of rulers to subjects) had been the predominant focus of political and ethical theory. However, at this point in history crucial new ideas were introduced, including the notion of universal "natural rights." These rights were thought to consist primarily of rights not to be interfered with, or liberty rights. Proclamations of such rights as those to life, liberty, property, safety, a speedy trial, and the pursuit of happiness subsequently formed the core of major political and legal documents.

Rights have since held a prominent place in political documents because they are powerful assertions of claims that demand respect and status. When someone appeals to rights, a response is demanded, and we must either accept the person's claim as valid, discredit the claim by countervailing considerations, or acknowledge the right but show how it can be overridden by competing moral claims. Yet the idea that certain moral rights exist prior to and independent of social conventions and laws had led philosophers to speculate about the nature and source of rights. They ask questions such as the following: Are there rights independent of laws and conventions, or are rights merely cultural fictions? If they exist, are they grounded purely in the obligations of others? Do moral rights exist prior to and independently of what governments recognize as rights? What are the limits on the scope of such rights? What does it mean to say that "X has a right to Y"?

Everyone would agree that legal rights exist, but the status of moral rights is more puzzling. Philosophers differ significantly in their accounts of the nature and grounding of such rights. Also, the language of moral rights is still greeted by some with scepticism. This scepticism emerged from theories of ethical relativism, from general doubts that human rights are "self-evident" and "inalienable," and from a widespread belief that rights can be translated into or reduced to obligations. Others find absurd the proliferation of and conflict among rights claims in recent political debates. For example, it has been claimed by some parties that there is a right to have an abortion, and claimed by different parties that there is a right to life that precludes a right to have an abortion. As seen repeatedly throughout this volume (Chapters 4–6, 8–12) rights language has been extended to include controversial rights to privacy, rights to health care, the rights of children, the rights of animals, the rights of the elderly, rights to confidential information, and the rights of other special groups. Even "smokers' rights" have been discussed—an alleged right that health officials have greeted with a noticeable lack of enthusiasm.

Some carefully drawn distinctions regarding the nature and types of moral rights have emerged in ethical theory, and it will prove useful to examine some of these distinctions.

Prima Facie and Absolute Rights. *Prima facie* duties were discussed earlier, in the section on Deontological Theories. It was noted there that moral philosophers generally regard duties not as absolute but rather as strong moral demands that may be validly overridden by more stringent competing demands in circumstances of competition. Such competition presumably occurs in the case of rights as well. Here the problem is whether rights may be overridden by competing rights. It has often been assumed, owing perhaps to political statements about fundamental human rights, that rights are absolute. Yet there appear to be many counterexamples to the thesis that they are absolute.

For example, it is sometimes assumed that the right to life is absolute, irrespective of competing claims or social conditions. This thesis is controversial, however, as evidenced by common moral judgments about capital punishment, international agreements about killing in war, and beliefs about the justifiability of killing in self-defense. Most writers in ethics agree that we have only a right not to have our life taken *without sufficient justification*. Although there is disagreement about which conditions are sufficient for taking another's life, most agree that some conditions—e.g., self-defense—can be specified. The right to life, then, according to this ethical view, is not absolute: The right can be legitimately exercised and can create actual duties on others only when the right has an overriding status. Thus, rights claims seem to be *prima facie* claims—ones that have to admit other rights claims as similarly valid. Rights such as a right to health care, a right to die, and a right to be saved from starvation must compete with other rights in many situations, which produces protracted controversy and a need to balance with great discretion the competing rights claims.

Moral and Legal Rights. There are substantial differences between moral and legal rights, for legal systems do not formally require reference to moral systems for their understanding or grounding, nor do moral systems formally require reference to legal systems. One may have a legal right to do something patently immoral, or have a moral right without any corresponding legal guarantee. Legal rights are derived from political constitutions, legislative enactments, case law, and the executive orders of the highest state official. Moral rights, by contrast, exist independently of and form a basis for criticizing or justifying legal rights. Finally, legal rights can be eliminated simply by lawful amendments to political constitutions, or even by a coup d'état, but moral rights cannot be eroded or banished by political votes, powers, or amendments.

Some rights are neither moral nor legal. Official organizations and professional societies such as nursing organizations and medical societies are two types of groups that offer declarations asserting rights for the special populations they represent. The rights of staffs in hospitals have, for example, been a persistent topic of discussion by such groups. Similarly, social practices and arrangements that define institutional roles and responsibilities often confer rights, as in the case of the physician-patient relationship. These conventional rights contrast with moral rights in that they do not exist independently of the set of conventions or rules governing the enterprise. They differ from legal rights in that they are not always recognized as rights within the law.

The Correlativity of Rights and Obligations. How are we to understand the language and basis of rights in moral discourse, and in what respect (if any) is there a relationship between one person's rights and another's obligations? A plausible approach to answering this question is to say that any right entails an obligation on others either not to interfere with one's liberty or to provide something. Thus, if a state promises or otherwise incurs an obligation to provide such goods as flu shots or therapeutic care to needy citizens, then citizens can claim an entitlement—a *positive* right—to the shots or therapy when they meet the relevant criteria of need. The right to die, the right to privacy, the right to a healthy environment, and all other so-called *negative* rights may be treated as entailing that someone is obligated to abstain from interfering with one's intended course in life. (The important distinction between positive and negative rights is analyzed in detail in the introduction to Chapter 9.)

If this general correlativity thesis is correct, there is perhaps little that is distinctive about rights as a moral category. The moral basis for their assertion rests in the obligations of others (though it is controversial whether rights are generated from obligations or obligations generated from rights). "X has a right to do or have Y" simply means that the moral system (or the legal or some other system) imposes an obligation on someone to act or to refrain from acting so that X is enabled to do or have Y (if X wishes Y). This analysis accords with the widely accepted idea that the language of rights is translatable into the language of obligations—that is, that rights and obligations are logically correlative: One person's right entails someone else's obligation to refrain from interfering or to provide some benefit, and all obligations similarly entail rights.[12] It is, of course, not always easy to track down the obligation entailed by an assertion of a right or the right that corresponds to an obligation, and there may be more than one obligation corresponding to any given right. Corresponding obligations may even derive from several different sources or persons.

This analysis of rights suggests—but does not prove—that rights are grounded in obligations. If so, a theory of rights would require a theory of obligations for its justification. The issue of whether there are rights to privacy, health care, or the like would thus turn on whether there are certain moral obligations to provide these benefits or to ensure these liberties. The basis of the required obligations—if there are such obligations—could, in theory, be justice, social utility, contractual agreement, or any of the ethical principles and theories studied previously.

LAW, AUTHORITY, AND LIBERTY

Various liberty rights are often said to be fundamental rights, perhaps because liberty is intimately connected to the nature and dignity of human beings. No right to liberty, however, is strong enough to entail a right to absolute freedom, for then no restrictions on liberty would ever be justified. The notion of "acceptable liberty" clearly refers to actions in which people *ought* to be free to engage. Although it would be difficult to determine a set of right and wrong exercises of liberty, some valid restrictions are surely appropriate.

Major ethical and social problems concerning liberty emerge when liberty intersects with law or with some other form of authority. By protecting rights or liberties for one group, the law creates obligations on or restricts the liberty of others. Even the most protective law or restrictive policy places a limit on what was formerly an open option. It is generally accepted that some liberties should be judiciously traded off for various forms of state protection or the protection of authorities, but in circumstances where no valid justification is forthcoming, authority can easily become an instrument of oppression.

Authorities in control can also be so lax as to permit foolish exercises of liberty—for example, when others use their freedom to engage in repulsive or degrading actions, or ones rooted in needless ignorance. Questions thus arise about the conditions under which it is justified to limit individual liberty, about which types of activities and behavior should be legally restricted, and about what sorts of liberties deserve protection.

Liberty-Limiting Principles. Various "moral" principles have been advanced in the attempt to stake out valid grounds for the limitation of individual human liberties. The following four "liberty-limiting principles" have been defended and have played a significant role in recent philosophical controversies:

1. *The Harm Principle*—A person's liberty is justifiably restricted to prevent *harm to others* caused by that person.
2. *The Principle of Paternalism*—A person's liberty is justifiably restricted to prevent *harm to self* caused by that person.
3. *The Principle of Legal Moralism*—A person's liberty is justifiably restricted to prevent that person's *immoral behavior*.
4. *The Offense Principle*—A person's liberty is justifiably restricted to prevent *offense to others* caused by that person.

Each of these four principles represents an attempt to balance liberty and other values. Although different people differently assess the weight of certain values in this balancing process, the harm principle is universally accepted as a valid liberty-limiting principle (despite certain unclarities that surround the notion of a harm). However, much controversy surrounds the other three liberty-limiting principles, and their general validity is widely doubted.

Each of these three "supplementary principles" proclaims that there is a valid limit on individual liberties, and therefore a valid limit on one's *right* to do something. Only one of these supplementary principles is pertinent to many controversies that arise in this volume: paternalism. Here the central problem is whether this form of justification for a restriction of liberty—even if highly qualified—may ever *validly* be invoked—and, if so, how the principle that stands behind this judgment is to be precisely formulated. In order to answer this question, it is necessary to look more closely at the nature of paternalism.

Paternalism. The word "paternalism" loosely refers to treating individuals in the way that a parent treats his or her child. But in ethical theory the word is more narrowly used to apply to treatment that restricts the liberty of individuals, without their consent, where the justification for such action is either the prevention of some harm they might do to themselves or the production of some benefit they might not otherwise secure. Although disagreement persists in philosophy concerning the precise meaning of "paternalism," the following definition should suffice for present purposes: Paternalism is the limitation of a person's liberty of action or liberty of information justified by reasons referring exclusively to the welfare or needs of the person whose liberty is limited.

Several writers have argued that paternalism is pervasively present in modern society; many actions, rules, and laws are commonly justified by appeal to a paternalistic principle. Examples in medicine include court orders for blood transfusions when patients have refused them, involuntary commitment to institutions for treatment, intervention to stop "rational" suicides, resuscitating patients who have asked not to be resuscitated, withholding medical information that patients have requested, denial of an innovative therapy to someone who wishes to try it, and some government efforts to promote health. Other health-related examples include laws requiring motorcyclists to wear helmets and motorists to wear seat belts and the regulations of governmental agencies such as the Food and Drug Administration that prevent people from purchasing possibly harmful or inefficacious drugs and chemicals. In all cases the motivation is the beneficent promotion of health and welfare.

In the case of *medical* paternalism, it is often said that the patient-physician relationship is essentially paternalistic. This view is held because patients can be so ill that their judgments or voluntary abilities are significantly affected, or because they may be incapable of grasping important information about their case, thus leaving them in no position to reach carefully reasoned decisions about their medical treatment. Illness, injury, depression, fear, the threat of death, and traditional staples of the medical profession such as drugs may overwhelm patients, so that their ability to ascertain their own best interests is in doubt. Moreover, every increase in illness, ignorance, and quantity of medication can increase the patient's dependence on his or her physician. Also, physicians commonly encourage patients with "innocent lies" intended to raise their spirits—when, in fact, matters are either hopeless or beyond the physician's capacities. Hospitals and the medical profession thus seem immersed in a paternalistic orientation.

The paternalism of the medical profession has been under attack in recent years, especially by defenders of patient autonomy. They hold that physicians intervene too often and assume too much control over their patients' choices. Many recent philosophical, legal, and medical writings have reflected this harsh judgment of the profession. Philosophers and lawyers have tended to support the view that patient autonomy is the decisive factor in the patient-physician relationship and that interventions can be valid only when patients are in some measure unable to make voluntary choices or to perform voluntary actions. Physicians too have increasingly criticized authoritarianism in their profession. In fact, a recent draft of principles of ethics of the American Medical Association asserted that "paternalism by the profession is no longer appropriate." It seems timely, then, to reflect on the nature of paternalism and the extent to which it is or is not justified.

Cases of paternalism are commonly distinguished as being one of two types, both of which fit the general definition. This distinction is between strong and weak forms of paternalism, where the weak form is understood as the liberty-limiting protection or benefit of a person when the person is substantially unable to make his or her own decisions. The strong form, by contrast, holds that it is proper to protect or benefit a person by liberty-limiting measures even when his or her contrary choices are informed and voluntary. A substantial problem surrounds this distinction. Virtually everyone acknowledges that some forms of so-called weak paternalism are justified—for example, preventing a person under the influence of a powerful drug from self-inflicted death. If, then, *some* forms of paternalism are justified, the problem of paternalism for ethical theory is that of deciding the conditions under which a principle of paternalism may be used and under what conditions it may not be used.

A conceptual problem plaguing these discussions is that weak paternalism does not clearly fit the foregoing definition of paternalism; because harm is *caused to* the person (not caused *by* a person's own voluntary actions), this form of "paternalism" may not be a liberty-limiting principle *independent* of the harm principle. For this reason some writers have restricted the meaning of the word "paternalism" to strong paternalism.

Any careful proponent of a principle of paternalism will specify precisely which goods and needs deserve paternalistic protection, and the conditions under which intervention is warranted. In most recent formulations, it has been argued that one is justified in interfering with a person's liberty only if the interference protects the person against his or her own actions where those actions are extremely and unreasonably risky (e.g., refusing a life-saving therapy in nonterminal situations) or are potentially dangerous and irreversible in effect (as some drugs and surgery are). Even among supporters of paternalism it is agreed that it takes a heavy burden of justification to limit free actions by competent persons when there is no informed consent (even if there might be a second-party or proxy consent). According to this position, paternalism is justified if and only if the evils prevented from occurring to the person are greater than the evils (if any) caused by interference with his or her liberty and if it can be universally justified, under relevantly similar circumstances, always to treat persons in this way. (Many but not all writers add a third condition requiring that the person's liberty is already restricted by some condition seriously encumbering autonomy; that is, the person's capacity to think or act must be substantially impaired in the circumstances.)

Gerald Dworkin and John Rawls have both argued that a cautious paternalism should be regarded as a form of "social insurance policy" that fully rational persons would take out in order to protect themselves. As Rawls puts it, such persons "will want to insure themselves against the possibility that their powers are undeveloped and they cannot rationally advance their interests, as in the case of children."[13] Such persons would know, for example, that they might be tempted at times to make decisions that are potentially dangerous and irreversible. They might at other times encounter social pressures to do something they honestly believe too risky, such as the social pressure involved in accepting a challenge to fight for one's honor.

Despite this fairly moderate formulation of paternalism, many remain firmly opposed to all possible uses of this principle. Their arguments against paternalism invariably turn on some defense of the importance of autonomy—for example, the autonomy of patients who might be treated paternalistically by physicians (see discussions of this problem in Chapters 4, 5, and 8) and the autonomy of citizens whose health behaviors are paternalistically regulated by their government (see the discussion of this problem in Chapter 10).

Three main arguments beyond mere appeals to the principle of autonomy have been offered in support of antipaternalism. The first argument is consequentialist: Even limited paternalistic rules or policies can easily be abused and will inevitably lead to serious adverse consequences when put into practice. Those concerned about paternalism in government, for example, mention the dangers of incompetent or authoritarian administrators, neglect of or failure of expertise in understanding individual and group needs, and political jockeying for power and position. The second argument challenges Rawls's claims that a rational individual who is informed of the risks and social pressures involved in community living would not object to a limited paternalism. As Mill repeatedly points out, the idea of "the informed rational individual" is often a mask for the will of a majority in society who may be unaffected, or least affected, by paternalistic social policies. Also, many rational persons would be justifiably sceptical of the ability of others both to know their interest better than would they and to act so as to promote those interests. It is precisely in circumstances under which paternalism would be most likely to flourish, such as the context of the patient-physician relationship, that antipaternalists are most reluctant to believe that others would be in a position to protect them against themselves. Finally, some antipaternalists will argue that if citizens *consent* to paternalistic powers that they *give* to authorities, then "paternalism" is freely consented to and not a matter of liberty limitation at all.

Even the severest critics of paternalism do not hold that patients and citizens should not be treated *beneficently* by authorities. They have therefore often argued for a severely limited version of what was referred to as *weak* paternalism. In particular, they have held that it is justifiable to protect a person from harm that might result directly from partially nonvoluntary acts—for example, acts due to serious illness or retardation. To the extent that one protects a person from causes beyond his or her knowledge and control, according to this argument, to that extent (subject perhaps to further specific qualifications) one justifiably intervenes. If a person genuinely has incapacitating "cloudy judgment" or is deceived because of ignorance about the situation in which he or she must make the choice, his or her choices are not entirely voluntary. Even some antipaternalists would say that intervention to restrict liberty is morally *required* if the person can be injured because of these "external" conditions, since disregard of the condition could imperil a person's future. This justification for intervention, however, is *not* truly in the end paternalistic, according to the critics of paternalism: once a person is informed of the dangers of an action and provided with a context in which voluntary choice is meaningfully possible, then, they hold, he or she cannot justifiably be further restrained. When persons become informed and capable of acting voluntarily, they believe that our obligations to them are altered and that limitation of their liberty is unjustified.

These three arguments used by antipaternalists indicate that one major source of the difference between supporters and opponents of paternalism rests on the emphasis each places on capabilities for autonomous action by patients making "choices." Supporters of paternalism tend to cite examples of persons of diminished or compromised capacity, for example, persons lingering on kidney dialysis, chronic alcoholics, compulsive smokers, and seriously depressed suicidal patients. Opponents of paternalism cite examples of persons who are capable of autonomous choice but have been socially restricted in exercising their capacities. Examples of this group include those involuntarily committed to institutions largely because of eccentric behavior, prisoners not permitted to volunteer for risky research, and those who might rationally elect to refuse treatment in life-threatening circumstances. One critical element of this controversy thus concerns the quality of consent or refusal by the persons whose liberty might be restricted by such policies.

Many articles reproduced in this volume deal with public policies that involve such substantive moral issues as liberty and liberty-limiting principles, and legal versus moral rights. These policies affect not only doctor and patient, lawyer and client, researcher and subject—they affect every individual in a society.

CONCLUSION

This chapter has surveyed some central themes in philosophical discussions of ethical theory. The objective has been to explore ethical theory in sufficient detail to provide a basis for reflecting critically on the readings in the ensuing eleven chapters. The aim of the chapter has not been to promote a particular point of view but rather to provide an understanding of the major options and distinctions in moral philosophy. Although none of the authors whose works are reprinted in the following chapters subscribes without qualification to the theories and principles discussed in this chapter, repeated appeals— either implicit or explicit—to most of these theories and principles are found in their essays.

Ethical theory alone will not prove sufficient as a tool of analysis for many of the problems and policies in medical practice and related fields dealt with in this volume. Some controversies are largely factual, and, as seen in the next two chapters, some controversies are more conceptual than moral. Nonetheless, the unifying theme in this collection is that of reflection on moral dilemmas, and ethical theory provides an indispensable means to this reflection.

T. L. B.

NOTES

1. *Tarasoff v. Regents of the University of California,* California Supreme Court (17 California Reports, 3d Series, 425. Decided July 1, 1976). Reprinted in Chapter 5.

2. These principles and their analysis by the National Commission for the Protection of Human Subjects of Biomedical and Behavioral Research have been published as *The Belmont Report: Ethical Principles and Guidelines for the Protection of Human Subjects of Research* (Washington, D.C.: Government Printing Office, DHEW Publication, 1978).

3. For a more developed discussion of levels of justification, see Tom L. Beauchamp and James F. Childress, *Principles of Biomedical Ethics* (New York: Oxford University Press, 1979), Chap. 1.

4. This idea of a "logical form" is somewhat obscure in Kant's philosophy, but on at least one interpretation Kant has a worthy point—whatever its limits. One of the clearest cases of an immoral action occurs when a person attempts to make an exception to a rule for himself or herself alone. For Kant such "excepting" actions are necessarily immoral, irrespective of circumstances, for they cannot be made universal.

5. 1953 and 1973 International Codes of Nursing Ethics of the International Council of Nurses.

6. Section 10 of the 1977 Principles of Medical Ethics of the American Medical Association.

7. The actual conditions for X's duty of beneficence to Y have been plausibly analyzed by Eric D'Arcy as follows. X has a duty of beneficence to Y if and only if: (1) Y is at risk of significant loss or damage; (2) X's action is necessary to prevent loss or damage; (3) X's action would probably prevent loss or damage; (4) X's own losses or damages would probably be minimal or negligible; (5) Benefit to Y will probably outweigh the harm to X. Eric D'Arcy, *Human Acts: An Essay in Their Moral Evaluation* (Oxford: Clarendon Press, 1963), pp. 56–57.

8. William Frankena, *Ethics,* 2nd Edition (Englewood Cliffs, N.J.: Prentice-Hall, 1973), p. 47.

9. The major issues are the following: Can Frankena's four elements (see note 8) be ranked in some order of priority; are all four actually statements of *obligation;* and is the final element merely an expression of a moral ideal? These issues are at present undecided.

10. Joel Feinberg, *Social Philosophy* (Englewood Cliffs, N.J.: Prentice-Hall, 1973), pp. 2–3.

11. This publication is cited in note 2.

12. A weaker version of the correlativity thesis holds that rights entail obligations, though not all obligations entail rights.

13. John Rawls, *A Theory of Justice* (Cambridge, Mass.: Harvard University Press, 1971), pp. 248–249.

SUGGESTED READINGS FOR CHAPTER 1

MORALITY AND MORAL PHILOSOPHY

Frankena, William K. *Ethics.* 2nd edition. Englewood Cliffs, N.J.: Prentice-Hall, 1973.

MacIntyre, Alasdair. *A Short History of Ethics.* New York: Macmillan, 1966.

Mackie, John. *Ethics: Inventing Right and Wrong.* Harmondsworth, Eng.: Penguin Books Ltd., 1977.

Nielsen, Kai. "Problems of Ethics." In Edwards, Paul, ed. *Encyclopedia of Philosophy.* New York: Macmillan and Free Press, 1967. Vol. 3, pp. 117–134.

Taylor, Paul W., ed. *Problems of Moral Philosophy,* 3rd edition. Belmont, Calif.: Dickenson Publishing Company, Inc., 1978. Chap. 1.

RELATIVISM AND DISAGREEMENT

Asch, Solomon E. *Social Psychology.* Englewood Cliffs, N.J.: Prentice-Hall, 1952. Chap. 13, "The Fact of Culture and the Problem of Relativism."

Beauchamp, Tom L. *Philosophical Ethics.* New York: McGraw-Hill, 1982. Chap. 2.

Brandt, Richard B. "Ethical Relativism." In Edwards, Paul, ed. *Encyclopedia of Philosophy.* New York: Macmillan and Free Press, 1967. Vol. 3, pp. 75–78.

Glover, Jonathan. *Causing Death and Saving Lives.* New York: Penguin Books, 1977. Chap. 2.

Ladd, John, ed. *Ethical Relativism.* Belmont, Calif.: Wadsworth Publishing Company, 1973.

Rachels, James. "Can Ethics Provide Answers?" *Hastings Center Report* 10 (June 1980), 32–40.

Wellman, Carl. "The Ethical Implications of Cultural Relativity." *Journal of Philosophy* 60 (1963), 169–184.

JUSTIFICATION

Beauchamp, Tom L. *Philosophical Ethics.* New York: McGraw-Hill, 1982. Chaps. 9 and 10.

————, and Childress, James F. *Principles of Biomedical Ethics.* New York: Oxford University Press, 1979. Chaps. 1 and 2.

Griffiths, A. Phillips. "Ultimate Moral Principles: Their Justification." In Edwards, Paul, ed. *Encyclopedia of Philosophy.* New York: Macmillan and Free Press, 1967. Vol. 8, pp. 177–182.

Held, Virginia. "Justification: Legal and Political." *Ethics* 86 (October 1975), 1–16.

UTILITARIANISM

Bayles, Michael D., ed. *Contemporary Utilitarianism.* Garden City, N.Y.: Doubleday & Co., Inc., 1968.

Bentham, Jeremy. *Introduction to the Principles of Morals and Legislation* (1789), ed. W. Harrison, with *A Fragment on Government.* Oxford: Hafner Press, 1948.

Gorovitz, Samuel, ed. *Mill: Utilitarianism, with Critical Essays.* New York: Bobbs-Merrill, 1971.

Mill, John Stuart. *On Liberty.* London: J. W. Parker, 1859. (Widely reprinted.)

DEONTOLOGY

Kant, Immanuel. *Foundations of the Metaphysics of Morals.* Trans. by Lewis White Beck. Indianapolis: Bobbs-Merrill, 1959.

Nell, Onora. *Acting on Principle, an Essay on Kantian Ethics.* New York and London: Columbia University Press, 1975.

Rawls, John. *A Theory of Justice*. Cambridge, Mass.: Harvard University Press, 1971.

Ross, William D. *The Right and the Good*. Oxford: Oxford University Press, 1930.

MORAL PRINCIPLES

Beauchamp, Tom L., and Childress, James F. *Principles of Biomedical Ethics*. New York: Oxford University Press, 1979. Chaps. 3–6.

Benn, Stanley I. "Justice." In Edwards, Paul, ed. *Encyclopedia of Philosophy*. New York: Macmillan and Free Press, 1967. Vol. 4, pp. 298–302.

Downie, R. S., and Telfer, Elizabeth. *Respect for Persons*. London: George Allen & Unwin, 1969.

Dworkin, Gerald. "Autonomy and Behavior Control." *Hastings Center Report* 6 (February 1976), 23–28.

———. "Moral Autonomy." In Engelhardt, H. Tristram, and Callahan, Daniel, eds. *Morals, Science, and Sociality*. Hastings-on-Hudson, N.Y.: The Hastings Center, 1978, pp. 156–171.

Feinberg, Joel. *Social Philosophy*. Englewood Cliffs, N.J.: Prentice-Hall, 1973. Chap. 7.

Jonsen, Albert. "Do No Harm: Axiom of Medical Ethics." In Spicker, Stuart F., and Engelhardt, H. Tristram, eds. *Philosophical Medical Ethics: Its Nature and Significance*. Boston: D. Reidel, 1977, pp. 27–41.

Mack, Eric. "Bad Samaritanism and the Causation of Harm." *Philosophy and Public Affairs* 9 (Spring, 1980), 230–259.

Singer, Marcus. "Is Beneficence a Duty?" In his *Generalization in Ethics*. New York: Alfred A. Knopf, 1963. Also in Frankena, William K., and Granrose, John, eds. *Introductory Readings in Ethics*. Englewood Cliffs, N.J.: Prentice-Hall, 1977, pp. 187–192.

Sterba, James, ed. *Justice: Alternative Political Perspectives*. Belmont, Calif.: Wadsworth Publishing Company, 1980.

U.S. National Commission for the Protection of Human Subjects of Biomedical and Behavioral Research. *The Belmont Report: Ethical Guidelines for the Protection of Human Subjects of Research*. DHEW Publication No. (OS) 78-0012. Washington, D.C.: Government Printing Office, 1978.

MORAL AND LEGAL RIGHTS

Dworkin, Ronald. *Taking Rights Seriously*. Cambridge, Mass.: Harvard University Press, 1977.

Feinberg, Joel. *Social Philosophy*. Englewood Cliffs, N.J.: Prentice-Hall, 1973. Chaps. 4–6.

———. "Rights: Systematic Analysis." In Reich, Warren T., ed. *Encyclopedia of Bioethics*. New York: Free Press, 1978. Vol. 4, pp. 1507–1511.

Golding, Martin P. "The Concept of Rights: A Historical Sketch." In Bandman, Elsie, and Bandman, Bertram, eds. *Bioethics and Human Rights*. Boston: Little, Brown & Co., 1978. Chap. 4.

Lyons, David, ed. *Rights*. Belmont, Calif.: Wadsworth Publishing Company, 1979.

Macklin, Ruth. "Rights: Rights in Bioethics." In Reich, Warren T., ed. *Encyclopedia of Bioethics*. New York: Free Press, 1978. Vol. 4, pp. 1511–1516.

LIBERTY, AUTHORITY, AND PATERNALISM

Bayles, Michael D. *Principles of Legislation: The Uses of Political Authority*. Detroit: Wayne State University Press, 1978.

Beauchamp, Tom L. "Paternalism." In Reich, Warren T., ed. *Encyclopedia of Bioethics*. New York: Free Press, 1978. Vol. 3, pp. 1194–1200.

Buchanan, A. "Medical Paternalism." *Philosophy and Public Affairs* 7 (1978), 370–390.

Dworkin, Gerald. "Paternalism." *The Monist* 56 (1972), 64–84.

Gert, Bernard, and Culver, Charles. "The Justification of Paternalism." In Robison, Wade, and Pritchard, Michael, eds. *Medical Responsibility*. Clifton, N.J.: Humana Press, 1979, pp. 1–14.

Wasserstrom, Richard, ed. *Morality and the Law*. Belmont, Calif.: Wadsworth Publishing Company, 1971.

BIBLIOGRAPHIES

Goldstein, Doris Mueller. *Bioethics: A Guide to Information Sources*. Detroit: Gale Research Company, 1982. See under "Ethics" and "Bioethics."

Lineback, Richard H., ed. *Philosopher's Index*. Vols. 1– . Bowling Green, Ohio: Philosophy Documentation Center, Bowling Green State University. Issued Quarterly. See under "Autonomy," "Bioethics," "Coercion," "Consequentialism," "Distributive Justice," "Duty," "Egalitarianism," "Equality," "Ethics," "Fairness," "Human Rights," "Justice," "Kant," "Law," "Medical Ethics," "Mill," "Moral(s)," "Morality," "Natural Rights," "Normative Ethics," "Obligations," "Paternalism," "Principles," "Public Policy," "Rawls," "Reasoning," "Respect," "Rights," "Situations," and "Utilitarianism."

2.
Concepts of Health and Disease

The controversies in every chapter of this book are either centrally or loosely connected with modern problems of disease treatment and prevention. Medical science, we often say, is dedicated to the restoration and maintenance of health. But precisely what is disease? And what constitutes health? To ask questions of this sort is to ask not only how disease and health are to be understood, but also how they are to be distinguished from other human conditions, such as misery and ecstasy or failure and achievement. The questions "What is health?" and "What is disease?" may be understood, then, as requests for comprehensive definitions or conceptual explications of health and disease.

An influential example examined in this chapter is the World Health Organization (WHO) definition of "health": "Health is a state of complete physical, mental, and social well-being and not merely the absence of disease or infirmity." This definition has important implications not only for our understanding of the role of medical practitioners but for public policy. If the goal of medicine is the maintenance and restoration of health, and if this term were understood broadly as complete well-being, then the scope of medical practice would include, for example, problems of social deviancy and all personal difficulties in adapting to new environments. Private and public health policies, such as insurance coverage, would then be adjusted to this (WHO) understanding of health.

To some, the analysis of health and disease is intrinsically interesting, for they would simply like to know for the sake of clarity and understanding what health and disease are. Others are interested in such knowledge as a means to the end of developing healthy persons. However, it is the implications such definitions have for both practical decisions and health policies that give the issue its urgency and direct relevance to ethics.

THE DEFINITION OF HEALTH AND DISEASE

There have been three prominent and competing ways of approaching the definition of health. The major controversy concerns how much ground the term "health" covers. Does it encompass merely treatment of the body? Also the mind? Also social adaptability? The WHO definition falls into the most inclusive class of definitions: "Health is a state of *complete physical, mental,* and *social* well-being." Sally Guttmacher, in her contribution to this chapter, also supports a definition of wide scope by arguing that broadly ranging concepts ("holistic concepts") of health and disease appear to be less misleading and more effective than narrowly oriented "biomedical concepts." (She does not, however, argue in favor of the expansive WHO definition.)

A second class of definitions excludes the social dimension while retaining the *physical and mental*. Daniel Callahan is tempted by this approach but eventually accepts a third and even more restrictive definition of health as "a state of *physical* well-being . . . without significant impairment of function." The approach taken by Callahan has the weight of tradition behind it, since in both the history of medicine and the history of philosophy (especially in the works of Plato, Aristotle, and Descartes) health is primarily regarded as physical well-being. This traditional support is not in itself decisive, of course. Several authors have pointed out that only recently have plausible reasons emerged for extending the scope of the concept. Joseph Margolis pursues precisely this line of investigation in his contribution by examining Freud's extension of the concepts of health and disease.

Controversies over the definition of *disease* have a rather different focus. Here one central issue is whether the term "disease" (and "illness," if different) refers to conditions objectively in nature or whether diseases are social constructions that are determined (wholly or partially) by our positive or negative evaluations—or whether some third alternative is correct. The so-called normativist thesis is bluntly exhibited in the following example and conclusion offered by Peter Sedgwick:

The blight that strikes at corn or at potatoes is a human invention, for if man wished to cultivate parasites (rather than potatoes or corn) there would be no blight, but simply the necessary foddering of the parasite-crop. . . . Outside the significances that man voluntarily attaches to certain conditions, *there are no illnesses or diseases in nature.*[1]

Not surprisingly, there has been a reaction to this normative, or evaluative, theory of disease. In this chapter Christopher Boorse argues for the objectivity of "disease" and the normativeness of "illness." Boorse is particularly opposed to such normative theses as the one developed by H. Tristram Engelhardt, who propounds his views in this chapter by analyzing the history of medical views of masturbation. Engelhardt argues explicitly against Boorse's objectivist theory in an essay following the Boorse selection.

Questions about whether "disease" is an inherently normative or evaluative concept may, of course, also be asked about "health." These controversies directly relate to the problem of whether "mental health" and "mental disease" are inherently evaluative notions. One could decide that "health" and "disease" should be defined as Callahan suggests (as exclusively concerned with *physical* well-being) and are *non-evaluative* notions as applied to physical health, while also claiming that such notions are either inherently evaluative or stretched beyond the bounds of normal objectivity when used in expressions such as "mental health" and "social disease." This problem is explored in the final two readings by Margolis and Thomas Szasz. Szasz regards the whole idea of "mental illness" as mythical and dangerous, but Margolis believes this issue turns on the plausibility of the analogy made between biomedically rooted understandings of health and those grounded in a theory of mental functioning.

This illustration of the interconnection between problems of defining health and problems of defining disease is only one indicator of the striking complexity and interrelatedness of the issues raised in this chapter.

TYPES OF DEFINITION

There are at least four different ways of defining terms, and it is important to distinguish them in attempting to define "health" and "disease." Since many other terms besides these two will be the subjects of definitional investigation in this book (prominent ones include "personhood," "death," "euthanasia," "behavior control," and "insanity"), it will prove worthwhile to discuss here the general nature of these four different types of definition.

1. *Descriptive definitions* attempt to report the usage of terms as people ordinarily employ them. All good dictionary definitions have this aim, since they inform us how the words of a particular language actually are used by those who speak the language. If there are different meanings or uses of the same term, they will be distinguished by such definitions. Sometimes dictionary definitions do little more than offer a synonym for the word being defined. The better formulated definitions, however, explicate the common

meaning of terms by specifying the conditions that must hold for the word to apply correctly. For example, Plato occasionally defines ''health'' in terms of the unimpeded natural functioning of the body. He seems to be attempting to describe the most general meaning of the term. Boorse similarly seems to believe that his analysis of disease eventuates in a descriptive definition. Such definitions are either true or false, since they are either correct or incorrect reports of common usage.

2. *Stipulative definitions* are ones that, instead of reporting actual usage, stipulate the meanings of terms, usually for purposes of clarity where the ordinary meaning is vague. Often the stipulation is only temporary and for a special purpose. For example, if the term ''health'' were defined as ''the state of successful adaptation to the pressures of city life,'' such a definition would be stipulative. There are reasons of convenience and clarity for using stipulative definitions such as this one (imagine a study of the pressures of city life being presented to a convention of social psychologists). It is not wrong to use such definitions as long as they are explicitly said to be stipulative and do not masquerade as descriptive. Unlike descriptive definitions, stipulative ones are neither true nor false, since they are simply proposals or announcements of usage. They might appear useless and misleading, since ordinary uses are excluded, but they cannot be mistaken.

3. *Reforming definitions* provide new meanings for old terms by suggesting new outlooks not incorporated in previous usage. But they are not simply stipulative, since they try to illuminate proper usage by giving a deeper insight into the meaning of a term. Also, they attempt to *reform* ordinary usage, whereas stipulative definitions often do not aim at reform (since they either introduce new meanings or are temporary and only for a special purpose). In the readings in this chapter, Daniel Callahan mentions an example of a reforming definition. He notes that the task of defining ''health'' is often not merely descriptive but (as in the case of the WHO definition) ''is nothing less than a way of deciding what should be valued, how life should be understood, and what principles should guide individual and social conduct.'' Joseph Margolis also explicates Freud's theory of mental illness as a value-laden reforming definition. If Callahan and Margolis are correct, it is clear that reforming definitions may be the bases of important and even programmatic attempts to change our actions and policies. Such definitions are usually the products of a theory—perhaps a social theory or a scientific theory. To assess the adequacy of the definition would thus probably require an assessment of the adequacy of the theory that generated it.

4. *Real definitions* are attempts to state what the real properties of something are. Such definitions are of special importance when (as in the case of reforming definitions) it is believed that ordinary usage is mistaken and therefore that descriptive definitions are necessarily inadequate. It might be, for example, that ordinary usage reflects Aristotle's belief that the term ''man'' means ''rational animal.'' But perhaps it is not truly necessary that man be rational, since human infants do not appear to be rational. (This topic is discussed in Chapter 6, Abortion.) If so, we would like to know what ''man'' *really is,* not just what the term might mean. Similarly in the case of ''mental illness,'' we want to know what such illness really is (if it is illness at all) and not simply what is commonly meant by the term. Such definitions are usually reforming definitions (though not necessarily, since the language might not need reformulation), but not all reforming definitions are real definitions. Many persons are now skeptical that real definitions can be given at all, since they are doubtful that language and theory are capable of grasping the real properties of things without recourse to an evaluative or theoretical perspective; whether or not this is so, attempts to provide real definitions recur frequently.

In the readings in this chapter, several authors provide definitions of ''health,'' ''disease,'' and ''illness.'' It is important to analyze what type or mixture of types of definition is being offered, for only then can one be prepared to judge the definition's acceptability. This is especially important where an author claims to be providing a descriptive or a real definition but is in fact providing a stipulative or a reforming one.

T.L.B.

NOTES

1. Peter Sedgwick, ''Illness—Mental and Otherwise,'' *Hastings Center Studies* I (3) (1973), pp. 19–40.

WORLD HEALTH ORGANIZATION

A Definition of Health

The States Parties to this Constitution declare, in conformity with the Charter of the United Nations, that the following principles are basic to the happiness, harmonious relations and security of all peoples:

Health is a state of complete physical, mental and social well-being and not merely the absence of disease or infirmity.

The enjoyment of the highest attainable standard of health is one of the fundamental rights of every human being without distinction of race, religion, political belief, economic or social condition.

The health of all peoples is fundamental to the attainment of peace and security and is dependent upon the fullest co-operation of individuals and States.

The achievement of any State in the promotion and protection of health is of value to all.

Unequal development in different countries in the promotion of health and control of disease, especially communicable disease, is a common danger.

Healthy development of the child is of basic importance; the ability to live harmoniously in a changing total environment is essential to such development.

The extension to all peoples of the benefits of medical, psychological and related knowledge is essential to the fullest attainment of health.

Informed opinion and active co-operation on the part of the public are of the utmost importance in the improvement of the health of the people.

Governments have a responsibility for the health of their peoples which can be fulfilled only by the provision of adequate health and social measures.

Accepting these principles, and for the purpose of co-operation among themselves and with others to promote and protect the health of all peoples, the Contracting Parties agree to the present Constitution and hereby establish the World Health Organization as a specialized agency within the terms of Article 57 of the Charter of the United Nations.

From the Preamble to the Constitution of the World Health Organization. Adopted by the International Health Conference held in New York from 19 June to 22 July 1946, and signed on 22 July 1946 by the representatives of sixty-one States *(Off. Rec. Wld Hlth Org.* 2, 100). Reprinted with permission of the publisher from *The First Ten Years of the World Health Organization, WHO,* 1958.

DANIEL CALLAHAN

The WHO Definition of "Health"

There is not much that can be called fun and games in medicine, perhaps because unlike other sports it is the only one in which everyone, participant and spectator, eventually gets killed playing. In the meantime, one of the grandest games is that version of king-of-the-hill where the aim of all players is to upset the World Health Organization (WHO) definition of "health." That definition, in case anyone could possibly forget it, is, "Health is a state of complete physical, mental, and social well-being and not merely the absence of disease or infirmity." Fair game, indeed. Yet somehow, defying all comers, the WHO definition endures, though literally every other aspirant to the crown has managed to knock it off the hill at least once. One possible reason for its presence is that it provides such an irresistible straw man; few there are who can resist attacking it in the opening paragraphs of papers designed to move on to more profound reflections.

But there is another possible reason which deserves some exploration, however unsettling the implications. It may just be that the WHO definition has more than a grain of truth in it, of a kind which is as profoundly frustrating as it is enticingly attractive. At the very least it is a definition which implies that there is some intrinsic relationship between the good of the body and the good of the self. The attractiveness of this relationship is obvious: it thwarts any movement toward a dualism of self and body, a dualism which in any event immediately breaks down when one drops a brick on one's toe; and it impels the analyst to work toward a conception of health which in the end is resistant to clear and distinct categories, closer to the felt experience. All that, naturally, is very frustrating. It seems simply impossible to devise a concept of health which is rich enough to be nutritious and yet not so rich as to be indigestible.

Reprinted with permission of the author and the Institute of Society, Ethics and the Life Sciences from *The Hastings Center Studies*, Vol. 1, No. 3 (1973).

One common objection to the WHO definition is, in effect, an assault upon any and all attempts to specify the meaning of very general concepts. Who can possibly define words as vague as "health," a venture as foolish as trying to define "peace," "justice," "happiness," and other systematically ambiguous notions? To this objection the "pragmatic" clinicians (as they often call themselves) add that, anyway, it is utterly unnecessary to know what "health" means in order to treat a patient running a high temperature. Not only that, it is also a harmful distraction to clutter medical judgment with philosophical puzzles.

Unfortunately for this line of argument, it is impossible to talk or think at all without employing general concepts: without them, cognition and language are impossible. More damagingly, it is rarely difficult to discover, with a bit of probing, that even the most "pragmatic" judgment (whatever *that* is) presupposes some general values and orientations, all of which can be translated into definitions of terms as general as "health" and "happiness." A failure to discern the operative underlying values, the conceptions of reality upon which they are based, and the definitions they entail, sets the stage for unexamined conduct and, beyond that, positive harm both to patients and to medicine in general.

But if these objections to any and all attempts to specify the meaning of "health" are common enough, the most specific complaint about the WHO definition is that its very generality, and particularly its association of health and general well-being as a positive ideal, has given rise to a variety of evils. Among them are the cultural tendency to define all social problems, from war to crime in the streets, as "health" problems; the blurring of lines of responsibility between and among the professions, and between the medical profession and the political order; the implicit denial of human freedom which results when failures to achieve social well-being are defined as forms of "sickness," somehow to be treated by medical means; and the general debasement of language which ensues upon the casual habit of labeling everyone from Adolf Hitler to student radicals to the brat next door as "sick." In short, the problem with the WHO definition is not that it represents an attempt to propose a general definition, but it is simply a bad one.

That is a valid line of objection, provided one can spell out in some detail just how the definition can or does entail some harmful consequences. Two lines of attack are possible against putatively hazardous social definitions of significant general concepts. One is by pointing out that the definition does not encompass all that a concept has commonly been taken to mean, either historically or at present, that it is a partial definition only. The task then is to come up with a fuller definition, one less subject to misuse. But there is still another way of objecting to socially significant definitions, and that is by pointing out some baneful effects of definitions generally accepted as adequate. Many of the objections to the WHO definition fall in the latter category, building upon the important insight that definitions of crucially important terms with a wide public use have ethical, social, and political implications; defining general terms is not an abstract exercise but a way of shaping the world metaphysically and structuring the world politically.

Wittgenstein's aphorism, "don't look for the meaning, look for the use," is pertinent here. The ethical problem in defining the concept of "health" is to determine what the implications are of the various uses to which a concept of "health" can be put. We might well agree that there are some uses of "health" which will produce socially harmful results. To carry Wittgenstein a step further, "don't look for the uses, look for the abuses." We might, then, examine some of the real or possible abuses to which the WHO definition leads, recognizing all the while that what we may term an "abuse" will itself rest upon some perceived *positive* good or value.

HEALTH AND HAPPINESS

Let us examine some of the principal objections to the WHO definition in more detail. One of them is that, by including the notion of "social well-being" under its rubric, it turns the enduring problem of human happiness into one more medical problem, to be dealt with by scientific means. That is surely an objectionable feature, if only because there exists no evidence whatever that medicine has anything more than a partial grasp of the sources of human misery. Despite [the optimism of Dr. Brock Chisholm, the first Director of WHO], medicine has not even found ways of dealing with more than a fraction of the whole range of physical diseases; campaigns, after all, are still being mounted against cancer and heart disease. Nor is there any special reason to think that future forays against those and other common diseases will bear rapid fruits. People will continue to die of disease for a long time to come, probably forever.

But perhaps, then, in the psychological and psychiatric sciences some progress has been made against what Dr. Chisholm called the "psychological ills," which lead to wars, hostility, and aggression. To be sure, there are many interesting psychological theories to be found about these "ills," and a few techniques which can, with some individuals, reduce or eliminate anti-social behavior. But so far as I can see, despite the mental health movement and the rise of the psychological sciences, war and human hostility are as much with us as ever. Quite apart from philosophical objections to the WHO definition, there was no empirical basis for the unbounded optimism which lay behind it at the time of its inception, and little has happened since to lend its limitless aspiration any firm support.

Common sense alone makes evident the fact that the absence of "disease or infirmity" by no means guarantees "social well-being." In one sense, those who drafted the WHO definition seem well aware of that. Isn't the whole point of their definition to show the inadequacy of negative definitions? But in another sense, it may be doubted that they really did grasp that point. For the third principle enunciated in the WHO Constitution says that "the health of all peoples is fundamental to the attainment of peace and security. . . ." Why is it fundamental, at least to peace? The worst wars of the twentieth century have been waged by countries with very high standards of health, by nations with superior life expectancies for individuals and with comparatively low infant mortality rates. The greatest present threats to world peace come in great part (though not entirely) from developed countries, those which have combated disease and illness most effectively. There seems to be no historical correlation whatever between health and peace, and that is true even if one includes "mental health."

How are human beings to achieve happiness? That

is the final and fundamental question. Obviously illness, whether mental or physical, makes happiness less possible in most cases. But that is only because they are only one symptom of a more basic restriction, that of human finitude, which sees infinite human desires constantly thwarted by the limitations of reality. "Complete" well-being might, conceivably, be attainable, but under one condition only: that people ceased expecting much from life. That does not seem about to happen. On the contrary, medical and psychological progress have been more than outstripped by rising demands and expectations. What is so odd about that, if it is indeed true that human desires are infinite? Whatever the answer to the question of human happiness, there is no particular reason to believe that medicine can do anything more than make a modest, finite contribution.

Another objection to the WHO definition is that, by implication, it makes the medical profession the gate-keeper for happiness and social well-being. Or if not exactly the gate-keeper (since political and economic support will be needed from sources other than medical), then the final magic-healer of human misery. Pushed far enough, the whole idea is absurd, and it is not necessary to believe that the organizers of the WHO would, if pressed, have been willing to go quite that far. But even if one pushes the pretension a little way, considerable fantasy results. The mental health movement is the best example, casting the psychological professional in the role of high priest.

At its humble best, that movement can do considerable good; people do suffer from psychological disabilities and there are some effective ways of helping them. But it would be sheer folly to believe that all, or even the most important, social evils stem from bad mental health: political injustice, economic scarcity, food shortages, unfavorable physical environments have a far greater historical claim as sources of a failure to achieve "social well-being." To retort that all or most of these troubles can, nonetheless, be seen finally as symptoms of bad mental health is, at best, self-serving and, at worst, just plain foolish.

A significant part of the objection that the WHO definition places, at least by implication, too much power and authority in the hands of the medical profession need not be based on a fear of that power as such. There is no reason to think that the world would be any worse off if health professionals made all decisions than if any other group did; and no reason to think it would be any better off. That is not a very important point. More significant is that cultural development which, in its skepticism about "traditional" ways of solving social problems, would seek a technological and specifically a medical solution for human ills of all kinds. There is at least a hint in early WHO discussions that, since politicians and diplomats have failed in maintaining world peace, a more expert group should take over, armed with the scientific skills necessary to set things right; it is science which is best able to vanquish that old Enlightenment bogey-man, "superstition." More concretely, such an ideology has the practical effect of blurring the lines of appropriate authority and responsibility. If all problems—political, economic, and social—reduce to matters of "health," then there ceases to be any ways to determine who should be responsible for what.

THE TYRANNY OF HEALTH

The problem of responsibility has at least two faces. One is that of a tendency to turn all problems of "social well-being" over to the medical professional, most pronounced in the instance of the incarceration of a large group of criminals in mental institutions rather than prisons. The abuses, both medical and legal, of that practice are, fortunately, now beginning to receive the attention they deserve, even if little corrective action has yet been taken. (Counterbalancing that development, however, are others, where some are seeking more "effective" ways of bringing science to bear on criminal behavior.)

The other face of the problem of responsibility is that of the way in which those who are sick, or purportedly sick, are to be evaluated in terms of their freedom and responsibility. Siegler and Osmond . . . discuss the "sick role," a leading feature of which is the ascription of blamelessness, of non-responsibility, to those who contract illness. There is no reason to object to this kind of ascription in many instances—one can hardly blame someone for contracting kidney disease—but, obviously enough, matters get out of hand when all physical, mental, and communal disorders are put under the heading of "sickness," and all sufferers (all of us, in the end) placed in the blameless "sick role." Not only are the concepts of "sickness" and "illness" drained of all content, it also becomes impossible to ascribe any freedom or responsibility to those caught up in the throes of sickness. The whole world is sick, and no one is responsible any longer for anything. That is determinism gone mad, a rather odd outcome of a development which began with attempts to bring unbenighted ''reason'' and free self-determination to bear for the release of the helpless captives of superstition and ignorance.

The final and most telling objection to the WHO definition has less to do with the definition itself than with one of its natural historical consequences. Thomas Szasz has been the most eloquent (and most single-minded) critic of that sleight-of-hand which has seen the concept of health moved from the medical to the moral arena. What can no longer be done in the name of ''morality'' can now be done in the name of ''health'': human beings labeled, incarcerated, and dismissed for their failure to toe the line of ''normalcy'' and ''sanity.''

At first glance, this analysis of the present situation might seem to be totally at odds with the tendency to put everyone in the blame-free ''sick role.'' Actually, there is a fine, probably indistinguishable, line separating these two positions. For as soon as one treats all human disorders—war, crime, social unrest—as forms of illness, then one turns health into a normative concept, that which human beings must and ought to have if they are to live in peace with themselves and others. Health is no longer an optional matter, but the golden key to the relief of human misery. We *must* be well or we will all perish. ''Health'' can and must be imposed; there can be no room for the luxury of freedom when so much is at stake. Of course the matter is rarely put so bluntly, but it is to Szasz's great credit that he has discerned what actually happens when ''health'' is allowed to gain the cultural clout which morality once had. (That he carries the whole business too far in his embracing of the most extreme moral individualism is another story, which cannot be dealt with here.) Something is seriously amiss when the ''right'' to have healthy children is turned into a further right for children not to be born defective, and from there into an obligation not to bring unhealthy children into the world as a way of respecting the right of those children to health! Nor is everything altogether lucid when abortion decisions are made a matter of ''medical judgment'' (see *Roe vs. Wade*); when decisions to provide psychoactive drugs for the relief of the ordinary stress of living are defined as no less ''medical judgment''; when patients are not allowed to die with dignity because of medical indications that they can, come what may, be kept alive; when prisoners, without their consent, are subjected to aversive conditioning to improve their mental health.

ABUSES OF LANGUAGE

In running through the litany of criticisms which have been directed at the WHO definition of ''health,'' and what seem to have been some of its long-term implications and consequences, I might well be accused of beating a dead horse. My only defense is to assert, first, that the spirit of the WHO definition is by no means dead either in medicine or society. In fact, because of the usual cultural lag which requires many years for new ideas to gain wide social currency, it is only now coming into its own on a broad scale. (Everyone now talks about everybody and everything, from Watergate to Billy Graham to trash in the streets, as ''sick.'') Second, I believe that we are now in the midst of a nascent (if not actual) crisis about how ''health'' ought properly to be understood, with much dependent upon what conception of health emerges in the near future.

If the ideology which underlies the WHO definition has proved to contain many muddled and hazardous ingredients, it is not at all evident what should take its place. The virtue of the WHO definition is that it tried to place health in the broadest human context. Yet the assumption behind the main criticisms of the WHO definition seem perfectly valid. Those assumptions can be characterized as follows: (1) health is only a part of life, and the achievement of health only a part of the achievement of happiness; (2) medicine's role, however important, is limited; it can neither solve nor even cope with the great majority of social, political, and cultural problems; (3) human freedom and responsibility must be recognized, and any tendency to place all deviant, devilish, or displeasing human beings into the blameless sick-role must be resisted; (4) while it is good for human beings to be healthy, medicine is not morality; except in very limited contexts (plagues and epidemics) ''medical judgment'' should not be allowed to become moral judgment; to be healthy is not to be righteous; (5) it is important to keep clear and distinct the different roles of different professions, with a clearly circumscribed role for medicine, limited to those domains of life where the contribution of medicine is appropriate. Medicine can save some lives; it cannot save the life of society.

These assumptions, and the criticisms of the WHO definition which spring from them, have some important implications for the use of the words "health," "illness," "sick," and the like. It will be counted an abuse of language if the word "sick" is applied to all individual and communal problems, if all unacceptable conduct is spoken of in the language of medical pathologies, if moral issues and moral judgments are translated into the language of "health," if the lines of authority, responsibility, and expertise are so blurred that the health profession is allowed to pre-empt the rights and responsibilities of others by redefining them in its own professional language.

Abuses of that kind have no possibility of being curbed in the absence of a definition of health which does not contain some intrinsic elements of limitation—that is, unless there is a definition which, when abused, is self-evidently *seen* as abused by those who know what health means. Unfortunately, it is in the nature of general definitions that they do not circumscribe their own meaning (or even explain it) and contain no built-in safeguards against misuse, e.g., our "peace with honor" in Southeast Asia— "peace," "honor"? Moreover, for a certain class of concepts—peace, honor, happiness, for example—it is difficult to keep them free in ordinary usage from a normative content. In our own usage, it would make no sense to talk of them in a way which implied they are not desirable or are merely neutral: by well-ingrained social custom (resting no doubt on some basic features of human nature) health, peace, and happiness are both desired and desirable—good. For those and other reasons, it is perfectly plausible to say the cultural task of defining terms, and settling on appropriate and inappropriate usages, is far more than a matter of getting our dictionary entries right. It is nothing less than a way of deciding what should be valued, how life should be understood, and what principles should guide individual and social conduct.

Health is not just a term to be defined. Intuitively, if we have lived at all, it is something we seek and value. We may not set the highest value on health— other goods may be valued as well—but it would strike me as incomprehensible should someone say that health was a matter of utter indifference to him; we would well doubt either his sanity or his maturity. The cultural problem, then, may be put this way. The acceptable range of uses of the term "health" should, at the minimum, capture the normative element in the concept as traditionally understood while, at the maximum, incorporating the insight (stemming from criticisms of the WHO definition) that the term "health" is abused if it becomes synonymous with virtue, social tranquility, and ultimate happiness. Since there are no instruction manuals available on how one would go about reaching a goal of that sort, I will offer no advice on the subject. I have the horrible suspicion, as a matter of fact, that people either have a decent intuitive sense on such matters (reflected in the way they use language) or they do not; and if they do not, little can be done to instruct them. One is left with the pious hope that, somehow, over a long period of time, things will change.

•   •   •

MODEST CONCLUSIONS

Two conclusions may be drawn. The first is that some minimal level of health is necessary if there is to be any possibility of human happiness. Only in exceptional circumstances can the good of self be long maintained in the absence of the good of the body. The second conclusion, however, is that one can be healthy without being in a state of "complete physical, mental, and social well-being." That conclusion can be justified in two ways: (a) because some degree of disease and infirmity is perfectly compatible with mental and social well-being; and (b) because it is doubtful that there ever was, or ever could be, more than a transient state of "complete physical, mental, and social well-being," for individuals or societies; that's just not the way life is or could be. Its attractiveness as an ideal is vitiated by its practical impossibility of realization. Worse than that, it positively misleads, for health becomes a goal of such all-consuming importance that it simply begs to be thwarted in its realization. The demands which the word "complete" entail set the stage for the worst false consciousness of all: the demand that life deliver perfection. Practically speaking, this demand has led, in the field of health, to a constant escalation of expectation and requirement, never ending, never satisfied.

What, then, would be a good definition of "health"? I was afraid someone was going to ask me that question. I suggest we settle on the following: "health is a state of physical well-being." That state need not be "complete," but it must be at least adequate, i.e., without significant impairment of function. It also need not encompass "mental" well-being; one can be healthy yet anxious, well yet depressed. And it surely ought not to encompass "social well-being,'' except insofar as that well-being will be impaired by the presence of large-scale, serious physical infirmities. Of course my definition is vague, but it would take some very fancy semantic footwork for it to be socially misused; that brat next door could not be called ''sick'' except when he is running a fever. This definition would not, though, preclude all social use of the language of ''pathology'' for other than physical disease. The image of a physically well body is a powerful one and, used carefully, it can be suggestive of the kind of wholeness and adequacy of function one might hope to see in other areas of life.

SALLY GUTTMACHER

Whole in Body, Mind, and Spirit: Holistic Health and the Limits of Medicine

Millions of North Americans have taken their health into their own hands. Those who are not jogging or mastering the intricate movements of T'ai Chi are consuming unprecedented amounts of whole bran, herbal teas, and assorted other ''natural'' substances in their quest for a healthy body. The intensity with which such regimens are pursued suggests that, for many, a healthy and vigorous body has become an end in itself rather than a means of pursuing other life goals. This new health consciousness manifests itself in forms ranging from the sensible and even puritanical to the frankly bizarre, but they can all be considered part of a larger movement—holistic health.

The terms ''holistic health'' and ''holistic medicine'' bring together very different theories and practices, but all who call themselves holistic healers share the notion that health is a positive state of functioning and not just the absence of symptoms or disease. While many of the concepts promoted by holistic medicine have ancient roots, the variety of practitioners makes it difficult to find any generally agreed-upon definitions, concepts, or practices. The central guiding principle, however, is that the *individual*—not the medical care system, not society—is responsible for the development and maintenance of health.[1]

From *The Hastings Center Report* 9 (April 1979), pp. 15–18, 20–21. Reprinted with permission of the Hastings Center: ©Institute of Society, Ethics and the Life Sciences, 360 Broadway, Hastings-on-Hudson, N.Y. 10706.

The holistic health movement has grown rapidly over the past decade, gathering adherents in its journey from the benevolent shores of California to the more skeptical enclaves of the Northeast. The diverse range of holistic practitioners reflects this journey: among them are segments of the now-faded counterculture; others are adherents of traditional healing practices like acupuncture; and still others use a variety of healing methods derived from psychologically and biochemically based theories, including meditation, massage, biofeedback, special diets, and esoteric forms of exercise. This latter group—perhaps due to its aura of scientific explanation and widespread publicity in magazines like *Psychology Today* and *Human Nature*—seems to be achieving for the whole movement a degree of legitimacy in the eyes of the public as well as the medical establishment. Even a past president of the American Medical Association, not known for its espousal of radical causes, publicly acknowledged the holistic health movement and recognized, perhaps because of its popular appeal, that it must be accommodated in some way.[2]

Whether as cause or effect, the development of the holistic health movement and the new health consciousness has been accompanied by an increasing dissatisfaction with certain aspects of medical care delivery.[3] Individuals complain about impersonal professional care and high fees. Economists and politicians inveigh against ever-spiraling costs.[4] Social critics point out the injustices of a medical care system in which, despite many reforms, access to care continues to vary by socioeconomic status and mode of payment.[5] Health analysts, including some medical practitioners, criticize the tenets of scientific medicine and the medical model of disease for the very limited notions of health and disease etiology that they promote.[6]

While the multitude of complaints come from diverse sectors of our society, they are grounded in a common perception: given the high level of intellectual, technical, and financial resources at its disposal, our current system of medical care has not produced a notably healthier population. . . .

MODELS OF HEALTH AND DISEASE

Holistic views of the concepts of health and disease differ in a number of important respects from the biomedical or allopathic model. Holistic practitioners are united in thinking that it is necessary to consider all dimensions of the person simultaneously and that the individual is ultimately responsible for his or her own state of health. In contrast, the biomedical model compares the body to a machine, made up of various organ systems, subsystems, and component parts. Disease manifests itself as a malfunction in a specific area; it can be corrected or ameliorated with proper diagnosis and reparative techniques. These techniques usually consist of a chemical or biological agent specifically suited to attack and render harmless the germ or biological malfunction that caused the disease.

These strong contrasts notwithstanding, the an-

Comparison of Biomedical and Holistic Concepts of Health and Disease

	Holistic concepts	Biomedical concepts
Health	A sense of well-being is the essential feature of the healthy individual. The precondition for health is the integration of the physiological, psychological, and spiritual dimensions of the individual.	Health is the absence of disease. It can be evaluated in relation to physical and physiological function within the normal range. Social, psychological, and spiritual dimensions are rarely considered as essential areas for intervention for a somatic problem. The preconditions for health are reasonably sanitary conditions, moderate exercise, and good eating and sleeping habits.
Disease	Disease is caused by more factors than a simple pathogenic agent. It should be viewed as an indicator of disharmony between the individual and his/her environment or a disintegration of the essential dimensions of the individual.	Disease can be thought of as "Deviations from the norm of measurable biological (somatic) variables."[†] It is commonly caused by a specific pathogenic agent, such as a chemical irritant or bacteria, and can be identified by distinctive symptoms. In essence, complex disease phenomena are ultimately derived from one or a few primary events such as contact with a pathogenic agent.
Healing	Healing must entail a reintegration of basic dimensions. The central factors in the process of successful healing are the intimacy of the patient-practitioner relationship, the quality of the spiritual experience, and the developing ability of the patient to deal with the problem independently.	The necessary prerequisite for healing is an attitude of cooperation with the physician. Disease can be "conquered" either by self-limitation of the pathogen or by a specific therapy. Steps in the healing process itself are congruent with our economic tradition. Prerequisites for cure are often presented to the patient as a set of consumable products (drugs, operations, days in the hospital, etc.)
Role of the Practitioner	The primary function of the practitioner is to teach the patient how to manage his/her illness and how to achieve and maintain a healthier state.	The physician possesses the necessary specialized technical knowledge and skill to cure the disease. His/her role is to develop the correct therapeutic measures to attack and conquer the disease.
Role of the Patient	The individual patient is essentially responsible for the outcome of an illness episode. The patient must engage in activities such as physical exercise, stress management, and nutritional awareness, which help maintain health as well as promote healing.[*]	The patient must cooperate with the physician and comply with instructions.

*Donald B. Ardell, *High Level Wellness* (Emmaus, Pa.: Rodale Press, 1977).

†George L. Engel, "The Need for a New Medical Model: A Challenge for Biomedicine," *Science* 196: 4286 (April 8, 1977), 130.

tagonism between the holistic and biomedical concepts may be more apparent than real. Holistic practitioners often propose the blending of some of modern Western medicine with practices from other cultures.[7] And since Virchow and the social medicine theorists of the mid-nineteenth century, many researchers and physicians have recognized that disease is rarely caused by a single factor, and that the body, psyche, and environment (which includes microorganisms) interact both to produce disease and to restore health.[8] Physicians trained in the biomedical model are, of course, capable in principle of appreciating the multidimensionality of holistic concepts. But to a significant extent their practice and habits have been constrained to a more narrow approach by the economic, social, and ideological framework within which they work. For example, conceptualizing the body as a highly sophisticated machine encourages the physician to view himself, in part, like an engineer with the ability and training to handle specialized information and technology.[9] The reliance upon specialists and experts, in conjunction with the rise of modern technology, fosters a hierarchical division of labor in medicine, much of which must take place within hospitals or research centers.

POTENTIAL BENEFITS OF THE HOLISTIC MOVEMENT

Although the holistic critique does not emphasize the influence of social-structural factors upon health, such as the bearing of our economic system upon the delivery of care, nonetheless, it stems in part from the observation that the received wisdom and conventional practice of biomedicine places untoward limits on what ought to be included in defining disease and in determining priorities of research and treatment.

The concepts and practices promoted by holistic healers merit close examination by those concerned about the continuing rise in the morbidity and mortality rates of specific chronic conditions. Cancer appears to be rising in the United States by about 1.6 percent annually.[10] Hypertension has become a serious and common health problem, especially among blacks.[11] In the wake of the inability of current medical practice to halt these increases, the costs of dealing with the symptoms and their sequelae continue to rise. Holistic medicine suggests approaching these problems in ways which may be well worth exploring and have not yet been complicated by extensive,

large-scale commercial momentum. For example, activities such as meditation, which help individuals "manage stress," may evolve into useful therapeutic practices. Even if such promises of holistic medicine are only partially realized, alternatives to the accepted mode of practice may infuse the health care consumer movement with momentum both to demand and to institute specific changes. For example, a fuller appreciation of the interpersonal aspects of healing could lead to the democratization and demystification of medical practice, patient-practitioner relations, and the institutional delivery of care. Challenges to the ever-increasing use of drugs, especially for chronic conditions, and to the emphasis upon drug-related research may encourage exploration of the efficacy of such alternative therapies as biofeedback, meditation, or traditional "home remedies."

In encouraging a new health consciousness, the holistic movement fosters a growing awareness of inadequacies in the current system of care. This awareness could lead to a deeper recognition of the relationship between the health of the individual and the way society is organized. Such an awareness might, in turn, promote an increase in resources allocated to preventive activities focused, for example, upon the stress-related causes of chronic disease. More important, the impact of the holistic movement could stimulate popular action challenging those conditions in our society that appear to generate stress or living conditions that lead to illness and disability.

THE LIMITATIONS OF HOLISTIC MEDICINE

Some of the social and political implications of holistic concepts, however, appear to present more cause for concern than reason for optimism. First, holistic ideology promotes a broadening of medicine into areas of life that have been considered inappropriate for medical intervention.[12] It raises specters of the therapeutic state and the threat of a social stratification system based on an individual's identity as patient or healer.[13] Second, the notion that disease is, in part, caused by disharmony within the individual reinforces the medical system's already strong tendency to deal with disorders chiefly at the personal level and largely to the exclusion of attacking other levels, such as economic or social organization.

Third, given the current climate of economic crisis and reaction against social welfare benefits, certain concepts of self-help promoted by the holistic movement lend themselves to cooptation by those who are mainly concerned with maintaining the present framework of medical care but cutting its costs. Fourth, if certain aspects of holistic concepts and practices prove preferable to the traditional model, it is likely that their acceptability and impact will vary by class. Finally, because holistic medicine would have to operate within the same political and economic constraints as the biomedical model, it is open to many of the same criticisms.

1. *Broadening the sphere of medicine.* In promoting a broader definition of health, holistic healers seem to be working hand-in-hand with those who think it necessary to expand the biomedical model into areas of life that had previously lain outside its control. There are even those who envisage a disease model framework for life cycle adjustment problems associated with development. Of course, the holistic movement cannot be held responsible for initiating that trend, but by viewing health as an end in itself, the holistic ideology pushes us further toward a life dominated by medical proscriptions and prescriptions. We may recoil from the extreme antitechnological position of social critics like Ivan Illich, but his warning about medicine should not be taken lightly[14]: the therapeutic invasion threatens the development of ever subtler measures of social control that will breed a passive population dependent upon medicine for the solutions to life's problems.

To take the clearest and most worrisome instance: chemical intervention, medicine's most advanced technology, is fast becoming the accepted mode for dealing with the daily problems of life, and in turn, dealing with a problem by pharmaceutical means gives strong impetus to thinking of it as a disease-like disorder. Instead of being provided with employment, a good education, or social supports, adolescents are prescribed drugs to help them cope with "Emancipation Disorder."[15] In lieu of dealing with the causes of depression, psychoactive drugs are increasingly prescribed for women who may in fact be reacting to "natural" events such as menopause or for those who feel unrewarded in their role of housewife or chief domestic consumer.[16]

2. *Individualistic focus.* At a time when a growing number of critics and researchers have begun to suggest that specific forms of morbidity and people's responses to them can be used as basic indicators of society's well-being, holistic ideology with its spiritual and metaphysical emphasis on illness, takes the opposite tack, calling upon the individual to gaze inward and focus upon the feelings or behavior that may be causing the disability. Such an emphasis supports the shallow notion of prevention common to biomedicine in which it is thought that we can stem the rise in rates of some chronic diseases by encouraging people to change the habits of a lifetime rather than working to change those aspects of our society that promote the development of such habits.[17]

A broader perspective than that of the biomedical or holistic mold views disease within an historical framework and calls into question not only the ministrations of care, but also the perceptions in which care is grounded. The particular course of a disease and, crucially, the way it is perceived and dealt with by the patient and healer is heavily influenced by its historical and environmental context. This is particularly obvious when one is dealing with "mental illness," where the criteria for identifying pathology are themselves suspect.[18]

Several researchers have argued that as the forms of economic activity and the social relations of a society change, so do the prevalence, virulence, and form of specific diseases.[19] This does not imply that the physical and biochemical laws that govern the working of disease mechanisms are not valid, but rather that the operation of these laws is inextricably linked to the social context. The type of potential diseases and the degree to which the "natural store" of disease expresses itself will shift in relation to this interaction. Evidence for this is abundantly clear in the changing patterns of disease noted by observers like Engels and Chadwick during the rise of the Industrial Revolution[20] or in the increase of stress-related chronic diseases associated with the modern period of industrialization.[21]

The mechanisms through which these relations operate are only now being studied in detail. In a few instances they are obvious: the occupational deaths, disease, and disability that only recently have begun to draw the attention—though not yet the action—they deserve; the fostering of poor nutrition and smoking habits by advertising.

From this perspective it follows that increased disease rates can be interpreted as a symptom of malfunction—sometimes peripheral, sometimes central—to the social structure. For example, the levels of certain chronic diseases endemic in our society are probably related to the stress generated by our form of economic and social practices. Researchers have suggested that the development of the "Type A personality" associated with heart disease is a product of the competitive and individualistic behavior pattern associated with the successful man in our society.[22] Others have shown that disease rates are closely tied to economic cycles.[23] A variety of factors such as job insecurity and unemployment during periods of recession or the increased demand on production lines during periods of economic boom may be correlated with the increase in stress-related disease. Finally, it is clear that the prevalence and incidence of certain conditions are associated with socioeconomic position.[24] That is, no matter how social class is measured, the risk of suffering from most of the chronic and infectious diseases is greater for the least-powerful members of our society. Furthermore, it has been well substantiated that the differences are not simply a reflection of differential access to care but are also related to basic differences in exposure to unhealthy environmental conditions and restricted opportunities for successfully dealing with stress.

In brief, understanding the cause and distribution of disease must take into account historical changes as well as social structure, and must recognize the continuities between injuries now treated as separate and discrete in the medical realm and the insults of day-to-day experience on the potential patient living in society. . . .

The holistic movement is unlikely to be any more effective than the biomedical model in reducing the high rates of morbidity and mortality from chronic diseases that characterize our society. Medicine, both holistic and biomedical, is structured, practiced, and embedded in our society in such a manner as to severely limit its perspectives. These limits stem not from the admittedly powerful science which informs medical diagnosis and treatment, but rather from other factors inseparably bound up with its current practice: from the settled interests and titled power of the medical profession; from related profit-making activities, such as the pharmaceutical industry; and from the pressures to seek technical solutions that avoid the necessity of confronting entrenched social relations where solutions can not be accomplished by technical tricks. As presently oriented, medicine is and will continue to be unable to grapple effectively with what are becoming the central health problems of advanced societies—disorders related to stress, to environmental hazard, to work, or to the self-indulgent

life styles fostered by powerful commercial and social interests. What is to be feared is that we create a medical system uniting the new focus on individual responsibility for illness with the technological biases of biomedicine, ignoring or underemphasizing the social, the preventive, and the deeper roots of health and disease.

NOTES

1. Richard B. Miles, "Humanistic Medicine and Holistic Health Care," in *The Holistic Health Handbook,* compiled by the Berkeley Holistic Health Center (Berkeley: AND/OR Press, 1978), pp. 20–24.

2. Malcolm C. Todd, "The Need for a New Health Program," in *The Holistic Health Handbook,* pp. 20–28. Todd was president of the AMA in 1975.

3. Boyce Rensberger, "Poll Shows Concern About Health Cost," *New York Times,* June 8, 1978, p. A16.

4. Alain C. Enthoven, "Consumer-Choice Health Plan," *The New England Journal of Medicine* 298: 12 (March 23, 1978), 650–58; and Barbara J. Culliton, "Health Care Economics: The High Cost of Getting Well," *Science* 200 (May 26, 1978), 883–85.

5. Karen Davis and Cathy Schoen, *Health and the War on Poverty* (Washington, DC: The Brookings Institution, 1978); and *The President's Commission on Mental Health* (Washington, DC: U.S. Government Printing Office, 1978).

6. Thomas McKeown, *The Modern Rise of Population* (New York: Academic Press, 1976); HMO Packets # 2 & 3, "The Social Etiology of Disease," *HMO* (New York: 1977), distributed by Health/Pac.

7. Jack LaPatra, *Healing: The Coming Revolution in Holistic Medicine* (New York: McGraw-Hill Book Co., 1978).

8. Howard S. Berliner and J. Warren Salmon, "Toward a Political Holistic Medicine," *Socialist Review* 43 (January–February 1979).

9. Thomas McKeown, "A Historical Appraisal of the Medical Task," *Medical History and Medical Care,* Gordon McLachlan and Thomas McKeown, eds. (London: Oxford University Press for the Nuffield Provincial Hospital Trust, 1971).

10. *Cancer Facts and Figures* (New York: American Cancer Society Inc., 1975).

11. J. Eyer, "Hypertension as a Disease of Modern Society," *International Journal of Health Services* 5:4 (1975), 539–58.

12. Rob Crawford, "Healthism and the Medicalization of Everyday Life," *International Journal of Health Services* 10:3 (1980), 365–88.

13. Ivan Illich, "Disabling Professions," in *Disabling Professions,* Ivan Illich, Irving K. Zola, John McKnight, Jonathan Caplan, Harley Shaiken (London: Marion Boyars Publishers Ltd., 1977).

14. Ivan Illich, *Medical Nemesis* (New York: Bantam Books, 1976).

15. *DSM III Operational Criteria,* American Psychiatric Association Task Force on Nomenclature and Statistics, January 15, 1978.

16. I. Waldron, "Increased Prescribers of Valium, Librium and Other Drugs—an Example of the Influence of Economic and Social Factors on the Practice of Medicine," *International Journal of Health Services* 7:1 (1977), 37–62.

17. John McKinlay, "A Case for Refocusing Upstream—The Political Economy of Illness," in *Applying Behavioral Science to*

Cardiovascular Risk, Proceedings of American Heart Association Conference, Seattle, Washington, June 17–19, 1974.

18. Kim Hopper and Sally Guttmacher, "Rethinking Suicide," *International Journal of Health Services;* A. Hollingshead and F. Redlich, *Social Class and Mental Illness* (New York: John Wiley and Sons, 1958).

19. Thomas McKeown, *The Role of Medicine: Dream, Mirage or Nemesis* (London: The Nuffield Provincial Hospitals Trust, 1976); John Powles, "On the Limitations of Modern Medicine"; Frank Feuner, "The Effects of Changing Social Organization on the Infectious Diseases of Man," in *The Impact of Civilization on the Biology of Man,* S. V. Boyden, ed. (Canberra: University Press, 1970), pp. 48–76.

20. Frederick Engels, *The Condition of the Working Class in England in 1844* (Moscow: Progress Publishers, 1973); Edwin Chadwick, *Report on an Inquiry into the Sanitary Conditions of the Laboring Population of Great Britain,* by W. M. Flinn, ed. (Scotland: Edinburgh University Press, 1965).

21. Joseph Eyer and Peter Sterling, "Stress-Related Mortality and Social Organization," *The Review of Radical Political Economics: Special Issue on the Political Economy of Health* (New York: Union of Radical Political Economists, 1977); Constantine A. Yeracaris and Jay H. Kim, "Socioeconomic Differentials in Selected Causes of Death," *American Journal of Public Health* 68:4 (April 1978), 342–51.

22. S. J. Zyzanski and C. D. Jenkins, "Basic Dimensions Within the Coronary-Prone Behavior Pattern," *Journal of Chronic Diseases* 22 (1970), 781–95; M. Friedman and R. H. Rosenman, *Type A Behavior and Your Heart* (New York: Alfred A. Knopf, 1973): Ingrid Waldron, "Type A Behavior Patterns and Coronary Heart Disease in Men and Women," *Social Science and Medicine* 12:3B (July 1978), 167–70.

23. M. Harvey Brenner, "Health Costs and the Benefits of Economic Policy," *International Journal of Health Services* 7:4 (1977), 581–624; Joseph Eyes, "Does Unemployment Cause the Death Rate Peak in Each Business Cycle? A Multifactor Model of Death Rate Changes," *International Journal of Health Services* 7:4 (1977), 625–62; D. S. Thomas, *Social Aspects of the Business Cycle* (New York: Alfred A. Knopf, 1927).

24. *Health of the Disadvantaged,* U.S. DHEW Public Health Service, Health Resources Administration, Office of Health Resources Opportunity, Washington, D.C., September 1977; Leonard Syme and Ira Berkman, "Social Class, Susceptibility and Sickness," *American Journal of Epidemiology* 104:1 (July 1976), 1–8.

The Concept of Disease

H. TRISTRAM ENGELHARDT, JR.

The Disease of Masturbation: Values and the Concept of Disease

Masturbation in the eighteenth and especially in the nineteenth century was widely believed to produce a spectrum of serious signs and symptoms, and was held to be a dangerous disease entity. Explanation of this phenomenon entails a basic reexamination of the concept of disease. It presupposes that one think of disease neither as an objective entity in the world nor as a concept that admits of a single universal definition: there is not, nor need there be, one concept of disease.[1] Rather, one chooses concepts for certain purposes, depending on values and hopes concerning the world.[2] The disease of masturbation is an eloquent example of the value-laden nature of science in general and of medicine in particular. In explaining the world, one judges what is to be significant or insignificant. For example, mathematical formulae are chosen in terms of elegance and simplicity, though elegance and simplicity are not attributes to be found in the world as such. The problem is even more involved in the case of medicine, which judges what the human organism should be (i.e., what counts as "health") and is thus involved in the entire range of human values. This paper will sketch the nature of the model of the disease of masturbation in the nineteenth century, particularly in America, and indicate the

Reprinted with permission of the author and the publisher from *Bulletin of the History of Medicine,* Vol. 48, No. 2 (Summer, 1974), pp. 234–248. ©1974 by The Johns Hopkins University Press.

scope of this "disease entity" and the therapies it evoked. The goal will be to outline some of the inter-relations between evaluation and explanation.

The moral offense of masturbation was transformed into disease with somatic not just psychological dimensions. Though sexual overindulgence generally was considered debilitating since at least the time of Hippocrates,[3] masturbation was not widely accepted as a disease until a book by the title *Onania* appeared anonymously in Holland in 1700 and met with great success.[4] This success was reinforced by the appearance of S. A. Tissot's book on onanism.[5] Tissot held that all sexual activity was potentially debilitating and that the debilitation was merely more exaggerated in the case of masturbation. The primary basis for the debilitation was, according to Tissot, loss of seminal fluid, one ounce being equivalent to the loss of forty ounces of blood.[6] When this loss of fluid took place in an other than recumbent position (which Tissot held often to be the case with masturbation), this exaggerated the ill effects.[7] In attempting to document his contention, Tissot provided a comprehensive monograph on masturbation, synthesizing and appropriating the views of classical authors who had been suspicious of the effects of sexual overindulgence. He focused these suspicions clearly on masturbation. In this he was very successful, for Tissot's book appears to have widely established the medical opinion that masturbation was associated with serious physical and mental maladies.[8]

There appears to have been some disagreement whether the effect of frequent intercourse was in any respect different from that of masturbation. The presupposition that masturbation was not in accordance with the dictates of nature suggested that it would tend to be more subversive of the constitution than excessive sexual intercourse. Accounts of this difference in terms of the differential effect of the excitation involved are for the most part obscure. It was, though, advanced that "during sexual intercourse the expenditure of nerve force is compensated by the magnetism of the partner."[9] Tissot suggested that a beautiful sexual partner was of particular benefit or was at least less exhausting.[10] In any event, masturbation was held to be potentially more deleterious since it was unnatural, and, therefore, less satisfying and more likely to lead to a disturbance or disordering of nerve tone.

At first, the wide range of illnesses attributed to masturbation is striking. Masturbation was held to be the cause of dyspepsia,[11] constrictions of the urethra,[12] epilepsy,[13] blindness,[14] vertigo, loss of hearing,[15] headache, impotency, loss of memory, "irregular action of the heart," general loss of health and strength,[16] rickets,[17] leucorrhea in women,[18] and chronic catarrhal conjunctivitis.[19] Nymphomania was found to arise from masturbation, occurring more commonly in blonds than in brunettes.[20] Further, changes in the external genitalia were attributed to masturbation: elongation of the clitoris, reddening and congestion of the labia majora, elongation of the labia minora,[21] and a thinning and decrease in size of the penis.[22] Chronic masturbation was held to lead to the development of a particular type, including enlargement of the superficial veins of the hands and feet, moist and clammy hands, stooped shoulders, pale sallow face with heavy dark circles around the eyes, a "draggy" gait, and acne.[23] Careful case studies were published establishing masturbation as a cause of insanity,[24] and evidence indicated that it was a cause of hereditary insanity as well.[25] Masturbation was held also to cause an hereditary predisposition to consumption.[26] Finally, masturbation was believed to lead to general debility. "From health and vigor, and intelligence and loveliness of character, they became thin and pale and cadaverous; their amiability and loveliness departed, and in their stead irritability, moroseness and anger were prominent characteristics. . . . The child loses its flesh and becomes pale and weak."[27] The natural history was one of progressive loss of vigor, both physical and mental.

In short, a broad and heterogeneous class of signs and symptoms were recognized in the nineteenth century as a part of what was tantamount to a syndrome, if not a disease: masturbation. If one thinks of a syndrome as the concurrence or running together of signs and symptoms into a recognizable pattern, surely masturbation was such a pattern. It was more, though, in that a cause was attributed to the syndrome, providing an etiological framework for a disease entity. That is, if one views the development of disease concepts as the progression from the mere collection of signs and symptoms to their interrelation in terms of a recognized causal mechanism, the disease of masturbation was fairly well evolved.

·   ·   ·

As mentioned, the concept of the disease of masturbation developed on the basis of a general suspicion that sexual activity was debilitating.[28] This development is not really unexpected: if one examines the world with a tacit presupposition of a parallelism between what is good for one's soul and what is good for one's health, then one would expect to find disease correlates for immoral sexual behavior.[29] Also, this was influenced by a concurrent inclination to translate a moral issue into medical terms and relieve it of the associated moral opprobrium in a fashion similar to the translation of alcoholism from a moral into a medical problem.[30] Further, disease as a departure from a state of stability due to excess or under excitation offered the skeleton of a psychosomatic theory of the somatic alterations attributed to the excitation associated with masturbation.

. . .

Those who held the disease of masturbation to be more than a culturally dependent phenomenon often employed somewhat drastic therapies. Restraining devices were devised,[31] infibulation or placing a ring in the prepuce was used to make masturbation painful,[32] and no one less than Jonathan Hutchinson held that circumcision acted as a preventive.[33] Acid burns or thermoelectrocautery[34] were utilized to make masturbation painful and, therefore, to discourage it. The alleged seriousness of this disease in females led, as Professor John Duffy has shown, to the employment of the rather radical treatment of clitoridectomy.[35] The classic monograph recommending clitoridectomy, written by the British surgeon Baker Brown, advocated the procedure to terminate the "long continued peripheral excitement, causing frequent and increasing losses of nerve force. . . ."[36] Brown recommended that "the patient having been placed completely under the influence of chloroform, the clitoris [be] freely excised either by scissors or knife—I always prefer the scissors."[37] The supposed sequelae of female masturbation, such as sterility, paresis, hysteria, dysmenorrhea, idiocy, and insanity, were also held to be remedied by the operation.

Male masturbation was likewise treated by means of surgical procedures. Some recommended vasectomy[38] while others found this procedure ineffective and employed castration.[39] One illustrative case involved the castration of a physician who had been confined as insane for seven years and who subsequently was able to return to practice.[40]

. . .

There were, though, more tolerant approaches, ranging from hard work and simple diet[41] to suggestions that "If the masturbator is totally continent,

sexual intercourse is advisable."[42] This latter approach to therapy led some physicians to recommend that masturbators cure their disease by frequenting houses of prostitution,[43] or acquiring a mistress.[44] Though these treatments would appear ad hoc, more theoretically sound proposals were made by many physicians in terms of the model of excitability. They suggested that the disease and its sequelae could be adequately controlled by treating the excitation and debility consequent upon masturbation. Towards this end, "active tonics" and the use of cold baths at night just before bedtime were suggested.[45] Much more in a "Brownian" mode was the proposal that treatment with opium would be effective. An initial treatment with $1/12$ of a grain of morphine sulfate daily by injection was followed after ten days by a dose of $1/16$ of a grain. This dose was continued for three weeks and gradually diminished to $1/30$ of a grain a day. At the end of the month the patient was dismissed from treatment "the picture of health, having fattened very much, and lost every trace of anaemia and mental imbecility."[46] The author, after his researches with opium and masturbation, concluded, *"We may find in opium a new and important aid in the treatment of the victims of the habit of masturbation by means of which their moral and physical forces may be so increased that they may be enabled to enter the true physiological path."*[47] This last example eloquently collects the elements of the concept of the disease of masturbation as a pathophysiological entity: excitation leads to physical debilitation requiring a physical remedy. Masturbation as a pathophysiological entity was thus incorporated within an acceptable medical model of diagnosis and therapy.

In summary, in the nineteenth century, biomedical scientists attempted to correlate a vast number of signs and symptoms with a disapproved activity found in many patients afflicted with various maladies. Given an inviting theoretical framework, it was very conducive to think of this range of signs and symptoms as having one cause. The theoretical framework, though, as has been indicated, was not value free but structured by the values and expectations of the times. In the nineteenth century, one was pleased to think that not "one bride in a hundred, of delicate, educated, sensitive women, accepts matrimony from any desire of sexual gratification: when she thinks of this at all, it is with shrinking, or even with horror, rather than with desire."[48] In contrast, in the twentieth century, articles are published for the instruction of women in the use of masturbation to overcome the disease of frigidity or orgasmic dysfunction.[49] In both cases, expectations concerning what should be significant structure the appreciation of reality by medicine. The variations are not due to mere fallacies of scientific method[50] but involve a basic dependence of the logic of scientific discovery and explanation upon prior evaluations of reality.[51] A sought-for coincidence of morality and nature gives goals to explanation and therapy.[52] Values influence the purpose and direction of investigations and treatment. Moreover, the disease of masturbation has other analogues. In the nineteenth century, there were such diseases in the South as "Drapetomania, the disease causing slaves to run away," and the disease "Dysaesthesia Aethiopis or hebetude of mind and obtuse sensibility of body—a disease peculiar to Negroes—called by overseers 'rascality'."[53] In Europe, there was the disease of *morbus democritus*.[54] Some would hold that current analogues exist in diseases such as alcoholism and drug abuse.[55] In short, the disease of masturbation indicates that evaluations play a role in the development of explanatory models and that this may not be an isolated phenomenon.

This analysis, then, suggests the following conclusion: although vice and virtue are not equivalent to disease and health, they bear a direct relation to these concepts. Insofar as a vice is taken to be a deviation from an ideal of human perfection, or "well-being," it can be translated into disease language. In shifting to disease language, one no longer speaks in moralistic terms (e.g., "You are evil"), but one speaks in terms of a deviation from a norm which implies a degree of imperfection (e.g., "You are a deviant"). The shift is from an explicitly ethical language to a language of natural teleology. To be ill is to fail to realize the perfection of an ideal type; to be sick is to be defective rather than to be evil. The concern is no longer with what is naturally, morally good, but what is naturally beautiful. Medicine turns to what has been judged to be naturally ugly or deviant, and then develops etiological accounts in order to explain and treat in a coherent fashion a manifold of displeasing signs and symptoms. The notion of the "deviant" structures the concept of disease, providing a purpose and direction for explanation and for action, that is, for diagnosis and prognosis, and for therapy. A "dis-

ease entity" operates as a conceptual form organizing phenomena in a fashion deemed useful for certain goals. The goals, though, involve choice by man and are not objective facts, data "given" by nature. They are ideals imputed to nature. The disease of masturbation is an eloquent example of the role of evaluation in explanation and the structure values give to our picture of reality.

NOTES

1. Alvan R. Feinstein, "Taxonomy and logic in clinical data," *Ann. N.Y. Acad. Sci.*, 1969, *161:* 450–459.

2. Horacio Fabrega, Jr., "Concepts of disease: logical features and social implications," *Perspect. Biol. Med.*, 1972, *15:* 583–616.

3. For example, Hippocrates correlated gout with sexual intercourse, *Aphorisms*, VI, 30. Numerous passages in the *Corpus* recommend the avoidance of overindulgence especially during certain illnesses.

4. René A. Spitz, "Authority and masturbation. Some remarks on a bibliographical investigation," *Yb. Psychoanal.*, 1953, *9:* 116. Also, Robert H. MacDonald, "The frightful consequences of onanism: notes on the history of a delusion." *J. Hist. Ideas*, 1967, *28:* 423–431.

5. Simon-André Tissot, *Tentamen de Morbis ex Manustrupatione* (Lausannae: M. M. Bousquet, 1758). An anonymous American translation appeared in the early 19th century: *Onanism* (New York: Collins & Hannay, 1832).

6. Simon-André Tissot, *Onanism* (New York: Collins & Hannay, 1832), p. 5.

7. *Ibid.*, p. 50.

8. E. H. Hare, "Masturbatory insanity: the history of an idea," *J. Mental Sco.*, 1962, *108:* 2–3.

9. Howe, *op. cit.* (n. 5 above), pp. 76–77.

10. Tissot, *op. cit.* (n. 6 above), p. 51.

11. J. A. Mayes, "Spermatorrhoea, treated by the lately invented rings," *Charleston Med. J. & Rev.*, 1854, *9:* 352.

12. Allen W. Hagenbach, "Masturbation as a cause of insanity," *J. Ner. Ment. Dis.*, 1879, *6:* 609.

13. Baker Brown, *On the Curability of Certain Forms of Insanity, Epilepsy, Catalepsy, and Hysteria in Females* (London: Hardwicke, 1866). Brown phrased the cause discreetly in terms of "peripheral irritation, arising originally in some branches of the pudic nerve, more particularly the incident nerve supplying the clitoris. . . ." (p. 7).

14. F. A. Burdem, "Self pollution in children," *Mass. Med. J.*, 1896, *16:* 340.

15. Weber Liel, "The influence of sexual irritation upon the diseases of the ear," *New Orleans Med. & Surg. J.*, 1884, *11:* 786–788.

16. Joseph Jones, "Diseases of the nervous system," *Trans. La. Med. Soc.* (New Orleans: L. Graham & Son, 1889), p. 170.

17. Howe, *op. cit.* (n. 5 above), p. 93.

18. J. Castellanos, "Influence of sewing machines upon the health and morality of the females using them," *South. J. Med. Sci.*, 1866–1867, *1:* 495–496.

19. Comment, "Masturbation and ophthalmia," *New Orleans Med. & Surg. J.*, 1881–1882, *9:* 67.

20. Howe, *op. cit.* (n. 5 above), pp. 108–111.

21. *Ibid.*, pp. 41, 72.

22. *Ibid.*, p. 68.

23. *Ibid.*, p. 73.

24. Hagenbach, *op. cit.* (n. 12 above), pp. 603–612.

25. Jones, *op. cit.* (n. 16 above), p. 170.

26. Howe, *op. cit.* (n. 5 above), p. 95.

27. Burdem, *op. cit.* (n. 14 above), pp. 339, 341.

28. Even Boerhaave remarked that "an excessive discharge of semen causes fatigue, weakness, decrease in activity, convulsions, emaciation, dehydration, heat and pains in the membranes of the brain, a loss in the acuity of the senses, particularly of vision, *tabes dorsalis,* simplemindedness, and various similar disorders." My translation of Hermanno Boerhaave's *Institutiones Medicae* (Viennae: J. T. Trattner, 1775), p. 315, paragraph 776.

29. "We have seen that masturbation is more pernicious than excessive intercourse with females. Those who believe in a special providence, account for it by a special ordinance of the Deity to punish this crime." Tissot, *op. cit.* (n. 6 above), p. 45.

30. ". . .the best remedy was not to tell the poor children that they were damning their souls, but to tell them that they might seriously hurt their bodies, and to explain to them the nature and purport of the functions they were abusing." Lawson Tait, "Masturbation. A clinical lecture," *Med. News,* 1888, *53:* 2.

31. C. D. W. Colby, "Mechanical restraint of masturbation in a young girl," *Med. Record in N.Y.,* 1897, *52:* 206.

32. Louis Bauer, "Infibulation as a remedy for epilepsy and seminal losses," *St. Louis Clin. Record,* 1879, *6:* 163–165. See also Gerhart S. Schwarz, "Infibulation, population control, and the medical profession," *Bull. N.Y. Acad. Med.,* 1970, *46:* 979, 990.

33. Jonathan Hutchinson, "On circumcision as preventive of masturbation," *Arch. Surg.,* 1890–1891, *2:* 267–269.

34. William J. Robinson, "Masturbation and its treatment," *Am. J. Clin. Med.,* 1907, *14:* 349.

35. John Duffy, "Masturbation and clitoridectomy. A nineteenth-century view," *J.A.M.A.,* 1963, *186:* 246–248.

36. Brown, *op. cit.* (n. 13 above), p. 11.

37. *Ibid.*, p. 17.

38. Timothy Haynes, "Surgical treatment of hopeless cases of masturbation and nocturnal emissions," *Boston Med. & Surg. J.,* 1883, *109:* 130.

39. J. H. Marshall, "Insanity cured by castration," *Med. & Surg. Reptr.,* 1865, *13:* 363–364.

40. "The patient soon evinced marked evidences of being a changed man, becoming quiet, kind, and docile." *Ibid.*, p. 363.

41. Editorial, "Review of European legislation for the control of prostitution," *New Orleans Med. & Surg. J.,* 1854–1855, *11:* 704.

42. Robinson, *op. cit.* (n. 34 above), p. 350.

43. Theophilus Parvin, "The hygiene of the sexual functions," *New Orleans Med. & Surg. J.,* 1884, *11:* 606.

44. Mayes, *op. cit.* (n. 11 above), p. 352.

45. Haynes, *op. cit.* (n. 38 above), p. 130.

46. B. A. Pope, "Opium as a tonic and alternative; with remarks upon the hypodermic use of the sulfate of morphia, and its use in the debility and amorosis consequent upon onanism," *New Orleans Med. & Surg. J.,* 1879, *6:* 725.

47. *Ibid.*, p. 727.

48. Parvin, *op. cit.* (n. 43 above), p. 607.

49. Joseph LoPiccolo and W. Charles Lobitz, "The role of masturbation in the treatment of orgasmic dysfunction," *Arch. Sexual Behavior,* 1972, *2:* 163–171.

50. E. Hare, *op. cit.* (n. 8 above), pp. 15–19.

51. Norwood Hanson, *Patterns of Discovery* (London: Cambridge University Press, 1965).

52. Tissot, *op. cit.* (n. 6 above), p. 45. As Immanuel Kant, a contemporary of S.-A. Tissot remarked, "Also, in all probability, it was through this moral interest [in the moral law governing the world] that attentiveness to beauty and the ends of nature was first aroused." *(Kants Werke,* Vol. 5, *Kritik der Urtheilskraft* [Berlin: Walter de Gruyter & Co., 1968], p. 459, A 439. My translation.) That is, moral values influence the search for goals in nature, and direct attention to what will be considered natural, normal, and non-deviant. This would also imply a relationship between the aesthetic, especially what was judged to be naturally beautiful, and what was held to be the goals of nature.

53. Samuel A. Cartwright, "Report on the diseases and physical peculiarities of the Negro race," *New Orleans Med. & Surg. J.,* 1850–1851, *7:* 707–709. An interesting examination of these diseases is given by Thomas S. Szasz, "The sane slave," *Am. J. Psychoth.,* 1971, *25:* 228–239.

54. Heinz Hartmann, "Towards a concept of mental health," *Brit. J. Med. Psychol.,* 1960, *33:* 248.

55. Thomas S. Szasz, "Bad habits are not diseases: a refutation of the claim that alcoholism is a disease," *Lancet,* 1972, *2:* 83–84; and Szasz, "The ethics of addiction," *Am. J. Psychiatry,* 1971, *128:* 541–546.

CHRISTOPHER BOORSE*

On the Distinction Between Disease and Illness

In this century a strong tendency has developed to debate social issues in psychiatric terms. Whether the topic is criminal responsibility, sexual deviance, feminism, or a host of others, claims about mental health are increasingly likely to be the focus of discussion. This growing preference for medicine over morals, which might be called the *psychiatric turn,* has an obvious appeal. In the paradigm health discipline, physiological medicine, judgments of health and disease are normally uncontroversial. The idea of reaching comparable certainty about difficult ethical problems is an inviting prospect. Unfortunately our grasp of the issues that surround the psychiatric turn continues to be impeded, as does psychiatric theory itself, by a fundamental misunderstanding of the concept of health. With few exceptions, clinicians and philosophers are agreed that health is an essentially evaluative notion. According to this consensus view, a value-free science of health is impossible. This thesis I believe to be entirely mistaken. I shall argue in this essay that it rests on a confusion between the theoretical and the practical senses of "health," or in other words, between disease and illness.

Two presuppositions of my whole discussion should be noted at the outset. The first is substantive: with Szasz and Flew, I shall assume that the idea of health ought to be analyzed by reference to physiological medicine alone.[1] It is a mistake to view physical and mental health as equally well-entrenched species of a single conceptual genus. In most respects, our institutions of mental health are recent offshoots from physiological medicine, and their nature and future are under continual controversy. In advance of a clear analysis of health in physiological

medicine, it seems an open question whether current applications of the health vocabulary to mental conditions have any justification at all. Such applications will therefore be put on probation in the first two sections below. The other presupposition of my discussion is terminological. For convenience in distinguishing theoretical from practical uses of "health," I shall adhere to the technical usage of "disease" found in textbooks of medical theory. In such textbooks "disease" is simply synonymous with "unhealthy condition." Readers who wish to preserve the much narrower ordinary usage of "disease" should therefore substitute "theoretically unhealthy condition" throughout.

NORMATIVISM ABOUT HEALTH

It is safe to begin any discussion of health by saying that health is normality, since the terms are interchangeable in clinical contexts. But this remark provides no analysis of health until one specifies the norms involved. The most obvious proposal, that they are pure statistical means, is widely recognized to be erroneous. On the one hand, many deviations from the average—e.g., unusual strength or vital capacity or eye color—are not unhealthy. On the other hand, practically everyone has some disease or other, and there are also particular diseases such as tooth decay and minor lung irritation that are nearly universal. Since statistical normality is therefore neither necessary nor sufficient for clinical normality, most writers take the following view about the norms of health: that they must be determined, in whole or in part, by acts of evaluation. More precisely, the orthodox view is that all judgments of health include value judgments as part of their meaning. To call a condition unhealthy is at least in part to condemn it; hence it is impossible to define health in nonevaluative terms. I shall refer to this orthodox view as *normativism.*

Normativism has many varieties, which are often not clearly distinguished from one another by the

*I thank the Delaware Institute for Medical Education and Research and the National Institute of Mental Health (Grant RO₃ MH 24621) for support in writing this essay.

Reprinted with permission of the publisher from *Philosophy and Public Affairs,* Vol. 5, No. 1 (Fall 1975), pp. 49–68. Copyright ©1975 by Princeton University Press.

clinicians who espouse them. The common feature of healthy conditions may, for example, be held to be either their desirability for the individual or their desirability for society. The gap between these two values is a persistent source of controversy in the mental-health domain. One especially common variety of normativism combines the thesis that health judgments are value judgments with ethical relativism. The resulting view that society is the final authority on what counts as disease is typical of psychiatric texts, as illustrated by the following quotation:

While professionals have a major voice in influencing the judgment of society, it is the collective judgment of the larger social group that determines whether its members are to be viewed as sick or criminal, eccentric or immoral.[2]

For the most part my arguments against normativism will apply to all versions indiscriminately. It will, however, be useful to make a minimal division of normativist positions into strong and weak. Strong normativism will be the view that health judgments are pure evaluations without descriptive meaning; weak normativism allows such judgments a descriptive as well as a normative component.[3]

As an example of a virtually explicit statement of strong normativism by a clinician, consider Dr. Judd Marmor's remark in a recent psychiatric symposium on homosexuality:

. . . to call homosexuality the result of disturbed sexual development really says nothing other than that you disapprove of the outcome of the development.[4]

If we may substitute "unhealthy" for "disturbed," Marmor is claiming that to call a condition unhealthy is *only* to express disapproval of it. In other words—to collapse a few ethical distinctions—for a condition to be unhealthy it is necessary and sufficient that it be bad. Now at least half of this view, the sufficiency claim, is demonstrably false of physiological medicine. It is undesirable to be moderately ugly or, for that matter, to lack the manual dexterity of Liszt, but neither of these conditions is a disease. In fact, there are undesirable conditions regularly corrected by physicians which are not diseases: Jewish nose, sagging breasts, adolescent fertility, and unwanted pregnancies are only a few of many examples. Thus strong normativism is an erroneous account of health judgments in their paradigm area of application, and its influence upon mental-health theorists is regrettable.

Unlike Marmor, however, many clinical writers take positions that can be construed as committing them merely to weak normativism. A good example is Dr. Marie Jahoda, who concludes her survey of current criteria of psychological health with these words:

Actually, the discussion of the psychological meaning of various criteria could proceed without concern for value premises. Only as one calls these psychological phenomena "mental health" does the problem of values arise in full force. By this label, one asserts that these psychological attributes are "good." And, inevitably, the question is raised: Good for what? Good in terms of middle class ethics? Good for democracy? For the continuation of the social *status quo?* For the individual's happiness? For mankind? . . . For the encouragement of genius or of mediocrity and conformity? The list could be continued.[5]

Jahoda may here mean to claim only that calling a condition healthy *involves* calling it good. Her remarks are at least consistent with the weak normativist thesis that healthy conditions are good conditions which satisfy some further descriptive property as well. On this view, "healthy" is a mixed normative-descriptive term of the same sort as "honest" and "courageous." The following passage by Dr. F. C. Redlich is likewise consistent with the weak view:

Most propositions about normal behavior refer implicitly or explicitly to ideal behavior. Deviations from the ideal obviously are fraught with value judgments; actually, all propositions on normality contain certain statements in various degrees.[6]

Redlich's term "contain" suggests that he too sees the goodness of something as merely one necessary condition of its healthiness, and similarly for badness and unhealthiness.

Yet even weak normativism runs into counterexamples within physiological medicine. It is obvious that a disease may be on balance desirable, as with the flat feet of a draftee or the mild infection produced by inoculation. It might be suggested in response that diseases must at any rate be prima facie undesirable. The trouble with this suggestion is that it is obscure. Consider the case of a disease that has infertility as its sole important effect. In what sense is infertility prima facie undesirable? Considered in abstraction from the actual effects of reproduction on human beings, it is hard to see how infertility is either desirable or undesirable. Possibly those who see it as "prima facie" undesirable assume that most people want to be able to have more children. But the corollary of this position will be that writers of medical texts must do an empirical survey of human preferences to be sure that a condition is a disease. No such considerations seem to enter into human physiological research, any more than they do into standard biological studies of the diseases of plants and animals. Here indeed is another difficulty for any normativist, weak or strong. It seems clear that one may speak of diseases in plants and animals without judging the conditions in question undesirable. Biologists who study the diseases of fruit flies or sharks need not assume that their health is a good thing for us. On the other hand, there is not much sense in talking about the best interests of, say, a begonia. So it seems that normativists must interpret health judgments about plants and lower animals as analogical, in the same way as would be statements about the courage or considerateness of wolves and rats.

If normativism about health is at once so influential and so objectionable, one must ask what persuasive arguments there are in its support. I know of only three arguments, of which one will be treated in the next section. A germ of an argument appears in the passage by Redlich just quoted. Health judgments involve a comparison to an ideal; hence, Redlich concludes, they are "fraught with value judgments." It seems evident, however, that Redlich is thinking of ideals such as beauty and holiness rather than the chemist's ideal gas or Weber's ideal bureaucrat. The fact that a gas or a bureaucrat deviates from the ideal type is nothing against the gas or the bureaucrat. There are normative and nonnormative ideals, as there are in fact normative and nonnormative norms. The question is which sort health is, and Redlich has here provided no grounds for an answer.

A second and equally incomplete argument for normativism is suggested by the first two chapters of Margolis' *Psychotherapy and Morality*.[7] Margolis argues in his first chapter that psychoanalysts have been mistaken in holding that their therapeutic activities can "escape moral scrutiny" (p. 13). From this he concludes that "it is reasonable to view therapeutic values as forming part of a larger system of moral values" (p. 37), and explicitly endorses normativism. But this inference is a non sequitur. From the fact that the promotion of health is open to moral review, it in

no way follows that health judgments are value judgments. Wealth and power are also "values" in the sense that people pursue them in a morally criticizable fashion; neither is a normative concept. The pursuit of any descriptively definable condition, if it has effects on persons, will be open to moral review.

These two arguments, like the health literature generally, do next to nothing to rule out the alternative view that health is a descriptively definable property which is usually valuable. Why, after all, may not health be a concept of the same sort as intelligence, or deductive validity? Though the idea of intelligence is certainly vague, it does not seem to be normative. Intelligence is the ability to perform certain intellectual tasks, and one would expect that these intellectual tasks could be characterized without presupposing their value.[8] Similarly, a valid argument may, for theoretical purposes, be descriptively defined[9] roughly as one that has a form no instance of which could have true premises and a false conclusion. Intelligence in people and validity in arguments being generally valued, the statement that a person is intelligent or an argument valid does tend to have the force of a recommendation. But this fact is wholly irrelevant to the employment of the terms in theories of intelligence or validity. To insist that evaluation is still part of the very meaning of the terms would be to make an implausible claim to which there are obvious counterexamples. Exactly the same may be true of the concept of health. At any rate, we have already seen some of the counterexamples.

Since the distinction between force and meaning in philosophy of language is in a rather primitive state, it is doubtful that weak normativism about health can be either decisively refuted or decisively established. But I suggest that its current prevalence is largely the result of two quite tractable causes. One is the lack of a plausible descriptive analysis; the other is a confusion between theoretical and practical uses of the health vocabulary. The required descriptive analysis I shall try to sketch in the next section. As for the second cause, one should always remember that a dual commitment to theory and practice is one of the features that distinguish a clinical discipline. Unlike chemists or astronomers, physicians and psychotherapists are professionally engaged in practical judgments about how certain people ought to be treated. It would not be surprising if the terms in which such practical judgments are formulated have normative content. One might contend, for example, that calling a cancer "inoperable" involves the value judgment that the results of operating will be worse than leaving the disease alone. But behind this conceptual framework of medical practice stands an autonomous framework of medical theory, a body of doctrine that describes the functioning of a healthy body, classifies various deviations from such functioning as diseases, predicts their behavior under various forms of treatment, etc. This theoretical corpus looks in every way continuous with theory in biology and the other natural sciences, and I believe it to be value-free.

The difference between the two frameworks emerges most clearly in the distinction between disease and illness. It is disease, the theoretical concept, that applies indifferently to organisms of all species. That is because, as we shall see, it is to be analyzed in biological rather than ethical terms. The point is that illnesses are merely a subclass of diseases, namely, those diseases that have certain normative features reflected in the institutions of medical practice. An illness must be, first, a reasonably *serious* disease with incapacitating effects that make it undesirable. A shaving cut or mild athlete's foot cannot be called an illness, nor could one call in sick on the basis of a single dental cavity, though all these conditions are diseases. Secondly, to call a disease an illness is to view its owner as deserving special treatment and diminished moral accountability. These requirements of "illness" will be discussed in some detail shortly, with particular attention to "mental illness." But they explain at once why the notion of illness does not apply to plants and animals. Where we do not make the appropriate normative judgments or activate the social institutions, no amount of disease will lead us to use the term "ill." Even if the laboratory fruit flies fly in listless circles and expire at our feet, we do not say they succumbed to an illness, and for roughly the same reasons as we decline to give them a proper funeral.

There are, then, two senses of "health." In one sense it is a theoretical notion, the opposite of "disease." In another sense it is a practical or mixed ethical notion, the opposite of "illness."[10] Let us now examine the relation between these two concepts more closely.

DISEASE AND ILLNESS

What is the theoretical notion of a disease? An admirable explanation of clinical normality was given thirty years ago by C. Daly King.

The normal . . . is objectively, and properly, to be defined as that which functions in accordance with its design.[11]

The root idea of this account is that the normal is the natural. The state of an organism is theoretically healthy, i.e., free of disease, insofar as its mode of functioning conforms to the natural design of that kind of organism. Philosophers have, of course, grown repugnant to the idea of natural design since its cooptation by natural-purpose ethics and the so-called argument from design. It is undeniable that the term "natural" is often given an evaluative force. Shakespeare as well as Roman Catholicism is full of such usages, and they survive as well in the strictures of state legislatures against "unnatural acts." But it is no part of biological theory to assume that what is natural is desirable, still less the product of divine artifice. Contemporary biology employs a version of the idea of natural design that seems ideal for the analysis of health.

The crucial element in the idea of a biological design is the notion of a natural function. I have argued elsewhere that a function in the biologist's sense is nothing but a standard causal contribution to a goal actually pursued by the organism.[12] Organisms are vast assemblages of systems and subsystems which, in most members of a species, work together harmoniously in such a way as to achieve a hierarchy of goals. Cells are goal-directed toward metabolism, elimination, and mitosis; the heart is goal-directed toward supplying the rest of the body with blood; and the whole organism is goal-directed both to particular activities like eating and moving around and to higher-level goals such as survival and reproduction. The specifically physiological functions of any component are, I think, its species-typical contributions to the apical goals of survival and reproduction. But whatever the correct analysis of function statements, there is no doubt that biological theory is deeply committed to attributing functions to processes in plants and animals. And the single unifying property of all recognized diseases of plants and animals appears to be this: that they interfere with one or more functions typically performed within members of the species.

The account of health thus suggested is in one sense thoroughly Platonic. The health of an organism consists in the performance by each part of its natural function. And as Plato also saw, one of the most interesting features of the analysis is that it applies without alteration to mental health as long as there are standard mental functions. In another way, however, the classical heritage is misleading, for it seems clear that biological function statements are descriptive rather than normative claims.[13] Physiologists obtain their functional doctrines without at any stage having to answer such questions as, What is the function of a man? or to explicate ''a good man'' on the analogy of ''a good knife.'' Functions are not attributed in this context to the whole organism at all, but only to its parts, and the functions of a part are its causal contributions to empirically given goals. What goals a type of organism in fact pursues, and by what functions it pursues them, can be decided without considering the value of pursuing them. Consequently health in the theoretical sense is an equally value-free concept. The notion required for an analysis of health is not that of a good man or a good shark, but that of a good specimen of a human being or shark.

All of this amounts to saying that the epistemology King suggested for health judgments is, at bottom, a statistical one. The question therefore arises how the functional account avoids our earlier objections to statistical normality. King did explain how to dissolve one version of the paradox of saying that everyone is unhealthy. Clearly all the members of a species can have some disease or other as long as they do not have the same disease. King somewhat grimly compares the job of extracting an empirical ideal of health from a set of defective specimens to the job of reconstructing the Norden bombsite from assorted aerial debris (p. 495). But this answer does not touch universal diseases such as tooth decay. Although King nowhere considers this objection, the natural-design idea nevertheless suggests an answer that I suspect is correct. If what makes a condition a disease is its deviation from the natural functional organization of the species, then in calling tooth decay a disease we are saying that it is not simply in the nature of the species—and we say this because we think of it as mainly due to environmental causes. In general, deficiencies in the functional efficiency of the body are diseases when they are unnatural, and they may be unnatural either by being atypical or by being attributable mainly to the action of a hostile environment. If this explanation is accepted,[14] then the functional account simultaneously avoids the pitfalls of statistical normality and also frees the idea of theoretical health of all normative content.

Theoretical health now turns out to be strictly analogous to the mechanical condition of an artifact.

Despite appearances, ''perfect mechanical condition'' in, say, a 1965 Volkswagen is a descriptive notion. Such an artifact is in perfect mechanical condition when it conforms in all respects to the designer's detailed specifications. Normative interests play a crucial role, of course, in the initial choice of the design. But what the Volkswagen design actually *is* is an empirical matter by the time production begins. Thenceforward a car may be in perfect condition regardless of whether the design is good or bad. If one replaces its stock carburetor with a high-performance part, one may well produce a better car, but one does not produce a Volkswagen in better mechanical condition. Similarly, an automatic camera may function perfectly and take wretched pictures; guided missiles and instruments of torture in perfect mechanical condition may serve execrable ends. Perfect working order is a matter not of the worth of the product but of the conformity of the process to a fixed design. In the case of organisms, of course, the ideal of health must be determined by empirical analysis of the species rather than by the intentions of a designer. But otherwise the parallel seems exact. A person who by mutation acquires a sixth sense, or the ability to regenerate severed limbs, is not thereby healthier than we are. Sixth senses and limb regeneration are not part of the human design, which at any given time, for better or worse, just is what it is.

We have been arguing that health is descriptively definable within medical theory, as intelligence is in psychological theory or validity in logical theory. Nevertheless medical theory is the basis of medical practice, and medical practice unquestioningly presupposes the value of health. We must therefore ask how the functional view explains this presumption that health is desirable.

In the case of physiological health, there are at least two general reasons why the functional normality that defines it is usually worth having. In the first place, most people do want to pursue the goals with respect to which physiological functions are isolated. Not only do we want to survive and reproduce, but we also want to engage in those particular activities, such as eating and sex, by which these goals are typically achieved. In the second place—and this is surely the main reason the value of physical health seems indisputable—physiological functions tend to contribute to all manner of activities neutrally. Whether it is desirable for one's heart to pump, one's stomach to digest, or one's kidneys to eliminate hardly depends at all on what one wants to do. It follows that essentially all serious physiological diseases will satisfy the first requirement of an illness, namely, undesirability for its bearer.

This explanation of the fit between medical theory and medical practice has the virtue of reminding us that health, though an important value, is conceptually a very limited one. Health is not unconditionally worth promoting, nor is what is worth promoting necessarily health. Although mental-health writers are especially prone to ignore these points, even the constitution of the World Health Organization seems to embody a similar confusion:

Health is a state of complete physical, mental, and social well-being, and not merely the absence of disease or infirmity.[15]

Unless one is to abandon the physiological paradigm altogether, this definition is far too wide. Health is functional normality, and as such is desirable exactly insofar as it promotes goals one can justify on independent grounds. But there is presumably no intrinsic value in having the functional organization typical of a species if the same goals can be better achieved by other means. A sixth sense, for example, would increase our goal-efficiency without increasing our health; so might the amputation of our legs at the knee and their replacement by a nuclear-powered air-cushion vehicle. Conversely, as we have seen, there is no a priori reason why ordinary diseases cannot contribute to well-being under appropriate circumstances.

In such cases, however, we will be reluctant to describe the person involved as ill, and that is because the term "ill" *does* have a negative evaluation built into it. Here again a comparison between health and other properties will be helpful. Disease and illness are related somewhat as are low intelligence and stupidity, or failure to tell the truth and speaking dishonestly. Sometimes the presumption that intelligence is desirable will fail, as in a discussion of qualifications for a menial job such as washing dishes or assembling auto parts. In such a context a person of low intelligence is unlikely to be described as stupid. Sometimes the presumption that truth should be told will fail, as when the Gestapo inquires about the Jews in your attic. Here the untruthful householder will not be described as speaking dishonestly. And sometimes the presumption that diseases are undesirable will fail, as with alcoholic intoxication or mild rubella intentionally contracted. Here the term "illness" is un-

likely to appear despite the presence of disease. One concept of each pair is descriptive; the other adds to the first evaluative content, and so may be withheld where the first applies.

If we supplement this condition of undesirability with two further normative conditions, I believe we have the beginning of a plausible analysis of "illness."

A disease is an *illness* only if it is serious enough to be incapacitating, and therefore is

    (i) undesirable for its bearer;
    (ii) a title to special treatment; and
    (iii) a valid excuse for normally criticizable behavior.

The motivation for condition (ii) needs no explanation. As for (iii), the connection between illness and diminished responsibility has often been argued,[16] and I shall mention here only one suggestive point. Our notion of illness belongs to the ordinary conceptual scheme of persons and their actions, and it was developed to apply to physiological diseases. Consequently the relation between persons and their illnesses is conceived on the model of their relation to their bodies. It has often been observed that physiological processes, e.g., digestion or peristalsis, do not usually count as actions of ours at all. By the same token, we are not usually held responsible for the results of such processes when they go wrong, though we may be blamed for failing to take steps to prevent malfunction at some earlier time. Now if this special relation between persons and their bodies is the reason for connecting disease with nonresponsibility, the connection may break down when diseases of the mind are at stake instead. I shall now argue, in fact, that conditions (i), (ii), and (iii) all present difficulties in the domain of mental health.

MENTAL ILLNESS

For the sake of discussion, let us simply assume that the mental conditions usually called pathological are in fact unhealthy by the theoretical standard sketched in the last section. That is, we shall assume both that there are natural mental functions and also that recognized types of psychopathology are unnatural interferences with these functions.[17] Is it reasonable to make a parallel extension of the vocabulary of medical practice by calling these mental diseases mental illnesses? Let us consider each condition on "illness."

Condition (i) was the undesirability of an illness for its bearer. Now there are obstacles to transferring our general arguments that physiological health is desirable to the psychological domain. Mental states are not nearly so neutral to the choice of actions as physiological states are. In particular, to evaluate the desirability of mental health we can hardly avoid consulting our desires; but in the mental-health context it could be those very desires that are judged unhealthy. From a theoretical standpoint desires must be assigned a motivational function in producing action. Thus our wants may or may not conform to the species design. But if our wants do not conform to the species design, it is not immediately obvious why we should want them to. If there is no good reason to want them to, then we have a disease which is not an illness. It is conceivable that this divergence between the two notions is illustrated by homosexuality. It can hardly be denied that one normal function of sexual desire is to promote reproduction. If one does not have a desire for heterosexual sex, however, the only good reason for wanting to have such a desire seems to be that one would be happier if one did. But this judgment needs to be supported by evidence. The desirability of having species-typical desires is not nearly so obvious on inspection as the desirability of having species-typical physiological functions.

One of the corollaries of this point is that recent debates over homosexuality and other disputable diagnoses usually ignore at least one important issue. Besides asking whether, say, homosexuality is a disease, one should also ask what difference it makes if it is. I have suggested that biological normality is an instrumental rather than an intrinsic good. We always have the right to ask, of normality, what is in it for us that we already desire. If it were possible, then, to maximize intrinsic goods such as happiness, for ourselves and others, with a psyche full of deviant desires and unnatural acts, it is hard to see what practical significance the theoretical judgment of unhealthiness would have. I do not actually have serious doubts that disorders such as neuroses and psychoses diminish human happiness. It is also true that what is desirable for a person need not coincide with what the person wants; though an anorectic may not wish to eat, it is desirable that he or she do so. But we must be clear that requests to justify the value of health in other terms are always in order, and there are reasons

to expect that such justification will require more evidence in the psychological domain than in the physiological.

We have been discussing the value of psychological normality for the individual, as dictated by condition (i) on illness, rather than its desirability for society at large. Since clinicians often assume that mental health involves social adjustment, it may be well to point out that the functional account of health shows this too to be a debatable assumption requiring empirical support. Certainly nothing in the mere statement that a person has a mental disease entails that he or she is contributing less to the social order than an arbitrary normal individual. There is no contradiction in calling van Gogh or Blake or Dostoyevsky mentally disturbed while admiring their work, even if they would have been less creative had they been healthier. Conversely, there is no a priori reason to assume that the healthy human personality will be morally worthy or socially acceptable. If Freud and Lorenz are right about the existence of an aggressive drive, there is a large component of the normal psyche that is less than admirable. Whether or not they are right, the suggestion clearly makes sense. Perhaps most psychiatrists would agree anyway that antisocial behavior is to be expected during certain developmental stages, e.g., the so-called anal-sadistic period or adolescence.

It must be conceded that *Homo sapiens* is a social species. Other organisms of this class, such as ants and bees, display elaborate fixed systems of social adaptations, and it would be remarkable if the human design included no standard functions at all promoting socialization. On the basis of the physiological paradigm, however, it is not at all clear that contributions to society can be viewed as requirements of health except when they also contribute to individual survival and reproduction. No matter how this issue is decided, the crucial point remains: the nature and extent of social functions in the human species can be discovered only empirically. Despite the contrary convictions of many clinicians, the concept of mental health itself provides no guarantee that healthy individuals will meet the standards or serve the interests of society at large. If it did, that would be one more reason to question the desirability of health for the individual.

Let us now go on to condition (ii) on a disease which is an illness: that it justify "special treatment" of its owner. It is this condition together with (iii) that gives some plausibility to the many recent attempts to explain mental illness as a "social status" or "role."[18] The idea that the "sick role" is a special one is consistent with the statistical normality of having some disease or other. Since illnesses are serious diseases that incapacitate at the level of gross behavior, everyone can be minimally diseased without being ill. In the realm of mental health, however, many psychiatrists suggest the stronger thesis that it is statistically normal to be significantly incapacitated by neurosis.[19] A similar problem may arise on Benedict's famous view that the characteristic personality type of some whole societies is clinically paranoid.[20] A statistically normal condition, according to our analysis, can be a disease only if it can be blamed on the environment. But one might plausibly claim that most or all existing *cultural* environments do injure children, filling their minds with excessive anxiety about sexual pleasure, grotesque role models, absurd prejudices about reality, etc. It is at least possible that some degree of neurosis or psychosis is a nearly universal environmental injury in our species. Only an empirical inquiry into the incidence and etiology of neurosis can show whether this possibility is a reality. If it is, however, one can maintain the idea that serious diseases are illnesses only by abandoning one of the presuppositions of the illness concept: that not everyone can be ill.[21]

The last and clearest difficulty with "mental illness" concerns condition (iii), the role of illness in excusing conduct. We said that the idea that serious diseases excuse conduct derives from the model of the relation of agents to their own physiology. Unfortunately the relation of agents to their own psychology is of a much more intimate kind. The puzzle about mental illness is that it seems to be an activity of the very seat of responsibility—the mind and character—and therefore to be beyond all hope of excuse.

This inference is hardly inescapable; there is room for considerable controversy to which I cannot do justice here. Strictly speaking, mental disorders are disturbances of the personality. It is persons, not personalities, who are held responsible for actions, and one central element in the idea of a person is certainly consciousness. This means that there may be some sense in contrasting responsible persons with their mental diseases insofar as these diseases lie outside their conscious personalities. Perhaps from a psychoanalytic standpoint this condition is often met in psychosis and neurosis. The unconscious processes that surface in these disorders seem at first sight more like things that happen within us, e.g., peristalsis, than like things we do. But several points make this classification look oversimplified. Unconscious ideas and wishes are still *our* ideas and wishes in a more compelling sense than movements of the gut are our movements. They may have been conscious at an earlier time or be made conscious in therapy, whereupon it becomes increasingly difficult to disclaim responsibility for them. It seems quite unclear that we are more responsible for many conscious desires and beliefs than for these unconscious ones. Finally, the hope for contrasting responsible people with their mental diseases grows vanishingly dim in the case of a character disorder, where the unhealthy condition seems to be integrated into the conscious personality.

In view of these points and the rest of the discussion, I think we must accept the following conclusion. While conditions (i), (ii), and (iii) apply fairly automatically to serious physical diseases, not one of them should be assumed to apply automatically to serious mental diseases. If the term "mental illness" is to be applied at all, it should probably be restricted to psychoses and disabling neuroses. But even this decision needs more analysis than I have provided in this essay. It seems doubtful that on any construal mental illness will ever be, in the mental-health movement's famous phrase, "just like any other illness."

What are the implications of our discussion for the social issues to which psychiatry is so frequently applied? As far as the criminal law is concerned, our results suggest that psychiatric theory alone should not be expected to define legal responsibility, e.g., in the insanity defense.[22] Although the notion of responsibility is a component of the notion of illness, it belongs not to medical theory but to ethics, and one can fix its boundaries only by rational ethical debate. It seems certain that such a simple responsibility test as that the act of the accused not be "the product of mental disease" is unsatisfactory. No doubt many of us have antisocial tendencies that derive from underlying psychopathology of an ordinary sort. When these tendencies erupt in a parking violation or negligent collision, it hardly seems inhumane or unjust to apply legal sanctions.[23] But this is not surprising, for no psychiatric concept is properly designed to answer moral questions. I am not saying that psychiatry is irrelevant to law and ethics. Anyone writing or applying a criminal code is certainly well advised to obtain the best available information about human nature, including the information about human nature that constitutes mental-health theory. The point is that one cannot expect to substitute psychiatry for moral debate, any more than moral evaluations can be substituted for psychiatric theory. Insofar as the psychiatric turn consists in such substitutions, it is fundamentally misconceived.

The other main implications of our discussion seem to me twofold. First, there is not the slightest warrant for the recurrent fantasy that what society or its professionals disapprove of is ipso facto unhealthy. This is not merely because society may disapprove of the wrong things. Even if ethical relativism were true, society still could not fix the functional organization of the members of a species. For this reason it could never be an infallible authority either on disease or on illness, which is a subclass of disease. Thus one main source of the tendency to call radical activists, Bohemians, feminists, and other unpopular deviants "sick" is nothing but a conceptual confusion.

The second moral suggested by our discussion is that it is always worth asking, in any particular case, how strong the presumption is that health is desirable. When the value of health is left both unquestioned and obscure, it has a tendency to undergo inflation. The diagnosis especially of a "mental illness" is then likely to become an amorphous and peculiarly repellent stigma to be removed at any cost. The use of muscle-paralyzing drugs to compel prisoners to participate in "group therapy" is a particularly gruesome example of this sort of thinking.[24] But there are many other situations in which everyone would profit by asking what exactly is wrong with being unhealthy. In a way liberal reformers tend to make the opposite mistake: in their zeal to remove the stigma of disease from conditions such as homosexuality, they wholly discount the possibility that these conditions, like most diseases, are somewhat unideal. If the value of health, as I have argued in this essay, is nothing but the value of conformity to a generally excellent species design, then by recognizing that fact we may improve both the clarity and the humanity of our social discourse.

NOTES

1. Thomas S. Szasz, *The Myth of Mental Illness* (New York,

1961); Antony Flew, *Crime or Disease?* (New York, 1973), pp. 40, 42.

2. Ian Gregory, *Fundamentals of Psychiatry* (Philadelphia, 1968), p. 32.

3. R. M. Hare, in *Freedom and Reason* (New York, 1963), Chap. 2, argues that no terms have prescriptive meaning alone. If this view is accepted, the difference between strong and weak normativism concerns the question of whether "healthy" is "primarily" or "secondarily" evaluative.

4. Judd Marmor, "Homosexuality and Cultural Value Systems," *American Journal of Psychiatry* 130 (1973): 1208.

5. Marie Jahoda, *Current Concepts of Positive Mental Health* (New York, 1958), pp. 76–77. See also her remark in *Interrelations Between the Social Environment and Psychiatric Disorders* (New York, 1953), p. 142: ". . . inevitably at some place there is a value judgement involved. I think that mental health or mental sickness cannot be conceived of without reference to some basic value."

6. F. C. Redlich, "The Concept of Normality," *American Journal of Psychotherapy* 6 (1952): 553.

7. Joseph Margolis, *Psychotherapy and Morality* (New York, 1966).

8. Exactly what intellectual abilities are included in intelligence is, of course, unclear and may vary from culture to culture. (See N. J. Block and Gerald Dworkin, "IQ. Heritability and Inequality, Part I," *Philosophy and Public Affairs* 3, no. 4 [Summer, 1974]: 333.) But this does not show that for any particular group of speakers "intelligent" is a normative term, i.e., has positive evaluation as part of its meaning.

9. The contrary view, which might be called normativism about validity, is defended by J. O. Urmson in "Some Questions Concerning Validity," *Revue Internationale de Philosophie* 25 (1953): 217–229.

10. Thomas Nagel has suggested that the adjective "ill" may have its own special opposite "well." Our thinking about health might be greatly clarified if "wellness" had some currency.

11. C. Daly King, "The Meaning of Normal," *Yale Journal of Biology and Medicine* 17 (1945): 493–494. Most definitions of health in medical dictionaries include some reference to functions. Almost exactly King's formulation also appears in Fredrick C. Redlich and Daniel X. Freedman, *The Theory and Practice of Psychiatry* (New York, 1966), p. 113.

12. "Wright on Functions," *The Philosophical Review*.

13. The view that function statements are normative generates the third argument for normativism. It is presented most fully by Margolis in "Illness and Medical Values," *The Philosophy Forum* 8 (1959): 55–76, section II. It is also suggested by Ronald B. de Sousa, "The Politics of Mental Illness," *Inquiry* 15 (1972): 187–201, p. 194, and possibly by Flew as well in *Crime or Disease?* pp. 39–40. I think philosophers of science have made too much progress in giving biological function statements a descriptive analysis for this argument to be very convincing.

14. For further discussion of environmental injuries and other details of the functional account of health sketched in this section, see my essay "Health as a Theoretical Concept."

15. Quoted by Flew, *Crime or Disease?* p. 46.

16. A good discussion of this point and of the undesirability condition (i) is provided by Flew in the extremely illuminating second chapter of *Crime or Disease?* Flew takes these conditions as part of the meaning of "disease" rather than "illness"; but since he seems to be working from the ordinary usage of "disease," there may be no real disagreement here.

17. The plausibility of these two claims is discussed at length in

my essay, "What a Theory of Mental Health Should Be," *Journal for the Theory of Social Behavior,* 6 (1976): 61–84.

18. An example of this approach is Robert B. Edgerton, "On The 'Recognition' of Mental Illness," in Stanley C. Plog and Robert B. Edgerton, *Changing Perspectives in Mental Illness* (New York, 1969), pp. 49–72.

19. Only one example of this suggestion is Dr. Reuben Fine's statement that neurosis afflicts 99 percent of the population. See Fine's "The Goals of Psychoanalysis," in *The Goals of Psychotherapy,* ed. Alvin R. Mahrer (New York, 1967), p. 95. I consider the issue of whether all neurosis can be called unhealthy in the essay cited in note 17.

20. See the descriptions of the Kwakiutl and the Dobu in Ruth Benedict, *Patterns of Culture* (Boston: Houghton Mifflin, 1934).

21. A number of clinicians have seriously suggested that people who are ill can be distinguished from those who are well by their presence in your office. One such author goes as far as to calculate an upper limit on the incidence of mental illness from the number of members in the American Psychiatric Association. On a literal reading, this patient-in-the-office test implies that one could wipe out mental illness once and for all by dissolving the APA and outlawing psychotherapy. But the whole idea seems silly anyway in the face of various studies that indicate that the population at large is, by the ordinary descriptive criteria for mental disorder, no less disturbed than the population of clinical patients.

22. The same conclusion is defended by Herbert Fingarette in "Insanity and Responsibility," *Inquiry* 15 (1972): 6–29.

23. Thus I disagree with H. L. A. Hart, among others, who writes: ". . .the contention that it is fair or just to punish those who have broken the law must be absurd if the crime is merely a manifestation of a disease." The quotation is from "Murder and the Principles of Punishment: England and the United States," reprinted in *Moral Problems,* ed. James Rachels (New York, 1975), p. 274.

24. For this and other "therapeutic" abuses in our prison system, see Jessica Mitford, *Kind and Usual Punishment* (New York, 1973), Chap. 8.

H. TRISTRAM ENGELHARDT, JR.

The Roles of Values in the Discovery of Illnesses, Diseases, and Disorders

Disease language, because it interweaves descriptive, evaluative, explanatory, and social interventional elements, raises philosophical questions about the interplay of values, facts, and explanatory accounts. There is the issue of whether the disease concepts used in characterizing diseases are created or discovered, of whether they reflect natural kinds or artificial groupings of signs, symptoms, and other medical findings. Moreover, if one could determine which constellations of findings are proper problems for medicine, one could on the basis of such ontological determinations decide the proper boundaries of medicine, and thus include or exclude such undertakings as nontherapeutic abortions and plastic surgery. There is also the question of whether medical descriptions are value-laden and the extent to which such values are relative to particular cultures, as well as the issue of the extent to which descriptions are theory-laden. Finally, if medicine is a social endeavor framing social roles, then the epistemic and axiological elements of medicine must be examined in social terms.

EVALUATIONS

Medicine is not undertaken in order simply to give explanations to or forward predictions, but to solve certain sorts of problems that people have with themselves or with others. Medicine is moved to fashion descriptions of certain phenomena out of interests in nonmoral values concerning what counts as pathology or well-being. That is, medicine does not describe clusters of phenomena because they form clusters of findings, or because they are failures to achieve species-typical levels of species-typical functions, but because they are clusters of findings associated with complaints about loss of function,[1] the presence of pain, or the failure to achieve certain minimum norms of human form and grace. Those states are, in short, disvalued.

Christopher Boorse has attempted to deny this

central role of values in the fashioning of concepts of disease by distinguishing between a value-laden and value-free dimension of disease language. Illness for Boorse is a state of affairs in which one has a disease which is serious enough to be incapacitating, and therefore is

(i) undesirable for its bearer;
(ii) a title to special treatment; and
(iii) a valid excuse for normally criticizable behavior.[2]

Disease, in contrast, is defined in terms of a failure to achieve a species-typical efficiency of a species-typical function. Or put more precisely,

1. The *reference class* is a natural class of organisms of uniform functional design; specifically, an age group of a sex of a species.
2. A *normal function* of a part or process within members of the reference class is a statistically typical contribution by it to their individual survival and reproduction. . .
3. A *disease* is a type of internal state which is either an impairment of normal functional ability, i.e., a reduction of one or more functional abilities below typical efficiency, or a limitation on functional ability caused by environmental agents.
4. *Health* is the absence of disease.

These definitions, however, involve a number of difficulties. First, Boorse appears to ignore the implications of variations within a species with different costs and benefits. Species may often develop a balance among various traits, as occurs in the case of sickle cell disease. Species design, insofar as one can speak of such, includes a strategic balance among numerous hemoglobin forms, each with its own advantages and disadvantages. It may, in short, be very difficult to speak of *a* species design, the more one discovers important variations within species. Second, many phenomena such as sickle cell disease may benefit species adaptation or maximize inclusive genetic fitness but not benefit the individual. This may be the case with universal diseases, such as those associated with aging, a point that Boorse acknowledges. Individuals may be programmed to become ill and die at a particular age and in a particular way, because such a trait maximizes inclusive genetic fitness though compromising the fitness of the individual and his or her own individual plans. Third,

new traits that may have new advantages but that lack the usual advantages of the established trait would, when they first appear, count as diseases, though members of the species might consider them on balance favorable mutations. Boorse's account, in short, depends upon the history of the species and its evolution, a dependence that appears irrelevant to the individually oriented concepts of disease employed by medicine. This point has been recognized by William Goosens.[3]

In short, it would appear that Boorse has not provided a reconstruction of the concept of disease as it is employed by medicine but a concept of species typicality, which may be of interest to biologists, though largely irrelevant to medicine. Boorse has failed to appreciate a point that would have been clear to physicians such as Sauvages and Cullen, namely, that medicine starts with patient complaints. That is, disease concepts are explanatory accounts fashioned to direct and illuminate therapy (i.e., in the broadest sense, including preventive treatment). It was the triumph of 19th-century patho-anatomy and patho-physiology, which distracted its inheritors from this seemingly obvious point, that medicine is a science developed to redress patient difficulties. Along with the success of 19th-century patho-anatomy and patho-physiology, there came as well the notion that diseases could be discovered, as Broussais suggested, by examining changes in organs.

However, insofar as medicine is not concerned to describe biological functions for their own sake but rather to fashion accounts that will aid in addressing the problems of patients, concepts of disease will be at least indirectly value laden. Such concepts are framed to account for phenomena that are disvalued as failures to reach minimum norms of physiological, psychological, and anatomical excellence (where this includes pain and distress). Which clusters of phenomena will be seen as failures depends upon particular environments and particular human goals. Thus, whether color blindness will be seen as a disease or a state of well-being will depend upon whether one esteems more highly the capacity to distinguish colors or to identify camouflage. Since many diseases impede the realization of so many important human goals, they are likely to be seen as diseases in nearly any foreseeable context or culture. That will not be the case due to a uniformity in value judgments but to the fact that certain processes or phenomena tend to preclude the realization of some values in nearly all contexts or environments.

Finally, Boorse's concept of illness appears to conflate those values that mark a state of affairs as one usually to be seen as a failure to achieve norms of physiological, psychological, or anatomical excellence and those values involved in a patient deciding, when he or she considers the secondary gains from an illness (e.g., sick pay, being excused from the draft), that the illness is worth his or her while. Illness possesses a prima facie disvalue which may be outweighed by other realizable goods. Boorse, in short, has failed to distinguish between those values that usually mark a cluster of phenomena as a disorder, and those values associated with the acceptance and use of particular social roles: sick roles or therapy roles.

THERAPY ROLES

Since medicine involves interventions in a social context, it regularly imposes various routinized social roles. That is, when individuals are seen to be suffering from a medical problem of a particular sort, there often is a range of established ways in which physicians respond, according to standards reflecting views of prudent canons for intervention. These canons develop because both illnesses and treatments carry risks of morbidity if not death. Treatments must be balanced against the risks of the illness. In this regard one must not only judge the merit of a particular treatment for a particular disease but recognize as well the likelihood of misdiagnosis. That is, standardized criteria for making a diagnosis should take into account the risk of false positive and false negative diagnosis, of overtreating or undertreating. As a result, standardized indications for a diagnosis establish a threshold that should express the balance among possible benefits and harms.

Different medical problems have as well different social costs. If one considers medical problems ranging from teething and athlete's foot to childbirth, acute schizophrenia, and active tuberculosis, one finds a range of complaints, some associated with value judgments about failures to meet norms of function, form, or grace and others simply associated with complaints of pain or distress. One finds as well a great variation in the extent to which such complaints involve an excuse from usual social responsibilities and in the extent to which they involve an imperative to seek medical care of a particular sort. There is not one sense of a sick role, to use Talcott Parsons' term[4] but rather a family of social roles within which individuals have their medical problems addressed, or seek to have medical problems prevented.

In short, therapy roles embrace individuals who are not clearly sick in the sense of being incapacitated or in the sense of being abnormal beyond being concerned with some present or future physiologically, anatomically, or psychologically based distress. Therapy roles focus on medical problems.

CONCLUSIONS

An examination of the concepts of disease reveals a rich interplay of descriptive, explanatory, evaluative, and social interventional elements. One may out of interests of analysis distinguish a descriptive pole concerned simply with characterizing disorders, an explanatory pole offering accounts and explanatory models, and a pole concerned with therapy roles. However, it is important to notice that all of these dimensions must be attended to in a characterization of medical problems, a term with greater scope than disease, illness, or sickness. Medicine traditionally aids individuals suffering from cancer, heart disease, unwanted pregnancy, and incapacity to reproduce. Medicine does so not out of pure scientific interests but rather in response to the complaints of patients or others about the problems of patients. As a result, medical problems are not amenable to characterization apart from the cultures and interests of individuals. Concepts of illness, disease, and disorder are as much cultural, and at times individual, creations as they are discoveries.

NOTES

1. By loss of function here I mean the loss of the ability to do things considered to be normal for individuals of a particular age or sex. I am not referring to dysfunctions as biological dysfunctions, which may underlie the production of pain, etc. Boorse appears not to have acknowledged this distinction. "Health as a Theoretical Concept," *Philosophy of Science* 44 (December, 1977), 560–561.

2. Christopher Boorse, "On the Distinction Between Disease and Illness," *Philosophy and Public Affairs* 5 (Fall, 1975), 61.

3. William Goosens, "Values, Health, and Medicine," *Philosophy of Science* 47 (March, 1980), 102.

4. See, for example, Talcott Parsons, *The Social System* (New York: Free Press, 1951); "The Mental Hospital as a Type of Organization," in M. Greenblatt *et al.* (eds.), *The Patient and the Mental Hospital* (Glencoe, Ill.: Free Press), pp. 108–129; "Definitions of Health and Illness in the Light of American Values and Social Structure," in E. G. Jaco (ed.), *Patients, Physicians, and Illness* (Glencoe, Ill.: Free Press), pp. 165–187.

THOMAS SZASZ

The Myth of Mental Illness

I

At the core of virtually all contemporary psychiatric theories and practices lies the concept of mental illness. A critical examination of this concept is therefore indispensable for understanding the ideas, institutions, and interventions of psychiatrists.

My aim in this essay is to ask if there is such a thing as mental illness, and to argue that there is not. Of course, mental illness is not a thing or physical object; hence it can exist only in the same sort of way as do other theoretical concepts. Yet, to those who believe in them, familiar theories are likely to appear, sooner or later, as "objective truths" or "facts." During certain historical periods, explanatory concepts such as deities, witches, and instincts appeared not only as theories but as *self-evident causes* of a vast number of events. Today mental illness is widely regarded in a similar fashion, that is, as the cause of innumerable diverse happenings.

As an antidote to the complacent use of the notion of mental illness—as a self-evident phenomenon, theory, or cause—let us ask: What is meant when it is asserted that someone is mentally ill? In this essay I shall describe the main uses of the concept of mental illness, and I shall argue that this notion has outlived whatever cognitive usefulness it might have had and that it now functions as a myth.

II

The notion of mental illness derives its main support from such phenomena as syphilis of the brain or delirious conditions—intoxications, for instance—in which persons may manifest certain disorders of thinking and behavior. Correctly speaking, however, these are diseases of the brain, not of the mind. According to one school of thought, *all* so-called mental illness is of this type. The assumption is made that some neurological defect, perhaps a very subtle one, will ultimately be found to explain all the disorders of thinking and behavior. Many contemporary physicians, psychiatrists, and other scientists hold this view, which implies that people's troubles cannot be caused by conflicting personal needs, opinions, social aspirations, values, and so forth. These difficulties—which I think we may simply call *problems in living*—are thus attributed to physicochemical processes that in due time will be discovered (and no doubt corrected) by medical research.

Mental illnesses are thus regarded as basically similar to other diseases. The only difference, in this view, between mental and bodily disease is that the former, affecting the brain, manifests itself by means of mental symptoms; whereas the latter, affecting other organ systems—for example, the skin, liver, and so on—manifests itself by means of symptoms referable to those parts of the body.

In my opinion, this view is based on two fundamental errors. In the first place, a disease of the brain, analogous to a disease of the skin or bone, is a neurological defect, not a problem in living. For example, a *defect* in a person's visual field may be explained by correlating it with certain lesions in the nervous system. On the other hand, a person's *belief*—whether it be in Christianity, in Communism, or in the idea that his internal organs are rotting and that his body is already dead—cannot be explained by a defect or disease of the nervous system. Explanations of this sort of occurrence—assuming that one is interested in the belief itself and does not regard it simply as a symptom or expression of something else that is more interesting—must be sought along different lines.

The second error is epistemological. It consists of interpreting communications about ourselves and the world around us as symptoms of neurological func-

From *American Psychologist*, 1960, *15*, pp. 113–118. Copyright 1960 by the American Psychological Association. Reprinted by permission of the publisher and author.

tioning. This is an error not in observation or reasoning, but rather in the organization and expression of knowledge. In the present case, the error lies in making a dualism between mental and physical symptoms, a dualism that is a habit of speech and not the result of known observations. Let us see if this is so.

In medical practice, when we speak of physical disturbances we mean either signs (for example, fever) or symptoms (for example, pain). We speak of mental symptoms, on the other hand, when we refer to a patient's communications about himself, others, and the world about him. The patient might assert that he is Napoleon or that he is being persecuted by the Communists. These would be considered mental symptoms only if the observer believed that the patient was *not* Napoleon or that he was *not* being persecuted by the Communists. This makes it apparent that the statement ''X is a mental symptom'' involves rendering a judgment that entails a covert comparison between the patient's ideas, concepts, or beliefs and those of the observer and the society in which they live. The notion of mental symptom is therefore inextricably tied to the social, and particularly the ethical, context in which it is made, just as the notion of bodily symptom is tied to an anatomical and genetic context.

To sum up: For those who regard mental symptoms as signs of brain disease, the concept of mental illness is unnecessary and misleading. If they mean that people so labeled suffer from diseases of the brain, it would seem better, for the sake of clarity, to say that and not something else.

III

The term ''mental illness'' is also widely used to describe something quite different from a disease of the brain. Many people today take it for granted that living is an arduous affair. Its hardship for modern man derives, moreover, not so much from a struggle for biological survival as from the stresses and strains inherent in the social intercourse of complex human personalities. In this context, the notion of mental illness is used to identify or describe some feature of an individual's so-called personality. Mental illness—as a deformity of the personality, so to speak—is then regarded as the cause of human disharmony. It is implicit in this view that social intercourse between people is regarded as something inherently harmonious, its disturbance being due solely to the presence of ''mental illness'' in many people. Clearly, this is faulty reasoning, for it makes the abstraction ''mental illness'' into a cause of, even though this abstraction was originally created to serve only as a shorthand expression for, certain types of human behavior. It now becomes necessary to ask: What kinds of behavior are regarded as indicative of mental illness, and by whom?

The concept of illness, whether bodily or mental, implies deviation from some clearly defined norm. In the case of physical illness, the norm is the structural and functional integrity of the human body. Thus, although the desirability of physical health, as such, is an ethical value, what health is can be stated in anatomical and physiological terms. What is the norm, deviation from which is regarded as mental illness? This question cannot be easily answered. But whatever this norm may be, we can be certain of only one thing: namely, that it must be stated in terms of psychosocial, ethical, and legal concepts. For example, notions such as ''excessive repression'' and ''acting out an unconscious impulse'' illustrate the use of psychological concepts for judging so-called mental health and illness. The idea that chronic hostility, vengefulness, or divorce are indicative of mental illness is an illustration of the use of ethical norms (that is, the desirability of love, kindness, and a stable marriage relationship). Finally, the widespread psychiatric opinion that only a mentally ill person would commit homicide illustrates the use of a legal concept as a norm of mental health. In short, when one speaks of mental illness, the norm from which deviation is measured is a *psychosocial and ethical* standard. Yet, the remedy is sought in terms of *medical* measures that—it is hoped and assumed—are free from wide differences of ethical value. The definition of the disorder and the terms in which its remedy are sought are therefore at serious odds with one another. The practical significance of this covert conflict between the alleged nature of the defect and the actual remedy can hardly be exaggerated.

Having identified the norms used for measuring deviations in cases of mental illness, we shall now turn to the question, Who defines the norms and hence the deviation? Two basic answers may be offered: First, it may be the person himself—that is, the patient—who decides that he deviates from a norm; for example, an artist may believe that he suffers from a work inhibition; and he may implement this conclusion by seeking help *for himself* from a psychotherapist. Second, it may be someone other than the ''patient'' who decides that the latter is deviant—for example, relatives, physicians, legal authorities, society generally; a psychiatrist may then be hired by persons other than the ''patient'' to do something *to him* in order to correct the deviation.

These considerations underscore the importance of asking the question, Whose agent is the psychiatrist? and of giving a candid answer to it. The psychiatrist (or non-medical mental health worker) may be the agent of the patient, the relatives, the school, the military services, a business organization, a court of law, and so forth. In speaking of the psychiatrist as the agent of these persons or organizations, it is not implied that his moral values, or his ideas and aims concerning the proper nature of remedial action, must coincide exactly with those of his employer. For example, a patient in individual psychotherapy may believe that his salvation lies in a new marriage; his psychotherapist need not share this hypothesis. As the patient's agent, however, he must not resort to social or legal force to prevent the patient from putting his beliefs into action. If his *contract* is with the patient, the psychiatrist (psychotherapist) may disagree with him or stop his treatment, but he cannot engage others to obstruct the patient's aspirations. Similarly, if a psychiatrist is retained by a court to determine the sanity of an offender, he need not fully share the legal authorities' values and intentions in regard to the criminal, nor the means deemed appropriate for dealing with him; such a psychiatrist cannot testify, however, that the accused is not insane but that the legislators are—for passing the law that decrees the offender's actions illegal. This sort of opinion could be voiced, of course—but not in a courtroom, and not by a psychiatrist who is there to assist the court in performing its daily work.

To recapitulate: In contemporary social usage, the finding of mental illness is made by establishing a deviance in behavior from certain psychosocial, ethical, or legal norms. The judgment may be made, as in medicine, by the patient, the physician (psychiatrist), or others. Remedial action, finally, tends to be sought in a therapeutic—or covertly medical—framework. This creates a situation in which it is claimed that psychosocial, ethical, and legal deviations can be corrected by medical action. Since medical interventions are designed to remedy only medical problems, it is logically absurd to expect that they will help solve problems whose very existence has been defined and established on non-medical grounds.

•   •   •

IV

The position outlined above, according to which contemporary psychotherapists deal with problems in living, not with mental illnesses and their cures, stands in sharp opposition to the currently prevalent position, according to which psychiatrists treat mental diseases, which are just as ''real'' and ''objective'' as bodily diseases. I submit that the holders of the latter view have no evidence whatever to justify their claim, which is actually a kind of psychiatric propaganda: their aim is to create in the popular mind a confident belief that mental illness is some sort of disease entity, like an infection or a malignancy. If this were true, one could *catch* or *get* a mental illness, one might *have* or *harbor* it, one might *transmit* it to others, and finally one could *get rid* of it. Not only is there not a shred of evidence to support this idea, but, on the contrary, all the evidence is the other way and supports the view that what people now call mental illnesses are, for the most part, *communications* expressing unacceptable ideas, often framed in an unusual idiom.

This is not the place to consider in detail the similarities and differences between bodily and mental illnesses. It should suffice to emphasize that whereas the term ''bodily illness'' refers to physico-chemical occurrences that are not affected by being made public, the term ''mental illness'' refers to sociopsychological events that are crucially affected by being made public. The psychiatrist thus cannot, and does not, stand apart from the person he observes, as the pathologist can and often does. The psychiatrist is committed to some picture of what he considers reality, and to what he thinks society considers reality, and he observes and judges the patient's behavior in the light of these beliefs. The very notion of ''mental symptom'' or ''mental illness'' thus implies a covert comparison, and often conflict, between observer and observed, psychiatrist and patient. Though obvious, this fact needs to be re-emphasized, if one wishes, as I do here, to counter the prevailing tendency to deny the moral aspects of psychiatry and to substitute for them allegedly value-free medical concepts and interventions.

Psychotherapy is thus widely practiced as though it entailed nothing other than restoring the patient from a state of mental sickness to one of mental health. While it is generally accepted that mental illness has something to do with man's social or interpersonal relations, it is paradoxically maintained that problems of values—that is, of ethics—do not arise in this process. Freud himself went so far as to assert: "I consider ethics to be taken for granted. Actually I have never done a mean thing."[1] This is an astounding thing to say, especially for someone who had studied man as a social being as deeply as Freud had. I mention it here to show how the notion of "illness"—in the case of psychoanalysis, "psychopathology," or "mental illness"—was used by Freud, and by most of his followers, as a means of classifying certain types of human behavior as falling within the scope of medicine, and hence, by fiat, outside that of ethics. Nevertheless, the stubborn fact remains that, in a sense, much of psychotherapy revolves around nothing other than the elucidation and weighing of goals and values—many of which may be mutually contradictory—and the means whereby they might best be harmonized, realized, or relinquished.

Because the range of human values and of the methods by which they may be attained is so vast, and because many such ends and means are persistently unacknowledged, conflicts among values are the main source of conflicts in human relations. Indeed, to say that human relations at all levels—from mother to child, through husband and wife, to nation and nation—are fraught with stress, strain, and disharmony is, once again, to make the obvious explicit. Yet, what may be obvious may be also poorly understood. This, I think, is the case here. For it seems to me that in our scientific theories of behavior we have failed to accept the simple fact that human relations are inherently fraught with difficulties, and to make them even relatively harmonious requires much patience and hard work. I submit that the idea of mental illness is now being put to work to obscure certain difficulties that at present may be inherent—not that they need to be unmodifiable—in the social intercourse of persons. If this is true, the concept functions as a disguise: instead of calling attention to conflicting human needs, aspirations, and values, the concept of mental illness provides an amoral and impersonal "thing"—an "illness"—as an explanation for problems in living. We may recall in this connection that not so long ago it was devils and witches that were held responsible for man's problems in living. The belief in mental illness, as something other than man's trouble in getting along with his fellow man, is the proper heir to the belief in demonology and witchcraft. Mental illness thus exists or is "real" in exactly the same sense in which witches existed or were "real."

· · ·

When I assert that mental illness is a myth, I am not saying that personal unhappiness and socially deviant behavior do not exist; what I am saying is that we categorize them as diseases at our own peril.

The expression "mental illness" is a metaphor that we have come to mistake for a fact. We call people physically ill when their body-functioning violates certain anatomical and physiological norms; similarly, we call people mentally ill when their personal conduct violates certain ethical, political, and social norms. This explains why many historical figures, from Jesus to Castro, and from Job to Hitler, have been diagnosed as suffering from this or that psychiatric malady.

NOTES

1. Quoted in E. Jones, *The Life and Work of Sigmund Freud* (New York: Basic Books, 1957), Vol. III, p. 247.

JOSEPH MARGOLIS

The Norms of Mental Health

The concept of mental health is, as a medical and professional category, of very recent vintage. It is a concept whose meaning is marked out by way of contrast with that of physical health; its acceptance is, for all practical purposes, the result of Freud's pioneer labors. There is no question, historically, that Freud modelled his discussion of mental disease and illness on concepts of physical disease. But Freud's norms represent an innovation in medicine and oblige us to ask quite pointedly, "How can we justify a change in the concept of health itself?"

The clue I see is the same that informs much of the philosophical work of John Wisdom. He spoke once of Christ's remark about a man's committing adultery *in his heart* as providing "a new geometry of adultery." The point is that the normative concept "adultery" was thereby enlarged to include cases not eligible in terms of overt act but sufficiently similar in other important respects—which, when once pointed out, are taken to "justify" the enlargement. Here is the only, and perfectly adequate, sense in which normative concepts (as well as other concepts—mere classificatory concepts, in fact) can be altered, reformed, enlarged. What we do to "justify" the change is to arrange a spectrum of cases, beginning with clearly eligible and indisputable cases and stretching back toward the doubtful ones. And to the extent that the new cases resemble the continuum of old ones, with comparatively little strain or leap, we allow the innovation to stand as a reasonable one.

This is the sense in which the concept of "mental health" can be justified. The substantive issue is a matter for professional physicians; we are here concerned only with the logical features of any attempt at justification. Let me cite Thomas Szasz . . . to exhibit the pertinence of these remarks. Szasz is a severe critic of the notion of psychiatric illness, and at one point in an extended polemic he says:

I maintain that Freud did not "discover" that hysteria was a mental illness. Rather, he advocated that so-called hysterics be declared "ill." The adjectives "mental," "emotional" and "neurotic" are simply devices to codify—and at the same time obscure—the differences between the two classes of disabilities, of "problems" in meeting life. One category consists of bodily diseases—say, leprosy, tuberculosis, or cancer—which, by rendering imperfect the functioning of the human body as a machine, produce difficulties in social adaptation. In contrast to the first, the second category is characterized by difficulties in social adaptation not attributable to malfunctioning machinery but "caused" rather by the purpose the machine was made to served by those who built it (e.g., parents, society), or by those who use it, i.e., individuals.[1]

Szasz is absolutely right in holding that Freud reclassified types of suffering. But what he fails to see is that this is a perfectly legitimate (and even necessary) maneuver. In fact, this enlargement of the concept of illness does not obscure the differences between physical and mental illness—and the differences themselves are quite gradual, as psychosomatic disorder and hysterical conversion attest. On the contrary, these differences are preserved and respected in the very idea of an *enlargement* of the concept of illness. Just so, . . . enlarging the legal concept of a "person" to include corporations (and "justifiably") does not obscure the difference between a corporation and an individual man.

Let me put the point this way. Szasz is in error in thinking that, if Freud were to justify his classification of hysteria as mental illness, he would have to do so by revealing certain scientific "discoveries." It is certainly true that the question of justification would concern his discoveries; but the justification could itself have been undertaken only *after* the relevant

From *Psychotherapy and Morality: A Study of Two Concepts* (New York: Random House, 1966), pp. 71–77, 80–82.

clinical facts had been supplied. The reason is apparent: the question at stake would have been, precisely, how to reclassify these clinical facts. If the category of mental health were already in currency in the required way, the question of whether hysteria was a mental illness would have been merely a straightforward factual question. But the question has to do rather with reasons for deciding to call hysteria an illness, in the light of the fact that the current usage of "illness" would preclude its being so called. The question concerns, that is, *the reasons for changing the classification*.

In short, if we ask for the justification for a change in normative models, we are bound to hold that naming—where it involves making use of established uses of names—is not an arbitrary matter but rather one that calls for defense. It is a matter for decision, but for decision with reasons. Consequently, though it is a concern of physicians, it is not a medical concern; that is, it is a question not of the facts, but of how to organize the facts.

Put in this way, our question becomes: Should mental "disorders" be allowed, in a medical sense, to count as diseases or illnesses? This is a difficult question. I wish it to be clear, before attempting an answer, that we are at least agreed as to what would count as affirmative evidence. If I were to describe a condition in which a patient suffers great pain in walking and is quickly overcome by fatigue, a condition which lasts for several years, and we were to find that there is an organic cause for this pattern, we should be strongly inclined to regard what we have before us as a *physical illness*. Now, if we have the same sort of pattern but are unable to find any organic cause, and begin to suspect that, in some unexplained way, the condition is due to the emotional or psychical life of the patient, we may have a reason for insisting that the pattern is still a *pattern of illness*.

What we should have done here is to *extend* the concept of illness to hitherto unclassified patterns and to *justify* the extension by showing the affinities between the new cases and the standard ones. We should not have shown that the patient was ill, but rather that what the patient exhibited could reasonably be called illness. It would, of course, always be possible to refuse to extend the use of the term in question. But the affinities drawn may be compared with other alleged affinities that are not so close—and in a way that does not depend on the new classificatory move at all. The issue is a general one, by no means confined to normative questions: for instance, I may see that the affinities between a coyote and a wolf are closer than those between a coyote and a bear, and whether I choose or refuse to call a coyote a wolf will not affect the discovery on which that very choice rests.

So *if* I succeed in making out significantly close affinities between so-called mental illnesses and standard physical illnesses, I shall oblige people (as Freud did) to construe the new judgments so facilitated in terms that are logically of the sort I have ascribed to findings. And this will be so even if people resist the new terminology—since they will be able, at any rate, to apply these categories in a way that is open to public confirmation and that does not depend on their personal tastes.

The defense of Freud's innovations, however, is rather more complicated than I have suggested. (I have, by the way, singled out Freud for reasons of convenience only. The issue at stake, as we shall see, is essentially the same for nearly all substantial contributions to the allied, but somewhat distinct, disciplines of psychiatry, psychotherapy, and psychoanalysis.) The defense of any would-be innovation in the medical concept of health would have to follow the plan of analogical extension already described. But the fact is that Freud mixed radically distinct elements in his normative models, so that it is not possible to provide a logically uniform defense for everything that falls under his extension of the concept of health.

The truth is that Freud's development of psychoanalytic medicine runs along two converging lines. In one, as in the studies of hysteria, Freud was extending case by case the medical concept of illness, by working out striking and undeniable affinities between physical illnesses and counterpart cases, for which the aetiology would have had to be radically different. And, in the other, Freud inevitably assimilated the concept of mental health to concepts of happiness—in particular, to his genital ideal. The result is that, *given* some version of this (or another such) ideal, deviation from the ideal tends to be viewed in terms of malady and disease, even though there are no strong analogical affinities between the pattern in question and clear-cut models of physical illness. Hence, patterns as significantly different as hysteria and homosexuality tend both to be assimilated to the concepts of health and disease.

In a word, in the psychotherapeutic setting, the relevant normative models move between the limits of health and happiness, between the limits set by physical medicine and those set by variable tastes of an ethical sort. The result is, as I have already suggested, that professional judgments do not always exhibit the logical form of medical findings and are in fact often appreciative judgments that take the form of findings.

Our problem is fairly illustrated by Freud's well-known analysis of so-called penis envy on the part of females. This involves, of course, the recasting of material about a late stage of sexual development in normative terms bearing primarily on happiness and self-fulfilment rather than on health. Freud notices the differences between male and female children in their reacting to the discovery of the different sexual organs and, in his strikingly fertile and ingenious way, links the contrast with the different points of view of the male and female. But among his comments, Freud speaks, not uncharacteristically, of ''the masculinity complex of women, which may put great difficulties in the way of their regular development towards femininity, if it cannot be got over soon enough.''[2] Similarly, speaking of a developing female child, he says:

She gives up her wish for a penis and puts in place of it a wish for a child: and *with this purpose in view* she takes her father as a love-object. Her mother becomes the object of her jealousy. The girl has turned into a little woman. If I am to credit a single exaggerated analytic instance, this new situation can give rise to physical sensations which would have to be regarded as a premature awakening of the female genital apparatus. If the girl's attachment to her father comes to grief later on and has to be abandoned, it may give place to an identification with him and the girl may thus return to her masculinity complex and perhaps remain fixated in it.[3]

Remarks of this sort, expressed in a noticeably neutral spirit, nevertheless look to the genital ideal and encourage the view that the girl in question is developing inappropriately. I do not wish to deny that the girl would be deviating from some ideal of femininity. But the crucial logical issue here is that the charge of deviation would be an appreciative judgment and not a medical finding. Furthermore, it is easy to see why the two are so readily confused, as well as actually fused, in the context of Freudian psychiatry. Deviation from the ideal of femininity tends to be construed in medical terms, precisely because the psychodynamics involved may show close affinities to patterns that, *in quite other circumstances,* result in mental illness.

•   •   •

It is clear that the psychotherapist, insofar as he interprets deviation from his maturational ideal in terms of malady, will be functioning as a moral critic of his society rather than as a medical specialist. He will not necessarily see this because he will tend to express himself in medical terms. Birnbach, for instance, in a striking passage, summarizes the social criticism of the neo-Freudians thus:

Neurosis or, to speak more broadly, mental illness, was shown to be the upshot of insecurity and anxiety (Sullivan); insecurity and anxiety were shown to be generated most frequently—almost infallibly—by competition (Horney); competition was shown to be the necessary consequence of the quest for individual self-validation in an egalitarian, competitive society of conflicting values (Alexander); and our egalitarian, competitive society was shown to be the product of a long-term evolution of social institutions (Kardiner). Neo-Freudian social philosophy therefore seems to point to the melancholy conclusion that an extensive incidence of mental illness is inherent in modern Western society, to say nothing of an unavoidable trend toward social breakdown.[4]

Here we have full-fledged social criticism presented as medicine; small wonder that some members of the neo-Freudian movement have found it necessary to construct or suggest visions of a utopian society.

The practical implications of seizing these contrasts between findings and appreciative judgments, between health and happiness, are quite serious. Both clients and therapists would be obliged to pay attention to two logically quite different kinds of value judgments that might be professionally supplied; and both the giving and the receiving of advice would inevitably be affected. This is not to criticize any particular advice. But a client who held distinct views about the meaning and fulfilment of his life could not possibly respond to his therapist's advice, if it were based on an alternative ideal, in the same way in which he received advice that was definitely medical in nature. And the therapist, for his part, could not possibly offer advice of these two sorts in the same spirit and with the same sense of professional responsibility.

My principal thesis here is both logical and historical. I am arguing that the model of health, in the setting of psychotherapy, is a mixed model that shows clear affinities with the models that obtain in physical medicine and at the same time with the models of happiness and well-being that obtain in the ethical domain. It need not be true (and doubtless it is not) that one could formulate a single, comprehensive model for the entire range of physical medicine. Perhaps there, too, in certain restricted areas (as with obesity), appreciative questions arise. But, generally speaking, to the extent that the concept of mental health bears close affinities with the concept of physical health, psychotherapeutic judgments behave as findings. On the other hand, to the extent that the concept of mental health really resembles alternative views of happiness and self-realization—which are inherently appreciative matters and thus have little or nothing to do with the medical conception of physical health—relevant psychotherapeutic judgments may

themselves be regarded as appreciative judgments. It follows from this contrast that the responsibility of both patient (or client) and therapist (or advisor) is seriously affected.

NOTES

1. Thomas S. Szasz, *The Myth of Mental Illness* (New York: 1961), pp. 41–42. Cf. also, John R. Reid, "The Myth of Doctor Szasz," *Journal of Nervous and Mental Disease* 135 (1962), pp. 381–386.
2. Cf. Sigmund Freud, "Some Psychological Consequences of the Anatomical Distinction Between the Sexes" (1923), in *Collected Papers,* Vol. V, edited by James Strachey (London, 1950), pp. 191–197.
3. *Ibid.,* p. 195.
4. Martin Birnbach, *Neo-Freudian Social Philosophy* (Stanford, 1961), p. 128.

HERBERT MORRIS

Thomas Szasz and the Manufacture of Madness

Though Szasz has a casual way of impugning the motives of psychiatrists, his most significant failing is that his way of looking at things idealizes the responsibility of the mad. He deprives the concept of responsibility of some of its discriminating power by refusing to distinguish between the responsibility of the mad—even the completely mad—and the sane.

There are two ways to make an all-out assault on a concept such as responsibility. One approach is to claim that the concept has no application. "No one is responsible." The other, more subtle way, is to claim that the concept applies to everything. "We are all responsible all the time." Szasz travels too far along the latter route and thereby makes less serviceable the very concept whose integrity it is his object to preserve. He does with responsibility, then, what he charges others with doing with sickness. This comes out clearly in one of his major arguments for abolition of the defense of insanity:

In the Anglo-American (and also Roman) philosophy of

From *On Guilt and Innocence* (Berkeley, Calif.: University of California Press, 1976), pp. 68–70, 72–73.

law, ignorance of the law is no excuse. How can a person ignorant of the law be held responsible for breaking it? How can he be blamed for committing an act that he did not know was prohibited? The answer is that the well-being of a free society is based on the assumption that every adult knows what he may and what he may not do. *Legal responsibility is an expectation:* first, that people will learn the laws of the land; second, that they will try to adhere to them. Thus, if they break the law, we consider them "blameworthy." If we apply this reasoning to offenders who are alleged to be mentally ill, similar conclusions will be reached. If mental illness resembles bodily illness, it will not excuse them from adherence to the law. If, on the other hand, mental illness is similar to ignorance (as indeed it is)—then again it is not a condition that excuses violation of the law. Just as the recognition of ignorance and its correction are the responsibility of the adult citizen, so also are the recognition of mental illness and its correction. Thus, from a purely logical point of view, there are no good grounds for the rule that there should be two types of laws, one for the mentally healthy and another for the mentally sick.[1]

At least two comments need to be made about this astounding passage. The first relates to its unquestioning acceptance of the principle "ignorance of the law is no excuse." If a man makes efforts to ascertain the law, efforts that we should judge those of a reasonable man in the circumstances and yet fails in his attempt, it would be a moral wrong to punish him for violating a law with which he believed in good faith he was complying. The principle of respect for individual freedom of choice, so venerated by Szasz, would be infringed if the man were punished. Second, Szasz places on all those whom we might classify as mentally ill the burden of discovering their condition and taking steps to correct it. This is weird. We might expect a blind man to realize his condition and take extra precautions in his social dealings because of it, but there would be something strange in expecting this of an idiot. Shall we impose upon him the burden of recognizing his idiocy and taking precautions appropriate to it? It is the same with certain classes of mental illness. To be sure, a person might feel himself inexplicably pulled toward doing harmful things to others despite his apparent desire not to do them. He might think, "I'm a kleptomaniac and I'd better get help." There is force in the claim that such a person should be held to the same degree of responsibility as one who suffers from some physical affliction and who because of it is expected to take appropriate precautionary steps. But surely there are others whose extraordinary habits of thought and feeling of long standing and pervasive effect have impaired their capacity to view accurately either themselves or the world around them. Are we guilty of some gross conceptual error and inhumanity when we seek to reflect sensitivity in our criminal law to those cases in which a man's capacity to appreciate what he is doing is substantially diminished? In the interest, then, of keeping within respectable limits the concept of illness, Szasz has so extended the boundaries of responsibility that he partially destroys the very thing he wishes to preserve, a meaningful concept of human responsibility. If mental illness is a myth, what shall we label the claim that all madmen are completely responsible?

.   .   .

A person may sometimes be blind to his own best interests and we are guilty of no lack of respect for him if we interfere, despite his protests, with what he wishes to do. Our friend's wine has been drugged and we observe him climbing out the twentieth-story window. Of course we stop him and do so despite his vehement protestations that he wants to die. Or, again, our friend may have drunk more than he can decently hold. He, not another, is responsible for his condition, but while in it, he is not himself as he climbs out the window, protesting he wants to die. Again, we may surely interfere. A person may also be blind to his own interests through lifelong habits of thought. May not interference also be justified in the case of such persons as it is with the drugged person? Can we not restrain in the hope that with time and talk—not limitless of course—some calm and rationality will gain ascendancy in such persons? We have, then, a difficult problem. It is always dangerous to substitute one's own judgment for that of another on the question of what is good for him. In some cases we believe that it is wrong to interfere even though we think the person blind to his own interests. In other cases we think it right to interfere. Where shall we place the blindness of the mad? Where shall we place it when their mistake may be irremediable as it is when life may be taken? Though I draw lines in these cases, I do not find it easy to do so. And I do not find particularly helpful observations such as: "—the individual must be free to abjure liberty; were he not, he would have no liberty to abjure."[2] What is absent in Szasz's treatment is a sufficiently sensitive appreciation of how difficult here is our choice between good and evil. In giving the impression that it is easy, he escapes full responsibility, one thing he knows we always do at too great a cost.

When we learn that a psychoanalyst believes that mental disease does not exist, that psychiatrists are power-hungry servants of the dominant elements in society, that the defense of insanity and involuntary commitment must be abolished to avoid crimes against humanity, we may find ourselves falling into a trap laid by the pervasive ideology condemned by Szasz. We may think: He must be mad. With that facile thought we can avoid seriously confronting what he has to say. The temptation must be withstood. Szasz's catalytic observations have thrown light where before there was too little or none. His great virtue, one that excuses for me all the exaggeration and seemingly deliberate perverseness, is his storming bastions of complacency and dogmatism, holding before us constantly the ideals of individual liberty and human dignity, and demanding of us reexamination of our ways of thinking, feeling, and acting in the light of these ideals.

HERBERT MORRIS **85**

NOTES

1. Thomas Szasz, *Law, Liberty, and Psychiatry* (New York: Macmillan Co., 1963), p. 14.

2. Thomas Szasz, *The Ethics of Psychoanalysis* (New York: Basic Books, 1965), p. 76.

SUGGESTED READINGS FOR CHAPTER 2

Boorse, Christopher. "What a Theory of Mental Health Should Be." *Journal for the Theory of Social Behaviour* 6 (April, 1976), 61–84.

———. "Health as a Theoretical Concept." *Philosophy of Science* 44 (December 1977), 542–573.

Breslow, Lester. "A Quantitative Approach to the World Health Organization Definition of Health: Physical, Mental, and Social Well-being." *International Journal of Epidemiology* 1 (Winter 1972), 347–355.

Clouser, K. Danner, Culver, Charles M., and Gert, Bernard. "Malady: A New Treatment of Disease." *Hastings Center Report* 11 (June 1981), 29–37.

Davis, Mary. "Disease and Its Treatment: Values in Medicine and Psychiatry." *Comprehensive Psychiatry* 18 (May/June 1977), 231–237.

"Defining 'Medical Care': The Key to Proper Application of the Medical Expense Deduction." Note in *Duke Law Journal* 1977 (October 1977), 909–932.

Dubos, René. *Mirage of Health*. New York: Harper & Row, 1959.

———. *Man, Medicine, and Environment*. New York: Frederick Praeger, 1968. Chap. 4.

Eisenberg, Leon. "What Makes Persons 'Patients' and Patients 'Well'?" *American Journal of Medicine* 69 (August 1980), 277–286.

Engelhardt, H. Tristram, Jr. "The Concepts of Health and Disease." In Engelhardt, H. Tristram, Jr., and Spicker, Stuart F., eds. *Evaluation and Explanation in the Biomedical Sciences*. Boston: D. Reidel, 1975, pp. 125–141.

———. "Ideology and Etiology." *The Journal of Medicine and Philosophy* 1 (September 1976), 256–258.

———. "Health and Disease: Philosophical Perspectives." In Reich, Warren T., ed. *Encyclopedia of Bioethics*. New York: Free Press, 1978. Vol. 2, pp. 599–606.

———. "Doctoring the Disease, Treating the Complaint, Helping the Patient." In Engelhardt, H. Tristram, and Callahan, Daniel, eds. *Knowing and Valuing*. Hastings-on-Hudson, N.Y.: The Hastings Center, 1980, pp. 225–249.

Fingarette, Herbert. *The Meaning of Criminal Insanity*. Berkeley, Calif.: University of California Press, 1972. Chap. 1.

Flew, Antony. *Crime or Disease?* New York: Barnes & Noble, 1973.

Fox, Renee C. "Illness." In Sills, David L., ed. *International Encyclopedia of the Social Sciences*. New York: Free Press, 1968. Vol. 7, pp. 90–95.

Gert, Bernard, and Culver, Charles. *Philosophy in Medicine*. New York: Oxford University Press, 1982. Chap. 4.

Hasker, William. "The Critique of 'Mental Illness': Conceptual and/or Ethical Crisis?" *Journal of Psychology and Theology* 5 (Spring 1977), 110–124.

Hoffman, Martin. "Philosophical Aspects of 'Mental Disease'." *Australian and New Zealand Journal of Psychiatry* 12 (March 1978), 29–33.

Journal of Medicine and Philosophy, Vol. 1 (September 1976). Special issue on "Concepts of Health and Disease"; Vol. 2 (September 1977). Special issue on "Mental Health"; Vol. 5 (June 1980). Special issue on "Social and Cultural Perspectives on Disease."

Kass, Leon. "Regarding the End of Medicine and the Pursuit of Health." *Public Interest* 40 (Summer 1975), 11–42.

———. "Medical Care and the Pursuit of Health." In Feldstein, Martin S., *et al. New Directions in Public Health Care*. San Francisco: Institute for Contemporary Studies, 1976, pp. 1–21.

Kendell, R. E. "The Concept of Disease and Its Implications for Psychiatry." *British Journal of Psychiatry* 127 (1975), 305–315.

Kopelman, Loretta. "On Disease. . . ." In Engelhardt, H. Tristram, and Spicker, Stuart F., eds. *Evaluation and Explanation in the Biomedical Sciences*. Boston: D. Reidel, 1974, pp. 143–150.

———, and Moskop, John. "The Holistic Health Movement: A Survey and Critique." *Journal of Medicine and Philosophy* 6 (May 1981), 209–235.

Macklin, Ruth. "Mental Health and Mental Illness: Some Problems of Definition and Concept Formation." *Philosophy of Science* 39 (September 1972), 341–365.

———. "The Medical Model in Psychoanalysis and Psychotherapy." *Comprehensive Psychiatry* 14 (January/February 1973), 49–69.

Margolis, Joseph. *Negativities: The Limits of Life*. Columbus, Ohio: Charles Merrill Publishing Co., 1975. Chaps. 7 and 8.

———. "The Concept of Disease." *The Journal of Medicine and Philosophy* 1 (September 1976), 238–255.

Mechanic, David. "The Concept of Illness Behavior." *Journal of Chronic Diseases* 15 (1962), 189–194.

Moore, Michael S. "Some Myths about 'Mental Illness'." *Inquiry* 18 (Autumn 1975), 233–265.

Osmond, Humphrey. "The Medical Model in Psychiatry: Love It or Leave It." *Medical Annals of the District of Columbia* 41 (March 1972), 171–175.

———, and Siegler, Miriam. *Models of Madness, Models of Medicine*. New York: Macmillan, 1974.

Parsons, Talcott. "Health and Disease: A Sociological and Action Perspective." In Reich, Warren T., ed. *Encyclopedia of Bioethics*. New York: Free Press, 1978. Vol. 2, pp. 590—599.

Pflanz, Manfred, and Keupp, Heinrich. "A Sociological Perspective on Concepts of Disease." *International Social Science Journal* 29 (1977), 386–396.

Polgar, Steven. "Health." In Sills, David L., ed. *International Encyclopedia of the Social Sciences*. New York: Free Press, 1968. Vol. 5, pp. 330–336.

Redlich, F. C. "The Concept of Health in Psychiatry." In Leighton, Alexander H., Claussen, John A., and Wilson, Robert N., eds. *Explorations in Social Psychiatry*. New York: Basic Books, 1957, pp. 138–158.

Reiss, S. "A Critique of Thomas S. Szasz's 'Myth of Mental Illness'." *American Journal of Psychiatry* 128 (March 1972), 1080–1084.

Risse, Guenter B. "Health and Disease: History of the Concepts."

In Reich, Warren T., ed. *Encyclopedia of Bioethics*. New York: Free Press, 1978. Vol. 2, pp. 579–585.

Scott, W. A. "Research Definitions of Mental Health and Illness." In Wechsler, H., Soloman, L., and Kramer, B. M., eds. *Social Psychology and Mental Health*. New York: Holt, Rinehart & Winston, Inc., 1970.

Szasz, Thomas. *The Manufacture of Madness*. New York: Harper & Row, 1970.

———. "Bad Habits Are Not Diseases." *Lancet* (July 8, 1972), 83–84.

———. *The Theology of Medicine: The Political-Philosophical Foundations of Medical Ethics*. New York: Harper & Row, 1977.

Temkin, Owsei. "Health and Disease." *Dictionary of the History of Ideas*. New York: Scribner's, 1973. Vol. 2, pp. 395–407.

Goldstein, Doris Mueller. *Bioethics: A Guide to Information Sources*. Detroit: Gale Research Company, 1982. See under "Philosophy of Medicine" and "Psychotherapy and Psychopharmacology."

Lineback, Richard H., ed. *Philosopher's Index*. Vols. 1–. Bowling Green, Ohio: Philosophy Documentation Center, Bowling Green State University. Issued quarterly. See under "Health," "Illness," "Mental Health," "Mental Illness," and "Physicians."

Walters, LeRoy, ed. *Bibliography of Bioethics*. Vols. 1–. New York: Free Press. Issued annually. See under "Genetic Defects," "Health," and "Mental Health." (The information contained in the annual *Bibliography of Bioethics* can also be retrieved from BIOETHICSLINE, an online data base of the National Library of Medicine.)

3.
Concepts of Personhood

Like concepts of health and disease, competing concepts of personhood have been the object of sustained philosophical debate. In biomedical ethics concepts of personhood have played a significant role in analyses of abortion (Chapter 6), the definition and determination of death (Chapter 7), euthanasia and the prolongation of life (Chapter 8), and, to a lesser extent, research involving children (Chapter 11).

Discussions of personhood frequently adopt a purely *descriptive* approach. They ask the question: "What sorts of beings are persons, and how are persons to be distinguished from other entities present in the universe, for example, dogs, trees, or rocks?" These discussions belong to the branch of philosophy called metaphysics, and more particularly to the part of metaphysics called ontology, or the study of that which exists.

As philosophers have reflected on the problem of personhood, they have usually found it quite easy to categorize nonliving objects (for example, rocks) and many types of living things (for example, bacteria, plants, and invertebrate animals) as nonpersons. However, beyond this point the search for what Joel Feinberg calls "the criterion of commonsense personhood" becomes much more complicated. Among the questions that have long puzzled philosophers are the following: Are some nonhuman beings—for example, chimpanzees—capable of becoming persons? Are all biologically human beings, including fetuses and the irreversibly comatose, persons? And can there be other types of beings—for example, residents of unknown planets, angels, or robots—who should also be designated persons?

The standard philosophical approach to solving these puzzles has been to devise a list of necessary, and possibly sufficient, conditions for being a person. These conditions are often expressed in terms of properties that must be possessed by the being in question if it is to qualify as a person. For example, in his essay in this chapter Joel Feinberg characterizes persons as beings that have the following properties: (a) consciousness; (b) possession of a self-concept; (c) self-awareness; (d) the capacity to experience emotions; (e) the capacity to reason and acquire understanding; (f) the capacity to plan ahead; (g) the capacity to act on one's plans; and (h) the capacity to feel pleasure and pain. Feinberg argues that possession of *all* these properties is a sufficient condition of personhood. To this argument he adds the more controversial claims that none of these eight properties is individually sufficient and that each of the eight is necessary.

Feinberg's list of the conditions of personhood faithfully reflects the two properties, or characteristes, that have figured most prominently in ontological notions of personhood—self-awareness and rationality. Other authors, however, have required a third characteristic, namely, the capacity to be a moral agent. That is, these authors explicitly identify moral characteristics, in addition to cognitive characteristics, as necessary conditions of personhood. As H. Tristram Engelhardt notes in his essay in this chapter, Immanuel Kant accented these moral characteristics of personhood, describing "moral personality" as "the freedom of a rational being under moral laws." In a similar vein, Roland Puccetti distinguishes between C-predicates, which apply to all conscious beings, and P-predicates, which apply only to persons. Among the predicates applied by Puccetti to the two groups of subjects are the following:

C is in pain	P wants to secure justice
C feels hungry	P summarized the point nicely
C is excited	P is an astute judge of character
C is afraid of you	P looks at everything abstractly
	P is a smug hypocrite[1]

According to Puccetti, the C-predicates in the left-hand column can be applied to conscious nonpersons like dogs, whereas the P-predicates in the right-hand column presuppose the possession of a conceptual scheme and the capacity to act as a moral agent. This latter capacity is for Puccetti the primary distinguishing feature of personhood, for persons are the only conscious entities who can adopt moral attitudes toward moral objects.

MORAL NOTIONS OF PERSONHOOD

It might seem that the preceding discussion has already crossed the line between ontological and moral notions of personhood. However, the authors cited to this point have only been involved in *describing* what sorts of beings persons are, not in *prescribing* how particular beings ought to be treated. Moral notions of personhood perform precisely this task. Ascribing moral personhood to an individual is tantamount to saying "I have moral obligations to this individual" or "This individual has moral rights." In the history of philosophy, Immanuel Kant was perhaps the most influential proponent of the moral personhood notion. Kant considered persons as beings whose rational nature "points them out as ends in themselves." Accordingly, Kant contended that the only appropriate attitude toward such beings is one of respect. (See the discussion of autonomy in Chapter 1. The difficulty inherent in specifying precisely what moral obligations are included in respect for persons is itself a complex philosophical problem. However, it need not detain us here. It is sufficient to observe the existence of at least minimal moral duties to all beings belonging to the category of persons.)

Given the moral obligations that are thought to be owed to persons, it is then an obvious strategy for anyone seeking to protect particular categories of beings to argue that those beings rightly belong to the category of (moral) persons. Conversely, it is sometimes thought that nonpersons do not deserve the same kind of respect, or even that any nonperson may be treated, in Kant's terms, merely as a means. In the present chapter, Puccetti and Feinberg explore whether beings classifiable as "potential persons," "beginning persons," or "former persons" are deserving of respect, while Engelhardt advocates the creation of a category of "social persons" to ensure that infants are protected until they develop into persons in the strict sense. On the other hand, Joseph Fletcher suggests that individuals lacking a minimal level of neocortical function are, in his words, "objects but not subjects." Fletcher does not clearly specify how such biologically human objects should be treated.

THE RELATIONSHIP BETWEEN ONTOLOGICAL AND MORAL
NOTIONS OF PERSONHOOD

Whether and how one can move logically from ontology to ethics, or from "is" to "ought," is one of the most vigorously contested questions in philosophy. The problem of the relationship between ontological and moral notions of personhood is, from one perspective, simply an instance of this more generic question.

Some philosophers, among them R. M. Hare, have argued that there is no necessary *logical* connection between ontological personhood and moral personhood. According to Hare, one cannot infer from the assertion "*X* is a person" that "I ought to be kind to *X*."[2] In contrast, Joel Feinberg sees an intimate connection between ontological personhood (or, in his words, "commonsense personhood") and moral personhood. Indeed, he argues that moral personhood is "conferred by the same characteristics that lead us to recognize personhood wherever we find it." Despite his strong assertion that the classes of actual commonsense and actual moral persons are identical, Feinberg might nonetheless concede that there is no *simple* way to make a logical move from is to ought.

Finally, there is an obverse side to the is-ought problem. The mere fact that a being is not ontologically a person does not logically entail the conclusion that we have no obligations to it or, correlatively, that it has no rights. Although Feinberg does not employ the language of obligation or rights in this connection, he notes that there are powerful arguments against infanticide, even if infants are not persons in the ontological sense. A similar question is explored in Chapter 12: "What moral obligations, if any, do we persons have toward animals which are not persons?"

L.W.

NOTES

1. Roland Puccetti, *Persons: A Study of Possible Moral Agents in the Universe* (New York: Herder and Herder, 1970), pp. 7–8. Puccetti's entire discussion of predicates builds upon P. F. Strawson's earlier work, *Individuals*. Whereas Strawson had distinguished only M-predicates (for material bodies) and P-predicates, Puccetti added the intermediate category of C-predicates.

2. R. M. Hare, *Freedom and Reason* (Oxford: Clarendon Press, 1963), pp. 212–213.

JOSEPH FLETCHER

Indicators of Humanhood: A Tentative Profile of Man

Mark Twain complained that people are always talking about the weather but they never do anything about it. The same is true of the humanhood agenda. In biomedical ethics writers constantly say that we need to explicate humanness or humaneness, what it means to be a truly human being, but they never follow their admission of the need with an actual inventory or profile, no matter how tentatively offered. Yet this is what must be done, or at least attempted.

Synthetic concepts such as *human* and *man* and *person* require operational terms, spelling out the which and what and when. Only in that way can we get down to cases—to normative decisions. There are always some people who prefer to be visceral and affective in their moral choices, with no desire to have any rationale for what they do. But *ethics* is precisely the business of rational, critical reflection (encephalic and not merely visceral) about the problems of the moral agent—in biology and medicine as much as in law, government, education or anything else.

To that end, then, for the purposes of biomedical ethics, I am suggesting a "profile of man" in concrete and discrete terms. As only one man's reflection on man, it will no doubt invite adding and subtracting by others, but this is the road to be followed if we mean business. As a dog is said to "worry" a bone, let me worry out loud and on paper, hoping for some agreement and, at the least, consideration. There is space only to itemize it, not to enlarge upon it, but I have fifteen positive propositions and five negative propositions. Let me set them out, in no rank order at all, and as hardly more than a list of criteria or indicators, by simple title.

From *Hastings Center Report* 2 (November, 1972), 1–4. Reprinted with permission of the Hastings Center: © Institute of Society, Ethics and the Life Sciences, 360 Broadway, Hastings-on-Hudson, N.Y. 10706.

POSITIVE HUMAN CRITERIA

MINIMAL INTELLIGENCE

Any individual of the species *homo sapiens* who falls below the I.Q. 40-mark in a standard Stanford-Binet test, amplified if you like by other tests, is questionably a person; below the 20-mark, not a person. *Homo* is indeed *sapiens*, in order to be *homo*. The *ratio*, in another turn of speech, is what makes a person of the *vita*. Mere biological life, before minimal intelligence is achieved or after it is lost irretrievably, is without personal status. This has bearing, obviously, on decision making in gynecology, obstetrics and pediatrics, as well as in general surgery and medicine.

SELF-AWARENESS

Self-consciousness, as we know, is the quality we watch developing in a baby; we watch it with fascination and glee. Its essential role in personality development is a basic datum of psychology. Its existence or function in animals at or below the primate level is debatable; it is clearly absent in the lower vertebrates, as well as in the nonvertebrates. In psychotherapy non-self-awareness is pathological; in medicine, unconsciousness when it is incorrigible at once poses quality-of-life judgments—for example, in neurosurgical cases of irreversible damage to the brain cortex.

SELF-CONTROL

If an individual is not only not controllable by others (unless by force) but not controllable by the individual himself or herself, a low level of life is reached about on a par with a paramecium. If the condition cannot be rectified medically, so that means-ends behavior is out of the question, the individual is not a person—not ethically, and certainly

A SENSE OF TIME

Time consciousness. By this is meant clock time or *chronos,* not timeliness or *kairos,* i.e., not the "fulness of time" or the pregnant moment (remember Paul Tillich?). A sense, that is, of the passage of time. A colleague of mine at the University of Virginia, Dr. Thomas Hunter, remarked recently, "Life is the allocation of time." We can disagree legitimately about how relatively important this indicator is, but it is hard to understand why anybody would minimize it or eliminate it as a trait of humanness.

A SENSE OF FUTURITY

How "truly human" is any man who cannot realize there is a time yet to come as well as the present? Subhuman animals do not look forward in time; they live only on what we might call visceral strivings, appetites. Philosophical anthropologies (one recalls William Temple's, for instance) commonly emphasize *purposiveness* as a key to humanness. Chesterton once remarked that we would never ask a puppy what manner of dog it wanted to be when it grows up. The assertion here is that men are typically teleological, although certainly not eschatological.

A SENSE OF THE PAST

Memory. Unlike other animals, men as a species have reached a unique level of neurologic development, particularly the cerebrum and especially its neo-cortex. They are linked to the past by conscious recall—not only, as with subhuman animals, by conditioning and the reactivation of emotions (reactivated, that is, externally rather than autonomously). It is this trait, in particular, that makes man, alone among all species, a cultural instead of an instinctive creature. An existentialist focus on "nowness" truncates the nature of man.

THE CAPABILITY TO RELATE TO OTHERS

Interpersonal relationships, of the sexual-romantic and friendship kind, are of the greatest importance for the fulness of what we idealize as being truly personal. (Medical piety in the past has always held its professional ethics to be only a one-to-one, physician-patient obligation.) However, there are also the more diffuse and comprehensive social relations of our vocational, economic and political life. Aristotle's characterization of man as a social animal, *zoon politikon,* must surely figure prominently in the inventory. It is true that even insects live in social systems, but the cohesion of all subhuman societies is based on instinct. Man's society is based on culture—that is, on a conscious knowledge of the system and on the exercise in some real measure of either consent or opposition.

CONCERN FOR OTHERS

Some people may be skeptical about our capacity to care about others (what in Christian ethics is often distinguished from romance and friendship as "neighbor love" or "neighbor concern"). The extent to which this capacity is actually in play is debatable. But whether concern for others is disinterested or inspired by enlightened self-interest it seems plain that a conscious extra-ego orientation is a trait of the species; the absence of this ambience is a clinical indication of psychopathology.

COMMUNICATION

Utter alienation or disconnection from others, if it is irreparable, is de-humanization. This is not so much a matter of not being disposed to receive and send "messages" as of the inability to do so. This criterion comes into question in patients who cannot hear, speak, feel or see others; it may come about as a result of mental or physical trauma, infection, genetic or congenital disorder, or from psychological causes. Completely and finally *isolated* individuals are subpersonal. The problem is perhaps most familiar in terminal illnesses and the clinical decision-making required.

CONTROL OF EXISTENCE

It is of the nature of man that he is not helplessly subject to the blind workings of physical or physiological nature. He has only finite knowledge, freedom and initiative, but what he has of it is real and effective. Invincible ignorance and total helplessness are the antitheses of humanness, and to the degree that a man lacks control he is not responsible, and to be irresponsible is to be subpersonal. This item in the agenda applies directly, for example, in psychiatric medicine, especially to severe cases of toxic and degenerative psychosis.

CURIOSITY

To be without affect, sunk in anomie, is to be not a person. Indifference is inhuman. Man is a learner and a knower as well as a tool maker and user. This raises a question, therefore, about demands to stop some kinds of biomedical inquiry. For example, an A.M.A. [American Medical Association] committee recently called a halt on *in vitro* reproduction and embryo transplants on the ground that they are dangerous. But dangerous ignorance is more dangerous than dangerous knowledge. It is dehumanizing to impose a moratorium on research. No doubt this issue arises, or will arise, in many other phases of medical education and practice.

CHANGE AND CHANGEABILITY

To the extent that an individual is unchangeable or opposed to change he denies the creativity of personal beings. It means not only the fact of biological and physiological change, which goes on as a condition of life, but the capacity and disposition for changing one's mind and conduct as well. Biologically, human beings are developmental: birth, life, health, and death are processes, not events, and are to be understood epigenetically, not episodically. All human existence is on a continuum, a matter of becoming. In this perspective, are we to regard potentials *als ob,* as if they were actual? I think not. The question arises prominently in abortion ethics.

BALANCE OF RATIONALITY AND FEELING

To be "truly human," to be a wholesome *person,* one cannot be either Apollonian or Dionysian. As human beings we are not "coldly" rational or cerebral, nor are we merely creatures of feeling and intuition. It is a matter of being both, in different combinations from one individual to another. To be one rather than the other is to distort the *humanum.*

IDIOSYNCRASY

The human being is idiomorphous, a distinctive individual. As Helmut Schoeck has shown, even the function of envy in human behavior is entirely consistent with idiosyncrasy. To be a person is to have an identity, to be recognizable and callable by name. It is this criterion which lies behind the fear that to replicate individuals by so-called "cloning" would be to make "carbon copies" of the parent source and thus dehumanize the clone by denying it its individuality. One or two writers have even spoken of a "right" to a "unique genotype," and while such talk is ethically and scientifically questionable it nonetheless reflects a legitimate notion of something essential to an authentic person.

NEO-CORTICAL FUNCTION

In a way, this is the cardinal indicator, the one all the others are hinged upon. Before cerebration is in play, or with its end, in the absence of the synthesizing function of the cerebral cortex, the *person* is nonexistent. Such individuals are objects but not subjects. This is so no matter how many other spontaneous or artificially supported functions persist in the heart, lungs, neurologic and vascular systems. Such noncerebral processes are not personal. Like the Harvard Medical School's *ad hoc* committee report on "brain death" the recent Kansas statute on defining death requires the absence of *brain* function. So do the guidelines recently adopted by the Italian Council of Ministers. But what is definitive in determining death is the loss of cerebration, not just of any or all brain function. Personal reality depends on cerebration and to be dead "humanly" speaking is to be ex-cerebral, no matter how long the *body* remains alive.

NEGATIVE HUMAN CRITERIA

The five negative points I have can be put even more briefly than the 15 positive ones, although I am inclined to believe that they merit just as much critical scrutiny and elaboration.

MAN IS NOT NON- OR ANTI-ARTIFICIAL

As [Willard] Gaylin says, men are characterized by technique, and for a human being to oppose technology is "self-hatred." We are often confused on this score, attitudinally. A "test tube baby," for example, although conceived and gestated *ex corpo,* would nonetheless be humanly reproduced and of human value. A baby made artificially, by deliberate and careful contrivance, would be more *human* than one resulting from sexual roulette—the reproductive mode of the subhuman species.

MAN IS NOT ESSENTIALLY PARENTAL

People can be fully personal without reproducing, as the religious vows of nuns, monks and celibate priests of the past have asserted, as the law has implied by refusing to annul marriages because of sterility, and as we see in the ethos-reversal of contemporary family and population control—and, more militantly, in the non-parental rhetoric of women's liberation and a growing rejection of the "baby trap."

MAN IS NOT ESSENTIALLY SEXUAL

Sexuality, a broader and deeper phenomenon than sex, is of the fulness but not of the essence of man. It is not even necessary to human species survival. I will not try here to indicate the psychological entailments of this negative proposition, but it is biologically apparent when we look at such nonsexual reproduction as cloning from somatic cells, and parthenogenetic reproduction by both androgenesis and gynogenesis. What light does this biology throw on the nature of man; what does a personistic view of man say about the ethics of such biology? (N.B. I do not refer here to personalism, which has more metaphysical freight than many of us want to carry.)

MAN IS NOT A BUNDLE OF RIGHTS

The notion of a human *nature* has served as a conceptual bucket, to contain "human rights" and certain other *given* things, like "original sin" and "the sense of oughtness" and "conscience." The idea behind this is that such things are objective, pre-existent phenomena, not contingent on biological or social relativities. People sometimes speak of rights to live, to die, to be healthy, to reproduce, and so on, as if they were absolute, eternal, intrinsic. But as the law makes plain, all rights are imperfect and may be set aside if human *need* requires it. We shall have to think through the relation of rights and needs, as it bears on clinical medicine's decision-making problems, as well as society's problems of health care delivery. One example: What is the "humane" policy if we should reach the point (I think we will) of deciding for or against compulsory birth control? Or, how are we to relate rights and needs if, to take only one example, an ethnic group protests against mass screening for sickle cell anemia? Or if after genetic counseling a couple elects to proceed with a predictably degenerate pregnancy?

MAN IS NOT A WORSHIPER

Faith in supernatural realities and attempts to be in direct association with them are choices some human beings make and others do not. Mystique is not essential to being truly a person. Like sexuality, it may arguably be of the fulness of humanness but it is not of the essence. This negative proposition is required by our basic guideline, the premise that a viable biomedical ethics is humanistic, whatever reasons we may have for putting human well-being at the center of concern.

MORE THINKING

How are we to go about testing such criteria as these? And how are we to compare and combine the results of our criticism? How are we to rank order or give priority to the items in our man-hood profile? Which are only optimal, which are essential? What are the applications of these or other indicators to the normative decisions of biologists and physicians? In my own list, here, which factors can be eliminated, in whole or in part, without lowering individuals and patients below the personal line? I trust that by this time it is plain that I do not claim to have produced the pure gospel of humanness. I remain open to correction.

The "nature of man" question is of such depth and sensitivity that it is bound to raise controversy, and our task is to welcome the controversy but try to reduce it through analysis and synthesis. Said Heraclitus: "Opposition brings concord. Out of discord comes the fairest harmony. It is by disease that health is pleasant; by evil that good is pleasant; by hunger, satiety; by weariness, rest."

As a final note, I rather suspect that we are more apt to find good answers inductively and empirically, from medical science and the clinicians, than by the necessarily syllogistic reasoning of the humanities, which proceeds deductively from abstract premises. Syllogisms always contain their conclusions in their major or first premises. Divorced from the laboratory and the hospital, talk about what it means to be human could easily become inhumane.

H . T R I S T R A M   E N G E L H A R D T

Medicine and the Concept of Person*

Recent advances in medicine and the biomedical sciences have raised a number of ethical issues that medical ethics or, more broadly, bioethics have treated. Ingredient in such considerations, however, are fundamentally conceptual and ontological issues. To talk of the sanctity of life, for example, presupposes that one knows (1) what life is, and (2) what makes for its sanctity. More importantly, to talk of the rights of persons presupposes that one knows what counts as a person. In this paper I will provide an examination of the concept of person and will argue that the terms "human life" and even "human person" are complex and heterogeneous terms. I will hold that human life has more than one meaning and that there is more than one sense of human person. I will then indicate how the recognition of these multiple meanings has important implications for medicine.

KINDS OF LIFE AND SANCTITY OF LIFE

Whatever is meant by life's being sacred, it is rarely held that all life is equally sacred. Most people would find the life of bacteria, for example, to be less valuable or sacred than the life of fellow humans. In fact, there appears to be a spectrum of increasing value to life (I will presume that the term sanctity of life signifies that life has either special values or rights). All else being equal, plants seem to be valued less than lower animals, lower animals less than higher animals (such as primates other than humans), and humans are usually held to have the highest value. Moreover, distinctions are made with respect to humans. Not all human life has the same sanctity.

*An earlier version of this paper was read as a part of the Matchette Foundation Series, "The Expanding Universe of Modern Medicine," The Kennedy Institute and the Department of Philosophy, Georgetown University, Washington, D.C., November 19, 1974. I wish to express my debt to George Agich, Thomas J. Bole, III, Edmund L. Erde, Laurence B. McCullough, and John Moskop for their discussion and criticism of the ancestral drafts of this paper.

The issue of brain-death, for example, turns on such a distinction. Brain-dead, but otherwise alive, human beings do not have the sanctity of normal adult human beings. That is, the indices of brain-death have been selected in order to measure the death of a person. As a legal issue, it is a question of when a human being ceases to be a person before the law. In a sense, the older definition of death measured the point at which organismic death occurred, when there was a complete cessation of vital functions.[1] The life of the human organism was taken as a necessary condition for being a person, and, therefore, such a definition allowed one to identify cases in which humans ceased to be persons.

The brain-oriented concept of death is more directly concerned with human *personal* life.[2] It makes three presuppositions: (1) that being a person involves more than mere vegetative life, (2) that merely vegetative life may have value but it has no rights, (3) that a sensory-motor organ such as the brain is a necessary condition for the possibility of experience and action in the world, that is, for being a person living in the world. Thus in the absence of the possibility of brain-function, one has the absence of the possibility of personal life—that is, the person is dead. Of course, the presence of some brain activity (or more than vegetative function) does not imply the presence of a person—a necessary condition for the life of a person is not a sufficient condition for the life of a person. The brain-oriented concept of death is of philosophical significance, for, among other things, it implies a distinction between human biological life and human personal life, between the life of a human organism and the life of a human person. That human biological life continues after brain death is fairly clear: the body continues to circulate blood, the kidneys function; in fact, there is no reason why the organism would not continue to be cross-fertile (e.g., produce viable sperm) and, thus, satisfy yet one more criterion for biological life. Such a body can be a biologically integrated reproductive unit even if the level of integration is very low. And, if such a body is an instance of human biological but not human personal life, then it is open to use merely as a subject of experimentation without the constraints of a second status as a person. Thus Dr. Willard Gaylin has argued that living but brain-dead bodies could provide an excellent source of subjects for medical experimentation and education[3] and recommends "sustaining life in the brain-dead."[4] To avoid what would otherwise be an oxymoronic position, he is legitimately pressed to distinguish, as he does in fact, between "aliveness" and "personhood,"[5] or, to use more precise terminology, between human biological and human personal life. In short, a distinction between the status of human biological and personal life is presupposed.

We are brought then to a set of distinctions: first, human life must be distinguished as human personal and human biological life. Not all instances of human biological life are instances of human personal life. Brain-dead (but otherwise alive) human beings, human gametes, cells in human cell cultures, all count as instances of human biological life. Further, not only are some humans not persons, there is no reason to hold that all persons are humans, as the possibility of extraterrestrial self-conscious life suggests.

Second, the concept of the sanctity of life comes to refer in different ways to the value of biological life and the dignity of persons. Probably much that is associated with arguments concerning the sanctity of life really refers to the dignity of the life of persons. In any event, there is no unambiguous sense of being simply "pro-life" or a defender of the sanctity of life—one must decide what sort of life one wishes to defend and on what grounds. To begin with, the morally significant difference between biological and personal life lies in the fact, to use Kant's idiom, that persons are ends in themselves. Rational, self-conscious agents can make claims to treatment as ends in themselves because they can experience themselves, can know that they experience themselves, and can determine and control the circumstances of such experience. Self-conscious agents are self-determining and can claim respect as such. That is, they can claim the right to be respected as free agents. Such a claim is to the effect that self-respect and mutual respect turn on self-determination, on the fact that self-conscious beings are necessary for the existence of a moral order—a kingdom of ends, a community based on mutual self-respect, not force. Only

self-conscious agents can be held accountable for their actions and thus be bound together solely in terms of mutual respect of each other's autonomy.

What I intend here is no more than an exegesis of what we could mean by "respecting persons." Kant, for example, argued that rational beings are "persons, because their very nature [as rational beings] points them out as ends in themselves."[6] In this fashion, Kant developed a distinction between things that have only "a worth *for us*" and persons "whose existence is an end in itself."[7] As a result, Kant drew a stark and clear distinction between persons and non-persons. "A person is [a] subject whose actions are capable of being imputed [that is, one who can act responsibly]. Accordingly, moral personality is nothing but the freedom of a rational being under moral laws (whereas psychological personality is merely the capacity to be conscious of the identity of one's self in the various conditions of one's existence). . . . [In contrast], a thing is that which is not capable of any imputation [that is, of acting responsibly]."[8] To be respected as a moral agent is precisely to be respected as a free self-conscious being capable of being blamed and praised, of being held responsible for its actions. The language of respect in the sense of recognizing others as free to determine themselves (i.e., as ends in themselves) rather than as beings to be determined by others (i.e., to be used as means, instruments to goods and values) turns upon acknowledging others as free, as moral agents.

This somewhat obvious exegesis (or tautological point) is an account of the nature of the language of obligation. Talk of obligation functions (1) to remind us that certain actions cannot be reconciled with the notion of a moral community, and (2) to enjoin others to pursue particular values or goods. The only actions that strictly contradict the notion of a moral community are those that are incompatible with the notion of such a community—actions that treat moral agents as if they were objects. Morality as mutual respect of autonomy (i.e., more than conjoint pursuit of particular goods or goals) can be consistently pursued only if persons in the strict sense (i.e., self-conscious agents, entities able to be self-legislative) are treated with respect for their autonomy. Though we may treat other entities with a form of respect, that respect is never central to the notion of a community of moral agents. Insofar as we identify persons with moral agents, we exclude from the range of the concept person those entities which are not self-conscious. Which is to say, only those beings are unqualified bearers of rights and duties who can both claim to be acknowledged as having a dignity beyond a value (i.e., as being ends in themselves) and can be responsible for their actions. Of course, this strict sense of person is not unlike that often used in the law.[9] And, as Kant suggests in the passage above, it requires as well an experience of self-identity through time.

It is only respect for persons in this strict sense that cannot be violated without contradicting the idea of a moral order in the sense of the living with others on the basis of a mutual respect of autonomy. The point to be emphasized is a distinction between value and dignity, between biological life and personal life. These distinctions provide a basis for the differentiation between biological or merely animal life, and personal life, and turn on the rather commonsense criterion of respect being given that which can be respected—that is, blamed or praised. Moral treatment comes to depend, not implausibly, on moral agency. The importance of such distinctions for medicine is that they can be employed in treating medical ethical issues. As arguments, they are attempts to sort out everyday distinctions between moral agents, other animals, and just plain things. They provide a conceptual apparatus based on the meaning of obligations as respect due that which can have obligations.

The distinctions between human biological life and human personal life, and between the value of human biological life and the dignity of human personal life, involve a basic conceptual distinction that modern medical science presses as an issue of practical importance. Medicine after all is not merely the enterprise of preserving human life—if that were the case, medicine would confuse human cell cultures with patients who are persons. In fact, a maxim "to treat patients as persons" presupposes that we do or can indeed know who the persons are. These distinctions focus not only on the newly problematic issue of the definition of death, but on the question of abortion as well: issues that turn on when persons end and when they begin. In the case of the definition of death, one is saying that even though genetic continuity, organic function, and reproductive capability may extend beyond brain death, personal life does not. Sentience in an appropriate embodiment is a necessary condition for being a person.[10] One, thus, finds that persons die when this embodiment is undermined.

With regard to abortion, many have argued similarly that the fetus is not a person, though it is surely an instance of human biological life. Even if the fetus is a human organism that will probably be genetically and organically continuous with a human person, it is not yet such a person.[11] Simply put, fetuses are not rational, self-conscious beings—that is, given a strict definition of persons, fetuses do not qualify as persons. One sees this when comparing talk about dead men with talk about fetuses. When speaking of a dead man, one knows of whom one speaks, the one who died, the person whom one knew before his death. But in speaking of the fetus, one has no such person to whom one can refer. There is not yet a person, a "who," to whom one can refer in the case of the fetus (compare: one can keep promises to dead men but not to men yet unborn). In short, the fetus in no way singles itself out as, or shows itself to be, a person. This conclusion has theoretical advantages, since many zygotes* never implant and some divide into two.[12] It offers as well a moral clarification of the practice of using intrauterine contraceptive devices and abortion. Whatever these practices involve, they do not involve the taking of the life of a person.[13] This position in short involves recurring to a distinction forged by both Aristotle and St. Thomas—between biological life and personal life,[14] between life that has value and life that has dignity.

But this distinction does too much, as the arguments by Michael Tooley on behalf of infanticide show.[15] By the terms of the argument, infants, as well as fetuses, are not persons—thus, one finds infants as much open to infanticide as fetuses are left open to abortion. The question then is whether one can recoup something for infants or perhaps even for fetuses. One might think that a counterargument, or at least a mitigating argument, could be made on the basis of potentiality—the potentiality of infants or the potentiality of fetuses. That argument, though, fails because one must distinguish the potentialities of a person from the potentiality to become a person. If, for example, one holds that a fetus has the potentiality of a person, one begs the very question at issue—whether fetuses are persons. But, on the other hand, if one succeeds in arguing that a fetus or infant has the potentiality to become a person, one has conceded the point that the fetus or infant is not a person. One may value a dozen eggs or a handful of acorns because

*Ed. note: A zygote is a one-celled embryo.

they can become chickens or oak trees. But a dozen eggs is not a flock of chickens, a handful of acorns is not a stand of oaks. In short, the potentiality of X's to become Y's may cause us to value X's very highly because Y's are valued very highly, but until X's are Y's they do not have the value of Y's.[16]

Which is to say, given our judgments concerning brain-dead humans and concerning zygotes, embryos, and fetuses, we are left in a quandary with regard to infants. How, if at all, are we to understand them to be persons, beings to whom we might have obligations? One should remember that these questions arise against the backdrop of issues concerning the disposition of deformed neonates—whether they should all be given maximal treatment, or whether some should be allowed to die, or even have their deaths expedited.[17]

In short, though we have sorted out a distinction between the value of human biological life and the dignity of human personal life, this distinction does not do all we want, or rather it may do too much. That is, it goes against an intuitive appreciation of children, even neonates, as not being open to destruction on request. We may not in the end be able to support that intuition, for it may simply be a cultural prejudice; but I will now try to give a reasonable exegesis of its significance.

TWO CONCEPTS OF PERSON

I shall argue in this section that a confusion arises out of a false presupposition that we have only one concept of person: we have at least two concepts (probably many more) of person. I will restrict myself to examining the two that are most relevant here. First, there is the sense of person that we use in identifying moral agents: individual, living bearers of rights and duties. That sense singles out entities who can participate in the language of morals, who can make claims and have those claims respected: the strict sense we have examined above. We would, for example, understand "person" in this sense to be used properly if we found another group of self-conscious agents in the universe and called them persons even if they were not human, though it is a term that usually applies to normal adult humans. This sense of person I shall term the strict sense, one which is used in reference to self-conscious, rational agents. But what of the respect accorded to infants and other examples of non-self-conscious or not-yet-self-conscious human life? How are such entities to be understood?

A plausible analysis can, I believe, be given in terms of a second concept or use of person—a social concept or social role of person that is invoked when certain instances of human biological life are treated as if they were persons strictly, even though they are not. A good example is the mother-child or parent-child relationship in which the infant is treated as a person even though it is not one strictly. That is, the infant is treated as if it had the wants and desires of a person—its cries are treated as a call for food, attention, care, etc., and the infant is socialized, placed within a social structure, the family, and becomes a child. The shift is from merely biological to social significance. The shift is made on the basis that the infant is a human and is able to engage in a minimum of social interaction. With regard to the latter point, severely anencephalic infants may not qualify for the role *person* just as brain-dead adults would fail to qualify; both lack the ability to engage in minimal social interaction.[18] This use of person is, after all, one employed with instances of human biological life that are enmeshed in social roles as if they were persons. Further, one finds a difference between the biological mother-fetus relation and the social mother-child relation. The first relation can continue whether or not there is social recognition of the fetus, the second cannot. The mother-child relation is essentially a social practice.[19]

This practice can be justified as a means of preserving trust in families, of nurturing important virtues of care and solicitude towards the weak, and of assuring the healthy development of children. Further, it has a special value because it is difficult to determine specifically when in human ontogeny persons strictly emerge. Socializing infants into the role *person* draws the line conservatively. Humans do not become persons strictly until some time after birth. Moreover, there is a considerable value in protecting anything that looks and acts in a reasonably human fashion, especially when it falls within an established human social role as infants do within the role *child*. This ascription of the role *person* constitutes a social practice that allows the rights of a person to be imputed to forms of human life that can engage in at least a minimum of social interaction. The interest is in guarding anything that could reasonably play the role *person* and thus to strengthen the social position of persons generally.

The social sense of person appears as well to

structure the treatment of the senile, the mentally retarded, and the otherwise severely mentally infirm. Though they are not moral agents, persons strictly, they are treated as if they were persons. The social sense of person identifies their place in a social relationship with persons strictly. It is, in short, a practice that gives to instances of human biological life the status of persons. Unlike persons strictly, who are bearers of both rights and duties, persons in the social sense have rights but no duties. That is, they are not morally responsible agents, but are treated with respect (i.e., rights are imputed to them) in order to establish a practice of considerable utility to moral agents: a society where kind treatment of the infirm and weak is an established practice. The central element of the utility of this practice lies in the fact that it is often difficult to tell when an individual is a person strictly (i.e., how senile need one be in order no longer to be able to be a person strictly), and persons strictly might need to fear concerning their treatment (as well as the inadvertent mistreatment of other persons strictly) were such a practice not established. The social sense of person is a way of treating certain instances of human life in order to secure the life of persons strictly.

To recapitulate, we value children and our feelings of care for them, and we seek ways to make these commitments perdure. That is, social roles are ways in which we give an enduring fabric to our often inconstant passions. This is not to say that the social role person is merely a convention. To the contrary, it represents a fabric of ways of nurturing the high value we place on human life, especially the life that will come to be persons such as we. That fabric constitutes a practice of giving great value to instances of human biological life that can in some measure act as if they were persons, so that (1) the dignity of persons strictly is guarded against erosion during the various vicissitudes of health and disease, (2) virtues of care and attention to the dependent are nurtured, and (3) important social goals such as the successful rearing of children (and care of the aged) succeed. In the case of infants, one can add in passing a special consideration (4) that with luck they will become persons strictly, and that actions taken against infants could injure the persons they will eventually become.[20]

It should be stressed that the social sense of person is primarily a utilitarian construct. A person in this sense is not a person strictly, and hence not an unqualified object of respect. Rather, one treats certain instances of human life as persons for the good of those individuals who are persons strictly. As a consequence, exactly where one draws the line between persons in the social sense and merely human biological life is not crucial as long as the integrity of persons strictly is preserved. Thus there is a somewhat arbitrary quality about the distinction between fetuses and infants. One draws a line where the practice of treating human life as human personal life is practical and useful. Birth, including the production of a viable fetus through an abortion procedure, provides a somewhat natural line at which to begin to treat human biological life as human personal life. One might retort, Why not include fetuses as persons in a social sense? The answer is, Only if there are good reasons to do so in terms of utility. One would have to measure the utility of abortions for the convenience of women and families, for the prevention of the birth of infants with serious genetic diseases, and for the control of population growth against whatever increased goods would come from treating fetuses as persons. In addition, there would have to be consideration of the woman's right to choose freely concerning her body, and this would weigh heavily against any purely utilitarian considerations for restricting abortions. Early abortions would probably have to be allowed in any case in order to give respect due to the woman as a moral agent. But if these considerations are met, the exact point at which the line is drawn between a fetus and an infant is arbitrary in that utility considerations rarely produce absolute lines of demarcation. The best that one can say is that treating infants as persons in a social sense supports many central human values that abortion does not undermine, and that allowing at least early abortions acknowledges a woman's freedom to determine whether or not she wishes to be a mother.

One is thus left with at least two concepts of person. On the one hand, persons strictly can and usually do identify themselves as such—they are self-conscious, rational agents, respect for whom is part of valuing freedom, assigning blame and praise, and understanding obligation. That is, one's duty to respect persons strictly is the core of morality itself. The social concept of person is, on the other hand, more mediate, it turns on central values but is not the same as respect for the dignity of persons strictly. It allows us to value highly certain but not all instances of human biological life, without confusing that value with the dignity of persons strictly. That is, we can maintain the distinction between human biological and human personal life. We must recognize, though, that some human biological life is treated as human personal life even though it does not involve the existence of a person in the strict sense.

CONCLUSIONS

I wish to conclude now with a number of reflections reviewing the implications of distinguishing between human biological and human personal life, and between social and strict senses of person. First, it would seem that one can appreciate the general value of human biological life as just that. Human sperm, human ova, human cell cultures, human zygotes, embryos, and fetuses can have value, but they lack the dignity of persons. They are thus, all else being equal, open to socially justifiable experimentation in a way persons in either the strict or social sense should never be. That is, they can be used as means merely.

With infants, one finds human biological life already playing the social role of person. An element of this is the propriety of parents' controlling the destiny of their very young children insofar as this does not undermine the role *child*. That is, parents are given broad powers of control over their children as long as they do not abuse them, because very young children do in fact live in and through their families. Very young children are more in the possession of their families than in their own possession—they are not self-possessed, they are not yet moral agents. They do not yet belong to themselves. In fact, though persons strictly have both rights and duties, persons in the social sense are given moral rights but have no duties. Moreover, others must act in their behalf, since they are not self-determining entities. And when they act in their behalf, they need not do so in a manner that respects them as moral agents (i.e., there is no moral autonomy to respect), but in terms of what in general would be their best interests. Further, the duty to pursue those best interests can be defeated.

At least some puzzles about parental choice with regard to the treatment of their deformed infants or experimentation on their very young children can be resolved in these terms. Parents become the obvious ones to decide concerning the treatment of their very young children as long as that choice does not erode the care of children generally, or injure the persons

strictly those children will become. And parents can properly refuse life-prolonging treatment for their deformed infants if such treatment would entail a substantial investment of their economic and psychological resources. They can be morally justified if they calculate expenses against the expected life-style of the child if treated, and the probability of success. Such a utility calculus is justified (i.e., it is in accord with general social interests in preserving the role child) insofar as it involves a sufficiently serious acknowledgment of the value of the role child (i.e., as long as such choices are not capricious and there is a substantial hardship involved so that such investment is "not worth it")[21] in order to maintain the practice of the social sense of person. Further, one can justify social intervention in the form of legal injunctions to treat where such calculations by the parents are not convincing.

As to using very young children in experiments, they can be used in a fashion that adults may not, since they are not persons strictly. By that I mean someone can consent on their behalf when the risk is minimal, the value pursued substantial, when such experiments cannot in fact be performed on adults, and when such treatment does not erode the use of the social sense of person. One might picture here the trial of rubella vaccine on children that was not intended to be of direct benefit to those children, especially those who would grow to be misanthropic bachelors and thus never want to protect fetuses from damage. Nor need one presume anything except that most small children who are vaccinated have in some fashion been coerced or coopted into being vaccinated.

Consequently, with very young children one need not respect caprice in order to maintain the social sense of person. With free agents that is a different matter. Part of the freedom of self-determination is the latitude to act with caprice. For example, adults should be able, all else being equal, to refuse life-prolonging treatment; very young children should not. Surely difficult issues arise with older children and adolescents.[22] But the problems of dealing with free choice on the part of older children and adolescents attest to the validity of the rule rather than defeating it. With adults one is primarily concerned with the dignity of free agents, and what is problematic with respect to adolescents is that they are very much free agents.[23] In contrast, with small children one is concerned with their value (and the value of the social sense of person) and with not damaging the persons the children will become. In intermediate cases (i.e., older children) one must respect what freedom and self-possession does exist.

In summary, fetuses appear in no sense to be persons, children appear in some sense to be persons, normal adult humans show themselves to be persons. Is anything lost by these distinctions? I would argue not and that only clarity is gained. For those who hold some variety of homunculus theory of potentiality, it may appear that something is lost, for example, by saying that infants are not persons strictly. But how they could be such is, on the view I have advanced, at best a mystery. In this respect I would like to add a caveat lest in some fashion my distinction between persons strictly and persons socially be taken to imply that those humans who are only (!) persons socially are somehow set in jeopardy. It is one thing to say that an entity lacks the dignity of being a person strictly, and another thing to say that it does not have great value. For example, the argument with regard to the social role *child* has been that a child is a person socially because it does indeed have great value and because the social sense of person has general value. Children receive the social sense of person because we value children, and moreover because the social sense of person has a general utility in protecting persons strictly. In short, there is no universal way of speaking of the sanctity of life; some life (personal life) has dignity, all life can have value, and human biological life that plays the social role person has a special value and is treated as human personal life.

What I have offered is, in short, an examination of the ways in which the biomedical sciences have caused the concept of person to be reexamined, and some of the conclusions of these examinations. These analyses lead us to speak not only of human biological versus human personal life, of strict versus social concepts of person, but to distinguish, with regard to the sanctity of life, the value of biological life, the dignity of strictly personal life, and the care due to human biological life that can assume the social role of a person.

NOTES

1. *Black's Law Dictionary*, 4th ed., rev., s.v. "death."

2. For the first such statutory definition of death see: "Definition of Death," Kan. Stat. Ann., secs. 77–202 (1970).

3. Willard Gaylin, "Harvesting the Dead," *Harper's Magazine*, 249 (September, 1974), 23–30.

4. *Ibid.*, p. 28.

5. *Ibid.*

6. Immanuel Kant, *Fundamental Principles of the Metaphysics of Morals*, in *Kant's Critique of Practical Reason and Other Works on the Theory of Ethics*, trans. Thomas K. Abbott, 6th ed. (1873; rpt. London: Longmans, Green and Co., 1909), p. 46; *Kants gesammelte Schriften*, 23 vols., Preussische Akademie der Wissenschaften, eds. (Berlin: Walter de Gruyter, 1902–1956), IV, 428.

7. *Ibid.*

8. Immanuel Kant, *The Metaphysical Principles of Virtue: Part II of The Metaphysics of Morals*, trans. James Ellington (New York: Bobbs-Merrill, 1964), p. 23; Akademie Textausgabe, VI, 223.

9. *Black's Law Dictionary*, 4th Ed., rev., s.v. "person."

10. Strictly, the present brain-oriented definition of death distinguishes between a vegetative level of biological life and all higher levels. Report of the Ad Hoc Committee of the Harvard Medical School to Examine the Definition of Brain Death, "A Definition of Irreversible Coma," *Journal of the American Medical Association*, 205 (August 5, 1968), 85–88; Report of the Ad Hoc Committee of the American Electroencephalographic Society on EEG Criteria for Determination of Cerebral Death, "Cerebral Death and the Electroencephalogram," *Journal of the American Medical Association*, 209 (September 8, 1969), 1505–10. The point of this definition (at least in part) is to be conservative, not to make the mistake of prematurely pronouncing someone dead. On that ground, it is better to draw the line between vegetative life and sentient life, rather than between sentient life and self-conscious life. Moreover, non-self-conscious human life can, as will be argued, be treated as a person in other than a strict sense of that concept.

11. I have treated these issues more fully elsewhere. H. Tristram Engelhardt, Jr., "The Ontology of Abortion," *Ethics*, 84 (April, 1974), 217–34.

12. If one held that zygotes were persons (i.e., that persons begin at conception), one would have to account for how persons can split into two (i.e., monozygous twins), and for the fact that perhaps half of all persons die *in utero*. That is, there is evidence to indicate that perhaps up to 50 percent of all zygotes never implant. Arthur T. Hertig, "Human Trophoblast: Normal and Abnormal," *American Journal of Clinical Pathology*, 47 (March, 1967), 249–68.

13. That is, even if such practices might involve some disvalue, it would surely not be that of taking the life of a person. Also, one must recognize that if intrauterine contraceptive devices act by preventing the implantation of the zygote, they would count as a form of abortion.

14. Both Aristotle and St. Thomas held that human persons developed at some point after conception. See Aristotle, *Historia Animalium*, Book II, Chapter 3, 583 b, and St. Thomas Aquinas, *Summa Theologica*, Part 1, Q 118, art. 2, reply to obj. 2. See also St. Thomas Aquinas, *Opera Omnia*, XXVI (Paris: Vives, 1875), in *Aristoteles Stagiritae: Politicorum seu de Rebus Civilibus*, Book II, Lectio XII, p. 484, and *Opera Omnia*, XI, *Commentum in Quartum Librum Sententiarium Magistri Petri Lombardi*, Distinctio XXXI, Expositio Textus, p. 127.

15. Michael Tooley, "A Defense of Abortion and Infanticide," in *The Problem of Abortion*, ed. Joel Feinberg (Belmont, Calif.: Wadsworth Publishing Company, 1973), pp. 51–91.

16. One might think that a counterexample exists in the case of sleeping persons. That is, a person while asleep is not self-conscious and rational, and would seem in the absence of a doctrine

of potentiality not to be a person and to be therefore open to being used by others. A sleeping person is, though, a person in three senses in which a fetus or infant is not. First, in speaking of the sleeping person, one can know of whom one speaks in the sense of having previously known him before sleep. One therefore can know whose rights would be violated should that "person" be killed while asleep. His right to his life would *in part* be analogous to a dead man's right to have a promise kept that had been made to him when he was a self-conscious living person. In contrast, the fetus is not yet a person, an entity to whom, for example, promises can be made in anything but a metaphorical sense. Second, the sleeping man has a concrete presence in the world that is uniquely his, a fully intact functioning brain. Though asleep, the fully developed physical presence of the person continues. Third, the gap of sleep will be woven together by the life of the person involved: he goes to sleep expecting to awake and awakes to bring those past expectations into his present life. In short, one is not dealing with the potentiality of something to become a person, but with the potentiality of a person to resume his life after sleep.

17. See, for example, John M. Freeman, "To Treat or Not to Treat," *Practical Management of Meningomyelocele,* ed. John Freeman (Baltimore: University Park Press, 1974), pp. 13–22, and John Lorber, "Selective Treatment of Myelomeningocele: To Treat or Not to Treat," *Pediatrics,* 53 (March 1974), 307–8. Arguments such as Professor Tooley's imply that one may fairly freely employ positive or negative euthanasia in such cases, in that infants are not yet persons. Tooley, "A Defense of Abortion and Infanticide," p. 91.

18. It is important to note that severely anencephalic infants and brain-dead adults fail to be persons in a social sense because they lack the ability for social interaction, not because they lack the potentiality to become persons. Markedly senile individuals can thus be persons socially long after they are no longer persons strictly.

19. H. Tristram Engelhardt, Jr., "The Ontology of Abortion," pp. 230–32.

20. That is, once one is committed to refraining from killing infants because of a general interest in the value of the role *child,* one is committed to caring for infants so as not to injure the persons (strict) who will develop out of those infants. If one were to treat infants poorly, one would set into motion a chain of events that would injure the persons who would come to exist in the future (i.e., the persons such injured infants would become). But this presupposes that one has already decided on other grounds that infants should not be subject to infanticide. S. I. Benn fails to make this point; see "Abortion, Infanticide, and Respect for Persons," in *The Problem of Abortion,* p. 102.

21. It is not merely that it is difficult to impose a positive duty upon parents when that positive duty would involve great hardship, but that the actual object of that duty is not a person strictly.

22. See, for example, John E. Schowalter *et al.,* "The Adolescent Patient's Decision to Die," *Pediatrics,* 51 (January, 1973), 97–103; and Robert M. Veatch, ed., "Case Studies in Bioethics, Case No. 315," *Hastings Center Report,* 4 (September, 1974), 8–10.

23. The issue with adolescents is not that they are not persons, but that special claims to act paternalistically can be made in their regard by parents.

R O L A N D   P U C C E T T I

The Life of a Person

When one reflects on the life of a person, it becomes immediately apparent that this can be done in two very different ways. One way is to look upon the person as a particular organism with a spatiotemporal history of its own; there the identity question is approached from the outside, so to speak, and differs not at all from questions about the identity of material

Reprinted with permission of the author and the publisher. Copyright © 1982 D. Reidel Publishing Company. The complete version of this essay is available in the volume *Abortion and the Status of the Fetus,* edited by William B. Bondeson, H. Tristram Engelhardt, Jr., Stuart F. Spicker and Daniel Winship. This entire volume is essential reading on the philosophical and legal aspects of personhood and abortion.

objects through time. The other way is to look upon the person's life history as the total span of conscious experience that this person has had; here identity is approached from the inside, whether it be your own life you are reflecting on, or that of another person. It was Lucretius' contention, in Book III of *De Rerum Natura,* that since good or harm can accrue only to a subject of conscious experiences, the latter is the correct view and the former leads to superstition.

I am inclined to think Lucretius was right about this, that personal life is ineluctably shorter at both ends than the life of the organism which is the biological substrate of the person, because developmental processes at the beginning and degenerative processes at the end of organic life are insufficient to support conscious functions, and without these nothing done to the living tissue has personal value or disvalue. But to bring out the intuitive force of Lucretius' position, consider the following parable.

THE GENIE'S BARGAIN

Suppose that one day a genie appears before you and convincingly displays magical powers. Now he tells you that he will, if you want, expand your brain so that you will have an IQ of 400. This means that whatever you are interested in achieving will come within easy grasp, whether it be leadership of state, heading a conglomerate, outpainting Picasso or getting a Nobel Prize in medicine. However, he explains, there is one hitch. If you want him to do this for you, you will at the moment of brain expansion cease forever to have conscious experience. No one will know this, for he will program your brain to make all the correct responses to questions, etc. Nevertheless the great future achiever will be an automaton and no more. Would you accept this offer?

I have tried this out on several groups of students and it is amazing how uniform the reaction has been. A few say they would accept the bargain, but upon probing it turns out they have in mind an altruistic act that might lead to discovering a cure for cancer or building world government. They, as well as the majority who refused, all agreed that accepting would be tantamount to personal annihilation, at least in this world, and that one could indeed doubt that wholly unconscious achieving automata with their bodies would still be *them*. But if this is correct, and given that the one and same living organism persists from conscious to permanently unconscious activity, it appears bodily continuity through time is not a sufficient condition of personal identity, whereas continuity of consciousness is, and that without even a capacity for conscious experience there is no person any more.

Let us now apply the same lesson to the other end of the life spectrum. Suppose the genie tells you that you are the reincarnation of Napoleon Bonaparte, whose life you happen to admire greatly. You protest that this cannot be, since you have no recollection of doing the things Napoleon did, or experiencing his triumphs and defeats. The genie replies that of course you do not, because as a young man Napoleon accepted his bargain and thus did all he is remembered for in the history books quite unconsciously. Just suppose you believed this, would you feel *proud* of Napoleon's deeds as if they had been yours? I think not, because without any sense of those deeds being included in your personal conscious history, they could just as well be the past deeds of anyone else around. Once again it is psychological continuity which underlies the strand of personal identity, and in its absence there is no clear notion of being one and the same person.

But if so, how vain it seems to extend personhood beyond the loss of a capacity for conscious experience, and equally so to thrust it back in time to a stage of organic life before that capacity existed. Yet, as we shall now see, this is exactly what many people tend to do.

POSSIBLE PERSONS

I begin with a notion Lucretius would certainly have found strange, namely that of *possible* persons. Here the reference is not to something so general as, say, persons who will live five generations from now, but to *specific* as yet unconceived humans. R. M. Hare,[1] for example, asks whether a life-saving operation for an abnormal child might not be denied so that the parents, facing the burden of caring for such an offspring, will not be discouraged from having normal, healthy children later on. He invites us to imagine "the next child in the queue," whom he christens "Andrew," and asks if a full, constructive and probably happy life for this possible person is not a better moral outcome than sustaining the abnormal child and risking Andrew's future nonexistence. Hare grants that since Andrew is only a possible person he cannot be *deprived* of life, but suggests that he can be harmed by *withholding* life from him. And Derek Parfit,[2] commenting on Hare's remarks, apparently concurs. He asks why, if it can be in a person's interest to have his life prolonged, it cannot be in his interest to have it started.

To this the Lucretian response would surely be that life cannot be *withheld* from a nonexistent subject any more than this nonexistent subject can be deprived of it. Similarly, a nonexistent subject cannot have his life *started* by anyone. To talk this way is to imagine there are ghostly persons somewhere just waiting to be given flesh and blood, but there are none. For suppose one agreed with Hare that it is unjust to withhold life from Andrew. In that case, how could one make restitution to him? Where would we go to find this possible person and give him, at last, the life he deserves? All one can do is imagine that the parents of the abnormal child, once it is gone, might conceive a healthy child two years down the road and, when it is born, baptize him "Andrew." It is only by retroactively predating this latter child's existence beyond the point of conception that we get the notion of him, quite illicitly, as a specific possible person awaiting conception. There are no such persons (except in the barren sense of a *logically* possible combination of genes occurring in the conceptus), and thus no harm can be done them.

POTENTIAL PERSONS

When I was writing on this topic many years ago,[3] I used the term *potential* persons to refer to human children, for reasons I shall make clear later. However, I now find the term has been preempted in the literature to refer to fetuses, and shall follow that usage here. Fetuses have an advantage over possible persons in that they exist; the question is whether they are really the sorts of entities that qualify as having a right to life (assuming there are such entities) by virtue of their potential for becoming human persons.

Michael Tooley[4] has argued strongly against the potentiality principle as follows. Most of us would agree that it is not morally wrong, or only slightly so, to destroy surplus newborn kittens. Now if a chemical were discovered that, when administered to newborn kittens, led to their developing into rational, language-using animals and hence candidate persons, would it become grossly immoral to continue destroying newborn kittens? If not, and if artificial vs. natural potentiality for becoming persons is not a morally relevant distinction, then naturally potential persons have no more right to life than such kittens would have.

What is it like to *be* a potential person, i.e., from the inside of that stage of life? None of us knows, not because we have forgotten what it is like, but because our conscious personal lives had not begun yet. I do not deny that is is possible a fetus has crude sensations of pressure, temperature, etc. But zygotes, morulae, blastocysts, embryos and even (in the technical sense) early "fetuses" do not have the neural complexes necessary to believably sustain a conscious and therefore, on Lucretius' criterion, a personal life. If not, no *person* begins his or her personal life before late term in the intrauterine environment, and only barely then. Terminating a human life before that stage is not, therefore, killing an innocent *person*. It is destruction of at most the organic blueprint of a future person.

For suppose we had the means, technically, of saving life and promoting normal development of a spontaneously aborted fetus at *any* stage whatever. Would the zygote have *more* of life ahead than a near neonate? Biologically, yes. Does that mean more personal value accrues to the saved zygote than to the premature baby? Surely not, for if they both lived a normal human life span and had equal enjoyment of it, it matters not at all that the zygote's organic life was saved seven or so months earlier; that was a time at which its personal life had not yet begun, and nothing in the events of those months adds to that future person's enjoyment of life. If so, can any event detract from it?

Many would say yes, for abortion constitutes an abrupt cancellation of the promise of a future personal life. My point is that cancellation of a promise is not cancellation of the thing promised. Take a young couple who have two healthy, happy children. It may be that at the time of the second pregnancy they gave serious thought to terminating it as inopportune but relented and now are glad they did, for he is a wonderful child who shows every sign of enjoying a long and prosperous life. The temptation is to say they are glad not only to have him as a son but glad they did not deprive him of his life. But on the Lucretian stance I am developing here, the latter source of self-contentment is confused. He did not exist as a *person* until shortly before his birth. Abortion of the fetus from which his personal life ensued would have prevented someone with his particular genetic throw of the dice from getting launched as a person but could not have ended a personal life, for this had not yet begun. Blueprints and miniature models are not edifices. What is more, all those early formative experiences in his personal life, comparable to the architect's dabbling with the original design to secure improvements as it actually takes shape, are indispensable ingredients in the individuation of the growing structure of a conscious human, and none of those could have taken place before extrauterine life, so the *particular person* he is would not have lost this actual life.

BEGINNING PERSONS

I will speak now of *beginning* persons, as a term to replace the pre-empted "potential persons" I used to designate human neonates and infants more than a decade ago. The reason I did this was that I then wanted to reserve "person" as co-extensive with *moral agent*. A moral agent, I said, is both moral subject and moral object, and while small human children are moral objects, as are other higher forms of animal life, by virtue of being able to suffer, they are not yet moral subjects but only potentially so. Adapting now to the terminological shift, I would say that potential persons, meaning fetuses before late term, are not even moral objects[5], whereas beginning persons are, and potential moral subjects as well.

But Tooley[4] has questioned even this. He holds that it is only when an organism becomes *self-conscious* and has a concept of itself as a continuing subject of experiences that it qualifies as a person with a right to life. Such a view, if correct, could be used to justify infanticide as well as feticide, on grounds that without linguistic abilities normally not developed before the second or third year of life, human infants do not have a self-concept. However, Tooley recognizes that it is possible a nonverbal concept of self emerges as early as a month after birth, pushing back the "cut-off point" between potential and actual personhood to the first few postnatal weeks; but then he worries that if there *is* such a nonverbal self-concept, all kinds of infrahuman species devoid of language functions might also qualify as persons whose right to life we humans routinely override.

Let us see what can be salvaged here. If it were true that without a verbal conceptual scheme no self-concept is possible, would this imply that beginning persons have no right to life (assuming, again, that any entity has this)? Consider, first, that there are some otherwise normal children who were raised in isolation by uncaring parents, cut off from human language, who if not rescued by age 10 or 12 are thereafter unable to learn language, even in an artificially enriched linguistic environment. Conversely, consider that some higher primate species who never develop symbolic language in natural conditions have been trained in similarly enriched environments to do so, using plastic cutouts, computer consoles, and American Sign Language. If what Tooley suggested were true, it follows that the isolated, otherwise normal human 12-year-old unable to learn to talk has no right to life, while the chimp who can sign "You take out cabbage and give me monkey chow" is a person with a right to life! Yet what morally relevant difference is there between the isolated child and the run-of-the-mill infant toddler? The fact that the former is

artificially speechless and the latter naturally so cannot serve to distinguish between them. And if not, the lack of a verbal self-concept in beginning persons cannot justify denying them whatever right to life anyone has.

ACTUAL PERSONS

Tooley's qualms about the person-status of languageless infrahuman species can now be addressed. The only solid evidence for a nonverbal self-concept comes from Gordon Gallup's[6] studies of self-recognition in a reflecting surface by higher apes, something lower apes such as monkeys cannot learn to do. Yet monkeys rely on recognition of *other* monkeys' faces to establish their place in the troop's dominance hierarchy. How can this be? After all, brain-damaged humans who lose the ability to recognize faces not only cannot identify their own but cannot recognize those of close friends or loved ones. Apparently it is because chimpanzees and other higher apes have a self-concept to begin with that they quickly learn to recognize their own faces and bodies in a mirror. Lacking this, lower apes such as the monkey can identify and react to other monkey faces appropriately but persist in seeing the reflected face and body as that of just another conspecific of similar age, sex and size. So if it were true that regarding oneself as a continuing subject of experiences is what qualifies an organism for personhood and the right to life, on present evidence only our closest phylogenetic relatives would make the grade.

But even this seems strained. According to many contemporary philosophers the kind of rude nonvocal but still verbal abilities demonstrated by chimpanzees after arduous human training, plus the evidence for a nonverbal self-concept already in place in such species, is a far cry from what *actual* persons like you and me are able to do. For example, H. Frankfurt[7] has influentially espoused the view that a necessary condition of being a person is the capacity for having what he calls "second-order volitions," i.e., the desire not to will what one wills and [to] will something else instead. And this clearly requires a rich verbal conceptual scheme, for how else is one going to think the equivalent of "I wish I were less ambitious" or "If only I could love her in return"? Beings that do not have this ability are simply characterized by Frankfurt as "wantons," and include nonhuman animal species, mental defectives, and the small children I called beginning persons.

More than a decade ago, I would have welcomed

Frankfurt's stipulation, because at that time I could not see how any entity could be a moral subject as well as a moral object, hence a moral agent and a full-blown person, without a complex verbal conceptual scheme. But since then I have come to distrust such maneuvers by philosophers, for the reason that they are dangerously exclusive. Who am I to say, for example, that someone with a lesion to Broca's area, a motor aphasic unable to think in propositional language anymore, is therefore a mere "wanton," a nonperson without a right to life? Except in the narrow legal sense that such a human may not sign a contract or witness a will because of linguistic incompetence subsequent to the brain damage, I might indeed prefer to regard such a human as a person with a language defect, no more and no less than that. And in that case I would have to conclude that moral agents are just a subclass of persons.

Then what is a person? I have come to share the skepticism of D. C. Dennett[8] over ever being able to give an exhaustive list of the necessary and sufficient conditions of being a person; as he says, it might turn out that the concept of a person is only a free-floating honorific that we all happily apply to ourselves, and to others as the spirit moves us, rather as those who are *chic* are all and only those who can get themselves considered *chic* by others who consider themselves *chic*. In any case it is not my task here to say exactly what a person is, but only to argue that a person is more than a living human organism[9]; it is a conscious entity that builds a personal life from agency and experience, and until and only for so long as it has a capacity for conscious experience does the notion of a right to life, if there is such a thing, take hold.

FORMER PERSONS

Probably there has been no time before this when philosophers have been more conscious of the brain dependence of the human mind. Yet and in spite of this, they sometimes talk of the brain as if it were a replaceable or substitutable organ a person has, on a par with the heart, a kidney, or the cornea of the eye. For example, John Perry[10] has suggested that some day it might be possible to make a duplicate "rejuvenated" brain exactly like the original except for having healthy arteries, etc., which could then be used to replace the latter when it starts to wear out. If the copy were exact enough, he argues, all the individuating psychological characteristics of the person, including the long-term memories he has, would persist, and exact similarity would, for all practical purposes, be

equivalent to one and the same person's surviving the operation. John Hick[11] has even extended this notion to the next world. He asks us to imagine that upon our earthly demise God will create a replica of each of us in a special Resurrection World, complete with an exactly similar brain containing the same memory traces, dispositions, etc., and holds that it would be unreasonable for these resurrectees not to regard themselves, and be regarded by others there, as continuants of the persons whose earthly pasts they recall as their own.

What such claims overlook is that for any future person to be me, any statement true of me now would have to be true of him as well, otherwise he is not me. Now it is true of me that I can really remember certain milestone events in my life, e.g., a delayed honeymoon on the island of Corfu. But the person with the duplicate of my brain came into existence as a subject of experiences only upon duplication, just as the replica of me in the Celestial City would come into existence upon my death, not before. But then neither the duplicatum nor the replicatum of me, given that the brain each has is what makes each a subject of experiences, could possibly have been a subject of experiences at the time of my honeymoon in Corfu, and so could not really remember the events there, but only seem to. If so, neither would be me and it would be vain for me to anticipate any experiences they are going to have as experiences I shall have. Duplication or replication of a brain cannot endow the resultant person with a retroactive personal history; not even God can change the past and tomorrow make true of it what was not true of it before. In sum, it is the spatiotemporal continuity of a particular living brain that is the anchor of personal identity through time.

If we have this straight, we may now ask when exactly does a person's life end and he or she become only a *former* person? At the beginning of this paper I suggested that on the Lucretian view personal life spans one's total conscious experience, and that this is necessarily shorter at both ends than the life of the organism supporting that conscious life. We have seen how this is probably so for the first several months of fetal development, but one might well wonder if it is true at the end of organic life in any more than a picayune sense. After all, if the organic basis for conscious life is the brain and if total brain infarction subsequent to, say, cardiac standstill or lung failure causes the death of masses of central neurons by oxygen deprivation within, normally, a matter of minutes, organic death of the brain follows very quickly upon loss of consciousness. It is true that electrical activity can persist in the spinal cord for hours, and some somatic cells may take up to two days to die, such as those composing cartilage in the knee, but these lingering signs of life are no obstacle to a medical finding that the person has died.

Such is indeed normally the sequence of events, but not always. Consider the following case reported by Ingvar *et al.*[12]

Case 8. The patient (Th. Sv.) was a female who had been born in 1936. In July 1960, at the age of 24, she suffered severe eclampsia during pregnancy, with serial epileptic attacks, followed by deep coma and transient respiratory and circulatory failure. In the acute phase, Babinski signs were present bilaterally and there was a transitory absence of pupillary, corneal and spinal reflexes. A left-sided carotid angiogram* showed a slow passage of contrast medium and signs of brain edema. An EEG taken during the acute stage did not reveal any electrical cerebral activity. The EEG remained isoelectric for the rest of the survival time (seventeen years). After the first three to four months the patient's state became stable, with complete absence of all higher functions.

Examination ten years after the initial anoxic episode showed the patient lying supine, motionless, and with closed eyes. Respiration was spontaneous, regular and slow with a tracheal cannula. The pulse was regular. The systolic blood pressure was 75–100 mm Hg. Severe flexion contractures had developed in all extremities. Stimulation with acoustic signals, touch or pain gave rise to primitive arousal reactions, including eye-opening, rhythmic movements of the extremities, chewing and swallowing, and withdrawal reflexes. The corneal reflex was present on the left side. . . . Pupillary reflexes were present and normal on both sides. On passive movements of the head, typical vestibulo-ocular reflexes were elicited. The spinal reflexes were symmetrical and hyperactive. Patellar clonus† was present bilaterally. Divergent strabismus‡ was found when the eyes were opened [by the examiner]. Measurement of the regional cerebral blood flow on the left side (ten years after the initial anoxic episode) showed a very low mean hemisphere flow of 9 ml/100 g/min. The distribution of the flow was also abnormal, high values being found over the brain stem. The patient's condition remained essentially un-

Ed. note: The angiogram measures blood circulation in the brain.

†*Ed. note:* Contraction and relaxation in rapid succession.

‡*Ed. note:* Lack of parallelism in the visual axes of the eyes, in this case walleye.

changed for seven more years and she died seventeen years after the anoxic episode after repeated periods of pulmonary edema.

Autopsy showed a highly atrophic brain weighing only 315 grams. The [cerebral] hemispheres were especially atrophied and they were in general transformed into thin-walled yellow-brown bags. The brain stem and cerebellum were sclerotic and shrunken. . . . Microscopically the cerebral cortex was almost totally destroyed. . . . (pp. 196–198).

This clinical picture, confirmed by the autopsy findings, goes by various titles in the literature: cerebral as opposed to whole brain death; neocortical death without brain stem death; and more recently and appropriately, as "the apallic syndrome," because the characteristic feature is selective destruction of the paleum, the cortical mantle of grey matter covering the cerebrum or telencephalon. As it happens, the neurons composing the paleum are the most vulnerable to oxygen deprivation during transient cardiac arrest or, as in the above case, asphyxiation. Whereas with whole brain death, therefore including the brain stem that mediates cardiopulmonary functions, the patient can be maintained on a respirator only up to a week in adults and two weeks in children before cardiac standstill, the apallic patient can breathe spontaneously and demonstrate cephalic reflexes, which are also brain stem mediated, for months and even years if fed intravenously and kept free of infection, thus allowing organic recovery after the top of the brain is gone.

I said "organic recovery" is possible with destruction of the cerebral cortex; but on the Lucretian model *personal* life thereupon comes to an end, for with the paleum gone the very capacity for conscious experience goes as well. That such was indeed the case with this patient is obvious from the time of stabilization a few months after the anoxic episode: how else can one explain the persistently flat EEG, the inability to move even the eyes voluntarily, the reduction of cerebral blood flow to less than 20% of normal, and the spastic flexions of extremities? Thus "the *patient*" was nonsentient and noncognitive for seventeen years, but the *person* was not, for she had died all that long ago, and what was left was a still breathing *former* person.

How can one be sure? Perhaps a homely analogy will help the medically uninitiated to understand this. Suppose we wanted to find out if anyone lives in an apparently abandoned house, on the top floor. But we dare not break into it to see, for legal and ethical reasons. So we stand outside, watching and listening. We can hear the furnace go on, but that could be due to an automatic thermostat. We also see the lights go on in the evening, but that could be the result of an automatic timer to thwart burglars. We dial the phone number and hear the instrument ringing, so the lines are still intact, but no one answers. We measure the heat flow from the furnace and find not enough is reaching that top floor to keep any occupants alive there in winter. Finally, we attach listening devices to the outer walls and videocameras to the windows, but absolutely no real activity is picked up. Surely at this juncture we would conclude it is pointless to go on fuelling the furnace and scrubbing the walls. Nobody is home upstairs.

Yet as things now stand, so long as the furnace goes on and the lights light up by themselves, we are supposed to be committed to heroic maintenance measures tying up scarce medical resources, even though there is *no one* being helped by these efforts. Lucretius would call this rank superstition and advise us to dispose of such former persons as reason dictates. After all, he would surely say, unconscious breathing and the beating of the heart have no intrinsic value to a departed person; you could do no more harm to *that* individual, now dead, than you could do by opening a grave and stabbing a corpse. And I think he would be right.

NOTES

1. R. M. Hare, "Survival of the Weakest," in S. Gorovitz, ed., *Moral Problems in Medicine* (Englewood Cliffs, N.J.: Prentice-Hall, 1976), pp. 364–369.

2. D. Parfit, "Rights, Interests, and Possible People," in S. Gorovitz, ed., *Moral Problems in Medicine* (Englewood Cliffs, N.J.: Prentice-Hall, 1976), pp. 369–375.

3. R. Puccetti, *Persons: A Study of Possible Moral Agents in the Universe* (London: Macmillan, 1968), Chap. 1.

4. M. Tooley, "Abortion and Infanticide," *Philosophy and Public Affairs,* 2 (1972), pp. 37–65.

5. However, Engelhardt, whose analysis is fully supported by my own, believes that there is sufficient evidence to indicate the aborted fetus feels pain (p. 334). If so, it would be a moral object and I am wrong to think otherwise. Yet being a moral object is obviously not a sufficient condition of being a person, as Tooley's example of surplus newborn kittens makes clear. The reason I hesitate to ascribe a "right to life" unreservedly even to human beings is that I cannot see how this follows from being a person. My concern is to argue against those who hold that, assuming persons do have a right to life, the early fetus has one because it is already a person. H. T. Engelhardt, Jr., "The Ontology of Abortion," *Ethics,* 84 (1974), 217–234.

6. G. Gallup, "Chimpanzees: Self-Recognition," *Science,* 167 (1970), pp. 86–87.

7. H. Frankfurt, "Freedom of the Will and the Concept of a Person," *Journal of Philosophy,* 68 (1971), pp. 5–20.

8. D. C. Dennett, "Conditions of Personhood," *Brainstorms* (Montgomery, Vermont: Bradford Books, 1978), Chap. 14.

9. I cannot exactly say what love is, but I would argue confidently nonetheless that it is more than sexual desire. For example, it includes caring about the desired person's happiness and state of mind.

10. J. Perry, *A Dialogue on Personal Identity and Immortality* (Indianapolis, Ind.: Hackett Publishing Company, 1978).

11. J. Hick, *Death and the Eternal Life* (London: Collins, 1976), Chap. 14.

12. D. H. Ingvar, *et al.,* "Survival after Severe Cerebral Anoxia with Destruction of the Cerebral Cortex: the Apallic Syndrome," in J. Korein, ed., *Brain Death: Interrelated Medical and Social Issues, Annals of the New York Academy of Sciences,* 315 (1978), pp. 184–214.

JOEL FEINBERG

The Problem of Personhood

HUMAN BEINGS AND PERSONS

The first step in coming to terms with the concept of a person is to disentangle it from a concept with which it is thoroughly intertwined in most of our minds, that of a human being. In an influential article, the young American social philosopher Mary Anne Warren has pointed out that the term "human" has two "distinct but not often distinguished senses."[1] In what she calls the "moral sense," a being is human provided that it is a "full-fledged member of the moral community," a being possessed (as Jefferson wrote of all "men"—did he mean men and women?) of inalienable rights to life, liberty, and the pursuit of happiness. For beings to be humans in this sense is precisely for them to be people, and the problem of the "humanity" of the fetus in this sense is that of determining whether the fetus is the sort of being—a person—who has such moral rights as the right to life. On the other hand, a being is human in what Warren calls the "genetic sense" provided he or she is a member of the species *Homo sapiens,* and *all* we mean in describing someone as a human in the genetic sense is that he or she belongs to that animal species. In this sense, when we say that Jones is a human being, we are making a statement of the same type as when we say that Fido is a dog (canine being). Any fetus conceived by human parents will of course be a human being in this sense, just as any fetus conceived by dogs will of course be canine in the analogous sense.

It is possible to hold, as no doubt many people do, that all human beings in the moral sense (persons) are human beings in the genetic sense (members of *Homo sapiens*) and *vice versa,* so that the two classes, while distinct in meaning, nevertheless coincide exactly in reality. In that case all genetically human beings, including fetuses from the moment of conception, have

From "Abortion," in Tom L. Regan, ed., *Matters of Life and Death* (New York: Random House, 1980), pp. 185–198, 201–202. Reprinted with permission of the publisher.

a right to life, the unjustified violation of which is homicide, and no beings who are genetically non-human are persons. But it is also possible to hold, as some philosophers do, that some genetically human beings (for example, zygotes and irreversibly comatose "human vegetables") are *not* human beings in the moral sense (persons), and/or that some persons (for example, God, angels, devils, higher animals, intelligent beings in outer space) are *not* members of *Homo sapiens*. Surely it is an open question to be settled, if at all, by argument or discovery, whether the two classes correspond exactly. It is not a question closed in advance by definition or appeals to word usage.

NORMATIVE *VERSUS* DESCRIPTIVE PERSONHOOD

Perhaps the best way to proceed from this point is to stick to the term "person" and avoid the term "human" except when we clearly intend the genetic sense, in that way avoiding the ever-present danger of being misunderstood. The term "person," however, is not without its own ambiguities. The one central ambiguity we should note is that between purely *normative* (moral or legal) uses of "person" and purely *descriptive* (conventional, commonsense) uses of the term.

When moralists or lawyers use the term "person" in a purely normative way they use it simply to ascribe moral or legal properties—usually rights or duties, or both—to the beings so denominated. To be a person in the normative sense is to have rights, or rights and duties, or at least to be the sort of being who could have rights and duties without conceptual absurdity. Most writers think that it would be sheer nonsense to speak of the rights or duties of rocks, or blades of grass, or sunbeams, or of historical events or abstract ideas. These objects are thought to be conceptually inappropriate subjects for the attribution of rights or duties. Hence we speak of them as "impersonal entities,'' the types of beings that are contrasted with objects that can stand in personal relationships to us, or make moral claims on us. The higher animals—our fellow mammalian species in particular—are borderline cases whose classification as persons or nonpersons has been a matter of controversy. Many of them are fit subjects of right-ascriptions but cannot plausibly be assigned duties or moral responsibilities. . . . In any case, when we attribute personhood in a purely normative way to any kind of being, we are attributing such moral qualities as rights or duties, but not (necessarily) any observable characteristics of any kind—for example, having flesh or blood, or belonging to a particular species. Lawyers have attributed (legal) personhood even to states and corporations, and their purely normative judgments say nothing about the presence or absence of body, mind, consciousness, color, etc.

In contrast to the purely normative use of the word ''person'' we can distinguish a purely empirical or descriptive use. There are certain characteristics that are fixed by a rather firm convention of our language such that the general term for any being who possesses them is ''person.'' Thus, to say of some being that he is a person, in this sense, is to convey some information about what the being is like. Neither are attributions of personhood of this kind essentially controversial. If to be a person *means* to have characteristics *a, b,* and *c,* then to say of a being who is known to have *a, b,* and *c* that he or she is a person (in the descriptive sense) is no more controversial than to say of an animal known to be a young dog that it is a puppy, or of a person known to be an unmarried man that he is a bachelor. What make these noncontroversial judgments true are conventions of language that determine what words mean. The conventions are often a bit vague around the edges but they apply clearly enough to central cases. It is in virtue of these reasonably precise linguistic conventions that the word ''person'' normally conveys the idea of a definite set of descriptive characteristics. I shall call the idea defined by these characteristics ''the commonsense concept of personhood.'' When we use the word ''person'' in this wholly descriptive way we are not attributing rights, duties, eligibility for rights and duties, or any other normative characteristics to the being so described. At most we are attributing characteristics that may be a *ground* for ascribing rights and duties.

These *purely* normative and *purely* descriptive uses of the word ''person'' are probably unusual. In most of its uses, the word both describes or classifies someone in a conventionally understood way *and* ascribes rights, etc., to him or her. But there is enough looseness or flexibility in usage to leave open the questions of whether the classes of moral and ''commonsense'' persons correspond in reality. Although some may think it obvious that all and only commonsense persons are moral persons, that identification of classes does not follow simply as a matter of word usage, and must, therefore, be supported independently by argument. Many learned writers, after all, have maintained that human zygotes and embryos are moral persons despite the fact that they are almost certainly not ''commonsense persons.'' Others have spoken of wicked murderers as ''monsters'' or ''fiends'' that can rightly be destroyed like ''wild beasts'' or eliminated like ''rotten apples.'' This seems to amount to holding that ''moral monsters'' are commonsense persons who are so wicked (only *persons* can be wicked) that they have lost their moral personhood, or membership in our moral community. The English jurist Sir William Blackstone (1723–1780) maintained that convicted murderers forfeit their rights to life. If one went further and maintained that moral monsters forfeit all their human rights, then one would be rejecting the view that the classes of moral and commonsense persons exactly coincide, for wicked persons who are answerable for their foul deeds must first of all be persons in the descriptive sense, but as beings without rights, they would not be moral persons.

THE CRITERION OF COMMONSENSE PERSONHOOD

A criterion of personhood in the descriptive sense would be a specification of those characteristics that are common and peculiar to commonsense persons and in virtue of which they are such persons. They are necessary conditions for commonsense personhood in the sense that no being who lacks any one of them can be a person. They are sufficient conditions in the sense that any being who possesses all of them is a person, whatever he or she may be like in other respects. How shall we formulate this criterion? If this question simply raises a matter of fixed linguistic convention, one might expect it to be easy enough to state the defining characteristics of personhood straight off. Surprisingly, the question is not quite that simple, and no mere dictionary is likely to give us a wholly satisfactory answer. What we must do is to think of the characteristics that come at least implicitly to mind when we hear or use such words as "person," "people," and the personal pronouns. We might best proceed by considering three different classes of cases: clear examples of beings whose personhood cannot be doubted, clear examples of beings whose nonpersonhood cannot be doubted, and actual or hypothetical examples of beings whose status is not initially clear. We probably will not be able to come up with a definitive list of characteristics if only because the word "person" may be somewhat loose, but we should be able to achieve a criterion that is precise enough to permit a definite classification of fetuses.

UNDOUBTED COMMONSENSE PERSONS

Who are undoubted persons? Consider first your parents, siblings, or friends. What is it about them that makes you so certain that they are persons? "Well, they look like persons," you might say; "They have human faces and bodies." But so do irreversibly comatose human vegetables, and we are, to put it mildly, not so certain that they are persons. "Well then, they are males and females and thus appropriately referred to by our personal pronouns, all of which have gender. We can't refer to any of them by use of the impersonal pronoun 'it,' because they have sex; so perhaps being gendered is the test of personhood." Such a reply has superficial plausibility, but is the idea of a "sexless person" logically contradictory? Perhaps any genetically human person will be predominately one sex or the other, but must the same be true of "intelligent beings in outer space," or spirits, gods, and devils?

Let's start again. "What makes me certain that my parents, siblings, and friends are people is that they give evidence of being conscious of the world and of themselves; they have inner emotional lives, just like me; they can understand things and reason about them, make plans, and act; they can communicate with me, argue, negotiate, express themselves, make agreements, honor commitments, and stand in relationships of mutual trust; they have tastes and values of their own; they can be frustrated or fulfilled, pleased or hurt." Now we clearly have the beginnings, at least, of a definitive list of person-making characteristics. In the commonsense way of thinking, persons are those beings who are conscious, have a concept and awareness of themselves, are capable of experiencing emotions, can reason and acquire understanding, can plan ahead, can act on their plans, and can feel pleasure and pain.

UNDOUBTED NONPERSONS

What of the objects that clearly are not persons? Rocks have none of the above characteristics; neither do flowers and trees; neither (presumably) do snails and earthworms. But perhaps we are wrong about that. Maybe rocks, plants, and lower animals are congeries of lower-level spirits with inner lives and experiences of their own, as primitive men and mystics have often maintained. Very well, that is possible. But if they do have these characteristics, contrary to all appearance, then it would seem natural to think of them as persons too, "contrary to all appearance." In raising the question of their possession of these characteristics at all, we seem to be raising by the same token the question of their commonsense personhood. Mere rocks are quite certainly not crowds of silent spirits, but if, contrary to fact, they are such spirits, then we must think of them as real people, quite peculiarly embodied.

HARD CASES

Now, what about the hard cases? Is God, as traditionally conceived, a kind of nonhuman—or better, superhuman—person? Theologians are divided about this, of course, but ordinary believers think of Him (note the personal pronoun) as conscious of self and world, capable of love and anger, eminently rational, having plans for the world, acting (if only through His creation), capable of communicating with humans, of issuing commands and making covenants, and of being pleased or disappointed in the use to which humans put their free will. To the extent that one believes that God has these various attributes, to that extent does one believe in a *personal* God. If one believes only in a God who is an unknown and unknowable First Cause of the world, or an obscure but powerful force sustaining the world, or the ultimate energy in the cosmos, then, it seems fair to say, one believes in an *impersonal* diety.

Now we come to the ultimate thought experiment. Suppose that you are a space explorer whose rocket ship has landed on a planet in a distant galaxy. The planet is inhabited by some very strange objects, so unlike anything you have previously encountered that at first you don't even know whether to classify them as animal, vegetable, mineral, or "none of the above.'' They are composed of a gelatinous sort of substance much like mucus except that it is held together by no visible membranes or skin, and it continually changes its shape from one sort of amorphous glob to another, sometimes breaking into smaller globs and then coming together again. The objects have no appendages, no joints, no heads or faces. They float mysteriously above the surface of the planet and move about in complex patterns while emitting eerie sounds resembling nothing so much as electronic music. The first thing you will wish to know about these strange objects is whether they are extraterrestrial *people* to be respected, greeted, and traded and negotiated with, or mere things or inferior animals to be chopped up, boiled, and used for food and clothing.

Almost certainly the first thing you would do is try to communicate with them by making approaches, gesturing by hand, voice, or radio signals. You might also study the patterns in their movements and sound emissions to see whether they have any of the characteristics of a language. If the beings respond even in a primitive way to early gestures, one might suspect at least that they are beings who are capable of perception and who can be *aware* of movements and sounds. If some sort of actual communication then follows, you can attribute to them at least the mentality of chimpanzees. If negotiations then follow and agreements are reached, then you can be sure that they are rational beings, and if you learn to interpret signs of worry, distress, anger, alarm, or friendliness, then you can be quite confident that they are indeed people, no matter how inhuman they are in biological respects.

A WORKING CRITERION OF COMMONSENSE PERSONHOOD

Suppose then that we agree that our rough list captures well the traits that are generally characteristic of commonsense persons. Suppose further (what is not quite as evident) that each trait on the list is necessary for commonsense personhood, that no one trait is by itself sufficient, but that the whole *collection* of traits is sufficient to confer commonsense personhood on any being that possesses it. Suppose, that is, that consciousness is necessary (no permanently unconscious being can be a person), but that it is not enough. The conscious being must also have a concept of a self and a certain amount of self-awareness. But although each of these last traits is necessary, they are still not enough even in conjunction, since a

self-aware, conscious being who was totally incapable of learning or reasoning would not be a person. Hence rationality is also necessary, though not by itself sufficient. And so on through our complete list of person-making characteristics, each one of which, let us suppose, is a necessary condition, and all of which are jointly a sufficient condition of being a person in the commonsense, descriptive sense of "person." Let us call our set of characteristics c. Now at last we can pose the most important and controversial question about the status of the fetus: What is the relation, if any, between having c and being a person in the normative (moral) sense, that is, a being who possesses, among other things, a right to life?

PROPOSED CRITERIA OF MORAL PERSONHOOD

It bears repeating at the outset of our discussion of this most important question that formulating criteria of personhood in the purely moral sense is not a scientific question to be settled by empirical evidence, not simply a question of word usage, not simply a matter to be settled by commonsense thought experiments. It is instead an essentially controversial question about the possession of moral rights that cannot be answered in these ways. That is not to say that rational methods of investigation and discussion are not available to us, but only that the methods of reasoning about morals do not often provide conclusive proofs and demonstrations. What rational methods can achieve for us, even if they fall short of producing universal agreement, is to list the various options open to us, and the strong and weak points of each of them. Every position has its embarrassments, that is, places where it appears to conflict logically with moral and commonsense convictions that even its proponents can be presumed to share. To point out these embarrassments for a given position is not necessarily to refute it but rather to measure the costs of holding it to the coherence of one's larger set of beliefs generally. Similarly, each position has its own peculiar advantages, respects in which it coheres uniquely well with deeply entrenched convictions that even its opponents might be expected to share. I shall try in the ensuing discussion to state and illustrate as vividly as I can the advantages and difficulties in all the major positions. Then I shall weigh the cases for and against the various alternatives. For those who disagree with my conclusion, the discussion will serve at least to locate the crucial issues in the controversy over the status of the fetus.

A proposed criterion for moral personhood is a statement of a characteristic (or set of characteristics) that its advocate deems both necessary and (jointly) sufficient for being a person in the moral sense. Such characteristics are not thought of as mere indexes, signs, or "litmus tests" of moral personhood, but as more basic traits that actually confer moral personhood on whoever possesses them. All and only those beings having these characteristics have basic moral rights, in particular the right to full and equal protection against homicide. Thus, fetuses must be thought of as having this right if they satisfy a proposed criterion of personhood. The main types of criteria of moral personhood proposed by philosophers can be grouped under one or another of five different headings, which we shall examine in turn. Four of the five proposed criteria refer to possession of c (the traits we have listed as conferring *commonsense* personhood). One of these four specifies actual possession of c; the other three refer to either actual or potential possession of c. The remaining criterion, which we shall consider briefly first, makes no mention of c at all.

THE SPECIES CRITERION

"All and only members of the biological species *Homo sapiens,* 'whoever is conceived by human beings,' are moral persons and thus are entitled to full and equal protection by the moral rule against homicide." The major advantage of this view (at least for some) is that it gives powerful support to those who would extend the protection of the rule against homicide to the fetus from the moment of conception. If this criterion is correct, it is not simply because of utilitarian reasons (such that it would usefully increase respect for life in the community) that we must not abort human zygotes and embryos, but rather because we owe it to these minute entities themselves not to kill them, for as members of the human species they are already possessed of a full right to life equal in strength to that of any adult person.

The species criterion soon encounters serious difficulties. Against the view that membership in the species *Homo sapiens* is a *necessary* condition of membership in the class of moral persons, we have the possibility of there being moral persons from other planets who belong to other biological species. Moreover, some human beings—in particular, those who are irreversibly comatose "vegetables"—are human beings but doubtfully qualify as moral persons, a fact that casts serious doubt on the view that membership in the species *Homo sapiens* is a *sufficient* condition of being a moral person. . . .

THE MODIFIED SPECIES CRITERION

"All and only members of species generally characterized by c, whether the species is *Homo sapiens* or another, and whether or not the particular individual in question happens to possess c, are moral persons entitled to full and equal protection by the moral rule against homicide." This modification is designed to take the sting out of the first objection (above) to the unmodified species criterion. If there are other species or categories of moral persons in the universe, it concedes, then they too have moral rights. Indeed, if there are such, then *all* of their members are moral persons possessed of such rights, even those individuals who happen themselves to lack c because they are not yet fully developed or because they have been irreparably damaged.

The major difficulty for the modified species criterion is that it requires further explanation why c should determine moral personhood when applied to *classes* of creatures rather than to individual cases. Why is a permanently unconscious but living body of a human or an extragalactic person (or for that matter, a chimpanzee, if we should decide that that species as a whole is characterized by c) a moral person when it lacks as an individual the characteristics that determine moral personhood? Just because opposable thumbs are a characteristic of *Homo sapiens,* it does not follow that this or that particular *Homo sapiens* has opposable thumbs. There appears to be no reason for regarding right-possession any differently, in this regard, from thumb-possession.

THE STRICT POTENTIALITY CRITERION

"All and only those creatures who either actually or potentially possess c (that is, who either have c now or would come to have c in the natural course of events) are moral persons now, fully protected by the rule against homicide." This criterion also permits one to draw the line of moral personhood in the human species right at the moment of conception, which will be counted by some as an advantage. It also has the undeniable advantage of immunity from one charge of arbitrariness since it will extend moral personhood to all beings in *any* species or category who possess $c,$ either actually or potentially. It may also cohere with our psychological attitudes, since it can explain why it is that many people, at least, think of unformed or unpretty fetuses as precious. Zygotes and embryos in particular are treasured not for what they are but for what they are biologically "programmed" to become in the fullness of time: real people fully possessed of c.

The difficulties of this criterion are of two general kinds, those deriving from the obscurity of the concept of "potentiality," which perhaps can be overcome, and the more serious difficulties of answering the charge that merely potential possession of any set of qualifications for a moral status does not logically ensure actual possession of that status. Consider just one of the problems raised by the concept of potentiality itself.[2] How, it might be asked, can a mere zygote be a potential person, whereas a mere spermatozoon or a mere unfertilized ovum is not? If the spermatozoon and ovum we are talking about are precisely those that will combine in a few seconds to form a human zygote, why are they not potential zygotes, and thus potential people, *now*? The defender of the potentiality criterion will reply that it is only at the moment of conception that any being comes into existence with exactly the same chromosomal makeup as the human being that will later emerge from the womb, and it is *that* chromosomal combination that forms the potential person, not anything that exists before it comes together. The reply is probably a cogent one, but uncertainties about the concept of potentiality might make us hesitate, at first, to accept it, for we might be tempted to think of both the germ cell (spermatozoon or ovum) and the zygote as potentially a particular person, while holding that the differences between their potentials, though large and significant to be sure, are nevertheless differences in degree rather than kind. It would be well to resist that temptation, however, for it could lead us to the view that some of the entities and processes that combined still earlier to form a given spermatozoon were themselves potentially that spermatozoon and hence potentially the person that spermatozoon eventually became, and so on. At the end of that road is the proposition that everything is potentially everything else, and thus the destruction of all utility in the concept of potentiality. It is better to hold this particular line at the zygote.

The remaining difficulty for the strict potentiality criterion is much more serious. It is a logical error, some have charged, to deduce *actual* rights from merely *potential* (but not yet actual) qualification for

those rights. What follows from potential qualification, it is said, is potential, not actual, rights; what entails actual rights is actual, not potential, qualification. As the Australian philosopher Stanley Benn puts it, "A potential president of the United States is not on that account Commander-in-Chief [of the U.S. Army and Navy]."[3] This simple point can be called "the logical point about potentiality." Taken on its own terms, I don't see how it can be answered as an objection to the strict potentiality criterion. It is is still open to an antiabortionist to argue that merely potential commonsense personhood is a ground for *duties* we may have toward the potential person. But he cannot argue that it is the ground for the potential person's *rights* without committing a logical error.

THE MODIFIED OR GRADUALIST POTENTIALITY CRITERION

"Potential possession of c confers not a right, but only a claim, to life, but that claim keeps growing stronger, requiring ever stronger reasons to override it, until the point when c is actually possessed, by which time it has become a full right to life." This modification of the potentiality criterion has one distinct and important advantage. It coheres with the widely shared feeling that the moral seriousness of abortion increases with the age of the fetus. It is extremely difficult to believe on other than very specific theological grounds that a zygote one day after conception is the sort of being that can have any rights at all, much less the whole armory of "human rights" including "the right to life." But it is equally difficult for a great many people to believe that a full-term fetus one day before birth does not have a right to life. Moreover, it is very difficult to find one point in the continuous development of the fetus before which it is utterly without rights and after which it has exactly the same rights as any adult human being. Some rights in postnatal human life can be acquired instantly or suddenly; the rights of citizenship, for example, come into existence at a precise moment in the naturalization proceedings after an oath has been administered and a judicial pronouncement formally produced and certified. Similarly, the rights of husbands and wives come into existence at just that moment when an authorized person utters the words "I hereby pronounce you husband and wife." But the rights of the fetus cannot possibly jump in this fashion from nonbeing to being at some precise moment in pregnancy. The alternative is to think of them as growing steadily and gradually throughout the entire nine-month period until they are virtually "mature" at parturition. There is, in short, a kind of growth in "moral weight" that proceeds in parallel fashion with the physical growth and development of the fetus.

• • •

The modified potentiality criterion has the attractiveness characteristic of compromise theories when fierce ideological quarrels rage between partisans of more extreme views. It shares one fatal flaw, however, with the strict potentiality criterion: Despite its greater flexibility, it cannot evade "the logical point about potentiality." A highly developed fetus is much closer to being a commonsense person with all the developed traits that qualify it for moral personhood than is the mere zygote. But being almost qualified for rights is not the same thing as being partially qualified for rights; nor is it the same thing as being qualified for partial rights, quasi-rights, or weak rights. The advanced fetus is closer to being a person than is the zygote, just as a dog is closer to personhood than a jellyfish, but that is not the same thing as being "more of a person." In 1930, when he was six years old, Jimmy Carter didn't know it, but he was a potential president of the United States. That gave him no claim *then,* not even a very weak claim, to give commands to the U.S. Army and Navy. Franklin D. Roosevelt in 1930 was only two years away from the presidency, so he was a potential president in a much stronger way (the potentiality was much less remote) than was young Jimmy. Nevertheless, he was not actually president, and he had no more of a claim to the prerogatives of the office than did Carter. The analogy to fetuses in different stages of development is of course imperfect. But in both cases it would seem to be invalid to infer the existence of a "weak version of a right" from an "almost qualification" for the full right. In summary, the modified potentiality criterion, insofar as it permits the potential possession of c to be a *sufficient condition* for the actual possession of claims, and in some cases of rights, is seriously flawed in the same manner as the strict potentiality criterion.

THE ACTUAL-POSSESSION CRITERION

"At any given time t, all and only those creatures who actually possess c are moral persons at t, what-

ever species or category they may happen to belong to." This simple and straightforward criterion has a number of conspicuous advantages. We should consider it with respect even before examination of its difficulties if only because the difficulties of its major rivals are so severe. Moreover, it has a certain tidy symmetry about it, since it makes the overlap between commonsense personhood and moral personhood complete—a total correspondence with no loose ends left over in either direction. There can be no actual commonsense persons who are not actual moral persons, nor can there be any actual moral persons who are not actual commonsense persons. Moral personhood is not established simply by species membership, associations, or potentialities. Instead, it is conferred by the same characteristics (c) that lead us to recognize personhood wherever we find it. It is no accident, no mere coincidence, that we use the moral term "person" for those beings, and only those beings, who have c. The characteristics that confer commonsense personhood are not arbitrary bases for rights and duties, such as race, sex, or species membership; rather they are the traits that make sense out of rights and duties and without which those moral attributes would have no point or function. It is because people are conscious; have a sense of their personal identities; have plans, goals, and projects; experience emotions; are liable to pains, anxieties, and frustrations; can reason and bargain, and so on—it is because of these attributes that people have values and interests, desires and expectations of their own, including a stake in their own futures, and a personal well-being of a sort we cannot ascribe to unconscious or nonrational beings. Because of their developed capacities they can assume duties and responsibilities and can have and make claims on one another. Only because of their sense of self, their life plans, their value hierarchies, and their stakes in their own futures, can they be ascribed fundamental rights. There is nothing arbitrary about these linkages.

Despite these impressive advantages, the actual-possession criterion must face a serious difficulty, namely that it implies that small infants (neonates) are not moral persons. There is very little more reason, after all, to attribute c to neonates than to advanced fetuses still *in utero.* Perhaps during the first few days after birth the infant is conscious and able to feel pain, but it is unlikely that it has a concept of its self or of its future life, that it has plans and goals, that it can think consecutively, and the like. In fact, the whole complex of traits that make up c is not *obviously* present until the second year of childhood. And that would seem to imply, according to the criterion we are considering, that the deliberate destruction of babies in their first year is no violation of their rights. And *that* might seem to entail that there is nothing wrong with infanticide (the deliberate killing of infants). But infanticide *is* wrong. Therefore, critics of the actual-possession criterion have argued that we ought to reject this criterion.

. . .

SUMMARY AND CONCLUSION

Killing human beings (homicide) is forbidden both by our criminal law and by the moral rules that are accepted in all civilized communities. If the fetus at any point in its development is a human being, then to kill it at that point is homicide, and if done without excuse or mitigation, murder. But the term "human being" is subtly ambiguous. The fetus at all stages is obviously human in the genetic sense, but that is not the sense of the term intended in the moral rule against homicide. For a genetically human entity to have a right to life it must be a human being in the sense of a person. But the term "person" is also ambiguous. In the commonsense descriptive meaning of the term, it refers to any being of any species or category who has certain familiar characteristics, of which consciousness of the world, self-concepts, and the capacity to plan ahead are prominent. In the purely normative (moral or legal) sense, a person is any being who has certain rights and/or duties, whatever his other characteristics. Whether or not abortion is homicide depends on what the correct criterion of moral personhood is.

We considered five leading formulations of the criterion of moral personhood and found that they are all subject to various embarrassments. One formulation in terms of species membership seemed both too broad and too narrow, and in the end dependent on an arbitrary preference for our own species. A more careful formulation escaped the charge of being too restrictive and the charge of arbitrariness but suffered from making the status of an individual derive from his membership in a group rather than from his own intrinsic characteristics. The two formulations in terms of potential possession of the characteristics definitive of commonsense personhood both stumbled on "the logical point about potentiality," that potential qualification for a right does not entail actual possession of that right. The modified or gradualist formulation of the potentiality criterion, however, does

have some attractive features, and could be reformulated as a more plausible answer to another question, that about the moral permissibility of abortion. Even if the fetus is not a person and lacks a right to life, ever stronger reasons might be required to justify aborting it as it grows older and more similar to a person.

The weaknesses of the first four proposed criteria of moral personhood create a strong presumption in favor of the remaining one, the "actual-possession" criterion. It is clear that fetuses are not "people" in the ordinary commonsense meaning of that term, hence according to our final criterion they are not moral persons either, since this criterion of moral personhood simply adopts the criteria of commonsense personhood. The very grave difficulty of this criterion is that it entails that infants are not people either, during the first few months or more of their lives. That is a genuine difficulty for the theory, but a far greater embarrassment can be avoided. Because there are powerful reasons against infanticide that apply even if the infant is not a moral person, the actual-possession criterion is not subject to the devastating objection that it would morally or legally justify infanticide on demand.

NOTES

1. Mary Anne Warren, "On the Moral and Legal Status of Abortion," *The Monist* 57 (1973), pp. 43–61. Reprinted in J. Feinberg and H. Gross (eds.), *Liberty: Selected Readings,* pp. 133–143. The quotation is from the latter source, p. 138.

2. These problems are discussed in more detail in Joel Feinberg, "The Rights of Animals and Future Generations" (Appendix: The Paradoxes of Potentiality), in W. T. Blackstone (ed.), *Philosophy and Environmental Crisis* (Athens, Ga.: University of Georgia Press, 1974), pp. 67–68.

3. Stanley I. Benn, "Abortion, Infanticide, and Respect for Persons," in J. Feinberg (ed.), *The Problem of Abortion* (Belmont, Cal.: Wadsworth Publishing Co., 1973), p. 102.

SUGGESTED READINGS FOR CHAPTER 3

Atkinson, Gary M. "Persons in the Whole Sense." *American Journal of Jurisprudence* 22 (1977), 86–117.

Ayer, A. J. *The Concept of a Person.* London: Macmillan, 1963. Chap. 4.

Becker, Lawrence C. "Human Being: The Boundaries of the Concept." *Philosophy and Public Affairs* 4 (Summer 1975), 334–358.

Bok, Sissela. "Who Shall Count as a Human Being? A Treacherous Question in the Abortion Discussion." In Perkins, Robert L., ed. *Abortion: Pro and Con.* Cambridge, Mass.: Schenkman, 1974, pp. 91–105.

Danto, Arthur C. "Persons." In Taylor, Paul, ed. *Encyclopedia of Philosophy*. New York: Free Press, 1967. Vol. 4, pp. 110–114.

Dennett, Daniel C. *Brainstorms: Philosophical Essays on Mind and Psychology*. Montgomery, Vt.: Bradford Books, 1978. Chap. 14.

Engelhardt, H. Tristram. "The Ontology of Abortion." *Ethics* 84 (April 1974), 217–234.

Fletcher, Joseph. "Four Indicators of Humanhood—The Enquiry Matures." *Hastings Center Report* 4 (December 1974), 4–7.

Frankfurt, Harry G. "Freedom of the Will and the Concept of a Person." *Journal of Philosophy* 68 (January 14, 1971), 5–20.

Margolis, Joseph. *Persons and Minds: The Prospects of Nonreductive Materialism*. Boston: D. Reidel, 1978.

Newton, Lisa. "Humans and Persons: A Reply to Tristram Engelhardt." *Ethics* 85 (July 1975), 332–336.

Puccetti, Roland. *Persons: A Study of Possible Moral Agents in the Universe*. London: Macmillan, 1968. New York: Herder and Herder, 1969.

Rorty, Amélie O. "Persons, Policies, and Bodies," *International Philosophical Quarterly* 13 (March 1973), 63–80.

Sellars, Wilfrid. "Metaphysics and the Concept of Person." In

Lambert, K., ed. *The Logical Way of Doing Things*. New Haven: Yale University Press, 1969.

Shaffer, Jerome A. *Philosophy of Mind*. Englewood Cliffs, N.J.: Prentice-Hall, 1968.

Strawson, P. F. *Individuals: An Essay in Descriptive Metaphysics*. London: Methuen and Company, 1959.

Weiss, Roslyn. "The Perils of Personhood." *Ethics* 89 (October 1978), 66–75.

BIBLIOGRAPHIES

Goldstein, Doris Mueller. *Bioethics: A Guide to Information Sources*. Detroit: Gale Research Company, 1982. See under "Philosophy of Medicine."

Lineback, Richard H., ed. *Philosopher's Index*. Vols. 1– . Bowling Green, Ohio: Philosophy Documentation Center, Bowling Green State University. Issued quarterly. See under "Humans," "Individuals," and "Person(s)."

Walters, LeRoy, ed. *Bibliography of Bioethics*. Vols. 1– . New York: Free Press. Issued annually. See under "Personhood." (The information contained in the annual *Bibliography of Bioethics* can also be retrieved from BIOETHICSLINE, an on-line data base of the National Library of Medicine.)

Part II

THE PATIENT-
PROFESSIONAL
RELATIONSHIP

4.
Patients' Rights and Professional Responsibilities

That the practice of medicine is an applied science none would deny. But it also involves the common human transactions of contracts and services. Interesting professional responsibilities and patients' rights emerge from this human side of medical practice. Professional obligations have long been recognized in medical codes, but only recently has much systematic thought been given to the moral and legal rights of patients. In this chapter both the traditional conceptions of and the emerging problems in the professional-patient relationship are explored.

CODES OF PROFESSIONAL ETHICS

The three codes of ethics included in this chapter are samples of numerous codes that have been developed by health professionals in both ancient and modern times. The Hippocratic Oath took the form of a series of religious vows. More recent codes, including those of the American Medical Association and American Nurses' Association, generally contain secular statements of moral rules. The central affirmation of such codes is that, in treating the (frequently vulnerable) patient, the health professional will not exploit his or her position of relatively controlling power and influence.

A comparison of the "Principles of Medical Ethics" adopted in 1980 by the American Medical Association and the 1976 code of the American Nurses' Association reveals several striking differences in emphasis. For example, the primary focus in the A.M.A. code is on the physician's duty to benefit the patient. In contrast, the Code for Nurses begins by vigorously affirming the "self-determination of clients." Each code is sufficiently nuanced to mention the theme emphasized by the other; however, a difference in accent is evident. The two codes also take divergent approaches to the questions of health care delivery. In the A.M.A. principles, the right of each physician to choose which patients he or she will serve is reaffirmed, except, of course, in emergency situations. By contrast, the Code for Nurses asserts a rather sweeping welfare right—the right to quality health care—for all citizens. (See Chapter 9 for a detailed discussion of issues in health care allocation.)

Two questions arise concerning the status of these codes of conduct: (1) What is their relation to law? and (2) What is their relation to general ethical principles? The codes, though quasi-legal in form, are self-legislative documents developed by particular professions. As such, they have only the force that the profession chooses to attribute to them. In most professions, including medicine and nursing, professional self-discipline or self-policing has usually been less than vigorous.

Two possible relationships between codes of professional ethics and general ethical principles can be envisioned. Professional codes may constitute autonomous, self-contained systems of ethics that are unrelated to external validating principles. On the other hand, the codes may be viewed as specific applications of universal ethical principles. According to the latter conception, the codes consist primarily of moral rules that implicitly appeal to general ethical principles, and perhaps even to particular ethical theories. On this view, the same canons of logical coherence and consistency that are applied to any other system of moral rules can also be employed in the critical evaluation of the professional codes. (See the discussion of moral rules and moral justification in Chapter 1.)

RIGHTS AND RESPONSIBILITIES

Most health-related codes of professional ethics—with the notable exception of the 1976 Code for Nurses—emphasize the duties of professionals rather than the rights of patients. However, in the 1970s explicit declarations of patients' rights began to be formulated. Perhaps the best-known and most widely distributed of these declarations is the American Hospital Association's "Patient's Bill of Rights," which was first formulated in 1972. This Bill of Rights can be interpreted as a statement of the moral rights that ought to be enjoyed by hospital patients. Some of the asserted rights are negative or noninterference rights, for example, the right to privacy and the right to refuse treatment. Other rights included in the Bill of Rights require positive action on the part of hospitals or health professionals; for example, patients have the right to "considerate and respectful care" or the right to various kinds of information. (See the detailed discussion of rights in Chapter 1 and of positive and negative rights in Chapter 9.)

The Patient's Bill of Rights provides an interesting test of the thesis that most rights of individuals and duties to individuals are correlative. (See Chapter 1.) One can envision how the assertions of patients' *rights* in the Bill could be translated without substantive loss into statements concerning the *obligations* of hospitals and/or health professionals to patients. For example, the assertion that "the patient has the right to considerate and respectful care" could also be formulated as "the hospital has the obligation to provide the patient decent and respectful care." Why the authors of the A.H.A. statement preferred the rhetoric of rights to the more traditional language of duty is not entirely clear. However, the patients' rights approach of the A.H.A. document may reflect the consumer participation—by representatives of the National Welfare Rights Organization—that occurred during the drafting process.

The Patient's Bill of Rights has been criticized from several perspectives. In his essay in this chapter Willard Gaylin questions whether hospitals are qualified to stipulate what rights patients have. Gaylin also argues that the list of rights included in the A.H.A. Bill of Rights is not sufficiently comprehensive. George Annas, a civil liberties lawyer, takes the further step of compiling a more expansive enumeration of patient rights. Annas recognizes that some of the rights he asserts on behalf of patients are moral rather than legal but argues that the most effective means of ensuring that patients' moral rights are respected is to enact them into law. (See Chapter 1 for a discussion of legal and moral rights.)

H. Tristram Engelhardt objects on both empirical and theoretical grounds to strong assertions of patients' rights, like those advanced by the American Hospital Association, Gaylin, and Annas. Empirically, Engelhardt argues, the patients'-rights model assumes a parity between health professionals and patients that seldom exists. According to him, the differential in knowledge between physicians and patients is usually significant; in addition, ill or depressed patients often have little choice but to enter a physician-patient relationship. At a more theoretical level, Engelhardt argues that in the private sphere of contractual relationships the physician has the right and perhaps even the responsibility to act in accordance with the patient's interests, as the physician interprets those interests, rather than in response to the rights-claims advanced by the patient.

As the preceding analysis of Engelhardt's essay suggests, the notion of contract has played a prominent role in discussions of the rights and responsibilities of patients and health professionals. Indeed, a contract may be viewed as a formal statement of mutually agreed-upon rights and duties. Both Engelhardt and Dan Brock employ the contract metaphor, but with distinctive applications. For Brock, the contractual negotiations are initiated by the patient, and the patient's terms ought to be accepted by the health professional—in his essay, the nurse—unless those terms are clearly unreasonable. In Engelhardt's view, the patient and the physician enter the free marketplace and seek to reach a mutually acceptable agreement. However, since the physician is less in need of a patient than *vice versa,* and since the physician has special expertise and participates in a venerable tradition, any contractual arrangement is likely to tilt in the physician's favor.

Both Brock and Engelhardt acknowledge that the professional-patient relationship is more complex than any one-to-one contractual model might suggest. Brock, for example, notes that a nurse may simultaneously have obligations to patients and obligations to physicians or hospitals that are contradictory. According to Engelhardt, the civil and political interest in medicine may impose obligations on physicians that conflict with their obligations to their patients, e.g., in the mandatory reporting of communicable diseases. Conversely, public support of medical education may provide a political basis for a right to health care that a simple contractarian model of the professional-patient relationship could not, by itself, sustain.

INVOLUNTARY COMMITMENT

The involuntary commitment of mentally ill persons represents an extreme boundary situation in the professional-patient relationship. Three distinct kinds of issues recur in the debate about involuntary commitment: conceptual, empirical, and normative issues.

1. *The conceptual problem of defining mental illness and dangerousness.* In Chapter 2 the difficulties involved in defining mental illness were explored in detail. In the present chapter Thomas Szasz repeats his charge that most alleged cases of mental illness are not illness at all but rather instances of moral or social deviancy; as such, they are beyond the realm of the health professional's expertise. Paul Chodoff, however, argues for a broader construal of mental illness as the inability to stop or change destructive behavior. The definition of dangerousness is similarly controverted. As Chodoff notes, "dangerousness" can either be interpreted narrowly—as the likelihood that a person will do physical damage to self or others—or broadly—as the likelihood that a person will perform foolish, uncontrolled acts that may result in serious damage to his or her reputation or fortune. In the *O'Connor v. Donaldson* decision excerpted in this chapter, the United States Supreme Court clearly subscribes to the narrower definition of dangerousness.

2. *Empirical questions concerning the results of involuntary hospitalization.* Szasz and Chodoff clash sharply in their descriptions of the results of involuntary hospitalization practices. For Szasz, the primary consequence is the imprisonment and involuntary treatment of thousands of harmless individuals by those in positions of power. In contrast, Chodoff argues that involuntary hospitalization is often a highly effective form of preventive medicine and that the indiscriminate deinstitutionalization of mental patients exposes them to severe risks of exploitation and irreparable damage. The extent to which each author's account is accurate is in part an empirical question that can be resolved by the systematic collection and analysis of data. Resolution of these empirical issues is, however, directly relevant to the normative questions surrounding involuntary commitment.

3. *Normative (ethical and legal) questions concerning involuntary commitment.* The appropriateness of involuntary commitment as a social practice or in a particular case can be assessed from the standpoint of both ethics and law. Ethically, the central question is: Under what circumstances is the commitment of another human being without his or her consent morally permissible—or even morally obligatory? Answers to this question will depend in part on the relative weight one assigns to the ethical principles of autonomy and beneficence. However, most of the normative discussion concerning involuntary commitment has been legal rather than ethical. Three questions have dominated the legal debate: (1) What grounds are sufficient to justify state action to confine the mentally ill? (2) What standards of due process should be established to protect citizens against arbitrary deprivation of liberty by the state? and (3) What types of treatment, if any, should the state be required to provide for those whom it confines on grounds of mental illness? The selections in this chapter by Szasz, Chodoff, and the United States Supreme Court present divergent—and often poignant—approaches to the resolution of these questions.

An innovative proposal for avoiding involuntary commitment in certain cases is suggested by Timothy Howell and associates in the final essay of this chapter. The authors' proposal is based on the well-documented fact that patients with recurrent psychiatric illness often have lucid intervals during which they can give informed consent to necessary therapy for their mental illness. Voluntary commitment contracts signed by such patients during periods of normal mental functioning would, in the authors' view, have the dual advantage of permitting timely therapeutic intervention (possibly including institutionalization) and of allowing *involuntary* commitment statutes to be narrowly drawn.

L. W.

The Hippocratic Oath

I swear by Apollo Physician and Asclepius and Hygieia and Panaceia and all the gods and goddesses, making them my witnesses, that I will fulfill according to my ability and judgment this oath and this covenant:

To hold him who has taught me this art as equal to my parents and to live my life in partnership with him, and if he is in need of money to give him a share of mine, and to regard his offspring as equal to my brothers in male lineage and to teach them this art—if they desire to learn it—without fee and covenant; to give a share of precepts and oral instruction and all the other learning to my sons and to the sons of him who has instructed me and to pupils who have signed the covenant and have taken an oath according to the medical law, but to no one else.

I will apply dietetic measures for the benefit of the sick according to my ability and judgment; I will keep them from harm and injustice.

I will neither give a deadly drug to anybody if asked for it, nor will I make a suggestion to this effect. Similarly I will not give to a woman an abortive remedy. In purity and holiness I will guard my life and my art.

I will not use the knife, not even on sufferers from stone, but will withdraw in favor of such men as are engaged in this work.

Whatever houses I may visit, I will come for the benefit of the sick, remaining free of all intentional injustice, of all mischief and in particular of sexual relations with both female and male persons, be they free or slaves.

What I may see or hear in the course of the treatment or even outside of the treatment in regard to the life of men, which on no account one must spread abroad, I will keep to myself holding such things shameful to be spoken about.

If I fulfill this oath and do not violate it, may it be granted to me to enjoy life and art, being honored with fame among all men for all time to come; if I transgress it and swear falsely, may the opposite of all this be my lot.

Reprinted with permission of the publisher from ''The Hippocratic Oath,'' in Ludwig Edelstein, *Ancient Medicine*, edited by Oswei Temkin and C. Lillian Temkin (Baltimore: Johns Hopkins University Press, 1967).

AMERICAN MEDICAL ASSOCIATION

Principles of Medical Ethics (1980)

PREAMBLE

The medical profession has long subscribed to a body of ethical statements developed primarily for the benefit of the patient. As a member of this profession, a physician must recognize responsibility not only to patients, but also to society, to other health professionals, and to self. The following Principles adopted by the American Medical Association are not laws, but standards of conduct which define the essentials of honorable behavior for the physician.

PRINCIPLES

I. A physician shall be dedicated to providing competent medical service with compassion and respect for human dignity.

II. A physician shall deal honestly with patients and colleagues, and strive to expose those physicians deficient in character or competence, or who engage in fraud or deception.

From *American Medical News*, August 1/8, 1980, p. 9. Reprinted with permission of the American Medical Association.

III. A physician shall respect the law and also recognize a responsibility to seek changes in those requirements which are contrary to the best interests of the patient.

IV. A physician shall respect the rights of patients, of colleagues, and of other health professionals, and shall safeguard patient confidences within the constraints of the law.

V. A physician shall continue to study, apply and advance scientific knowledge, make relevant information available to patients, colleagues, and the public, obtain consultation, and use the talents of other health professionals when indicated.

VI. A physician shall, in the provision of appropriate patient care, except in emergencies, be free to choose whom to serve, with whom to associate, and the environment in which to provide medical services.

VII. A physician shall recognize a responsibility to participate in activities contributing to an improved community.

AMERICAN NURSES' ASSOCIATION

Code for Nurses (1976)

POINT 1

The nurse provides services with respect for human dignity and the uniqueness of the client unrestricted by considerations of social or economic status, personal attributes, or the nature of health problems.

1.1 SELF-DETERMINATION OF CLIENTS

Whenever possible, clients should be fully involved in the planning and implementation of their own health care. Each client has the moral right to determine what will be done with his/her person; to be given the information necessary for making informed judgments; to be told the possible effects of care; and to accept, refuse, or terminate treatment. These same rights apply to minors and others not legally qualified and must be respected to the fullest degree permissible under the law. The law in these areas may differ from state to state; each nurse has an obligation to be knowledgeable about and to protect and support the moral and legal rights of all clients under state laws and applicable federal laws, such as the 1974 Privacy Act.

The nurse must also recognize those situations in which individual rights to self-determination in health care may temporarily be altered for the common good. The many variables involved make it imperative that each case be considered with full awareness of the need to provide for informed judgments while preserving the rights of clients.

1.2 SOCIAL AND ECONOMIC STATUS OF CLIENTS

The need for nursing care is universal, cutting across all national, ethnic, religious, cultural, political, and economic differences, as does nursing's responses to this fundamental need. Nursing care should be determined solely by human need, irrespective of background, circumstances, or other indices of individual social and economic status.

Reprinted with permission of the publisher, the American Nurses' Association.

1.3 PERSONAL ATTRIBUTES OF CLIENTS

Age, sex, race, color, personality, or other personal attributes, as well as individual differences in background, customs, attitudes, and beliefs, influence nursing practice only insofar as they represent factors the nurse must understand, consider, and respect in tailoring care to personal needs and in maintaining the individual's self-respect and dignity. Consideration of individual value systems and life-styles should be included in the planning of health care for each client.

1.4 THE NATURE OF HEALTH PROBLEMS

The nurse's respect for the worth and dignity of the individual human being applies irrespective of the nature of the health problem. It is reflected in the care given the person who is disabled as well as the normal; the patient with the long-term illness as well as the one with the acute illness, or the recovering patient as well as the one who is terminally ill or dying. It extends to all who require the services of the nurse for the promotion of health, the prevention of illness, the restoration of health, and the alleviation of suffering.

The nurse's concern for human dignity and the provision of quality nursing care is not limited by personal attitudes or beliefs. If personally opposed to the delivery of care in a particular case because of the nature of the health problem or the procedures to be used, the nurse is justified in refusing to participate. Such refusal should be made known in advance and in time for other appropriate arrangements to be made for the client's nursing care. If the nurse must knowingly enter such a case under emergency circumstances or enters unknowingly, the obligation to provide the best possible care is observed. The nurse withdraws from this type of situation only when assured that alternative sources of nursing care are available to the client. If a client requests information or counsel in an area that is legally sanctioned but contrary to the nurse's personal beliefs, the nurse may refuse to provide these services but must advise the client of sources where such service is available.

1.5 THE SETTING FOR HEALTH CARE

The nurse adheres to the principle of non-discriminatory, non-prejudicial care in every employment setting or situation and endeavors to promote its acceptance by others. The nurse's readiness to accord respect to clients and to render or obtain needed services should not be limited by the setting, whether nursing care is given in an acute care hospital, nursing home, drug or alcoholic treatment center, prison, patient's home, or other setting.

1.6 THE DYING PERSON

As the concept of death and ways of dealing with it change, the basic human values remain. The ethical problems posed, however, and the decision-making responsibilities of the patient, family, and professional are increased.

The nurse seeks ways to protect these values while working with the client and others to arrive at the best decisions dictated by the circumstances, the client's rights and wishes, and the highest standards of care. The measures used to provide assistance should enable the client to live with as much comfort, dignity, and freedom from anxiety and pain as possible. The client's nursing care will determine to a great degree how this final human experience is lived and the peace and dignity with which death is approached.

POINT 2

The nurse safeguards the client's right to privacy by judiciously protecting information of a confidential nature.

2.1 DISCLOSURE TO THE HEALTH TEAM

It is an accepted standard of nursing practice that data about the health status of clients be accessible, communicated, and recorded. Provision of quality health services requires that such data be available to all members of the health team. When knowledge gained in confidence is relevant or essential to others involved in planning or implementing the client's care, professional judgment is used in sharing it. Only information pertinent to a client's treatment and welfare is disclosed and only to those directly concerned with the client's care. The rights, well-being, and safety of the individual client should be the determining factors in arriving at this decision.

2.2 DISCLOSURE FOR QUALITY ASSURANCE PURPOSES

Patient information required to document the appropriateness, necessity, and quality of care that is required for peer review, third party payment, and other quality assurance mechanisms must be disclosed only under rigidly defined policies, mandates, or protocols. These written guidelines must assure that the confidentiality of client information is maintained.

2.3 DISCLOSURE TO OTHERS NOT INVOLVED IN THE CLIENT'S CARE

The right of privacy is an inalienable right of all persons, and the nurse has a clear obligation to safeguard any confidential information about the client acquired from any source. The nurse-client relationship is built on trust. This relationship could be destroyed and the clients' welfare and reputation jeopardized by injudicious disclosure of information provided in confidence. Since the concept of confidentiality has legal as well as ethical implications, an inappropriate breach of confidentiality may also expose the nurse to liability.

2.4 DISCLOSURE IN A COURT OF LAW

Occasionally, the nurse may be obligated to give testimony in a court of law in relation to confidential information about a client. This should be done only under proper authorization or legal compulsion. Privilege in relation to the disclosure of such information is a legal right that only the patient or his representative may claim or waive. The statutes governing privilege and the exceptions to them vary from state to state, and the nurse may wish to consult legal counsel before testifying in court to be fully informed about professional rights and responsibilities.

2.5 ACCESS TO RECORDS

If, in the course of providing care, there is need for access to the records of persons not under the nurse's care, as may be the case in relation to the records of the mother of a newborn, the person should be notified and permission first obtained whenever possible. Although records belong to the agency where collected, the individual maintains the right of control over the information provided by him, his family, and his environment. Similarly, professionals may exercise the right of control over information generated by them in the course of health care.

If the nurse wishes to use a client's treatment record for research or nonclinical purposes in which confidential information may be identified, the client's consent must first be obtained. Ethically, this insures the client's right to privacy; legally, it serves to protect the client against unlawful invasion of privacy and the nurse against liability for such action.

POINT 3

The nurse acts to safeguard the client and the public when health care and safety are affected by incompetent, unethical, or illegal practice of any person.

ROLE OF ADVOCATE

The nurse's primary commitment is to the client's care and safety. Hence, in the role of client advocate, the nurse must be alert to and take appropriate action regarding any instances of incompetent, unethical, or illegal practice(s) by any member of the health care team or the health care system itself, or any action on the part of others that is prejudicial to the client's best interests. To function effectively in the role, the nurse should be fully aware of the state laws governing practice in the health care field and the employing institution's policies and procedures in relation to incompetent, unethical, or illegal practice.

. . .

POINT 4

The nurse assumes responsibility and accountability for individual nursing judgments and actions.

. . .

POINT 5

The nurse maintains competence in nursing.

. . .

POINT 6

The nurse exercises informed judgment and uses individual competence and qualifications as criteria in seeking consultation, accepting responsibilities, and delegating nursing activities to others.

. . .

POINT 7

The nurse participates in activities that contribute to the ongoing development of the profession's body of knowledge.

7.1 THE NURSE AND RESEARCH

Every profession must engage in systematic inquiry to identify, verify, and continually enlarge the body of knowledge which forms the foundations for its practice. A unique body of verified knowledge provides both framework and direction for the profession in all of its activities and for the practitioner in the provision of nursing care. The accrual of knowledge promotes the advancement of practice and with it the well-being of the profession's clients. Ongoing research is thus indispensable to the full discharge of a profession's obligations to society. Each nurse has a role in this area of professional activity, whether involved as an investigator in the furthering of knowledge, as a participant in research, or as a user of research results.

7.2 GENERAL GUIDELINES FOR PARTICIPATING IN RESEARCH

Before participating in research the nurse has an obligation:

1. To ascertain that the study design has been approved by an appropriate body.
2. To obtain information about the intent and the nature of the research.
3. To determine whether the research is consistent with professional goals.

Research involving human subjects should be conducted only by scientifically qualified persons or under such supervision. The nurse who participates in research in any capacity should be fully informed about both nurse and client rights and responsibilities as set forth in the publication *Human Rights Guidelines for Nurses in Clinical and Other Research* prepared by the ANA Commission on Nursing Research.

7.3 THE PROTECTION OF HUMAN RIGHTS IN RESEARCH

The individual rights valued by society and by the nursing profession have been fully outlined and discussed in *Human Rights Guidelines for Nurses in Clinical and Other Research;* namely, the right to freedom from intrinsic risks of injury and the rights of privacy and dignity. Inherent in these rights is respect for each individual to exercise self-determination, to choose to participate, to have full information, to terminate participation without penalty.

It is the duty of both the investigator and the nurse participating in research to maintain vigilance in protecting the life, health, and privacy of human subjects from unanticipated as well as anticipated risks. The subjects' integrity, privacy, and rights must be especially safeguarded if they are unable to protect themselves because of incapacity or because they are in a dependent relationship to the investigator. The investigation should be discontinued if its continuance might be harmful to the subject.

7.4 THE PRACTITINER'S RIGHTS AND RESPONSIBILITIES IN RESEARCH

Practitioners of nursing providing care to clients who serve as human subjects for research have a special need to clearly understand in advance how the research can be expected to affect treatment and their own moral and legal responsibilities to clients. Here, as in other problematic situations, the practitioner has the right not to participate or to withdraw under the circumstances described in paragraph 1.4 of this document. More detailed guidance about the rights and responsibilities of nurses in relation to research activities may be found in *Human Rights Guidelines for Nurses in Clinical and Other Research.*

POINT 8

The nurse participates in the profession's efforts to implement and improve standards of nursing.

•   •   •

POINT 9

The nurse participates in the profession's efforts to establish and maintain conditions of employment conducive to high quality nursing care.

•   •   •

POINT 10

The nurse participates in the profession's effort to protect the public from misinformation and misrepresentation and to maintain the integrity of nursing.

•   •   •

POINT 11

The nurse collaborates with members of the health professions and other citizens in promoting community and national efforts to meet the health needs of the public.

11.1 QUALITY HEALTH CARE AS A RIGHT

Quality health care is mandated as a right to all citizens. Availability and accessibility to quality health services for all citizens require collaborative planning by health providers and consumers at both the local and national level. Nursing care is an integral part of quality health care, and nurses have a responsibility to help ensure that citizens' rights to health care are met.

11.2 RESPONSIBILITY TO THE CONSUMER OF HEALTH CARE

The nurse is a member of the largest group of health providers, and therefore the philosophies and goals of the nursing profession should have a significant impact on the consumer of health care. An effective way of ensuring that nurses' views regarding health care and nursing service are properly represented is by involvement of nurses in political decision making.

11.3 RELATIONSHIPS WITH OTHER DISCIPLINES

The complexity of the delivery of health care service demands an interdisciplinary approach to delivery of health services as well as strong support from allied health occupations. The nurse should actively seek to promote collaboration needed for ensuring the quality of health services to all persons.

11.4 RELATIONSHIP WITH MEDICINE

The interdependent relationship of the nursing and medical professions requires collaboration around the need of the client. The evolving role of the nurse in the health delivery system requires joint practice as colleagues, deliberations in determining functional relationships, and differentiating areas of practice between the two professions.

11.5 CONFLICT OF INTEREST

Nurses who provide public service and who have financial or other interests in health care facilities or services should avoid a conflict of interest by refraining from casting a vote on any deliberation affecting the public's health care needs in those areas.

AMERICAN HOSPITAL ASSOCIATION

A Patient's Bill of Rights

The American Hospital Association presents a Patient's Bill of Rights with the expectation that observance of these rights will contribute to more effective patient care and greater satisfaction for the patient, his physician, and the hospital organization. Further, the Association presents these rights in the expectation that they will be supported by the hospital on behalf of its patients, as an integral part of the healing process. It is recognized that a personal relationship between the physician and the patient is essential for the provision of proper medical care. The traditional physician-patient relationship takes on a new dimension when care is rendered within an organizational structure. Legal precedent has established that the institution itself also has a responsibility to the patient. It is in recognition of these factors that these rights are affirmed.

1. The patient has the right to considerate and respectful care.

2. The patient has the right to obtain from his physician complete current information concerning his diagnosis, treatment, and prognosis in terms the patient can be reasonably expected to understand. When it is not medically advisable to give such information to the patient, the information should be made available to an appropriate person in his behalf. He has the right to know, by name, the physician responsible for coordinating his care.

3. The patient has the right to receive from his physician information necessary to give informed consent prior to the start of any procedure and/or treatment. Except in emergencies, such information for informed consent should include but not necessarily be limited to the specific procedure and/or treatment, the medically significant risks involved, and the probable duration of incapacitation. Where medi-

cally significant alternatives for care or treatment exist, or when the patient requests information concerning medical alternatives, the patient has the right to such information. The patient also has the right to know the name of the person responsible for the procedures and/or treatment.

4. The patient has the right to refuse treatment to the extent permitted by law and to be informed of the medical consequences of his action.

5. The patient has the right to every consideration of his privacy concerning his own medical care program. Case discussion, consultation, examination, and treatment are confidential and should be conducted discreetly. Those not directly involved in his care must have the permission of the patient to be present.

6. The patient has the right to expect that all communications and records pertaining to his care should be treated as confidential.

7. The patient has the right to expect that within its capacity a hospital must make reasonable response to the request of a patient for services. The hospital must provide evaluation, service, and/or referral as indicated by the urgency of the case. When medically permissible, a patient may be transferred to another facility only after he has received complete information and explanation concerning the needs for and alternatives to such a transfer. The institution to which the patient is to be transferred must first have accepted the patient for transfer.

8. The patient has the right to obtain information as to any relationship of his hospital to other health care and educational institutions insofar as his care is concerned. The patient has the right to obtain information as to the existence of any professional relationships among individuals, by name, who are treating him.

9. The patient has the right to be advised if the hospital proposes to engage in or perform human experimentation affecting his care or treatment. The

patient has the right to refuse to participate in such research projects.

10. The patient has the right to expect reasonable continuity of care. He has the right to know in advance what appointment times and physicians are available and where. The patient has the right to expect that the hospital will provide a mechanism whereby he is informed by his physician or a delegate of the physician of the patient's continuing health care requirements following discharge.

11. The patient has the right to examine and receive an explanation of his bill regardless of source of payment.

12. The patient has the right to know what hospital rules and regulations apply to his conduct as a patient.

No catalog of rights can guarantee for the patient the kind of treatment he has a right to expect. A hospital has many functions to perform, including the prevention and treatment of disease, the education of both health professionals and patients, and the conduct of clinical research. All these activities must be conducted with an overriding concern for the patient, and, above all, the recognition of his dignity as a human being. Success in achieving this recognition assures success in the defense of the rights of the patient.

WILLARD GAYLIN

The Patient's Bill of Rights

A stay in a hospital exposes an individual to a condition of passivity and impotence unparalleled in adult life, this side of prison. You are dressed in an uncomfortable garment, leaving you exposed and ludicrous; told when you must sleep and when you must rise; informed of what you may eat and when you have to eat it; notified as to when you can have visitors, who they shall be, and how long they can stay. You are discussed in the third person in your presence as though you were some idiot child or inanimate object. If you are unfortunate enough to have an interesting case, you will be presented to a group of strangers who may take the invasion of your privacy as their privilege. Your chart, at the foot of the bed, will contain all the vital information that you would seem to be entitled to have; yet, should you attempt to examine it, you will be treated like a prepubescent caught with a copy of *Portnoy's Complaint*.

Some of this may be necessary for health and some for convenience, but most of it is simply the inevitable result of an authoritative person dealing with people who unquestionably accept his authority.

Hospital regulations are endured by a patient conditioned to seeing his physician as a benevolent father in whose reassuring presence he is prepared to play the role of the child. Beyond this, however, more serious rights are violated under the numbing atmosphere of the same paternalism.

Modern scientific medicine, as exemplified in complex teaching hospitals, has advanced technical skill at the cost of personal warmth. Often there is no one physician rendering care, rather a battery of specialists, and while "treatment" may be superior, "care" is absent. This depersonalization of medicine is having a predictable effect on the patient, causing him to abandon his tendency to romanticize the physician, and, by extension, the medical community. For this and other reasons the patient is now pressing for a reevaluation of the medical contract.

In response to this, the American Hospital Association recently presented, with considerable fanfare, a "Patient's Bill of Rights." It is a document worth examining, for nothing indicates the low estate of

Reprinted with permission of the publisher from *Saturday Review of the Sciences*, Vol. 1, No. 2 (February 24, 1973), p. 22.

current hospital care (as distinguished from treatment) more graphically than the form of the proffered cure.

The substance of the document is amazingly innocent of controversy. It affirms that "the patient has the right to considerate and respectful care" and, beyond that, the right to "reasonable continuity of care." He is told that he may expect a modicum of personal privacy; that the usual medical concern for confidentiality should be respected; that he has a right to expect "a reasonable response" to his request for service; and, as in any other commercial transaction, that he has a right to receive an explanation of his bill.

In addition, he will be relieved to hear that, as a patient in a hospital, knowledge of the "rules and regulations" that apply to him is manifestly his due—just as it would be if he were a participant in a poker game. Similarly, the right to obtain information "concerning his diagnosis, treatment and prognosis" seems perfectly straightforward—no more than the minimum required of any standard commercial transaction. On the other hand, the patient's right to "obtain information as to any relationship of his hospital to other health care and educational institutions in so far as his care is concerned" is disquieting, for it anxiously suggests that while his exclusive reason for being in the hospital is his personal health, the hospital may have multiple, unstated other reasons influencing its treatment of him.

Finally, when the bill affirms the patient's right to "give informed consent prior to the start of any procedure," his "right to refuse treatment to the extent permitted by law," and his right to be advised "if the hospital proposes to engage in or perform human experimentation" on him, it seems to be merely belaboring the obvious. It says no more than that the hospital is subject to the same laws concerning assault and battery as any other institution or member of society.

The objection to this well-intended, though timid, document is that it perpetuates the very paternalism that precipitated the abuses. By presenting its considerations as a "Patient's Bill of Rights," it creates the impression that the hospital is "granting" these rights to the patient. The hospital has no power to grant these rights. They were vested in the patient to begin with. If the rights have been violated, they have been violated by the hospital and its hirelings. The title a "Patient's Bill of Rights" therefore seems not only pretentious but deceptive. In effect, all that the document does is return to the patient, with an air of largess, some of the rights hospitals have previously stolen from him. It is the thief lecturing his victim on self-protection—i.e., the hospital instructs the patient to make sure that the hospital treats him according to the rules of decency and law to which he is entitled. It would be more appropriate if the association addressed its 7,000 member hospitals, cautioning them that for years they have violated patient rights, some of which have the mandate of law, and warning them they must no longer presume on the innocence of their customers or the indifference of judicial authorities.

Since this is a patently decent document, the fact that the American Hospital Association takes the circuitous route of speaking to the patient of his rights, rather than to the hospital of its duties, reveals the essential weakness of such professional organizations. The AHA, like the American Medical Association and similar groups, is designed to be the servant of its constituent members—and not of the general public. A servant does not lay down the law to his master. In this regard the AHA can only state that it "presents these rights in the expectation that they will be supported" by the member hospitals. The fact that it feels the need to alert the patient indicates how insecure that "expectation" is.

A reevaluation of patient rights—one that goes beyond the old rights reaffirmed in this bill—is greatly needed. The public should not look to the professional association for leadership here. It is not for the hospital community to outline the rights it will offer, but rather for the patient consumer to delineate and then demand those rights to which he feels entitled, by utilizing all the instruments of society designed for that purpose—including the legislature and the courts.

GEORGE J. ANNAS

A Model Patients' Bill of Rights

In late 1972 the American Hospital Association issued a twelve-point Patient Bill of Rights and encouraged its 7,000 member hospitals to adopt it or a similar declaration. As one could probably guess from the source, the document's provisions were a vague restatement of the law involving such concepts as informed consent and the right to refuse treatment.

• • •

In Minnesota a bill of rights similar to the AHA model has been enacted into law, and all health care institutions are required to post it in conspicuous places in their facilities. This trend toward publishing rights is important because it not only reminds people that they have rights, it also encourages them to assert them and to make further demands. To be really significant, however, such bills should deal with the fundamental problems that patients encounter in trying to retain self-determination and privacy in health care facilities. I offer the following model bill which contains a minimal listing of the rights that should be accorded all patients both as a matter of policy by hospitals and as law by state legislatures.

In talking about "rights" here, the term is used in three senses: (1) rights that a citizen clearly or probably can claim as a matter of law under the Constitution, existing statutes, or judicial doctrines; (2) rights that a person probably can claim as judicially enforceable because of his or her relationship with another party, such as a doctor or hospital administrator; and (3) rights that a growing body of people believe should be recognized as the moral rights of individuals and the obligations of authorities, even though courts would probably not recognize them as such yet. Though some would like to see the emphasis placed on enforceable legal rights only, at this stage in the development of the patients' rights concept such a

From *Civil Liberties Review* 1 (Fall 1974), pp. 20–22. Reprinted with permission of the publisher.

limitation would be both conceptually and strategically unwise; humanizing the hospital will require a movement that joins the legal and moral aspects of the cause into one campaign, and buttresses the arguments from legal precedent and logic with the spirit of the moral cause. This was the manner of the civil rights and women's movements, and it would be useful for patients as well. Therefore, where the phrase "legal right" is used in the model bill, the right is one well recognized by case law or statute. The term "right" refers to one that probably would be recognized if the case were brought to court, and "we recognize the right" refers to a statement of what "ought to be." Once these rights are recognized, some mechanism for hearing complaints and enforcing rules must also, of course, be established. If enacted into law in the future, all of the rights would then be legal rights.

The model bill is set out as it would apply to a patient in his or her chronological relations with the hospital: sections 1–4 for a person not hospitalized but a *potential* patient; 5 for emergency admission; 6–15 for in-patients; 16–22 for discharge and after discharge; and 23 relating back to all 22 rights.

A MODEL PATIENTS' BILL OF RIGHTS

Preamble: As you enter this health care facility, it is our duty to remind you that your health care is a cooperative effort between you as a patient and the doctors and hospital staff. During your stay a patients' rights advocate will be available to you. The duty of the advocate is to assist you in all the decisions you must make and in all situations in which your health and welfare are at stake. The advocate's first responsibility is to help you understand the role of all who will be working with you, and to help you understand what your rights as a patient are. Your advocate can be reached at any time of the day by dialing _____. The following is a list of your rights as a patient. Your advocate's duty is to see to it that you are afforded these rights. You should call your advocate whenever you have any questions or concerns about any of these rights.

1. The patient has a legal right to informed participation in all decisions involving his/her health care program.
2. We recognize the right of all potential patients to know what research and experimental protocols are being used in our facility and what alternatives are available in the community.
3. The patient has a legal right to privacy regarding the source of payment for treatment and care. This right includes access to the highest degree of care without regard to the source of payment for that treatment and care.
4. We recognize the right of a potential patient to complete and accurate information concerning medical care and procedures.
5. The patient has a legal right to prompt attention, especially in an emergency situation.
6. The patient has a legal right to a clear, concise explanation in layperson's terms of all proposed procedures, including the possibilities of any risk of mortality or serious side effects, problems related to recuperation, and probability of success, and will not be subjected to any procedure without his/her voluntary, competent and understanding consent. The specifics of such consent shall be set out in a written consent form, signed by the patient.
7. The patient has a legal right to a clear, complete, and accurate evaluation of his/her condition and prognosis without treatment before being asked to consent to any test or procedure.
8. We recognize the right of the patient to know the identity and professional status of all those providing service. All personnel have been instructed to introduce themselves, state their status, and explain their role in the health care of the patient. Part of this right is the right of the patient to know the identity of the physician responsible for his/her care.
9. We recognize the right of any patient who does not speak English to have access to an interpreter.
10. The patient has a right to all the information contained in his/her medical record while in the health care facility, and to examine the record on request.
11. We recognize the right of a patient to discuss his/her condition with a consultant specialist, at the patient's request and expense.
12. The patient has a legal right not to have any test or procedure, designed for educational purposes rather than his/her direct personal benefit, performed on him/her.
13. The patient has a legal right to refuse any particular drug, test, procedure, or treatment.
14. The patient has a legal right to privacy of both person and information with respect to: the hospital staff, other doctors, residents, interns and medical students, researchers, nurses, other hospital personnel, and other patients.
15. We recognize the patient's right of access to people outside the health care facility by means of visitors and the telephone. Parents may stay with their children and relatives with terminally ill patients 24 hours a day.
16. The patient has a legal right to leave the health care facility regardless of his/her physical condition or financial status, although the patient may be requested to sign a release stating that he/she is leaving against the medical judgment of his/her doctor or the hospital.
17. The patient has a right not to be transferred to another facility unless he/she has received a complete explanation of the desirability and need for the transfer, the other facility has accepted the patient for transfer, and the patient has agreed to transfer. If the patient does not agree to transfer, the patient has the right to a consultant's opinion on the desirability of transfer.
18. A patient has a right to be notified of his/her impending discharge at least one day before it is accomplished, to insist on a consultation by an expert on the desirability of discharge, and to have a person of the patient's choice notified in advance.
19. The patient has a right, regardless of the source of payment, to examine and receive an itemized and detailed explanation of the total bill for services rendered in the facility.
20. The patient has a right to competent counseling from the hospital staff to help in obtaining

financial assistance from public or private sources to meet the expense of services received in the institution.

21. The patient has a right to timely prior notice of the termination of his/her eligibility for reimbursement by any third-party payer for the expense of hospital care.

22. At the termination of his/her stay at the health care facility we recognize the right of a patient to a complete copy of the information contained in his/her medical record.

23. We recognize the right of all patients to have 24-hour-a-day access to a patient's rights advocate who may act on behalf of the patient to assert or protect the rights set out in this document.

As is apparent from the preamble of this document, it is my view that a statement of rights alone is insufficient. What is needed in addition is someone, whom I term an advocate, to assist patients in asserting their rights. As indicated previously, this advocate is necessary because a sick person's first concern is to regain health, and in pursuit of health patients are willing to give up rights that they otherwise would vigorously assert.

Rights and Responsibilities

H . T R I S T R A M   E N G E L H A R D T

Rights and Responsibilities of Patients and Physicians

Patients and physicians are involved in a social fabric which includes medicine as a corporate endeavor, as well as society in general as a political structure. In the course of this paper, I will briefly describe the complexity of this fabric of rights and responsibilities which binds patients and physicians in the enterprises of medicine. I will argue that the physician-patient relationship is not merely one of patients and physicians. Rather, in order to understand the claims of rights and responsibilities as well as interests by patients and physicians, account must be taken of medicine as a profession and society as a political structure. In particular, most talk of patients' rights to health care, to knowledge of their prognoses, to refusing treatment, including life-prolonging

From Michael D. Bayles and Dallas M. High, eds., *Medical Treatment of the Dying: Moral Issues* (Cambridge, Mass.: Schenkman Publishing Co., 1978), pp. 9–28. Reprinted with permission of the publisher.

treatment, can be fully accounted for only as claims to civil or political rights. In point of fact, such rights can rarely be secured contractually because patients are often too disadvantaged by disease itself, and because physicians have reasonable grounds for wanting to pursue treatment on their own terms. I will pursue these considerations with a focus on the dying patient, though the issues raised concern medicine generally.

In doing this, I will first sketch circumstances which usually disadvantage patients and review historically some of the central leitmotifs of physician-patient claims and counterclaims. I will then briefly analyze the nature of this fabric of rights and duties which binds patients and physicians. The thrust is that claims such as those to a "right to health care," or to a "right to death with dignity," develop out of a civil or political interest in medicine, a recent development which has in part transmogrified medicine. To put it another way, I will argue that a theoretical account of such claims is best accomplished by an appeal to social or civil rights and duties which transcend individual contractual claims.

THE FABRIC

DISEASE AND DEATH: THE SETTING OF MEDICINE

Death is a universal reality, a central structure of the human condition. The fact of death invites men to enlist physicians in the postponement of death and in making death easier. But, physicians obviously cannot prevent death; at best, they can substitute one cause of death for another, one time of death for another, one manner of death for another. Hence, ultimately medicine cares, it does not cure. The medical profession makes the passage through life more successful or more pleasant, often overcoming certain difficulties (i.e., curing particular diseases). But in the end, medicine must fail to cure, though there is no similar restraint on the possibilities for care. While death is beyond cure, the dying are usually capable of being cared for. Physicians, though, may be committed to cure when the patient is interested only in care. Moreover, there are circumstances which disadvantage the patient in choosing what care and/or cure he wishes, particularly if he is dying.

The physician-patient relationship is likely to be assumed under circumstances that compromise the integrity of the patient. Disease, injury, and the approach of death can disable and overwhelm freedom. At the very moments when much must be decided by the ill or dying person, he is often least able to decide with full competence. Disease not only places the patient at a general disadvantage, creating a need for the service of another, it also makes the patient dependent upon the physician for continued health and perhaps survival. Though patients may claim openness and participation in decisions concerning their own therapy as far as possible, such claims are countered by inescapable themes of paternalism, insofar as disease often involves a natural need for regression and dependence on the part of the patient. Concepts of informed consent seem to guide, yet these, too, always involve weighing different goods. There often exists a need *not* to be overly informed. For example, an anxious patient who has just sustained a serious myocardial infarction may not need, at that time, to be informed *precisely* of his prognosis because information might itself adversely change the prognosis. In short, one often enters into the arms of medicine as one might enter passionately into the arms of a lover—with great haste and need, but little forethought. And it often makes little sense to look for informed or voluntary consent in either case, if one wishes to understand consent in a rigorous and pure fashion. Patient and physician are thrown together because of the exigencies of nature. Other relations (e.g., the lawyer-client relation) rarely have their focus so immediately upon one's very presence in the world.

Disease, which is the occasion of the social interactions of medicine, imposes peculiar restrictions and reveals unique needs for trust and keeping trust. Though we all maintain basic rights, still we find ourselves in the grip of natural forces, the control of which often presupposes the intrusion of medicine in circumstances when our freedom is blunted.

Moreover, medicine, as all technical endeavors, has become increasingly less open to well-informed decision-making on the part of the general public. One of the most pervading consequences of modern technological society is the social distribution of knowledge (i.e., groups of experts possess various portions of society's store of knowledge; the knowledge explosion precludes all from full possession of our current stock of knowledge)[1] which prevents fully informed individual, and to some extent societal, decisions and consent concerning the directions of medicine. The accrual of a special stock of skills and knowledge by a particular group of individuals, with consequent peculiar social duties, rights, powers, and expectations, in part defines medicine as a profession and distinguishes the physician from the layman, his actual or potential patient. It establishes not only divisions of labor but of power due to the possession of special knowledge bearing on the life and death of laymen. It also establishes a social sub-group defined by its interest in the preservation and maintenance of its skills and knowledge, and thus by special interests and goals.

However, to talk of rights and responsibilities of patients and physicians in the absence of any reference to the goals of society in general or of the medical profession in particular, is to prescind artificially from the actual context of patients and physicians. Physicians have civil duties *to* society and *to* their profession *regarding* patients that extend beyond the rights that patients have with respect to physicians.[2] Physicians have a duty to society to report communicable diseases, for example, which is not a duty to any particular patient. Moreover, patients possess certain duties *to* society *regarding* physicians and the medical professions which they do not have strictly to physicians. Patients with communicable diseases have a duty to society to follow the advice of their physicians with regard to preventing their spread.

Further, modern medicine is the creation of society; public investment in the education of physicians and medical research has produced it. Medicine has become part of society's explicit political response to the general predicament of man. That is, society has begun to invest in and use medicine for the general political purposes of the community. Private individuals no longer provide the major support for medical research and education.[3] Rather, medicine has become a social or civil instrument, and in this sense has become socialized. Medicine has been employed to affect the conditions of society, e.g., change infant mortality rates, enable a population explosion, provide contraception, make life in cities possible without frequent fatal epidemics, etc., and it has thereby become an instrument of society in the sense of a publicly supported means of effecting publicly chosen goals.

This thesis of the social or civil nature of medicine is stronger and more complex than the more general maxim of "he who pays the piper calls the tune." The relation of society and medicine is no longer merely a contractual one. The compass of modern medicine is a political creation. As a result, physicians accrue both rights and duties. They acquire duties to society regarding particular patients. Members of society also acquire social duties to have immunizations, blood tests, special examinations for certain occupations (food handlers, airplane pilots, etc.). These are civil duties of "patients" to society regarding medicine. It is in this broader social context that citizens have a civil right to health care. Their right is one from society regarding medicine, one in virtue of modern medicine existing as a social product. We will return to this issue when discussing the socialization of medicine.

HISTORICAL LEITMOTIFS

In talking about physicians and patients, one must view the issues in terms which transcend relations between particular physicians and patients, and concern general social or civil structures. Further, the interests and enterprises shared by physicians and patients is such that duties and rights are never unilateral; rather, they are mutually implicatory and asymmetrical. Patients trade money and freedom for care and cure. A brief sketch of attitudes expressed in the Hippocratic corpus and the first A.M.A. code is illustrative.

The Hippocratic corpus is a diverse collection of writings on medicine, which has been imputed to Hippocrates (circa 460–379 B.C.), but which reflects more than one tradition. It contains at least four treatises with significant focus on values in medicine: "The Oath," "Law," "The Physician," and "Decorum." Though other treatises in the corpus refer to medical ethical issues, only these have a primary focus on the ethical conduct of medicine. They are central to the lore of medicine. The Oath in particular concerns both physician and patient rights.[4] From physicians, the Oath requires loyalty and support of their teachers and an esoteric attitude towards medical knowledge. Medical knowledge was to be communicated to the initiate but not to others, an attitude still prevalent today. Patient-directed concerns included the duty to give proper treatment, to avoid taking advantage of the special intimacies of the physician-patient relationship and, in particular, to maintain confidentiality.[5]

The Oath evidences a recognition of the peculiar nature of the physician-patient relationship as established on the basis of the vicissitudes of nature. Because of a person's vulnerability to disease, he is forced to the physician for aid. The physician, moreover, is a part of a community of physicians. Patients, on the other hand, apart from some social recognition, are not a social body but merely an aggregate of persons gathered together by chance, indeed, bad luck. By the nature of the circumstances and the relationship, the patient is disadvantaged, if not disabled, and is at the mercy of the physician. Beyond that, the process of cure requires disclosure of the patient's body, his way of life, and his habits to the physician. In the process, the physician gains a unique and privileged knowledge of the patient. But the intimacy is one-sided. The physician is not constrained to reciprocate except with competent therapy, confidentiality, and restraint from using the relationship for clearly self-interested motives. The Oath requires the physician to be circumspect and not to seduce his patients.

To put it another way, the Oath recognizes that the physician and the patient meet in circumstances structured by the difficulties of the patient and by the art of medicine. There are always at least four elements involved: the physician, the patient, the disease, and medicine. In modern communities, one must add a fifth element: society in the form of a political structure. As stated in the Hippocratic corpus, "The art has three factors, the disease, the patient, the physician. The physician is the servant of the art. The patient must co-operate with the physician in combating the disease."[6] The physician, as servant of the art (i.e., the profession of medicine), brings interests peculiar to himself: the goals and pleasures of medicine. An art well practiced is an end in itself, which is no less the case with medicine. Diagnosis and consequent explanation and prediction, or prognosis, are intellectual goals which can lead to social approval even in the absence of therapy. And again, importantly, the corpus suggests that the physician's duty regarding the patient is to the profession: "The physician is the servant of the art."[7]

This fabric of interests (i.e., those of patients, of individual physicians, and of the profession of medicine) structured the development of the present concept of medical ethics. In America, the historical development shows the evolution of a fabric of social concerns. Initial interest in medical ethics centered upon establishing the etiquette of proper medical practice. This emphasis is reflected in the "Boston Medical Police" of 1808, and the numerous early codes of "Medical Etiquette" which followed.[8] These codes were in great proportion focused on regulating consultations, interactions of physicians, and setting a schedule of fees.

The current term "medical ethics" gained currency and one of its meanings was fixed in the United States when the American Medical Association adopted its "Code of Medical Ethics" at its first meeting in May, 1847.[9] This code dealt explicitly with duties of different kinds: duties of physicians to patients, of patients to physicians, of physicians to their profession and fellow physicians, of the profession to society, and of society to the profession. Duties of physicians to patients included offering treatment to the ill; keeping confidentiality; giving adequate care; not giving gloomy prognoses (in particular, not informing a patient of his impending death); not abandoning a patient when only care, not cure, was possible; and consulting other physicians when necessary. In other words, the physician was to give care and treatment while keeping trust with his patient and recognizing his own limitations. The patient, on the other hand, was to respond by selecting

only bona fide physicians (not quacks), being open and complete in giving the history of his diseases, following the orders of the physician "promptly and implicit[ly]" and not leaving one physician for another without first giving the reasons for this action, etc. Patients, in short, were to submit almost unquestioningly to the treatment of their physicians. In addition, as in the Oath, there was a recognition of duties of physicians to their fellows and to the profession itself. Finally, there was an acknowledgment of duties of physicians to society and of society to physicians and medicine: physicians were seen to have an obligation to aid the development of social policy in matters of public health, while the community was seen to have the duty to encourage and facilitate medical education, etc.

In short, the history of Western medicine places the physician-patient relationship in the context of the community of physicians, if not that of society generally. Finally, even in the absence of historical argument, there is a somewhat obvious development of the social nature of medicine. In Greek times, the author of "Law" could assert: "Medicine is the only art which our states have made subject to no penalty save that of dishonour. . . ."[10] But in 1847, the same year in which the A.M.A. code was written, Salomon Neumann was arguing for "the social nature of the healing art."[11] And shortly thereafter, that argument was assumed by Rudolf Virchow, who finally contended that medicine should deal with the basic laws of social structure.[12] Any account of patient and physician rights and responsibilities must therefore sort out different levels and kinds of claims and counterclaims, social and individual.

THE MEANING OF THE FABRIC

How then are we to understand the complex fabric of rights and duties binding patients and physicians? What is its nature? The conclusion seems to be that the rights and duties are not only complex but heterogeneous in nature. Some historically more basic ones are in part contractual and in part imposed by the circumstance that most patients are in some sense disabled. The rights and duties are contractual in the sense of arising out of the therapeutic contract between physicians and patients: the patient can always refuse any treatment, or the treatment of a particular physician, though the consequences may be severe. Physicians can, on the other hand, refuse to treat particular patients, but with less dire consequences. A physician is not usually in as pressing a need for a patient, at a particular time, as a patient is for a physician. Yet, there are circumstances when the patient determines the direction of the relationship rather than leaving it to a physician's judgment, as for example when a rhinoplasty or an abortion is sought. But the constraints of nature (e.g., fever, fear, delirium, pain, simple weakness), constraints of the social distribution of knowledge, and the interests of the profession of medicine in pursuing its own goals usually curtail full patient knowledge about the significance of treatment and thus curtail participation in determining the course of treatment. Physicians as members of an independent enterprise may simply refuse to make such participation an element of the therapeutic relationship.

Thus to a great extent the relation of physicians and patients arises out of the state of things, just as marriage arises out of the mutual needs of the sexes, or a family out of the mutual needs and abilities of its members. When ill, one is often simply dependent on a physician, as a small child is on its parents; the physician's paternalism is in this sense a natural one born out of the constraints of nature. That is, in this context, physician and patient rights arise as much out of the status of the individuals involved as out of any contract.

The contractual relations of physicians and patients are thus usually unequal because patients enter such contracts under duress, while physicians are supported by a strong profession with independent goals. How then are we to understand the character and place of patient rights such as those of the Patient's Bill of Rights of the American Hospital Association? What is the basis of claims such as "the right to obtain from [one's] physician complete current information concerning [one's] diagnosis, treatment and prognosis in terms the patient can be reasonably expected to understand [or] when it is not medically advisable to give such information to the patient [to have that] information . . . made available to an appropriate person in [the patient's] behalf," or "the right to refuse treatment to the extent permitted by law . . ."?[13] These strong statements of patient rights imply a parity between physician and patient not usually possible in the situations under which therapeutic contracts, physician-patient relationships, are developed, Nor are such claims to rights claims to

contractual rights, for it is difficult to argue that physicians would generally agree to physician-patient relationships that are contrary to the interests of physicians in care and cure. Further it is difficult to see how patients have a prima facie right such that physicians would have a duty to agree to therapeutic contracts which physicians find to collide with the aims and purposes of medicine.

PATIENT INTERESTS AND RIGHTS VERSUS THE PHYSICIAN

Patients have an interest in gaining cure and care, and in avoiding loss of freedom or privacy. But since disease and death involve partial or total loss of liberty, patients are usually willing to cede some freedom in order to maintain liberty from illness and death. Claims to privacy are often withdrawn in order to secure cure and care. Conflicts arise when a patient decides that the sacrifice of freedom and privacy is not justified by the cure or care offered, while others, physicians in particular, hold such cure or care to be in that person's best interests. Such conflicts are likely to arise in cases of incurable diseases and are often articulated in terms of rights to refuse treatment, especially extraordinary treatment. Conflicts also arise in terms of claims that it is in the best interests of a patient not to know the true severity of his illness.

The strongest general arguments on behalf of the patient are those with regard to the patient as a free agent. If respect is due to persons as free agents, then to preempt another's freedom to choose in his own behalf is precisely not to treat that person as free. Freedom to decide one's own best interests is, in the end, the core of self-determination. Yet, there is a dilemma, for it is illness and approaching death which are likely to overwhelm a patient and make self-determination difficult, if not impossible. The issue of patient rights is then, as has been argued, to be weighed against a paternalism required because of the intrusions of disease. It has been accepted by some (though more so in the past than in the present) that the patient's right to consent to his treatment and to knowledge concerning its significance is suspended when such knowledge and decisions might unduly stress the patient. I have in mind a situation in which a physician would say to a patient, "If you want me to treat you, trust me, follow my orders, I will take care of you, there is nothing more you need to know about your heart attack than that I will treat you well and in your best interests."[14]

But not only does the patient have a right to expect

that the physician will act only in the patient's best interest, he also has a right to attempt to negotiate with the physician the bounds of such paternalism. Yet when such paternalism is accepted by the profession of medicine and by society as usually being beneficial, it becomes a generally established social practice. In such circumstances, what claims can the patient succeed in making against medicine? Or, rather, how can such claims be framed? Medicine as an independent social enterprise sets its own standards, and the patient can at best demand that the physician not abuse the powers that come into his hands as a result of the physician's following the established mode of giving treatment. All things being equal, persons may become physicians in order to cure and care, and may hold that (1) this is their prime goal, and (2) too much information conveyed to the patient may thwart that goal. Insofar as medicine can act as an independent social enterprise, physicians may simply say—take it or leave it.

The situation is one in which the physician can see himself as the agent of cure and care, not the agent of the patient, who must therefore accept cure and care on the physician's terms. Physicians, moreover, can bolster such stances by appeals that anything less than resolute, unwavering dedication to cure will (1) cause patients to be abandoned prematurely as hopeless when more resolute physicians would have effected a cure, and (2) lead patients to lose confidence in their physicians. That is, physicians can appeal to a policy of "dedication to cure at all costs" as being the best policy for most patients in the long run.

There are two axes along which the success of such arguments can be plotted. One is the mental competence of the patient and the second is the likelihood of survival given persistent therapy. Thus, the more a patient is overwhelmed by the disease process itself and the greater the likelihood of cure given persistent therapy, the easier it is to justify a physician's paternalism by an argument in terms of those best interests which the patient himself would pursue, were he clear of intellect. One should imagine here a patient suffering miserably from a painful but easily curable disease who is ready to abandon all hope. Given the pain and exhaustion involved in illness, a patient is liable to despair prematurely.

This is similar to the account of Odysseus given by Dworkin. Odysseus' crew is justified in not freeing him from the mast, even if he so requests, because that was the reason he had himself bound in the first place—so he could resist the Sirens.[15] Often an argument similar to that of Odysseus' crew can be made by the physician—namely, to secure the patient against the Sirens of depression and despair. In such cases, the physician's dedication to cure and care and against allowing euthanasia or suicide provides a "social insurance" policy.[16] There is a good case for the physician's treating as far as possible and being as persuasive as possible in obtaining the patient's consent to treatment, when there is a reasonable chance for cure of a patient who is not in a position to decide on the significance of his chances. The physician can then presume that when the patient entered into the physician-patient relationship, he wanted the assurance of such action and gave implicit consent to "benign coercion."

Claims to such paternalism, though, are weakened when the patient is relatively clear of mind and his chances of survival are minimal, if not nil. In the imminence of death, neither the patient nor society can gain anything from further prolongation of life. In such cases, the patient may make a presumptively valid claim that any and all further treatment should cease and he be free to commit suicide. I will leave the issue of assisted suicide in the imminence of death, i.e., euthanasia, unexamined because it raises more issues than are pertinent here. It is enough here to indicate that the imminence of death, along with physical incapacitation, excuses one from most duties. In short, there rarely are good grounds under which a dying person with severe physical incapacitation can be constrained to live further because of duties to others or society.[17] It should be noted that this point is made without reference to extraordinary or ordinary means of therapy: when there is no need to constrain the present freedom of an individual as a rational insurance that in the future he can act freely, constraint is not justified. While one often prevents irrevocable decisions that would seriously undercut one's ability to choose freely in order to maintain freedom in the future, the imminence of death removes the need for such calculations.

So-called living wills, instructions to one's physician regarding what the physician's actions should be if the patient is incapacitated, are designed to provide a clear notion of the will of the patient in some of these circumstances. Living wills are doubly conditional physician-patient contracts. Most physician-patient relationships are conditional upon the continued consent of both partners. A living will (among other things) can explicitly condition the patient's consent upon a significant chance of survival as a conscious agent. So, for example, a living will could provide that, if in the future the patient is unconscious with no likely chance of regaining consciousness, there would be no consent to further treatment.

But there are other grounds in terms of which medicine and physicians may still find reasons to constrain patients to submit to treatment, even when there is little likelihood of cure and it only prolongs dying. Physicians might argue, for example, that such a course provides a patient comfort built on a hope, albeit a vain hope. Further, physicians might hold that one should never stop treatment as long as there is any hope, however remote. Such attitudes are of long standing in American medicine, especially with regard to the physician never being the person to tell a patient that his condition is fatal. "For the physician should be the minister of hope and comfort to the sick; that, by such cordials to the drooping spirit, he may smooth the bed of death, revive expiring life, and counteract the depressing influence of those maladies which often disturb the tranquillity of the most resigned in their last moments. The life of a sick person can be shortened not only by the acts, but also by the words or the manner of the physician. It is, therefore, a sacred duty to guard himself carefully in this respect, and to avoid all things which have a tendency to discourage the patient and to depress his spirits."[18]

The point is that the physician should attempt to act in the best interests of the patient, which include living as long and as free from suffering and anxiety as possible. This view of course conflicts with the notion that some patients may choose a life lived on their own terms, even if shorter and more marked by anxiety derived from a true knowledge of their impending death. The issue is the extent to which a patient, in particular a dying patient, has rights to full knowledge concerning his condition and to participate in decisions concerning his treatment.

On the other hand, the physician has independent claims and interests. The physician has presumably entered into the practice of a particular profession because he or she enjoys the activities of that art and science. He has an interest and indeed a *prima facie* right not to be forced to do things which he holds to be against good medical judgment, thereby making a claim for intellectual integrity. In fact, the physician can make such strong claims as, "If you want me to

treat you, then you will have to follow my directions for therapy." The physician has a proper interest in the patient following the prescribed treatment beyond merely having the patient pay his bills. The physician makes a claim for the integrity of his art and science as a condition of his practice. Finally, one should remember that medicine can be practiced independently of goals of cure, as the history of therapeutic nihilism attests.[19] Medicine can be satisfying to the physician as a purely intellectual undertaking, the parody of which are statements such as "the operation was a success but the patient died." But even in such statements of derision, a legitimate claim is made to pursue an art with integrity of judgment and purpose.

Further, the profession of medicine presupposes the acquisition of skill and its transmission from one practitioner to another. Insofar as medicine has as its goal the cure of disease and the care of man in illness and dying, and insofar as medicine always fails to cure and care fully, there arises a basic nisus* to research, observation, and the development of further knowledge of skills in treatment and care. Patients are thus also subjects of at least clinical observations. They are always possible contributors to medical knowledge as well as patients, recipients of medical care. Further, as a science and technology, medicine has its own independent interest in knowledge which can exceed that of society—to which past disapproval of anatomical dissection and present opposition to the study of *in vitro* fertilization attest.[20]

Unlike society at large, the medical profession has a special investment in the goals of medical progress. Increase in medical knowledge and technology represents an increase in the abilities and prestige of the medical profession and its individual members. It represents, as well, the achievement of an intrinsic goal of medicine: the better understanding and treatment of disease. Though for society in general, a certain high level of health might be sufficient, medicine always has an implicit commitment to advance and, therefore, to further experimentation and investment of resources in the expansion of medical knowledge and technology. There is a conflict implicit in this goal, for the progress of medical knowledge requires the use of large numbers of human beings in medical research and experimentation. In particular, these internal interests of medicine can lead to conflicts with medicine's more general interests in cure and care. These conflicts can become acute with

Ed. note: Impulse.

regard to special groups such as the dying, who may be asked to submit to research which may not benefit their cure or care, though the dying may vainly and falsely so hope.

In summary, against these claims by physicians and the medical profession, patients can make only relatively weak counterclaims, if the physician-patient relationship is only a narrowly construed contractual one. While patients can refuse to contract with particular physicians, they may be forced by disease to contract with physicians on terms for the most part set by nature and by the paternalistic judgments of medicine. A patient can demand the care and cure and to withdraw at will from the relationship, but he cannot, without further negotiation, demand that treatment, if given, be given in any way except in terms of medical judgment of the treating physician. That is, the physician as expert makes a claim to know best and, if engaged, to be allowed to act upon that better knowledge. There is also a paternalistic element to this position, that at a future time (i.e., after being cured), the patient will agree that it was good to have been induced to follow the physician's advice. Thus, modern claims such as those to a right to health care or to full knowledge concerning the course of one's treatment and therefore full participation in decisions concerning it, must arise, if they are to arise at all, from sources other than a physician-patient contract.

THE SOCIALIZATION OF MEDICINE

My use of the phrase, "socialization of medicine," is somewhat idiosyncratic; it is meant to focus on a general shift in the significance of patient rights with regard to medicine. In particular, the social nature of medicine augments the otherwise circumscribed rights of patients, providing a context in terms of which the physician-patient contract can be renegotiated, giving the patient more parity with the physician by sustaining his claims to knowledge and decision, even if sustaining such claims is not conducive to effective treatment.

The point is that, because of societal investment in the development of medical research and education, public health care programs, and individual health care (e.g., Medicare), medicine has become an element of social or civil policy. Medicine, once an enterprise of private citizens, has now become an extension of those citizens through the development of medicine within a political structure. The force of this development is that medicine as a social or political enterprise can legitimately be required to temper its interests in cure and care and make them accord with basic claims of citizens to self-determination and choice. In this sense, rights to health care and the rights listed in patients' bills of rights are civil rights, rights which accrue to an individual in virtue of his membership in a political structure of a certain character. One begins thus to speak of a new quality of patient freedom, even though its quantity, its scope, can never (because of the restraints of disease and the social distribution of knowledge) be comparable to that of the physician. Patient bills of rights involve bringing the pursuit of cure and care on medicine's terms into a social context of basic non-medical concerns for self-determination, so that such concerns are less likely to be overridden.

It is worth remarking again that the patient is probably most disadvantaged in the imminence of death, when there will not be a future time in which the social insurance of a medical paternalism could be evaluated by that patient. Moreover, choices of the point at which further treatment ceases to make sense are probably much more an issue of what makes sense for that patient; they are more idiosyncratic and less amenable to judgments made on the basis of medical paternalism. The point at which further pain incurred to prolong life is no longer justified by the quality of life achieved is an issue best determined by the person suffering the pain and living that life. One might think here of a patient with disseminated carcinoma, deciding against further treatment on the basis that further investment of pain and effort is not worth the likely return. Again, if present paternalistic constraint is to be justified on the basis of protection of future freedom of the patient, the justification fails in the case of the dying patient. There will be no future of any material significance. The issue here is in part that of allowing the patient to decide what counts as a meaningful extension of his future, given the fact of his imminent death. The patient here would need a clear notion of his prognosis to decide intelligently when further treatment is no longer justified. Such claims, though, can conflict with an interest physicians have in deciding when further treatment should be forgone. However, the social nature of modern medicine provides a political context in which such claims by patients can be raised as general civil rights and thus as prior yet complementary to any particular physician-patient contracts. Such claims by patients are basically claims to a general civil right to liberty—even to the point of caprice.

The socialization of medicine paradoxically implies both less and more freedom. On the one hand, it provides an arena in which general claims to greater parity in physician-patient relationships can be made. That is, patients as citizens can constrain medicine, an enterprise of their society, to allow patients to share in the responsibility for treatment and diagnosis. On the other hand, the socialization of medicine (i.e., the placing of medicine within a political structure and thus in terms of civil policies) implies that an element of general societal concern will extend to general treatment of the population—fluoridation and chlorination of water supplies, the requirement of vaccinations, etc. The socialization of medicine can not only give all persons a civil right to health care and to participation in decisions concerning their treatment, but it can also impose on them civil duties to participate in health maintenance, even in programs which cannot be directly in their self-interest (e.g., rubella vaccinations). In short, the socialization of medicine involves the placing of individual concerns about disease, health, care and cure in terms of general civil goals. It provides a domain within which talk about general rights and duties with regard to health care can take place.

In particular, talk of patients' rights to health care, to full knowledge concerning their prognosis, to terminating life-prolonging therapy, can gain a meaning in terms of duties to society by medicine regarding those patients. They can be viewed as rights from society, as a political institution, regarding medicine. It is not as if a particular physician had a duty to accept a particular patient as his and discharge his general duty to provide health care in the instance of that particular patient. Nor is it really the case that, all things being equal, a physician, *qua* physician, has a duty to let a patient determine the criteria for informing the patient concerning his prognosis or for terminating his treatment. It is rather, I suggest, that such issues arise in terms of the scope of the patients' basic civil rights. Otherwise puzzling talk about rights to health care can thus be given a sense, a social one. Patients' rights, including the rights of the dying patient, are, if they are to be rights at all, civil rights. They are claims that must be formally recognized by society.

This development should not be unexpected. The claim of patients to bills of rights is the claim to have the right to develop a social policy which will structure the practice of medicine. Claims to patient rights and liberties grow out of general civil claims to rights and liberties, which is to say that patients form the larger society within which physicians and medicine are finally placed. Until general society comes to terms with the rights of patients, patients suffer from an anomie, to which physicians as members of a uniting enterprise (i.e., medicine) are not subject. Patients are merely isolated patients until society addresses the status of medicine and patients. Only then can a patient receive special standing as a free citizen with rights with respect to health care.

This point is not unlike that made by Plato concerning the difference between free and slave physicians. "A physician of this kind [a slave] never gives a servant any account of his complaint, nor asks him for any . . . [But], the free practitioner . . . treats [his patients'] diseases by going into things thoroughly from the beginning in a scientific way, and takes the patient and his family into his confidence."[21] To develop this point with broad brushstrokes yet one further step, in a society of free men, claims can be made not only to a right to knowledge concerning one's illness and to a right to consent knowingly to therapy, but to a right to refuse life-prolonging therapy as well. Concepts of death with dignity thus become more the notion of a death chosen under circumstances most in accord with the wishes of the patient as a free citizen. Since disease and the imminence of death can make full, voluntary, and informed consent impossible, such participation becomes an ideal more than a completely realizable goal. Attempts to articulate patients' bills of rights and to provide for living wills are attempts to extend personal freedom into the relationships of physicians and patients, to provide ideals for citizen participation. Such bills of rights act to bring elements of general human freedom into circumstances otherwise structured only by the forces of nature and the interests of medicine. In particular, it may be necessary for society to protect a patient's right to choose death rather than a prolonged dying that an over-dedication to cure might entail. One sees at play here a general role of political structures, namely, to place the legitimate concerns of special interest groups within the context of the interests of society at large. Medicine is the special interest group of cure and care. However, citizens may not always have an interest in cure and may instead desire care on their own terms.

NOTES

I am indebted to Laurence McCullough for criticism and discussion of the ancestral drafts of this paper.

1. Alfred Schutz and Thomas Luckmann, *The Structures of the Life-World,* trans. Richard M. Zaner and H. Tristram Engelhardt, Jr. (Evanston: Northwestern University Press, 1973), pp. 324–326.

2. A good discussion of duties one has *to A regarding B* is given by Marcus G. Singer in his article "On Duties to Oneself," *Ethics* 69 (1959): 204.

3. Report by the Committee on the Financing of Medical Education of the Association of American Medical Colleges, "Current Funding Patterns: Medical School Programs," *Journal of Medical Education* 49 (1974): 1097–1102.

4. The document, though, is probably of Pythagorean origin, representing the views of that particular philosophico-religious sect and not that of the general medical community of the time. Ludwig Edelstein, *The Hippocratic Oath: Text, Translation and Interpretation,* Supplement No. 1, *The Bulletin of the History of Medicine* (Baltimore: The Johns Hopkins Press, 1943), pp. 14–38.

5. Further, in a somewhat religious tone, the Oath required one to conduct one's medical practice in purity and holiness. It was this latter leitmotif which led to its unique proscriptions of abortion, euthanasia, and surgery—practices which violated Pythagorean religious prohibitions, but which were otherwise fairly widely practiced in the Graeco-Roman world prior to the Christian era. I will pass over these latter issues, which are still primarily religious, and focus on the broader context of physician and patient interests.

6. Epidemics I, xi. *Hippocrates,* Vol. 1, trans. W.H.S. Jones (London: William Heinemann Ltd., 1923), p. 165.

7. *Ibid.*

8. Donald E. Konold, *A History of American Medical Ethics, 1847–1912* (Madison: The State Historical Society of Wisconsin for the Department of History, University of Wisconsin, 1962), p. 2.

9. *Ibid.,* p. 9, and *Code of Medical Ethics Adopted by the American Medical Association* (New York: New York Academy of Medicine, 1848).

10. Law i. *Hippocrates,* Vol. 2, p. 263.

11. Salomon Neumann, *Die öffentliche Gesundheitspflege und das Eigenthum* (Berlin: Adolph Riess, 1847), p. 65.

12. Rudolf Virchow, "Über die Standpunkte in der wissenschaftlichen Medicin," *Archiv für pathologische Anatomie und Physiologie* 70 (1847): 1–10.

13. American Hospital Association, "Statement on a Patient's Bill of Rights, Affirmed by the Board of Trustees, November 17, 1972," *Hospitals* 47 (February 16, 1973): 41.

14. One should remember that such bold paternalism is almost all medicine had to offer until the late nineteenth century. Further, such a demeanor, when accepted, probably itself has a beneficial, placebo effect.

15. Gerald Dworkin, "Paternalism," *Monist* 56 (1972): 77.

16. *Ibid.,* p. 78.

17. Marcus G. Singer in "On Duties to Oneself" provides an interesting argument against the possibility of talking, in any strict sense, of duties to oneself, and thus indirectly against duties not to commit suicide, pp. 202–205.

18. "Code of Medical Ethics of the American Medical Association," Sec. 4, pp. 2–3.

19. Owsei Temkin, "Medicine in 1847—Continental Europe," in "One Hundred Years Ago: A Symposium Presented by the Johns Hopkins Institute of the History of Medicine," *Bulletin of the History of Medicine* 21 (1947): 475–476.

20. A.M. Lassek, *Human Dissection: Its Drama and Struggle* (Springfield, Ill.: Charles C. Thomas, 1958). There have been a number of attempts, for example, to prohibit by law potentially harmful experimentation on fetuses, such as the law enacted by the state of Minnesota, Minn. Sess. Law ch. 562, § 145.42 (1973), and to prosecute physicians who engage in experimentation on fetal material. See Donald Day, "Fetal Study Stirs Grand Jury in Abortion Debate," *Hospital Tribune,* April 8, 1974, 1, 28.

21. Plato, *Laws* 720 c–d, *The Collected Dialogues of Plato,* ed. Edith Hamilton and Huntington Cairns, trans. A.E. Taylor (Princeton: Princeton University Press, 1963), pp. 1310–11.

DAN W. BROCK

The Nurse-Patient Relation: Some Rights and Duties

NURSE-PATIENT RELATIONSHIP

There are at least two sorts of moral considerations relevant to a full understanding of the moral relationship between the nurse and the patient. First, there are general moral considerations, rights and duties, that the nurse and patient would have simply as individuals, apart from their roles as nurse or patient (e.g., on most any moral theory it is prima facie wrong to kill or seriously injure another human being, and this holds for persons generally, not merely for nurses and patients). Second, there are moral considerations that arise only out of the particular relationship that exists between a nurse and patient, just as there are in other relationships such as parent and child, public official and citizen, and so forth. A complete account of the nurse's moral situation must include both sorts of considerations, and would be far too complex and lengthy to attempt here.

I shall emphasize considerations of the second sort, and even then my discussion will not be at all comprehensive. On virtually any account of the nurse-patient relationship, the nurse owes at least some care to the patient and the patient has a right to expect that care. However, this is not an obligation that the nurse has to just anyone, but only to the patient, nor a right a person has toward just anyone, or even toward any nurse, but rather only toward his or her nurse. How then do nurse and patient get into this relationship at all? If we pose the question in this way, I think it is clear that the common alternative accounts of the nurse-patient relationship cannot all be plausibly construed as even possible answers to this question, and that more generally, they address two different questions—some speak to the origin of the relation-

ship, how it comes about, while others speak to the nature or content of the relationship. I think a clearer understanding of the relationship is gained if we separate these two issues, because the account of the origin of the relationship will affect in turn the account of its content. Consider six of the more common accounts of the relationship of the role of the nurse vis-à-vis the patient:[1]

1. The nurse as parent surrogate
2. The nurse as physician surrogate
3. The nurse as healer
4. The nurse as patient advocate or protector
5. The nurse as health educator
6. The nurse as contracted clinician

I do not want to deny that nurses do at times, and at times justifiably so, fill each of the first five of these roles. And at least most of these first five roles refer to professional duties a nurse assumes in entering the profession of nursing. But how is it that a nurse has any duty to perform in any of these roles toward a particular person (patient), and how is it that a person (patient) has any right to expect a particular nurse to perform in these roles? Only the last model, the nurse as contracted clinician, can explain that. We must be able to make reference to a contract, or better an agreement, between the two to explain these roles. This point may be obscured somewhat by the fact that what a nurse would do for a patient in any of the first five roles can be generally assumed to be beneficial for the patient, or at least intended to be beneficial. If it is for the patient's good, why must the patient agree before the nurse is permitted to act? But just imagine someone coming up to you on the street and giving you an injection, even one intended to be, and in fact, beneficial to you. A natural response would be, "You have no right to do that," and underlying that response would likely be some belief that each person

From Dan W. Brock. ''The Nurse-Patient Relation: Some Rights and Duties,'' pp. 108–124. In Stuart F. Spicker and Sally Gadow, eds., *Nursing: Images and Ideals*. Copyright © 1980 by Stuart F. Spicker. Published by Springer Publishing Company, Inc., New York. Used by permission.

has a moral right to determine what is done to his or her body, however difficult it may be to determine the precise nature, scope, and strength of that right. Or, imagine a strange person in a white uniform coming up to you and lecturing you about the health hazards of your smoking or lack of exercise. Well-intentioned though it might be, a natural response again might be, "What business is it of yours, what right do you have to lecture me about my health habits?" Again, the point would be that it is a person's right to act in ways detrimental to his health if he chooses to do so and bears the consequences of doing so. This particular right usually derives from some more general and basic right to privacy, liberty, or self-determination (autonomy). Yet both these actions, are, of course, of the sort frequently performed by nurses toward their patients. Likewise, any duties of a nurse to provide care to a particular person cannot derive simply from the duties she assumes in the nurse's role, nor can the right of a particular patient to nursing care from a specific nurse.

If we think of the nurse-patient relationship as arising from a contract or agreement between the nurse and her patient, then these otherwise problematic rights and duties become readily explicable. The patient contracts to have specified care provided by the nurse, in return for payment by the patient, and the patient in so doing grants permission to the nurse to perform actions (injections, tests, and the like) that she would otherwise have no right or duty to do. In agreeing to perform these duties, the nurse incurs an obligation to the patient to do so, as well as a right to be paid for doing so.

A natural objection to such an account is that it appears to rest on a fiction, since in the great majority of cases nurses and patients never in fact make any such agreement; rather, the patient finds himself in a physician's office, or in a hospital, where the nurse as a matter of course performs certain tasks, while the nurse, if she makes any such agreements at all, makes them with the physician or the hospital that employs her. This reflects the fact that the provision of health care is considerably more complex and institutionalized than any simple nurse-patient account would suggest, but it does not, in my view, show the contract or agreement model to be mistaken. The patient makes the agreement generally with the physician or the hospital's representative, and that agreement is to have a complex of services performed by a variety of health-care professionals. The nurse is an indirect

party to this agreement, and can become committed to it, by having contracted or agreed with the employing physician or hospital to perform a particular role in the health-care process.

A related objection to this account is that at these intervening agreement points, it is still often the case that the contract or agreement never takes place, certainly not to the extent that what is to be done is spelled out in any detail, and so the account still rests on a fiction. But these agreements can and do have implicit terms, terms which can be just as binding on the parties as if they had been explicitly spelled out. These implicit terms are to be found primarily in the generally known and accepted understanding of the nature of such health-care relationships, and in the warranted social expectations the involved parties have concerning who will do what in such relationships. The content of such expectations will in large part derive from the nature of the training of various health-care professionals, the professional codes and legal requirements governing their conduct, as well as more general public understandings of their roles.

Why insist on a contract or agreement model of the nurse-patient relationship that requires an appeal to agreements between intervening parties, as well as to implicit terms that are generally not spelled out? The reason is that such an account makes one fundamental point very clear. That is, that the right to determine what is done to and for the patient, and to control, within broad limits, the course of the patient's treatment and care, originates and generally remains with the patient. One important reason for insisting on this is that it is insufficiently appreciated and respected by health-care professionals. Many health-care professionals hold that if they reasonably believe that what they are doing is in the best interests of the patient, that is sufficient justification for doing it. However, in my view, this is a serious mistake because it does not take an adequate account of the patient's right to control the course of treatment.

An important part of at least one common understanding of the physician-patient relationship, and in turn of the patient's other health-care professional relationships (including, but not limited to, the nurse), is that the health-care professional will, with limited exceptions (e.g. public health problems arising from highly contagious diseases), act to promote the best interests of his or her patient. Treatment recommendations and decisions are to be made solely according to how they affect the interests of the patient, and ought not be influenced by the interests or convenience of others.[2] The patient's confidence that the health professional will act in this way is especially important because of the extreme vulnerability and apprehension the ill patient often feels, the patient's inability to provide his or her own necessary health care, and the patient's often very limited capacity to evaluate for himself whether a proposed course of treatment and care is in fact for the best. This focus on the patient's interests to the exclusion of others, however, is different from, and should not be confused with, physicians' or nurses' being justified in acting in whichever manner they reasonably believe to be in the patient's best interest.

The right of the physician or nurse to act in the patient's interest is *created* and *limited* by the permission or consent (from the patient-nurse/physician agreement) that the patient has given. To take two extremes, a patient might say to the physician or nurse, ''I want you to do whatever you think best, and don't bother me with the details,'' or the patient might insist on being fully informed about all factors and alternatives concerning the treatment and on retaining the right to reject any aspect of that treatment. In my view, should the patient desire it, either of these arrangements can be justifiable, as well as, of course, many modified versions of them. This has the important implication that the various expectations concerning what the health professional will do, which generally give content to the nurse-patient relationship, only partially determine that relationship. It is also subject to modification that is determined principally by what the patient desires of the relationship, and how he or she in turn constructs it. This is the other difficulty, besides their failure to explain how the relationship comes into being between particular persons, of the five alternatives mentioned above to the contract or agreement model of the nurse-patient relation. One cannot speak generally about the extent to which the nurse ought to act or has a duty to act, for example, as health educator or parent surrogate, because it ought to be the patient's right to determine in large part the extent to which the nurse is to take those roles. What the patient wants will often become clear only in the course of treatment, but to put the point in obligation language, the nurse's obligation is in large

part to accommodate herself to the patient's desires in these matters.

•   •   •

Consider the following cases:

Case 1. Patient A has requested his nurse to inform him fully of the nature of his condition and of the course of treatment prescribed for it. However, the treatment called for, and which the nurse believes will be most effective in his case, is such that given her knowledge of the patient, she believes that fully informing the patient will reduce his ability and willingness to cooperate in the treatment and so will significantly reduce the likely effectiveness of the treatment. What should she tell him?

Case 2. Patient B instructs his nurse that if his condition deteriorates beyond a specified point, he considers life no longer worth living and wishes all further life-sustaining treatment withdrawn. The nurse believes that life still has value even in such a deteriorated state, that it would be wrong for the patient deliberately to bring about his own death in this way, and, in turn, wrong for her to aid him in doing so. Should she follow his instructions?

Case 3. Patient C, after being fully informed of principal alternative treatments for his condition, has insisted on a course of treatment that the nurse has good reason to believe is effective in a substantially smaller proportion of cases than an alternative treatment procedure would be. She considers the additional risk in the rejected treatment, which seems to have affected the patient's choice, completely insignificant. Should she insist on the more effective treatment, for example, even by surreptitiously substituting it, if she is able to do so?

Each of these cases lacks sufficient detail to allow a full discussion of it, and in particular, each artificially ignores the presence and role of other health-care practitioners, most notably the physician, who is generally prominent if not paramount in such decision making. I shall bring the physician into the picture shortly, but the cases are instructive even in this over-simplified form. Case 3 is perhaps the least difficult. It would be permissible for any interested party, and a duty of the nurse according to her roles as health educator and healer, to discuss the treatment decision with her patient, and to attempt to convince him that he has made a serious mistake in his choice of treatments. But just as the patient should be free to refuse any treatment for his condition if he is competent and so decides, he is likewise entitled to select and have the treatment that the nurse (or physician, for that matter) would not choose if it were her choice; the point simply is that it is not her treatment and so not her choice. She has no moral (or professional) right to insist on a treatment the patient does not want, even if it is clearly the ''best'' treatment, and it would be still more seriously wrong to surreptitiously and deceptively substitute the treatment she prefers.

Case 2 can be somewhat more difficult because it may at least involve action in conflict with the nurse's moral views rather than a conflict over what course of action is, all things considered, medically advisable, as in Case 3. Case 2, of course, raises the controversial issue of euthanasia and the so-called right to die. This is a complex question that I have considered elsewhere, and here I only want to note that Case 2 involves only fully voluntary euthanasia, generally accepted to be the least morally controversial form of euthanasia.[3] I shall suppose here that a patient's right to control his treatment, and to refuse treatment he does not want, can include the right to order withdrawal of treatment even when that will have the known and intended consequence of terminating his life. If we interpret the nurse's view that life under the circumstances in question would still be worth living as merely her own view about what she would do in similar circumstances, then her view is relevant only to what she would do if she were the patient and nothing more; it entails nothing about what should be done where it is another's life and his attitude to it that is in question. She would not waive her right not to be killed in these circumstances, but the patient would and does, and it is his life and so his right that is in question. I would suggest as well that a mere difference over what it is best to do in the circumstances (apart from moral considerations) does not morally justify the nurse's refusal to honor the patient's expressed wishes. However, her difference with the patient may be a moral one; in particular she may hold as a basic moral principle that she has an inviolable moral duty not to kill deliberately an innocent human being. In that case, to assist in the withdrawal of treatment in order to bring about the patient's death will be according to her moral view a serious wrong, a serious evil. The nurse's professional obligations to provide care should not, in my view, be understood to

require her to do such, just as she should not be required to assist in abortions if she believes that fetuses are protected by a duty not to take deliberately an innocent human life. While there should be no requirement in general for her to participate in medical procedures that violate important moral principles that she holds, that of course in no way implies that another nurse who does not hold such duty-based views about killing should not assist in the withdrawal of treatment. (Of course, if she holds killing to be wrong because it violates a person's right not to be killed, then she will correctly reason that the patient in Case 2 has waived that right, and so no conflict between her moral views and what the patient wants will arise.)

Finally, consider Case 1. The ''Patient Bill of Rights'' proposed by the American Hospital Association specifically allows that ''when it is not medically advisable to give . . . information to the patient'' concerning his diagnosis, treatment, and prognosis, such information need only ''be made available to an appropriate person in his behalf'' but need not be given to the patient himself. This would seem clearly to permit the nurse to withhold the information from the patient in Case 1. However, I believe the Patient's Bill of Rights is mistaken on this point. This is a particular instance of a general overemphasis on and consequent overenlargement of the area in which health professionals should be permitted to act toward patients on the basis of their own judgment of the ''medical advisability'' of their action toward the patient. It is perhaps natural that health professionals, who are trained to provide medical care for patients and who undertake professional responsibilities to do so, should consider medical advisability a sufficient condition generally for acting contrary to a patient's wishes, and here for withholding relevant information from the patient. But once again, as long as we are dealing with patients who satisfy minimal conditions of competence to make decisions about their treatment, unless the patient has explicitly granted the nurse the right to withhold information he seeks when she considers it medically advisable to do so, medical advisability is not sufficient justification for doing so. Our moral right to control what is done to our body, and our right, in turn, not to be denied relevant available information for decisions about the exercise of that right, do not end at the point where others decide, even with good reason, that it is medically advisable for us not to be free to exercise that right. In general, one element of the moral respect owed competent adults is to respect, in the sense of honor, their right to make decisions of this sort even when their doing so may not be deemed medically advisable by others, and even when those others are health professionals generally in a better position to make an informed decision. When other health professionals are in a better position to make an informed decision, a patient may have good reason to transfer his rights to decide to them, or to allow himself to be strongly influenced by what they think best, but he is not required to do so, and so they have no such rights to decide for him what his treatment will be when he has not done so.

I want to emphasize that, in my view, moral rights generally, and in particular the rights of the patient relevant in the three cases above, are not absolute in the sense that they can never justifiably be overridden by competing moral considerations. But such justifiable overriding requires a special justification, and that human welfare generally, or the welfare of the person whose right is at issue, will be better promoted by violation of the right is *not* such a special justification.[4] Thus, rights need not be absolute in order to have an important place in moral reasoning. Cases involving young children and noncompetent adults are important instances where specifically paternalistic interference with a person's exercise of his rights can be justified.

Perhaps the point of emphasizing the contract or agreement between the patient and the health care professional is now a bit clearer. That contract model emphasizes the basis for and way in which the right to control the direction one's care will take ought to rest with the patient. It is not, of course, that the nurse is mistaken in taking her role to be a healer, or health educator, for these are important professional services she performs, but rather that her performance in these roles ought to be significantly constrained and circumscribed by the rights of her patients to control what is done to them and their bodies.

NURSE-PHYSICIAN/HOSPITAL RELATION

Until now, my discussion of the nurse's situation has focused on her relations with her patient, and this narrowed focus has made the discussion unrealistic in at least one important respect. Specifically, the fact that the nurse generally operates in a hierarchic, institutional setting in which she is in the employ of others—hospitals, physicians, and the like—has been ignored. Many of the moral uncertainties and conflicts that nurses experience concerning their duties and responsibilities derive from their role in this hierarchical structure, and from questions about their consequent authority to decide and act in particular matters. The patient has a place in such issues, but the issues do not arise when only the nurse and patient are considered. Now I want to fill in the picture some by considering briefly this nurse-physician/hospital relation. It might seem tempting to maintain that since the physician's and hospital's relation to the patient ought to be understood in terms of the same agreement or contract model as the nurse's, it ought to be possible to talk generally of the patient-health-care professional relationship. Differences in specific duties and rights of nurses as opposed to other health-care professionals would derive only from the division of labor and differentiation of function within the health-care setting. Since all health-care professionals ought equally to be constrained by the rights of the patient, and since all ought to advise, decide, and act on the basis of the interests and rights of the patient, there should be no conflict among health-care professionals in general, and among nurses and other health-care professionals in particular. There is, in principle, an important truth in this point, but I doubt that any nurse would recognize this as an accurate or realistic account, however oversimplified, of her situation, and so we must see where it goes wrong. The basic point is an obvious one. Conflicts arise because the nurse has conflicting roles, as agent for the patient but also as employee of the hospital or physician. These roles can conflict in at least two significantly different sorts of ways. First, the nurse can find herself in disagreement with other health-care professionals, in whose employ she is, over what is in fact best for the patient. Second, physicians, hospital administrators, and the like, as well as the nurse herself, have other roles and in turn other interests besides that of acting to serve the patient's health needs, and these interests can come into conflict with the patient's interests.

The potential for conflicts of both sorts for the nurse is probably increased by the relatively low degree of autonomy nurses currently possess in comparison with many other professionals. One aspect of the notion of a profession and professional is the assumption that there is a body of knowledge the professional has mastered, which others generally do not possess; this has contributed to the idea that professionals ought to be able to decide jointly with their clients how they will practice their profession with a high degree of autonomy and freedom from control and regulation by others outside the profession. Nurses, however, generally work for a hospital or physician, and so are largely under the direction and authority of that employer. This is unlike many other professionals like architects, lawyers, and physicians, who are either self-employed, or in the employ of the client whose interests are to be served. I suspect that this fact about the current status of nursing—a profession with an increasingly large body of technical knowledge that has been mastered, but with quite limited autonomy in acting on that professional knowledge without control and direction from others—contributes importantly to the uncertainty about its role and status to which nursing as a profession seems to be subject.

.   .   .

Consider a case similar to Case 1 above where a nurse is explicitly instructed by the attending physician to withhold certain information from the patient concerning his condition on the grounds that he believes it would be medically detrimental to the course of treatment for the patient to be fully informed. Suppose now that the patient asks the nurse for the withheld information. What kinds of considerations are relevant to the nurse's decision about what to do?

1. Is this physician's decision within accepted medical and hospital practice in this case? Is the nurse's following the physician's directive in cases of this sort required by accepted standards of professional nursing practice?

Only if the answer to one or both of these questions is negative will she be able to protest (e.g., to others in the hospital or medical hierarchy) about this particular order of the physician as opposed to general medical practice in such cases, or to be within her professional rights in acting contrary to his directive. If the answer is affirmative to both questions, then the nurse will have a professional duty to withhold the information as directed, though that will not fully settle the moral question.

2. Who ought to make decisions of this sort concerning withholding of information from patients?

The nurse may or may not believe that the existing decision-making process for such questions should be changed, quite apart from her views about what the content of the decisions made should be. Nurses commonly, and in my view rightly, argue that their role in health-care decision making should be increased from what it now is, and so this may be an area where appropriate action includes protest of and attempts to change the way such decisions are made; how such protest would most effectively be made, and to whom, depends on the context. However, change of the decision-making process is likely to be a long-term matter and so not helpful to her with the case at hand. Alternatively, she may not believe the decision-making process requires change at all, despite her disagreement with this particular decision.

3. What alternative courses of action are open to the nurse in the case at hand if she remains convinced the physician's directive is wrong, despite its accordance with existing medical practice?

Relevant alternatives include: discussing the issue with the physician in an attempt to get him to change his decision; protesting this decision to others in the medical hierarchy; acting on the physician's order while trying to change the decision process; acting contrary to the physician's directive with the likely personal loss involved, such as disciplinary action or loss of job; attempting to withdraw from the case; resigning her position, perhaps coupled with protests concerning the physician's action to others (e.g., the hospital and media). Which of these alternatives, or combinations of them, is the most advisable will depend on a variety of considerations such as the likelihood of her protest being effective, the personal cost to her in making it, the likely effect of her withdrawal from the case on what is done to the patient, and so forth.

Notice that none of the above depends directly on the issue being about withholding of information—these are considerations and alternatives that arise independently of what the specific conflict in roles concerns. However, the seriousness of the harm done to the patient by the action she has been ordered to perform will, of course, also be relevant to the nurse's overall decision. For example, if what had been ordered was "not to resuscitate," without the knowledge and against the will of the patient, a more serious wrong to the patient would be in prospect than in the case at hand, and a more serious obligation would fall on the nurse to attempt to prevent that wrong.

This very brief sketch of some morally relevant considerations in the decision about what to do in role conflicts and conflicts of duty that nurses face, does not take us very far toward resolutions of such conflicts. However, I believe no general, authoritative principles or pronouncements indicating how such conflicts should be resolved would be both helpful and defensible. Instead, once we recognize the pervasiveness of such role conflicts in nursing practice, the next step must be the detailed consideration of the concrete instances of these role conflicts in their full complexity and diversity.

1. I have drawn these from the very helpful paper by Sally Gadow, "Humanistic Issues at the Interface of Nursing and the Community." See *Connecticut Medicine*, Vol. 41, No. 6, June, 1977, pp. 357–361.

2. Such a view, with specific reference to the dying patient, is advocated in, among other places, Leon Kass, "Death as an Event: A Commentary on Robert Morrison," *Science*, 173, August 20, 1971, pp. 698–702. To what extent this account of the physician-patient relationship is defensible, or is in fact adhered to in practice by physicians, is problematic.

3. I have discussed some implications of a rights-based view for euthanasia in my "Moral Rights and Permissible Killing," in *Ethical Issues Relating to Life and Death*, (ed.) John Ladd, New York: Oxford University Press, 1979. See also the paper by Michael Tooley, "The Termination of Life: Some Moral Issues," in the same volume.

4. For one attempt to specify the general limits of such special justifications, see Ronald Dworkin, *Taking Rights Seriously*, Chap. 7 (Cambridge, 1977).

Involuntary Commitment

T H O M A S   S .   S Z A S Z

Involuntary Mental Hospitalization: A Crime Against Humanity

I

For some time now I have maintained that commitment—that is, the detention of persons in mental institutions against their will—is a form of imprisonment;[1] that such deprivation of liberty is contrary to the moral principles embodied in the Declaration of Independence and the Constitution of the United States;[2] and that it is a crass violation of contemporary concepts of fundamental human rights.[3] The practice of "sane" men incarcerating their "insane" fellow men in "mental hospitals" can be compared to that of white men enslaving black men. In short, I consider commitment a crime against humanity.

Existing social institutions and practices, espe-

cially if honored by prolonged usage, are generally experienced and accepted as good and valuable. For thousands of years slavery was considered a "natural" social arrangement for the securing of human labor; it was sanctioned by public opinion, religious dogma, church, and state;[4] it was abolished a mere one hundred years ago in the United States; and it is still a prevalent social practice in some parts of the world, notably in Africa.[5] Since its origin, approximately three centuries ago, commitment of the insane has enjoyed equally widespread support; physicians, lawyers, and the laity have asserted, as if with a single voice, the therapeutic desirability and social necessity of institutional psychiatry. My claim that commitment is a crime against humanity may thus be countered—as indeed it has been—by maintaining, first, that the practice is beneficial for the mentally ill, and second, that it is necessary for the protection of the mentally healthy members of society.

Illustrative of the first argument is Slovenko's assertion that "Reliance solely on voluntary hospital admission procedures ignores the fact that some persons may desire care and custody but cannot communicate their desire directly."[6] Imprisonment in mental hospitals is here portrayed—by a professor of law!—as a service provided to persons by the state because they "desire" it but do not know how to ask for it. Felix defends involuntary mental hospitalization by asserting simply, "We *do* [his italics] deal with illnesses of the mind."[7]

Illustrative of the second argument is Guttmacher's characterization of my book *Law, Liberty, and Psychiatry* as ". . .a pernicious book . . . certain to produce intolerable and unwarranted anxiety in the families of psychiatric patients."[8] This is an admission of the fact that the families of "psychiatric patients" frequently resort to the use of force in order to control their "loved ones," and that when attention is directed to this practice it creates embarrassment and guilt. On the other hand, Felix simply defines the psychiatrist's duty as the protection of society: "Tomorrow's psychiatrist will be, as is his counterpart today, one of the gatekeepers of his community."[9]

These conventional explanations of the nature and uses of commitment are, however, but culturally accepted justifications for certain quasi-medical forms of social control, exercised especially against individuals and groups whose behavior does not violate criminal laws but threatens established social values.

II

What is the evidence that commitment does not serve the purpose of helping or treating people whose behavior deviates from or threatens prevailing social norms or moral standards; and who, because they inconvenience their families, neighbors, or superiors, may be incriminated as "mentally ill"?

1. *The medical evidence.* Mental illness is a metaphor. If by "disease" we mean a disorder of the physiochemical machinery of the human body, then we can assert that what we call functional mental diseases are not diseases at all.[10] Persons said to be suffering from such disorders are socially deviant or inept, or in conflict with individuals, groups, or institutions. Since they do not suffer from disease, it is impossible to "treat" them for any sickness.

Although the term "mentally ill" is usually applied to persons who do not suffer from bodily disease, it is sometimes applied also to persons who do (for example, to individuals intoxicated with alcohol or other drugs, or to elderly people suffering from degenerative disease of the brain). However, when patients with demonstrable diseases of the brain are involuntarily hospitalized, the primary purpose is to exercise social control over their behavior;[11] treatment of the disease is, at best, a secondary consideration. Frequently, therapy is non-existent, and custodial care is dubbed "treatment."

In short, the commitment of persons suffering from "functional psychoses" serves moral and social, rather than medical and therapeutic, purposes. Hence, even if, as a result of future research, certain conditions now believed to be "functional" mental illnesses were to be shown to be "organic," my argument against involuntary mental hospitalization would remain unaffected.

2. *The moral evidence.* In free societies, the relationship between physician and patient is predicated on the legal presumption that the individual "owns" his body and his personality.[12] The physician can examine and treat a patient only with his consent; the latter is free to reject treatment (for example, an operation for cancer).[13] After death, "ownership" of the person's body is transferred to his heirs; the physician must obtain permission from the patient's relatives for a postmortem examination. John Stuart Mill explicitly affirmed that ". . . each person is the proper guardian of his own health, whether bodily, or mental and spiritual."[14] Commitment is incompatible with this moral principle.

3. *The historical evidence.* Commitment practices flourished long before there were any mental or psychiatric "treatments" of "mental diseases." Indeed, madness or mental illness was not always a necessary condition for commitment. For example, in the seventeenth century, "children of artisans and other poor inhabitants of Paris up to the age of 25, . . . girls who were debauched or in evident danger of being debauched, . . ." and other "misérables" of the community, such as epileptics, people with venereal diseases, and poor people with chronic diseases of all sorts, were all considered fit subjects for confinement in the Hôpital Général.[15] And, in 1860, when Mrs. Packard was incarcerated for disagreeing with her minister-husband,[16] the commitment laws of the State of Illinois explicitly proclaimed that ". . .

married women . . . may be entered or detained in the hospital at the request of the husband of the woman or the guardian. . ., without the evidence of insanity required in other cases.''[17] It is surely no coincidence that this piece of legislation was enacted and enforced at about the same time that Mill published his essay *The Subjection of Women*.[18]

4. *The literary evidence*. Involuntary mental hospitalization plays a significant part in numerous short stories and novels from many countries. In none that I have encountered is commitment portrayed as helpful to the hospitalized person; instead, it is always depicted as an arrangement serving interests antagonistic to those of the so-called patient.[19]

III

The claim that commitment of the "mentally ill" is necessary for the protection of the "mentally healthy" is more difficult to refute, not because it is valid, but because the danger that "mental patients" supposedly pose is of such an extremely vague nature.

1. *The medical evidence*. The same reasoning applies as earlier: If "mental illness" is not a disease, there is no medical justification for protection from disease. Hence, the analogy between mental illness and contagious disease falls to the ground: The justification for isolating or otherwise constraining patients with tuberculosis or typhoid fever cannot be extended to patients with "mental illness."

Moreover, because the accepted contemporary psychiatric view of mental illness fails to distinguish between illness as a biological condition and as a social role,[20] it is not only false, but also dangerously misleading, especially if used to justify social action. In this view, regardless of its "causes"—anatomical, genetic, chemical, psychological, or social—mental illness has "objective existence." A person either has or has not a mental illness; he is either mentally sick or mentally healthy. Even if a person is cast in the role of mental patient against his will, his "mental illness" exists "objectively"; and even if, as in the cases of the Very Important Person, he is never treated as a mental patient, his "mental illness" still exists "objectively"—apart from the activities of the psychiatrist.[21]

The upshot is that the term "mental illness" is perfectly suited for mystification: It disregards the crucial question of whether the individual assumes the role of mental patient voluntarily, and hence wishes to engage in some sort of interaction with the psychiatrist; or whether he is cast in that role against his will, and hence is opposed to such a relationship. This obscurity is then usually employed strategically, either by the subject himself to advance *his* interests, or by the subject's adversaries to advance *their* interests.

In contrast to this view, I maintain, first, that the involuntarily hospitalized mental patient is, by definition, the occupant of an ascribed role; and, second, that the "mental disease" of such a person—unless the use of this term is restricted to demonstrable lesions or malfunctions of the brain—is always the product of interaction between psychiatrist and patient.

2. *The moral evidence*. The crucial ingredient in involuntary mental hospitalization is coercion. Since coercion is the exercise of power, it is always a moral and political act. Accordingly, regardless of its medical justification, commitment is primarily a moral and political phenomenon—just as, regardless of its anthropological and economic justifications, slavery was primarily a moral and political phenomenon.

Although psychiatric methods of coercion are indisputably useful for those who employ them, they are clearly not indispensable for dealing with the problems that so-called mental patients pose for those about them. If an individual threatens others by virtue of his beliefs or actions, he could be dealt with by methods other than "medical"; if his conduct is ethically offensive, moral sanctions against him might be appropriate; if forbidden by law, legal sanctions might be appropriate. In my opinion, both informal, moral sanctions, such as social ostracism or divorce, and formal, judicial sanctions, such as fine and imprisonment, are more dignified and less injurious to the human spirit than the quasi-medical psychiatric sanction of involuntary mental hospitalization.[22]

3. *The historical evidence*. To be sure, confinement of so-called mentally ill persons does protect the community from certain problems. If it didn't, the arrangement would not have come into being and would not have persisted. However, the question we ought to ask is not *whether* commitment protects the community from "dangerous mental patients," but rather from precisely *what danger* it protects and by *what means?* In what way were prostitutes or vagrants dangerous in seventeenth-century Paris? Or married women in nineteenth-century Illinois?

It is significant, moreover, that there is hardly a prominent person who, during the past fifty years or so, has not been diagnosed by a psychiatrist as suffering from some type of "mental illness." Barry Goldwater was called a "paranoid schizophrenic";[23] Whittaker Chambers, a "psychopathic personality";[24] Woodrow Wilson, a "neurotic" frequently "very close to psychosis";[25] and Jesus, "a born degenerate" with a "fixed delusional system," and a "paranoid" with a "clinical picture [so typical] that is is hardly conceivable that people can even question the accuracy of the diagnosis."[26] The list is endless.

Sometimes, psychiatrists declare the same person sane *and* insane, depending on the political dictates of their superiors and the social demand of the moment. Before his trial and execution, Adolph Eichmann was examined by several psychiatrists, all of whom declared him to be normal; after he was put to death, "medical evidence" of his insanity was released and widely circulated.

According to Hannah Arendt, "Half a dozen psychiatrists had certified him [Eichmann] as 'normal.' " One psychiatrist asserted, ". . . his whole psychological outlook, his attitude toward his wife and children, mother and father, sisters and friends, was 'not only normal but most desirable.'. . ." And the minister who regularly visited him in prison declared that Eichmann was "a man with very positive ideas."[27] After Eichmann was executed, Gideon Hausner, the Attorney General of Israel, who had prosecuted him, disclosed in an article in *The Saturday Evening Post* that psychiatrists diagnosed Eichmann as " 'a man obsessed with a dangerous and insatiable urge to kill,' 'a perverted, sadistic personality.' "[28]

Whether or not men like those mentioned above are considered "dangerous" depends on the observer's religious beliefs, political convictions, and social situation. Furthermore, the "dangerousness" of such persons—whatever we may think of them—is not analogous to that of a person with tuberculosis or typhoid fever; nor would rendering such a person "non-dangerous" be comparable to rendering a patient with a contagious disease noninfectious.

In short, I hold—and I submit that the historical evidence bears me out—that people are committed to mental hospitals neither because they are "dangerous," nor because they are "mentally ill," but rather because they are society's scapegoats, whose persecution is justified by psychiatric propaganda and rhetoric.[29]

4. *The literary evidence.* No one contests that involuntary mental hospitalization of the so-called dangerously insane "protects" the community. Dis-

agreement centers on the nature of the threat facing society, and on the methods and legitimacy of the protection it employs. In this connection, we may recall that slavery, too, "protected" the community: it freed the slaveowners from manual labor. Commitment likewise shields the non-hospitalized members of society: first, from having to accommodate themselves to the annoying or idiosyncratic demands of certain members of the community who have not violated any criminal statutes; and, second, from having to prosecute, try, convict, and punish members of the community who have broken the law but who either might not be convicted in court, or, if they would be, might not be restrained as effectively or as long in prison as in a mental hospital. The literary evidence cited earlier fully supports this interpretation of the function of involuntary mental hospitalization.

IV

I have suggested that commitment constitutes a social arrangement whereby one part of society secures certain advantages for itself at the expense of another part. To do so, the oppressors must possess an ideology to justify their aims and actions; and they must be able to enlist the police power of the state to impose their will on the oppressed members. What makes such an arrangement a "crime against humanity"? It may be argued that the use of state power is legitimate when law-abiding citizens punish lawbreakers. What is the difference between this use of state power and its use in commitment?

In the first place, the difference between committing the "insane" and imprisoning the "criminal" is the same as that between the rule of man and the rule of law:[30] whereas the "insane" are subjected to the coercive controls of the state because persons more powerful than they have labeled them as "psychotic," "criminals" are subjected to such controls because because they have violated legal rules applicable equally to all.

The second difference between these two proceedings lies in their professed aims. The principal purpose of imprisoning criminals is to protect the liberties of the law-abiding members of society.[31] Since the individual subject to commitment is not considered a threat to liberty in the same way as the accused criminal is (if he were, he would be prosecuted), his removal from society cannot be justified on the same grounds. Justification for commitment must thus rest on its therapeutic promise and potential: it will help restore the "patient" to "mental health." But if this can be accomplished only at the cost of robbing the individual of liberty, "involuntary mental hospitalization" becomes only a verbal camouflage for what is, in effect, punishment. This "therapeutic" punishment differs, however, from traditional judicial punishment, in that the accused criminal enjoys a rich panoply of constitutional protections against false accusation and oppressive prosecution, whereas the accused mental patient is deprived of these protections.[32]

.   .   .

V

A basic assumption of American slavery was that the Negro was racially inferior to the Caucasian. "There is no malice toward the Negro in Ulrich Phillips' work," wrote Stanley Elkins about the author's book *American Negro Slavery,* a work sympathetic with the Southern position. "Phillips was deeply fond of the Negroes as a people; it was just that he could not take them seriously as men and women; they were children."[33]

Similarly, the basic assumption of institutional psychiatry is that the mentally ill person is psychologically and socially inferior to the mentally healthy. He is like a child: he does not know what is in his best interests and therefore needs others to control and protect him.[34] Psychiatrists often care deeply for their involuntary patients, whom they consider—in contrast with the merely "neurotic" persons—"psychotic," which is to say, "very sick." Hence, such patients must be cared for as the "irresponsible children" they are considered to be.

The perspective of paternalism has played an exceedingly important part in justifying both slavery and involuntary mental hospitalization. Aristotle defined slavery as "an essentially domestic relationship"; in so doing, wrote Davis, he "endowed it with the sanction of paternal authority, and helped to establish a precedent that would govern discussions of political philosophers as late as the eighteenth century."[35] The relationship between psychiatrists and mental patients has been and continues to be viewed in the same way. "If a man brings his daughter to me from California," declares Braceland, "because she is in manifest danger of falling into vice or in some way disgracing herself, he doesn't expect me to let her loose in my hometown for that same thing to happen."[36] Indeed,

almost any article or book dealing with the "care" of involuntary mental patients may be cited to illustrate the contention that physicians fall back on paternalism to justify their coercive control over the uncooperative patient. "Certain cases" [not individuals!]—writes Solomon in an article on suicide— ". . . must be considered irresponsible, not only with respect to violent impulses, but also in all medical matters." In this class, which he labels "The Irresponsible," he places "Children," "The Mentally Retarded," "The Psychotic," and "The Severely or Terminally Ill." Solomon's conclusion is that "Repugnant though it may be, he [the physician] may have to act against the patient's wishes in order to protect the patient's life and that of others."[37] The fact that, as in the case of slavery, the physician needs the police power of the state to maintain his relationship with his involuntary patient does not alter this self-serving image of institutional psychiatry.

Paternalism is the crucial explanation for the stubborn contradiction and conflict about whether the practices employed by slaveholders and institutional psychiatrists are "therapeutic" or "noxious." Masters and psychiatrists profess their benevolence; their slaves and involuntary patients protest against their malevolence. As Seymour Halleck puts it: ". . . the psychiatrist experiences himself as a helping person, but his patient may see him as a jailer. Both views are partially correct."[38] Not so. Both views are completely correct. Each is a proposition about a different subject: the former, about the psychiatrist's self-image; the latter, about the involuntary mental patient's image of his captor.

NOTES

1. Szasz, T. S.: "Commitment of the mentally ill: Treatment or social restraint?" *J. Nerv. & Ment. Dis.* 125:293–307 (Apr.-June) 1957.

2. Szasz, T. S.: *Law, Liberty, and Psychiatry: An Inquiry into the Social Uses of Mental Health Practices* (New York: Macmillan, 1963), pp. 149–90.

3. *Ibid.*, pp. 223–55.

4. Davis, D. B.: *The Problem of Slavery in Western Culture* (Ithaca, N.Y.: Cornell University Press, 1966).

5. See Cohen, R.: "Slavery in Africa." *Trans-Action* 4:44–56 (Jan.–Feb.), 1967; Tobin, R.L.: "Slavery still plagues the earth." *Saturday Review,* May 6, 1967, pp. 24–25.

6. Slovenko, R.: "The psychiatric patient, liberty, and the law." *Amer. J. Psychiatry,* 121:534–39 (Dec.), 1964, p. 536.

7. Felix, R. H.: "The image of the psychiatrist: Past, present, and future." *Amer. J. Psychiatry,* 121:318–22 (Oct.), 1964, p. 320.

8. Guttmacher, M. S.: "Critique of views of Thomas Szasz on legal psychiatry." *AMA Arch. Gen. Psychiatry,* 10:238–45 (March), 1964, p. 244.

9. Felix, op. cit., p. 231.

10. See Szasz, T. S.: "The myth of mental illness." This volume [original source] pp. 12–24; *The Myth of Mental Illness: Foundations of a Theory of Personal Conduct* (New York: Hoeber-Harper, 1961); "Mental illness is a myth." *The New York Times Magazine,* June 12, 1966, pp. 30 and 90–92.

11. See, for example, Noyes, A. P.: *Modern Clinical Psychiatry,* 4th ed. (Philadelphia: Saunders, 1956), p. 278.

12. Szasz, T. S.: "The ethics of birth control; or, who owns your body?" *The Humanist,* 20:332–36 (Nov.–Dec.) 1960.

13. Hirsch, B. D.: "Informed consent to treatment," in Averbach, A. and Belli, M. M., eds., *Tort and Medical Yearbook* (Indianapolis: Bobbs-Merrill, 1961), Vol. I, pp. 631–38.

14. Mill, J.S.: *On Liberty* [1859] (Chicago: Regnery, 1955), p. 18.

15. Rosen, G.: "Social attitudes to irrationality and madness in 17th and 18th century Europe." *J. Hist. Med. & Allied Sciences,* 18:220–40 (1963), p. 223.

16. Packard, E. W. P.: *Modern Persecution, or Insane Asylums Unveiled,* 2 Vols. (Hartford: Case, Lockwood, and Brainard, 1873).

17. Illinois Statute Book, Sessions Laws 15, Section 10, 1851. Quoted in Packard, E. P. W.: *The Prisoner's Hidden Life* (Chicago: published by the author, 1868), p. 37.

18. Mill, J. S.: *The Subjection of Women* [1869] (London: Dent, 1965).

19. See, for example, Chekhov, A.P.: *Ward No. 6,* [1892], in *Seven Short Novels by Chekhov* (New York: Bantam Books, 1963), pp. 106–57; De Assis, M.: *The Psychiatrist* [1881–82], in De Assis, M., *The Psychiatrist and Other Stories* (Berkeley and Los Angeles: University of California Press, 1963), pp. 1–45; London, J.: *The Iron Heel* [1907] (New York: Sagamore Press, 1957); Porter, K. A.: *Noon Wine* [1937], in Porter, K. A., *Pale Horse, Pale Rider: Three Short Novels* (New York: Signet, 1965), pp. 62–112; Kesey, K.: *One Flew Over the Cuckoo's Nest* (New York: Viking, 1962); Tarsis, V.: *Ward 7: An Autobiographical Novel* (London and Glasgow: Collins and Harvill, 1965).

20. See Szasz, T. S.: "Alcoholism: A socio-ethical perspective." *Western Medicine,* 7:15–21 (Dec.) 1966.

21. See, for example, Rogow, A. A.: *James Forrestal: A Study of Personality, Politics, and Policy* (New York: Macmillan, 1964); for a detailed criticism of this view, see Szasz, T. S.: "Psychiatric classification as a strategy of personal constraint." This volume [original source] pp. 190–217.

22. Szasz, T. S.: *Psychiatric Justice* (New York: Macmillan, 1965).

23. "The Unconscious of a Conservative: A Special Issue on the Mind of Barry Goldwater." *Fact,* Sept.–Oct. 1964.

24. Zeligs, M. A.: *Friendship and Fratricide: An Analysis of Whittaker Chambers and Alger Hiss* (New York: Viking, 1967).

25. Freud, S., and Bullitt, W. C.: *Thomas Woodrow Wilson: A Psychological Study* (Boston: Houghton Mifflin, 1967).

26. Quoted in Schweitzer, A.: *The Psychiatric Study of Jesus* [1913] transl. by Charles R. Joy (Boston: Beacon Press, 1956), pp. 37, 40–41.

27. Arendt, H.: *Eichmann in Jerusalem: A Report on the Banality of Evil* (New York: Viking, 1963), p. 22.

28. *Ibid.,* pp. 22–23.

29. For a full articulation and documentation of this thesis, see Szasz, T. S.: *The Manufacture of Madness: A Comparative Study of the Inquisition and the Mental Health Movement* (New York: Harper & Row, 1970).

30. Hayek, F.A.: *The Constitution of Liberty* (Chicago: University of Chicago Press, 1960), especially pp. 162–92.

31. Mabbott, J.D.: "Punishment" [1939], in Olafson, F.A., ed., *Justice and Social Policy: A Collection of Essays* (Englewood Cliffs, N.J.: Prentice-Hall, 1961), pp. 39–54.

32. For documentation, see Szasz, T. S.: *Law, Liberty, and Psychiatry: An Inquiry into the Social Uses of Mental Health Practices* (New York: Macmillan, 1963); *Psychiatric Justice* (New York: Macmillan, 1965).

33. Elkins, S. M.: *Slavery: A Problem in American Institutional and Intellectual Life* [1959] (New York: Universal Library, 1963), p. 10.

34. See, for example, Linn, L.: *A Handbook of Hospital Psychiatry* (New York: International Universities Press, 1955), pp. 420–22; Braceland, F. J.: Statement, in *Constitutional Rights of the Mentally Ill* (Washington, D.C.: U. S. Government Printing Office, 1961), pp. 63–74; Rankin, R. S. and Dallmayr, W. B.: "Rights of Patients in Mental Hospitals," in *Constitutional Rights of the Mentally Ill, supra,* pp. 329–70.

35. Davis, op. cit., p. 69.

36. Braceland, op. cit., p. 71.

37. Solomon, P.: "The burden of responsibility in suicide." *JAMA,* 199:321–24 (Jan. 30), 1967.

38. Halleck, S.L.: *Psychiatry and the Dilemmas of Crime* (New York: Harper & Row, 1967), p. 230.

PAUL CHODOFF

The Case for Involuntary Hospitalization of the Mentally Ill

I will begin this paper with a series of vignettes designed to illustrate graphically the question that is my focus: under what conditions, if any, does society have the right to apply coercion to an individual to hospitalize him against his will, by reason of mental illness?

Case 1. A woman in her mid 50s, with no previous overt behavioral difficulties, comes to believe that she is worthless and insignificant. She is completely preoccupied with her guilt and is increasingly unavailable for the ordinary demands of life. She eats very little because of her conviction that the food should go to others whose need is greater than hers, and her physical condition progressively deteriorates. Although she will talk to others about herself, she insists that she is not sick, only bad. She refuses medication, and when hospitalization is suggested she also refuses that on the grounds that she would be taking up space that otherwise could be occupied by those who merit treatment more than she.

Case 2. For the past 6 years the behavior of a 42-year-old woman has been disturbed for periods of 3 months or longer. After recovery from her most recent episode she has been at home, functioning at a borderline level. A month ago she again started to withdraw from her environment. She pays increasingly less attention to her bodily needs, talks very little, and does not respond to questions or attention from those about her. She lapses into a mute state and lies in her bed in a totally passive fashion. She does not respond to other people, does not eat, and does not void. When her arm is raised from the bed it remains for several minutes in the position in which it is left. Her medical history and a physical examination reveal no evidence of primary physical illness.

Case 3. A man with a history of alcoholism has been on a binge for several weeks. He remains at

home doing little else than drinking. He eats very little. He becomes tremulous and misinterprets spots on the wall as animals about to attack him, and he complains of "creeping" sensations in his body, which he attributes to infestation by insects. He does not seek help voluntarily, insists there is nothing wrong with him, and despite his wife's entreaties he continues to drink.

Case 4. Passersby and station personnel observe that a young woman has been spending several days at Union Station in Washington, D.C. Her behavior appears strange to others. She is finally befriended by a newspaper reporter who becomes aware that her perception of her situation is profoundly unrealistic and that she is, in fact, delusional. He persuades her to accompany him to St. Elizabeths Hospital, where she is examined by a psychiatrist who recommends admission. She refuses hospitalization and the psychiatrist allows her to leave. She returns to Union Station. A few days later she is found dead, murdered, on one of the surrounding streets.

Case 5. A government attorney in his late 30s begins to display pressured speech and hyperactivity. He is too busy to sleep and eats very little. He talks rapidly, becomes irritable when interrupted, and makes phone calls all over the country in furtherance of his political ambitions, which are to begin a campaign for the Presidency of the United States. He makes many purchases, some very expensive, thus running through a great deal of money. He is rude and tactless to his friends, who are offended by his behavior, and his job is in jeopardy. In spite of his wife's pleas he insists that he does not have the time to seek or accept treatment, and he refuses hospitalization. This is not the first such disturbance for this individual; in fact, very similar episodes have been occurring at roughly 2-year intervals since he was 18 years old.

Case 6. Passersby in a campus area observe two young women standing together, staring at each

Reprinted with permission of the author and the publisher from *American Journal of Psychiatry,* Vol. 133, No. 5 (May 1976), pp. 496–501. Copyright 1976, the American Psychiatric Association.

other, for over an hour. Their behavior attracts attention, and eventually the police take the pair to a nearby precinct station for questioning. They refuse to answer questions and sit mutely, staring into space. The police request some type of psychiatric examination but are informed by the city attorney's office that state law (Michigan) allows persons to be held for observation only if they appear obviously dangerous to themselves or others. In this case, since the women do not seem homicidal or suicidal, they do not qualify for observation and are released.

Less than 30 hours later the two women are found on the floor of their campus apartment, screaming and writhing in pain with their clothes ablaze from a self-made pyre. One woman recovers; the other dies. There is no conclusive evidence that drugs were involved.[1]

Most, if not all, people would agree that the behavior described in these vignettes deviates significantly from even elastic definitions of normality. However, it is clear that there would not be a similar consensus on how to react to this kind of behavior and that there is a considerable and increasing ferment about what attitude the organized elements of our society should take toward such individuals. Everyone has a stake in this important issue, but the debate about it takes place principally among psychiatrists, lawyers, the courts, and law enforcement agencies.

Points of view about the question of involuntary hospitalization fall into the following three principal groups: the "abolitionists," medical model psychiatrists, and civil liberties lawyers.

THE ABOLITIONISTS

Those holding this position would assert that in none of the cases I have described should involuntary hospitalization be a viable option because, quite simply, it should never be resorted to under any circumstances. As Szasz[2] has put it, "we should value liberty more highly than mental health no matter how defined" and "no one should be deprived of his freedom for the sake of his mental health." Ennis[3] has said that the goal "is nothing less than the abolition of involuntary hospitalization."

Prominent among the abolitionists are the "antipsychiatrists," who, somewhat surprisingly, count in their ranks a number of well-known psychiatrists. For them mental illness simply does not exist in the field of psychiatry.[4] They reject entirely the medical model of mental illness and insist that acceptance of it relies on a fiction accepted jointly by the state and by psychiatrists as a device for exerting social control over annoying or unconventional people. The antipsychiatrists hold that these people ought to be afforded the dignity of being held responsible for their behavior and required to accept its consequences. In addition, some members of this group believe that the phenomena of "mental illness" often represent essentially a tortured protest against the insanities of an irrational society.[5] They maintain that society should not be encouraged in its oppressive course by affixing a pejorative label to its victims.

Among the abolitionists are some civil liberties lawyers who both assert their passionate support of the magisterial importance of individual liberty and react with repugnance and impatience to what they see as the abuses of psychiatric practice in this field—the commitment of some individuals for flimsy and possibly self-serving reasons and their inhuman warehousing in penal institutions wrongly called "hospitals."

The abolitionists do not oppose psychiatric treatment when it is conducted with the agreement of those being treated. I have no doubt that they would try to gain the consent of the individuals described earlier to undergo treatment, including hospitalization. The psychiatrists in this group would be very likely to confine their treatment methods to psychotherapeutic efforts to influence the aberrant behavior. They would be unlikely to use drugs and would certainly eschew such somatic therapies as ECT*. If efforts to enlist voluntary compliance with treatment failed, the abolitionists would not employ any means of coercion. Instead, they would step aside and allow social, legal, and community sanctions to take their course. If a human being should be jailed or a human life lost as a result of this attitude, they would accept it as a necessary evil to be tolerated in order to avoid the greater evil of unjustified loss of liberty for others.[6]

THE MEDICAL MODEL PSYCHIATRISTS

I use this admittedly awkward and not entirely accurate label to designate the position of a substantial number of psychiatrists. They believe that mental illness is a meaningful concept and that under certain conditions its existence justifies the state's exercise, under the doctrine of *parens patriae*, of its right and obligation to arrange for the hospitalization of the sick

*Ed. note: Electroconvulsive therapy.

individual even though coercion is involved and he is deprived of his liberty. I believe that these psychiatrists would recommend involuntary hospitalization for all six of the patients described earlier.

THE MEDICAL MODEL

There was a time, before they were considered to be ill, when individuals who displayed the kind of behavior I described earlier were put in "ships of fools" to wander the seas or were left to the mercies, sometimes tender but often savage, of uncomprehending communities that regarded them as either possessed or bad. During the Enlightenment and the early nineteenth century, however, these individuals gradually came to be regarded as sick people to be included under the humane and caring umbrella of the Judeo-Christian attitude toward illness. This attitude, which may have reached its height during the era of moral treatment in the early nineteenth century, has had unexpected and ambiguous consequences. It became overextended and partially perverted, and these excesses led to the reaction that is so strong a current in today's attitude toward mental illness.

However, reaction itself can go too far, and I believe that this is already happening. Witness the disastrous consequences of the precipitate dehospitalization that is occurring all over the country. To remove the protective mantle of illness from these disturbed people is to expose them, their families, and their communities to consequences that are certainly maladaptive and possibly irreparable. Are we really acting in accordance with their best interests when we allow them to "die with their rights on"[1] or when we condemn them to a "preservation of liberty which is actually so destructive as to constitute another form of imprisonment"[7]? Will they not suffer "if [a] liberty they cannot enjoy is made superior to a health that must sometimes be forced on them"[8]?

Many of those who reject the medical model out of hand as inapplicable to so-called "mental illness" have tended to oversimplify its meaning and have, in fact, equated it almost entirely with organic disease. It is necessary to recognize that it is a complex concept and that there is a lack of agreement about its meaning. Sophisticated definitions of the medical model do not require only the demonstration of unequivocal organic pathology. A broader formulation, put forward by sociologists and deriving largely from Talcott Parsons' description of the sick role,[9] extends the domain of illness to encompass certain forms of social deviance as well as biological disorders. According to this definition, the medical model is characterized not only by organicity but also by being negatively valued by society, by "non-voluntariness," thus exempting its exemplars from blame, and by the understanding that physicians are the technically competent experts to deal with its effects.[10]

Except for the question of organic disease, the patients I described earlier conform well to this broader conception of the medical model. They are all suffering both emotionally and physically, they are incapable by an effort of will of stopping or changing their destructive behavior, and those around them consider them to be in an undesirable sick state and to require medical attention.

Categorizing the behavior of these patients as involuntary may be criticized as evidence of an intolerably paternalistic and antitherapeutic attitude that fosters the very failure to take responsibility for their lives and behavior that the therapist should uncover rather than encourage. However, it must also be acknowledged that these severely ill people are not capable at a conscious level of deciding what is best for themselves and that in order to help them examine their behavior and motivation, it is necessary that they be alive and available for treatment. Their verbal message that they will not accept treatment may at the same time be conveying other more covert messages—that they are desperate and want help even though they cannot ask for it.[11]

Although organic pathology may not be the only determinant of the medical model, it is of course an important one and it should not be avoided in any discussion of mental illness. There would be no question that the previously described patient with delirium tremens is suffering from a toxic form of brain disease. There are a significant number of other patients who require involuntary hospitalization because of organic brain syndrome due to various causes. Among those who are not overtly organically ill, most of the candidates for involuntary hospitalization suffer from schizophrenia or one of the major affective disorders. A growing and increasingly impressive body of evidence points to the presence of an important genetic-biological factor in these conditions; thus, many of them qualify on these grounds as illnesses.

Despite the revisionist efforts of the anti-psychiatrists, mental illness *does* exist. It does not by any means include all of the people being treated by psychiatrists (or by nonpsychiatrist physicians), but it does encompass those few desperately sick people for whom involuntary commitment must be considered. In the words of a recent article. "The problem is that mental illness is not a myth. It is not some palpable falsehood propagated among the populace by power-mad psychiatrists, but a cruel and bitter reality that has been with the human race since antiquity."[12]

CRITERIA FOR INVOLUNTARY HOSPITALIZATION

Procedures for involuntary hospitalization should be instituted for individuals who require care and treatment because of diagnosable mental illness that produces symptoms, including marked impairment in judgment, that disrupt their intrapsychic and interpersonal functioning. All three of these criteria must be met before involuntary hospitalization can be instituted.

1. Mental Illness. This concept has already been discussed, but it should be repeated that only a belief in the existence of illness justifies involuntary commitment. It is a fundamental assumption that makes aberrant behavior a medical matter and its care the concern of physicians.

2. Disruption of functioning. This involves combinations of serious and often obvious disturbances that are both intrapsychic (for example, the suffering of severe depression) and interpersonal (for example, withdrawal from others because of depression). It does not include minor peccadilloes or eccentricities. Furthermore, the behavior in question must represent symptoms of the mental illness from which the patient is suffering. Among these symptoms are actions that are imminently or potentially dangerous in a physical sense to self or others, as well as other manifestations of mental illness such as those in the cases I have described. This is not to ignore dangerousness as a criterion for commitment but rather to put it in its proper place as one of a number of symptoms of the illness. A further manifestation of the illness, and indeed, the one that makes involuntary rather than voluntary hospitalization necessary, is impairment of the patient's judgment to such a degree that he is unable to consider his condition and make decisions about it in his own interests.

3. Need for care and treatment. The goal of physicians is to treat and cure their patients; however, sometimes they can only ameliorate the suffering of their patients and sometimes all they can offer is care. It is not possible to predict whether someone will respond to treatment; nevertheless, the need for treatment and the availability of facilities to carry it out constitute essential preconditions that must be met to justify requiring anyone to give up his freedom. If mental hospital patients have a right to treatment, then psychiatrists have a right to ask for treatability as a front-door as well as a back-door criterion for commitment.[7] All of the six individuals I described earlier could have been treated with a reasonable expectation of return to a more normal state of functioning.

I believe that the objections to this formulation can be summarized as follows:

1. The whole structure founders for those who maintain that mental illness is a fiction.

2. These criteria are also untenable to those who hold liberty to be such a supreme value that the presence of mental illness per se does not constitute justification for depriving an individual of his freedom; only when such illness is manifested by clearly dangerous behavior may commitment be considered. For reasons to be discussed later, I agree with those psychiatrists[13,14] who do not believe that dangerousness should be elevated to primacy above other manifestations of mental illness as a *sine qua non* for involuntary hospitalization.

3. The medical model criteria are "soft" and subjective and depend on the fallible judgment of psychiatrists. This is a valid objection. There is no reliable blood test for schizophrenia and no method for injecting grey cells into psychiatrists. A relatively small number of cases will always fall within a grey area that will be difficult to judge. In those extreme cases in which the question of commitment arises, competent and ethical psychiatrists should be able to use these criteria without doing violence to individual liberties and with the expectation of good results. Furthermore, the possible "fuzziness" of some aspects of the medical model approach is certainly no greater than that of the supposedly "objective" criteria for dangerousness, and there is little reason to believe that lawyers and judges are any less fallible than psychiatrists.

4. Commitment procedures in the hands of psychiatrists are subject to intolerable abuses. Here, as Peszke said, "It is imperative that we differentiate between the principle of the process of civil commitment and the practice itself."[13] Abuses can contaminate both the medical and the dangerousness approaches, and I believe that the abuses stemming from the abolitionist view of no commitment at all are even greater. Measures to abate abuses of the medical ap-

proach include judicial review and the abandonment of indeterminate commitment. In the course of commitment proceedings and thereafter, patients should have access to competent and compassionate legal counsel. However, this latter safeguard may itself be subject to abuse if the legal counsel acts solely in the adversary tradition and undertakes to carry out the patient's wishes even when they may be destructive.

COMMENT

The criteria and procedures outlined will apply most appropriately to initial episodes and recurrent attacks of mental illness. To put it simply, it is necessary to find a way to satisfy legal and humanitarian considerations and yet allow psychiatrists access to initially or acutely ill patients in order to do the best they can for them. However, there are some involuntary patients who have received adequate and active treatment but have not responded satisfactorily. An irreducible minimum of such cases, principally among those with brain disorders and process schizophrenia, will not improve sufficiently to be able to adapt to even a tolerant society.

The decision of what to do at this point is not an easy one, and it should certainly not be in the hands of psychiatrists alone. With some justification they can state that they have been given the thankless job of caring, often with inadequate facilities, for badly damaged people and that they are now being subjected to criticism for keeping these patients locked up. No one really knows what to do with these patients. It may be that when treatment has failed they exchange their sick role for what has been called the impaired role,[15] which implies a permanent negative evaluation of them coupled with a somewhat less benign societal attitude. At this point, perhaps a case can be made for giving greater importance to the criteria for dangerousness and releasing such patients if they do not pose a threat to others. However, I do not believe that the release into the community of these severely malfunctioning individuals will serve their interests even though it may satisfy formal notions of right and wrong.

It should be emphasized that the number of individuals for whom involuntary commitment must be considered is small (although, under the influence of current pressures, it may be smaller than it should be). Even severe mental illness can often be handled by securing the cooperation of the patient, and certainly one of the favorable effects of the current ferment has been to encourage such efforts. However, the distinction between voluntary and involuntary hospitalization is sometimes more formal than meaningful. How "voluntary" are the actions of an individual who is being buffeted by the threats, entreaties, and tears of his family?

I believe, however, that we are at a point (at least in some jurisdictions) where, having rebounded from an era in which involuntary commitment was too easy and employed too often, we are now entering one in which it is becoming very difficult to commit anyone, even in urgent cases. Faced with the moral obloquy that has come to pervade the atmosphere in which the decision to involuntarily hospitalize is considered, some psychiatrists, especially younger ones, have become, as Stone[16] put it, "soft as grapes" when faced with the prospect of committing anyone under any circumstances.

THE CIVIL LIBERTIES LAWYERS

I use this admittedly inexact label to designate those members of the legal profession who do not in principle reject the necessity for involuntary hospitalization but who do reject or wish to diminish the importance of medical model criteria in the hands of psychiatrists. Accordingly, the civil liberties lawyers, in dealing with the problem of involuntary hospitalization, have enlisted themselves under the standard of dangerousness, which they hold to be more objective and capable of being dealt with in a sounder evidentiary manner than the medical model criteria. For them the question is not whether mental illness, even of disabling degree, is present, but only whether it has resulted in the probability of behavior dangerous to others or to self. Thus they would scrutinize the cases previously described for evidence of such dangerousness and would make the decision about involuntary hospitalization accordingly. They would probably feel that commitment is not indicated in most of these cases, since they were selected as illustrative of severe mental illness in which outstanding evidence of physical dangerousness was not present.

The dangerousness standard is being used increasingly not only to supplement criteria for mental illness but, in fact, to replace them entirely. The recent Supreme Court decision in *O'Connor v. Donaldson*[17] is certainly a long step in this direction. In addition, "dangerousness" is increasingly being understood to refer to the probability that the individual will inflict harm on himself or others in a specific physical manner rather than in other ways. This tendency has perhaps been carried to its ultimate in the *Lessard v. Schmidt* case[18] in Wisconsin, which restricted suitability for commitment to the "extreme likelihood that if the person is not confined, he will do immediate harm to himself or others." (This decision was set aside by the U.S. Supreme Court in 1974.) In a recent Washington, D.C., Superior Court case[19] the instructions to the jury stated that the government must prove that the defendant was likely to cause "substantial physical harm to himself or others in the reasonably foreseeable future."

For the following reasons, the dangerousness standard is an inappropriate and dangerous indicator to use in judging the conditions under which someone should be involuntarily hospitalized. Dangerousness is being taken out of its proper context as one among other symptoms of the presence of severe mental illness that should be the determining factor.

1. To concentrate on dangerousness (especially to others) as the sole criterion for involuntary hospitalization deprives many mentally ill persons of the protection and treatment that they urgently require. A psychiatrist under the constraints of the dangerousness rule, faced with an out-of-control manic individual whose frantic behavior the psychiatrist truly believes to be a disguised call for help, would have to say, "Sorry, I would like to help you but I can't because you haven't threatened anybody and you are not suicidal." Since psychiatrists are admittedly not very good at accurately predicting dangerousness to others, the evidentiary standards for commitment will be very stringent. This will result in mental hospitals becoming prisons for a small population of volatile, highly assaultive, and untreatable patients.[14]

2. The attempt to differentiate rigidly (especially in regard to danger to self) between physical and other kinds of self-destructive behavior is artificial, unrealistic, and unworkable. It will tend to confront psychiatrists who want to help their patients with the same kind of dilemma they were faced with when justification for therapeutic abortion on psychiatric grounds depended on evidence of suicidal intent. The advocates of the dangerousness standard seem to be more comfortable with and pay more attention to the factor of dangerousness to others even though it is a much less frequent and much less significant consequence of mental illness than is danger to self.

3. The emphasis on dangerousness (again, especially to others) is a real obstacle to the right-to-treatment movement since it prevents the hospitalization and therefore the treatment of the population most amenable to various kinds of therapy.

4. Emphasis on the criterion of dangerousness to others moves involuntary commitment from a civil to a criminal procedure, thus, as Stone[14] put it, imposing the procedures of one terrible system on another. Involuntary commitment on these grounds becomes a form of preventive detention and makes the psychiatrist a kind of glorified policeman.

5. Emphasis on dangerousness rather than mental disability and helplessness will hasten the process of deinstitutionalization. Recent reports[20,21] have shown that these patients are not being rehabilitated and reintegrated into the community, but rather, that the burden of custodialism has been shifted from the hospital to the community.

6. As previously mentioned, emphasis on the dangerousness criterion may be a tactic of some of the abolitionists among the civil liberties lawyers[22] to end involuntary hospitalization by reducing it to an unworkable absurdity.

DISCUSSION

It is obvious that it is good to be at liberty and that it is good to be free from the consequences of disabling and dehumanizing illness. Sometimes these two values are incompatible, and in the heat of the passions that are often aroused by opposing views of right and wrong, the partisans of each view may tend to minimize the importance of the other. Both sides can present their horror stories—the psychiatrists, their dead victims of the failure of the involuntary hospitalization process, and the lawyers, their Donaldsons. There is a real danger that instead of acknowledging the difficulty of the problem, the two camps will become polarized, with a consequent rush toward extreme and untenable solutions rather than working toward reasonable ones.

The path taken by those whom I have labeled the abolitionists is an example of the barren results that ensue when an absolute solution is imposed on a complex problem. There are human beings who will suffer greatly if the abolitionists succeed in elevating an abstract principle into an unbreakable law with no exceptions. I find myself oppressed and repelled by their position, which seems to stem from an ideological rigidity which ignores that element of the contingent immanent in the structure of human existence. It is devoid of compassion.

The positions of those who espouse the medical model and the dangerousness approaches to commitment are, one hopes, not completely irreconcilable. To some extent these differences are a result of the vantage points from which lawyers and psychiatrists view mental illness and commitment. The lawyers see and are concerned with the failures and abuses of the process. Furthermore, as a result of their training, they tend to apply principles to classes of people rather than to take each instance as unique. The psychiatrists, on the other hand, are required to deal practically with the singular needs of individuals. They approach the problem from a clinical rather than a deductive stance. As physicians, they want to be in a position to take care of and to help suffering people whom they regard as sick patients. They sometimes become impatient with the rules that prevent them from doing this.

I believe we are now witnessing a pendular swing in which the rights of the mentally ill to be treated and protected are being set aside in the rush to give them their freedom at whatever cost. But is freedom defined only by the absence of external constraints? Internal physiological or psychological processes can contribute to a throttling of the spirit that is as painful as any applied from the outside. The "wild" manic individual without his lithium, the panicky hallucinator without his injection of fluphenazine hydrochloride and the understanding support of a concerned staff, the sodden alcoholic—are they free? Sometimes, as Woody Guthrie said, "Freedom means no place to go."

Today the civil liberties lawyers are in the ascendancy and the psychiatrists on the defensive to a degree that is harmful to individual needs and the public welfare. Redress and a more balanced position will not come from further extension of the dangerousness doctrine. I favor a return to the use of medical criteria by psychiatrists—psychiatrists, however, who have been chastened by the buffeting they have received and are quite willing to go along with even strict legal safeguards as long as they are constructive and not tyrannical.

NOTES

1. Treffert, D. A.: "The practical limits of patients' rights." *Psychiatric Annals* 5(4):91–96, 1971.

2. Szasz T.: *Law, Liberty and Psychiatry,* New York, Macmillan Co., 1963.

3. Ennis, B.: *Prisoners of Psychiatry,* New York, Harcourt Brace Jovanovich, 1972.

4. Szasz, T.: *The Myth of Mental Illness,* New York, Harper & Row, 1961.

5. Laing, R.: *The Politics of Experience,* New York, Ballantine Books, 1967.

6. Ennis, B.: "Ennis on 'Donaldson'." *Psychiatric News,* Dec. 3, 1975, pp. 4, 19, 37.

7. Peele, R., Chodoff, P., Taub, N.: "Involuntary hospitalization and treatability. Observations from the DC experience." *Catholic University Law Review* 23:744–753, 1974.

8. Michels, R.: "The right to refuse psychotropic drugs." *Hastings Center Report,* Hastings-on-Hudson, NY, 1973.

9. Parsons, T.: *The Social System.* New York, Free Press, 1951.

10. Veatch, R. M.: "The medical model: its nature and problems." *Hastings Center Studies* 1(3):59–76, 1973.

11. Katz, J.: "The right to treatment—an enchanting legal fiction?" *University of Chicago Law Review* 36:755–783, 1969.

12. Moore, M. S.: "Some myths about mental illness." *Arch Gen Psychiatry* 32:1483–1497, 1975.

13. Peszke, M. A.: "Is dangerousness an issue for physicians in emergency commitment?" *Am J Psychiatry* 132:825–828, 1975.

14. Stone, A. A.: "Comment on Peszke, M.A.: Is dangerousness an issue for physicians in emergency commitment?" *Ibid.,* 829–831.

15. Siegler, M., Osmond, H.: *Models of Madness, Models of Medicine.* New York, Macmillan Co., 1974.

16. Stone, A.: Lecture for course on The Law, Litigation, and Mental Health Services. Adelphi, Md., Mental Health Study Center, September 1974.

17. O'Connor v Donaldson, 43 USLW 4929 (1975).

18. Lessard v Schmidt, 349 F Supp 1078, 1092 (ED Wis 1972).

19. In re Johnnie Hargrove, Washington, D.C., Superior Court Mental Health number 506–75, 1975.

20. Rachlin, S., Pam, A., Milton, J.: "Civil liberties versus involuntary hospitalization." *Am J Psychiatry* 132:189–191, 1975.

21. Kirk, S. A., Therrien, M. E.: "Community mental health myths and the fate of former hospitalized patients." *Psychiatry* 38:209–217, 1975.

22. Dershowitz, A. A.: "Dangerousness as a criterion for confinement." *Bulletin of the American Academy of Psychiatry and the Law* 2:172–179, 1974.

UNITED STATES SUPREME COURT

O'Connor v. Donaldson

MR. JUSTICE STEWART delivered the opinion of the Court.

The respondent, Kenneth Donaldson, was civilly committed to confinement as a mental patient in the Florida State Hospital at Chattahoochee in January 1957. He was kept in custody there against his will for nearly 15 years. The petitioner, Dr. J. B. O'Connor, was the hospital's superintendent during most of this period. Throughout his confinement Donaldson repeatedly, but unsuccessfully, demanded his release, claiming that he was dangerous to no one, that he was not mentally ill, and that, at any rate, the hospital was not providing treatment for his supposed illness. Finally, in February 1971, Donaldson brought this lawsuit . . . alleging that O'Connor and other members of the hospital staff, named as defendants, had intentionally and maliciously deprived him of his constitutional right to liberty. After a four-day trial, the jury returned a verdict assessing both compensatory and punitive damages against O'Connor and a codefendant. The Court of Appeals for the Fifth Circuit affirmed the judgment. We granted O'Connor's petition for certiorari because of the important constitutional questions seemingly presented.

I

Donaldson's commitment was initiated by his father, who thought that his son was suffering from "delusions." After hearings before a county judge of Pinellas County, Fla., Donaldson was found to be suffering from "paranoid schizophrenia" and was committed for "care, maintenance, and treatment" pursuant to Florida statutory provisions that have since been repealed. The state law was less than clear in specifying the grounds necessary for commitment, and the record is scanty as to Donaldson's condition at the time of the judicial hearing. These matters are, however, irrelevant, for this case involves no challenge to the initial commitment, but is focused, instead, upon the nearly 15 years of confinement that followed.

The evidence at the trial showed that the hospital staff had the power to release a patient, not dangerous to himself or others, even if he remained mentally ill and had been lawfully committed. Despite many requests, O'Connor refused to allow that power to be exercised in Donaldson's case. At the trial, O'Connor indicated that he had believed that Donaldson would have been unable to make a "successful adjustment outside the institution," but could not recall the basis for that conclusion. O'Connor retired as superintendent shortly before the suit was filed. A few months thereafter, and before the trial, Donaldson secured his release and a judicial restoration of competency, with the support of the hospital staff.

The testimony at the trial demonstrated, without contradiction, that Donaldson had posed no danger to others during his long confinement, or indeed at any point in his life. O'Connor himself conceded that he had no personal or secondhand knowledge that Donaldson had ever committed a dangerous act. There was no evidence that Donaldson had ever been suicidal or been thought likely to inflict injury upon himself. One of O'Connor's codefendants acknowledged that Donaldson could have earned his own living outside the hospital. He had done so for some 14 years before his commitment, and immediately upon his release he secured a responsible job in hotel administration.

Furthermore, Donaldson's frequent requests for release had been supported by responsible persons willing to provide him any care he might need on release. In 1963, for example, a representative of Helping Hands, Inc., a halfway house for mental patients, wrote O'Connor asking him to release Donaldson to its care. The request was accompanied by a supporting letter from the Minneapolis Clinic of Psychiatry and Neurology, which a codefendant con-

From 422 *United States Reports* 563, pp. 565–570, 573–576.

ceded was a "good clinic." O'Connor rejected the offer, replying that Donaldson could be released only to his parents. That rule was apparently of O'Connor's own making. At the time, Donaldson was 55 years old, and, as O'Connor knew, Donaldson's parents were too elderly and infirm to take responsibility for him. Moreover, in his continuing correspondence with Donaldson's parents, O'Connor never informed them of the Helping Hands offer. In addition, on four separate occasions between 1964 and 1968, John Lembcke, a college classmate of Donaldson's and a longtime family friend, asked O'Connor to release Donaldson to his care. On each occasion O'Connor refused. The record shows that Lembcke was a serious and responsible person, who was willing and able to assume responsibility for Donaldson's welfare.

The evidence showed that Donaldson's confinement was a simple regime of enforced custodial care, not a program designed to alleviate or cure his supposed illness. Numerous witnesses, including one of O'Connor's codefendants, testified that Donaldson had received nothing but custodial care while at the hospital. O'Connor described Donaldson's treatment as "milieu therapy." But witnesses from the hospital staff conceded that, in the context of this case, "milieu therapy" was a euphemism for confinement in the "milieu" of a mental hospital. For substantial periods, Donaldson was simply kept in a large room that housed 60 patients, many of whom were under criminal commitment. Donaldson's requests for ground privileges, occupational training, and an opportunity to discuss his case with O'Connor or other staff members were repeatedly denied.

At the trial, O'Connor's principal defense was that he had acted in good faith and was therefore immune from any liability for monetary damages. His position, in short, was that state law, which he had believed valid, had authorized indefinite custodial confinement of the "sick," even if they were not given treatment and their release could harm no one.

• • •

II

As we view it, this case raises a single, relatively simple, but nonetheless important question concerning every man's constitutional right to liberty.

The jury found that Donaldson was neither dangerous to himself nor dangerous to others, and also found that, if mentally ill, Donaldson had not received treatment. That verdict, based on abundant evidence, makes the issue before the Court a narrow one. We need not decide whether, when, or by what procedures, a mentally ill person may be confined by the State on any of the grounds which, under contemporary statutes, are generally advanced to justify involuntary confinement of such a person—to prevent injury to the public, to ensure his own survival or safety, or to alleviate or cure his illness. For the jury found that none of the above grounds for continued confinement was present in Donaldson's case.

Given the jury's findings, what was left as justification for keeping Donaldson in continued confinement? The fact that state law may have authorized confinement of the harmless mentally ill does not itself establish a constitutionally adequate purpose for the confinement. Nor is it enough that Donaldson's original confinement was founded upon a constitutionally adequate basis, if in fact it was, because even if his involuntary confinement was initially permissible, it could not constitutionally continue after that basis no longer existed.

A finding of "mental illness" alone cannot justify a State's locking a person up against his will and keeping him indefinitely in simple custodial confinement. Assuming that that term can be given a reasonably precise content and that the "mentally ill" can be identified with reasonable accuracy, there is still no constitutional basis for confining such persons involuntarily if they are dangerous to no one and can live safely in freedom.

May the State confine the mentally ill merely to ensure them a living standard superior to that they enjoy in the private community? That the State has a proper interest in providing care and assistance to the unfortunate goes without saying. But the mere presence of mental illness does not disqualify a person from preferring his home to the comforts of an institution. Moreover, while the State may arguably confine a person to save him from harm, incarceration is rarely if ever a necessary condition for raising the living standards of those capable of surviving safely in freedom, on their own or with the help of family or friends.

May the State fence in the harmless mentally ill solely to save its citizens from exposure to those whose ways are different? One might as well ask if the State, to avoid public unease, could incarcerate all who are physically unattractive or socially eccentric. Mere public intolerance or animosity cannot constitutionally justify the deprivation of a person's physical liberty.

In short, a State cannot constitutionally confine without more cause a nondangerous individual who is capable of surviving safely in freedom by himself or with the help of willing and responsible family members or friends. Since the jury found, upon ample evidence, that O'Connor, as an agent of the State, knowingly did so confine Donaldson, it properly concluded that O'Connor violated Donaldson's constitutional right to freedom.

. . .

TIMOTHY HOWELL
RONALD J. DIAMOND
DANIEL WIKLER

Is There a Case for Voluntary Commitment?

Recurrent psychotic illnesses, which affect thousands of Americans, are a problem often seen in the practice of psychiatry.[1] One common dilemma confronting the mental health professional is how to best care for those patients who refuse all treatment at the onset of a relapse. The situation is even more complex and poignant in the case of patients who, while well, implored their therapists to treat them when they again became ill—even to impose treatment, if necessary—to minimize the destructive impact of the relapses on their lives. Under the laws of many states, such patients cannot be involuntarily committed for treatment, despite their relapses, if they are neither incompetent nor a danger to themselves or others.

It is painful for a clinician to be unable to intervene as previously requested because the patient refuses treatment at the time of the relapse. The therapist must watch and wait while these patients strain personal, family, and community resources, until they either recover, agree to therapy, or, as often happens, their psychotic behavior escalates until they meet legal criteria for involuntary commitment. Current law mandates that a patient's present wishes not to be treated, irrational as they may seem, take priority even though the patient had previously expressed a desire to be treated during relapse.

We believe the current mental health laws are inadequate to deal effectively with such instances of recurrent psychotic illnesses. Because they are unable to voluntarily commit themselves in advance in a truly binding fashion to psychiatric treatment, these patients fall through a gap in the present medical–legal system. The patients, their families, and their communities suffer needless psychological, social, and financial hardships as a consequence. Opinions about how best to accommodate such difficult situations seem to be polarizing; some wish to loosen existing standards for involuntary commitment, whereas others argue that commitment proceedings be restricted even more tightly.

We propose an addition to the present set of legal options, which would enable patients with recurrent psychotic illnesses to voluntarily, during periods of remission, enter into agreements with their physicians that would commit them to treatment during a relapse. We offer this proposal as an invitation for discussion about whether persons with recurrent psychotic illnesses should be able, while free of their illnesses, to bind themselves legally to arrangements that would ensure treatment if a relapse occurred. Culver and Gert,[2] as well as Elster,[3] have suggested such arrangements. We suggest describing these agreements as "voluntary commitment contracts." By the term "commitment" we mean, not simply coercive hospitalization, but commitment to treatment, whether it involves hospitalization or not.

Restrictions on the personal liberties of some mentally ill persons have generally been based wholly or in part on the principle of paternalism. Paternalism for our purposes can be described as justifying an interference with a person's freedom of action as being in that person's best interests. Thus the state may invoke the doctrine of *parens patriae* to justify restricting the liberties of individuals who have become incompetent through mental illness. The state may also invoke its police powers to justify coercive restraint of individuals who become a substantial danger to themselves because of mental illness. Using the state's police powers to restrict the freedom of the mentally ill who pose a significant danger to others is usually defended on the basis of the need to protect others in society. But these arguments can be buttressed by the paternalistic claim that, given the social consequences of violent behavior, it is in the interest of the mentally ill individual to be restrained from harming others.

A misguided, overreaching paternalism has been at the root of much of the past abuse of involuntary commitment procedures. Mental health professionals who believed they were acting in their clients' best interests often deprived patients of liberties in clinical situations that involved neither dangerousness nor incompetence and that were not grave enough to warrant such serious intervention. This practice was a major impetus behind the movement to restrict the application of involuntary commitment laws solely to those cases involving incompetency or dangerousness. We applaud refinements of mental health law designed to better preserve individual liberties, and it is not our intention to revive or extend psychiatric paternalism by our proposal. We feel instead that voluntary commitment contracts would increase the autonomy of patients with recurrent psychotic illnesses by providing them an option for greater self-determination that they do not presently have. Under current law patients may make agreements with their physicians in an attempt to ensure best treatment if a relapse occurs; informal arrangements of this type are not uncommon. But these agreements are not legally binding where patients refuse treatment during relapse, for the powers of the state may not be employed to enforce them.

The issue we wish to raise for debate is: should not these individuals be allowed to make binding restrictions on their own liberties if these restrictions would be in their own best interests? Or, on the contrary, should the state continue to refuse to enforce such arrangements on the grounds of protecting these individuals from "inappropriately" limiting their own freedom? Before addressing these questions, we need first to look more closely at a typical clinical situation that may give rise to this dilemma, and the medical–legal background that frames it.

Consider an individual with a bipolar affective disorder, whose manic-depressive mood swings have reached psychotic proportions. During a period of remission, realizing how destructive his psychotic episodes can be to all involved, he has reviewed the likelihood of a recurrence with his psychiatrist. He has instructed her to do whatever she reasonably can to thwart another relapse, even to treat him against his will at the time should he then need but refuse medications or hospitalization.

A few months later, as he progresses from a normal, euthymic state toward a full-blown manic psychosis, he passes through a hypomanic stage, much as they had foreseen. He gradually becomes more energetic and requires less sleep. His speech grows more rapid and pressured, reflecting his increasingly racing thoughts. His mood expands and is alternately euphoric and irritable, and he becomes more and more grandiose and reckless in his actions, much to the distress of his family, friends, and co-workers. He spends large sums of money on things he does not need and would not normally purchase, seriously depleting family resources. He makes sexual advances toward female neighbors and co-workers.

When family and friends attempt to intervene and to persuade him to seek psychiatric care, he resists. His mood has become still more expansive and irritable, and he denies even having the illness for which he has been regularly taking a prophylactic medication, lithium carbonate. Instead, he throws away his medication, refuses to see his psychiatrist, and dismisses the possibility of any treatment to help him through the manic episode. Nonetheless, at no time does he represent, as defined by the law, a danger to himself or to others, nor is he incompetent or so gravely disabled as to prevent him from being able to meet his biological needs for food, clothing, and shelter. Thus he does not meet the grounds for involuntary civil commitment.

How can this patient's psychiatrist best act under these circumstances? An optimum therapeutic plan would include medication and brief hospitalization. Yet she cannot obtain the assistance of the state to implement such a course of action, because the patient does not meet the criteria for involuntary commitment. In such a clinical situation the potential benefits of treatment are currently lost, even where the patient foresaw that he might refuse assistance during a relapse and requested that his physician treat him despite any protests.

We appreciate the need to define narrowly the criteria for involuntary commitment, and we do not recommend a general loosening of these criteria. Rather, we suggest that a new legal mechanism may provide a better way to assist patients with recurrent psychoses to obtain the psychiatric care that they need and have desired.

Our proposal is that individuals with recurrent psychotic illnesses be allowed to commit themselves by a binding legal agreement before relapse to treatment during a relapse. Just as Odysseus instructed his crew to bind him to the mast before they sailed past the irresistible Sirens and to ignore his requests for release, such patients should be able to contract with their physicians to disregard certain specified instructions they might issue during relapse (such as refusing needed treatment) for a limited period of time. To minimize the potential for abuse, these agreements would be limited by specified conditions and restrictions. We will expand briefly on these conditions and the rationales for them.

The opportunity to make binding voluntary commitment contracts would be limited to individuals with specific types of mental illness, namely, those which involve psychosis, are recurrent, and are amenable to treatment. Major affective disorders (such as bipolar and manic-depressive affective disorders, recurrent mania, and psychotic depression) and certain forms of schizophrenia are examples of psychiatric disorders that might qualify. The requirement that the illness be a psychosis stems from our belief that only illnesses in which behavior reaches serious psychotic proportions are sufficiently severe to warrant this type of intervention if the legal criteria for involuntary commitment have not been met. The illness must be recurrent, with periods of remission during which the individual is relatively symptom-free; such contracts would be unnecessary for patients who experienced only a single psychotic episode, and

would be more difficult to justify for persons constantly under the duress of an unremitting illness. It might be useful to specify a minimum number of psychotic episodes (e.g., two or three) to establish the likelihood of a pattern of relapses and remissions and hence the need for such a contract. (Patients with bipolar affective disorders experience, on the average, a total of five manic and seven depressive episodes over the course of their illness.[4]) Of course, a binding contract for treatment would be pointless if the illness were refractory to any form of therapeutic intervention.

Several additional prerequisites are needed to justify an agreement with the treating physician. First, the patient must be competent when the contract is made, since a contract made by an incompetent person would not be valid. Second, patients must be in remission when the agreement is made; this will then protect them from being persuaded to make contracts under the stress of illness. Third, patients must enter into contracts voluntarily and without coercion. Although the physician might suggest a contract, arrangements for drawing it up would depend upon the initiative of the patient. Discussions with patients about a contract should make clear that opportunities for future treatment will not be contingent on the patient's making such an agreement. In addition, a third party—the individual's lawyer, for example, or a court-appointed lawyer—should participate to assure that the patient's best interests are served. Finally, the agreement should be drawn up with a physician (either a psychiatrist or a nonpsychiatrist in consultation with a psychiatrist) who knows the patient well and is familiar with the unique aspects of his clinical situation. Once drawn up, contracts might also be subject to review by medical–legal boards as an additional safeguard.

To prevent legal difficulties arising from vagueness, a contract would clearly specify the conditions for invoking it and the actions then to be taken. It would define a relapse in terms of certain criteria (a minimum number of specified signs and symptoms of the patient's psychotic illness), and would indicate what treatments could be imposed even if the patient refused. It should further elaborate a number of treatment plans, and specify that the least restrictive alternative consistent with sound clinical judgment of need be used. Contracts would automatically expire after a certain time (e.g., one year) but would be open to renewal; thus, they would be self-limiting in their capacity to bind. The patient would also retain the right to renegotiate the agreement or to revoke it unilaterally on two or three weeks' notice, at any time other than during a relapse as defined in the contract.

When the patient showed signs and symptoms suggesting a relapse, the physician would be obligated to assess them and, if he diagnosed a relapse (as opposed to a new or different illness), to begin treatment. If the patient refused treatment it could be imposed, employing the assistance of the state if needed, as previously arranged. As an additional safeguard, the period of commitment to treatment (and hospitalization, if also necessary) would be limited to a specified brief time span, perhaps three weeks at most. Most patients who are likely to respond to therapy will have begun to do so by that time. If the patient still insisted that he not be treated after this interval, he would be allowed to decline treatment. Of course, if a patient had by then become a clear and convincing danger to himself or others or had become gravely disabled, he could still be involuntarily committed according to existing mental health laws in most states. As a further protection, a patient could be coercively treated according to the terms of a voluntary commitment contract for only a single three-week period during each psychotic relapse. Finally, patients who voluntarily committed themselves in advance to treatment would retain the right to a hearing within seventy-two hours of commitment. This hearing would review the implementation of the contract to determine whether its terms regarding both the occurrence of a relapse and the appropriateness of the therapy has been honored.

This proposed addition to mental health law would facilitate the delivery of improved psychiatric care to many individuals with recurrent psychotic illnesses who presently suffer without treatment during relapses until they reach the point of grave disability or dangerousness to themselves or others. More timely and effective psychiatric intervention through voluntary commitment would significantly reduce the mental anguish experienced by these patients and their families, the disruption of their social environment, and the depletion of personal and community resources. Furthermore, the opportunity to make such contracts would enhance patients' ability to plan their

lives and put into effect their prior decisions, and would thus broaden the scope of their autonomy.

What objections might opponents to this proposal raise? They might point out that difficulties in assessing exactly when a relapse had occurred could open a potential for abuse through fraudulent implementation of these contracts (as well as through honest mistakes in clinical judgment). We believe, though, that clear specification of diagnostic criteria for a relapse would minimize the frequency of invalid commitments. Some might object that persons committed under a voluntary commitment contract would be socially stigmatized. Yet surely being treated under the terms of such a contract would be less stigmatizing than having one's psychotic behavior reach the extreme and reckless levels described in our example earlier, or being hospitalized involuntarily under emergency detention as dangerous or gravely disabled.

Those who have opposed past abuse of involuntary commitment procedures have rightly objected to the overreaching paternalism that contributed to that abuse. One advantage of the proposed voluntary commitment contract is that it can redress some of the imbalance of authority that lies at the root of medical paternalism. One way to ameliorate the asymmetry between mental health professionals and patients is through patient education. While preparing such a contract with a professional, each patient can acquire a better understanding of the nature of his illness, its signs and symptoms, diagnosis, course, and treatment. This greater knowledge of their conditions would help patients approach more equal status with their therapists. Furthermore, by working out the terms of their contracts with their physicians as consultants, they would actively participate in determining their own treatment programs. In binding themselves they achieve greater autonomy and a therapeutic alliance in which power is shared more equally.

A central philosophical problem raised by this proposal is how much value to assign to liberty. How much interference with present freedom is acceptable in this context? Should one be allowed to waive the right to change one's mind about receiving treatment and being hospitalized? John Stuart Mill, in his classic defense of liberty, argued that society should impose no restrictions on exercising personal freedom in ways not harmful to others except to prohibit people from selling themselves into slavery. ''The principle of freedom cannot require that he should be free not to be free. It is not freedom to be allowed to alienate his freedom.''[5] Commentators on Mill have noted his inconsistent paternalism on this point. Civil libertarians hold that individuals are free to bind themselves in a variety of contracts involving property and services, yet many would disallow a contract that abrogates personal freedom and might lead to physical coercion. The question highlighted here is whether those with recurrent psychotic illnesses should have a qualified right to place some restrictions on their own personal liberties in return for significant benefits. These restrictions would be quite limited in scope and duration, and the tradeoff seems eminently reasonable. We are not proposing that patients be empowered to sell themselves into slavery; the amount of freedom one might lose under a voluntary commitment contract is far more modest.

Those who would oppose such contracts must address the question whether the same principles on which they base their attacks on paternalistic abuses of involuntary commitment do not logically require giving patients the freedom to make voluntary commitment contracts. Given the nature of their predicament, these patients might argue that to refuse them the opportunity and resources to make such arrangements to protect themselves and others from their psychotic behavior would itself be an unwarranted, paternalistic infringement on their liberties.

A more extended discussion of the ethical and legal dimensions of this issue—namely, whether it is justifiable to permit certain patients to relinquish voluntarily the future exercise of some of their civil rights for a brief period—will be the occasion for another paper. The point we wish to make here is that perhaps patients with recurrent psychotic illnesses should be allowed to decide for themselves whether they wish to briefly surrender their right to refuse treatment in order to avoid needless suffering. Given the substantial benefits that might be gained through voluntary commitment contracts, the burden of proof must rest on those who would deny patients the right to make such contracts.

We see this proposal as neither a relaxation nor a tightening of current involuntary commitment procedures but rather as an adjustment of existing mental health law. It is an adjustment designed to accommodate the needs of a specific group of patients in a way that augments rather than diminishes their autonomy and power. We offer this proposal for consideration by interested members of the legal and mental health professions, philosophers, and also by patients, their families, and others affected by their dilemma. We invite them all to address the issues involved in a difficult clinical situation that affects thousands of Americans.

NOTES

1. Medical Practice Information Demonstration Project, Bipolar Disorder: A-State-of-the-Science Report (Baltimore: Policy Research, Inc., 1979,), p. 3.

2. Culver, C. M. and Gert, B., ''The Morality of Involuntary Hospitalization,'' in Spicker, S. F. *et al.,* eds. *The Law-Medicine Relation: A Philosophical Exploration* (Boston: Reidel, 1981).

3. Elster, J., *Ulysses and the Sirens* (Cambridge: Cambridge University Press, 1978), p. 38.

4. Medical Practice Information Demonstration Project, *op. cit.,* p. 27.

5. Mill, J. S., ''On Liberty,'' in *Essential Works of John Stuart Mill,* Lerner, M., ed. (New York: Bantam, 1965), p. 348.

SUGGESTED READINGS FOR CHAPTER 4

GENERAL ISSUES

Annas, George J. *The Rights of Hospital Patients.* New York: Avon Books, 1975.

Benjamin, Martin, and Curtis, Joy. *Ethics in Nursing.* New York: Oxford University Press, 1981.

Bloom, Samuel W. ''Therapeutic Relationship: Sociohistorical Perspectives.'' In Reich, Warren T., ed. *Encyclopedia of Bioethics.* New York: Free Press, 1978. Vol. 4, pp. 1663–1668.

Branson, Roy, ''The Secularization of American Medicine.'' *Hastings Center Studies* 1 (No. 2, 1973), 17–28.

Davis, Anne J., and Aroskar, Mila A. *Ethical Dilemmas and Nursing Practice.* New York: Appleton-Century Crofts, 1978.

Ennis, Bruce J., and Emery, Richard D. *The Rights of Mental Patients.* New York: Avon Books, 1978.

Etziony, M.B., comp. *The Physician's Creed: An Anthology of Medical Prayers, Oaths and Codes of Ethics Written and Recited by Medical Practitioners through the Ages.* Springfield, Ill.: Charles C Thomas, 1973.

Gass, Ronald S. ''Appendix: Codes and Statements Related to Medical Ethics.'' In Reich, Warren T., ed. *Encyclopedia of Bioethics.* New York: Free Press, 1978. Vol. 4, pp. 1721–1815.

Gorovitz, Samuel, and MacIntyre, Alasdair. ''Toward a Theory of Medical Fallibility.'' *Journal of Medicine and Philosophy* 1 (March 1976), 51–71.

Jameton, Andrew. ''The Nurse: When Roles and Rules Conflict.'' *Hastings Center Report* 7 (August 1977), 22–23.

Kass, Leon. ''Ethical Dilemmas in the Care of the Ill.'' *Journal of the American Medical Association* 244 (October 17 and 24/31, 1980), 1811–1816, 1946–1949.

Margolis, Joseph. ''Conceptual Aspects of a Patients' Bill of Rights.'' *Journal of Value Inquiry* 11 (Summer 1977), 126–135.

Masters, Roger D. ''Is Contract an Adequate Basis for Medical Ethics?'' *Hastings Center Report* 5 (December 1975), 24–28.

May, William F. "Code, Covenant, Contract, or Philanthropy." *Hastings Center Report* 5 (December 1975), 29–38.

Mechanic, David. *Future Issues in Health Care: Social Policy and the Rationing of Medical Services*. New York: Free Press, 1979. Chap. 9.

Ramsey, Paul. *The Patient as Person*. New Haven: Yale University Press, 1970.

Stanley, Theresa. "Nursing." In Reich, Warren T., ed. *Encyclopedia of Bioethics*. New York: Free Press, 1978. Vol. 3, pp. 1138–1146.

Veatch, Robert M. *A Theory of Medical Ethics*. New York: Basic Books, 1981.

———. *Case Studies in Medical Ethics*. Cambridge, Mass.: Harvard University Press, 1977.

———. "Models for Ethical Medicine in a Revolutionary Age." *Hastings Center Report* 2 (June 1972), 5–7.

———. "Professional Medical Ethics: The Grounding of Its Principles." *Journal of Medicine and Philosophy* 4 (March 1979), 1–19.

INVOLUNTARY COMMITMENT

Annas, George J. "O'Connor v. Donaldson: Insanity Inside Out." *Hastings Center Report* 6 (August 1976), 11–12.

Bazelon, David. "Institutionalization, Deinstitutionalization, and the Adversary Process." *Columbia Law Review* 75 (June 1975), 897–912.

Brock, Dan W. "Involuntary Commitment of the Mentally Ill: Some Moral Issues." In Davis, John W., *et al.*, eds. *Contemporary Issues in Biomedical Ethics*. Clifton, N.J.: Humana Press, 1978, pp. 213–226.

Culver, Charles M., and Gert, Bernard. "The Morality of Involuntary Hospitalization." In Spicker, Stuart F., *et al.*, eds. *The Law-Medicine Relation: A Philosophical Exploration*. Boston: D. Reidel, 1981, pp. 159–175.

Curran, William J. "The Supreme Court and Madness: A Middle Ground on Proof of Mental Illness for Commitment." *New England Journal of Medicine* 301 (August 9, 1979), 317–318.

"Developments in the Law: Civil Commitment of the Mentally Ill." *Harvard Law Review* 87 (April 1974), 1190–1406.

Katz, Jay. "The Right to Treatment—An Enchanting Legal Fiction?" *University of Chicago Law Review* 36 (Summer 1969), 755–783.

Kittrie, Nicholas N. *The Right to Be Different: Deviance and Enforced Therapy*. Baltimore: Johns Hopkins University Press, 1971.

Peszke, Michael A. *Involuntary Treatment of the Mentally Ill: The Problem of Autonomy*. Springfield, Ill.: Charles C Thomas, 1975.

Szasz, Thomas. *Law, Liberty, and Psychiatry: An Inquiry into the Social Uses of Mental Health Practices*. New York: Macmillan, 1963.

———. *Psychiatric Slavery*. New York: Free Press, 1977.

BIBLIOGRAPHIES

American Nurses' Association, Committee on Ethics. *Ethics in Nursing: References and Resources*. Kansas City, Mo.: American Nurses' Association, 1979.

Goldstein, Doris Mueller. *Bioethics: A Guide to Information Sources*. Detroit. Gale Research Company, 1982. See under "Codes of Ethics," "Professional-Patient Relationship," and "Behavior Control."

Lineback, Richard H., ed. *Philosopher's Index*. Vols. 1– . Bowling Green, Ohio: Philosophy Documentation Center, Bowling Green State University. Issued quarterly. See under "Codes," "Physicians," "Rights," and "Therapy."

Walters, LeRoy, ed. *Bibliography of Bioethics*. Vols. 1– . New York: Free Press. Issued annually. See under "Involuntary Commitment," "Medical Ethics," "Nursing Ethics," "Patient Care," "Patients' Rights," "Professional Patient Relationship," and "Voluntary Admission." (The information contained in the annual *Bibliography of Bioethics* can also be retrieved from BIOETHICSLINE, an online data base of the National Library of Medicine.)

5.
The Disclosure of Information

In Chapter 4 an interesting array of professional obligations and patients' rights emerged. Professional obligations to patients have long been recognized in codes of medical and nursing ethics, where the central affirmation has been that health professionals must not exploit their position of controlling influence. As we shall explore in this chapter, systematic thought has recently been given to what moral and legal rights patients should have to information in the possession of health professionals. The basic problem is that of determining under what conditions patients and related parties should have an overriding right to nondeceptive information that they can use to make choices about their future.

The right of a patient to autonomous choice (as discussed in Chapter 1) is widely recognized in medical practice, but its meaning and practical implications remain uncertain. Documents such as the American Hospital Association's "Patient's Bill of Rights" (see Chapter 4) and numerous court cases have brought attention to a need to specify the conditions under which full or at least accurate disclosure should be given to patients, and also when they should be free to use such information in order to control their treatment or even the time of their own death. The rights most frequently asserted as fundamental rights are the right to be told the truth and the right to receive adequate information so that a responsible decision may be made. We shall consider in turn each of these asserted rights.

TRUTH-TELLING

In modern medicine the nature and quality of the physician-patient relationship may vary with the duration of prior contact, the mental or physical state of the patient, the style the physician chooses for relating to the family, and problems of patient-family interaction. The patient's right to know the truth and the physician's obligation to tell it have traditionally been thought to turn on such factors. Most physicians believe that some pressing circumstances justify departures from the general principle of truth-telling, and few moral philosophers have regarded truth-telling as an absolute obligation, especially where telling the truth may itself cause someone's condition to worsen.

Physicians have been especially sensitive to the Hippocratic principle that they should do no harm to patients by revealing too starkly what their condition is. Thus, one common argument is that where risks of harm from nondisclosure are low and benefits of nondisclosure to the patient substantial, a physician may legitimately lie, deceive, or underdisclose. A physician might decide, for example, that the use of a placebo would be in a patient's best interest, even though the patient would never consent to a placebo. Similarly, a physician might decide it is necessary gradually to withdraw medication used to control pain, whereas the patient would not agree to this gradual withdrawal. In still other cases, the physician might decide that it is in the patient's best interest not to know facts that may induce a negative psychological reaction or lead to suicide, and so may suppress the facts. The article by Sissela Bok in this chapter starts from precisely this professional viewpoint and then criticizes it from "the patient's perspective."

Deception that does not involve lying is commonly believed less difficult to justify than lying, because such deception does not so deeply threaten the relationship of trust as does lying; many philosophers have held that the way intentional deception undermines trust and cooperation is the fundamental problem with such practices. Similarly, underdisclosure and nondisclosure are thought still less difficult to justify in many contexts. Those who take this point of view argue that it is important not to conflate duties of nonlying, nondeception, and disclosure. They note that much of the literature on truth-telling, however, treats these duties as if they were a single duty of veracity.

Some philosophers have argued, by contrast, that, except for patients who do not want the truth, all intentional suppression of truth violates a patient's rights and violates fundamental physician duties. This view has been especially characteristic of certain deontological writers. Kant, for example, strongly condemns lying. W. D. Ross argues, far less severely, that a requirement not to lie is implicit in the act of entering into conversation but that it is sometimes right to tell a lie. As Ross seems to recognize, even a broad principle of veracity (truth-telling) construed to condemn lying is not an unconditional or exceptionless principle. We are all familiar with cases outside of medicine where nondisclosure, deception, and even lying can be justified, for veracity can easily conflict with other moral objectives or principles. Thus, the question of the limits of justified deception and nondisclosure is the central issue. In this chapter, this question is specifically addressed in the context of clinical medicine by Alexander Guiora, who argues that the art of balancing what and how much information should be provided is "part and parcel of the therapeutic process."

Children have posed special problems in the area of truth-telling. Increasingly, it has seemed desirable to develop environments for children in which questions can be asked and answers provided as a means of helping a child cope with informational problems about procedures, serious illness, and death. In many situations the child is old enough to question the purpose and nature of a procedure or treatment but too young to give legal consent and too young to grasp the significance of much that is said. This problem leads to the general topic of informed consent (and to related issues about children discussed in Chapter 11).

INFORMED CONSENT

It is widely believed that the physician has a moral obligation to make it possible for patients to decide important matters that affect their health. However, the ability to "make a decision" is largely dependent upon the information available to the patient. A patient's consent to a medical procedure would be insignificant in the absence of relevant information. For example, suppose it is believed but not well confirmed that a patient has cancer. If this patient is asked to submit to dangerous exploratory surgery, it may be of fundamental importance that he or she understands that the cancer is likely before consenting to the surgery. If the patient is only informed that exploratory surgery is needed, a piece of true but incomplete information has been provided. Unless additional information is supplied, the consent will probably be invalid from a moral standpoint. Moreover, even if the consent were genuinely informed, it would have to be voluntary to be valid. Hence, it is often said that before a physician performs a medical procedure on a competent patient, he or she has an obligation to obtain the patient's voluntary informed consent. In recent years this principle has become virtually an axiom of medical ethics, but in many ways it is unclear what it means.

There are at least three major problems of informed consent. The first problem is both conceptual and moral. What is the proper meaning of informed consent and what are the conditions of a valid consent? The *consent* element is relatively unproblematic, but what is it to give *informed* consent, as distinct from either partially informed or uninformed consent? Physicians are hardly in a position to give patients a course in medicine as a way of explaining the patient's problem. But how can patients make an informed decision if they incompletely comprehend their medical condition? Moreover, most medical decisions are made by doctors under conditions of uncertainty on what *they* know to be incomplete information, for the simple reason that not all the desired information can be obtained. Since neither the patient nor the doctor can in most situations have full information, the notion of informed consent might be regarded as an ideal that is not fully realizable but ought to be approximated. Still, even if "informed consent" functions as an ideal, the question remains as to what constitutes a *valid* consent, and how much information is required for validity. Virtually every essay on informed consent in this chapter treats this issue—but it is the special focus of the essay by Charles Culver and Bernard Gert. (The conclusions in this essay contrast sharply to those reached by Franz Ingelfinger in Chapter 11.)

Despite unclarity over the precise meaning of "informed consent" and the conditions of valid consent, there has emerged a clear (though rough) consensus of the critical elements involved in the process of obtaining and proffering consent. In addition to (a) disclosure and (b) voluntariness, virtually all writers are agreed that there must be (c) cognitive information-processing steps required for the subject to respond effectively to material information. Finally, it is agreed that central to the concept of informed consent is (d) subject competence, which is often treated as a presupposition of informed consent rather than as an element. That is, competence is regarded as a necessary condition of both effective information processing and voluntariness, not an element distinct from them.

The second problem of informed consent is that of specifying the proper function or objective of consent, or, as it is sometimes put, the purpose and justification of informed consent. Two positions have dominated the literature. One maintains that the purpose and justification for obtaining informed consent is to protect persons from various harms that might be done to them. Those who subscribe to a justification that turns on *protection from harm* are inclined to protect patients whether or not it is the patient's choice that leads to an "unwise" taking of a risk. The other maintains that the purpose and justification for obtaining informed consent is to respect the autonomy of patients by granting them the right to choose what shall happen to them. Those who subscribe to a justification that turns on *protection of autonomy* are not inclined to protect patients against their own choices, on grounds that such constraint would be an overprotection that violates their autonomy. Jay Katz argues in this chapter that Anglo-American law is caught in a conflict between roughly these two "visions."

The third problem has to do with standards of disclosure in informed consent contexts. These standards are not at present well articulated in either biomedical ethics or case law, and much of the material in the informed consent section of this chapter focuses on this problem. The foundations of the so-called "legal doctrine" of informed consent are ultimately to be found in tort law of assault and battery, which holds that a person can be validly "touched" only when properly authorized. Legal history reveals an evolving doctrine—from a 1767 case *(Slater v. Baker and Stapleton)* of a failure to adhere to customary professional standards of disclosure to the 1972 *Canterbury v. Spence* case (and its aftermath) found in this chapter.

The *Canterbury* case was the first and most influential of the recent landmark informed consent cases, and for this reason is featured in this chapter. This case involved a form of surgery on the back (laminectomy) that led to unexpected paralysis, the possibility of which had not been disclosed. Judge Spottswood Robinson's opinion focuses on the right to self-determination: "The root premise is the concept, fundamental in American juris- prudence, that '[e]very human being of adult years and sound mind has a right to deter- mine what shall be done with his own body'. . . ." True consent is held in this case to be contingent upon the informed exercise of a choice, and thus the physician's disclosure must provide the patient an opportunity to assess available options and attendant risks. As to sufficiency of information, the court holds: "The patient's right of self-decision shapes the boundaries of the duty to reveal. That right can be effectively exercised only if the patient possesses enough information to enable an intelligent choice."[1]

The specific focus in *Canterbury* and similar subsequent cases has been on the de- velopment of an adequate *standard* for adequate disclosure. In case law two general standards or rules for defining adequate disclosures are in competition as a result of these cases and the history that preceded them: the "professional practice standard" and the "reasonable person standard." In addition, a third alternative legal standard has been proposed, commonly called the "subjective standard," or sometimes the "individual standard." These standards deserve careful scrutiny, since so much in contemporary law turns on which of them is accepted.

THE PROFESSIONAL PRACTICE STANDARD

The first standard holds that adequate disclosure is determined by the customary rules or traditional practices of a professional community—e.g., a community of physicians, psychologists, or anthropologists. The custom in a profession establishes both the topics to be discussed and the amount and kinds of information to be disclosed about each topic. The 1972 *ZeBarth* case reprinted in this chapter provides an example of this standard. This case, which involved radiation therapy for Hodgkin's disease that led to paralysis, invokes the professional practice standard as follows: "The duty of the physician to inform and the extent of the information required should be established by expert medical testimony." By this standard only expert testimony from members of such professional groups could count as evidence that there has been a violation of a right to information.

Many problems, however, attend this professional practice standard for disclosure. First, it is unclear that there even exists a customary standard of disclosure for a particular situation within the medical profession. Indeed, how much consensus—and within which of the fields of medicine—is necessary to establish that a professional practice standard for disclosure does, in fact, exist? Second, if custom alone is taken as conclusive, then pervasively negligent care can be perpetuated with impunity, for relevant professionals will jointly offer the same inferior information and precautions. Finally, a third and the principal objection to the professional practice standard is that this standard undermines patient autonomy, the promotion of which many hold to be the primary function and justification of informed consent requirements. From this perspective, the weighing of risks against patient welfare is not an expert skill to be measured through a professional standard but rather is a nonprofessional judgment reserved to the affected person alone.

THE REASONABLE PERSON STANDARD

In the aftermath of *Canterbury* the reasonable person standard has gradually emerged as a substantial legal criterion. Approximately 25 percent of the legal jurisdictions in the United States now accept this criterion, while the remaining 75 percent adhere to the more traditional professional practice standard. According to this newer standard, information to be disclosed is determined by reference to a hypothetical reasonable person, and the materiality of a piece of information is measured by the significance a reasonable person would attach to a risk in deciding whether to submit to a procedure. Most proponents of the reasonable person standard believe that considerations of autonomy generally outweigh those of beneficence and that (all things considered) the reasonable person standard better serves the individual than does the professional practice standard.

Unfortunately, the reasonable person standard harbors conceptual, moral, and practical difficulties. The concept of ''materiality'' is only ambiguously defined in *Canterbury* and related cases, and the central concept of ''the reasonable person'' goes altogether undefined. Second, as Katz argues, no broad duty of disclosure follows from such a standard anyway, and thus the ''new'' standard expressed in *Canterbury* gives a false sense of an advance over the older standard. Finally, because application of the abstract reasonable person standard to a concrete case would require reference to specific facts of the case, a pressing conceptual puzzle is how to understand what information the reasonable person would want ''under the same or similar circumstances'' as those of the patient. When, for example, a patient argues that a physician failed to inform him or her of the risk of cancer associated with a therapy, the question to be asked is whether a reasonable person in this patient's *precise* position would have wanted to be told of the cancer risk. But how is that position to be described?

THE SUBJECTIVE STANDARD

In the reasonable person model developed in *Canterbury,* sufficiency of information is to be judged by reference to the informational needs of the ''objective'' reasonable person, and *not* by reference to the specific informational needs of the individual subject—as proposed by the third, or subjective, standard. Individual informational needs can differ, because the subject may have highly personal or unorthodox beliefs, unusual health problems, or a unique family history that require a different informational base than that required by most persons. For example, a female employee with a family history of reproductive problems might have a need for information that no other person would wish to obtain before becoming involved in research on sexual and familial relations or accepting employment in some industries. Such special circumstances clearly can be relevant to the process of making a decision; if a physician knows or has reason to believe that a person needs the information, then withholding it may deprive the patient of the opportunity to give an informed consent, and thus may undermine autonomy. The issue here is the extent to which the reasonable person standard should be tailored to the individual patient (i.e., made ''subjective''). Whereas *Canterbury* rejects the subjective interpretation, many critics have thought that the very autonomy-based arguments found in *Canterbury* support a subjective standard. Some arguments to this effect are found in Katz and are also suggested by the analysis of Culver and Gert.

It remains undecided in contemporary writings which of these three proposed standards will ultimately prevail—or whether they should somehow be combined into a fourth standard that includes components from each.

CONFIDENTIALITY

Unlike informed consent, which is a relatively recent topic in codes of professional ethics, confidentiality was a significant theme in some of the earliest codes, including the Hippocratic Oath. There the physician vowed: ''What I may see or hear in the course of treatment or even outside of the treatment in regard to the life of men, . . . I will keep to myself. . . .''

Two general types of justifications have been proposed for the confidentiality principle in health care relationships. The first type of justification is that the health professional does not show proper respect for the patient's autonomy and privacy if he or she does not uphold the confidentiality of the professional-patient relationship. A variant of this approach asserts that there is an implied promise of confidentiality inherent in the professional-patient relationship—a promise that ought to be honored just because it is a promise. A second type of justification is that violations of confidentiality will make patients unwilling to reveal sensitive information to health professionals; this unwillingness, in turn, will render diagnosis and cure more difficult and will, in the long run, be highly detrimental to the health of patients.

Even if one accepts the principle of medical confidentiality as important, there remains the question whether it states an absolute duty, and if not, under what conditions it is permissible to reveal otherwise confidential information. Perhaps the most difficult test cases come in situations paralleling the one described in *Tarasoff v. Regents of the University of California*. In this case a patient confided to his psychologist that he intended to kill a third party. The psychologist then faced the choice of preserving the confidentiality of the patient or of breaching the principle of confidentiality to warn a young woman that her life might be in danger. (In addition to the analysis of this case by William J. Curran in this chapter, see the analysis of *Tarasoff* in Chapter 1—in the section on moral dilemmas.) Of course, not all examples of the problem of confidentiality are so dramatic. More common problems concern how much of a patient's medical record can be fed into a relatively "public" data bank and how much information about a patient's genetic makeup may be revealed to a sexual partner when there is a substantial likelihood of the couple's producing genetically handicapped children.

The readings in this chapter provide only a few samples of the rich literature on the relationship between patients and health professionals. In the past, much of this literature was written by health professionals for health professionals. It therefore highlighted their own sense of their *obligations* to the patient. In the foreseeable future, it seems likely that much of the literature on this topic will have its origin outside the health professions and will emphasize the *rights* of patients.

T. L. B.

NOTES

1. Two other 1972 landmark cases (which are not included in this chapter) make similar demands to those found in *Canterbury*. *Cobbs v. Grant,* an ulcer surgery case, requires disclosure of *"all* significant perils pertaining to death or serious harm," and *Wilkinson v. Vesey* rejects the view that decisions whether to proceed with a therapy are medical determinations. It insists that "all the known material risks peculiar to the proposed procedure" must be divulged, as judged by what "a reasonable person, in what the physician knows or should know is his patient's position" would want to know.

SISSELA BOK

Lies to the Sick and Dying

DECEPTION AS THERAPY

A forty-six-year-old man, coming to a clinic for a routine physical check-up needed for insurance purposes, is diagnosed as having a form of cancer likely to cause him to die within six months. No known cure exists for it. Chemotherapy may prolong life by a few extra months, but will have side effects the physician does not think warranted in this case. In addition, he believes that such therapy should be reserved for patients with a chance for recovery or remission. The patient has no symptoms giving him any reason to believe that he is not perfectly healthy. He expects to take a short vacation in a week.

For the physician, there are now several choices involving truthfulness. Ought he to tell the patient what he has learned, or conceal it? If asked, should he deny it? If he decides to reveal the diagnosis, should he delay doing so until after the patient returns from his vacation? Finally, even if he does reveal the serious nature of the diagnosis, should he mention the possibility of chemotherapy and his reasons for not recommending it in this case? Or should he encourage every last effort to postpone death?

In this particular case, the physician chose to inform the patient of his diagnosis right away. He did not, however, mention the possibility of chemotherapy. A medical student working under him disagreed; several nurses also thought that the patient should have been informed of this possibility. They tried, unsuccessfully, to persuade the physician that this was the patient's right. When persuasion had failed, the student elected to disobey the doctor by informing the patient of the alternative of chemotherapy. After consultation with family members, the patient chose to ask for the treatment.

Doctors confront such choices often and urgently.

What they reveal, hold back, or distort will matter profoundly to their patients. Doctors stress with corresponding vehemence their reasons for the distortion or concealment: not to confuse a sick person needlessly, or cause what may well be unnecessary pain or discomfort, as in the case of the cancer patient; not to leave a patient without hope, as in those many cases where the dying are not told the truth about their condition; or to improve the chances of cure, as where unwarranted optimism is expressed about some form of therapy. Doctors use information as part of the therapeutic regimen; it is given out in amounts, in admixtures, and according to timing believed best for patients. Accuracy, by comparison, matters far less.

Lying to patients has, therefore, seemed an especially excusable act. Some would argue that doctors, and *only* doctors, should be granted the right to manipulate the truth in ways so undesirable for politicians, lawyers, and others.[1] Doctors are trained to help patients; their relationship to patients carries special obligations, and they know much more than laymen about what helps and hinders recovery and survival.

Even the most conscientious doctors, then, who hold themselves at a distance from the quacks and the purveyors of false remedies, hesitate to forswear all lying. Lying is usually wrong, they argue, but less so than allowing the truth to harm patients. B. C. Meyer echoes this very common view:

[O]urs is a profession which traditionally has been guided by a precept that transcends the virtue of uttering truth for truth's sake, and that is, "so far as possible, do no harm."[2]

Truth, for Meyer, may be important, but not when it endangers the health and well-being of patients. This has seemed self-evident to many physicians in the past—so much so that we find very few mentions of veracity in the codes and oaths and writings by

From *Lying: Moral Choice in Public and Private Life* (New York: Pantheon Books, 1978), pp. 221–231, 234–240.

physicians through the centuries. This absence is all the more striking as other principles of ethics have been consistently and movingly expressed in the same documents.

The two fundamental principles of doing good and not doing harm—of beneficence and nonmaleficence—are the most immediately relevant to medical practitioners, and the most frequently stressed. To preserve life and good health, to ward off illness, pain, and death—these are the perennial tasks of medicine and nursing. These principles have found powerful expression at all times in the history of medicine. In the Hippocratic Oath physicians promise to:

use treatment to help the sick . . . but never with a view to injury and wrong-doing.[3]

And a Hindu oath of initiation says:

Day and night, however thou mayest be engaged, thou shalt endeavor for the relief of patients with all thy heart and soul. Thou shalt not desert or injure the patient even for the sake of thy living.[4]

But there is no similar stress on veracity. It is absent from virtually all oaths, codes, and prayers. The Hippocratic Oath makes no mention of truthfulness to patients about their condition, prognosis, or treatment. Other early codes and prayers are equally silent on the subject. To be sure, they often refer to the confidentiality with which doctors should treat all that patients tell them; but there is no corresponding reference to honesty toward the patient. One of the few who appealed to such a principle was Amatus Lusitanus, a Jewish physician widely known for his skill, who, persecuted, died of the plague in 1568. He published an oath which reads in part:

If I lie, may I incur the eternal wrath of God and of His angel Raphael, and may nothing in the medical art succeed for me according to my desires.[5]

Later codes continue to avoid the subject. Not even the Declaration of Geneva, adopted in 1948 by the World Medical Association, makes any reference to it. And the Principles of Medical Ethics of the American Medical Association[6] still leave the matter of informing patients up to the physician.

Given such freedom, a physician can decide to tell as much or as little as he wants the patient to know, so long as he breaks no law. In the case of the man mentioned at the beginning of this chapter, some physicians might feel justified in lying for the good of the patient, others might be truthful. Some may conceal alternatives to the treatment they recommend; others not. In each case, they could appeal to the A.M.A. Principles of Ethics. A great many would choose to be able to lie. They would claim that not only can a lie avoid harm for the patient, but that it is also hard to know whether they have been right in the first place in making their pessimistic diagnosis; a "truthful" statement could therefore turn out to hurt patients unnecessarily. The concern for curing and for supporting those who cannot be cured then runs counter to the desire to be completely open. This concern is especially strong where the prognosis is bleak; even more so when patients are so affected by their illness or their medication that they are more dependent than usual; perhaps more easily depressed or irrational.

Physicians know only too well how uncertain a diagnosis or prognosis can be. They know how hard it is to give meaningful and correct answers regarding health and illness. They also know that disclosing their own uncertainty or fears can reduce those benefits that depend upon faith in recovery. They fear, too, that revealing grave risks, no matter how unlikely it is that these will come about, may exercise the pull of the "self-fulfilling prophecy." They dislike being the bearers of uncertain or bad news as much as anyone else. And last, but not least, sitting down to discuss an illness truthfully and sensitively may take much-needed time away from other patients.

These reasons help explain why nurses and physicians and relatives of the sick and dying prefer not to be bound by rules that might limit their ability to suppress, delay, or distort information. This is not to say that they necessarily plan to lie much of the time. They merely want to have the freedom to do so when they believe it wise. And the reluctance to see lying prohibited explains, in turn, the failure of the codes and oaths to come to grips with the problems of truth-telling and lying.

But sharp conflicts are now arising. Doctors no longer work alone with patients. They have to consult with others much more than before; if they choose to lie, the choice may not be met with approval by all who take part in the care of the patient. A nurse expresses the difficulty which results as follows:

From personal experience I would say that the patients who aren't told about their terminal illness have so many verbal and mental questions unanswered that many will begin to realize that their illness is more serious than they're being told. . . .

Nurses care for these patients twenty-four hours a day compared to a doctor's daily brief visit, and it is the nurse many times that the patient will relate to, once his underlying fears become overwhelming. . . . This is difficult for us nurses because being in constant contact with patients we can see the events leading up to this. The patient continually asks you, "Why isn't my pain decreasing?" or "Why isn't the radiation treatment easing the pain?" . . . We cannot legally give these patients an honest answer as a nurse (and I'm sure I wouldn't want to) yet the problem is still not resolved and the circle grows larger and larger with the patient alone in the middle.[7]

The doctor's choice to lie increasingly involves co-workers in acting a part they find neither humane nor wise. The fact that these problems have not been carefully thought through within the medical profession, nor seriously addressed in medical education, merely serves to intensify the conflicts.[8] Different doctors then respond very differently to patients in exactly similar predicaments. The friction is increased by the fact that relatives often disagree even where those giving medical care to a patient are in accord on how to approach the patient. Here again, because physicians have not worked out to common satisfaction the question of whether relatives have the right to make such requests, the problems are allowed to be haphazardly resolved by each physician as he sees fit.

THE PATIENT'S PERSPECTIVE

The turmoil in the medical profession regarding truth-telling is further augmented by the pressures that patients themselves now bring to bear and by empirical data coming to light. Challenges are growing to the three major arguments for lying to patients: that truthfulness is impossible; that patients do not want bad news; and that truthful information harms them.

The first of these arguments . . . confuses "truth" and "truthfulness" so as to clear the way for occasional lying on grounds supported by the second and third arguments. At this point, we can see more clearly that it is a strategic move intended to discourage the question of truthfulness from carrying much weight in the first place, and thus to leave the choice of what to say and how to say it up to the physician. To claim that "since telling the truth is impossible, there can be no sharp distinction between what is true

and what is false"[9] is to try to defeat objections to lying before even discussing them. One need only imagine how such an argument would be received, were it made by a car salesman or a real estate dealer, to see how fallacious it is.

In medicine, however, the argument is supported by a subsidiary point: even if people might ordinarily understand what is spoken to them, patients are often not in a position to do so. This is where paternalism enters in. When we buy cars or houses, the paternalist will argue, we need to have all our wits about us; but when we are ill, we cannot always do so. We need help in making choices, even if help can be given only by keeping us in the dark. And the physician is trained and willing to provide such help.

It is certainly true that some patients cannot make the best choices for themselves when weakened by illness or drugs. But most still can. And even those who are incompetent have a right to have someone—their guardian or spouse perhaps—receive the correct information.

The paternalistic assumption of superiority to patients also carries great dangers for physicians themselves—it risks turning to contempt. The following view was recently expressed in a letter to a medical journal:

As a radiologist who has been sued, I have reflected earnestly on advice to obtain Informed Consent but have decided to "take the risks without informing the patient" and trust to "God, judge, and jury" rather than evade responsibility through a legal gimmick. . . .

[I]n a general radiologic practice many of our patients are uninformable and we would never get through the day if we had to obtain their consent to every potentially harmful study.

. . . We still have patients with language problems, the uneducated and the unintelligent, the stolid and the stunned who cannot form an Informed Opinion to give an Informed Consent; we have the belligerent and the panicky who do not listen or comprehend. And then there are the Medicare patients who comprise 35 percent of general hospital admissions. The bright ones wearily plead to be left alone. . . . As for the apathetic rest, many of them were kindly described by Richard Bright as not being able to comprehend because "their brains are so poorly oxygenated."[10]

The argument which rejects informing patients because adequate truthful information is impossible in itself or because patients are lacking in understanding must itself be rejected when looked at from the point of view of patients. They know that liberties granted to the most conscientious and altruistic doctors will be exercised also in the "Medicaid Mills"; that the choices thus kept from patients will be exercised by not only competent but incompetent physicians; and that even the best doctors can make choices patients would want to make differently for themselves.

The second argument for deceiving patients refers specifically to giving them news of a frightening or depressing kind. It holds that patients do not, in fact, generally want such information, that they prefer not to have to face up to serious illness and death. On the basis of such a belief, most doctors in a number of surveys stated that they do not, as a rule, inform patients that they have an illness such as cancer.

When studies are made of what patients desire to know, on the other hand, a large majority say that they *would* like to be told of such a diagnosis.[11] All these studies need updating and should be done with larger numbers of patients and non-patients. But they do show that there is generally a dramatic divergence between physicians and patients on the factual question of whether patients want to know what ails them in cases of serious illness such as cancer. In most of the studies, over 80 percent of the persons asked indicated that they would want to be told.

Sometimes this discrepancy is set aside by doctors who want to retain the view that patients do not want unhappy news. In reality, they claim, the fact that patients say they want it has to be discounted. The more someone asks to know, the more he suffers from fear which will lead to the denial of the information even if it is given. Informing patients is, therefore, useless; they resist and deny having been told what they cannot assimilate. According to this view, empirical studies of what patients say they want are worthless since they do not probe deeply enough to uncover this universal resistance to the contemplation of one's own death.

This view is only partially correct. For some patients, denial is indeed well established in medical experience. A number of patients (estimated at between 15 percent and 25 percent) will give evidence of denial of having been told about their illness, even when they repeatedly ask and are repeatedly informed. And nearly everyone experiences a period of denial at some point in the course of approaching death.[12] Elisabeth Kübler-Ross sees denial as result-

ing often from premature and abrupt information by a stranger who goes through the process quickly to "get it over with." She holds that denial functions as a buffer after unexpected shocking news, permitting individuals to collect themselves and to mobilize other defenses. She describes prolonged denial in one patient as follows:

> She was convinced that the X-rays were "mixed up"; she asked for reassurance that her pathology report could not possibly be back so soon and that another patient's report must have been marked with her name. When none of this could be confirmed, she quickly asked to leave the hospital, looking for another physician in the vain hope "to get a better explanation for my troubles." This patient went "shopping around" for many doctors, some of whom gave her reassuring answers, others of whom confirmed the previous suspicion. Whether confirmed or not, she reacted in the same manner; she asked for examination and reexamination. . . .[13]

But to say that denial is universal flies in the face of all evidence. And to take any claim to the contrary as "symptomatic" of deeper denial leaves no room for reasoned discourse. There is no way that such universal denial can be proved true or false. To believe in it is a metaphysical belief about man's condition, not a statement about what patients do and do not want. It is true that we can never completely understand the possibility of our own death, any more than being alive in the first place. But people certainly differ in the degree to which they can approach such knowledge, take it into account in their plans, and make their peace with it.

Montaigne claimed that in order to learn both to live and to die, men have to think about death and be prepared to accept it.[14] To stick one's head in the sand, or to be prevented by lies from trying to discern what is to come, hampers freedom—freedom to consider one's life as a whole, with a beginning, a duration, an end. Some may request to be deceived rather than to see their lives as thus finite; others reject the information which would require them to do so; but most say that they want to know. Their concern for knowing about their condition goes far beyond mere curiosity or the wish to make isolated personal choices in the short time left to them; their stance toward the entire life they have lived, and their ability to give it meaning and completion, are at stake.[15] In lying or withholding the facts which permit such discernment, doctors may reflect their own fears (which, according to one study,[16] are much stronger than those of laymen) of facing questions about the meaning of one's life and the inevitability of death.

Beyond the fundamental deprivation that can result from deception, we are also becoming increasingly aware of all that can befall patients in the course of their illness when information is denied or distorted. Lies place them in a position where they no longer participate in choices concerning their own health, including the choice of whether to be a "patient" in the first place. A terminally ill person who is not informed that his illness is incurable and that he is near death cannot make decisions about the end of his life: about whether or not to enter a hospital, or to have surgery; where and with whom to spend his last days; how to put his affairs in order—these most personal choices cannot be made if he is kept in the dark, or given contradictory hints and clues.

· · ·

The reason why even doctors who recognize a patient's right to have information might still not provide it brings us to the third argument against telling all patients the truth. It holds that the information given might hurt the patient and that the concern for the right to such information is therefore a threat to proper health care. A patient, these doctors argue, may wish to commit suicide after being given discouraging news, or suffer a cardiac arrest, or simply cease to struggle, and thus not grasp the small remaining chance for recovery. And even where the outlook for a patient is very good, the disclosure of a minute risk can shock some patients or cause them to reject needed protection such as a vaccination or antibiotics.

The factual basis for this argument has been challenged from two points of view. The damages associated with the disclosure of sad news or risks are rarer than physicians believe; and the *benefits* which result from being informed are more substantial, even measurably so. Pain is tolerated more easily, recovery from surgery is quicker, and cooperation with therapy is greatly improved. The attitude that "what you don't know won't hurt you" is proving unrealistic; it is what patients do not know but vaguely suspect that causes them corrosive worry.

It is certain that no answers to this question of harm from information are the same for all patients. If we look, first, at the fear expressed by physicians that informing patients of even remote or unlikely risks connected with a drug prescription or operation might shock some and make others refuse the treatment that

would have been best for them, it appears to be unfounded for the great majority of patients. Studies show that very few patients respond to being told of such risks by withdrawing their consent to the procedure and that those who do withdraw are the very ones who might well have been upset enough to sue the physician had they not been asked to consent beforehand.[17] It is possible that on even rarer occasions especially susceptible persons might manifest physical deterioration from shock; some physicians have even asked whether patients who die after giving informed consent to an operation, but before it actually takes place, somehow expire because of the information given to them.[18] While such questions are unanswerable in any one case, they certainly argue in favor of caution, a real concern for the person to whom one is recounting the risks he or she will face, and sensitivity to all signs of distress.

The situation is quite different when persons who are already ill, perhaps already quite weak and discouraged, are told of a very serious prognosis. Physicians fear that such knowledge may cause the patients to commit suicide, or to be frightened or depressed to the point that their illness takes a downward turn. The fear that great numbers of patients will commit suicide appears to be unfounded.[19] And if some do, is that a response so unreasonable, so much against the patient's best interest that physicians ought to make it a reason for concealment or lies? Many societies have allowed suicide in the past; our own has decriminalized it; and some are coming to make distinctions among the many suicides which ought to be prevented if at all possible, and those which ought to be respected.[20]

Another possible response to very bleak news is the triggering of physiological mechanisms which allow death to come more quickly—a form of giving up or of preparing for the inevitable, depending on one's outlook. Lewis Thomas, studying responses in humans and animals, holds it not unlikely that:

. . . there is a pivotal movement at some stage in the body's reaction to injury or disease, maybe in aging as well, when the organism concedes that it is finished and the time for dying is at hand, and at this moment the events that lead to death are launched, as a coordinated mechanism. Functions are then shut off, in sequence, irreversibly, and, while this is going on, a neural mechanism, held ready for this occasion, is switched on. . . .[21]

Such a response may be appropriate, in which case it makes the moments of dying as peaceful as those who have died and been resuscitated so often testify. But it may also be brought on inappropriately, when the organism could have lived on, perhaps even induced malevolently, by external acts intended to kill. Thomas speculates that some of the deaths resulting from "hexing" are due to such responses. Lévi-Strauss describes deaths from exorcism and the casting of spells in ways which suggest that the same process may then be brought on by the community.[22]

It is not inconceivable that unhappy news abruptly conveyed, or a great shock given to someone unable to tolerate it, could also bring on such a "dying response," quite unintended by the speaker. There is every reason to be cautious and to try to know ahead of time how susceptible a patient might be to the accidental triggering—however rare—of such a response. One has to assume, however, that most of those who have survived long enough to be in a situation where their informed consent is asked have a very robust resistance to such accidental triggering of processes leading to death.

. . .

Apart from the possible harm from information, we are coming to learn much more about the benefits it can bring patients. People follow instructions more carefully if they know what their disease is and why they are asked to take medication; any benefits from those procedures are therefore much more likely to come about. Similarly, people recover faster from surgery and tolerate pain with less medication if they understand what ails them and what can be done for them.

RESPECT AND TRUTHFULNESS

Taken all together, the three arguments defending lies to patients stand on much shakier ground as a counterweight to the right to be informed than is often thought. The common view that many patients cannot understand, do not want, and may be harmed by, knowledge of their condition, and that lying to them is either morally neutral or even to be recommended, must be set aside. Instead, we have to make a more complex comparison. Over against the right of patients to knowledge concerning themselves, the medical and psychological benefits to them from this

knowledge, the unnecessary and sometimes harmful treatment to which they can be subjected if ignorant, and the harm to physicians, their profession, and other patients from deceptive practices, we have to set a severely restricted and narrowed paternalistic view—that *some* patients cannot understand, *some* do not want, and *some* may be harmed by, knowledge of their condition, and that they ought not to have to be treated like everyone else if this is not in their best interest.

Such a view is persuasive. A few patients openly request not to be given bad news. Others give clear signals to that effect, or are demonstrably vulnerable to the shock or anguish such news might call forth. Can one not in such cases infer implied consent to being deceived?

Concealment, evasion, withholding of information may at times be necessary. But if someone contemplates lying to a patient or concealing the truth, the burden of proof must shift. It must rest, here, as with all deception, on those who advocate it in any one instance. They must show why they fear a patient may be harmed or how they know that another cannot cope with the truthful knowledge. A decision to deceive must be seen as a very unusual step, to be talked over with colleagues and others who participate in the care of the patient. Reasons must be set forth and debated, alternatives weighed carefully. At all times, the correct information must go to *someone* closely related to the patient.

The law already permits doctors to withhold information from patients where it would clearly hurt their health. But this privilege has been sharply limited by the courts. Certainly it cannot be interpreted so broadly as to permit a general practice of deceiving patients "for their own good." Nor can it be made to include cases where patients might calmly decide, upon hearing their diagnosis, not to go ahead with the therapy their doctor recommends.[23] Least of all can it justify silence or lies to large numbers of patients merely on the grounds that it is not always easy to tell what a patient wants.

For the great majority of patients, on the contrary, the goal must be disclosure, and the atmosphere one of openness. But it would be wrong to assume that patients can therefore be told abruptly about a serious diagnosis—that, so long as openness exists, there are no further requirements of humane concern in such communication. Dr. Cicely Saunders, who runs the well-known St. Christopher's Hospice in England, describes the sensitivity and understanding which are needed:

> Every patient needs an explanation of his illness that will be understandable and convincing to him if he is to cooperate in his treatment or be relieved of the burden of unknown fears. This is true whether it is a question of giving a diagnosis in a hopeful situation, or of confirming a poor prognosis.
>
> The fact that a patient does not ask does not mean that he has no questions. One visit or talk is rarely enough. It is only by waiting and listening that we can gain an idea of what we should be saying. Silences and gaps are often more revealing than words as we try to learn what a patient is facing as he travels along the constantly changing journey of his illness and his thoughts about it.
>
> . . .So much of the communication will be without words or given indirectly. This is true of all real meeting with people but especially true with those who are facing, knowingly or not, difficult or threatening situations. It is also particularly true of the very ill.
>
> The main argument against a policy of deliberate, invariable denial of unpleasant facts is that it makes such communication extremely difficult, if not impossible. Once the possibility of talking frankly with a patient has been admitted, it does not mean that this will always take place, but the whole atmosphere is changed. We are then free to wait quietly for clues from each patient, seeing them as individuals from whom we can expect intelligence, courage, and individual decisions. They will feel secure enough to give us these clues when they wish.[24]

Above all, truthfulness with those who are suffering does not mean that they should be deprived of all hope: hope that there is a chance of recovery, however small; nor of reassurance that they will not be abandoned when they most need help.

Much needs to be done, however, if the deceptive practices are to be eliminated, and if concealment is to be restricted to the few patients who ask for it or those who can be shown to be harmed by openness. The medical profession has to address this problem.

NOTES

1. Plato, *The Republic,* 389 b.

2. B. C. Meyer, "Truth and the Physician," *Bulletin of the New York Academy of Medicine* 45 (1969): 59–71.

3. W. H. S. Jones, trans., *Hippocrates,* Loeb Classical Library (Cambridge, Mass.: Harvard University Press, 1923), p. 164.

4. Reprinted in M. B. Etziony, *The Physician's Creed: An Anthology of Medical Prayers, Oaths and Codes of Ethics* (Springfield, Ill.: Charles C Thomas, 1973), pp. 15–18.

5. See Harry Friedenwald, "The Ethics of the Practice of Medicine from the Jewish Point of View," *Johns Hopkins Hospital Bulletin,* no. 318 (August 1917), pp. 256–61.

6. "Ten Principles of Medical Ethics," *Journal of the American Medical Association* 164 (1957): 1119–20.

7. Mary Barrett, letter, *Boston Globe,* 16 November 1976, p. 1.

8. Though a minority of physicians have struggled to bring them to our attention. See Thomas Percival, *Medical Ethics,* 3d ed. (Oxford: John Henry Parker, 1849), pp. 132–41; Worthington Hooker, *Physician and Patient* (New York: Baker and Scribner, 1849), pp. 357–82; Richard C. Cabot, "Teamwork of Doctor and Patient Through the Annihilation of Lying," in *Social Service and the Art of Healing* (New York: Moffat, Yard & Co., 1909), pp. 116–70; Charles C. Lund, "The Doctor, the Patient, and the Truth," *Annals of Internal Medicine* 24 (1946): 955; Edmund Davies, "The Patient's Right to Know the Truth," *Proceedings of the Royal Society of Medicine* 66 (1973): 533–36.

9. Lawrence Henderson, "Physician and Patient as a Social System," *New England Journal of Medicine* 212 (1955).

10. Nicholas Demy, Letter to the Editor, *Journal of the American Medical Association* 217 (1971): 696–97.

11. For the views of physicians, see Donald Oken, "What to Tell Cancer Patients," *Journal of the American Medical Association* 175 (1961): 1120–28; and tabulations in Robert Veatch, *Death, Dying, and the Biological Revolution* (New Haven and London: Yale University Press, 1976), pp. 229–38. For the view of patients, see Veatch, *ibid.;* Jean Aitken-Swan and E. C. Easson, "Reactions of Cancer Patients on Being Told Their Diagnosis," *British Medical Journal,* 1959, pp. 779–83; Jim McIntosh, "Patients' Awareness and Desire for Information About Diagnosed but Undisclosed Malignant Disease," *The Lancet* 7 (1976): 300–303; William D. Kelly and Stanley R. Friesen, "Do Cancer Patients Want to Be Told?," *Surgery* 27 (1950): 822–26.

12. See Avery Weisman, *On Dying and Denying* (New York: Behavioral Publications, 1972); Elisabeth Kübler-Ross, *On Death and Dying* (New York: The Macmillan Co., 1969); Ernest Becker, *The Denial of Death* (New York: Free Press, 1973); Philippe Ariès, *Western Attitudes Toward Death,* trans. Patricia M. Ranum (Baltimore and London: Johns Hopkins University Press, 1974); and Sigmund Freud, "Negation," *Collected Papers,* ed. James Strachey (London: Hogarth Press, 1950), 5: 181–85.

13. Kübler-Ross, *On Death and Dying,* p. 34.

14. Michel de Montaigne, *Essays,* bk. I, chap. 20.

15. It is in literature that these questions are most directly raised. Two recent works where they are taken up with striking beauty and simplicity are May Sarton, *As We Are Now* (New York: W. W. Norton & Co., 1973); and Freya Stark, *A Peak in Darien* (London: John Murray, 1976).

16. Herman Feifel et al., "Physicians Consider Death," *Proceedings of the American Psychoanalytical Association,* 1967, pp. 201–2.

17. See Ralph Alfidi, "Informed Consent: A Study of Patient Reaction," *Journal of the American Medical Association* 216 (1971): 1325–29.

18. See Steven R. Kaplan, Richard A. Greenwald, and Arvey I. Rogers, Letter to the Editor, *New England Journal of Medicine* 296 (1977): 1127.

19. Oken, "What to Tell Cancer Patients"; Veatch, *Death, Dying, and the Biological Revolution;* Weisman, *On Dying and Denying.*

20. Norman L. Cantor, "A Patient's Decision to Decline Life-Saving Treatment: Bodily Integrity Versus the Preservation of

Life," *Rutgers Law Review* 26: 228–64; Danielle Gourevitch, "Suicide Among the Sick in Classical Antiquity," *Bulletin of the History of Medicine* 18 (1969): 501–18; for bibliography, see Bok, "Voluntary Euthanasia."

21. Lewis Thomas, "A Meliorist View of Disease and Dying," *The Journal of Medicine and Philosophy* 1 (1976): 212–21.

22. Claude Lévi-Strauss, *Structural Anthropology* (New York:

Basic Books, 1963), p. 167; See also Eric Cassell, "Permission to Die," in John Behnke and Sissela Bok, eds., *The Dilemmas of Euthanasia* (New York: Doubleday, Anchor Press, 1975), pp. 121–31.

23. See Charles Fried, *Medical Experimentation: Personal Integrity and Social Policy* (Amsterdam and Oxford: North Holland Publishing Co., 1974), pp. 20–24.

24. Cicely M. S. Saunders, "Telling Patients," in Reiser, Dyck, and Curran, *Ethics in Medicine*, pp. 238–40.

A L E X A N D E R   Z .   G U I O R A

Freedom of Information vs. Freedom from Information

Not too surprisingly perhaps, I am likely to approach the problem [of a right to know] from a perspective other than [a philosopher's]. . . . Instead, I wish to offer the observations of a clinician, a clinician much sobered by a rich experience of poor judgment calls.

First of all, I would suggest that the conceptual framework as posited in . . . "the right of the patient to know" is the wrong question. As a matter of fact it is worse than that, it is a bad question. And, once you are willing to answer a bad question, you are being led down the garden path of somebody else's choosing. Accordingly, I don't intend to address the question of the "right of the patient to know," and certainly not in the conceptual frame of reference created by the freedom of information act. Rather, I shall argue that information relating to the process of illness and recovery is very much part of that very process, influencing it significantly. It is not an entity independent of it. Consequently, information is to be conceived as part and parcel of the medical intervention, and has to be examined using the same criteria one would in scrutinizing any other aspect of the medical intervention equation.

Now, I believe that many practitioners of the healing arts, experienced in the ways of patients, would not disagree with this position, especially if they stop to think of their own actual clinical be-

haviors. The traditionally and formally articulated position however is quite another matter. This traditional response treats the patient in the most patronizing fashion, reinforcing dependence and regression, if you will. The illness, in this view, is not the patient's business, it is the proprietary domain of the physician. The sick person must not intrude himself into this relationship either by his conduct or by his curiosity. Doctor will take care of everything, patient has only to follow orders. You don't tell the patient anything, he wouldn't understand, and he needs to know nothing anyway; all he needs is the reassuring hand of the physician. There are entire medical cultures subscribing to this view and to this set.

On the other hand, you have another extreme response, couched in the language of freedom of information, holding that the patient has the right to all knowledge about him (it is his property as it were), and it is the duty of the physician to share all he knows (as if he and the patient were discussing something outside of the situation).

Both extreme positions are very convenient for the physician: they represent socially sanctioned freedom from decision making.

What I am suggesting here is that neither of these positions is correct. Information is medicine, very potent medicine indeed, that has to be titrated, properly dosaged based on proper diagnosis. Diagnosis, of course, in this context means an assessment of how information will affect the course of illness, how much and what kind of information is the most

From *Ethics, Humanism, and Medicine*, ed. Marc D. Basson (New York: Alan R. Liss, Inc., 1980), pp. 31–34.

therapeutic in face of the patient's preferred modes of coping. The plea I am making here parenthetically is for the physician to include a rudimentary (but not just intuitive) personality assessment in the total intervention equation.

Now let me illustrate my point, using a hypothetical clinical situation of the kind that I am most familiar with. Let us take a daily occurrence in the emergency room. Somebody is brought in by friends or relatives, in an obviously agitated, perhaps even in a violent state. He is telling about experiences that do not seem reasonable. He is hearing voices that you the examining physician cannot hear. He presents you with a system of logic that you, brought up in the Aristotelian tradition, cannot share. In short, you have a patient who is hallucinating and has delusions. All evidence seems to point to an acute psychotic state. Now what do you tell him? Are you going to tell him, in keeping with the simplistic interpretation of freedom of information, that the voices he is hearing are in his head, he is hearing them because he is crazy? Are you going to tell him that no electricity is coming out of the wall, and he has those strange notions only because he is sick in the head, or are you considering what is most conducive to the patient's well-being? If so, then I suggest that you make a therapeutic decision and tell him something like, "you seem to be upset, you seem to be experiencing all kinds of things that you are not entirely in control of, and I think it would be a good idea for you to stay here now for a while, until things straighten themselves out." The idea, of course, is that information, what, how much, and when, is part and parcel of the therapeutic process.

Some of you might argue that I had set up a straw man, in the above example, only to knock it down. Some of you might say that in the case of an obviously deranged person, the freedom of information concept doesn't apply. I could respond, of course, that "obviously deranged" is a matter of judgment, but will not press the point for the moment.

Let's take another example, when there is no suspicion of psychosis, where the patient is clearly in "possession of his faculties." Let us take the patient who comes in a state of extreme agitation. He is tense, anxious, ready to climb the wall. After a care-

ful and patient assessment you come to the conclusion that the patient is in an acute homosexual panic. Homosexual panic means that the person is in the throes of acute panic that he might become a practicing homosexual. Now, what do you tell him? The simplistic advocates of the "freedom of information" concept would undoubtedly argue that it is his truth, and you must share it with him. The rigid adherents of the paternalistic medical tradition will tell you that it is none of the patient's business, your task is to reassure him, to reduce his anxiety. I would suggest that they are both wrong. What you tell this hypothetical patient is part of the therapeutic process based on clinical judgment. In some cases confrontation might be the most therapeutic course, in others careful circumlocution, in still others outright withholding. The point is that whatever you do and say must have a good, defensible therapeutic reason.

I would like to conclude with a final illustration taken from my daily work. The reference is to uncovering psychotherapy and the role of the interpretive process in it. Uncovering, insight oriented, or psychoanalytic psychotherapy is a delicate and slow process, in the course of which connections are made between past and present, the conscious and the unconscious, symptom and conflict, behavior and motivation. A delicate and intensive process, in which the therapist is usually ahead of the patient in making connections, in discovering the link-ups. This moment of discovery and the sharing of it with the patient is what we call interpretation. The very curative process in psychotherapy rests on a system of *properly* timed interpretations. I always tell my residents it is not enough for an interpretation to be correct, it must be right, because if it is not timed right it can be more harmful than helpful. Here, perhaps more than in any other clinical circumstance, the absolute irrelevance of both the freedom of information position and the traditional paternalistic position is clearly demonstrated.

It is my suggestion that the interpretive process in psychotherapy can serve as a paradigm for all clinical situations regarding information disclosure and withholding.

CHARLES CULVER AND BERNARD GERT

Valid Consent

In any situation in which someone contracts for services with a professional with whom he has a fiduciary relationship, the notion of valid consent may come into play. If a lawyer or an accountant suggests a particular course of action to a client, and the client authorizes this action on his behalf, then in order for the authorization to be valid, the same features must be present as are necessary for valid consent in medicine. It is important to make this point, since if one believes that valid consent is required only in medicine, one may not only distort the concept, one may also foster the incorrect view that ethical considerations are different for doctors.

There are, of course, reasons why the concept of valid consent has come to play a larger role in medicine than in any of the other professions, but these are matters of degree, not of kind. First, medical patients often know less about the alternatives to, and consequences of, the courses of treatment suggested to them than do the clients in other professions. Second, because of their condition it is often more difficult for them to understand the information provided. Third, the consequences of these courses of treatment are often more serious than are the consequences of actions involving other professions. Fourth, the medical profession has a history of making decisions for patients without their valid consent to a much greater degree than the other professions. We can summarize these points as follows: In medicine, it is often more difficult to achieve valid consent because of the amount of information needed and the condition of the patient; it is often more important to obtain it because of the serious consequences to the patient; and often little attempt has been made to obtain it

because of the paternalistic attitude of the medical profession.

Ideally, a patient should know everything that would affect his decision concerning which of the courses of treatment available to him he should choose. This means, first, that he should be informed of everything that all rational persons would want to know: all of the goods and evils involved in the various alternatives, including their severity and probability. In addition, each patient should know of anything else that might affect his *personal* decision. He may have religious beliefs, or cultural beliefs, or even superstitions that would influence which alternative he would choose. Ideally, he should know of any facts that would lead him to decide one way or another, even on the basis of these superstitions. What he does not need to know, unless he happens to have some special interest in the matter, are technical details concerning the treatment.

Thus the adequate information component of valid consent does not demand, even ideally, that the patient know the chemical formulae of his medications, the internal location of any incisions, or even the location of the various affected internal organs, for example, the spleen or the liver. Though these are appropriate objects of patients' curiosity, and providing such information often relieves a patient's anxiety, they normally have no relationship to valid consent. Adequate information must include only those facts that all rational persons would want to know, namely, the various goods and evils that result from the alternative modes of treatment, including their severity and probability. However, in some cases, it must also include those facts that would affect the decisions of persons with idiosyncratic views; for example, if a patient has views that prohibit being seen nude by members of the opposite sex, then he must be told if a procedure requires being thus seen.

One may object that medicine is an inexact field, that we do not know with any precision the goods and evils which might result from alternative treatments, that we do not even know the probabilities except in the vaguest fashion. But this objection has little force, for one who puts it forward is subject to the following dilemma. If knowledge is as inexact as you say, then how can you rationally decide which of the various alternative treatments to recommend? Whatever estimates you make of the risks and benefits involved, including the knowledge that the probability estimates are not reliable, can be conveyed to the patient. Unless one wishes to defend purely intuitive judgments that cannot be rationally justified even to colleagues, then it must be possible to convey the grounds of one's judgment to the patient. Further, making the risks and benefits of the various alternatives explicit helps counter the various biases that enter into making one's judgments. To guard further against the effects of these biases, patients must be told if there is legitimate disagreement among medical practitioners about the value of the different treatment alternatives.

Except in unusual circumstances, it is not difficult to determine what should be told to a patient: namely, everything that one has any reason to believe would affect his decision. It is the patient's life, health, time, money, and so on that are most directly affected by his decision, and thus he is entitled to make the decision on the basis of the most complete and personally relevant information possible.

But even though the kind of information a patient must have is limited to information about the goods and evils, their severity and probability, and to information relevant to a patient's special values, it is still impossible to give complete information. There are an indefinite number of very small risks, say of the magnitude of one in ten million, about which it does not seem morally required to inform the patient. This has been recognized by almost everyone writing on the subject of consent. However, most justify not providing this information on the somewhat questionable grounds that the patient probably already knows, for example, that there is some extremely small but finite risk in taking diagnostic blood samples. We justify not telling about very small risks on the grounds that rational persons would not find them relevant to their decision. This justification also explains why it is not just the probability that determines if the patient should be told, but also the severity of the evil if it should occur. Thus, one need not tell about a one in

one thousand risk of a severe but temporary pain, but should tell if there were a one in one thousand risk of death.

It is very important that a patient be informed of the risks and benefits of all aspects of a proposed course of treatment. For example, a patient confronting possible surgery should be given adequate information with regard to not only surgery but also anesthesia, if there are any significant differences in risks and benefits among the possible alternative methods. Pregnant women are often told of the various possible forms of anesthesia and allowed to choose among them, but other surgical patients are frequently not presented any such alternatives. This is often true for parents of children who are confronting surgery. It is often true that these children can be sedated preparatory to anesthesia by giving them either an injection or an oral medication. There is no question that almost all children prefer a pill to an injection, though some anesthesiologists prefer the injection. However, except in rare cases in which oral medication is contraindicated, parents should be informed of the alternatives and allowed to make the choice. The anesthesiologist may certainly make recommendations, but he should not make the decision unilaterally without even informing the parents of the alternatives.

Another instance of information that is generally not given, but that is clearly relevant, is the mortality and morbidity rate for the contemplated type of procedure in one's specific hospital or medical center, especially if there is a significant difference between local results and those of medical centers where a particular kind of procedure is performed more often. There is now substantial evidence that some kinds of surgery are volume-sensitive to a rather high degree.[1] Thus, all candidates for volume-sensitive operations at low-volume hospitals should be told that they are at a somewhat greater risk than they might be elsewhere. Any rational person who is advised to undergo a major operation, for example cardiac or major vascular surgery, would want to know that traveling fifty miles (or five blocks) might lessen his chances of dying during or after the surgery. . . .

One should also know the mortality and morbidity rate of one's surgeon, especially if it is significantly different from that of other surgeons in the same hospital, or in the same vicinity, who operate on cases of comparable severity and complexity. This assumes that such knowledge is available.

It is also relevant for the patient to know if the particular kind of surgery being suggested is performed far more often in the patient's area of the state or country than elsewhere, because this at least raises the possibility that the suggested surgery may be unnecessary, and that a second opinion from outside the area may be desirable. There is now strong evidence that the frequency with which particular kinds of surgery are performed (e.g., hysterectomy, tonsillectomy, and prostatectomy) varies widely from area to area.[2], [3] Because individual physicians are often unaware of these kinds of epidemiological data, we would recommend that such data be collected and published by public health agencies and be made prominently available through local libraries, consumers' groups, and so on.

Some of the above-mentioned kinds of information go beyond what is now required by law. The fact that our account of valid consent requires a physician to tell patients of this information may seem evidence of the lack of practical impact of philosophy. However, one should note that what counts as information the patient should have before giving consent has usually been determined not by legislation but by court decision (see *Cobbs v. Grant*, 1972). A patient who was not given some of the information mentioned above and who suffered an unfortunate complication due to the surgery might decide to bring suit against his physician. If it were plausible that he might have made a different decision if he had obtained the information, and if it were established that the information was indeed available but was not given to the patient, there is a genuine possibility that the jury decision would be in his favor. It has already been determined by some courts that the information required for valid consent is determined not by the standard practice of physicians to tell, but by what reasonable persons would want to know (for example, *Cobbs v. Grant*, 1972). Thus, it may be only a matter

of time before the law enforces what we believe is morally required.

It is clearly a historical accident that consent forms are required for surgery and not for most nonsurgical procedures. Side effects from drugs can result in complications as great as those from surgery. Clearly, these problems should be discussed as fully as the risks of surgery. There are also risks in nontreatment, and the patient should be informed if other qualified physicians would advise more aggressive treatment, whether surgical or medical. Some persons seem automatically to think that when both conservative treatment and surgery are possible, the former is better, but that choice, just like the choice to refuse surgery, is up to the patient. Patients should be told of all of the legitimate alternative courses of treatment. All these issues simply make explicit the consequences of the view that the patient should make the decision, not the doctor. . . .

We do not question the practical difficulties in having physicians provide adequate information to their patients. It is possible that many physicians will not want to take the time to provide the kind of information required. Objections to providing adequate information to the patient, though often stated as impossible, are not impossible in any important sense; they simply demand a change in the system of providing information for valid consent. Quite possibly the provision of information should no longer be regarded as the sole responsibility of the physician. Instead, in many in-patient settings, it could become one of the major responsibilities of the nursing profession. As we noted earlier, the information that a patient should have is not technical; it is information about the severity and probability of the goods and evils of the recommended course of treatment compared to no treatment or other treatments. For almost all standard treatments, nurses could be trained to provide such information. Indeed, nurses are often as well suited as doctors to provide the information required for valid consent. They are possibly less likely to overwhelm the patient with irrelevant technical details and more likely to concentrate on that information which the patient really needs, for example, how much pain and risk of disability are involved, how long a hospital stay is anticipated, and how high the chances are of a successful outcome. Nurses could then determine that the patient did indeed have all of the relevant information required for valid consent.

1. H.S. Luft, et al., *New England Journal of Medicine* 301 (1979), 1364–9.
2. J.E. Wennberg, *Hospital Practice* 14 (September 1979), 115–21, 126–7.
3. J.E. Wennberg, et al., *Annual Review of Public Health* 1 (1980), 277–95.

WASHINGTON STATE SUPREME COURT

ZeBarth v. Swedish Hospital Medical Center

Defendant hospital administered to plaintiff [Donald ZeBarth] a course of radiation therapy in treating him for Hodgkin's disease. About a year after the treatments had ended, plaintiff became paralyzed from injury to his spinal cord. He brought this action against the hospital alleging negligence in the treatment, and a jury returned a verdict in the sum of $450,280.

. . .

Altogether there was the testimony of experts in an esoteric field, one of exceptional complexity and scientific sophistication, from which it could be inferred that paralysis does not ordinarily result from radiation therapy unless the therapy has been somehow negligently administered, and additionally there were the general and ordinary experiences of mankind that people do not emerge from a course of radiation therapy paralyzed from the waist down unless there has been negligence in the treatment. . . .

The next assignment of error [concerns] what has become known in medical malpractice cases as "informed consent." Informed consent, an obvious misnomer, identifies a principle covering situations where medical treatment involves a grave risk of collateral injury and puts the physician under a duty to advise the patient of such risks before initiating the treatment. Informed consent, therefore, is the name for a general principle of law that a physician has a duty to disclose what a reasonably prudent physician in the medical community in the exercise of reasonable care would disclose to his patient as to whatever grave risks of injury may be incurred from a proposed course of treatment so that a patient, exercising ordinary care for his own welfare, and faced with a choice of undergoing the proposed treatment, or alternative treatment, or none at all, can, in reaching a decision,

intelligently exercise his judgment by reasonably balancing the probable risks against the probable benefits. . . .

What proof is necessary to establish a duty to inform? From time to time cases may arise where the obligation upon the physician to inform his patient of the risks of treatment is so manifest that a layman, even without the benefit of medical testimony, could reasonably find that the benefits from the proposed therapy would be so slight in relation to the gravity of the risks of harm from it that no medical testimony would be required to prove the duty to inform. For example, high voltage, heavy dosage radiation therapy utilized to treat a wholly benign wart would undoubtedly call for a duty to inform without expert medical testimony to prove it. But in most instances, and as a general rule, the duty to inform the patient must be established by expert medical testimony or reasonable inferences to be drawn from it. Thus, as stated by Waltz & Scheuneman (64 NW UL Rev 628, 636), "The great majority of courts follow some professional standard, variously worded. The largest group within this majority would measure the duty according to the custom and practice of physicians within the 'community'." Some courts within the majority group require the disclosure that a reasonable practitioner would make under the circumstances; others require disclosure consistent with "good medical practice." Whatever may be the verbal formula, however, these courts generally require expert testimony to prove a duty to inform.

We deem it to be the prevailing view and one which should be followed by this court that generally the duty of the physician to inform and the extent of the information required should be established by expert medical testimony. . . .

This duty, however, is limited to those disclosures which, according to the recognized medical standards of that specialty, should be given by a reasonable

From *American Law Reports* 52, 3d series (1972), pp. 1069, 1075–1078, 1080.

doctor practicing the same specialty, in the same or similar circumstances. The standards must be proven by testimony of members of the medical profession practicing the same specialty.

•   •   •

The duty of a medical doctor to inform his patient of the risks of harm reasonably to be expected from a proposed course of treatment does not place upon the physician a duty to elucidate upon all of the possible risks, but only those of a serious nature. Nor does it contemplate that the patient or those in whose charge he may be are completely ignorant of medical matters. A patient is obliged to exercise the intelligence and act on the knowledge which an ordinary person would bring to the doctor's office. The law does not contemplate that a doctor need conduct a short course in anatomy, medicine, surgery and therapeutics nor that he do anything which in reasonable standards for practice of medicine in the community might be inimical to the patient's best interests. The doctrine of informed consent does not require the doctor to risk frightening the patient out of a course of treatment which sound medical judgment dictates the patient should undertake, nor does the rule assume that the patient possesses less knowledge of medical matters than a person of ordinary understanding could reasonably be expected to have or by law should be charged with having. Nor should the rule declaring a duty to inform be so stated or applied that a physician, in the interest of protecting himself from an overburden of law suits and the attendant costs upon his time and purse, will always follow the most conservative therapy—which, while of doubtful benefit to the patient, exposes the patient to no affirmative medical hazards and the doctor to no risks of litigation. Thus, the information required of the doctor by the general rule is that information which a reasonably prudent physician or medical specialist of that medical community should or would know to be essential to enable a patient of ordinary understanding to intelligently decide whether to incur the risk by accepting the proposed treatment or avoid that risk by forgoing it. A doctor or specialist who fails to discharge this duty to inform would thus be liable as for negligence to the patient for the harm proximately resulting from the treatment to which the patient submitted. Whether the information should have been given at all and the nature, kind and extent of the disclosure thus must in most instances be established by expert medical testimony.

•   •   •

Dr. Orliss Wildermuth, a highly trained specialist in radiation therapy, practicing on the staff of defendant tumor institute, said that from a medical standpoint a patient about to undergo radiation therapy should be advised in terms of ordinary understanding by his physician of the nature and effect of radiation therapy and the nature and effect of possible alternative treatments, and that the patient needed this medical information in order to reach an intelligent decision as to whether he would undergo the risks. Dr. Frederick Exner, a physician specialist in radiology, called by plaintiff, was more emphatic as to this duty and said in effect that the duty to inform the patient was specifically imposed by the very essence of good practice; and that this was done as a time-honored custom as well as a duty required of a physician in the practice of medicine.

•   •   •

At trial, the court first had to determine whether the evidence warranted an instruction on the subject of informed consent, i.e., whether the evidence showed a duty upon the doctors to inform the patient (*Watkins v. Parpala,* 2 Wash App 484, 469 P2d 974 [1970]), and then, assuming that the circumstances shown generally supported such an instruction, whether it, nevertheless, should have been refused because the plaintiff did not testify directly that had he known the risks he would not have accepted the proposed treatment. See *Mason v. Ellsworth,* 3 Wash App 298, 474 P2d 909 (1970).

Plaintiff professed little knowledge of the possible harmful effects of radiation therapy. He testified that he received no advice or information whatever from defendant institute or the treating physicians as to the hazards of radiation therapy or the harm that might result from it. Neither was the amount, duration and degree of fractionation mentioned to him. He realized that Hodgkin's is regarded as a fatal disease if unarrested; he was in no position to decline radiation therapy despite the hazards of treatment. He thus had no effective choice between some radiation treatment and the almost certain death without it.

But there was a vital choice open to him, had he been informed of the alternative: the initial large dose with the dangers of myelopathy, or a markedly lesser fractionated dose with its attendant danger of swelling. The totality of evidence permits an inference that, had plaintiff been informed that a massive initial dose carried with it a possible danger of a paralysis-inducing myelopathy, in contrast to the usual and

lesser dosages so fractionated that the ultimate total amounted to the same, he would have chosen the latter course.

UNITED STATES COURT OF APPEALS

Canterbury v. Spence

SPOTTSWOOD W. ROBINSON, III,
Circuit Judge

Suits charging failure by a physician adequately to disclose the risks and alternatives of proposed treatment are not innovations in American law. They date back a good half-century, and in the last decade they have multiplied rapidly. There is, nonetheless, disagreement among the courts and the commentators on many major questions, and there is no precedent of our own directly in point. For the tools enabling resolution of the issues on this appeal, we are forced to begin at first principles.

The root premise is the concept, fundamental in American jurisprudence, that "[e]very human being of adult years and sound mind has a right to determine what shall be done with his own body. . . ." True consent to what happens to one's self is the informed exercise of a choice, and that entails an opportunity to evaluate knowledgeably the options available and the risks attendant upon each. The average patient has little or no understanding of the medical arts, and ordinarily has only his physician to whom he can look for enlightenment with which to reach an intelligent decision. From these almost axiomatic considerations springs the need, and in turn the requirement, of a reasonable divulgence by physician to patient to make such a decision possible.

• • •

Once the circumstances give rise to a duty on the physician's part to inform his patient, the next inquiry

No. 22099, U.S. Court of Appeals, District of Columbia Circuit, May 19, 1972. 464 Federal Reporter, 2nd Series, 772.

is the scope of the disclosure the physician is legally obliged to make. The courts have frequently confronted this problem, but no uniform standard defining the adequacy of the divulgence emerges from the decisons. Some have said "full" disclosure,[1] a norm we are unwilling to adopt literally. It seems obviously prohibitive and unrealistic to expect physicians to discuss with their patients every risk of proposed treatment—no matter how small or remote—and generally unnecessary from the patient's viewpoint as well. Indeed, the cases speaking in terms of "full" disclosure appear to envision something less than total disclosure,[2] leaving unanswered the question of just how much.

The larger number of courts, as might be expected, have applied tests framed with reference to prevailing fashion within the medical profession. Some have measured the disclosure by "good medical practice," others by what a reasonable practitioner would have bared under the circumstances, and still others by what medical custom in the community would demand. We have explored this rather considerable body of law but are unprepared to follow it. The duty to disclose, we have reasoned, arises from phenomena apart from medical custom and practice. The latter, we think, should no more establish the scope of the duty than its existence. Any definition of scope in terms purely of a professional standard is at odds with the patient's prerogative to decide on projected therapy himself. That prerogative, we have said, is at the very foundation of the duty to disclose, and both the patient's right to know and the physician's correlative obligation to tell him are diluted to the extent that its compass is dictated by the medical profession.

In our view, the patient's right of self-decision shapes the boundaries of the duty to reveal. That right can be effectively exercised only if the patient possesses enough information to enable an intelligent choice. The scope of the physician's communications to the patient, then, must be measured by the patient's need, and that need is the information material to the decision. Thus the test for determining whether a particular peril must be divulged is its materiality to the patient's decision: all risks potentially affecting the decision must be unmasked. And to safeguard the patient's interest in achieving his own determination on treatment, the law must itself set the standard for adequate disclosure.

Optimally for the patient, exposure of a risk would be mandatory whenever the patient would deem it significant to his decision, either singly or in combination with other risks. Such a requirement, however, would summon the physician to second-guess the patient, whose ideas on materiality could hardly be known to the physician. That would make an undue demand upon medical practitioners, whose conduct, like that of others, is to be measured in terms of reasonableness. Consonantly with orthodox negligence doctrine, the physician's liability for nondisclosure is to be determined on the basis of foresight, not hindsight; no less than any other aspect of negligence, the issue of nondisclosure must be approached from the viewpoint of the reasonableness of the physician's divulgence in terms of what he knows or should know to be the patient's informational needs. If, but only if, the fact-finder can say that the physician's communication was unreasonably inadequate is an imposition of liability legally or morally justified.

Of necessity, the content of the disclosure rests in the first instance with the physician. Ordinarily it is only he who is in position to identify particular dangers; always he must make a judgment, in terms of materiality, as to whether and to what extent revelation to the patient is called for. He cannot know with complete exactitude what the patient would consider important to his decision, but on the basis of his medical training and experience he can sense how the average, reasonable patient expectably would react. Indeed, with knowledge of, or ability to learn, his patient's background and current condition, he is in a position superior to that of most others—attorneys, for example—who are called upon to make judg-

ments on pain of liability in damages for unreasonable miscalculation.

From these considerations we derive the breadth of the disclosure of risks legally to be required. The scope of the standard is not subjective as to either the physician or the patient; it remains objective with due regard for the patient's informational needs and with suitable leeway for the physician's situation. In broad outline, we agree that "[a] risk is thus material when a reasonable person, in what the physician knows or should know to be the patient's position, would be likely to attach significance to the risk or cluster of risks in deciding whether or not to forgo the proposed therapy."[3]

The topics importantly demanding a communication of information are the inherent and potential hazards of the proposed treatment, the alternatives to that treatment, if any, and the results likely if the patient remains untreated. The factors contributing significance to the dangerousness of a medical technique are, of course, the incidence of injury and the degree of the harm threatened. A very small chance of death or serious disablement may well be significant; a potential disability which dramatically outweighs the potential benefit of the therapy or the detriments of the existing malady may summon discussion with the patient.

There is no bright line separating the significant from the insignificant; the answer in any case must abide a rule of reason. Some dangers—infection, for example—are inherent in any operation; there is no obligation to communicate those of which persons of average sophistication are aware. Even more clearly, the physician bears no responsibility for discussion of hazards the patient has already discovered, or those having no apparent materiality to patients' decision on therapy. The disclosure doctrine, like others marking lines between permissible and impermissible behavior in medical practice, is in essence a requirement of conduct prudent under the circumstances. Whenever nondisclosure of particular risk information is open to debate by reasonable-minded men, the issue is for the finder of the facts.

Two exceptions to the general rule of disclosure have been noted by the courts. Each is in the nature of a physician's privilege not to disclose, and the reasoning underlying them is appealing. Each, indeed, is but a recognition that, as important as is the patient's right to know, it is greatly outweighed by the magnitudinous circumstances giving rise to the privilege. The first comes into play when the patient is unconscious or otherwise incapable of consenting, and harm from a failure to treat is imminent and outweighs any harm threatened by the proposed treatment. When a genuine emergency of that sort arises, it is settled that the impracticality of conferring with the patient dispenses with need for it. Even in situations of that character the physician should, as current law requires, attempt to secure a relative's consent if possible. But if time is too short to accommodate discussion obviously the physician should proceed with the treatment.

The second exception obtains when risk-disclosure poses such a threat of detriment to the patient as to become unfeasible or contraindicated from a medical point of view. It is recognized that patients occasionally become so ill or emotionally distraught on disclosure as to foreclose a rational decision, or complicate or hinder the treatment, or perhaps even pose psychological damage to the patient. Where that is so, the cases have generally held that the physician is armed with a privilege to keep the information from the patient, and we think it clear that portents of that type may justify the physician in action he deems medically warranted. The critical inquiry is whether the physician responded to a sound medical judgment that communication of the risk information would present a threat to the patient's well-being.

The physician's privilege to withhold information for therapeutic reasons must be carefully circumscribed, however, for otherwise it might devour the disclosure rule itself. The privilege does not accept the paternalistic notion that the physician may remain silent simply because divulgence might prompt the patient to forgo therapy the physician feels the patient really needs. That attitude presumes instability or perversity for even the normal patient, and runs counter to the foundation principle that the patient should and ordinarily can make the choice for himself. Nor does the privilege contemplate operation save where the patient's reaction to risk information, as reasonably foreseen by the physician, is menacing. And even in a situation of that kind, disclosure to a close relative with a view to securing consent to the proposed treatment may be the only alternative open to the physician.

NOTES

1. *E.g.,* Salgo v. Leland Stanford Jr. Univ. Bd. of Trustees, 154 Cal. App. 2d 560, 317 P.2d 170, 181 (1957); Woods v. Brumlop, *supra* note 13 [in original text], 377 P.2d at 524–525.

2. See, Comment, Informed Consent in Medical Malpractice, 55 Calif. L. Rv. 1396, 1402–03 (1967).

3. Waltz and Scheuneman, Informed Consent to Therapy, 64, Nw. U.L. Rev. 628, 640 (1970).

J A Y   K A T Z

Informed Consent—A Fairy Tale?

INTRODUCTION

Fairy tales are so appealing because ultimately they reduce complex human encounters to enchanting simplicity. In listening to them we suspend judgment and believe that once upon a time it was, and maybe even today it is, possible to utter magic words or perform magic deeds which transform frogs into princes or punish greedy fishermen's wives. The phrase ''informed consent'' evokes the same magic

From *University of Pittsburgh Law Review* 39 (Winter 1977), pp. 137, 139–142, 145–147, 155–160, 162–164, 174.

expectations. Its protagonists often convey that once kissed by the doctrine, frog-patients will become autonomous princes. Its antagonists warn that all the gold of good medical care which physicians now so magnanimously bestow on patients will turn to worthless metal if the curse of informed consent were to remain with us.

• • •

The common law's vision of informed consent is confusing and confused. Its frequently articulated underlying purpose—to promote patients' decisional authority over their medical fate—has been severely compromised from the beginning. The wish that patients can or should be allowed to make their own decisions, based on the fullest disclosure possible, runs through most of the opinions. But once the wish has been given its separate due, the rest of the opinion ignores that dream and instead defers to those realities of legal, medical, and human life which are opposed to fostering patients' decision-making. Thus the doctrine of informed consent remains a symbol which despite widespread currency has had little impact on patients' decision-making, either in legal theory or medical practice.

Anglo-American law is caught up in a conflict between its vision of human beings as autonomous persons and its deference to paternalism, another powerful vision of man's interaction with man. The conflict created by uncertainties about the extent to which individual and societal well-being is better served by encouraging patients' self-determination or supporting physicians' paternalism is the central problem of informed consent. This fundamental conflict, reflecting a thoroughgoing ambivalence about human beings' capacities for taking care of themselves and need for care-taking, has shaped judicial pronouncements on informed consent more decisively than is commonly appreciated. The assertion of a "need" for physicians' discretion—for a professional expert's rather than a patient's judgment as to what constitutes well-being—reveals this ambivalence. Other oft-invoked impediments to fostering patients' self-determination, such as patients' medical ignorance, doctors' precious time, the threat of increased litigation, or the difficulty of proving what actually occurred in the dialogue between physician and patient are, substantially, rationalizations which obscure the basic conflict over whose judgment is to be respected.

This ambivalence also reflects conflicting legal views about the psychological nature of human beings. In jurisprudential theory, man is said to be autonomous, self-determining and responsible for his actions. Yet law-makers do not place complete faith in such theoretical constructs once man comes into living contact with law. The never-ending debates over criminal responsibility and civil commitment are telling examples of this conflict in other areas of law. It extends, however, from encounters with persons tainted by attributes of "mental illness" to interactions with "normal" persons where, as in most informed consent disputes, no considerations of mental abnormality enter.

Medical law in the United States is a clear case of institutionalized paternalism. In the last fifty years allopathic physicians have been awarded virtually a complete monopoly over the licensure and practice of the healing arts. Similarly, for the "protection" of citizens, the most rigid drug laws in the world have been promulgated, sequestering most of the pharmacopaeia under the control of experts. When judges began to consider the issue of patients' autonomy in medical decision-making, it took place in a climate where the question of self-determination had been neglected by law for centuries. Lawmakers had reduced patients' personal freedom to the right of vetoing unwanted procedures and even this veto power is not always respected.[1]

As will be developed below, the courts' dicta on self-determination as the fundamental principle underlying the informed consent doctrine are misleading if taken to imply a broad duty of physicians to disclose pertinent medical information or to invite active patients' participation in medical decison-making. Such dicta give the unwary reader of informed consent opinions a false sense that they shaped the doctrine's development, when instead other considerations, including strong doubts about the dicta themselves, were more important. There may, however, have been wisdom in judges' reluctance to give full support to patients' self-determination, once having made a symbolic bow to its supposed supremacy. Disclosure and consent may well be deleterious to a patient if, for example, as a consequence of medicine's ubiquitous uncertainties about risks and benefits, physicians' *and* patients' unexamined faith in the curative power of medical interventions contributes significantly to therapeutic success. Even partial awareness of such uncertainties, which an informed consent doctrine based on thoroughgoing self-determination would bring to consciousness, thus could prove detrimental to recovery. Judges, having been patients themselves, may intuitively have appreciated this crucial, though unexplored, issue and decided to avoid it. They focused instead on individual physicians' "transgressions" and ignored the fact that such "transgressions" are guided by all-embracing Hippocratic convictions about the "anti-therapeutic" consequences of disclosure and consent. These convictions have gained unquestioned acceptance by the way medicine has been taught to students since ancient times, though it is not at all clear that they can pass the test of careful examination. One thing is clear, however—traditional medical practices, indeed all professional practices, would be radically altered if courts were to enforce patients' rights to disclosure and consent.

Underlying this problem, however, rests another: Who decides what, if any, medical intervention should be undertaken? Justice Bray gave an equivocal response. He said that disclosure was a matter for physicians' "discretion . . . consistent with the full disclosure of facts necessary to an informed consent."[2] Subsequent judges stated more forcefully the patient's right to decide, but their opinions, read as a whole, are much more qualified.

Courts have not acknowledged their failure to place effective authority in patients' hands. Though judges have felt morally bound to announce that patients ought to be enabled to guide their medical fate, they considered this position unsatisfactory in application and subjected it to extensive modifications. That such modifications significantly tampered with the basic posit of patients' self-determination and that altogether judicial commitment to individual decision-making was not very firm, were never clearly admitted. Judicial concern about patients' capacity to make medical decisions and about the detrimental impact of disclosure on patients proved to be more influential than self-determination in shaping the informed consent doctrine, even though the validity of these concerns rests more on conjecture than fact.

Physicians, while in recent decades increasingly confused as to what law expected them to do, have continued to exercise their traditional discretion in deciding what to and what not to disclose to patients. They have done so out of a felt necessity that unites most professionals in society. At the same time the fear of malpractice suits has led to an increased flow of words between physicians and patients. But this has not altered greatly the nature of the "informed consent" dialogue, because the information was not conveyed in the spirit of extending greater freedom of choice to patients. To accomplish that objective would have required a significant modification of the physician's deeply held convictions that he must make the ultimate decision about his patient's medical fate and this has not happened. Instead, the "dialogue" between them continues to be subtly and not so subtly punctuated with crucial distortions, not so much guided by enlightenment in order to facilitate patients'

participation in decision-making, but by a conviction that doctors' orders should be followed.

• • •

THE LAW OF CONSENT

The courts' dicta have been quoted frequently in case and commentary in support of the proposition that the judges had established a patient's right to thoroughgoing self-decision-making.[3] A careful reading of the cases, however, does not bear out this contention. These declamations addressed only the absolute duty of doctors to advise their patients of what is going to be done to them and to obtain their consent. It is this basic disclosure duty which courts underscored with their broad statements on self-determination. Their inquiry, for purposes of analysis of this quite limited, but rigorously enforced, duty did not invite or require a sophisticated examination of the consent process; for consent sufficient to obviate a claim of battery, the doctor only need relate in lay language what he intends to do to his patient.

The recent pronouncements on "informed consent" have not altered this simple requirement for valid consent. The label "informed consent" is misleading, since violation of the new duty to disclose risks and alternative treatments does not invalidate the patients' consent to the procedure in the great majority of jurisdictions. Rather the law of "informed consent" denotes a cause of action based on negligent failure to warn, i.e., failure to disclose pertinent medical information. While concern over patients' right to self-determination has led judges to entertain the need for greater disclosure of medical information, it did not prompt them to expand the requisites for valid consent. It is important to appreciate this lack of development, for it raises the question: Can patients' right to self-decision-making be safeguarded by merely modifying requirements for disclosure without at the same time expanding the requirement for valid consent? Or put another way, since there is a reciprocal relationship between disclosure and consent, how extensively and substantively must the informational needs of patients be satisfied to insure greater self-decision-making if it is to be accomplished within the matrix of the traditional consent requirement? In theory there is perhaps nothing wrong with leaving consent as it has always been, since self-determination could be protected by amplifying the requirements for mandatory disclosure. In practice, however, judges' sole focus on disclosure, to the exclusion of consent, tends to perpetuate physicians' disengaged monologues and to discourage a meaningful dialogue between doctors and patients. While it is difficult to compel change in the discourse between human beings where so much depends on the spirit in which it is carried on, a focus on the consent process would highlight the need for being mindful not only of physicians' conduct, standing alone, but of their conduct in relation to their patient. Questions would then arise as to whether physicians have explored what a patient wishes to know by inviting him to ask further questions about treatment options and by ascertaining whether a patient's informational needs have been met to his satisfaction. Consent is more responsive to inquiries into the care taken for facilitating understanding, while disclosure is less so; for the temptation is great to emphasize what is said rather than how it is communicated. Not only was nothing done about consent but, as we shall see, judges have been exceedingly reluctant even to require significant disclosure.

THE LEGAL LIFE OF "INFORMED CONSENT"

In the last two decades, judges have begun to ask whether patients are entitled not only to know what the doctor proposes to do, but also to decide whether an intervention is acceptable in light of its risks and benefits and the available alternatives, including no treatment. . . .

I. HYBRID STANDARD OF CARE

The new rule of law laid down in *Canterbury,* however, is far from clear. Judge Robinson, returning to basic principles of expert testimony, had simply said, there is "no basis for operation of the special medical standard whenever the physician's activity does not bring his medical knowledge and skills peculiarly into play,"[4] and that ordinarily disclosure was not such a situation. But Judge Robinson left room for such situations, with respect to disclosure: "When medical judgment enters the picture and for that reason the special standard controls, prevailing medical practice must be given its *just due*."[5] He did not spell out his meaning. In this case, the defendant claimed that "communication of that risk (of paralysis) to the patient is not good medical practice because it might deter patients from undergoing needed

surgery and might produce adverse psychological reactions which could preclude the success of the operation."[6] Such claims, we shall see, will almost invariably be raised by physicians since they derive from widely held tenets of medical practice. "Just due," Judge Robinson's enigmatic phrase, in context certainly suggests that the medical professional standard would be applicable in such a case. If so, the plaintiff's failure to produce an expert witness to contradict the defendant's proposed applicable standard of care, expressing an exercise of professional judgment, will demand or strongly invite a directed verdict. Alternatively, the defense of medical judgment could be treated under the "therapeutic privilege" not to disclose, admitted by Judge Robinson and other courts.[7] "It is recognized," he said, "that patients occasionally become so ill or emotionally distraught on disclosure as to foreclose a rational decision, or complicate or hinder the treatment, or perhaps even pose psychological damage to the patient. . . . The critical inquiry is, whether the physician responded to a sound medical judgment that communication of the risk information would present a threat to the patient's well-being."[8]

At the same time the court paid no deference to the medical judgment, that disclosure of a one percent risk of paralysis is generally unwise where a laminectomy is considered medically necessary; instead the "just due" of that judgment is to be treated like any other testimony. Thus, on what may have seemed to be an easy fact situation, the court did not face the trial problems of respecting medical judgment raised by its statement of the law. Neither did the plaintiff, since on retrial he came equipped with an expert witness to establish the plaintiff's version of the standard of disclosure.

Finally, despite the court's dictum that medical judgment, where it "enters the picture," must be given its just due by applying the professional standard of disclosure, the court later suggested that questions of medical judgment must be raised in defense by means of the therapeutic privilege: "With appellant's prima facie case of violation of duty to disclose, the burden of introducing evidence showing a privilege was on Dr. Spence."[9] The court did not specify the legal consequences of invoking such a privilege.

The therapeutic privilege not to disclose, as Judge Robinson recognized, is merely a procedurally different way of invoking the professional standard of care. The burden of proof of course remains on the plaintiff. Only if a prima facie case of negligent nondisclosure has been made, does the burden of going forward shift to the defendant, to produce evidence that failure to disclose represented a reasonable exercise of medical judgment. The effect of such evidence is as yet unclear. It may be given the status of medical professional evidence, so that failure to produce contralateral expert testimony will demand a directed verdict. If so, there is virtually no difference between the *Natanson* and *Canterbury* lines of cases, since the plaintiff will almost always be obliged to produce expert testimony that non-disclosure was unreasonable. Alternatively, the defendant-doctor's evidence of the therapeutic appropriateness of nondisclosure could be given no special status, and the question of reasonableness of disclosure could be sent to the jury on the testimony of the plaintiff that it was unreasonable to withhold the information at issue. If so, then the therapeutic privilege becomes merely a description of reasonableness, and not a true legal privilege; it would then have no role at trial except as a basis for jury instruction.

The ambiguous status of the standard of care and the therapeutic privilege in informed consent case law brings to surface judges' ambivalence toward both patients' self-determination and medical paternalism. In attempting to resolve their ambivalance, however, courts favored the traditional wisdom of the medical profession. For if there is meaning in Judge Robinson's support for the professional standard in cases where "medical judgment enters the picture," then the touted *Canterbury* "rule," that the duty to disclose is to be found in the language of judges rather than in the customary practice of physicians, means much less than previously imagined. Like *Salgo* and *Natanson, Canterbury* exhibits unresolved conflict in its attraction for both openness of communication and "discretion." Even though the court appeared to lay down a rule of mandatory disclosure, it excused doctors from compliance where "medical judgment," based on professional standards of disclosure, was involved. Yet Hippocratic physicians will find such medical judgment involved in virtually every case. Thus, the abrogation by the *Canterbury* court of the professional standard of disclosure in favor of a judge-made rule was much more ambiguous than a cursory reading would indicate. The ambiguity about the weight to be given to expert evidence on professional disclosure practices has not been resolved in the jurisdictions which follow *Canterbury*.

2. "MATERIALITY" OF RISKS AND ALTERNATIVES

The *Canterbury* court, in elaborating its judge-made standard for disclosure, went further than previous courts in tracing the ramifications of that standard. Since the court departed from medical custom as the standard, it had to give some indication as to the information it expected physicians to disclose. The court said "the test for determining whether a particular peril must be divulged is its materiality to the patient's decision: all risks potentially affecting the decision must be unmasked."[10] And it added that physicians similarly must disclose alternatives to the proposed treatment and the "results likely if the patient remains untreated."[11] The court adopted the language of Waltz and Scheuneman, that a risk "is thus material when a reasonable person in what the physician knows or should know to be the patient's position, would be likely to attach significance to the risk or cluster of risks in deciding whether or not to forgo the proposed therapy."[12] The court rejected a "subjective" test of materiality for disclosure of risks and alternatives. While appreciating that a "subjective" test of materiality to the particular patient would more ideally comply with self-determination, it felt that such a test would unfairly burden the physician by requiring him to guess the needs of this particular patient; thus a physician should be compelled to divulge only that information which would be required by a reasonable patient. The court stated:

Optimally for the patient, exposure of a risk would be mandatory whenever the patient would deem it significant to his decision, either singly or in combination with other risks. Such a requirement, however, would summon the physician to second-guess the patient, whose ideas on materiality could hardly be known to the physician. That would make an undue demand upon medical practitioners, whose conduct, like that of others, is to be measured in terms of reasonableness. . . .

Of necessity, the content of the disclosure rests in the first instance with the physician. Ordinarily it is only he who is in position to identify particular dangers; always he must make a judgment, in terms of materiality, as to whether and to what extent revelation to the patient is called for. He cannot know with complete exactitude what the patient would consider important to his decision, but on the basis of his medical training and experience he can sense how the average, reasonable patient expectably would react. Indeed, with knowledge of, or ability to learn, his patient's background and current condition, he is in a position superior to that of most others—attorneys, for example—who are called upon to make judgments on pain of liability in damages for unreasonable miscalculation.[13]

The court's preoccupation with physicians' plight in determining what to disclose prevented it from considering the patient's plight and proceeding further to protect his right of choice, by requiring the physician to ascertain what his patient's concerns, doubts and misconceptions are about the treatment—its risks, benefits and alternatives. The physician cannot know with exactitude what the patient would consider important; and little in his medical training and experience has as yet prepared him, if it ever can, to sense how patients will react to disclosures. Moreover, patients differ widely in their informational needs. For all these reasons, safeguarding self-determination requires asking the patient whether he understands what has been explained to him in order to assess whether his informational needs have been satisfied. Physicians need not "sense" how the patient will react or "second-guess" him; instead, they should explore what questions need further explanation.

Indeed the court's sole emphasis on specific disclosures, particularly material risks, overlooks the crucial significance of the unsatisfactory climate in which specific disclosures are now being made. To be sure, satisfying a patient's informational needs demands knowledge of risks. But such information, if it is to serve the patient as data for decision, can only begin to become meaningful to him if he is viewed as an active and not passive participant in the medical decision-making process. The court quite correctly singled out risks and alternatives as most important facts which patients may wish to know. However, its discussion on materiality—*e.g.*, that the physician "must make a judgment in terms of materiality"[14]—strongly implies that courts wish to leave decisional control with physicians. Thus wittingly or unwittingly the court gave powerful support to the traditional paternalistic pattern of physician-patient interaction.

The court also ignored the crucial problem of how much a physician needs to know concerning risks, *e.g.*, the frequency of their occurrence in his, as contrasted to general, experience, and the problems with alternative treatments of which he is unlikely to be a practitioner.[15] Unless judges are willing to articulate standards in this area, expert witnesses will be required to detail the extent of learning reasonably to be expected under a professional standard of competency, even where *Canterbury* is followed.[16]

3. PROXIMATE CAUSE: THE REQUIREMENT OF ALTERED CONDUCT

The *Canterbury* court, following *Natanson*, accepted the traditional requirement, that the injury to the plaintiff be proximately caused by the negligence of the defendant. Therefore, the plaintiff must prove that he would not have agreed to the proposed therapy, if disclosure had been adequate.[17] . . .

Judge Robinson . . . reasoned that the question for the jury is not what the patient would have decided to do, had the physician adequately informed him, but "what a prudent person in the patient's position would have decided if suitably informed of all perils bearing significance."[18] Such an "objective" standard, the court said, will prevent the patient's testimony, perhaps influenced by "hindsight and bitterness,"[19] from threatening "to dominate the findings,"[20] and will "ease the fact-finding process and better assure the truth as its product."[21]

Self-determination is given unnecessarily short shrift. The whole point of the inquiry, and the potential liability, is to safeguard the right of *individual* choice, even where it may appear idiosyncratic. The "objective" standard of "causality" contradicts the right of each individual to decide what will be done with his body by denying the patient recovery whenever his hypothetical decision is out of step with the judgment of a prudent person. The belief that there is one "reasonable" or "prudent" response to every situation inviting medical intervention is nonsense, both from the point of view of the physician as well as that of the patient. Since different doctors approach similar cases in diametrically opposed ways, equally varying responses by patients ought to be considered "reasonable." The aim of the doctrine is not to encourage uniformity in medical treatment, but to preserve individual choice.

•   •   •

INFORMED CONSENT—FAIRY TALE AND MYTH

The law of informed consent has undergone little analytic development since *Canterbury*. In the twenty years following its birth in *Salgo*, legal protection for patients' freedom of choice was not significantly expanded. Whatever promise *Salgo* and the first *Natan-*

son opinion held out to secure such rights faded in subsequent constructions of the doctrine.

JAY KATZ   197

• • •

At present the law of informed consent is substantially mythic and fairy tale-like as far as advancing patients' rights to self-decision-making is concerned. It conveys in its dicta about such rights a fairy tale-like optimism about human capacities for "intelligent" choice and for being respectful of other persons' choices; yet in its implementation of dicta, it conveys a mythic pessimism of human capacities to be choice-makers. The resulting tensions have had a significant impact on the law of informed consent which only has made a bow toward a commitment to patients' self-determination, perhaps in an attempt to resolve these tensions by a belief that it is "less important that this commitment be total than that we believe it to be there."[22] It is premature to decide whether society is better served by proclaiming a commitment to patients' autonomy, even though we do not wish to implement it, or by a frank acknowledgment that it is a fairy tale, at least to a considerable extent; but it is not at all clear whether in interactions between physicians and patients both fairy tale and myth cannot be reconciled much more satisfactorily with reality.

NOTES

1. *See, e.g.,* Application of President and Directors of Georgetown College, 331 F. 2d 1000, *rehearing denied,* 331 F. 2d 1010 (D.C. Cir.), *cert. denied,* 337 U.S. 978 (1964); Petition of Nemser, 51 Misc. 2d 616, 273 N.Y.S. 2d 624 (Sup. Ct. 1966).

2. Salgo v. Leland Stanford, Jr., University Board of Trustees, 154 Cal. App. 2d 560, 578, 317 P. 2d 170, 181 (Dist. Ct. of App. 1957).

3. *See, e.g.,* Canterbury v. Spence, 464 F. 2d 772, 780 (D.C. Cir. 1972); Shack v. Holland, 389 N.Y. Supp. 2d 988, 991 (1976); 1 D. Louisell, H. Williams and J. Kalisch, Medical Malpractice Para. 8.09, at 221 (1973); Capron, *Informed Consent in Catastrophic Disease Research and Treatment,* 123 U. Pa. L. Rev. 340, 346–347 (1974); Note, *Restructuring Informed Consent: Legal Therapy for the Doctor-Patient Relationship,* 79 Yale L.J. 1533, 1555 (1970).

4. 464 F. 2d at 785 (footnote omitted).

5. *Id.* (emphasis added).

6. *Id.* at 778.

7. *Id.* at 789. The idea of a "therapeutic privilege" originated with Dr. Hubert Smith. *Therapeutic Privilege to Withhold Specific Diagnosis from Patient Sick with Serious or Fatal Illness,* 19 Tenn. L. Rev. 349 (1946), to sanction the practice of doctors in not telling patients they have cancer. Smith recognized that there was "no legal authority" for such a privilege. *Id.* at 351.

8. 464 F. 2d at 789 (footnote omitted).

9. 464 F. 2d at 794, n. 138.

10. 464 F. 2d at 786–87 (footnote omitted).

11. *Id.* at 788.

12. *Id.* at 787, *citing* Waltz and Scheuneman, *Informed Consent to Therapy,* 64 Nw. U. L. Rev. 628, 640 (1970). *See also,* Wilkinson v. Vesey, 295 A. 2d 676, 689 (R.I. 1972).

13. 464 F. 2d at 787 (footnote omitted).

14. 464 F. 2d at 787.

15. *See id.* n. 84.

16. Cf., e.g., Miller v. Kennedy, 11 Wash. App. 272, 284, 522 P. 2d 852, 861 (1974), *aff'd per curiam,* 85 Wash. 2d 151, 530 P. 2d 334 (1975).

17. 464 F. 2d at 789.

18. 464 F. 2d at 791 (footnote omitted), *citing* Waltz and Scheuneman, *Informed Consent to Therapy,* 64 Nw. U. L. Rev. 628, 646 (1970).

19. 464 F. 2d at 791.

20. *Id.*

21. *Id.*

22. G. Calabresi, *Reflections on Medical Experimentation in Humans,* Daedalus, 387, 388 (Spring 1969).

LEROY WALTERS

Ethical Aspects of Medical Confidentiality

I. THE PRINCIPLE OF MEDICAL CONFIDENTIALITY: HISTORICAL SKETCH

Within the history of ethics the most extensive and detailed references to the principle of medical confidentiality occur within codes of professional ethics. The ancient works of Hindu medicine mention the obligation of medical secrecy.[1] For the Western tradition of medical ethics, however, the fundamental statement concerning medical confidentiality occurs in the Hippocratic Oath. There we read:

What I may see or hear in the course of the treatment or even outside of the treatment in regard to the life of men, which on no account one must spread abroad, I will keep to myself, holding such things shameful to be spoken about.[2]

This affirmation of the principle of confidentiality in the Hippocratic Oath exerted a strong influence on the formulation of subsequent codes of medical ethics. The principle recurs in the first great modern textbook of professional ethics for physicians, Thomas Percival's *Medical Ethics,* published in 1803. Percival noted:

Secrecy and delicacy, when required by peculiar circumstances, should be strictly observed. And the familiar and confidential intercourse, to which the faculty are admitted in their professional visits, should be used with discretion and with the most scrupulous regard to fidelity and honour.[3]

Percival's statement was reproduced practically verbatim in the first major American code, *The Code of Medical Ethics,* adopted by the American Medical Association in 1847.[4]

In more recent times the principle of medical confidentiality has been reaffirmed in numerous codes of professional ethics. The International Code of Medi-

cal Ethics adopted by the World Medical Association contains a strong statement of the principle:

A doctor owes to his patient absolute secrecy on all which has been confided to him or which he knows because of the confidence entrusted in him.[5]

The most recent version of the AMA's ''Principles of Medical Ethics'' devotes a separate section to the topic of medical confidentiality.[6]

In addition to appearing in codes of professional ethics for physicians, the principle of confidentiality also plays a prominent role in the ethical codes of various other health professionals, including nurses, medical social workers, and medical record librarians.[7] Of particular interest is a statement in the Code of Ethics of the American Association of Medical Record Librarians:

As a member of one of the paramedical professions [the librarian] shall . . . (2) Preserve and protect the medical records in his custody and hold inviolate the privileged contents of the records and any other information of a confidential nature obtained in his official capacity, taking due account of applicable status and of regulations and policies of his employer.[8]

Professional codes of ethics have been the main locus of ethical discussion concerning the principle of medical confidentiality. However, there are two other nonlegal sources which should at least be mentioned in passing. The first is the tradition of Western religious ethics. The literature of various religious groups, particularly Jews and Roman Catholics, has devoted substantial attention to questions of medical ethics.[9] On the specific issue of medical confidentiality Jewish religious ethics is totally silent.[10] In contrast, Catholic textbooks of moral theology frequently include detailed discussions of confidentiality in the physician-patient relationship, perhaps in part be-

This essay is a revised version of an article originally published in the *Journal of Clinical Computing,* Vol. 4 (1974), pp. 9–20. Copyright 1974 by LeRoy Walters.

cause of its obvious parallels with the confidential relationship of priest and penitent.[11] Within the moral-theology textbooks are extended analyses of the nature of a secret, mental reservation, and the circumstances under which professional secrets may or may not be revealed.[12]

The other major nonprofessional source of ethical discussion concerning medical confidentiality is the emergent patient's rights movement. Probably the most important document resulting from pressures generated by the movement is the "Patient's Bill of Rights," published by the American Hospital Association in 1973. In that document one reads:

The patient has the right to expect that all communications and records pertaining to his care should be treated as confidential.[13]

The legal tradition has also wrestled at length with the problem of medical confidentiality. In many cases, the law has simultaneously discussed the analogous questions of confidential communications between attorneys and clients and between ministers or rabbis and persons who solicit their advice. Two kinds of legal protection for medical confidentiality can be distinguished: positive protection and negative protection. Positive protection refers to legal sanctions which can be applied against physicians who reveal confidential information about their patients. In English and American law the patient injured by such a breach can seek a remedy at law by bringing suit. In contrast, on the European continent, the violation of medical secrecy by the physician is punishable or punished according to provisions of the criminal law.[14]

Negative protection of medical confidentiality is provided by laws which establish communications between physician and patient as privileged communications and which thereby exempt the physician from the normal obligation to testify before a court of law. The English Common Law did not consider as privileged the communications which pass between physicians and patients. Since the common law formed the basis for American jurisprudence, it was to be expected that early American law would also lack any provision protecting communication between physicians and patients. However, in 1828, New York State by statute made physician-patient communication privileged. The New York State statute, which became the model for similar statutes adopted in many other states of the Union, read as follows:

No person duly authorized to practice physic or surgery, shall be allowed to disclose any information which he may have acquired in attending any patient, in a professional character, and which information was necessary to enable him to prescribe for such patient as a physician, or to do any act for him as a surgeon.[15]

As of 1973, forty-three states and the District of Columbia, had enacted general physician-patient privilege statutes. In addition, at least seventeen states have recently adopted laws which protect psychiatrist-patient or psychologist-client communications.[16]

II. THE PRINCIPLE OF MEDICAL CONFIDENTIALITY: PHILOSOPHICAL JUSTIFICATION

We turn now from history to philosophy, from the question of when and how the principle of medical confidentiality was formulated to the question of why it is important. There are two primary philosophical arguments in favor of preserving medical confidentiality. The first argument is utilitarian and refers to possible long-term consequences. The second argument is non-utilitarian and speaks of respect for the rights of persons.

The utilitarian argument for the preservation of medical confidentiality is that without such confidentiality the physician-patient relationship would be seriously impaired. More specifically, the promise of confidentiality encourages the patient to make a full disclosure of his symptoms and their causes, without fearing that an embarrassing condition will become public knowledge.[17] Among medical professionals, psychotherapists have been particularly concerned to protect the confidentiality of their relationship with patients. In the words of one psychiatrist:

The patient in analysis must learn to free associate and to break down resistances to deal with unconscious threatening thoughts and feelings. To revoke secrecy after encouraging such risk-taking is to threaten all future interaction.[18]

A second argument for the principle of medical confidentiality is that the right to a sphere of privacy is a basic human right. In what is perhaps the classic essay concerning the right of privacy, Samuel Warren and Louis Brandeis wrote in 1890 that the common law secured "to each individual the right of determining, ordinarily, to what extent his thoughts, sentiments, and emotions shall be communicated to others.''[19] Present-day advocates of the right of privacy frequently employ the imagery of concentric circles or spheres. In the center is the "core self," which shelters the individual's "ultimate secrets"—"those hopes, fears, and prayers that are beyond sharing with anyone unless the individual comes under such stress that he must pour out these ultimate secrets to secure emotional release.''[20] According to this image, the next largest circle contains intimate secrets which can be shared with close relatives or confessors of various kinds. Successively larger circles are open to intimate friends, to casual acquaintances, and finally to all observers.

The principle of medical confidentiality can be based squarely on this general right of privacy. The patient, in distress, shares with the physician detailed information concerning problems of body or mind. To employ the imagery of concentric circles, the patient admits the physician to an inner circle. If the physician, in turn, were to make public the information imparted by the patient—that is, if he were to invite scores or thousands of other persons into the same inner circle—we would be justified in charging that he had violated the patient's right of privacy and that he had shown disrespect to the patient as a human being.

These two arguments for the principle of medical confidentiality—the argument based on probable consequences of violation and the argument based on the right of privacy—seem to constitute a rather strong case for the principle. However, we have not yet faced the question whether the principle of confidentiality is a moral absolute, or whether it can be overridden by other considerations.

III. THE PRINCIPLE OF CONFIDENTIALITY: POSSIBLE GROUNDS FOR VIOLATING THE PRINCIPLE.

There are, in my view, three general reasons which might conceivably justify violating the principle of confidentiality.[21] The first is that the principle may come into conflict with the rights of the patient himself. To illustrate, one can envision a situation in which a patient, in a temporary fit of depression, threatens to kill himself or herself or to perform an irrational act which will almost certainly destroy the patient's reputation. In the case of threatened suicide, one finds oneself weighing a secret vs. a life. Perhaps the physician should feel free, in such a case, to violate the principle of confidentiality and to involve a third party for the protection of the patient himself or herself.

A second possible ground for violating the principle of confidentiality is that it may conflict with the right of an innocent third party. In older textbooks of moral theology, one can discover hypothetical cases constructed to illustrate this dilemma. Often the case involved a physician and a young couple about to be married. Because of his professional relationship with the husband-to-be, the physician knows that the man is concealing a condition of infective syphilis or permanent impotence from his future wife. The question then arises whether the physician should violate the principle of confidentiality in order to warn the unsuspecting innocent party.[22]

In our own time the physician's dilemma is more likely to concern the case of a "battered child." If the abused child is brought to the physician by the battering parents, the physician faces an immediate conflict of loyalties. Does he or she owe it to his adult patients to keep confidential the fact that they have abused the child? Or, is the physician under the obligation to protect the child from further harm by disclosing the child's injuries to the proper public authorities? It should perhaps be noted in passing that most states require that the physician report child-abuse cases to the appropriate governmental agency.[23]

A third possible ground for violating the principle of confidentiality is a serious conflict between the principle and the rights or interests of society in general. The possibility of such a conflict was formally recognized in 1912, when the American Medical Association revised its code of ethics. A new clause was introduced into the confidentiality section of the code, specifically authorizing the physician to report communicable diseases, even if such reports were based on confidential information. The justification for this type of disclosure was, of course, the protection of society at large from the spread of infectious disease.[24]

At present, various states require reports of particular types of contagious disease. Almost universally, the physician is legally obligated to report cases of venereal disease to the proper government authorities. The reporting of tuberculosis is also frequently required. State provisions for protecting the confidentiality of such public health reports vary widely, with about half of the states taking measures to prevent public disclosure of the data.[25] Whenever states require physicians to report such data concerning communicable diseases, the general justification for the violation of physician-patient confidentiality is that society at large must be protected.

There is a second type of situation in which the principle of confidentiality and the public good seem to come into sharp conflict. In these cases the physician discovers a serious medical problem in a patient whose occupation makes him responsible for the lives of many other persons. Two standard examples are a railroad signalman who is discovered to be subject to attacks of epilepsy, or an airline pilot with failing eyesight. A case reported in a recent essay on medical secrecy reads as follows:

Last year, 30 people were killed when a bus driver had a heart attack and plunged his bus into the East River in New York City. The driver's physician had known about the bad heart, had cautioned him not to drive, but felt he could not report it to the company since the patient might lose his job.[26]

In cases involving such critical occupations, some would argue that the physician's duty to protect the lives of many persons overrides his obligation to observe the principle of medical confidentiality.

In the future we are likely to see vigorous battles waged over the question of medical confidentiality vs. the public good. Three examples can be briefly cited. Already one hears rhetoric which implies that genetic disorders are quasi-contagious diseases.[27] According to this viewpoint, members of future generations will be "infected" if decisive action is not taken now. Is it possible that such pressures will lead to the requirement that physicians routinely report genetic defects to public health authorities? To cite a second example, epidemiologists constantly pursue new correlations between chronic diseases and particular environmental factors or medical conditions. Their studies frequently require surveys of total populations or random samples of such populations.[28] Will the desire of patients to keep their medical records confidential and their refusal to take part in such epidemiological studies come to be seen as an antisocial act or as a failure to perform a civic duty? Third, it is at least conceivable that the concept of public health could be expanded to include "economic contamination." According to this view, any disease which prevents a person from being a fully productive member of the labor force would be seen as a hazard to the society's overall economic health, particularly if public funds were being used to defray the expenses of

the illness. Cost-benefit analysis would indicate that because of the illness, other persons in the society would need to work to subsidize the relatively less-productive ill person. As one economist put it, well persons would become, at least partially, the "economic slaves" of the patient.[29] If the concept of public health is expanded in this economic direction, it seems likely that there will be tremendous pressure directed against maintaining the medical confidentiality of patients whose treatment is subsidized by public funds.

My own view is that the physician has a prima facie obligation to preserve the principle of medical confidentiality.[30] This obligation is based on the two considerations mentioned in Part II above, a concern for protecting the physician-patient relationship and a desire to respect the patient's right of privacy. Thus, the burden of proof must be assumed by anyone who wishes to argue that the principle of medical confidentiality should be violated. However, there are some cases in which this prima facie obligation can be overridden because of other very weighty considerations, for example, the desire to protect the patient's own life or the lives of other persons. According to this view, then, the physician's duty to observe the principle of medical confidentiality is a very important moral obligation, but not an absolute obligation or one's only obligation.

IV. THE PRINCIPLE OF MEDICAL CONFIDENTIALITY AND COMPUTERIZED HEALTH-DATA SYSTEMS

In a sense, computers introduce only a quantitative change into the traditional physician-patient relationship. Thus, it would seem at first glance that no fundamentally new challenges to the principle of medical confidentiality are raised by the development of computerized health data systems.

The increasing participation of subspecialists and allied-health personnel in medical care has meant that an ever-widening circle of persons has access to the medical records of patients, particularly the records of hospital patients. We have noted that each new group with access has tended to develop a professional code which includes a pledge to preserve the confidentiality of the record. Automation does not fundamentally change this situation, provided that access is restricted to the same circle of persons. At most, the new situation would seem to require that the persons managing the computerized health data system adopt a similar code of confidentiality.

Similarly, the gathering of the patient's disparate medical records into a single comprehensive file does not seem to raise qualitatively new problems, any more than a manual operation of photocopying, cutting, and pasting scattered records into a single master record would. So long as the rules of access to particular parts of the file remain the same, the medical-confidentiality issue remains fundamentally the same.

However, the quantitative difference is perhaps significant. Because of the efficiency of automated systems, violations of medical confidentiality may appear to be easier. Because of the amount of data which may be included in a comprehensive patient file, the damage to the patient whose confidentiality is violated may be proportionately greater.

In addition, the transition from manual to automated health-data systems provides us with an occasion to think through ethical issues which we should perhaps have confronted before this point but which we have largely ignored. Three issues merit brief consideration.

The first is the issue of patient access to his or her own confidential medical record. This question has been the subject of considerable debate since the early 1970s.[31] In my view, the development of comprehensive health records in computerized health-data systems makes it more important than ever for the patient to have a way to correct misinformation in his or her file. If lifetime records are compiled, information more than several years old may be badly outdated and therefore convey a false impression of the patient's current medical condition. Moreover, since many subspecialists do not know the patient personally, there is no built-in check against serious misinformation about the patient. The precise mechanism for patient access remains to be worked out. Majority opinion seems to favor access through an intermediary, perhaps a lawyer or an ombuds-person.[32]

A second issue which merits thorough discussion is the grading of confidential information according to different levels of sensitivity. The effort to determine degrees of sensitivity is reminiscent of our earlier discussion of concentric circles of privacy. It is perhaps Sweden which has gone furthest in attempting to deal with the question of assessing the relative sensitivity of medical data. In the Stockholm district, several hospitals are linked to a central data bank which stores all medical data on every patient. This information is graded for sensitivity into three categories; details are decided upon by a reference committee. The most sensitive grade of information includes data concerning psychiatric problems, venereal disease, and gynecological problems. Users of the system are assigned codes which provide access only to particular grades of confidential information.[33]

A final issue is the question of *guaranteeing* medical confidentiality. Until now, the primary positive protection for patients against unwarranted disclosure of medical data has been the development of various codes of professional ethics. In effect, various professional groups have solemnly promised not to violate the principle of medical confidentiality. Professional self-regulation has been the primary sanction against abuse; legal remedies have been, except in cases of gross abuse, relatively unavailable. Now that more complete data files are being stored in automated systems, it is perhaps time to go beyond codes of ethics and to seek more precise legal guarantees for medical confidentiality. One scholar has proposed, for example, that the patient should be expressly protected by law against injuries resulting from a "breach of [medical] confidence."[34]

In summary, the principle of medical confidentiality has a long history. The primary arguments in favor of the principle are that it preserves the physician-patient relationship and that it expresses respect for the patient's right of privacy. I have argued that the principle of medical confidentiality should be adhered to in most cases but that it may be violated when an important value—for example, human life—would be threatened by such adherence. Finally, we have noted that the development of computerized health-data systems throws into sharp relief a series of critical issues which urgently require further attention and discussion.

NOTES

1. See the English translation of the *"Charaka Samhita"* in M. B. Etziony, *The Physician's Creed* (Springfield, Ill.: Charles C Thomas, 1973), pp. 15–17.

2. Translated in Ludwig Edelstein, "The Hippocratic Oath: Text, Translation and Interpretation," in Owsei Temkin and C. Lillian Temkin, eds., *Ancient Medicine: Selected Papers of Ludwig Edelstein* (Baltimore: Johns Hopkins University Press, 1967), p. 6.

3. Thomas Percival, *Medical Ethics,* edited by Chauncey D. Leake (Baltimore: Williams & Wilkins, 1927), p. 90.

4. American Medical Association, *Code of Medical Ethics* (New York: H. Ludwig & Co., 1848), p. 13.

5. Quoted by Etziony, *Physician's Creed*, p. 88.

6. American Medical Association, Judicial Council, *Opinions and Reports* (Chicago: American Medical Association, 1968), p. VII.

7. See Etziony, *Physician's Creed*, pp. 120–122, 127–128, 135–137.

8. *Ibid.*, p. 136.

9. For a survey of the professional and religious sources of medical ethics see LeRoy Walters, "Medical Ethics," in David Eggenberger, ed., *New Catholic Encyclopedia*. Vol. 16: Supplement 1967–1974 (New York: McGraw-Hill, 1974), pp. 290–291. Two standard textbooks of religious thought concerning medical ethics are Immanuel Jakobovits, *Jewish Medical Ethics* (2nd ed.; New York: Bloch Publishing Company, 1975) and Charles J. McFadden, *Medical Ethics* (6th ed.; Philadelphia: F. A. Davis Co., 1967).

10. Jakobovits, *Jewish Medical Ethics*, p. 210.

11. On this point see Ralph Slovenko, *Psychiatry and Law* (Boston: Little Brown and Company, 1973), p. 435. Within Catholic moral theology textbooks, discussion of medical confidentiality usually appears at one of three points: in the treatment of the Eighth Commandment (vs. lying) or of justice and right *(de justitia et jure)*, or in the consideration of special duties which attach to particular professions or states in life (Robert E. Regan, *Professional Secrecy in the Light of Moral Principles: with an Application to Several Important Professions* [Washington, D.C.: Augustinian Press, 1943, p. 124]).

12. See Regan's comprehensive survey in *Professional Secrecy*, pp. 114–48.

13. American Hospital Association, "Statement on a Patient's Bill of Rights," Hospitals 47(4): 41, 16 February 1973.

14. Regan, *Professional Secrecy*, p. 119.

15. New York Revised Statutes, 1828, II, 406, Part III, c. vii, art. 8, paragraph 3; quoted by Elyce Zenoff, "Confidential and Privileged Communications," *Journal of the American Medical Association* 182(6): 657, 10 November 1962. For a comprehensive discussion of the physician-patient privilege see Clinton DeWitt, *Privileged Communications Between Physician and Patient* (Springfield, Ill.: Charles C Thomas, 1958).

16. Dennis Helfman *et al.*, "Access to Medical Records" in the *Appendix* to U.S. Department of Health, Education and Welfare, *Report of the Secretary's Commission on Medical Malpractice* (Washington, D.C.: U.S. Government Printing Office, 1973), pp. 178–179. The authors of this report note that in the 1971 draft of the Proposed Federal Rules of Evidence, the physician-patient privilege is abolished but a psychotherapist-patient privilege is retained *(ibid., p. 182)*.

17. A similar line or argument was advanced in favor of testimonial privilege for physicians in *Randa v. Bear,* 50 Wash. 2d 415, 312 P. 2d 640 (1957); cited by William J. Curran and E. Donald Shapiro, *Law, Medicine, and Forensic Science* (2nd ed.; Boston: Little, Brown and Company, 1970), p. 377.

18. Harvey L. Ruben and Diane D. Ruben, "Confidentiality and Privileged Communications: The Psychotherapeutic Relationship Revisited," *Medical Annals of the District of Columbia* 41(6): 365, June 1972.

19. The Warren-Brandeis article appeared in the *Harvard Law Review*, vol. 4, 1890, at p. 193. This quotation is taken from Susan

Beggs-Baker *et al.*, "Individual Privacy Considerations for Computerized Health Information Systems," *Medical Care* 12 (1): 79, January 1974. For a perceptive recent treatment of the right to privacy see Charles Fried, *An Anatomy of Values: Problems of Personal and Social Choice* (Cambridge, Mass.: Harvard University Press, 1970), Chap. 9. The constitutional right of privacy has recently been affirmed by the U.S. Supreme Court in the cases *Griswold v. Connecticut* [381 U.S. 479, 85 S. Ct. 1678 (1965) and *Katz v. United States* (389 U.S. 347, 88 S. Ct. 507 (1967)].

20. Alan F. Westin, *Privacy and Freedom* (New York: Atheneum, 1967), p. 33.

21. The following analysis parallels, in part, Regan's discussion of "various conflicts between the duty of medical secrecy and other rights and duties" *(Professional Secrecy,* pp. 138–148).

22. This illustration is drawn from Regan, *Professional Secrecy,* pp. 143–147.

23. Helfman *et al.*, "Access to Medical Records," pp. 180–181.

24. Regan, *Professional Secrecy,* p. 116. A similar, although more general, exception to the confidentiality obligation is included in the current AMA "Principles of Medical Ethics" (Judicial Council, *Opinions and Reports,* p. VII).

25. Helfman *et al.*, "Access to Medical Records," p. 181. State laws requiring that cases of drug addiction be reported would be justified by means of analogous arguments *(ibid.).*

26. Henry A. Davidson, "Professional Secrecy," in E. Fuller Torrey, ed., *Ethical Issues in Medicine: the Role of the Physician in Today's Society* (Boston: Little, Brown and Company, 1968), p. 194.

27. See for example, Amitai Etzioni, *Genetic Fix* (New York: Macmillan, 1973), especially Chap. 4.

28. Great Britain, Medical Research Council, "Responsibility in the Use of Medical Information for Research," *British Medical Journal* 1 (5847): 213–216, 27 January 1973.

29. See the comments of the economist Lester Thurow on a related issue in Betty Cochran, "Conference Report: Conception, Coercion, and Control," *Hospital and Community Psychiatry* 25 (5), 287, May 1974.

30. William Frankena, *Ethics* (2nd ed.; Englewood Cliffs, N.J.: Prentice-Hall, 1973), p. 26–28.

31. See U.S. Department of Health, Education, and Welfare, *Medical Malpractice: Report of the Secretary's Commission on Medical Malpractice,* pp. 75–77; and Budd N. Shenkin and David C. Warner, "Giving the Patient His Medical Record: a Proposal to Improve the System," *New England Journal of Medicine* 289 (13): 688–692, 27 September 1973.

32. U.S. Department of Health, Education, and Welfare, *Medical Malpractice,* p. 77.

33. "Research and Confidentiality," *C.M.A. Journal* 108 (11): 1351, 2 June 1973.

34. Roedersheimer, "Action for Breach of Medical Secrecy Outside the Courtroom," *University of Cincinnati Law Review* 36 (1966), 103; cited by Helfman *et al.*, "Access to Medical Records," p. 183.

CALIFORNIA SUPREME COURT

Tarasoff v. Regents of the University of California

TOBRINER, Justice.

On October 27, 1969, Prosenjit Poddar killed Tatiana Tarasoff. Plaintiffs, Tatiana's parents, allege that two months earlier Poddar confided his intention to kill Tatiana to Dr. Lawrence Moore, a psychologist employed by the Cowell Memorial Hospital at the University of California at Berkeley. They allege that on Moore's request, the campus police briefly detained Poddar, but released him when he appeared rational. They further claim that Dr. Harvey Powelson, Moore's superior, then directed that no further action be taken to detain Poddar. No one warned plaintiffs of Tatiana's peril.

. . .

We shall explain that defendant therapists cannot escape liability merely because Tatiana herself was not their patient. When a therapist determines, or pursuant to the standards of his profession should determine, that his patient presents a serious danger of violence to another, he incurs an obligation to use reasonable care to protect the intended victim against such danger. The discharge of this duty may require the therapist to take one or more of various steps, depending upon the nature of the case. Thus it may call for him to warn the intended victim or others likely to apprise the victim of the danger, to notify the police, or to take whatever other steps are reasonably necessary under the circumstances.

. . .

1. PLAINTIFFS' COMPLAINTS

Plaintiffs, Tatiana's mother and father, filed separate but virtually identical second amended complaints. The issue before us on this appeal is whether those complaints now state, or can be amended to

131 California Reporter 14. Decided July 1, 1976. All footnotes and numerous references in the text of the decision and a dissent have been omitted.

state, causes of action against defendants. We therefore begin by setting forth the pertinent allegations of the complaints.

Plaintiffs' first cause of action, entitled "Failure to Detain a Dangerous Patient," alleges that on August 20, 1969, Poddar was a voluntary outpatient receiving therapy at Cowell Memorial Hospital. Poddar informed Moore, his therapist, that he was going to kill an unnamed girl, readily identifiable as Tatiana, when she returned home from spending the summer in Brazil. Moore, with the concurrence of Dr. Gold, who had initially examined Poddar, and Dr. Yandell, assistant to the director of the department of psychiatry, decided that Poddar should be committed for observation in a mental hospital. Moore orally notified Officers Atkinson and Teel of the campus police that he would request commitment. He then sent a letter to Police Chief William Beall requesting the assistance of the police department in securing Poddar's confinement.

Officers Atkinson, Brownrigg, and Halleran took Poddar into custody, but, satisfied that Poddar was rational, released him on his promise to stay away from Tatiana. Powelson, director of the department of psychiatry at Cowell Memorial Hospital, then asked the police to return Moore's letter, directed that all copies of the letter and notes that Moore had taken as therapist be destroyed, and "ordered no action to place Prosenjit Poddar in 72-hour treatment and evaluation facility."

Plaintiffs' second cause of action, entitled "Failure to Warn On a Dangerous Patient," incorporates the allegations of the first cause of action, but adds the assertion that defendants negligently permitted Poddar to be released from police custody without "notifying the parents of Tatiana Tarasoff that their daughter was in grave danger from Prosenjit Poddar." Poddar persuaded Tatiana's brother to share an apartment with him near Tatiana's residence; shortly after her return from Brazil, Poddar went to her residence and killed her.

CALIFORNIA SUPREME COURT   205

. . .

2. PLAINTIFFS CAN STATE A CAUSE OF ACTION AGAINST DEFENDANT THERAPISTS FOR NEGLIGENT FAILURE TO PROTECT TATIANA.

The second cause of action can be amended to allege that Tatiana's death proximately resulted from defendants' negligent failure to warn Tatiana or others likely to apprise her of her danger. Plaintiffs contend that as amended, such allegations of negligence and proximate causation, with resulting damages, establish a cause of action. Defendants, however, contend that in the circumstances of the present case they owed no duty of care to Tatiana or her parents and that, in the absence of such duty, they were free to act in careless disregard of Tatiana's life and safety.

In analyzing this issue, we bear in mind that legal duties are not discoverable facts of nature, but merely conclusory expressions that, in cases of a particular type, liability should be imposed for damage done. As stated in *Dillion v. Legg* (1968): "The assertion that liability must . . . be denied because defendant bears no 'duty' to plaintiff 'begs the essential question—whether the plaintiff's interests are entitled to legal protection against the defendant's conduct . . . [Duty] is not sacrosanct itself, but only an expression of the sum total of those considerations of policy which lead the law to say that the particular plaintiff is entitled to protection.' (Prosser, Law of Torts [3d ed. 1964] at pp. 332–333.)"

In the landmark case of *Rowland v. Christian* (1968), Justice Peters recognized that liability should be imposed "for an injury occasioned to another by his want of ordinary care or skill" as expressed in section 1714 of the Civil Code. Thus, Justice Peters, quoting from *Heaven v. Pender* (1883) stated: " 'whenever one person is by circumstances placed in such a position with regard to another . . . that if he did not use ordinary care and skill in his own conduct . . . he would cause danger of injury to the person or property of the other, a duty arises to use ordinary care and skill to avoid such danger.' "

We depart from "this fundamental principle" only upon the "balancing of a number of considerations"; major ones "are the foreseeability of harm to the plaintiff, the degree of certainty that the plaintiff suffered injury, the closeness of the connection between the defendant's conduct and the injury suffered, the moral blame attached to the defendant's conduct, the policy of preventing future harm, the extent of the burden to the defendant and consequences to the community of imposing a duty to exercise care with resulting liability for breach, and the availablity, cost and prevalence of insurance for the risk involved."

The most important of these considerations in establishing duty is foreseeability. As a general principle, a "defendant owes a duty of care to all persons who are foreseeably endangered by his conduct, with respect to all risks which make the conduct unreasonably dangerous."

As we shall explain, however, when the avoidance of foreseeable harm requires a defendant to control the conduct of another person, or to warn of such conduct, the common law has traditionally imposed liability only if the defendant bears some special relationship to the dangerous person or to the potential victim. Since the relationship between a therapist and his patient satisfies this requirement, we need not here decide whether foreseeability alone is sufficient to create a duty to exercise reasonable care to protect a potential victim of another's conduct.

Although, as we have stated above, under the common law, as a general rule, one person owed no duty to control the conduct of another, . . . nor to warn those endangered by such conduct, the courts have carved out an exception to this rule in cases in which the defendant stands in some special relationship to either the person whose conduct needs to be controlled or in a relationship to the foreseeable victim of that conduct. Applying this exception to the present case, we note that a relationship of defendant therapists to either Tatiana or Poddar will suffice to establish a duty of care; as explained in section 315 of the Restatement Second of Torts, a duty of care may arise from either "(a) a special relation . . . between the actor and the third person which imposes a duty upon the actor to control the third person's conduct, or (b) a special relation . . . between the actor and the other which gives to the other a right of protection."

Although plaintiffs' pleadings assert no special relation between Tatiana and defendant therapists, they establish as between Poddar and defendant therapists the special relation that arises between a patient and his doctor or psychotherapist. Such a relationship may support affirmative duties for the benefit of third persons. Thus, for example, a hospital must exercise reasonable care to control the behavior of a patient which may endanger other persons. A doctor must also warn a patient if the patient's condition or medication renders certain conduct, such as driving a car, dangerous to others.

Although the California decisions that recognize this duty have involved cases in which the defendant stood in a special relationship *both* to the victim and to the person whose conduct created the danger, we do not think that the duty should logically be constricted to such situations. Decisions of other jurisdictions hold that the single relationship of a doctor to his patient is sufficient to support the duty to exercise reasonable care to protect others against dangers emanating from the patient's illness. The courts hold that a doctor is liable to persons infected by his patient if he negligently fails to diagnose a contagious disease, or, having diagnosed the illness, fails to warn members of the patient's family.

Since it involved a dangerous mental patient, the decision in *Merchants Nat. Bank & Trust Co. of Fargo v. United States* (1967) comes closer to the issue. The Veterans Administration arranged for the patient to work on a local farm, but did not inform the farmer of the man's background. The farmer consequently permitted the patient to come and go freely during nonworking hours; the patient borrowed a car, drove to his wife's residence and killed her. Notwithstanding the lack of any "special relationship" between the Veterans Administration and the wife, the court found the Veterans Administration liable for the wrongful death of the wife.

In their summary of the relevant rulings Fleming and Maximov conclude that the "case law should dispel any notion that to impose on the therapists a duty to take precautions for the safety of persons threatened by a patient, where due care so requires, is in any way opposed to contemporary ground rules on the duty relationship. On the contrary, there now seems to be sufficient authority to support the conclusion that by entering into a doctor-patient relationship the therapist becomes sufficiently involved to assume some responsibility for the safety, not only of the patient himself, but also of any third person whom the doctor knows to be threatened by the patient." (Fleming & Maximov, *The Patient or His Victim: The Therapist's Dilemma* [1974] 62 Cal.L.Rev. 1025, 1030.)

Defendants contend, however, that imposition of a duty to exercise reasonable care to protect third persons is unworkable because therapists cannot accurately predict whether or not a patient will resort to violence. In support of this argument amicus representing the American Psychiatric Association and other professional societies cites numerous articles which indicate that therapists, in the present state of the art, are unable reliably to predict violent acts; their forecasts, amicus claims, tend consistently to overpredict violence, and indeed are more often wrong than right. Since predictions of violence are often erroneous, amicus concludes, the courts should not render rulings that predicate the liability of therapists upon the validity of such predictions.

The role of the psychiatrist, who is indeed a practitioner of medicine, and that of the psychologist who performs an allied function, are like that of the physician who must conform to the standards of the profession and who must often make diagnoses and predictions based upon such evaluations. Thus the judgment of the therapist in diagnosing emotional disorders and in predicting whether a patient presents a serious danger of violence is comparable to the judgment which doctors and professionals must regularly render under accepted rules of responsibility.

We recognize the difficulty that a therapist encounters in attempting to forecast whether a patient presents a serious danger of violence. Obviously we do not require that the therapist, in making that determination, render a perfect performance; the therapist need only exercise "that reasonable degree of skill, knowledge, and care ordinarily possessed and exercised by members of [that professional specialty] under similar circumstances." Within the broad range of reasonable practice and treatment in which professional opinion and judgment may differ, the therapist is free to exercise his or her own best judgment without liability; proof, aided by hindsight, that he or she judged wrongly is insufficient to establish negligence.

In the instant case, however, the pleadings do not raise any question as to failure of defendant therapists to predict that Poddar presented a serious danger of violence. On the contrary, the present complaints allege that defendant therapists did in fact predict that Poddar would kill, but were negligent in failing to warn.

Amicus contends, however, that even when a therapist does in fact predict that a patient poses a serious danger of violence to others, the therapist should be absolved of any responsibility for failing to act to protect the potential victim. In our view, however, once a therapist does in fact determine, or under applicable professional standards reasonably should have determined, that a patient poses a serious danger of violence to others, he bears a duty to exercise reasonable care to protect the foreseeable victim of that danger. While the discharge of this duty of due care will necessarily vary with the facts of each case, in each instance the adequacy of the therapist's conduct must be measured against the traditional negligence standard of the rendition of reasonable care under the circumstances. As explained in Fleming and Maximov, *The Patient or His Victim: The Therapist's Dilemma* (1974) 62 Cal.L.Rev. 1025, 1067: ". . . the ultimate question of resolving the tension between the conflicting interests of patient and potential victim is one of social policy, not professional expertise. . . . In sum, the therapist owes a legal duty not only to his patient, but also to his patient's would-be victim and is subject in both respects to scrutiny by judge and jury."

Contrary to the assertion of amicus, this conclusion is not inconsistent with our recent decision in *People v. Burnick* (1975). Taking note of the uncertain character of therapeutic prediction, we held in *Burnick* that a person cannot be committed as a mentally disordered sex offender unless found to be such by proof beyond a reasonable doubt. The issue in the present context, however, is not whether the patient should be incarcerated, but whether the therapist should take any steps at all to protect the threatened victim; some of the alternatives open to the therapist, such as warning the victim, will not result in the drastic consequences of depriving the patient of his liberty. Weighing the uncertain and conjectural character of the alleged damage done the patient by such a warning against the peril to the victim's life, we conclude that professional inaccuracy in predicting violence cannot negate the therapist's duty to protect the threatened victim.

The risk that unnecessary warnings may be given is a reasonable price to pay for the lives of possible victims that may be saved. We would hesitate to hold that the therapist who is aware that his patient expects to attempt to assassinate the President of the United States would not be obligated to warn the authorities because the therapist cannot predict with accuracy that his patient will commit the crime.

Defendants further argue that free and open communication is essential to psychotherapy, that "Unless a patient . . . is assured that . . . information [revealed by him] can and will be held in utmost confidence, he will be reluctant to make the full disclosure upon which diagnosis and treatment . . . depends." The giving of a warning, defendants contend, constitutes a breach of trust which entails the revelation of confidential communications.

We recognize the public interest in supporting effective treatment of mental illness and in protecting the rights of patients to privacy, and the consequent public importance of safeguarding the confidential character of psychotherapeutic communication. Against this interest, however, we must weigh the public interest in safety from violent assault. The Legislature has undertaken the difficult task of balancing the countervailing concerns. In Evidence Code section 1014, it established a broad rule of privilege to protect confidential communications between patient and psychotherapist. In Evidence Code section 1024, the Legislature created a specific and limited exception to the psychotherapist-patient privilege: "There is no privilege . . . if the psychotherapist has reasonable cause to believe that the patient is in such mental or emotional condition as to be dangerous to himself or to the person or property of another and that disclosure of the communication is necessary to prevent the threatened danger."

We realize that the open and confidential character of psychotherapeutic dialogue encourages patients to express threats of violence, few of which are ever executed. Certainly a therapist should not be encouraged routinely to reveal such threats; such disclosures could seriously disrupt the patient's relationship with his therapist and with the persons threatened. To the contrary, the therapist's obligations to his patient require that he not disclose a confidence unless such disclosure is necessary to avert danger to others, and even then that he do so discreetly, and in a fashion that would preserve the privacy of his patient to the fullest extent compatible with the prevention of the threatened danger.

The revelation of a communication under the above circumstances is not a breach of trust or a violation of professional ethics; as stated in the Principles of Medical Ethics of the American Medical Association (1957), section 9: "A physician may not reveal the confidence entrusted to him in the course of medical attendance . . . *unless he is required to do so by law or unless it becomes necessary in order to protect the welfare of the individual or of the community.*"

(Emphasis added.) We conclude that the public policy favoring protection of the confidential character of patient-psychotherapist communications must yield to the extent to which disclosure is essential to avert danger to others. The protective privilege ends where the public peril beings.

Our current crowded and computerized society compels the interdependence of its members. In this risk-infested society we can hardly tolerate the further exposure to danger that would result from a concealed knowledge of the therapist that his patient was lethal. If the exercise of reasonable care to protect the threatened victim requires the therapist to warn the endangered party or those who can reasonably be expected to notify him, we see no sufficient societal interest that would protect and justify concealment. The containment of such risks lies in the public interest. For the foregoing reasons, we find that plaintiffs' complaints can be amended to state a cause of action against defendants Moore, Powelson, Gold, and Yandell and against the Regents as their employer, for breach of a duty to exercise reasonable care to protect Tatiana.

· · ·

CLARK, Justice (dissenting).

Until today's majority opinion, both legal and medical authorities have agreed that confidentiality is essential to effectively treat the mentally ill, and that imposing a duty on doctors to disclose patient threats to potential victims would greatly impair treatment. Further, recognizing that effective treatment and society's safety are necessarily intertwined, the Legislature has already decided effective and confidential treatment is preferred over imposition of a duty to warn.

The issue whether effective treatment for the mentally ill should be sacrificed to a system of warnings is, in my opinion, properly one for the Legislature, and we are bound by its judgment. Moreover, even in the absence of clear legislative direction, we must reach the same conclusion because imposing the majority's new duty is certain to result in a net increase in violence.

· · ·

COMMON LAW ANALYSIS

Entirely apart from the statutory provisions, the same result must be reached upon considering both general tort principles and the public policies favoring effective treatment, reduction of violence, and justified commitment.

Generally, a person owes no duty to control the conduct of another. Exceptions are recognized only in limited situations where (1) a special relationship exists between the defendant and injured party, or (2) a special relationship exists between defendant and the active wrongdoer, imposing a duty on defendant to control the wrongdoer's conduct. The majority does not contend the first exception is appropriate to this case.

Policy generally determines duty. Principal policy considerations include foreseeability of harm, certainty of the plaintiff's injury, proximity of the defendant's conduct to the plaintiff's injury, moral blame attributable to defendant's conduct, prevention of future harm, burden on the defendant, and consequences to the community.

Overwhelming policy considerations weigh against imposing a duty on psychotherapists to warn a potential victim against harm. While offering virtually no benefit to society, such a duty will frustrate psychiatric treatment, invade fundamental patient rights and increase violence.

The importance of psychiatric treatment and its need for confidentiality have been recognized by this court. "It is clearly recognized that the very practice of psychiatry vitally depends upon the reputation in the community that the psychiatrist will not tell." (Slovenko, *Psychiatry and a Second Look at the Medical Privilege* (1960) 6 Wayne L.Rev. 175, 188.)

Assurance of confidentiality is important for three reasons.

DETERRENCE FROM TREATMENT

First, without substantial assurance of confidentiality, those requiring treatment will be deterred from seeking assistance. It remains an unfortunate fact in our society that people seeking psychiatric guidance tend to become stigmatized. Apprehension of such stigma—apparently increased by the propensity of people considering treatment to see themselves in the worst possible light—creates a well-recognized reluctance to seek aid. This reluctance is alleviated by the psychiatrist's assurance of confidentiality.

FULL DISCLOSURE

Second, the guarantee of confidentiality is essential in eliciting the full disclosure necessary for effective treatment. The psychiatric patient approaches treatment with conscious and unconscious inhibitions against revealing his innermost thoughts. "Every person, however well-motivated, has to overcome resistances to therapeutic exploration. These resistances seek support from every possible source and the possibility of disclosure would easily be employed in the service of resistance." (Goldstein & Katz, 36 Conn. Bar J. 175, 179.) Until a patient can trust his psychiatrist not to violate their confidential relationship, "the unconscious psychological control mechanism of repression will prevent the recall of past experiences." (Butler, *Psychotherapy and Griswold: Is Confidentiality a Privilege or a Right?* (1971) 3 Conn.L.Rev. 599, 604.)

SUCCESSFUL TREATMENT

Third, even if the patient fully discloses his thoughts, assurance that the confidential relationship will not be breached is necessary to maintain his trust in his psychiatrist—the very means by which treatment is effected. "[T]he essence of much psychotherapy is the contribution of trust in the external world and ultimately in the self, modelled upon the trusting relationship established during therapy." (Dawidoff, *The Malpractice of Psychiatrists,* 1966 Duke L.J. 696, 704.) Patients will be helped only if they can form a trusting relationship with the psychiatrist. All authorities appear to agree that if the trust relationship cannot be developed because of collusive communication between the psychiatrist and others, treatment will be frustrated.

Given the importance of confidentiality to the practice of psychiatry, it becomes clear the duty to warn imposed by the majority will cripple the use and effectiveness of psychiatry. Many people, potentially violent—yet susceptible to treatment—will be deterred from seeking it; those seeking it will be inhibited from making revelations necessary to effective treatment; and, forcing the psychiatrist to violate the patient's trust will destroy the interpersonal relationship by which treatment is effected.

VIOLENCE AND CIVIL COMMITMENT

By imposing a duty to warn, the majority contributes to the danger to society of violence by the mentally ill and greatly increases the risk of civil commitment—the total deprivation of liberty—of those who should not be confined. The impairment of treatment and risk of improper commitment resulting from the new duty to warn will not be limited to a few patients but will extend to a large number of the men-

tally ill. Although under existing psychiatric procedures only a relatively few receiving treatment will ever present a risk of violence, the number making threats is huge, and it is the latter group—not just the former—whose treatment will be impaired and whose risk of commitment will be increased.

Both the legal and psychiatric communities recognize that the process of determining potential violence in a patient is far from exact, being fraught with complexity and uncertainty. In fact precision has not even been attained in predicting who of those having already committed violent acts will again become violent, a task recognized to be of much simpler proportions.

This predictive uncertainty means that the number of disclosures will necessarily be large. As noted above, psychiatric patients are encouraged to discuss all thoughts of violence, and they often express such thoughts. However, unlike this court, the psychiatrist does not enjoy the benefit of overwhelming hindsight in seeing which few, if any, of his patients will ultimately become violent. Now, confronted by the majority's new duty, the psychiatrist must instantaneously calculate potential violence from each patient on each visit. The difficulties researchers have encountered in accurately predicting violence will be heightened for the practicing psychiatrist dealing for brief periods in his office with heretofore nonviolent patients. And, given the decision not to warn or commit must always be made at the psychiatrist's civil peril, one can expect most doubts will be resolved in favor of the psychiatrist protecting himself.

Neither alternative open to the psychiatrist seeking to protect himself is in the public interest. The warning itself is an impairment of the psychiatrist's ability to treat, depriving many patients of adequate treatment. It is to be expected that after disclosing their threats, a significant number of patients, who would not become violent if treated according to existing practices, will engage in violent conduct as a result of unsuccessful treatment. In short, the majority's duty to warn will not only impair treatment of many who would never become violent but worse, will result in a net increase in violence.

The second alternative open to the psychiatrist is to commit his patient rather than to warn. Even in the absence of threat of civil liability, the doubts of psychiatrists as to the seriousness of patient threats have led psychiatrists to overcommit to mental institutions. This overcommitment has been authoritatively documented in both legal and psychiatric studies. This practice is so prevalent that it has been estimated that "as many as twenty harmless persons are incarcerated for every one who will commit a violent act." (Steadman & Cocozza, *Stimulus/*

Response: We Can't Predict Who Is Dangerous (Jan. 1975) 8 Psych. Today 32, 35.)

Given the incentive to commit created by the majority's duty, this already serious situation will be worsened, contrary to Chief Justice Wright's admonition "that liberty is no less precious because forfeited in a civil proceeding than when taken as a consequence of a criminal conviction."

WILLIAM J. CURRAN

Confidentiality and the Prediction of Dangerousness in Psychiatry: The Tarasoff Case

The California Supreme Court continues to make financial awards to patients in suits against physicians with seemingly little regard for the effect of these awards and decisions upon the practice of medicine and the availability of insurance to cover this largesse of the judiciary, and without regard for the social consequences of this "money-for-everything" attitude.

The particular case, *Tarasoff vs. Regents of the University of California,*[1] has already become infamous among mental health programs in California and among college and university student medical programs all over the country as it has taken its course through the various levels of trial and appeals courts in the Golden State.

The facts of the situation are undisputed. A student at the University of California's Berkeley campus was in psychotherapy with the student health service on an outpatient basis. He told his therapist, a psychologist, that he wanted to kill an unmarried girl who lived in Berkeley but who was then on a summer trip to Brazil. The psychologist, with the concurrence of another therapist and the assistant director of the Department of Psychiatry, reported the matter orally to the campus police and on their suggestion sent them a letter requesting detention of the student and his

From *New England Journal of Medicine* Vol. 293, No. 6 (August 7, 1975), pp. 285–286.

commitment for observation to a mental hospital. The campus police picked up the student for questioning but "satisfied" that he was "rational," released him on his "promise to stay away" from Miss Tarasoff. The police reported back to the director of psychiatry, Dr. Powelson. Dr. Powelson asked for the return of the psychologist's letter to the police and directed that all copies of the letter be destroyed. Nothing more was done at the health service about the matter. Two months later, shortly after Miss Tarasoff's return, the student went to her home and killed her.

The parents of Miss Tarasoff brought suit for damages against the University and against the therapists and the campus police, as employees of the University and individually. In suing Dr. Powelson, the plaintiffs sought not only general money damages for negligence in failure to warn the girl and her parents and to confine the student, but exemplary or punitive damages (which could be assessed in huge amounts as multiples of the general damages or in any amount at the determination of the jury) for malicious and oppressive abandonment of a dangerous patient.

The Superior Court dismissed all these grounds for legal action against the defendants. The Supreme Court, in a four-to-two decision, reversed the decision and found that on these facts a cause of action was stated for general damages against all the therapists involved in the case and the assistant director and the director of psychiatry and against the University as their employer for breach of the duty to warn Miss Tarasoff. The Court dismissed the claim for exemplary damages against the therapists. It also dismissed the action against the police as protected from a suit by a statutory immunity, as well as the suit against the therapists for failure to confine the student under a commitment order, again because of a statutory immunity. The Court implied that without the immunity, both these actions might have been meritorious.

It seems to me most physicians would throw up their hands in dismay over this result and the massive contradictions in the assessment of who was and who was not legally responsible for this death. If I were to describe in detail the reasoning of the Court, the confusion of the medical mind would be compounded a thousand times.

The Court asserted that the *Principles of Medical Ethics of the American Medical Association,* Section 9, did not bar breaching the confidentiality of this patient ''in order to protect the welfare of this individual [the patient] or the community.'' From this premise the Court jumped wholeheartedly to a positive duty to warn Miss Tarasoff. This is not what the *Principles* said. The traditional code of medical ethics allows a physician in his sound discretion to breach the confidentiality, but does not require it. It is almost impossible to draft an ethical principle to force a duty on physicians to breach confidences. Must they always warn of death threats, but have discretion on less dangerous threats? Must they warn if the patient is psychotic, but not if he is less disturbed? Does this case mean that every time a patient makes a threat against an unnamed person, the therapist must take steps to find out who it is and warn him (of anything at all, from vague threats to murder) or suffer money damages in the thousands or tens of thousands if the threat, or an aspect of the threat, is carried out?

This case was greatly confused by the array of immunities from suits created under California law. It can be strongly argued that the thrust of these immunity statutes regarding the duty to warn should also have been applied to the therapists, since the statutes were intended to encourage police and mental-health personnel to release patients and not confine them on the basis of unreliable diagnoses of dangerousness. In the past it was thought that too many mental patients were confined for years and years because of their threats to other people, rarely carried out, and because of the conservatism of mental-health personnel in exercising any doubt about dangerousness in favor of confinement as the safest way to prevent harm to third parties.

It seems clear that the therapists here thought that they had done all they could to protect their patient and the community by reporting the case to the police. They had exercised their discretion to warn the community and to breach the confidence of the patient, for his own sake, and that of the unknown girl. They could hardly warn her, since she was not even in the country at the time. Also, the threat to Miss Tarasoff might actually have been vaguely directed. The student could well have turned his anger and violence toward another person or toward himself. The only basic recourse was to recommend temporary observational commitment. The practice was to make this known to the campus police. It was the police who acted, and they decided to release the student with a warning and a promise to stay away from the girl. How many thousands of such warnings—and releases—do police departments make every year? How many people then proceed to kill? The immunity statute was established to encourage release in these circumstances. But the statutory armor had a hole in it. The director of psychiatry was found by the Court to have a 'duty' to warn the girl, irrespective of the police action. The Court utilized some precedents, none clearly applicable to this case, to justify its decision. It seems, however, that the real rationale was the aggravated nature of the case—a killing—in which the family was left without someone else to sue. The therapists, particularly Dr. Powelson, could have warned the girl if they had wanted to go against the police action and if they had thought the specific threat to Miss Tarasoff so serious as to warrant that action. The Court did not apply any test to ascertain the custom of psychiatrists and mental-health programs actually in such situations. The Court declared the duty as a matter of law, regardless of the accepted practices of the profession. As in the *Helling* decision[2] discussed in an earlier column,[3] the Court made the physician a guarantor against harm to this party, here not even a patient, on the basis of its own concept of monetary justice.

NOTES

1. 529 P. 2d 553.

2. *Helling vs. Carey and Laughlin,* 519 P.2d 981.

3. Curran W J: Glaucoma and streptococcal pharyngitis: diagnostic practices and malpractice liability. N Engl J Med 291: 508–509, 1974.

SUGGESTED READINGS FOR CHAPTER 5

TRUTH-TELLING

Beachamp, Tom L., and Perlin, Seymour, eds. *Ethical Issues in Death and Dying*. Englewood Cliffs, N.J.: Prentice-Hall, 1978. Part III.

Bok, Sissela. *Lying: Moral Choice in Public and Private Life*. New York: Pantheon Books, 1978.

———. "Truth-Telling: Ethical Aspects." In Reich, Warren T., ed. *Encyclopedia of Bioethics*. New York: Free Press, 1978. Vol. 4, pp. 1682–1688.

Cabot, Richard C. "The Use of Truth and Falsehood in Medicine," as edited by Jay Katz from the 1909 version. *Connecticut Medicine* 42 (1978), 189–194.

Cousins, Norman. "A Layman Looks at Truth Telling in Medicine." *Journal of the American Medical Association* 244 (October 24, 1980), 1929–1930.

Isenberg, Arnold. "Deontology and the Ethics of Lying." *Philosophy and Phenomenological Research* 24 (June 1964), 465–480.

Vandeveer, Donald. "The Contractual Argument for Withholding Medical Information." *Philosophy and Public Affairs* 9 (Winter 1980), 198–205.

Veatch, Robert M. *Case Studies in Medical Ethics*. Cambridge, Mass.: Harvard University Press, 1977. Chaps. 6 and 12.

———. "Truth-Telling: Attitudes of Patients and Health-Care Professionals." In Reich, Warren T., ed. *Encyclopedia of Bioethics*. New York: Free Press, 1978. Vol. 4, pp. 1677–1682.

Weir, Robert. "Truthtelling in Medicine." *Perspectives in Biology and Medicine* 24 (Autumn 1980), 95–112.

INFORMED CONSENT

Beauchamp, Tom L., and Childress, James F. *Principles of Biomedical Ethics*. New York: Oxford University Press, 1979. Chap. 3.

Canada Law Reform Commission. *Consent to Medical Care*. A Monograph prepared by Margaret A. Somerville. Ottawa: Canadian Government Publication, 1979.

Capron, Alexander. "Informed Consent in Catastrophic Disease Research and Treatment." *University of Pennsylvania Law Review* 123 (December 1974), 340–438.

Faden, Ruth R., and Beauchamp, Tom L. "Decision-Making and Informed Consent: A Study of the Impact of Disclosed Information." *Social Indicators Research* 7 (January 1980), 313–336.

———., et al. "Disclosure of Information to Patients in Medical Care." *Medical Care* XIX (July 1981), 718–733.

Freedman, Benjamin. "A Moral Theory of Informed Consent." *Hastings Center Report* 5 (August 1975), 32–39.

Katz, Jay. "Informed Consent in the Therapeutic Relationship: Legal and Ethical Aspects." In Reich, Warren T., ed. *Encyclopedia of Bioethics*. New York: Free Press, 1978. Vol. 2, pp. 770–778.

Ludlam, James E. *Informed Consent*. Chicago: American Hospital Association, 1978.

Meisel, Alan. "Expansion of Liability for Medical Accidents: From Negligence to Liability by way of Informed Consent." *Nebraska Law Review* 56 (1977), 51–152.

———. "The 'Exceptions' to the Informed Consent Doctrine: Striking a Balance Between Competing Values in Medical Decisionmaking." *Wisconsin Law Review* 1979 (2) (July 1979), 413–488.

Miller, Leslie J. "Informed Consent: I, II, III, IV." *Journal of the American Medical Association* 244 (November 7, 1980–December 12, 1980), 2100–2103, 2347–2350, 2556–2558, 2661–2662.

Montange, Charles H. "Informed Consent and the Dying Patient." *Yale Law Journal* 83 (July 1974), 1632–1664.

Murphy, Jeffrie G. "Therapy and the Problem of Autonomous Consent." *International Journal of Law and Psychiatry* 2 (1979), 415–430.

Plante, Marcus. "The Decline of 'Informed Consent'." *Washington and Lee Law Review* 35 (Winter 1978), 91–105.

Robison, Wade L., and Pritchard, Michael S., eds. *Medical Responsibility: Paternalism, Informed Consent, and Euthanasia*. Clifton, N.J.: Humana Press, 1979.

Rosoff, Arnold. *Informed Consent*. Rockville, Md.: Aspen Systems Corporation, 1981.

Roth, Loren, Meisel, Alan, and Lidz, Charles. "Tests of Competency to Consent to Treatment." *American Journal of Psychiatry* 134 (1977), 279–284.

Tancredi, Laurence R. "The Right to Refuse Psychiatric Treatment: Some Legal and Ethical Considerations." *Journal of Health Politics, Policy and Law* 5 (Fall 1980), 514–522.

Veatch, Robert M. "Three Theories of Informed Consent: Philosophical Foundations and Policy Implications." In *Appendix B* to *The Belmont Report: Ethical Guidelines for the Protection of Human Subjects of Research*. DHEW Publication No. (OS) 78-0014. Washington, D.C.: Government Printing Office, 1978. Vol. II, pp. (26-1)–(26-66).

CONFIDENTIALITY AND PRIVACY

Beauchamp, Tom L., and Childress, James F. *Principles of Biomedical Ethics*. New York: Oxford University Press, 1979. Chap. 7.

Beigler, Jerome S. American Psychiatric Association. Committee on Confidentiality. "Statement of the American Psychiatric Association Before the Subcommittee on Government Information and Individual Rights." *New York State Journal of Medicine* 79 (December 1979), 2088–2092.

Everstine, Louis, et al. "Privacy and Confidentiality in Psychotherapy." *American Psychologist* 35 (September, 1980), 828–840.

Freedman, Alfred M. "Threats to Confidentiality." *Journal of the American Academy of Psychoanalysis* 7 (January 1979), 1–5.

Gordis, Leon, and Gold, Ellen. "Privacy, Confidentiality, and the Use of Medical Records in Research." *Science* 207 (January 11, 1980).

Kelsey, Jennifer L. "Privacy and Confidentiality in Epidemiological Research Involving Patients." *IRB: A Review of Human Subjects Research* 3 (February 1981), 1–4.

Lindenthal, Jacob J., and Claudewell, S. Thomas. "A Comparative Study of the Handling of Confidentiality." *Journal of Nervous and Mental Disease* 168 (June 1980), 361–369.

Marsh, Frank H. "The 'Deeper Meaning' of Confidentiality Within the Physician-Patient Relationship." *Ethics in Science and Medicine* 6 (1979), 131–136.

Nesbitt, Nancy A. "*Tarasoff v. Regents of the University of California:* Psychotherapist's Obligation of Confidentiality versus the Duty to Warn." *Tulsa Law Journal* 12 (1977), 747–757.

Rosner, Bennett L. "Psychiatrists, Confidentiality, and Insurance Claims." *Hastings Center Report* 10 (December 1980), 5–7.

Samuels, Alec. "The Duty of the Doctor to Respect the Confidence of the Patient." *Medicine, Science, and the Law* 20 (January 1980), 58–66.

Veatch, Robert M. *Case Studies in Medical Ethics.* Cambridge, Mass.: Harvard University Press, 1977. Chap. 5.

Wexler, David B. "Patients, Therapists, and Third Parties: The Victimological Virtues of Tarasoff." *International Journal of Law and Psychiatry* 2 (1979), 1–28.

BIBLIOGRAPHIES

Goldstein, Doris Mueller. *Bioethics: A Guide to Information Sources.* Detroit: Gale Research Company, 1982. See under "Physician-Patient Communication and Truth-Telling," "Confidentiality," "Informed Consent" and "Refusal of Treatment."

Lineback, Richard H., ed. *Philosopher's Index.* Vols. 1– . Bowling Green, Ohio: Philosophy Documentation Center, Bowling Green State University. Issued quarterly. See under "Coercion," "Deception," "Informed Consent," "Lie(s)," "Lying," and "Paternalism."

Walters, LeRoy, ed. *Bibliography of Bioethics.* Vols. 1– . New York: Free Press. Issued annually. See under "Confidentiality," "Disclosure," "Informed Consent," "Patient Care," "Patients' Rights," "Physician-Patient Relationship" and "Treatment Refusal." (The information contained in the annual *Bibliography of Bioethics* can also be retrieved from BIOETHICSLINE, an online data base of the National Library of Medicine.)

6.
Abortion

Recently laws that restrict abortion have either been sharply modified or struck down by courts in several Western nations, including the United States. While abortion is legally permitted in these nations, questions of its ethical acceptability continue to be widely debated. In addition, the adequacy of court decisions that have rendered highly restrictive abortion laws unconstitutional is also debated. In this chapter these contemporary ethical and legal issues will be examined.

THE PROBLEM OF JUSTIFICATION

Among the many reasons why abortions are commonly sought are cardiac complications, a suicidal condition of mind, psychological trauma, pregnancy caused by rape, the inadvertent use of fetus-deforming drugs, and many personal and family reasons such as the financial burden or intrusiveness of a child. Such reasons certainly *explain* why abortions are often viewed as an available way to extricate a woman or a family from difficult circumstances. But the primary ethical issue remains: Are any such reasons sufficient to *justify* the act of aborting a human fetus? An ethicist concerned to defend abortion seeks a principled justification where ethical reasons are advanced for one's conclusions. It might be decided, of course, that in only some of the above mentioned circumstances would an abortion be warranted, whereas in others it would not be justified. Even so, such a decision presupposes some set of general criteria that enables one to discriminate ethically justified abortions from ethically unjustified ones.

The central moral problem of abortion may be stated in the following general form: Under what conditions, if any, is abortion ethically permissible? Some contend that abortion is never aceptable, or at most is permissible only if abortion is required to save the pregnant woman's life or for some other similarly serious reason. This view is commonly called the *conservative* theory of abortion. Roman Catholics have traditionally been among the leading exponents of the conservative approach, but they are by no means its only advocates. Baruch Brody (who is neither Roman Catholic nor even Christian) and Philip Devine present some conservative arguments in this chapter, though neither is a conservative without qualification. Others hold that abortion is always permissible, whatever the state of fetal development. This view is commonly termed the *liberal* theory of abortion and has frequently been advocated by those adherents of women's rights who emphasize the right of a woman to make decisions that affect her own body, but again the position is advocated by others as well. Mary Anne Warren defends such a liberal theory in this chapter. Finally, many defend *intermediate* or *moderate* theories, according to which abortion is ethically permissible up to a certain stage of fetal development or for some limited set of moral reasons that is sufficient to warrant the taking of fetal life in this or that special circumstance. In the present chapter Brody and Devine discuss possible intermediate theories leaning toward conservatism, while Judith Thomson's essay may be interpreted as suggesting an intermediate theory that leans toward liberalism. (While the traditional terminology of ''liberal'' and ''conservative'' is here employed, this terminology can be both distracting and inaccurate. Whether or not one considers the fetus to be a person, for example, is an issue not at all clearly linked to political liberalism and conservatism.)

FACTS OF HUMAN BIOLOGICAL DEVELOPMENT

Since one immediate goal of some articles in this chapter is to establish the conditions under which human life begins, it is advisable first to explain the biological facts of human development, including the terminology used to designate different stages of human growth. Some important features of these biological facts, as related to abortion, are discussed in this chapter by a physician, André Hellegers.

Pregnancy does not begin with intercourse, since the earliest point at which it can be dated is during the fertilization of the female egg (the ovum) by the sperm of the male. Once fertilization has occurred, a new genetic entity results from the combination of the genetic contributions of the male and the female. This new unit is a single cell capable, under normal conditions, of a constant process of alteration and growth. This single cell has twenty-three pairs of chromosomes (each parent contributes one chromosome in each pair). It quickly divides into two cells, four cells, then eight cells—reaching sixteen at approximately the third day after fertilization. Organ systems gradually appear before the eighth week of growth, roughly the point at which brain waves can be detected. Between approximately the nineteenth and twenty-eighth week of growth, the fetus reaches the stage known as "viability," the point at which it is capable of survival outside the womb.

There exists a small but useful body of terminology frequently used by embryologists and others who discuss human biological development. *Conception* is said to occur when the male sperm and the female egg combine; during this process, the resultant entity is spoken of as a *conceptus* and is referred to in this way until its implantation, at the wall of the uterus. It is also referred to as a *zygote* until the completion of implantation, which occurs roughly two weeks after conception. Thereafter the term *embryo* is used to designate the developing entity, until about eight weeks, when it is referred to as a *fetus*. However, the term "fetus" is frequently used to designate the unborn entity in *any* state of development, and in the readings in this chapter the latter is the most common way of using the term.

THE ONTOLOGICAL STATUS OF THE FETUS

Recent controversies about abortion focus on ethical problems of how we ought and ought not to treat fetuses and on what rights, if any, are possessed by fetuses. But a more basic issue is that of *what kind of entities fetuses are*. Following current usage, we shall refer to this as the problem of *ontological status*. An account of what kind of entities fetuses are will, of course, have important implications for all issues of the permissible treatment of fetuses. But the two issues are distinct, and we must first attempt to resolve the preliminary question.

Although there is no single problem of ontological status, several layers of questions may be distinguished: (1) whether the fetus is *an individual organism,* (2) whether the fetus is *biologically a human being,* (3) whether the fetus is *psychologically a human being,* and (4) whether the fetus is a *person.* Some who write on problems of ontological status attempt to develop a theory that specifies the conditions under which the fetus can be said to be independent, individual, and alive, while others focus on the conditions, if any, under which the fetus is in some sense human, and still others are concerned to explain the conditions, if any, under which the fetus is a person. It would be generally agreed that one attributes a more significant status to the fetus by saying that it is a fully human being rather than by simply saying that it is an individual organism, and also that one enhances its status still further by claiming that it is a person.

Many would be willing to concede that an individual life begins at fertilization without conceding that there is a human being or a person at fertilization. Others would upgrade the fetus's status by claiming that the fetus is a human being at fertilization, but not a person. Still others would grant full personhood at fertilization. Those who espouse these views sometimes differ only because they define one or the other of these terms differently, but most of the differences come from serious theoretical disagreements about what constitutes either life or humanity or personhood, including disagreements over which category correctly applies to the fetus.

THE CONCEPT OF HUMANITY

The concept of human life is an especially perplexing one, for it can mean at least two very different things. On the one hand, it can mean (a) *biological human life,* that set of biological classificatory characteristics (e.g., genetic ones) that set the human species apart from nonhuman species. (This sense *may* be coextensive with "individual organism.") On the other hand, "human life" can also be used to mean (b) *life that is distinctively human*—that is, a life that is characterized by those properties which define the essence of humanity. These are largely psychological, as contrasted with biological properties. It is often said, for example, that the ability to use symbols, to imagine, to love, and to perform various higher intellectual skills are the most distinctive human properties, those that define humans as human. To have these properties, we sometimes say, is to be a "human being."

A simple example will illustrate the differences between these two senses. Infants with various exotic diseases are often born and die after a short period of time. They are born of human parents and certainly are classifiable in all relevant biological ways as human. However, they never exhibit any distinctively human traits, and do not have the potential for doing so. For such individuals it is not possible to make human life in the "biological" sense human in the "distinctively human" or "psychological" sense. We do not differentiate these two levels of life in discourse about any other animal species. We do not, for example, speak of making feline life feline. But we do meaningfully speak of making human life human, and this usage makes sense precisely because there exists in the language the dual meaning just discussed. In discussions of abortion, it is imperative that one be specific about which meaning is being employed when using an expression like the "taking of human life." A great many proponents of abortion, and opponents as well, would agree that while biological human life is taken by abortions, human life in the second or psychological sense is not.

THE CONCEPT OF PERSONHOOD

The concept of personhood was discussed in detail in Chapter 3. Here it need only be observed that personhood may or may not be different from either the biological sense or the psychological sense of "human life" just discussed. That is, one might claim that what it means to be a person is simply to have some properties that make an organism human in one or both of these senses. But other writers have suggested a list of rather more demanding criteria for being a person. A list of conditions for being a person, similar to the following, is advanced by Mary Anne Warren in this chapter and has been put forward by several recent writers:

(a) consciousness

(b) self-consciousness

(c) freedom to act on one's own reasons

(d) capacity to communicate with other persons

(e) capacity to make moral judgments

(f) rationality

Sometimes it is said by those who propose such a list that in order to be a person an entity need only satisfy some one criterion on the list—e.g., it must be conscious (a) but need not also satisfy the other conditions (b-f). Others say that all of these conditions must be satisfied in order to be a person. We shall see that it makes a major difference which of these two views one accepts. But the dominant and prior question is whether one needs to accept anything like this list at all—a question raised in the present chapter by Philip Devine and (at least elliptically) by Baruch Brody.

Two issues have emerged concerning the proper analysis of the concept of person. First, there is considerable dispute concerning the *range of factual characteristics* an entity must possess in order to be a person. One might analyze personhood in terms of a rather abbreviated list of factual, though not necessarily biological characteristics—e.g., in terms of physical characteristics such as genetic structure, characteristics of consciousness such as rationality and free choice, and perhaps characteristics that can at present be applied only to human developmental histories such as having learned a language. If personhood can be explicated in this way by listing only *elementary* properties such as genetic structure, then fetuses might well qualify as persons. But one might also analyze personhood in terms of a more demanding list of presumably factual properties, such as *b–f* above. Clearly one would be under a heavy burden of argument to show that a fetus is a person if criteria such as these must be satisfied. In any event, the first controversy is over precisely this issue of whether any of these more demanding properties must be present in order to be a person, and if so which such properties.

A second dispute has emerged in connection with this first one. Several writers have suggested that the concept of personhood must be analyzed in terms of properties bestowed by human *evaluation* as well as in terms of factual properties possessed by persons. For example, it has been argued that in order to be a person one must be the bearer of legal rights and social responsibilities, and must be capable of being judged by others as morally praiseworthy or blameworthy. The central question in this controversy is whether fetuses are the sort of entity that it is appropriate to value in this way. This issue is closely related to what we shall discuss momentarily as the moral status of the fetus.

It is certainly not self-evident that a fetus either is or is not a person in any of the above senses. Anyone who claims to have resolved these controversies about persons must be prepared either to defend a particular theory of personhood or to show that these issues have somehow been wrongly conceived.

The problem of ontological status is complicated by a further factor related to the biological development of the fetus. It is important to state at what point of development an entity is to be distinguished as fully individual, or fully human, or fully a person. This involves specifying at what point full ontological status is gained. This issue turns directly on when fetuses achieve important ontological status and only indirectly concerns what status they have. But—as both Devine and Warren urge—it is imperative that any theory be specific regarding whether it is status as an individual entity, a human being, or a person that is in question.

THE PROBLEM OF LINE-DRAWING

The problem of ontological status is complicated by a further factor related to the biological development of the fetus. It is important to state at what *point of development* an entity is to be distinguished as fully individual, or fully human, or fully a person. This involves specifying at what point *full ontological status* is gained. This issue turns directly on *when* fetuses achieve important ontological status and only indirectly concerns *what* status they have. But it is imperative that any theory be specific regarding whether it is status as an individual entity, a human being, or a person that is in question.

This problem is sometimes referred to as the problem of drawing the line between that which has full status and that which does not. One polar position (said to be the extreme liberal position) is that the fetus never achieves status in terms of any of the categories mentioned above, and therefore has *no ontological status* of any importance. Warren defends this view. The polar opposite position (often said to be the extreme conservative position) is that the fetus always has *full ontological status* in regard to all of the categories discussed above. Those who hold this view claim that the line must be drawn at conception, in which case the fetus is always an individual human person. Obviously there can be many intermediate positions. These are generally defended by drawing the line somewhere between the two extremes of conception and birth. For example, the line may be drawn at quickening or viability—or perhaps when brain waves are first present. Whichever point is chosen, it is essential that any theory be clear on two crucial matters: (1) It should be specified whether the ontological status of persons or human beings or some other category is under discussion; and (2) Whatever the point at which the line is drawn (viability, conception, birth, etc.), it should be argued that the line can be justifiably drawn at that point so that the theory is a nonarbitrary one.

As we saw previously, it remains controversial precisely what *ontological* status the fetus has. We shall now see that the fetus's *moral* status is equally controversial.

THE MORAL STATUS OF THE FETUS

The notion of moral status might be explicated in several ways but probably is most easily understood in abortion contexts in terms of *rights*.[1] Accordingly, to say that a fetus possesses moral status is to say that it possesses rights. But which rights, if any? Conservatives hold that unborn fetuses possess the same rights as those who are born and therefore have *full moral status*. Devine and Brody hold such a thesis for at least most stages of fetal development. At least some moderates contend that fetuses have only some rights and therefore have only a *partial moral status*. (Thomson's article might be so interpreted.) Liberals, on the other hand, maintain that fetuses possess no rights and therefore *no moral status,* as Warren maintains. If this liberal account is accepted, then the unborn have no more right to life than a bodily cell or a tumor, and an abortion would seem to be no more morally objectionable than surgery to remove the tumor. On the other hand, if the conservative account is accepted, then the unborn possess all the rights possessed by other human beings, and an abortion would appear to be as objectionable as any common killing—except perhaps those killings committed in self-defense.

Theories of moral status are usually closely connected with theories of ontological status. The conservative holds that since the line between the human and the nonhuman must be drawn at conception, the fetus has full ontological status and therefore full moral status. The liberal may contend that since the line between the human and the nonhuman must be drawn at birth, the fetus has no significant ontological status and therefore no moral status. However, recently a rather different approach has been more popular. Liberals have argued that even though the fetus is biologically human, and thus has full ontological status as biologically human, it nonetheless is not human in a morally significant sense and hence has no significant moral status. (Compare the second sense of human life previously mentioned.) This claim is usually accompanied by the thesis that only persons constitute the moral community, and since fetuses are not persons they do not have a moral status (*cf.* Warren). Moderates, on the other hand, use a wide mixture of arguments, which sometimes do and sometimes do not combine an ontological account with a moral one. Typical of moderate views is the claim that the line between the human and the nonhuman or the line between persons and nonpersons should be drawn at some point between conception and birth, and therefore that the fetus has no significant moral status during some stages of growth but does have significant moral status beginning at some later stage (*cf.* the discussions in Devine and Brody). In many recent theories viability has been an especially popular point at which to draw the line, with the result that the fetus is given either full moral status or partial moral status at viability (*cf.* the Supreme Court opinion delivered by Justice Blackmun). Baruch Brody, however, rejects this criterion and attempts to substitute the more conservative standard of the development of a functional brain.

THE PROBLEM OF CONFLICTING RIGHTS

If either the liberal or the conservative view of the moral status of the fetus is adopted, the problem of morally justifying abortion may appear to admit of rather easy resolution. If one endorses the liberal theory—that a fetus does not enjoy an ethically significant claim to treatment as a human being—the problem may seem to disappear quickly, for it is then arguable that abortions are not morally reprehensible and are prudentially justified much as other surgical procedures are. On the other hand, if one endorses the conservative theory—that a fetus at any stage of development is a human life with full moral status, and possibly a person—the equation "abortion is murder" might be accepted. By this reasoning abortion is never justified under any conditions, or at least could be permitted only if it were an instance of "justified homicide." Many conservative theories would not accept the claim that homicide in such circumstances is ever justified. Killing of the innocent, they would argue, is never permitted. Since intended abortion is a case of the deliberate destruction of innocent human life, it must under no circumstances be permitted and cannot be correctly classified as justifiable homicide.

A conservative theory, however, is not committed by its account of the fetus (as a human being with full moral status) to take precisely this latter ethical position. Instead, it may be argued that there are cases of justified homicide involving the unborn. For example, it might be argued that a pregnant woman may legitimately "kill" the fetus in "self-defense" if only one of the two may survive or if both will die unless the life of the fetus is terminated. In order to claim that abortion is always wrong, conservatives must justify maintaining the position that the fetus's "right to life" *always* overrides (or at least is equal to) all the pregnant woman's rights, including *her* rights to life and liberty.

Even if the conservative theory is construed so that it entails that human fetuses have equal rights because of their moral status, nothing in the theory requires that these moral rights always override all other moral rights. Here a defender of the conservative theory confronts the problem of the morality of abortion on the level of conflicting rights: the unborn possess some rights (including a right to life) and pregnant women also possess rights (including a right to life). Those who possess the rights have a *(prima facie)* moral claim to be treated in accordance with their rights. But what is to be done when these rights conflict?

This problem is in some respects even greater for those who hold a moderate theory of the moral status of the fetus. These theories provide moral grounds against arbitrary termination of fetal life (the fetus has some claim to protection against the actions of others) yet do not grant to the unborn (at least in some stages) the same right to life possessed by those already born. Accordingly, advocates of these theories are faced with the problem of specifying which rights or claims are sufficiently weighty to take precedence over other rights or claims. More precisely, one must decide which rights or claims justify or fail to justify abortions. Is the woman's right to decide what happens to her body sufficient to justify abortion? Is pregnancy as a result of rape sufficient? Is the likely death of the mother sufficient? Is psychological damage (sometimes used to justify "therapeutic abortion") sufficient? Is knowledge of a grossly deformed fetus, which produces severe mental suffering to the pregnant woman, sufficient? These issues of conflicting rights are raised in a striking manner by Thomson, who in turn is criticized by both Brody and Warren.

Finally, it could be argued that problems of the moral status of the fetus and problems of conflicting rights are irresolvable and thus fail to grasp the central issue in the abortion dispute. One could take the position that abortion is a practice whose justification is a *social* issue. From a utilitarian perspective, for example, the permissibility of abortion must be judged in terms of the consequences it has for society as a whole: If the consequences are generally better than the consequences of not allowing abortion then it should be permitted, either as a rule or in particular cases, depending on the kind of utilitarian argument being advanced.

T. L. B.

NOTES

1. The notion of moral status could be explicated in ways other than by reference to rights. To say that a fetus possesses some form of moral status might be simply to say that it is *wrong* to do certain things to it. This is important since some who deny that fetuses have rights still believe that certain ways of treating fetuses are wrong, just as some who believe that animals do not have rights nonetheless believe that it is wrong to do certain things to them.

ANDRÉ E. HELLEGERS

Fetal Development ✓

No [treatment of] abortion would be complete without a chapter on the fetus. He or she (in the absence of knowledge of the sex, we shall use the neutral ''it'') is, after all, one of the subjects in the debate. Frequently in the discussions on abortion, the physician is asked when life begins. Some seem to imply that there would be no problem of abortion if only a definitive statement could be made about the beginning of human life. This, however, is far from so, for the presence of human life has never precluded our taking it if we felt justified in doing so. In this [treatment of] abortion the question (when life begins) is therefore asked not to endorse or prohibit abortion, but rather because the layman is baffled by the fetus, since he cannot see it.

Since society has imagery and definitions of its own, which it has inherited from the past, it may be well in the description which follows to highlight those stages of development to which, for one reason or another, men have attached importance in the past.[1]

I

First, let us ask in what way the ovum, or female egg, and the sperm, or male eggs, differ from the fertilized ovum. The essential difference is that an ovum or a sperm will inevitably die unless they are combined together in the process of fertilization, while the fertilized egg will automatically develop unless untoward events occur. The first definition of life, then, could be the ability to reproduce oneself, and this the fertilized egg has while the individual ovum and sperm do not.

How is this process of fertilization brought about? At intercourse, about 300,000,000 sperm are deposited in the vagina and will begin their journey upwards through the uterus, or womb, and up into the

Reprinted with permission of the author and the publisher from *Theological Studies*, Vol. 31, No. 1 (March, 1970), pp. 3–9.

tube leading from the uterus towards the ovary. If an ovum has been released from the woman's ovary, it in turn will pass from the ovary down the same tube towards the uterus. The survival time of this ovum will be about twenty-four hours. If fertilization has not occurred in that time, both the ovum and the sperm will die. From a variety of mammalian species it has been learned that the sperm, as ejaculated, are not capable of immediately fertilizing an ovum. They must undergo a chemical change called ''capacitation,'' without which they cannot fertilize the ovum.[2] The process is as yet little understood, but it is thought that a substance in the female uterus or tube changes the sperm in such a way that they gain the ability to fertilize. In most species this process occurs in a matter of hours, say six or eight. Although the process has not yet been proven in the human, it is commonly assumed to exist, since it occurs in other mammalian species studied. Following intercourse, there would therefore be a period of several hours in which interference with reproduction would fall under the generally recognized heading of contraception rather than abortion, since no ovum would yet have been fertilized. Several hours after intercourse, then, fertilization may occur. The significance of this event lies in the fact that a totally new genetic package is now produced. The fertilized ovum contains genetic information brought from the father through the sperm, and from the mother through the ovum, so that a new combination of genetic information is created. This newly fertilized egg, sometimes called a zygote, has within it the hereditary characteristics of both the father and the mother, one half from each. The characteristics are derived from the genetic thread of life called DNA, contained in each.

This single fertilized cell will then proceed to divide into two cells, then four, then eight, etc., and this it will do at a rate of almost one division per day.[3]

It is well known that in this early stage of development the sphere of cells may split into identical parts to form identical twins. Twinning in the human may occur until the fourteenth day, when conjoined twins can still be produced. Less well known is the fact that it is also in these first few days that twins or triplets may be recombined into one single individual.

Experiments carried out in mice by Mintz showed that it was possible to recombine the early dividing cell stages from black parents and from white parents into a single black-and-white-striped mouse.[4] The significance of this phenomenon would seem to be that up until this stage the new individual mammal is not as yet irreversibly an individual, since it still may be recombined with others into one new, final being.

In the last few years this phenomenon has also been found in man. From the genetic make-up of these human individuals and from the make-up of their red blood cells it is clear that these human so-called chimeras, whose genetic type is XX-XY, are in fact recombinations into one human being of the products of more than one fertilization. The subject has recently been extensively reviewed by Benirschke,[5] and a prototype case can be found in the report of Myhre et al.[6] It is not as yet clear up to precisely what stage of development this can occur in the human, but in mice the recombination can still be performed at the 32-cell stage. The diagnostic criteria for such cases are that their genetic karyotype is XX-XY, that they are gonadally disturbed, consisting as they do of a genetic mixture of male and female, that they can contain two different populations of red blood cells, and that they may have heterochromia of the eyes. Six human cases meeting these requirements have been reported up to the present time.

The initial stages of cell division of the fertilized egg do not seem to be dependent on any paternal genetic material brought to the fertilized egg by the sperm. It would seem as if genetic material brought to the fertilized egg in the mother's ovum suffices to take the fertilized egg through the earliest stages of cell division.

All these matters are brought forth to point out that, although at fertilization a new genetic package is brought into being within the confines of one cell, this anatomical fact does not necessarily mean that all of the genetic material in it becomes crucially activated at that point, or that final irreversible individuality has been achieved.

Modern genetic studies therefore suggest that, in old standard Catholic language, one could say: "If by means of two fertilizations two souls are infused, and if a single body only contains one soul, then we are beginning to see cases in which one of the two souls must have disappeared without any fertilized egg having died."

It is also important to realize that in these first few days of life it is quite impossible for the woman to know that she is pregnant, or for the doctor to diagnose the condition by a pregnancy test.

The fact that the first seven days of the reproductive process take place entirely in the tube, and not in the uterus itself, has several major implications for the subject of abortion. These should be fully understood. If within seven days of intercourse, as for instance following rape, the lining of the uterus is removed by curettage, abortion, in its legal sense, has not taken place. It would be impossible to prove that an abortion have been performed when all pregnancy tests were shown to be negative and the lining of the uterus was shown, under the microscope, to have contained no pregnancy. Indeed the operation of curettage is a common gynecological one, which is frequently carried out in the second half of the menstrual cycle, when a fertilized ovum may well be present in the tube. There has never been a medical tradition to perform the curettage only immediately following menstruation, in order to assure that no fertilized egg could be present in the tube (since ovulation would not as yet have occurred). By the same token, women scheduled to undergo a curettage are not instructed to forgo intercourse lest there be present in the tube a fertilized ovum which would be unable to implant into the uterus due to the removal of its lining. Moreover, there is some evidence that modern "contraceptive" techniques such as the intrauterine loop, and even some of the steroid pills, may well exert their effect in pregnancy prevention by acting after fertilization of the ovum has occurred, but before implantation in the uterus.[7] Although the action of these agents is not yet fully understood, there has never been a suggestion that they would be considered abortifacient under the civil law, since no evidence of pregnancy could possibly be obtained.

II

After approximately six or seven days of this cell-division process (all of which occurs in the tube), the next critical stage of development starts. The sphere of cells will now enter the uterus and implant itself into the uterine lining. This process of implantation is highly critical, for it is during these days that one pole of the sphere of cells, the trophoblast (later to become the placenta), burrows its way into the lining of the uterus. The opposite pole of this sphere will become the fetus. The part which becomes the placenta produces hormones. These enter the maternal blood stream and serve a critical function in preventing the mother from menstruating. Since the time interval between ovulation and menstruation is approximately fourteen days, and since the first seven days of the new life have been passed in the tube, it is obvious that the implanting trophoblast only has about seven days to produce enough hormone to stop the mother from menstruating and thus sloughing off the fetal life. These same hormones, circulating in the mother, form the basis for the chemical tests which enable us to diagnose pregnancy. After this second week of pregnancy the zygote rapidly becomes more complex and is now called the embryo. Somewhere between the third and fourth week the differentiation of the embryo will have been sufficient for heart pumping to occur,[8] although the heart will by no means yet have reached its final configuration. At the end of six weeks all of the internal organs of the fetus will be present, but as yet in a rudimentary stage. The blood vessels leading from the heart will have been fully deployed, although they too will continue to grow in size with growth of the fetus. By the end of seven weeks tickling of the mouth and nose of the developing embryo with a hair will cause it to flex its neck, while at the end of eight weeks there will be readable electrical activity coming from the brain.[9] The meaning of the activity cannot be interpreted. By now also the fingers and toes will be fully recognizable. Sometime between the ninth and the tenth week local reflexes appear such as swallowing, squinting, and tongue retraction. By the tenth week spontaneous movement is seen, independent of stimulation. By the eleventh week thumb-sucking has been observed, and X rays of the fetus at this time show clear details of the skeleton. After twelve weeks the fetus, now 3½ inches in size, will have completed its brain structure, although growth of course will continue. By this time also it has become possible to pick up the fetal heart by modern electrocardiographic techniques, via the mother.

The twelve-week stage is also important for an entirely different reason. It is after this stage that the performance of an abortion by the relatively simple D&C (scraping of the womb) becomes dangerous. Thereafter abortion must be performed either by abdominal operation or by the more recently developed technique of the injection of a concentrated fluid into the amniotic cavity.

Some time between the twelfth and sixteenth week "quickening" will occur. This event, long considered important in law, denotes the fact that fetal movements are first felt by the mother. Quickening, therefore, is a phenomenon of maternal perception rather than a fetal achievement. It is subjective and varies with the degree of experience and obesity of the mother.

Some time between the sixteenth and twentieth week it will also become possible to hear the fetal heart, not just by the refined EKG, but also by the simple stethoscope.

The twentieth-week stage again has definite importance. Before this date delivery of the product of conception is called an abortion in medical terminology. After this date we no longer speak of abortion but of premature delivery. The fetus at this stage will weigh about one pound. Between the twentieth and twenty-eighth week fetuses born have an approximately 10% chance of survival. At twenty-eight weeks the fetus will weigh slightly over two pounds. In former days the medical profession defined fetuses of less than twenty-eight weeks of age as abortions, but this was impossible to maintain when 10% of such infants might survive. As a consequence, a discrepancy may now exist between possible definitions of viability in legal and in medical circles; at least the ability to ensure survival of fetuses has progressively occurred at earlier stages.

After the twenty-eighth week little change in outward appearance of the fetus occurs, although growth obviously continues, and with this growth the chances of survival also increase.

These, then, are the major stages of fetal development in the order of their occurrence. Grouped systematically, and therefore rather arbitrarily, by genetic factors, by cardiovascular or nervous system development, and by chances of survival, they can be summarized as in the accompanying Table.

Throughout the analysis of the beginning of life it is important to bear several factors in mind. First, the understanding of the processes described is the understanding of today. The eliciting of fetal responses depends on the methods available today. Second, it is not a function of science to prove, or disprove, where in this process *human* life begins, in the sense that those discussing the abortion issue so frequently use the word "life," i.e., human dignity, human personhood, or human inviolability. Such entities do not pertain to the science or art of medicine, but are rather a societal judgment. Science cannot prove them; it can only describe the biological development and predict what will occur to it with an accuracy that depends on the stage of development of the particular science. In the ultimate analysis the question is not just to forecast when life begins, but rather: How should one behave when one does not know whether dignity is or is not present in the fetus?

NOTES

1. I shall stress heavily the new biology on the developmental processes in the first seven days, while the "fetus" is in the tube. This is crucial, I believe, (1) by reason of its own biological interest; (2) because of the action of the pill and intrauterine devices, which may act during these seven days; (3) because this stage precedes the period when a diagnosis of pregnancy can be made, i.e., it is the stage commonly described as "the normal second half of the normal menstrual cycle"; (4) because it is the stage when the "morning-after pill" may act; (5) because it is not presently covered under abortion laws, inasmuch as it precedes the stage when the woman knows she is pregnant (for she has not yet missed a period) and precedes the stage when a diagnosis can be made; (6) because it is a stage upon which the Catholic Hospital Association

TABLE 1   SOME MAJOR NORMAL STAGES IN FETAL DEVELOPMENT

Time	Cardiovascular system	Nervous system	Other criteria
Some hours	—	—	Intercourse followed by "capacitation"
0 hours	—	—	Fertilization; 1 cell, often called zygote
About 22 hours	—	—	2 cell ⎫ Possible recombination
About 44 hours	—	—	4 cell ⎬ until day ?
About 66 hours	—	—	8 cell ⎰ Possible twinning
About 4 days	—	—	16 cell ⎭ until day 14 "Morula" stage
About 6–7 days	—	—	Implantation—often called "blastocyst" stage
2 weeks	—	—	Name changed from zygote to embryo
3–4 weeks	Heart Pumping	—	—
6 weeks	—	—	All organs present
7–8 weeks	—	Mouth or nose tickling–neck flexing	—
8 weeks	—	Readable brain electric activity	Name change from embryo to fetus. Length 3 cm.
9–10 weeks	—	Swallowing, squinting, local reflexes	—
10 weeks	—	Spontaneous movement	—
11 weeks	—	—	Thumb sucking
12 weeks	Fetal EKG via mother	—	Brain structure complete Length 10 cm.
13 weeks*	—	—	D&C contraindicated hereafter
12–16 weeks*	—	—	"Quickening." Length 18 cm. at 16 weeks
16–20 weeks*	Fetal heart heard	—	Length 25 cm. at 20 weeks
20 weeks*	—	—	Name change from abortus to premature infant
20–28 weeks*	—	—	10% survive
28 weeks*	—	—	Fetus said to be "viable" in some definitions
40 weeks*	—	—	Birth

*Calculated from the first day of the last menstrual period.

has not yet reflected, since we frequently do operations after ovulation but before a period is missed, i.e., during these seven days.

2. Cf. C. E. Adams, "The Influence of Maternal Environment on Preimplantation Stages of Pregnancy in the Rabbit," in *Preimplantation Stages of Pregnancy,* ed. G. E. W. Wolstenholme and M. O'Connor (Boston, 1965) p. 345; K. A. Rafferty, "The Beginning of Development," in *Intrauterine Development,* ed. A. C. Barnes (Philadelphia, 1968).

3. Cf. Rafferty, *op. cit.*

4. Cf. B. Mintz, "Experimental Genetic Mosaicism in the Mouse," in *Preimplantation Stages of Pregnancy* (n. 2 above) p. 194.

5. Cf. K. Benirschke, *Current Topics in Pathology* 1 (1969) 1.

6. Cf. A. Myhre, T. Meyer, J. N. Opitz, R. R. Race, R. Sanger, and T. J. Greenwalt, "Two Populations of Erythrocytes Associated with XX-XY Mosaicism," *Transfusion* 5 (1965) 501.

7. Cf. P. A. Corfman and S. J. Segal, "Biologic Effects of Intrauterine Devices," *American Journal of Obstetrics and Gynecology* 100 (1968) 448; also "Hormonal Steroids in Contraception," *WHO Technical Report Series, 1968* (Geneva, 1968) p. 386.

8. Cf. J. W. C. Johnson, "Cardio-Respiratory Systems," in *Intrauterine Development* (n. 2 above).

9. Cf. D. Goldblatt, "Nervous System and Sensory Organs," in *Intrauterine Development* (n. 2 above).

UNITED STATES SUPREME COURT

Roe v. Wade: Majority Opinion and Dissent

[Mr. Justice Blackmun delivered the opinion of the Court.]

It is . . . apparent that at common law, at the time of the adoption of our Constitution, and throughout the major portion of the nineteenth century, abortion was viewed with less disfavor than under most American statutes currently in effect. Phrasing it another way, a woman enjoyed a substantially broader right to terminate a pregnancy than she does in most states today. At least with respect to the early stage of pregnancy, and very possibly without such a limitation, the opportunity to make this choice was present in this country well into the nineteenth century. Even later, the law continued for some time to treat less punitively an abortion procured in early pregnancy. . . .

Three reasons have been advanced to explain historically the enactment of criminal abortion laws in the nineteenth century and to justify their continued existence.

It has been argued occasionally that these laws were the product of a Victorian social concern to discourage illicit sexual conduct. Texas, however, does

Reprinted from 410 *United States Reports* 113; decided January 22, 1973.

not advance this justification in the present case, and it appears that no court or commentator has taken the argument seriously. . . .

A second reason is concerned with abortion as a medical procedure. When most criminal abortion laws were first enacted, the procedure was a hazardous one for the woman. This was particularly true prior to the development of antisepsis. Antiseptic techniques, of course, were based on discoveries by Lister, Pasteur, and others first announced in 1867, but were not generally accepted and employed until about the turn of the century. Abortion mortality was high. Even after 1900, and perhaps until as late as the development of antibiotics in the 1940s, standard modern techniques such as dilation and curettage were not nearly so safe as they are today. Thus it has been argued that a state's real concern in enacting a criminal abortion law was to protect the pregnant woman, that is, to restrain her from submitting to a procedure that placed her life in serious jeopardy.

Modern medical techniques have altered this situation. Appellants and various *amici* refer to medical data indicating that abortion in early pregnancy, that is, prior to the end of first trimester, although not without its risk, is now relatively safe. Mortality rates for women undergoing early abortions, where the procedure is legal, appear to be as low as or lower than the rates for normal childbirth. Consequently, any interest of the state in protecting the woman from an inherently hazardous procedure, except when it would be equally dangerous for her to forgo it, has largely disappeared. Of course, important state interests in the area of health and medical standards do remain. The state has a legitimate interest in seeing to it that abortion like any other medical procedure, is performed under circumstances that insure maximum safety for the patient. This interest obviously extends at least to the performing physician and his staff, to the facilities involved, to the availability of after-care, and to adequate provision for any complication or emergency that might arise. The prevalence of high mortality rates at illegal ''abortion mills'' strengthens, rather than weakens, the state's interest in regulating the conditions under which abortions are performed. Moreover, the risk to the woman increases as her pregnancy continues. Thus the state retains a definite interest in protecting the woman's own health and safety when an abortion is performed at a late stage of pregnancy.

The third reason is the state's interest—some phrase it in terms of duty—in protecting prenatal life. Some of the argument for this justification rests on the theory that a new human life is present from the moment of conception. The state's interest and general obligation to protect life then extends, it is argued, to prenatal life. Only when the life of the pregnant mother herself is at stake, balanced against the life she carries within her, should the interest of the embryo or fetus not prevail. Logically, of course, a legitimate state interest in this area need not stand or fall on acceptance of the belief that life begins at conception or at some other point prior to live birth. In assessing the state's interest, recognition may be given to the less rigid claim that as long as at least *potential* life is involved, the state may assert interests beyond the protection of the pregnant woman alone.

Parties challenging state abortion laws have sharply disputed in some courts the contention that a purpose of these laws, when enacted, was to protect prenatal life. Pointing to the absence of legislative history to support the contention, they claim that most state laws were designed solely to protect the woman. Because medical advances have lessened this concern, at least with respect to abortion in early pregnancy, they argue that with respect to such abortions the laws can no longer be justified by any state interest. There is some scholarly support for this view of

original purpose. The few states courts called upon to interpret their laws in the late nineteenth and early twentieth centuries did focus on the state's interest in protecting the woman's health rather than in preserving the embryo and fetus. . . .

The Constitution does not explicitly mention any right of privacy. In a line of decisions, however, going back perhaps as far as *Union Pacific R. Co. v. Botsford* (1891), the Court has recognized that a right of personal privacy, or a guarantee of certain areas or zones of privacy, does exist under the Constitution. In varying contexts the Court or individual Justices have indeed found at least the roots of that right in the First Amendment, . . . in the Fourth and Fifth Amendments, . . . in the penumbras of the Bill of Rights, . . . in the Ninth Amendment, . . . or in the concept of liberty guaranteed by the first section of the Fourteenth Amendment. . . . These decisions make it clear that only personal rights that can be deemed ''fundamental'' or ''implicit in the concept of ordered liberty'' . . . are included in this guarantee of personal privacy. They also make it clear that the right has some extension to activities relating to marriage, . . . procreation, . . . contraception, . . . family relationships, . . . and child rearing and education. . . .

This right of privacy, whether it be founded in the Fourteenth Amendment's concept of personal liberty and restrictions upon state action, as we feel it is, or, as the District Court determined, in the Ninth Amendment's reservation of rights to the people, is broad enough to encompass a woman's decision whether or not to terminate her pregnancy. . . .

Appellants and some *amici* argue that the woman's right is absolute and that she is entitled to terminate her pregnancy at whatever time, in whatever way, and for whatever reason she alone chooses. With this we do not agree. Appellants' arguments that Texas either has no valid interest at all in regulating the abortion decision, or no interest strong enough to support any limitation upon the woman's sole determination, is unpersuasive. The Court's decisions recognizing a right of privacy also acknowledge that some state regulation in areas protected by that right is appropriate. As noted above, a state may properly assert important interests in safeguarding health, in maintaining medical standards, and in protecting potential life. At some point in pregnancy, these respective interests become sufficiently compelling to sustain regulation of the factors that govern the abortion decision. The privacy right involved, therefore, cannot be said to be absolute. . . .

We therefore conclude that the right of personal privacy includes the abortion decision, but that this right is not unqualified and must be considered against important state interests in regulation.

We note that those federal and state courts that have recently considered abortion law challenges have reached the same conclusion. . . .

Although the results are divided, most of these courts have agreed that the right of privacy, however based, is broad enough to cover the abortion decision; that the right, nonetheless, is not absolute and is subject to some limitations; and that at some point the state interests as to protection of health, medical standards, and prenatal life, become dominant. We agree with this approach. . . .

The appellee and certain *amici* argue that the fetus is a ''person'' within the language and meaning of the Fourteenth Amendment. In support of this they outline at length and in detail the well-known facts of fetal development. If this suggestion of personhood is established, the appellant's case, of course, collapses, for the fetus's right to life is then guaranteed specifically by the Amendment. The appellant conceded as much on reargument. On the other hand, the appellee conceded on reargument that no case could be cited that holds that a fetus is a person within the meaning of the Fourteenth Amendment. . . .

All this, together with our observation, *supra,* that throughout the major portion of the nineteenth century prevailing legal abortion practices were far freer than they are today, persuades us that the word ''person,'' as used in the Fourteenth Amendment, does not include the unborn. . . . Indeed, our decision in *United States v. Vuitch* (1971), inferentially is to the same effect, for we there would not have indulged in statutory interpretation favorable to abortion in specified circumstances if the necessary consequence was the termination of life entitled to Fourteenth Amendment protection.

. . . As we have intimated above, it is reasonable and appropriate for a state to decide that at some point in time another interest, that of health of the mother or that of potential human life, becomes significantly involved. The woman's privacy is no longer sole and any right of privacy she possesses must be measured accordingly.

Texas urges that, apart from the Fourteenth Amendment, life begins at conception and is present throughout pregnancy, and that, therefore, the state has a compelling interest in protecting that life from and after conception. We need not resolve the difficult question of when life begins. When those trained in the respective disciplines of medicine, philosophy, and theology are unable to arrive at any consensus, the judiciary, at this point in the development of man's knowledge, is not in a position to speculate as to the answer.

It should be sufficient to note briefly the wide divergence of thinking on this most sensitive and difficult question. There has always been strong support for the view that life does not begin until live birth. This was the belief of the Stoics. It appears to be the predominant, though not the unanimous, attitude of the Jewish faith. It may be taken to represent also the position of a large segment of the Protestant community, insofar as that can be ascertained; organized groups that have taken a formal position on the abortion issue have generally regarded abortion as a matter for the conscience of the individual and her family. As we have noted, the common law found greater significance in quickening. Physicians and their scientific colleagues have regarded that event with less interest and have tended to focus either upon conception or upon live birth or upon the interim point at which the fetus becomes ''viable,'' that is, potentially able to live outside the mother's womb, albeit with artificial aid. Viability is usually placed at about seven months (28 weeks) but may occur earlier, even at 24 weeks. . . .

In areas other than criminal abortion the law has been reluctant to endorse any theory that life, as we recognize it, begins before live birth or to accord legal rights to the unborn except in narrowly defined situations and except when the rights are contingent upon live birth. . . . In short, the unborn have never been recognized in the law as persons in the whole sense.

In view of all this, we do not agree that, by adopting one theory of life, Texas may override the rights of the pregnant woman that are at stake. We repeat, however, that the state does have an important and legitimate interest in preserving and protecting the health of the pregnant woman, whether she be a resident of the state or a nonresident who seeks medical consultation and treatment there, and that it has still *another* important and legitimate interest in protecting the potentiality of human life. These interests are separate and distinct. Each grows in substantiality as the woman approaches term and, at a point during pregnancy, each becomes "compelling."

With respect to the state's important and legitimate interest in the health of the mother, the "compelling" point, in the light of present medical knowledge, is at approximately the end of the first trimester. This is so because of the now established medical fact . . . that until the end of the first trimester mortality in abortion is less than mortality in normal childbirth. It follows that, from and after this point, a state may regulate the abortion procedure to the extent that the regulation reasonably relates to the preservation and protection of maternal health. Examples of permissible state regulation in this area are requirements as to the qualifications of the person who is to perform the abortion; as to the licensure of that person; as to the facility in which the procedure is to be performed, that is, whether it must be a hospital or may be a clinic or some other place of less-than-hospital status; as to the licensing of the facility; and the like.

This means, on the other hand, that, for the period of pregnancy prior to this "compelling" point, the attending physician, in consultation with his patient, is free to determine, without regulation by the state, that in his medical judgment the patient's pregnancy should be terminated. If that decision is reached, the judgment may be effectuated by an abortion free of interference by the state.

With respect to the state's important and legitimate interest in potential life, the "compelling" point is at viability. This is so because the fetus then presumably has the capability of meaningful life outside the mother's womb. State regulation protective of fetal life after viability thus has both logical and biological justifications. If the state is interested in protecting fetal life after viability, it may go so far as to proscribe abortion during that period except when it is necessary to preserve the life or health of the mother. . . .

To summarize and repeat:

1. A state criminal abortion statute of the current Texas type, that excepts from criminality only a *lifesaving* procedure on behalf of the mother, without regard to pregnancy stage and without recognition of the other interests involved, is violative of the Due Process Clause of the Fourteenth Amendment.

(a) For the stage prior to approximately the end of the first trimester, the abortion decision and its effectuation must be left to the medical judgment of the pregnant woman's attending physician.

(b) For the stage subsequent to approximately the end of the first trimester, the state, in promoting its interest in the health of the mother, may, if it chooses, regulate the abortion procedure in ways that are reasonably related to maternal health.

(c) For the stage subsequent to viability the state, in promoting its interest in the potentiality of human life, may, if it chooses, regulate, and even proscribe, abortion except where it is necessary, in appropriate medical judgment, for the preservation of the life or health of the mother.

2. The state may define the term "physician" . . . to mean only a physician currently licensed by the state, and may proscribe any abortion by a person who is not a physician as so defined.

. . . The decision leaves the state free to place increasing restrictions on abortion as the period of pregnancy lengthens, so long as those restrictions are tailored to the recognized state interests. The decision vindicates the right of the physician to administer medical treatment according to his professional judgment up to the points where important state interests provide compelling justifications for intervention. Up to those points the abortion decision in all its aspects is inherently, and primarily, a medical decision, and basic responsibility for it must rest with the physician. If an individual practitioner abuses the privilege of exercising proper medical judgment, the usual remedies, judicial and intraprofessional, are available. . . .

[Mr. Justice White, with whom Mr. Justice Rehnquist joins, dissenting.]

At the heart of the controversy in these cases are those recurring pregnancies that pose no danger whatsoever to the life or health of the mother but are, nevertheless, unwanted for any one or more of a variety of reasons—convenience, family planning, economics, dislike of children, the embarrassment of illegitimacy, etc. The common claim before us is that for any one of such reasons, or for no reason at all, and without asserting or claiming any threat to life or health, any woman is entitled to an abortion at her request if she is able to find a medical advisor willing to undertake the procedure.

The Court for the most part sustains this position: During the period prior to the time the fetus becomes viable, the Constitution of the United States values the convenience, whim, or caprice of the putative mother more than the life or potential life of the fetus; the Constitution, therefore, guarantees the right to an abortion as against any state law or policy seeking to protect the fetus from an abortion not prompted by more compelling reasons of the mother.

With all due respect, I dissent. I find nothing in the language or history of the Constitution to support the Court's judgment. The Court simply fashions and announces a new constitutional right for pregnant mothers and, with scarcely any reason or authority for its action, invests that right with sufficient substance to override most existing state abortion statutes. The upshot is that the people and the legislatures of the 50 states are constitutionally disentitled to weigh the relative importance of the continued existence and development of the fetus, on the one hand, against a spectrum of possible impacts on the mother, on the other hand. As an exercise of raw judicial power, the Court perhaps has authority to do what it does today; but in my view its judgment is an improvident and extravagant exercise of the power of judicial review that the Constitution extends to this Court.

The Court apparently values the convenience of the pregnant mother more than the continued existence and development of the life or potential life that she carries. Whether or not I might agree with that marshaling of values, I can in no event join the Court's judgment because I find no constitutional warrant for imposing such an order of priorities on the people and legislatures of the states. In a sensitive area such as this, involving as it does issues over which reasonable men may easily and heatedly differ, I cannot accept the Court's exercise of its clear power of choice by interposing a constitutional barrier to state efforts to protect human life and by investing mothers and doctors with the constitutionally protected right to exterminate it. This issue, for the most part, should be left with the people and to the political processes the people have devised to govern their affairs.

It is my view, therefore, that the Texas statute is not constitutionally infirm because it denies abortions to those who seek to serve only their convenience rather than to protect their life or health. Nor is this plaintiff, who claims no threat to her mental or physical health, entitled to assert the possible rights of those women whose pregnancy assertedly implicated their health. This, together with *United States v. Vuitch,* 402 U.S. 62 (1971), dictates reversal of the judgment of the District Court.

JUDITH JARVIS THOMSON

A Defense of Abortion[1]

Most opposition to abortion relies on the premise that the fetus is a human being, a person, from the moment of conception. The premise is argued for, but, as I think, not well. Take, for example, the most common argument. We are asked to notice that the development of a human being from conception through birth into childhood is continuous; then it is said that to draw a line, to choose a point in this development and say "before this point the thing is not a person, after this point it is a person" is to make an arbitrary choice, a choice for which in the nature of things no good reason can be given. It is concluded that the fetus is, or anyway that we had better say it is, a person from the moment of conception. But this conclusion does not follow. Similar things might be said about the development of an acorn into an oak tree, and it does not follow that acorns are oak trees, or that we had better say they are. Arguments of this form are sometimes called "slippery slope arguments"—the phrase is perhaps self-explanatory—and it is dismaying that opponents of abortion rely on them so heavily and uncritically.

I am inclined to agree, however, that the prospects for "drawing a line" in the development of the fetus look dim. I am inclined to think also that we shall probably have to agree that the fetus has already become a human person well before birth. Indeed, it comes as a surprise when one first learns how early in its life it begins to acquire human characteristics. By the tenth week, for example, it already has a face, arms and legs, fingers and toes; it has internal organs, and brain activity is detectable.[2] On the other hand, I think that the premise is false, that the fetus is not a person from the moment of conception. A newly fertilized ovum, a newly implanted clump of cells, is no more a person than an acorn is an oak tree. But I shall not discuss any of this. For it seems to me to be of

great interest to ask what happens if, for the sake of argument, we allow the premise. How, precisely, are we supposed to get from there to the conclusion that abortion is morally impermissible? Opponents of abortion commonly spend most of their time establishing that the fetus is a person, and hardly any time explaining the step from there to the impermissibility of abortion. Perhaps they think the step too simple and obvious to require much comment. Or perhaps instead they are simply being economical in argument. Many of those who defend abortion rely on the premise that the fetus is not a person, but only a bit of tissue that will become a person at birth; and why pay out more arguments than you have to? Whatever the explanation, I suggest that the step they take is neither easy nor obvious, that it calls for closer examination than it is commonly given, and that when we do give it this closer examination we shall feel inclined to reject it.

I propose, then, that we grant that the fetus is a person from the moment of conception. How does the argument go from here? Something like this, I take it. Every person has a right to life. So the fetus has a right to life. No doubt the mother has a right to decide what shall happen in and to her body; everyone would grant that. But surely a person's right to life is stronger and more stringent than the mother's right to decide what happens in and to her body, and so outweighs it. So the fetus may not be killed; an abortion may not be performed.

It sounds plausible. But now let me ask you to imagine this. You wake up in the morning and find yourself back to back in bed with an unconscious violinist. A famous unconscious violinist. He has been found to have a fatal kidney ailment, and the Society of Music Lovers has canvassed all the available medical records and found that you alone have the right blood type to help. They have therefore kidnapped you, and last night the violinist's circulatory system was plugged into yours, so that your kidneys

Reprinted with permission of the publisher from *Philosophy and Public Affairs*, Vol. 1, No. 1 (1971), pp. 47–66. Copyright © 1971 by Princeton University Press.

can be used to extract poisons from his blood as well as your own. The director of the hospital now tells you, "Look, we're sorry the Society of Music Lovers did this to you—we would never have permitted it if we had known. But still, they did it, and the violinist now is plugged into you. To unplug you would be to kill him. But never mind, it's only for nine months. By then he will have recovered from his ailment, and can safely be unplugged from you." Is it morally incumbent on you to accede to this situation? No doubt it would be very nice of you if you did, a great kindness. But do you *have* to accede to it? What if it were not nine months, but nine years? Or longer still? What if the director of the hospital says, "Tough luck, I agree, but you've now got to stay in bed, with the violinist plugged into you, for the rest of your life. Because remember this. All persons have a right to life, and violinists are persons. Granted you have a right to decide what happens in and to your body, but a person's right to life outweighs your right to decide what happens in and to your body. So you cannot ever be unplugged from him." I imagine you would regard this as outrageous, which suggests that something really is wrong with that plausible-sounding argument I mentioned a moment ago.

In this case, of course, you were kidnapped; you didn't volunteer for the operation that plugged the violinist into your kidneys. Can those who oppose abortion on the ground I mentioned make an exception for a pregnancy due to rape? Certainly. They can say that persons have a right to life only if they didn't come into existence because of rape; or they can say that all persons have a right to life, but that some have less of a right to life than others, in particular, that those who came into existence because of rape have less. But these statements have a rather unpleasant sound. Surely the question of whether you have a right to life at all, or how much of it you have, shouldn't turn on the question of whether or not you are the product of a rape. And in fact the people who oppose abortion on the ground I mentioned do not make this distinction, and hence do not make an exception in case of rape.

Nor do they make an exception for a case in which the mother has to spend the nine months of her pregnancy in bed. They would agree that would be a great pity, and hard on the mother; but all the same, all persons have a right to life, the fetus is a person, and so on. I suspect, in fact, that they would not make an exception for a case in which, miraculously enough, the pregnancy went on for nine years, or even the rest of the mother's life.

Some won't even make an exception for a case in which continuation of the pregnancy is likely to shorten the mother's life; they regard abortion as impermissible even to save the mother's life. Such cases are nowadays very rare, and many opponents of abortion do not accept this extreme view. All the same, it is a good place to begin: a number of points of interest come out in respect to it.

1. Let us call the view that abortion is impermissible even to save the mother's life "the extreme view." I want to suggest first that it does not issue from the argument I mentioned earlier without the addition of some fairly powerful premises. Suppose a woman has become pregnant, and now learns that she has a cardiac condition such that she will die if she carries the baby to term. What may be done for her? The fetus, being a person, has a right to life, but as the mother is a person too, so has she a right to life. Presumably they have an equal right to life. How is it supposed to come out that an abortion may not be performed? If mother and child have an equal right to life, shouldn't we perhaps flip a coin? Or should we add to the mother's right to life her right to decide what happens in and to her body, which everybody seems to be ready to grant—the sum of her rights now outweighing the fetus's right to life?

The most familiar argument here is the following. We are told that performing the abortion would be directly killing[3] the child, whereas doing nothing would not be killing the mother, but only letting her die. Moreover, in killing the child, one would be killing an innocent person, for the child has committed no crime, and is not aiming at his mother's death. And then there are a variety of ways in which this might be continued. (a) But as directly killing an innocent person is always and absolutely impermissible, an abortion may not be performed. Or, (b) as directly killing an innocent person is murder, and murder is always and absolutely impermissible, an abortion may not be performed.[4] Or, (c) as one's duty to refrain from directly killing an innocent person is more stringent than one's duty to keep a person from dying, an abortion may not be performed. Or, (d) if one's only options are directly killing an innocent person or letting a person die, one must prefer letting the person die, and thus an abortion may not be performed.[5]

Some people seem to have thought that these are

not further premises which must be added if the conclusion is to be reached, but that they follow from the very fact that an innocent person has a right to life.[6] But this seems to me to be a mistake, and perhaps the simplest way to show this is to bring out that while we must certainly grant that innocent persons have a right to life, the theses in (a) through (d) are all false. Take (b), for example. If directly killing an innocent person is murder, and thus is impermissible, then the mother's directly killing the innocent person inside her is murder, and thus is impermissible. But it cannot seriously be thought to be murder if the mother performs an abortion on herself to save her life. It cannot seriously be said that she *must* refrain, that she *must* sit passively by and wait for her death. Let us look again at the case of you and the violinist. There you are, in bed with the violinist, and the director of the hospital says to you, ''It's all most distressing, and I deeply sympathize, but you see this is putting an additional strain on your kidneys, and you'll be dead within the month. But you *have* to stay where you are all the same. Because unplugging you would be directly killing an innocent violinist, and that's murder, and that's impermissible.'' If anything in the world is true, it is that you do not commit murder, you do not do what is impermissible, if you reach around to your back and unplug yourself from that violinist to save your life.

The main focus of attention in writings on abortion has been on what a third party may or may not do in answer to a request from a woman for an abortion. This is in a way understandable. Things being as they are, there isn't much a woman can safely do to abort herself. So the question asked is what a third party may do, and what the mother may do, if it is mentioned at all, is deduced, almost as an afterthought, from what it is concluded that third parties may do. But it seems to me that to treat the matter in this way is to refuse to grant to the mother that very status of person which is so firmly insisted on for the fetus. For we cannot simply read off what a person may do from what a third party may do. Suppose you find yourself trapped in a tiny house with a growing child. I mean a very tiny house, and a rapidly growing child—you are already up against the wall of the house and in a few minutes you'll be crushed to death. The child on the other hand won't be crushed to death; if nothing is done to stop him from growing he'll be hurt, but in the end he'll simply burst open the house and walk out a free man. Now I could well understand it if a bystander were to say, ''There's nothing we can do for

you. We cannot choose between your life and his, we cannot be the ones to decide who is to live, we cannot intervene.'' But it cannot be concluded that you too can do nothing, that you cannot attack it to save your life. However innocent the child may be, you do not have to wait passively while it crushes you to death. Perhaps a pregnant woman is vaguely felt to have the status of house, to which we don't allow the right of self-defense. But if the woman houses the child, it should be remembered that she is a person who houses it.

I should perhaps stop to say explicitly that I am not claiming that people have a right to do anything whatever to save their lives. I think, rather, that there are drastic limits to the right of self-defense. If someone threatens you with death unless you torture someone else to death, I think you have not the right, even to save your life, to do so. But the case under consideration here is very different. In our case there are only two people involved, one whose life is threatened, and one who threatens it. Both are innocent: the one who is threatened is not threatened because of any fault, the one who threatens does not threaten because of any fault. For this reason we may feel that we bystanders cannot intervene. But the person threatened can.

In sum, a woman surely can defend her life against the threat to it posed by the unborn child, even if doing so involves its death. And this shows not merely that the theses in (a) through (d) are false; it shows also that the extreme view of abortion is false, and so we need not canvass any other possible ways of arriving at it from the argument I mentioned at the outset.

2. The extreme view could of course be weakened to say that while abortion is permissible to save the mother's life, it may not be performed by a third party, but only by the mother herself. But this cannot be right either. For what we have to keep in mind is that the mother and the unborn child are not like two tenants in a small house which has, by an unfortunate mistake, been rented to both: the mother *owns* the house. The fact that she does adds to the offensiveness of deducing that the mother can do nothing from the supposition that third parties can do nothing. But it does more than this: it casts a bright light on the supposition that third parties can do nothing. Certainly it lets us see that a third party who says ''I cannot choose between you'' is fooling himself if he

thinks this is impartiality. If Jones has found and fastened on a certain coat, which he needs to keep him from freezing, but which Smith also needs to keep him from freezing, then it is not impartiality that says "I cannot choose between you" when Smith owns the coat. Women have said again and again "This body is *my* body!" and they have reason to feel angry, reason to feel that it has been like shouting into the wind. Smith, after all, is hardly likely to bless us if we say to him, "Of course it's your coat, anybody would grant that it is. But no one may choose between you and Jones who is to have it."

We should really ask what it is that says "no one may choose" in the face of the fact that the body that houses the child is the mother's body. It may be simply a failure to appreciate this fact. But it may be something more interesting, namely, the sense that one has a right to refuse to lay hands on people, even where it would be just and fair to do so, even where justice seems to require that somebody do so. Thus justice might call for somebody to get Smith's coat back from Jones, and yet you have a right to refuse to be the one to lay hands on Jones, a right to refuse to do physical violence to him. This, I think, must be granted. But then what should be said is not "no one may choose," but only "*I* cannot choose," and indeed not even this, but "*I* will not *act*," leaving it open that somebody else can or should, and in particular that anyone in a position of authority, with the job of securing people's rights, both can and should. So this is no difficulty. I have not been arguing that any given third party must accede to the mother's request that he perform an abortion to save her life, but only that he may.

I suppose that in some views of human life the mother's body is only on loan to her, the loan not being one which gives her any prior claim to it. One who held this view might well think it impartiality to say "I cannot choose." But I shall simply ignore this possibility. My own view is that if a human being has any just, prior claim to anything at all, he has a just, prior claim to his own body. And perhaps this needn't be argued for here anyway, since, as I mentioned, the arguments against abortion we are looking at do grant that the woman has a right to decide what happens in and to her body.

But although they do grant it, I have tried to show that they do not take seriously what is done in grant-

ing it. I suggest the same thing will reappear even more clearly when we turn away from cases in which the mother's life is at stake, and attend, as I propose we now do, to the vastly more common cases in which a woman wants an abortion for some less weighty reason than preserving her own life.

3. Where the mother's life is not at stake, the argument I mentioned at the outset seems to have a much stronger pull. "Everyone has a right to life, so the unborn person has a right to life." And isn't the child's right to life weightier than anything other than the mother's own right to life, which she might put forward as ground for an abortion?

This argument treats the right to life as if it were unproblematic. It is not, and this seems to me to be precisely the source of the mistake.

For we should now, at long last, ask what it comes to, to have a right to life. In some views having a right to life includes having a right to be given at least the bare minimum one needs for continued life. But suppose that what in fact *is* the bare minimum a man needs for continued life is something he has no right at all to be given. If I am sick unto death, and the only thing that will save my life is the touch of Henry Fonda's cool hand on my fevered brow, then all the same, I have no right to be given the touch of Henry Fonda's cool hand on my fevered brow. It would be frightfully nice of him to fly in from the West Coast to provide it. It would be less nice, though no doubt well meant, if my friends flew out to the West Coast and carried Henry Fonda back with them. But I have no right at all against anybody that he should do this for me. Or again, to return to the story I told earlier, the fact that for continued life that violinist needs the continued use of your kidneys does not establish that he has a right to be given the continued use of your kidneys. He certainly has no right against you that *you* should give him continued use of your kidneys. For nobody has any right to use your kidneys unless you give him such a right; and nobody has the right against you that you shall give him this right—if you do allow him to go on using your kidneys, this is a kindness on your part, and not something he can claim from you as his due. Nor has he any right against anybody else that *they* should give him continued use of your kidneys. Certainly he had no right against the Society of Music Lovers that they should plug him into you in the first place. And if you now start to unplug yourself, having learned that you will otherwise have to spend nine years in bed with him, there is nobody in the world who must try to prevent you, in order to see to it that he is given something he has a right to be given.

Some people are rather stricter about the right to life. In their view, it does not include the right to be given anything, but amounts to, and only to, the right not to be killed by anybody. But here a related difficulty arises. If everybody is to refrain from killing that violinist, then everybody must refrain from doing a great many different sorts of things. Everybody must refrain from slitting his throat, everybody must refrain from shooting him—and everybody must refrain from unplugging you from him. But does he have a right against everybody that they shall refrain from unplugging you from him? To refrain from doing this is to allow him to continue to use your kidneys. It could be argued that he has a right against us that *we* should allow him to continue to use your kidneys. That is, while he had no right against us that we should give him the use of your kidneys, it might be argued that he anyway has a right against us that we shall not now intervene and deprive him of the use of your kidneys. I shall come back to third-party interventions later. But certainly the violinist has no right against you that *you* shall allow him to continue to use your kidneys. As I said, if you do allow him to use them, it is a kindness on your part, and not something you owe him.

The difficulty I point to here is not peculiar to the right to life. It reappears in connection with all the other natural rights; and it is something which an adequate account of rights must deal with. For present purposes it is enough just to draw attention to it. But I would stress that I am not arguing that people do not have a right to life—quite to the contrary, it seems to me that the primary control we must place on the acceptability of an account of rights is that it should turn out in that account to be a truth that all persons have a right to life. I am arguing only that having a right to life does not guarantee having either a right to be given the use of or a right to be allowed continued use of another person's body—even if one needs it for life itself. So the right to life will not serve the opponents of abortion in the very simple and clear way in which they seem to have thought it would.

4. There is another way to bring out the difficulty. In the most ordinary sort of case, to deprive someone of what he has a right to is to treat him unjustly. Suppose a boy and his small brother are jointly given a box of chocolates for Christmas. If the older boy takes the box and refuses to give his brother any of the chocolates, he is unjust to him, for the brother has been given a right to half of them. But suppose that, having learned that otherwise it means nine years in bed with that violinist, you unplug yourself from him. You surely are not being unjust to him for you gave him no right to use your kidneys, and no one else can have given him any such right. But we have to notice that in unplugging yourself, you are killing him; and violinists, like everybody else, have a right to life, and thus in the view we were considering just now, the right not to be killed. So here you do what he supposedly has a right you shall not do, but you do not act unjustly to him in doing it.

The emendation which may be made at this point is this: the right to life consists not in the right not to be killed, but rather in the right not to be killed unjustly. This runs a risk of circularity, but never mind: it would enable us to square the fact that the violinist has a right to life with the fact that you do not act unjustly toward him in unplugging yourself, thereby killing him. For if you do not kill him unjustly, you do not violate his right to life, and so it is no wonder you do him no injustice.

But if this emendation is accepted, the gap in the argument against abortion stares us plainly in the face: It is by no means enough to show that the fetus is a person, and to remind us that all persons have a right to life—we need to be shown also that killing the fetus violates its right to life, i.e., that abortion is unjust killing. And is it?

I suppose we may take it as a datum that in a case of pregnancy due to rape the mother has not given the unborn person a right to the use of her body for food and shelter. Indeed, in what pregnancy could it be supposed that the mother has given the unborn person such a right? It is not as if there were unborn persons drifting about the world, to whom a woman who wants a child says "I invite you in."

But it might be argued that there are other ways one can have acquired a right to the use of another person's body than by having been invited to use it by that person. Suppose a woman voluntarily indulges in intercourse, knowing of the chance it will issue in pregnancy, and then she does become pregnant; is she not in part responsible for the presence, in fact the very existence, of the unborn person inside her? No doubt she did not invite it in. But doesn't her partial responsibility for its being there itself give it a right to the use of her body?[7] If so, then her aborting it would be more like the boy's taking away the chocolates, and less like your unplugging yourself from the violinist—doing so would be depriving it of what it does have a right to, and thus would be doing it an injustice.

And then, too, it might be asked whether or not she can kill it even to save her own life: If she voluntarily called it into existence, how can she now kill it, even in self-defense?

The first thing to be said about this is that it is something new. Opponents of abortion have been so concerned to make out the independence of the fetus, in order to establish that it has a right to life, just as its mother does, that they have tended to overlook the possible support they might gain from making out that the fetus is *dependent* on the mother, in order to establish that she has a special kind of responsibility for it, a responsibility that gives it rights against her which are not possessed by any independent person—such as an ailing violinist who is a stranger to her.

On the other hand, this argument would give the unborn person a right to its mother's body only if her pregnancy resulted from a voluntary act, undertaken in full knowledge of the chance a pregnancy might result from it. It would leave out entirely the unborn person whose existence is due to rape. Pending the availability of some further argument, then, we would be left with the conclusion that unborn persons whose existence is due to rape have no right to the use of their mothers' bodies, and thus that aborting them is not depriving them of anything they have a right to and hence is not unjust killing.

And we should also notice that it is not at all plain that this argument really does go even as far as it purports to. For there are cases and cases, and the details make a difference. If the room is stuffy, and I therefore open a window to air it, and a burglar climbs in, it would be absurd to say, ''Ah, now he can stay, she's given him a right to the use of her house—for she is partially responsible for his presence there, having voluntarily done what enabled him to get in, in full knowledge that there are such things as burglars, and that burglars burgle.'' It would be still more absurd to say this if I had had bars installed outside my windows, precisely to prevent burglars from getting in, and a burglar got in only because of a defect in the bars. It remains equally absurd if we imagine it is not a burglar who climbs in, but an innocent person who blunders or falls in. Again, suppose it were like this: people-seeds drift about in the air like pollen, and if you open your windows, one may drift in and take root in your carpets or upholstery. You don't want children, so you fix up your windows with fine mesh screens, the very best you can buy. As can happen, however, and on very, very rare occasions does happen, one of the screens is defective; and a seed drifts in and takes root. Does the person-plant who now develops have a right to the use of your house? Surely not—despite the fact that you voluntarily opened your windows, you knowingly kept carpets and upholstered furniture, and you knew that screens were sometimes defective. Someone may argue that you are responsible for its rooting, that it does have a right to your house, because after all you *could* have lived out your life with bare floors and furniture, or with sealed windows and doors. But this won't do—for by the same token anyone can avoid a pregnancy due to rape by having a hysterectomy, or anyway by never leaving home without a (reliable!) army.

It seems to me that the argument we are looking at can establish at most that there are *some* cases in which the unborn person has a right to the use of its mother's body, and therefore *some* cases in which abortion is unjust killing. There is room for much discussion and argument as to precisely which, if any. But I think we should sidestep this issue and leave it open, for at any rate the argument certainly does not establish that all abortion is unjust killing.

5. There is room for yet another argument here, however. We surely must all grant that there may be cases in which it would be morally indecent to detach a person from your body at the cost of his life. Suppose you learn that what the violinist needs is not nine years of your life, but only one hour: All you need do to save his life is to spend one hour in that bed with him. Suppose also that letting him use your kidneys for that one hour would not affect your health in the slightest. Admittedly you were kidnapped. Admittedly you did not give anyone permission to plug him into you. Nevertheless it seems to me plain you *ought* to allow him to use your kidneys for that hour—it would be indecent to refuse.

Again, suppose pregnancy lasted only an hour, and constituted no threat to life or health. And suppose that a woman becomes pregnant as a result of rape. Admittedly she did not voluntarily do anything to bring about the existence of a child. Admittedly she did nothing at all which would give the unborn person a right to the use of her body. All the same it might well be said, as in the newly emended violinist story, that she *ought* to allow it to remain for that hour—that it would be indecent in her to refuse.

Now some people are inclined to use the term "right" in such a way that it follows from the fact that you ought to allow a person to use your body for the hour he needs, that he has a right to use your body for the hour he needs, even though he has not been given that right by any person or act. They may say that it follows also that if you refuse, you act unjustly toward him. This use of the term is perhaps so common that it cannot be called wrong; nevertheless it seems to me to be an unfortunate loosening of what we would do better to keep a tight rein on. Suppose that box of chocolates I mentioned earlier had not been given to both boys jointly, but was given only to the older boy. There he sits, stolidly eating his way through the box, his small brother watching enviously. Here we are likely to say "You ought not to be so mean. You ought to give your brother some of those chocolates." My own view is that it just does not follow from the truth of this that the brother has any right to any of the chocolates. If the boy refuses to give his brother any, he is greedy, stingy, callous—but not unjust. I suppose that the people I have in mind will say it does follow that the brother has a right to some of the chocolates, and thus that the boy does act unjustly if he refuses to give his brother any. But the effect of saying this is to obscure what we should keep distinct, namely the difference between the boy's refusal in this case and the boy's refusal in the earlier case, in which the box was given to both boys jointly, and in which the small brother thus had what was from any point of view clear title to half.

A further objection to so using the term "right" that from the fact that A ought to do a thing for B, it follows that B has a right against A that A do it for him, is that it is going to make the question of whether or not a man has a right to a thing turn on how easy it is to provide him with it; and this seems not merely unfortunate, but morally unacceptable. Take the case of Henry Fonda again. I said earlier that I had no right to the touch of his cool hand on my fevered brow, even though I needed it to save my life. I said it would be frightfully nice of him to fly in from the West Coast to provide me with it, but that I had no right against him that he should do so. But suppose he isn't on the West Coast. Suppose he has only to walk across the room, place a hand briefly on my brow—

and lo, my life is saved. Then surely he ought to do it, it would be indecent to refuse. Is it to be said "Ah well, it follows that in this case she has a right to the touch of his hand on her brow, and so it would be an injustice in him to refuse"? So that I have a right to it when it is easy for him to provide it, though no right when it's hard? It's rather a shocking idea that anyone's rights should fade away and disappear as it gets harder and harder to accord them to him.

So my own view is that even though you ought to let the violinist use your kidneys for the one hour he needs, we should not conclude that he has a right to do so—we would say that if you refuse, you are, like the boy who owns all the chocolates and will give none away, self-centered and callous, indecent in fact, but not unjust. And similarly, that even supposing a case in which a woman pregnant due to rape ought to allow the unborn person to use her body for the hour he needs, we should not conclude that he has a right to do so; we should conclude that she is self-centered, callous, indecent, but not unjust, if she refuses. The complaints are no less grave; they are just different. However, there is no need to insist on this point. If anyone does wish to deduce "he has a right" from "you ought," then all the same he must surely grant that there are cases in which it is not morally required of you that you allow that violinist to use your kidneys, and in which he does not have a right to use them, and in which you do not do him an injustice if you refuse. And so also for mother and unborn child. Except in such cases as the unborn person has a right to demand it—and we were leaving open the possibility that there may be such cases—nobody is morally *required* to make large sacrifices, of health, of all other interests and concerns, of all other duties and commitments, for nine years, or even for nine months, in order to keep another person alive.

6. We have in fact to distinguish between two kinds of Samaritan: the Good Samaritan and what we might call the Minimally Decent Samaritan. The story of the Good Samaritan, you will remember, goes like this:

A certain man went down from Jerusalem to Jericho, and fell among thieves, which stripped him of his raiment, and wounded him, and departed, leaving him half dead.

And by chance there came down a certain priest that way; and when he saw him, he passed by on the other side.

And likewise a Levite, when he was at the place, came and looked on him, and passed by on the other side.

But a certain Samaritan, as he journeyed, came where he was; and when he saw him he had compassion on him.

And went to him, and bound up his wounds, pouring in oil and wine, and set him on his own beast, and brought him to an inn, and took care of him.

And on the morrow, when he departed, he took out two pence, and gave them to the host, and said unto him, "Take care of him; and whatsoever thou spendest more, when I come again, I will repay thee."

(Luke 10:30–35)

The Good Samaritan went out of his way, at some cost to himself, to help one in need of it. We are not told what the options were, that is, whether or not the priest and the Levite could have helped by doing less than the Good Samaritan did, but assuming they could have, then the fact they did nothing at all shows they were not even Minimally Decent Samaritans, not because they were not Samaritans, but because they were not even minimally decent.

These things are a matter of degree, of course, but there is a difference, and it comes out perhaps most clearly in the story of Kitty Genovese, who, as you will remember, was murdered while thirty-eight people watched or listened, and did nothing at all to help her. A Good Samaritan would have rushed out to give direct assistance against the murderer. Or perhaps we had better allow that it would have been a Splendid Samaritan who did this, on the ground that it would have involved a risk of death for himself. But the thirty-eight not only did not do this, they did not even trouble to pick up a phone to call the police. Minimally Decent Samaritanism would call for doing at least that, and their not having done it was monstrous.

After telling the story of the Good Samaritan, Jesus said "Go, and do thou likewise." Perhaps he meant that we are morally required to act as the Good Samaritan did. Perhaps he was urging people to do more than is morally required of them. At all events it seems plain that it was not morally required of any of the thirty-eight that he rush out to give direct assistance at the risk of his own life, and that it is not morally required of anyone that he give long stretches of his life—nine years or nine months—to sustaining the life of a person who has no special right (we were leaving open the possibility of this) to demand it.

Indeed, with one rather striking class of exceptions, no one in any country in the world is *legally* required to do anywhere near as much as this for anyone else. The class of exceptions is obvious. My main concern here is not the state of the law in respect to abortion, but it is worth drawing attention to the fact that in no state in this country is any man compelled by law to be even a Minimally Decent Samaritan to any person; there is no law under which charges could be brought against the thirty-eight who stood by while Kitty Genovese died. By contrast, in most states in this country women are compelled by law to be not merely Minimally Decent Samaritans, but Good Samaritans to unborn persons inside them. This doesn't by itself settle anything one way or the other, because it may well be argued that there should be laws in this country—as there are in many European countries—compelling at least Minimally Decent Samaritanism.[8] But it does show that there is a gross injustice in the existing state of the law. And it shows also that the groups currently working against liberalization of abortion laws, in fact working toward having it declared unconstitutional for a state to permit abortion, had better start working for the adoption of Good Samaritan laws generally, or earn the charge that they are acting in bad faith.

I should think, myself, that Minimally Decent Samaritan laws would be one thing, Good Samaritan laws quite another, and in fact highly improper. But we are not here concerned with the law. What we should ask is not whether anybody should be compelled by law to be a Good Samaritan, but whether we must accede to a situation in which somebody is being compelled—by nature, perhaps—to be a Good Samaritan. We have, in other words, to look now at third-party interventions. I have been arguing that no person is morally required to make large sacrifices to sustain the life of another who has no right to demand them, and this even where the sacrifices do not include life itself; we are not morally required to be Good Samaritans or anyway Very Good Samaritans to one another. But what if a man cannot extricate himself from such a situation? What if he appeals to us to extricate him? It seems to me plain that there are cases in which we can, cases in which a Good Samaritan would extricate him. There you are, you were kidnapped, and nine years in bed with that violinist lie ahead of you. You have your own life to lead. You are sorry, but you simply cannot see giving up so much of your life to the sustaining of his. You cannot extricate yourself, and ask us to do so. I should have thought that—in light of his having no right to the use of your body—it was obvious that we do not have to accede to your being forced to give up so much. We can do what you ask. There is no injustice to the violinist in our doing so.

7. Following the lead of the opponents of abortion, I have throughout been speaking of the fetus merely as a person, and what I have been asking is whether or not the argument we began with, which proceeds only from the fetus's being a person, really does establish its conclusion. I have argued that it does not.

But of course there are arguments and arguments, and it may be said that I have simply fastened on the wrong one. It may be said that what is important is not merely the fact that the fetus is a person, but that it is a person for whom the woman has a special kind of responsibility issuing from the fact that she is its mother. And it might be argued that all my analogies are therefore irrelevant—for you do not have that special kind of responsibility for that violinist, Henry Fonda does not have that special kind of responsibility for me. And our attention might be drawn to the fact that men and women both *are* compelled by law to provide support for their children.

I have in effect dealt (briefly) with this argument in section 4 above; but a (still briefer) recapitulation now may be in order. Surely we do not have any such "special responsibility" for a person unless we have assumed it, explicitly or implicitly. If a set of parents do not try to prevent pregnancy, do not obtain an abortion, and then at the time of birth of the child do not put it out for adoption, but rather take it home with them, then they have assumed responsibility for it, they have given it rights, and they cannot *now* withdraw support from it at the cost of its life because they now find it difficult to go on providing for it. But if they have taken all reasonable precautions against having a child, they do not simply by virtue of their biological relationship to the child who comes into existence have a special responsibility for it. They may wish to assume responsibility for it, or they may not wish to. And I am suggesting that if assuming responsibility for it would require large sacrifices, then they may refuse. A Good Samaritan would not refuse—or anyway, a Splendid Samaritan, if the sacrifices that had to be made were enormous. But then so would a Good Samaritan assume responsibility for that violinist; so would Henry Fonda, if he is a Good Samaritan, fly in from the West Coast and assume responsibility for me.

8. My argument will be found unsatisfactory on two counts by many of those who want to regard abortion as morally permissible. First, while I do argue that abortion is not impermissible, I do not argue that it is always permissible. There may well be cases in which carrying the child to term requires only Minimally Decent Samaritanism of the mother, and this is a standard we must not fall below. I am inclined to think it a merit of my account precisely that it does *not* give a general yes or a general no. It allows for and supports our sense that, for example, a sick and desperately frightened fourteen-year-old school-girl, pregnant due to rape, may *of course* choose abortion, and that any law which rules this out is an insane law. And it also allows for and supports our sense that in other cases resort to abortion is even positively indecent. It would be indecent in the woman to request an abortion, and indecent in a doctor to perform it, if she is in her seventh month and wants the abortion just to avoid the nuisance of postponing a trip abroad. The very fact that the arguments I have been drawing attention to treat all cases of abortion, or even all cases of abortion in which the mother's life is not at stake, as morally on a par ought to have made them suspect at the outset.

Secondly, while I am arguing for the permissibility of abortion in some cases, I am not arguing for the right to secure the death of the unborn child. It is easy to confuse these two things in that up to a certain point in the life of the fetus it is not able to survive outside the mother's body; hence removing it from her body guarantees its death. But they are importantly different. I have argued that you are not morally required to spend nine months in bed, sustaining the life of that violinist; but to say this is by no means to say that if, when you unplug yourself, there is a miracle and he survives, you then have a right to turn round and slit his throat. You may detach yourself even if this costs him his life; you have no right to be guaranteed his death, by some other means, if unplugging yourself does not kill him. There are some people who will feel dissatisfied by this feature of my argument. A woman may be utterly devastated by the thought of a child, a bit of herself, put out for adoption and never seen or heard of again. She may therefore want not merely that the child be detached from her, but more, that it die. Some opponents of abortion are inclined to regard this as beneath contempt—thereby showing insensitivity to what is surely a powerful source of despair. All the same, I agree that the desire for the child's death is not one which anybody may gratify, should it turn out to be possible to detach the child alive.

At this place, however, it should be remembered that we have only been pretending throughout that the fetus is a human being from the moment of conception. A very early abortion is surely not the killing of a person, and so is not dealt with by anything I have said here.

NOTES

1. I am very much indebted to James Thomson for discussion, criticism, and many helpful suggestions.

2. Daniel Callahan, *Abortion: Law, Choice and Morality* (New York, 1970), p. 373. This book gives a fascinating survey of the available information on abortion. The Jewish tradition is surveyed in David M. Feldman, *Birth Control in Jewish Law* (New York, 1968), Part 5; the Catholic tradition in John T. Noonan, Jr., "An Almost Absolute Value in History," in *The Morality of Abortion*, ed. John T. Noonan, Jr. (Cambridge, Mass., 1970).

3. The term "direct" in the arguments I refer to is a technical one. Roughly, what is meant by "direct killing" is either killing as an end in itself, or killing as a means to some end, for example, the end of saving someone else's life. See note 6, below, for an example of its use.

4. Cf. *Encyclical Letter of Pope Pius XI on Christian Marriage*, St. Paul Editions (Boston, n.d.), p. 32: "however much we may pity the mother whose health and even life is gravely imperiled in the performance of the duty allotted to her by nature, nevertheless what could ever be a sufficient reason for excusing in any way the direct murder of the innocent? This is precisely what we are dealing with here." Noonan *(The Morality of Abortion,* p. 43) reads this as follows: "What cause can ever avail to excuse in any way the direct killing of the innocent? For it is a question of that."

5. The thesis in (d) is in an interesting way weaker than those in (a), (b), and they rule out abortion even in cases in which both mother *and* child will die if the abortion is not performed. By contrast, one who held the view expressed in (d) could consistently say that one needn't prefer letting two persons die to killing one.

6. Cf. the following passage from Pius XII, *Address to the Italian Catholic Society of Midwives:* "The baby in the maternal breast has the right to life immediately from God.—Hence there is no man, no human authority, no science, no medical, eugenic, social, economic or moral 'indication' which can establish or grant a valid juridical ground for a direct deliberate disposition of an innocent human life, that is a disposition which looks to its destruction either as an end or as a means to another end perhaps in itself not illicit.—The baby, still not born, is a man in the same degree and for the same reason as the mother" (quoted in Noonan, *The Morality of Abortion,* p. 45).

7. The need for a discussion of this argument was brought home to me by members of the Society for Ethical and Legal Philosophy, to whom this paper was originally presented.

8. For a discussion of the difficulties involved, and a survey of the European experience with such laws, see *The Good Samaritan and the Law,* ed. James M. Ratcliffe (New York, 1966).

BARUCH BRODY

The Morality of Abortion*

THE WOMAN'S RIGHT TO HER BODY

It is a common claim that a woman ought to be in control of what happens to her body to the greatest

From *Abortion and the Sanctity of Human Life: A Philosophical View* (Cambridge, Mass.: MIT Press, 1975), pp. 26–32, 37–39, 44–47, 123–129, 131, and "Fetal Humanity and the Theory of Essentialism," in *Philosophy and Sex,* Robert Baker and Frederick Elliston, eds. (Buffalo, N.Y.: Prometheus Books, 1975), pp. 348–352. (Some parts of these essays were later revised by Professor Brody.)

Ed. note: This selection from the writings of Professor Brody is divided into five sections. Section 1 discusses whether abortions can be justified on the grounds that the woman owns her own body if the fetus is a human being; section 2 discusses whether abortions can be justified by a wide variety of special circumstances if the fetus is a human being. Both sections conclude that on this assumption abortions cannot be justified. Section 3 justifies the claim that, from an early stage after conception, the fetus is a human being. The last two sections discuss the implications of this position for the law, focusing on a criticism of the Supreme Court's opinion.

extent possible, that she ought to be able to use her body in ways that she wants to and refrain from using it in ways that she does not want to. This right is particularly pressed where certain uses of her body have deep and lasting effects upon the character of her life, personal, social, and economic. Therefore, it is argued, a woman should be free either to carry her fetus to term, thereby using her body to support it, or to abort the fetus, thereby not using her body for that purpose.

In some contexts in which this argument is advanced, it is clear that it is not addressed to the issue of the morality of abortion at all. Rather, it is made in opposition to laws against abortion on the ground that the choice to abort or not is a moral decision that should belong only to the mother. But that specific direction of the argument is irrelevant to our present purposes; I will consider it [later] when I deal with the issues raised by laws prohibiting abortions. For the moment, I am concerned solely with the use of this principle as a putative ground tending to show the permissibility of abortion, with the claim that because it is the woman's body that carries the fetus and upon which the fetus depends, she has certain rights to abort the fetus that no one else may have.

We may begin by remarking that it is obviously correct that, as carrier of the fetus, the mother has it within her power to choose whether or not to abort the fetus. And, as an autonomous and responsible agent, she must make this choice. But let us notice that this in no way entails either that whatever choice she makes is morally right or that no one else has the right to evaluate the decision that she makes.

· · ·

At first glance, it would seem that this argument cannot be used by anyone who supposes, as we do for the moment, that there is a point in fetal development from which time on the fetus is a human being. After all, people do not have the right to do anything whatsoever that may be necessary for them to retain control over the uses of their bodies. In particular, it would seem wrong for them to kill another human being in order to do so.

In a recent article,[1] Professor Judith Thomson has, in effect, argued that this simple view is mistaken. How does Professor Thomson defend her claim that the mother has a right to abort the fetus, even if it is a human being, whether or not her life is threatened and whether or not she has consented to the act of intercourse in which the fetus is conceived? At one point,[2] discussing just the case in which the mother's life is threatened, she makes the following suggestion:

In [abortion], there are only two people involved, one whose life is threatened and one who threatens it. Both are innocent: the one who is threatened is not threatened because of any fault, the one who threatens does not threaten because of any fault. For this reason, we may feel that we bystanders cannot intervene. But the person threatened can.

But surely this description is equally applicable to the following case: A and B are adrift on a lifeboat, B has a disease that he can survive, but A, if he contracts it, will die, and the only way that A can avoid that is by killing B and pushing him overboard. Surely, A has no right to do this. So there must be some special reason why the mother has, if she does, the right to abort the fetus.

There is, to be sure, an important difference between our lifeboat case and abortion, one that leads us to the heart of Professor Thomson's argument. In the case that we envisaged, both A and B have equal rights to be in the lifeboat, but the mother's body is hers and not the fetus's and she has first rights to its use. The primacy of these rights allow an abortion whether or not her life is threatened. Professor Thomson summarizes this argument in the following way:[3]

I am arguing only that having a right to life does not guarantee having either a right to be given the use of, or a right to be allowed continued use of, another person's body—even if one needs it for life itself.

One part of this claim is clearly correct. I have no duty to X to save X's life by giving him the use of my body (or my life savings, or the only home I have, and so on), and X has no right, even to save his life, to any of those things. Thus, the fetus conceived in the laboratory that will perish unless it is implanted into a woman's body has in fact no right to any woman's body. But this portion of the claim is irrelevant to the abortion issue, for in abortion of the fetus that is a human being the mother must kill X to get back the sole use of her body, and that is an entirely different matter.

This point can also be put as follows: . . . we must distinguish the taking of X's life from the saving of X's life, even if we assume that one has a duty not to do the former and to do the latter. Now that latter duty, if it exists at all, is much weaker than the first duty; many circumstances may relieve us from the latter duty that will not relieve us from the former one. Thus, I am certainly relieved from my duty to save X's life by the fact that fulfilling it means the loss of my life savings. It may be noble for me to save X's life at the cost of everything I have, but I certainly have no duty to do that. And the same observation may be made about cases in which I can save X's life by giving him the use of my body for an extended period of time. However, I am not relieved of my duty not to take X's life by the fact that fulfilling it means the loss of everything I have and not even by the fact that fulfilling it means the loss of my life. . . .

At one point in her paper, Professor Thomson does consider this objection. She has previously imagined the following case: a famous violinist, who is dying from a kidney ailment, has been, without your consent, plugged into you for a period of time so that his body can use your kidneys:

Some people are rather stricter about the right to life. In their view, it does not include the right to be given anything, but amounts to, and only to, the right not to be killed by anybody. But here a related difficulty arises. If everybody is to refrain from killing that violinist, then everybody must refrain from doing a great many different sorts of things . . . everybody must refrain from unplugging you from him. But does he have a right against everybody that they shall refrain from unplugging you from him? To refrain from doing this is to allow him to continue to use your kidneys . . . certainly the violinist has no right against you that you shall allow him to continue to use your kidneys.

Applying this argument to the case of abortion, we can see that Professor Thomson's argument would run as follows:

    a. Assume that the fetus's right to life includes the right not to be killed by the woman carrying him.
    b. But to refrain from killing the fetus is to allow him the continued use of the woman's body.
    c. So our first assumption entails that the fetus's right to life includes the right to the continued use of the woman's body.
    d. But we all grant that the fetus does not have the right to the continued use of the woman's body.
    e. Therefore, the fetus's right to life cannot include the right not to be killed by the woman in question.

And it is also now clear what is wrong with this argument. When we granted that the fetus has no right to the continued use of the woman's body, all that we meant was that he does not have this right merely because the continued use saves his life. But, of course, there may be other reasons why he has this right. One would be that the only way to take the use of the woman's body away from the fetus is by killing him, and that is something that neither she nor we have the right to do. So, I submit, the way in which Assumption d is true is irrelevant, and cannot be used by Professor Thomson, for Assumption d is true only in cases where the saving of the life of the fetus is at stake and not in cases where the taking of his life is at stake.

I conclude therefore that Professor Thomson has not established the truth of her claims about abortion, primarily because she has not sufficiently attended to the distinction between our duty to save X's life and our duty not to take it. Once one attends to that distinction, it would seem that the mother, in order to regain control over her body, has no right to abort the fetus from the point at which it becomes a human being.

It may also be useful to say a few words about the larger and less rigorous context of the argument that the woman has a right to her own body. It is surely true that one way in which women have been oppressed is by their being denied authority over their own bodies. But it seems to me that, as the struggle is carried on for meaningful amelioration of such oppression, it ought not to be carried so far that it violates the steady responsibilities all people have to one another. Parents may not desert their children, one class may not oppress another, one race or nation may not exploit another. For parents, powerful groups in society, races or nations in ascendancy, there are penalties for refraining from these wrong actions, but those penalties can in no way be taken as the justification for such wrong actions. Similarly, if the fetus is a human being, the penalty of carrying it cannot, I believe, be used as the justification for destroying it.

        •   •   •

THE MODEL PENAL CODE CASES

All of the arguments that we have looked at so far are attempts to show that there is something special about abortion that justifies its being treated differently from other cases of the taking of human life. We shall now consider claims that are confined to certain special cases of abortion: the case in which the mother has been raped, the case in which bearing the child would be harmful to her health, and the case in which having the child may cause a problem for the rest of her family (the latter case is a particular case of the societal argument). In addressing these issues, we shall see whether there is any point to the permissibility of abortions in some of the cases covered by the Model Penal Code[4] proposals.

When the expectant mother has conceived after being raped, there are two different sorts of considerations that might support the claim that she has the right to take the life of the fetus. They are the following: (A) the woman in question has already suffered immensely from the act of rape and the physical and/or psychological aftereffects of that act. It would be particularly unjust, the argument runs, for her to have to live through an unwanted pregnancy owing to that act of rape. Therefore, even if we are at a stage at which the fetus is a human being, the mother has the right to abort it; (B) the fetus in question has no right to be in that woman. It was put there as a result of an act of aggression upon her by the rapist, and its continued presence is an act of aggression against the mother. She has a right to repel that aggression by aborting the fetus.

The first argument is very compelling. We can all agree that a terrible injustice has been committed on the woman who is raped. The question that we have to consider, however, is whether it follows that it is morally permissible for her to abort the fetus. We must make that consideration reflecting that, however unjust the act of rape, it was not the fetus who committed or commissioned it. The injustice of the act, then, should in no way impinge upon the rights of the fetus, for it is innocent. What remains is the initial misfortune of the mother (and the injustice of her having to pass through the pregnancy, and, further, to assume responsibility of at least giving the child over for adoption or assuming the burden of its care). However unfortunate that circumstance, however unjust, the misfortune and the injustice are not sufficient cause to justify the taking of the life of an innocent human being as a means of mitigation.

It is at this point that Argument B comes in, for its whole point is that the fetus, by its mere presence in the mother, is committing an act of aggression against her, one over and above the one committed by the rapist, and one that the mother has a right to repel by abortion. But . . . (1) the fetus is certainly innocent (in the sense of not responsible) for any act of aggression against the mother and that (2) the mere presence of the fetus in the mother, no matter how unfortunate for her, does not constitute an act of aggression by the fetus against the mother. Argument B fails then at just that point at which Argument A needs its support, and we can therefore conclude that the fact that pregnancy is the result of rape does not give the mother the right to abort the fetus.

We turn next to the case in which the continued existence of the fetus would threaten the mental and/or physical health but not necessarily the life of the mother. Again, . . . the fact that the fetus's continued existence poses a threat to the life of the mother does not justify her aborting it.* It would seem to be true, a fortiori, that the fact that the fetus's continued existence poses a threat to the mental and/or physical health of the mother does not justify her aborting it either.

We come finally to those cases in which the continuation of the pregnancy would cause serious problems for the rest of the family. There are a variety of cases that we have to consider here together. Perhaps the health of the mother will be affected in such a way that she cannot function effectively as a wife and mother during, or even after, the pregnancy. Or perhaps the expenses incurred as a result of the pregnancy would be utterly beyond the financial resources of the family. The important point is that the continuation of the pregnancy raises a serious problem for other innocent people involved besides the mother and the fetus, and it may be argued that the mother has the right to abort the fetus to avoid that problem.

By now, the difficulties with this argument should be apparent. We have seen earlier that the mere fact that the continued existence of the fetus threatens to harm the mother does not, by itself, justify the aborting of the fetus. Why should anything be changed by the fact that the threatened harm will accrue to the other members of the family and not to the mother? Of course, it would be different if the fetus were committing an act of aggression against the other members of the family. But, once more, this is certainly not the case.

We conclude, therefore, that none of these special

*Ed. note: Professor Brody provided a lengthy argument to this effect in a chapter not here excerpted. His summary of that argument is as follows: "Is it permissible, as an act of killing a pursuer, to abort the fetus in order to save the mother? The first thing that we should note is that Pope Pius's objection to aborting the fetus as a permissible act of killing a pursuer is mistaken. His objection is that the fetus shows no knowledge or intention in his attempt to take the life of the mother, that the fetus is, in a word, innocent. But that only means that the condition of guilt is not satisfied, and we have seen that its satisfaction is not necessary.

"Is, then, the aborting of the fetus, when necessary to save the life of the mother, a permissible act of killing a pursuer? It is true that in such cases the fetus is a danger to the mother. But it is also clear that the condition of attempt is not satisfied. The fetus has neither the beliefs nor the intention to which we have referred. Furthermore, there is on the part of the fetus no action that threatens the life of the mother. So not even the condition of action is satisfied. It seems to follow, therefore, that aborting the fetus could not be a permissible act of killing a pursuer."

circumstances justifies an abortion from that point at which the fetus is a human being.

. . .

FETAL HUMANITY AND BRAIN FUNCTION

The question which we must now consider is the question of fetal humanity. Some have argued that the fetus is a human being with a right to life (or, for convenience, just a human being) from the moment of conception. Others have argued that the fetus only becomes a human being at the moment of birth. Many positions in between these two extremes have also been suggested. How are we to decide which is correct?

The analysis which we will propose here rests upon certain metaphysical assumptions which I have defended elsewhere. These assumptions are: (a) the question is when has the fetus acquired all the properties essential (necessary) for being a human being, for when it has, it is a human being; (b) these properties are such that the loss of any one of them means that the human being in question has gone out of existence and not merely stopped being a human being; (c) human beings go out of existence when they die. It follows from these assumptions that the fetus becomes a human being when it acquires all those characteristics which are such that the loss of any one of them would result in the fetus's being dead. We must, therefore, turn to the analysis of death.

. . .

We will first consider the question of what properties are essential to being human if we suppose that death and the passing out of existence occur only if there has been an irreparable cessation of brain function (keeping in mind that that condition itself, as we have noted, is a matter of medical judgment). We shall then consider the same question on the supposition that [Paul] Ramsey's more complicated theory of death (the modified traditional view) is correct.

According to what is called the brain-death theory, as long as there has not been an irreparable cessation of brain function the person in question continues to exist, no matter what else has happened to him. If so, it seems to follow that there is only one property—leaving aside those entailed by this one property—that is essential to humanity, namely, the possession of a brain that has not suffered an irreparable cessation of function.

Several consequences follow immediately from this conclusion. We can see that a variety of often advanced claims about the essence of humanity are false. For example, the claim that movement, or perhaps just the ability to move, is essential for being human is false. A human being who has stopped moving, and even one who has lost the ability to move, has not therefore stopped existing. Being able to move, and a fortiori moving, are not essential properties of human beings and therefore are not essential to being human. Similarly, the claim that being perceivable by other human beings is essential for being human is also false. A human being who has stopped being perceivable by other humans (for example, someone isolated on the other side of the moon, out of reach even of radio communication) has not stopped existing. Being perceivable by other human beings is not an essential property of human beings and is not essential to being human. And the same point can be made about the claims that viability is essential for being human, that independent existence is essential for being human, and that actual interaction with other human beings is essential for being human. The loss of any of these properties would not mean that the human being in question had gone out of existence, so none of them can be essential to that human being and none of them can be essential for being human.

Let us now look at the following argument: (1) A functioning brain (or at least, a brain that, if not functioning, is susceptible of function) is a property that every human being must have because it is essential for being human. (2) By the time an entity acquires that property, it has all the other properties that are essential for being human. Therefore, when the fetus acquires that property it becomes a human being. It is clear that the property in question is, according to the brain-death theory, one that is had essentially by all human beings. The question that we have to consider is whether the second premise is true. It might appear that its truth does follow from the brain-death theory. After all, we did see that the theory entails that only one property (together with those entailed by it) is essential for being human. Nevertheless, rather than relying solely on my earlier argument, I shall adopt an alternative approach to strengthen the conviction that this second premise is true: I shall note the important ways in which the fetus resembles and differs from an ordinary human being by the time it definitely has a functioning brain (about the end of the sixth week of development). It shall then be evident, in light of our theory of essentialism, that none of these differences involves the lack of some property in the fetus that is essential for its being human.

Structurally, there are few features of the human being that are not fully present by the end of the sixth week. Not only are the familiar external features and all the internal organs present, but the contours of the body are nicely rounded. More important, the body is functioning. Not only is the brain functioning, but the heart is beating sturdily (the fetus by this time has its own completely developed vascular system), the stomach is producing digestive juices, the liver is manufacturing blood cells, the kidney is extracting uric acid from the blood, and the nerves and muscles are operating in concert, so that reflex reactions can begin.

What are the properties that a fetus acquires after the sixth week of its development? Certain structures do appear later. These include the fingernails (which appear in the third month), the completed vocal chords (which also appear then), taste buds and salivary glands (again, in the third month), and hair and eyelashes (in the fifth month). In addition, certain functions begin later than the sixth week. The fetus begins to urinate (in the third month), to move spontaneously (in the third month), to respond to external stimuli (at least in the fifth month), and to breathe (in the sixth month). Moreover, there is a constant growth in size. And finally, at the time of birth the fetus ceases to receive its oxygen and food through the placenta and starts receiving them through the mouth and nose.

I will not examine each of these properties (structures and functions) to show that they are not essential for being human. The procedure would be essentially the one used previously to show that various essentialist claims are in error. We might, therefore, conclude, on the supposition that the brain-death theory is correct, that the fetus becomes a human being about the end of the sixth week after its development.

There is, however, one complication that should be noted here. There are, after all, progressive stages in the physical development and in the functioning of the brain. For example, the fetal brain (and nervous system) does not develop sufficiently to support spontaneous motion until some time in the third month after conception. There is, of course, no doubt that that stage of development is sufficient for the fetus to be human. No one would be likely to maintain that a spontaneously moving human being has died; and similarly, a spontaneously moving fetus would seem

to have become human. One might, however, want to claim that the fetus does not become a human being until the point of spontaneous movement. So then, on the supposition that the brain-death theory of death is correct, one ought to conclude that the fetus becomes a human being at some time between the sixth and twelfth week after its conception.

But what if we reject the brain-death theory, and replace it with its equally plausible contender, Ramsey's theory of death? According to that theory—which we can call the brain, heart, and lung theory of death—the human being does not die, does not go out of existence, until such time as the brain, heart and lungs have irreparably ceased functioning naturally. What are the essential features of being human according to this theory?

Actually, the adoption of Ramsey's theory requires no major modifications. According to that theory, what is essential to being human, what each human being must retain if he is to continue to exist, is the possession of a functioning (actually or potentially) heart, lung, or brain. It is only when a human being possesses none of these that he dies and goes out of existence; and the fetus comes into humanity, so to speak, when he acquires one of these.

On Ramsey's theory, the argument would now run as follows: (1) The property of having a functioning brain, heart, or lungs (or at least organs of the kind that, if not functioning, are susceptible of function) is one that every human being must have because it is essential for being human. (2) By the time that an entity acquires that property it has all the other properties that are essential for being human. Therefore, when the fetus acquires that property it becomes a human being. There remains, once more, the problem of the second premise. Since the fetal heart starts operating rather early, it is not clear that the second premise is correct. Many systems are not yet operating, and many structures are not yet present. Still, following our theory of essentialism, we should conclude that the fetus becomes a human being when it acquires a functioning heart (the first of the organs to function in the fetus).

There is, however, a further complication here, and it is analogous to the one encountered if we adopt the brain-death theory: When may we properly say that the fetal heart begins to function? At two weeks, when occasional contractions of the primitive fetal heart are present? In the fourth to fifth week, when the heart, although incomplete, is beating regularly and pumping blood cells through a closed vascular system, and when the tracings obtained by an ECG exhibit the classical elements of an adult tracing? Or after the end of the seventh week, when the fetal heart is functionally complete and "normal"?

We have not reached a precise conclusion in our study of the question of when the fetus becomes a human being. We do know that it does so some time between the end of the second week and the end of the third month. But it surely is not a human being at the moment of conception and it surely is one by the end of the third month. Though we have not come to a final answer to our question, we have narrowed the range of acceptable answers considerably.

[In summary] we have argued that the fetus becomes a human being with a right to life some time between the second and twelfth week after conception. We have also argued that abortions are morally impermissible after that point except in rather unusual circumstances. What is crucial to note is that neither of these arguments appeal to any theological considerations. We conclude, therefore, that there is a human-rights basis for moral opposition to abortions.

· · ·

LAW AND SOCIETY IN A DEMOCRACY

Before turning to such considerations, however, we must first examine several important assertions about law and society that, if true, would justify the joint assertion of the principles that abortion is murder but nevertheless should be or remain legal. The first is the assertion that citizens of a pluralistic society must forgo the use of the law as a method of enforcing what are their private moralities. It might well be argued that in our pluralistic society, in which there are serious disagreements about the status of the fetus and about the rightness and wrongness of abortion in consequence, it would be wrong (or inappropriate) to legislate against abortion.

Such assertions about a pluralistic society are difficult to evaluate because of their imprecision. So let us first try to formulate some version of them more carefully. Consider the following general principle: Principle [1]. When the citizens of a society strongly disagree about the rightness and wrongness of a given action, and a considerable number think that such an action is right (or, at least, permissible), then it is wrong (or inappropriate) for that society to prohibit that action by law, even if the majority of citizens believe such an action to be wrong.

There are a variety of arguments that can be offered in support of the principle. One appeals to the right of the minority to follow its own conscience rather than being compelled to follow the conscience of the majority. That right has a theoretical political justification, but it also is practically implicit in the inappropriateness in the members of the majority imposing this kind of enforcement upon the minority that would be opposed were they the minority and were the enforcement being imposed upon them. Another argument appeals to the detrimental consequences to a society of the sense on the part of a significant minority that the law is being used by the majority to coerce. Such considerations make it seem that a principle like [1] is true.

If Principle [1] is true, it is easy to offer a defense of the joint assertion of the principles that abortion is murder but nevertheless should be or remain legal. All we need are the additional obvious assumptions that the citizens of our society strongly disagree about the morality of abortion and that at least a significant minority of individuals believe that there are many cases in which abortion is permissible. From these assumptions and Principle [1] it follows that abortions should be or remain legal even if they are murders.

The trouble with this argument is that it depends upon Principle [1]. I agree that, because of the considerations mentioned already, something like Principle [1] must be true. But Principle [1] as formulated is much too broad to be defensible. Consider, after all, a society in which a significant number of citizens think that it is morally permissible, and perhaps even obligatory, to kill Blacks or Jews, for example, because they are seen as being something less than fully human. It would seem to follow from Principle [1] that the law should not prohibit such actions. Surely this consequence of Principle [1] is wrong. Even if a pluralistic society should forgo passing many laws out of deference to the views of those who think that the actions that would thereby be prevented are not wrong, there remain some cases in which the force of the law should be applied because of the evil of the actions it is intended to prevent. If such actions produce very harmful results and infringe upon the rights of a sufficiently large number of individuals, then the possible benefits that may be derived from passing and enforcing a law preventing those actions may well override the rights of the minority (or even of the majority) to follow its conscience.

Principle [1] must therefore be modified as follows: Principle [2]. When the citizens of a society strongly disagree about the rightness and wrongness of a given action, and a considerable number think that such an action is right (or, at least, permissible), then it is wrong (or inappropriate) for that society to prohibit that action by law, even if the majority of citizens believe such an action to be wrong, unless the action in question is so evil that the desirability of legal prohibition outweighs the desirability of granting to the minority the right to follow its own conscience.

Principle [2] is, of course, rather vague. In particular, its last clause needs further clarification. But Principle [2] is clear enough for us to see that it cannot be used to justify the joint assertibility of the principles that abortion is murder but should nevertheless be or remain legal. Principle [2], conjoined with the obvious truths that the citizens of our society strongly disagree about the rightness and wrongness of abortion and that a significant number of citizens believe that, in certain circumstances, the right (or, at least, a permissible) thing to do is to have an abortion, does not yield the conclusion that abortion should be or remain legal if abortion is murder. After all, if abortion is murder, then the action in question is the unjustifiable taking of a human life and may well fall under the last clause of Principle [2]. The destruction of a fetus may not be unlike the killing of a Black or Jew. They may all be cases of the unjust taking of a human life.

•   •   •

THE DECISION IN *ROE V. WADE*

Two decisions were announced by the [United States Supreme] Court on January 22 [1973]. The first *(Roe v. Wade)* involved a challenge to a Texas law prohibiting all abortions not necessary to save the life of the mother. The second *(Doe v. Bolton)* tested a Georgia law incorporating many of the recommendations of the Model Penal Code as to the circumstances under which abortion should be allowed (in the case of rape and of a defective fetus, as well as when the pregnancy threatens the life or health of the mother), together with provisions regulating the place where abortions can be performed, the number of doctors that must concur, and other factors.

Of these two decisions, the more fundamental was *Roe v. Wade.* It was in this case that the Court came to grips with the central legal issue, namely, the extent to which it is legitimate for the state to prohibit or regulate abortion. In *Doe v. Bolton,* the Court was more concerned with subsidiary issues involving the legitimacy of particular types of regulations.

The Court summarized its decision in *Roe v. Wade* as follows:[5]

(a) For the stage prior to approximately the end of the first trimester/three months/the abortion decision and its effectuation must be left to the medical judgment of the pregnant woman's attending physician.

(b) For the stage subsequent to approximately the end of the first trimester, the state, in promoting its interest in the health of the mother, may, if it chooses, regulate the abortion procedure in ways that are reasonably related to maternal health.

(c) For the stage subsequent to viability, the state, in promoting its interest in the potentiality of human life, may, if it chooses, regulate, and even proscribe, abortion except where it is necessary, in appropriate medical judgment, for the preservation of the life or health of the mother.

In short, the Court ruled that abortion can be prohibited only after viability and then only if the life or health of the mother is not threatened. Before viability, abortions cannot be prohibited, but they can be regulated after the first trimester if the regulations are reasonably related to maternal health. This last clause is taken very seriously by the Court. In *Doe v. Bolton,* instances of regulation in the Georgia code were found unconstitutional on the ground that they were not reasonably related to maternal health.

How did the Court arrive at this decision? In Sections V and VII of the decision, it set out the claims on both sides. Jane Roe's argument was summarized in these words:[6]

The principal thrust of appellant's attack on the Texas statutes is that they improperly invade a right, said to be possessed by the pregnant woman, to choose to terminate her pregnancy.

On the other hand, the Court saw as possible legitimate interests of the state the regulation of abortion, like other medical procedures, so as to ensure maximum safety for the patient and the protection of prenatal life. At this point in the decision, the Court added the following very significant remark:[7]

Logically, of course, a legitimate state interest in this area need not stand or fall on acceptance of the belief that life begins at conception or at some other point prior to live birth. In assessing the state's interest, recognition may be given to the less rigid claim that as long as at least potential life is involved, the state may assert interests beyond the protection of the pregnant woman alone.

In Sections VIII to X, the Court stated its conclusion. It viewed this case as one presenting a conflict of interests, and it saw itself as weighing these interests. It began by agreeing that the woman's right to privacy did encompass her right to decide whether or not to terminate her pregnancy. But it argued that this right is not absolute, since the state's interests must also be considered:[8]

We therefore conclude that the right of personal privacy includes the abortion decision, but that this right is not unqualified and must be considered against important state interests in regulation.

The Court had no hesitation in ruling that the woman's right can be limited after the first trimester because of the state's interest in preserving and protecting maternal health. But the Court was less prepared to agree that the woman's right can be limited because of the state's interest in protecting prenatal life. Indeed, the Court rejected Texas's strong claim that life begins at conception, and that the state therefore has a right to protect such life by prohibiting abortion. The first reason advanced for rejecting that claim was phrased in this way:[9]

We need not resolve the difficult question of when life begins. When those trained in the respective disciplines of medicine, philosophy, and theology are unable to arrive at any consensus, the judiciary, at this point in the development of man's knowledge, is not in a position to speculate as to the answer.

Its second reason was that[10]

In areas other than criminal abortion, the law has been reluctant to endorse any theory that life, as we recognize it, begins before live birth or to accord legal rights to the unborn except in narrowly defined situations and except when the rights are contingent upon live birth.

The Court accepted the weaker claim that the state has an interest in protecting the potential of life. But when does that interest become compelling enough to enable the state to prohibit abortion? The Court said:[11]

. . . the compelling point is at viability. This is so because the fetus then has the capacity of meaningful life outside the mother's womb. State regulation protective of fetal life after viability thus has both logical and biological justifications. If the state is interested in protecting fetal life after viability, it may go so far as to proscribe abortion during that period except where it is necessary to preserve the life or health of the mother.

THE COURT ON POTENTIAL LIFE

I want to begin by considering that part of the Court's decision that allows Texas to proscribe abortions after viability so as to protect its interest in potential life. I note that it is difficult to evaluate that important part of the decision because the Court had little to say in defense of it other than the paragraph just quoted.

There are three very dubious elements of this ruling:

1. Why is the state prohibited from proscribing abortions when the life or health of the mother is threatened? Perhaps the following argument may be offered in the case of threat to maternal life: the mother is actually alive but the fetus is only potentially alive, and the protection of actual life takes precedence over the protection of potential life. Even if we grant this argument, why is the state prevented from prohibiting abortion when only maternal health is threatened? What is the argument against the claim that protecting potential life takes precedence in that case?

2. Why does the interest in potential life become compelling only when the stage of viability is reached? The Court's whole argument for this claim is[12]

This is so because the fetus then presumably has the capacity of meaningful life outside the mother's womb.

There is, no doubt, an important type of potential for life, the capacity of meaningful life outside the mother's womb, that the fetus acquires only at the time of viability. But there are other types of potential for life that it acquires earlier. At conception, for example, the fertilized cell has the potential for life in the sense that it will, in the normal course of events, develop into a human being. A six-week-old fetus has the potential for life in the stronger sense that all of the major organs it needs for life are already functioning. Why then does the state's interest in protecting potential life become compelling only at the point of viability? The Court failed to answer that question.

3. It can fairly be said that those trained in the respective disciplines of medicine, philosophy, and theology are unlikely to be able to arrive at any consensus on the question of when the fetus becomes potentially alive and when the state's interest in protecting this potential life becomes compelling enough to outweigh the rights of the mother. Why then did not the court conclude, as it did when it considered the question of fetal humanity, that the judiciary cannot rule on such a question?

In pursuit of this last point, we approach the Court's more fundamental arguments against prohibiting abortion before viability.

THE COURT ON ACTUAL LIFE

The crucial claim in the Court's decision is that laws prohibiting abortion cannot be justified on the ground that the state has an interest in protecting the life of the fetus who is a human being. The Court offered two reasons for this claim: that the law has never yet accorded the fetus this status, and that the matter of fetal humanity is not one about which it is appropriate for the courts to speculate.

The first of the Court's reasons is not particularly strong. Whatever force we want to ascribe to precedent in the law, the Court has in the past modified its previous decisions in light of newer information and insights. In a matter as important as the conflict between the fetus's right to life and the rights of the mother, it would have seemed particularly necessary to deal with the issues rather than relying upon precedent.

In its second argument, the Court did deal with those issues by adopting the following principle:

1. It is inappropriate for the Court to speculate about the answer to questions about which relevant professional specialists cannot arrive at a consensus. This principle seems irrelevant. The issue before the Court was whether the Texas legislature could make a determination in light of the best available evidence and legislate on the basis of it. Justice White, in his dissent, raised this point:[13]

The upshot is that the people and legislatures of the fifty states are constitutionally disentitled to weigh the relative importance of the continued existence and development of the fetus on the one hand against the spectrum of possible impacts on the mother on the other hand.

This objection could be met, however, if we modified the Court's principle in the following way:

2. It is inappropriate for a legislature to write law upon the basis of its best belief when the relevant professional specialists cannot agree that that belief is correct.

On the basis of such a principle, the Court could argue that Texas had no right to protect by law the right of the fetus to life, thereby acknowledging it to be a human being with such a right, because the relevant specialists do not agree that the fetus has that right. As it stands, however, Principle 2 is questionable. In a large number of areas, legislatures regularly do (and must) act upon issues upon which there is a wide diversity of opinion among professional specialists. So Principle 2 has to be modified to deal with only certain cases, and the obvious suggestion is:

3. It is inappropriate for the legislature, on the ground of belief, to write law in such a way as to violate the basic rights of some individuals, when professional specialists do not agree that that belief is correct.

This principle could be used to defend the Court's decision. But is there any reason to accept it as true? Two arguments for this principle immediately suggest themselves: (a) If the relevant professional specialists do not agree, then there cannot be any proof that the answer in question is the correct one. But a legislature should not infringe the rights of people on the basis of unproved belief. (b) When the professional specialists do not agree, there must be legitimate and reasonable alternatives of belief, and we ought to respect the rights of believers in each of these alternatives to act on their own judgments.

. . .

We have already discussed . . . the principles that lie behind these arguments. We saw . . . that neither of these arguments, as applied to abortion, is acceptable if the fetus is a human being. To employ these arguments correctly, the Court must presuppose that the fetus is not a human being. And that, of course, it cannot do, since the aim of its logic is the view that courts and legislatures, at least at this juncture, should remain neutral on the issue of fetal humanity.

There is a second point that should be noted about Principles 1 to 3. There are cases in which, by failing to deal with an issue, an implicit, inevitable decision is in fact reached. We have before us such a case. The Court was considering Texas's claim that it had the right to prohibit abortion in order to protect the fetus.

The Court conceded that if the fetus had a protectable right to life, Texas could prohibit abortions. But when the Court concluded that it (and, by implication, Texas) could not decide whether the fetus is a human being with the right to life, Texas was compelled to act as if the fetus had no such right that Texas could protect. Why should Principles like 1 to 3 be accepted if the result is the effective endorsement of one disputed claim over another?[14]

There is an alternative to the Court's approach. It is that each of the legislatures should consider the vexing problems surrounding abortions, weigh all of the relevant factors, and write law on the basis of its conclusions. The legislature would, undoubtedly, have to consider the question of fetal humanity, but, I submit, the Court is wrong in supposing that there is a way in which that question can be avoided.

· · ·

CONCLUSION

The Supreme Court has ruled, and the principal legal issues in this country are, at least for now, resolved. I have tried to show, however, that the Court's ruling was in error, that it failed to grapple with the crucial issues surrounding the laws prohibiting abortion. The serious public debate about abortion must, and certainly will, continue.

NOTES

1. J. Thomson, "A Defense of Abortion," *Philosophy and Public Affairs*, Vol. 1 (1971), pp. 47–66.

2. *Ibid.*, p. 53.

3. *Ibid.*, p. 56.

4. On the Model Penal Code provisions, see American Law Institute, *Model Penal Code:* Tentative Draft No. 9 (1959).

5. *Roe v. Wade*, 41 *LW* 4229.

6. *Roe*, 41 *LW* 4218.

7. *Roe*, 41 *LW* 4224.

8. *Roe*, 41 *LW* 4226.

9. *Roe*, 41 *LW* 4227.

10. *Roe*, 41 *LW* 4228.

11. *Roe*, 41 *LW* 4228–4229.

12. *Ibid.*

13. *Roe*, 41 *LW* 4246.

14. This argument is derived from one used (for very different purposes) by William James in *The Will to Believe*, reprinted in William James, *The Will to Believe and Other Essays on Popular Philosophy* (New York: Dover, 1956), pp. 1–31.

MARY ANNE WARREN

On the Moral and Legal Status of Abortion

We will be concerned with both the moral status of abortion, which for our purposes we may define as the act which a woman performs in voluntarily terminating, or allowing another person to terminate, her pregnancy, and the legal status which is appropriate for this act. I will argue that, while it is not possible to produce a satisfactory defense of a woman's right to obtain an abortion without showing that a fetus is not a human being, in the morally relevant sense of that term, we ought not to conclude that the difficulties involved in determining whether or not a fetus is

Reprinted from *The Monist*, Vol. 57, No. 1 (January 1973) with the permission of the author and the publisher.

human make it impossible to produce any satisfactory solution to the problem of the moral status of abortion. For it is possible to show that, on the basis of intuitions which we may expect even the opponents of abortion to share, a fetus is not a person, and hence not the sort of entity to which it is proper to ascribe full moral rights.

Of course, while some philosophers would deny the possibility of any such proof,[1] others will deny that there is any need for it, since the moral permissibility of abortion appears to them to be too obvious to require proof. But the inadequacy of this attitude should be evident from the fact that both the friends and the foes of abortion consider their position to be morally self-evident. Because proabortionists have never adequately come to grips with the conceptual issues surrounding abortion, most, if not all, of the arguments which they advance in opposition to laws restricting access to abortion fail to refute or even weaken the traditional antiabortion argument, i.e., that a fetus is a human being, and therefore abortion is murder.

These arguments are typically of one of two sorts. Either they point to the terrible side effects of the restrictive laws, e.g., the deaths due to illegal abortions, and the fact that it is poor women who suffer the most as a result of these laws, or else they state that to deny a woman access to abortion is to deprive her of her right to control her own body. Unfortunately, however, the fact that restricting access to abortion has tragic side effects does not, in itself, show that the restrictions are unjustified, since murder is wrong regardless of the consequences of prohibiting it; and the appeal to the right to control one's body, which is generally construed as a property right, is at best a rather feeble argument for the permissibility of abortion. Mere ownership does not give me the right to kill innocent people whom I find on my property, and indeed I am apt to be held responsible if such people injure themselves while on my property. It is equally unclear that I have any moral right to expel an innocent person from my property when I know that doing so will result in his death.

Furthermore, it is probably inappropriate to describe a woman's body as her property, since it seems natural to hold that a person is something distinct from her property, but not from her body. Even those who would object to the identification of a person with his body, or with the conjunction of his body and his mind, must admit that it would be very odd to describe, say, breaking a leg, as damaging one's property, and much more appropriate to describe it as injuring one*self*. Thus it is probably a mistake to argue that the right to obtain an abortion is in any way derived from the right to own and regulate property.

But however we wish to construe the right to abortion, we cannot hope to convince those who consider abortion a form of murder of the existence of any such right unless we are able to produce a clear and convincing refutation of the traditional antiabortion argument, and this has not, to my knowledge, been done. With respect to the two most vital issues which that argument involves, i.e., the humanity of the fetus and its implication for the moral status of abortion, confusion has prevailed on both sides of the dispute.

Thus, both proabortionists and antiabortionists have tended to abstract the question of whether abortion is wrong to that of whether it is wrong to destroy a fetus, just as though the rights of another person were not necessarily involved. This mistaken abstraction has led to the almost universal assumption that if a fetus is a human being, with a right to life, then it follows immediately that abortion is wrong (except perhaps when necessary to save the woman's life), and that it ought to be prohibited. It has also been generally assumed that unless the question about the status of the fetus is answered, the moral status of abortion cannot possibly be determined.

Two recent papers, one by B. A. Brody,[2] and one by Judith Thomson,[3] have attempted to settle the question of whether abortion ought to be prohibited apart from the question of whether or not the fetus is human. Brody examines the possibility that the following two statements are compatible: (1) that abortion is the taking of innocent human life, and therefore wrong; and (2) that nevertheless it ought not to be prohibited by law, at least under the present circumstances.[4] Not surprisingly, Brody finds it impossible to reconcile these two statements since, as he rightly argues, none of the unfortunate side effects of the prohibition of abortion is bad enough to justify legalizing the *wrongful* taking of human life. He is mistaken, however, in concluding that the incompatibility of (1) and (2), in itself, shows that "the legal problem about abortion cannot be resolved independently of the status of the fetus problem" (p. 369).

What Brody fails to realize is that (1) embodies the questionable assumption that if a fetus is a human being, then of course abortion is morally wrong, and that an attack on *this* assumption is more promising, as a way of reconciling the humanity of the fetus with the claim that laws prohibiting abortion are unjustified, than is an attack on the assumption that if abortion is the wrongful killing of innocent human beings then it ought to be prohibited. He thus overlooks the possibility that a fetus may have a right to life and abortion still be morally permissible, in that the right of a woman to terminate an unwanted pregnancy might override the right of the fetus to be kept alive. The immorality of abortion is no more demonstrated by the humanity of the fetus, in itself, than the immorality of killing in self-defense is demonstrated by the fact that the assailant is a human being. Neither is it demonstrated by the *innocence* of the fetus, since there may be situations in which the killing of innocent human beings is justified.

It is perhaps not surprising that Brody fails to spot this assumption, since it has been accepted with little or no argument by nearly everyone who has written on the morality of abortion. John Noonan is correct in saying that "the fundamental question in the long history of abortion is, How do you determine the humanity of a being?"[5] He summarizes his own anti-abortion argument, which is a version of the official position of the Catholic Church, as follows:

. . . it is wrong to kill humans, however poor, weak, defenseless, and lacking in opportunity to develop their potential they may be. It is therefore morally wrong to kill Biafrans. Similarly, it is morally wrong to kill embryos.[6]

Noonan bases his claim that fetuses are human upon what he calls the theologians' criterion of humanity: that whoever is conceived of human beings is human. But although he argues at length for the appropriateness of this criterion, he never questions the assumption that if a fetus is human then abortion is wrong for exactly the same reason that murder is wrong.

Judith Thomson is, in fact, the only writer I am aware of who has seriously questioned this assumption; she has argued that, even if we grant the antiabortionist his claim that a fetus is a human being, with the same right to life as any other human being, we can still demonstrate that, in at least some and perhaps most cases, a woman is under no moral obligation to complete an unwanted pregnancy.[7] Her argument is worth examining, since if it holds up it may enable us to establish the moral permissibility of abortion without becoming involved in problems about what entitles an entity to be considered human, and accorded full moral rights. To be able to do this would be a great gain in the power and simplicity of the pro-abortion position, since, although I will argue that these problems can be solved at least as decisively as can any other moral problem, we should certainly be pleased to be able to avoid having to solve them as part of the justification of abortion.

On the other hand, even if Thomson's argument does not hold up, her insight, i.e., that it requires *argument* to show that if fetuses are human then abortion is properly classified as murder, is an extremely valuable one. The assumption she attacks is particularly invidious, for it amounts to the decision that it is

appropriate, in deciding the moral status of abortion, to leave the rights of the pregnant woman out of consideration entirely, except possibly when her life is threatened. Obviously, this will not do; determining what moral rights, if any, a fetus possesses is only the first step in determining the moral status of abortion. Step two, which is at least equally essential, is finding a just solution to the conflict between whatever rights the fetus may have, and the rights of the woman who is unwillingly pregnant. While the historical error has been to pay far too little attention to the second step, Ms. Thomson's suggestion is that if we look at the second step first we may find that a woman has a right to obtain an abortion *regardless* of what rights the fetus has.

Our own inquiry will also have two stages. In Section I, we will consider whether or not it is possible to establish that abortion is morally permissible even on the assumption that a fetus is an entity with a full-fledged right to life. I will argue that in fact this cannot be established, at least not with the conclusiveness which is essential to our hopes of convincing those who are skeptical about the morality of abortion, and that we therefore cannot avoid dealing with the question of whether or not a fetus really does have the same right to life as a (more fully developed) human being.

In Section II, I will propose an answer to this question, namely, that a fetus cannot be considered a member of the moral community, the set of beings with full and equal moral rights, for the simple reason that it is not a person, and that it is personhood, and not genetic humanity, i.e., humanity as defined by Noonan, which is the basis for membership in this community. I will argue that a fetus, whatever its stage of development, satisfies none of the basic criteria of personhood, and is not even enough *like* a person to be accorded even some of the same rights on the basis of this resemblance. Nor, as we will see, is a fetus's *potential* personhood a threat to the morality of abortion, since, whatever the rights of potential people may be, they are invariably overridden in any conflict with the moral rights of actual people.

I

We turn now to Professor Thomson's case for the claim that even if a fetus has full moral rights, abortion is still morally permissible, at least sometimes, and for some reasons other than to save the woman's life. Her argument is based upon a clever, but I think faulty, analogy. She asks us to picture ourselves waking up one day, in bed with a famous violinist. Imagine that you have been kidnapped, and your bloodstream hooked up to that of the violinist, who happens to have an ailment which will certainly kill him unless he is permitted to share your kidneys for a period of nine months. No one else can save him, since you alone have the right type of blood. He will be unconscious all that time, and you will have to stay in bed with him, but after the nine months are over he may be unplugged, completely cured, that is, provided that you have cooperated.

Now then, she continues, what are your obligations in this situation? The antiabortionist, if he is consistent, will have to say that you are obligated to stay in bed with the violinist: for all people have a right to life, and violinists are people, and therefore it would be murder for you to disconnect yourself from him and let him die (p. 49). But this is outrageous, and so there must be something wrong with the same argument when it is applied to abortion. It would certainly be commendable of you to agree to save the violinist, but it is absurd to suggest that your refusal to do so would be murder. His right to life does not obligate you to do whatever is required to keep him alive; nor does it justify anyone else in forcing you to do so. A law which required you to stay in bed with the violinist would clearly be an unjust law, since it is no proper function of the law to force unwilling people to make huge sacrifices for the sake of other people toward whom they have no such prior obligation.

Thomson concludes that, if this analogy is an apt one, then we can grant the antiabortionist his claim that a fetus is a human being, and still hold that it is at least sometimes the case that a pregnant woman has the right to refuse to be a Good Samaritan towards the fetus, i.e., to obtain an abortion. For there is a great gap between the claim that x has a right to life, and the claim that y is obligated to do whatever is necessary to keep x alive, let alone that he ought to be forced to do so. It is y's duty to keep x alive only if he has somehow contracted a *special* obligation to do so; and a woman who is unwillingly pregnant, e.g., who was raped, has done nothing which obligates her to make the enormous sacrifice which is necessary to preserve the conceptus.

This argument is initially quite plausible, and in the extreme case of pregnancy due to rape it is probably conclusive. Difficulties arise, however, when we try to specify more exactly the range of cases in which abortion is clearly justifiable even on the assumption

that the fetus is human. Professor Thomson considers it a virtue of her argument that it does not enable us to conclude that abortion is *always* permissible. It would, she says, be "indecent" for a woman in her seventh month to obtain an abortion just to avoid having to postpone a trip to Europe. On the other hand, her argument enables us to see that "a sick and desperately frightened schoolgirl pregnant due to rape may *of course* choose abortion, and that any law which rules this out is an insane law" (p. 65). So far, so good; but what are we to say about the woman who becomes pregnant not through rape but as a result of her own carelessness, or because of contraceptive failure, or who gets pregnant intentionally and then changes her mind about wanting a child? With respect to such cases, the violinist analogy is of much less use to the defender of the woman's right to obtain an abortion.

Indeed, the choice of a pregnancy due to rape, as an example of a case in which abortion is permissible even if a fetus is considered a human being, is extremely significant; for it is only in the case of pregnancy due to rape that the woman's situation is adequately analogous to the violinist case for our intuitions about the latter to transfer convincingly. The crucial difference between a pregnancy due to rape and the *normal* case of an unwanted pregnancy is that in the normal case we cannot claim that the woman is in no way responsible for her predicament; she could have remained chaste, or taken her pills more faithfully, or abstained on dangerous days, and so on. If on the other hand, you are kidnapped by strangers, and hooked up to a strange violinist, then you are free of any shred of responsibility for the situation, on the basis of which it would be argued that you are obligated to keep the violinist alive. Only when her pregnancy is due to rape is a woman clearly just as nonresponsible.[8]

Consequently, there is room for the antiabortionist to argue that in the normal case of unwanted pregnancy a woman has, by her own actions, assumed responsibility for the fetus. For if x behaves in a way which he could have avoided, and which he knows involves, let us say, a 1 percent chance of bringing into existence a human being, with a right to life, and does so knowing that if this should happen then that human being will perish unless x does certain things to keep him alive, then it is by no means clear that when it does happen x is free of any obligation to what he knew in advance would be required to keep that human being alive.

The plausibility of such an argument is enough to show that the Thomson analogy can provide a clear and persuasive defense of a woman's right to obtain an abortion only with respect to those cases in which the woman is in no way responsible for her pregnancy, e.g., where it is due to rape. In all other cases, we would almost certainly conclude that it was necessary to look carefully at the particular circumstances in order to determine the extent of the woman's responsibility, and hence the extent of her obligation. This is an extremely unsatisfactory outcome, from the viewpoint of the opponents of restrictive abortion laws, most of whom are convinced that a woman has a right to obtain an abortion regardless of how and why she got pregnant.

Of course a supporter of the violinist analogy might point out that it is absurd to suggest that forgetting her pill one day might be sufficient to obligate a woman to complete an unwanted pregnancy. And indeed it *is* absurd to suggest this. As we will see, the moral right to obtain an abortion is not in the least dependent upon the extent to which the woman is responsible for her pregnancy. But unfortunately, once we allow the assumption that a fetus has full moral rights, we cannot avoid taking this absurd suggestion seriously. Perhaps we can make this point more clear by altering the violinist story just enough to make it more analogous to a normal unwanted pregnancy and less to a pregnancy due to rape, and then seeing whether it is still obvious that you are not obligated to stay in bed with the fellow.

Suppose, then, that violinists are peculiarly prone to the sort of illness the only cure for which is the use of someone else's bloodstream for nine months, and that because of this there has been formed a society of music lovers who agree that whenever a violinist is stricken they will draw lots and the loser will, by some means, be made the one and only person capable of saving him. Now then, would you be obligated to cooperate in curing the violinist if you had voluntarily joined this society, knowing the possible consequences, and then your name had been drawn and you had been kidnapped? Admittedly, you did not promise ahead of time that you would, but you did deliberately place yourself in a position in which it might happen that a human life would be lost if you did not. Surely this is at least a prima facie reason for

supposing that you have an obligation to stay in bed with the violinist. Suppose that you had gotten your name drawn deliberately; surely *that* would be quite a strong reason for thinking that you had such an obligation.

It might be suggested that there is one important disanalogy between the modified violinist case and the case of an unwanted pregnancy, which makes the woman's responsibility significantly less, namely, the fact that the fetus *comes into existence* as the result of the woman's actions. This fact might give her a right to refuse to keep it alive, whereas she would not have had this right had it existed previously, independently, and then as a result of her actions become dependent upon her for its survival.

My own intuition, however, is that x has no more right to bring into existence, either deliberately or as a foreseeable result of actions he could have avoided, a being with full moral rights (y), and then refuse to do what he knew beforehand would be required to keep that being alive, than he has to enter into an agreement with an existing person, whereby he may be called upon to save that person's life, and then refuse to do so when so called upon. Thus, x's responsibility for y's existence does not seem to lessen his obligation to keep y alive, if he is also responsible for y's being in a situation in which only he can save him.

Whether or not this intuition is entirely correct, it brings us back once again to the conclusion that once we allow the assumption that a fetus has full moral rights it becomes an extremely complex and difficult question whether and when abortion is justifiable. Thus the Thomson analogy cannot help us produce a clear and persuasive proof of the moral permissibility of abortion. Nor will the opponents of the restrictive laws thank us for anything less; for their conviction (for the most part) is that abortion is obviously *not* a morally serious and extremely unfortunate, even though sometimes justified act, comparable to killing in self-defense or to letting the violinist die, but rather is closer to being a morally neutral act, like cutting one's hair.

The basis of this conviction, I believe, is the realization that a fetus is not a person, and thus does not have a full-fledged right to life. Perhaps the reason why this claim has been so inadequately defended is that it seems self-evident to those who accept it. And so it is, insofar as it follows from what I take to be perfectly obvious claims about the nature of personhood, and about the proper grounds for ascribing moral rights, claims which ought, indeed, to be obvi-

ous to both the friends and foes of abortion. Nevertheless, it is worth examining these claims, and
showing how they demonstrate the moral innocuous-
ness of abortion, since this apparently has not been
adequately done before.

II

The question which we must answer in order to
produce a satisfactory solution to the problem of the
moral status of abortion is this: How are we to define
the moral community, the set of beings with full and
equal moral rights, such that we can decide whether a
human fetus is a member of this community or not?
What sort of entity, exactly, has the inalienable rights
to life, liberty, and the pursuit of happiness? Jefferson
attributed these rights to all *men*, and it may or may
not be fair to suggest that he intended to attribute them
only to men. Perhaps he ought to have attributed them
to all human beings. If so, then we arrive, first, at
Noonan's problem of defining what makes a being
human, and second, at the equally vital question
which Noonan does not consider, namely, What reason is there for identifying the moral community with
the set of all human beings, in whatever way we have
chosen to define that term?

ON THE DEFINITION OF "HUMAN"

One reason why this vital second question is so
frequently overlooked in the debate over the moral
status of abortion is that the term "human" has two
distinct, but not often distinguished, senses. This fact
results in a slide of meaning, which serves to conceal
the fallaciousness of the traditional argument that
since (1) it is wrong to kill innocent human beings,
and (2) fetuses are innocent human beings, then (3) it
is wrong to kill fetuses. For if "human" is used in the
same sense in both (1) and (2) then, whichever of the
two senses is meant, one of these premises is
question-begging. And if it is used in two different
senses, then of course the conclusion doesn't follow.

Thus, (1) is a self-evident moral truth,[9] and avoids
begging the question about abortion, only if "human
being" is used to mean something like "a full-fledged
member of the moral community." (It may or may
not also be meant to refer exclusively to members of
the species *Homo sapiens*.) We may call this the
moral sense of "human." It is not to be confused
with what we will call the *genetic* sense, i.e., the
sense in which *any* member of the species is a human
being, and no member of any other species could be.
If (1) is acceptable only if the moral sense is intended,

(2) is non-question-begging only if what is intended is
the genetic sense.

In "Deciding Who is Human," Noonan argues for
the classification of fetuses with human beings by
pointing to the presence of the full genetic code, and
the potential capacity for rational thought (p.135). It
is clear that what he needs to show, for his version of
the traditional argument to be valid, is that fetuses are
human in the moral sense, the sense in which it is
analytically true that all human beings have full moral
rights. But, in the absence of any argument showing
that whatever is genetically human is also morally
human, and he gives none, nothing more than genetic
humanity can be demonstrated by the presence of the
human genetic code. And, as we will see, the *potential* capacity for rational thought can at most show that
an entity has the potential for *becoming* human in the
moral sense.

DEFINING THE MORAL COMMUNITY

Can it be established that genetic humanity is sufficient for moral humanity? I think that there are very
good reasons for not defining the moral community in
this way. I would like to suggest an alternative way of
defining the moral community, which I will argue for
only to the extent of explaining why it is, or should
be, self-evident. The suggestion is simply that the
moral community consists of all and only *people*,
rather than all and only human beings;[10] and probably
the best way of demonstrating its self-evidence is by
considering the concept of personhood, to see what
sorts of entity are and are not persons, and what the
decision that a being is or is not a person implies
about its moral rights.

What characteristics entitle an entity to be considered a person? This is obviously not the place to attempt a complete analysis of the concept of personhood, but we do not need such a fully adequate
analysis just to determine whether and why a fetus is
or isn't a person. All we need is a rough and approximate list of the most basic criteria of personhood, and
some idea of which, or how many, of these an entity
must satisfy in order to properly be considered a person.

In searching for such criteria, it is useful to look
beyond the set of people with whom we are acquainted, and ask how we would decide whether a
totally alien being was a person or not. (For we have
no right to assume that genetic humanity is necessary

for personhood.) Imagine a space traveler who lands on an unknown planet and encounters a race of beings utterly unlike any he has ever seen or heard of. If he wants to be sure of behaving morally toward these beings, he has to somehow decide whether they are poeple, and hence have full moral rights, or whether they are the sort of thing which he need not feel guilty about treating as, for example, a source of food.

How should he go about making this decision? If he has some anthropological background he might look for such things as religion, art, and the manufacturing of tools, weapons, or shelters, since these factors have been used to distinguish our human from our prehuman ancestors, in what seems to be closer to the moral than the genetic sense of "human." And no doubt he would be right to consider the presence of such factors as good evidence that the alien beings were people, and morally human. It would, however, be overly anthropocentric of him to take the absence of these things as adequate evidence that they were not, since we can imagine people who have progressed beyond, or evolved without ever developing, these cultural characteristics.

I suggest that the traits which are most central to the concept of personhood, or humanity in the moral sense, are, very roughly, the following:

1. Consciousness (of objects and events external and/or internal to the being), and in particular the capacity to feel pain;
2. Reasoning (the *developed* capacity to solve new and relatively complex problems);
3. Self-motivated activity (activity which is relatively independent of either genetic or direct external control);
4. The capacity to communicate, by whatever means, messages of an indefinite variety of types, that is, not just with an indefinite number of possible contents, but on indefinitely many possible topics;
5. The presence of self-concepts, and self-awareness, either individual or racial, or both.

Admittedly, there are apt to be a great many problems involved in formulating precise definitions of these criteria, let alone in developing universally valid behavioral criteria for deciding when they apply. But I will assume that both we and our explorer know approximately what (1)–(5) mean, and that he is also able to determine whether or not they apply. How,

then, should he use his findings to decide whether or not the alien beings are people? We needn't suppose that an entity must have *all* of these attributes to be properly considered a person; (1) and (2) alone may well be sufficient for personhood, and quite probably (1)–(3) are sufficient. Neither do we need to insist that any one of these criteria is *necessary* for personhood, although once again (1) and (2) look like fairly good candidates for necessary conditions, as does (3), if "activity" is construed so as to include the activity of reasoning.

All we need to claim, to demonstrate that a fetus is not a person, is that any being which satisfies *none* of (1)–(5) is certainly not a person. I consider this claim to be so obvious that I think anyone who denied it, and claimed that a being which satisfied none of (1)–(5) was a person all the same, would thereby demonstrate that he had no notion at all of what a person is—perhaps because he had confused the concept of a person with that of genetic humanity. If the opponents of abortion were to deny the appropriateness of these five criteria, I do not know what further arguments would convince them. We would probably have to admit that our conceptual schemes were indeed irreconcilably different, and that our dispute could not be settled objectively.

I do not expect this to happen, however, since I think that the concept of a person is one which is very nearly universal (to people), and that it is common to both proabortionists and antiabortionists, even though neither group has fully realized the relevance of this concept to the resolution of their dispute. Furthermore, I think that on reflection even the antiabortionists ought to agree not only that (1)–(5) are central to the concept of personhood, but also that it is a part of this concept that all and only people have full moral rights. The concept of a person is in part a moral concept; once we have admitted that x is a person we have recognized, even if we have not agreed to respect, x's right to be treated as a member of the moral community. It is true that the claim that x is a *human being* is more commonly voiced as part of an appeal to treat x decently than is the claim that x is a person, but this is either because "human being" is here used in the sense which implies personhood, or because the genetic and moral senses of "human" have been confused.

Now if (1)–(5) are indeed the primary criteria of personhood, then it is clear that genetic humanity is neither necessary nor sufficient for establishing that an entity is a person. Some human beings are not people, and there may well be people who are not human beings. A man or woman whose consciousness has been permanently obliterated but who remains alive is a human being which is no longer a person; defective human beings, with no appreciable mental capacity, are not and presumably never will be people; and a fetus is a human being which is not yet a person, and which therefore cannot coherently be said to have full moral rights. Citizens of the next century should be prepared to recognize highly advanced, self-aware robots or computers, should such be developed, and intelligent inhabitants of other worlds, should such be found, as people in the fullest sense, and to respect their moral rights. But to ascribe full moral rights to an entity which is not a person is as absurd as to ascribe moral obligations and responsibilities to such an entity.

FETAL DEVELOPMENT AND THE RIGHT TO LIFE

Two problems arise in the application of these suggestions for the definition of the moral community to the determination of the precise moral status of a human fetus. Given that the paradigm example of a person is a normal adult being, then (1) How like this paradigm, in particular how far advanced since conception, does a human being need to be before it begins to have a right to life by virtue, not of being fully a person as of yet, but of being *like* a person? and (2) To what extent, if any, does the fact that a fetus has the *potential* for becoming a person endow it with some of the same rights? Each of these questions requires some comment.

In answering the first question, we need not attempt a detailed consideration of the moral rights of organisms which are not developed enough, aware enough, intelligent enough, etc., to be considered people, but which resemble people in some respects. It does seem reasonable to suggest that the more like a person, in the relevant respects, a being is, the stronger is the case for regarding it as having a right to life, and indeed the stronger its right to life is. Thus we ought to take seriously the suggestion that, insofar as "the human individual develops biologically in a continuous fashion . . . the rights of a human person might develop in the same way."[11] But we must keep in mind that the attributes which are relevant in determining whether or not an entity is enough like a person to be regarded as having some of the same moral rights are no different from those which are relevant to determining whether or not it is fully a person—i.e., are no different from (1)–(5)—and that

being genetically human, or having recognizably human facial and other physical features, or detectable brain activity, or the capacity to survive outside the uterus, are simply not among these relevant attributes.

Thus it is clear that even though a seven- or eight-month fetus has features which make it apt to arouse in us almost the same powerful protective instinct as is commonly aroused by a small infant, nevertheless it is not significantly more personlike than is a very small embryo. It is *somewhat* more personlike; it can apparently feel and respond to pain, and it may even have a rudimentary form of consciousness, insofar as its brain is quite active. Nevertheless, it seems safe to say that it is not fully conscious, in the way that an infant of a few months is, and that it cannot reason, or communicate messages of indefinitely many sorts, does not engage in self-motivated activity, and has no self-awareness. Thus, in the *relevant* respects, a fetus, even a fully developed one, is considerably less personlike than is the average mature mammal, indeed the average fish. And I think that a rational person must conclude that if the right to life of a fetus is to be based upon its resemblance to a person, then it cannot be said to have any more right to life than, let us say, a newborn guppy (which also seems to be capable of feeling pain), and that a right of that magnitude could never override a woman's right to obtain an abortion, at any stage of her pregnancy.

There may, of course, be other arguments in favor of placing legal limits upon the stage of pregnancy in which an abortion may be performed. Given the relative safety of the new techniques of artificially inducing labor during the third trimester, the danger to the woman's life or health is no longer such an argument. Neither is the fact that people tend to respond to the thought of abortion in the later stages of pregnancy with emotional repulsion, since mere emotional responses cannot take the place of moral reasoning in determining what ought to be permitted. Nor, finally, is the frequently heard argument that legalizing abortion, especially late in the pregnancy, may erode the level of respect for human life, leading, perhaps to an increase in unjustified euthanasia and other crimes. For this threat, if it is a threat, can be better met by educating people to the kinds of moral distinctions which we are making here than by limiting access to abortion (which limitation may, in its disregard for the rights of women, be just as damaging to the level of respect for human rights).

Thus, since the fact that even a fully developed fetus is not personlike enough to have any significant right to life on the basis of its person-likeness shows that no legal restrictions upon the stage of pregnancy in which an abortion may be performed can be justified on the grounds that we should protect the rights of the older fetus; and since there is no other apparent justification for such restrictions, we may conclude that they are entirely unjustified. Whether or not it would be *indecent* (whatever that means) for a woman in her seventh month to obtain an abortion just to avoid having to postpone a trip to Europe, it would not, in itself, be *immoral,* and therefore it ought to be permitted.

POTENTIAL PERSONHOOD AND THE RIGHT TO LIFE

We have seen that a fetus does not resemble a person in any way which can support the claim that it has even some of the same rights. But what about its *potential,* the fact that if nurtured and allowed to develop naturally it will very probably become a person? Doesn't that alone give it at least some right to life? It is hard to deny that the fact that an entity is a potential person is a strong prima facie reason for not destroying it; but we need not conclude from this that a potential person has a right to life, by virtue of that potential. It may be that our feeling that it is better, other things being equal, not to destroy a potential person is better explained by the fact that potential people are still (felt to be) an invaluable resource, not to be lightly squandered. Surely, if every speck of dust were a potential person, we would be much less apt to conclude that every potential person has a right to become actual.

Still, we do not need to insist that a potential person has no right to life whatever. There may well be something immoral, and not just imprudent, about wantonly destroying potential people, when doing so isn't necessary to protect anyone's rights. But even if a potential person does have some prima facie right to life, such a right could not possibly outweigh the right of a woman to obtain an abortion, since the rights of any actual person invariably outweigh those of any potential person, whenever the two conflict. Since this may not be immediately obvious in the case of a human fetus, let us look at another case.

Suppose that our space explorer falls into the hands of an alien culture, whose scientists decide to create a few hundred thousand or more human beings, by breaking his body into its component cells, and using these to create fully developed human beings, with, of course, his genetic code. We may imagine that each of these newly created men will have all of the original man's abilities, skills, knowledge, and so on, and also have an individual self-concept, in short that each of them will be a bona fide (though hardly unique) person. Imagine that the whole project will take only seconds, and that its chances of success are extremely high, and that our explorer knows all of this, and also knows that these people will be treated fairly. I maintain that in such a situation he would have every right to escape if he could, and thus to deprive all of these potential people of their potential lives; for his right to life outweighs all of theirs together, in spite of the fact that they are all genetically human, all innocent, and all have a very high probability of becoming people very soon, if only he refrains from action.

Indeed, I think he would have a right to escape even if it were not his life which the alien scientists planned to take, but only a year of his freedom, or, indeed, only a day. Nor would he be obligated to stay if he had gotten captured (thus bringing all these people-potentials into existence) because of his own carelessness, or even if he had done so deliberately, knowing the consequences. Regardless of how he got captured, he is not morally obligated to remain in captivity for *any* period of time for the sake of permitting any number of potential people to come into actuality, so great is the margin by which one actual person's right to liberty outweighs whatever right to life even a hundred thousand potential people have. And it seems reasonable to conclude that the rights of a woman will outweigh by a similar margin whatever right to life a fetus may have by virtue of its potential personhood.

Thus, neither a fetus's resemblance to a person, nor its potential for becoming a person provides any basis whatever for the claim that it has any significant right to life. Consequently, a woman's right to protect her health, happiness, freedom, and even her life,[12] by terminating an unwanted pregnancy will always override whatever right to life it may be appropriate to ascribe to a fetus, even a fully developed one. And thus, in the absence of any overwhelming social need for every possible child, the laws which restrict the right to obtain an abortion, or limit the period of pregnancy during which an abortion may be performed, are a wholly unjustified violation of a woman's most basic moral and constitutional rights.[13]

POSTSCRIPT ON INFANTICIDE

Since the publication of this article, many people have written to point out that my argument appears to justify not only abortion, but infanticide as well. For a new-born infant is not significantly more person-like than an advanced fetus, and consequently it would seem that if the destruction of the latter is permissible so too must be that of the former. Inasmuch as most people, regardless of how they feel about the morality of abortion, consider infanticide a form of murder, this might appear to represent a serious flaw in my argument.

Now, if I am right in holding that it is only people who have a full-fledged right to life, and who can be murdered, and if the criteria of personhood are as I have described them, then it obviously follows that killing a new-born infant isn't murder. It does *not* follow, however, that infanticide is permissible, for two reasons. In the first place, it would be wrong, at least in this country and in this period of history, and other things being equal, to kill a new-born infant, because even if its parents do not want it and would not suffer from its destruction, there are other people who would like to have it, and would, in all probability, be deprived of a great deal of pleasure by its destruction. Thus, infanticide is wrong for reasons analogous to those which make it wrong to wantonly destroy natural resources, or great works of art.

Secondly, most people, at least in this country, value infants and would much prefer that they be preserved, even if foster parents are not immediately available. Most of us would rather be taxed to support orphanages than allow unwanted infants to be destroyed. So long as there are people who want an infant preserved, and who are willing and able to provide the means of caring for it, under reasonably humane conditions, it is, *certeris paribus,* wrong to destroy it.

But, it might be replied, if this argument shows that infanticide is wrong, at least at this time and in this country, doesn't it also show that abortion is wrong? After all, many people value fetuses, are disturbed by their destruction, and would much prefer that they be preserved, even at some cost to themselves. Furthermore, as a potential source of pleasure to some foster family, a fetus is just as valuable as an infant. There is, however, a crucial difference between the two cases: so long as the fetus is unborn, its preservation, contrary to the wishes of the pregnant woman, violates her rights to freedom, happiness, and self-determination. Her rights override the rights of those who would like the fetus preserved, just as if someone's life or limb is threatened by a wild animal, his right to protect himself by destroying the animal overrides the rights of those who would prefer that the animal not be harmed.

The minute the infant is born, however, its preservation no longer violates any of its mother's rights, even if she wants it destroyed, because she is free to put it up for adoption. Consequently, while the moment of birth does not mark any sharp discontinuity in the degree to which an infant possesses the right to life, it does mark the end of its mother's right to determine its fate. Indeed, if abortion could be performed without killing the fetus, she would never possess the right to have the fetus destroyed, for the same reasons that she has no right to have an infant destroyed.

On the other hand, it follows from my argument that when an unwanted or defective infant is born into a society which cannot afford and/or is not willing to care for it, then its destruction is permissible. This conclusion will, no doubt, strike many people as heartless and immoral; but remember that the very existence of people who feel this way, and who are willing and able to provide care for unwanted infants, is reason enough to conclude that they should be preserved.

NOTES

1. For example, Roger Wertheimer, who in "Understanding the Abortion Argument" (*Philosophy and Public Affairs,* 1, No. 1 [Fall, 1971], 67–95), argues that the problem of the moral status of abortion is insoluble, in that the dispute over the status of the fetus is not a question of fact at all, but only a question of how one responds to the facts.

2. B. A. Brody, "Abortion and the Law," *The Journal of Philosophy,* 68, No. 12 (June 17, 1971), 357–69.

3. Judith Thomson, "A Defense of Abortion," *Philosophy and Public Affairs,* 1, No. 1 (Fall, 1971), 47–66.

4. I have abbreviated these statements somewhat, but not in a way which affects the argument.

5. John Noonan, "Abortion and the Catholic Church: A Summary History," *Natural Law Forum,* 12 (1967), 125.

6. John Noonan, "Deciding Who Is Human," *Natural Law Forum,* 13 (1968), 134.

7. "A Defense of Abortion."

8. We may safely ignore the fact that she might have avoided getting raped, e.g., by carrying a gun, since by similar means you might likewise have avoided getting kidnapped, and in neither case does the victim's failure to take all possible precautions against a highly unlikely event (as opposed to reasonable precautions against a rather likely event) mean that he is morally responsible for what happens.

9. Of course, the principle that it is (always) wrong to kill innocent human beings is in need of many other modifications, e.g., that it may be permissible to do so to save a greater number of other innocent human beings, but we may safely ignore these complications here.

10. From here on, we will use "human" to mean genetically human, since the moral sense seems closely connected to, and perhaps derived from, the assumption that genetic humanity is sufficient for membership in the moral community.

11. Thomas L. Hayes, "A Biological View," *Commonweal*, 85 (March 17, 1967), 677–78; quoted by Daniel Callahan, in *Abortion, Law, Choice, and Morality* (London: Macmillan & Co., 1970).

12. That is, insofar as the death rate, for the woman, is higher for childbirth than for early abortion.

13. My thanks to the following people, who were kind enough to read and criticize an earlier version of this paper: Herbert Gold, Gene Glass, Anne Lauterbach, Judith Thomson, Mary Mothersill, and Timothy Binkley.

PHILIP E. DEVINE

Abortion

I shall assume here that infants are protected by the moral rule against homicide. From this assumption it seems to follow immediately that fetuses, and other instances of human life from conception onward, are also so protected, so that, unless justified or mitigated, abortion is murder. For there seem to be only two possible grounds for asserting the humanity of the infant: (1) The infant is a member of the human species (species principle). (2) The infant will, in due course, think, talk, love, and have a sense of justice (potentiality principle). And both (1) and (2) are true of fetuses, embryos, and zygotes, as well as of infants. A zygote is alive (it grows) and presumably is an instance of the species *Homo sapiens* (of what other species might it be?), and it will, if nothing goes wrong, develop into the kind of creature which is universally conceded to be a person.

But a number of arguments still have to be answered before the humanity or personhood of the fetus can be asserted with confidence. All of them are reflected in, and lend plausibility to, Joel Feinberg's remark: "To assert that a single-cell zygote, or a tiny cluster of cells, as such, is a complete human being already possessed of all the rights of a developed per-

From *The Ethics of Homicide* (Ithaca, NY: Cornell University Press, 1978), pp. 74–90, 203–204.

son seems at least as counter-intuitive as the position into which some liberals [defenders of abortion] are forced, that newly born infants have no right to continue living."[1] These arguments are (1) that if a fetus is a person because of its potential and its biological humanity, spermatozoa and ova must also be considered persons, which is absurd; (2) that personhood is something one acquires gradually, so that a fetus is only imperfectly a person; (3) that there is an adequately defensible dividing point between the human and the nonhuman, the personal and the nonpersonal, which enables us to defend abortion (or "early" abortion) without being committed to the defense of infanticide; and finally (4) that the opponent of abortion himself does not take seriously the humanity of the fetus, an argument *ad hominem*. Insofar as one relies on intuition to establish the wrongness of infanticide, one must come to terms with the contention that the assertion that a fetus is a person is itself counter-intuitive.

1. Michael Tooley argues that if it is seriously wrong to kill infants or fetuses because they potentially possess human traits, it must also be seriously wrong to prevent systems of objects from developing into an organism possessing self-consciousness, so that artificial contraception will be just as wrong as infanticide. But only organisms can have a right to

life, although something more like an organism than a mere concatenation of sperm and egg might have a right to something like life. And the same point can be reached if we speak not in terms of a right to life but of a moral rule against certain kinds of killing, for only an organism can be killed.

There is another, more complicated, argument against the contention that a spermatozoon and an ovum, not united, might be protected by the moral rule against homicide (or would be if infants and fetuses were). Since the moral rule against homicide is a rule that protects rights, it cannot obtain unless there is some specifiable individual[2] whose rights would be violated were it breached. A sperm conjoined with an ovum in this way is not in any sense an individual; therefore it cannot have any rights. For this reason the prevention of such a combination's being fruitful cannot be a violation of the moral rule against homicide. An ejaculation contains many more spermatozoa than could possibly be united with ova, and it is difficult to see the sperm-plus-ovum combinations which do not prevail as somehow deprived of something on which they have a claim.

. . .

Spermatozoa and ova might be said to be living individuals in a sense. But it is clear that a spermatozoon cannot be considered a member of the human species or a being potentially possessing the traits we regard as distinctively human in the way a fetus or infant can. A developed human being issuing from a sperm alone is a possibility far outside the normal powers of the spermatozoon in the way a developed human being issuing from a fetus or infant is not outside the normal powers of those creatures.

The case of the ovum is more complicated, since parthenogenesis, reproduction from ovum alone, takes place in at least some species. But, apart from considerations involving twinning and recombination (to be discussed below), fertilization still remains a relatively bright line available for distinguishing prehuman organic matter from the developing human organism. Finally, we must remember that sperm and ovum are biologically parts of *other* human individuals (the parents).

2. Perhaps, however, it is a mistake to look for a bright line between prehuman organic matter and a developing human being or person. Perhaps personhood is a quality the developing human creature acquires gradually. This suggestion will always have a considerable appeal to the moderate-minded. For it avoids the harshness, or seeming harshness, of those who would require great suffering on the part of the woman carrying a fetus for the sake of that fetus's rights, while avoiding also the crudity of those who regard abortion as of no greater moral significance than cutting one's toenails, having a tooth pulled, or swatting a fly. Moreover, that abortion is morally less desirable the closer it is to birth—and not simply because a late abortion is more likely to harm the woman—is one of the few intuitions widely shared on all sides of the abortion controversy, and thus not to be despised. That abortion should become harder and harder to justify as pregnancy proceeds, without being ever as hard to justify as is the killing of a person, is a suggestion which ought therefore to be given the most serious attention.

The gradualist suggestion raises a problem of quite general scope. Not only as regards the distinction between prehuman organic matter and a human person, but also as regards that between human beings and brute animals,[3] and that between a dying person and a corpse,[4] our thought is pulled in two different directions. On the one hand, we find it natural to look for sharp, if not radical, breaks between different kinds of being, for evolutionary quanta so to speak. On the other hand, we are suspicious of sharp breaks and look for continuities at every point in nature. . . .

There seems to be no stable, nonarbitrary way of correlating stages of fetal development with justifying grounds. At the stage of development when the embryo most closely resembles a fish, the moderate on the abortion question will want to ascribe it stronger rights than he does fish, but weaker rights than he does full human beings. And the moderate, as I conceive him, regards an infant as a human person, though the difference between a human infant and an infant ape is not palpable. . . .

If personhood or humanity admits of degrees before birth, then it would seem that it must admit of degrees after birth as well. And even if we can manage to block such inferences as that kings are more persons than peasants, Greeks than barbarians, men than women (or women than men), or those with Ph.D.'s than those with M.A.'s, according to this theory we should still expect that adults will be considered more fully human than children. But few hold and fewer still teach that a ten-year-old child[5] can be killed on lighter grounds than an adult. Indeed the killing of small children is often considered worse than the killing of adults. (Although a parent who kills his child is likely to receive a less severe sentence than someone who kills an adult, this remnant of the *patria potestas* is the result of excuse or mitigation rather than of justification.)[6]

Some philosophers, it is true, might contend that there are degrees of humanity, but that full-fledged humanity is attained well before the age of ten. The question then is at what point full-fledged humanity is attained. Tooley's suggestion—twenty-four hours after birth—is clearly dictated by considerations of convenience rather than by the nature of the newborn. Some might say that first use of speech is a plausible criterion, but the development of linguistic capacities is a process, if anything is, not completed, if ever, until much later in a human being's development than his tenth birthday. If one wishes to fix a point after birth when someone becomes a full-fledged person, it could seem plausible to some thinkers to choose a point after the age of ten—when the nervous system is fully developed, at puberty, or at the conventional age of majority. In any case, the gradualist does not avoid the central problem—that of determining when we have a person in the full sense on our hands.

It has also been argued that a graduation from personhood into nonpersonhood can be observed at the end of life.[7] But the consequences of such a view are scarcely tolerable. For what the analogy with abortion leads to is the killing of old people (1) without their consent, and (2) for the sake of relieving *others* of the burden they pose. Whatever our conclusion might be concerning voluntary euthanasia, and whatever difficulties there might be in fixing a precise moment of death, we cannot admit that anyone who is humanly conscious, or will or may regain human consciousness, is anything but a full-fledged person. This point can be restated in more technical terms as follows. The concept of a person is normally both open-textured and flexible in its application—a corporation for instance may be treated legally as a person for some purposes and not for others. But when the concept of a person is given one particular use, to mark out those creatures whose existence and interests are to be given special protection in the court of morality, there are special reasons weighing in the direction of clarity and rigidity. Whatever the extent to which the interest of a given person might legitimately be sacrificed for the good of the community, it seems intolerable that a creature should be regarded as not a person—and hence of next to no account in moral deliberation—simply because it is or appears to be in the interest of others to so regard that creature. At any rate, to proceed in such a manner would be to overthrow some of the most fundamental elements of our moral tradition.

The difference between early and late abortion is best accounted for, I believe, not by the more nearly human status of the mature fetus as compared with the younger one, but rather by the closer imaginative and emotional link between the mature fetus and a born child and hence between such a creature and an adult human than is the case of a young fetus or embryo.

. . .

3. We are now prepared to address the question of the homicidal character of abortion head on. If we assume the personhood of the human infant when born, is there a point later than fertilization when the life of a human person may be said to begin?

a. One possible dividing point is that stage at which twinning, and the combination of two developing zygotes to form one organism, is no longer possible. If something which we could not help but regard as a person were to split, or merge with another person, in such a manner, we would be compelled, in order to ascertain what (if anything) was the continuation of our original person, to rely on such criteria as memory and character. Bodily continuity would not give an unambiguous result. But since a developing zygote has neither memory nor character, we are left without means of resolving questions of personal identity. The potentiality of acquiring memory or character may suffice to ground a claim of personhood, but only with an organism whose unity and uniqueness is firmly secured.

One can hardly leave the question in this state, however, since the question of dividing (and fusing) selves cuts very deeply into the contested question of personal identity. Faced with the possibility of a dividing self, there are, I think, three different possible responses. One can employ such a possibility to undermine our idea of a person, of one being persisting throughout the human life span.[8] Such a course would seem to overthrow a great deal of our moral universe, not least our ethics of homicide. A second strategy is the heroic course of regarding the self before a division as in fact two selves, so that each subsequent self will have the whole pre-split history as part of its past. The implausibility of this position need hardly be labored. The third possibility treats the question of who a given person is (in split cases) as relative to the temporal perspective from which the question is asked. Asked from before the split, the question leads us to pick out a *Y*-shaped "lifetime," including the pre-split self, and both subsequent branches. Asked from the perspective of afterwards, the question leads us to pick out one of the post-split selves, including the pre-split self as part of its history. The labored quality of this solution means that it can coexist with our concept of a person only when splits remain extraordinary (or a mere possibility): it is a precondition of the kind of language of selves that we have that selves normally neither split nor fuse.[9] Hence there is a legitimate presumption against positions which require us to admit splitting or fusing selves, and hence also the capacity for fission and fusion enjoyed by the one-celled zygote is a legitimate moral difference between it and an infant or older embryo which warrants our regarding it as not a person. It hardly seems plausible to regard a distinction linked to our very concept of a person as arbitrary.

If this cut-off point is accepted, we are committed to the existence of bits of human biological material which are neither human organisms, nor parts of human organisms, but things which are becoming human organisms. But this of itself provides no warrant for extending the category of "human becoming" to embryos and fetuses generally.[10] For the behavior of the zygote is quite clearly an anomaly, and any way we choose to deal with it is going to produce some degree of conceptual discomfort. At least where the context is an ethical one, the category of "human becoming" seems to be the least uncomfortable way of dealing with the problem. But being an embryo can still be part of the life cycle of members of the human species, as being a caterpillar is part of the life cycle of members of various species of butterfly. For the justification present in the zygotic case for introducing an anomalous concept is not present in the embryonic one.

b. A plausible but troublesome dividing point is suggested by a difficulty of persuasion which the opponent of abortion commonly faces: the invisibility of his client, the fetus. (Consider the frequent occurrence of abortion in lists of crimes without victims.) This difficulty is met, at least in part, by photographs of fetuses *in utero* and of the results of abortion now widely available. But such persuasive devices have a very important limitation: they are of use only when the unborn creature has some semblance of human form.

This line of reasoning suggests that a necessary criterion of personhood is the possibility that the creature regarded as a person be the object of at least a modicum of human sympathy, and that such sympathy cannot in principle be extended to embryonic life lacking any semblance of human form even when the standard of comparison is an infant rather than an adult. . . .

On the other hand, it is essential that the limitation on human sympathy in question be in some sense intrinsic and inherent. To allow merely contingent limitations upon our sympathy to delimit those who are entitled to rights would be to sanction every kind of prejudice. One cannot for instance justify—though one can of course *explain*—the difficulty many people have in regarding the fetus as an object of serious moral concern by appealing to the limited nature of the encounters mature humans have with it.[11] At least, when such concern is *possible,* sufficient basis for regarding such concern as appropriate is provided by the consideration that the fetus is a member of the human species which will in due course do the things we normally think of as human. And I know of no way of proving that fellow-feeling for zygotes is impossible, apart from a showing (not available without independent reasons for not regarding the nascent human organism as a person) that such sympathy is so radically inappropriate as to be humanly unintelligible. Certainly some people have believed, if only because the logic of their argument required (or appeared to require) it, that zygotes were human persons.

Supposing fellow-feeling for zygotes to be impossible (in the relevant sense of "impossible"), we are faced with the question of at what point fellow-feeling for the nascent human organism becomes a possibility. And the answer to this question may well depend on the mood in which we approach the data (in particular the photographs). In any case, the latest cut-off point which seems at all defensible on this kind of ground is six weeks. After that point, while one might have difficulty feeling sympathy for a fetus (or indeed an infant or an adult of another race), there seems to be no way of maintaining that such sympathy is impossible or unintelligible.

c. None of the other proposed intrauterine dividing points is in the end credible. The beginning of heart or brain activity gains its plausibility from the criteria of death, but the cessation of such activity is a criterion of death only because it is irreversible: when, as in the embryonic case, such activity will begin in due course, there is no reason to regard its absence as decisive on the personhood issue. Growth alone, combined with the possibility of future activity, seems sufficient to justify the finding that the distinctively human kind of life is present, unless we are able to find some other reason for denying the immature embryo the status of a person, or are prepared to revert to the present enjoyment principle and treat infants as well as fetuses as subpersonal.

Writing in defense of a brain-activity criterion, Baruch Brody asks:

Imagine the following science-fiction case: imagine that medical technology has reached the stage at which, when brain death occurs, the brain is removed, "liquefied," and "recast" into a new functioning brain. The new brain bears no relation to the old one (it has none of its memory traces and so on). If the new brain were put back into the old body, would the same human being exist or a new human being who made use of the body of the old one? I am inclined to suppose the latter. But consider the entity whose body has died. Is he not like the fetus? Both have the potential for developing into an entity with a functioning brain (we shall call this a weak potential) but neither now has the structure of a functioning brain.[12]

The answer is that there is this crucial distinction between the two sorts of "weak potential." The weak potential of the fetus includes genetic information, with which the fetus will, in due course, generate a brain of its own. The weak potential of a brain-dead individual is merely the capacity to sustain a brain which can be imposed upon it from the outside.

Of course the absence of brain activity means that the unborn organism is not conscious, but once again this lack of consciousness, being merely temporary, has no decisive moral weight. Conversely, the responses to stimuli observed in very young embryos do not of themselves establish personhood—that must rest on the capacity for distinctively human development—whether or not these responses indicate consciousness in the usual sense. They do, however, like human form, provide a possible basis for sympathy.

d. Quickening has moral relevance of a secondary sort, since it affects the way a woman perceives the life within her, and hence also the social results of the widespread practice of abortion. But it does not represent any biologically or morally significant stage in the development of the fetus itself.

The decisive objection to viability is not that it is unclear precisely when a given fetus is capable of prolonged life outside the womb—with the result that legal definitions of viability are often too late. It is not necessary to demand that the line between persons and nonpersons be perfectly precise, so long as it is clear enough to enable us to make intelligent decisions regarding abortion and other such issues; it is necessary to demand only that it not be arbitrary. Nor is it decisive that viability is relative to medical technology. (So, on many views, is death.) The decisive objection to viability is that there is no reason to suppose that the fact that a given creature cannot live outside a given environment provides a reason why depriving it of that environment should be morally acceptable. (And the independent viability of even a born human being is of course a highly relative matter.) The moral significance of viability, like that of quickening, is secondary. It results from our ability to relieve a woman of burdensome pregnancy while preserving the fetus alive—by premature birth rather than abortion in the usual sense. But the relevance of this point is limited, since prematurity has its hazards.

e. Although birth is given considerable significance by our law and conventional morality (otherwise this section would not have to be written), it is still difficult to see how it can be treated as morally decisive. Considered as a shift from one sort of dependency to another, I believe it has little moral importance. The severance of the umbilical cord removes the child, not from the body of his mother, but from the placenta, an organ of his own for which he has no further use. The social and administrative importance of birth is well accounted for in terms of practicality and discretion irrelevant to the abortion issue. One example is the reckoning of United States citizenship from birth rather than conception; another is the practice of not counting fetuses in the census.

And the grounds given by H. Tristram Engelhardt for distinguishing between fetus and infant, "that the mother-fetus relationship is not an instance of a generally established social relation," whereas "the infant, in virtue of being able to assume the role 'child,' is socialized in terms of this particular role, and a personality is *imputed* to it,"[13] are in fact an argument for drawing the line some time, say twenty-four hours, after birth. It would be possible to postpone the imputation of personality (signalized by naming) for such a period in order to look for defects and decide whether to kill the infant or spare it. On the assumption . . . that newborn infants are persons, Engelhardt's argument must therefore be rejected.

Finally, treating birth as the dividing point between the human and the nonhuman places a rationally indefensible premium on modes of abortion designed to kill the unborn infant within the womb, since once removed from the womb a fetus is born, and thus human by the suggested criterion, and is therefore entitled to be kept alive if prospects of success exist. Some might try to get around this by stipulating that whether a creature of the human species counts as an infant (with a right to life) or an abortus (which doesn't have one) depends on the intentions with which it is delivered. This kind of proposal seems quite arbitrary, however.

4. A final objection to the claim that abortion is homicide is the argument *ad hominem*. Ralph B. Potter, Jr., phrases this objection:

> Neither the church nor the state nor the family actually carries out the practices logically entailed by the affirmation that the fetus is fully human. The church does not baptize the outpouring spontaneously aborted soon after conception. Extreme unction is not given. Funeral rites are not performed. The state calculates age from date of birth, not of conception, and does not require a death or a burial or a birth certificate nor even a report of the demise of a fetus aborted early in pregnancy. Convicted abortionists are not subjected to penalities for murder. The intensity of grief felt within a family over a miscarriage is typically less than that experienced upon the loss of an infant, an older child, or an adult.[14]

But alongside the indications of a less than personal status for the fetus in our laws and customs listed by defenders of abortion, there have been many indications of fetal personhood. Since Potter mentions baptism, it is worth remarking that the Roman Catholic Church ordains the baptism of embryos of whatever degree of maturity, although problems of feasibility naturally arise in cases close to conception because the nascent organism is so small. And Protestants who do not baptize fetuses need not be expressing a lesser evaluation of unborn life, but only a non-Catholic baptismal theology. (Certainly many Protestants have condemned abortion, as have many non-Christians, who of course do not baptize anyone.)

There have been many indications that the fetus has been considered a person in the law of torts and the law of property. One might also notice the holding of a New York court that a fetus is a patient for the purposes of the doctor-patient testimonial privilege,[15] as well as the traditional reluctance to execute a pregnant woman and the accompanying feeling that the killing of a pregnant woman is a peculiarly reprehensible act. And men and women sometimes feel significant grief over the loss of an unborn child. Even contemporary sensibility has little difficulty personalizing a fetus—calling it a ''baby,'' and using the pronouns ''he'' and ''she''—in the context, say, of instruction in the facts of reproduction or in the techniques of prenatal care. Finally, the existence of inherited norms forbidding abortion itself testifies to a recognition of fetal rights.[16]

Some (although hardly all) of the above features of our laws and customs might be explained in other terms. A fetus might be treated as a person with a condition subsequent,[17] in other words as having rights (now), subject to the rebuttable expectation that it will mature. So artificial a concept—while no doubt acceptable in law—should not be introduced into morality without very compelling justification. A few might tend to think of a fetus as a person when its interests and those of its mother work together (for instance in the getting of food stamps),[18] while doubting its status only when the mother herself desires to be rid of her child. But it is difficult to see how this could be justified.

Moreover, the practices that seem to point away from fetal personhood can be explained in other ways. To the extent that funeral practices are designed to deal with a severed relationship, they are not necessary when no such relationship has been established. The same can be said of the rule of inheritance cited by Joel Feinberg as counting against fetal personhood: ''A posthumous child . . . may inherit; but if he dies in the womb, or is stillborn, his inheritance fails to take effect, and no one can claim through him, though it would have been different if he lived for an hour after birth.''[19] It can be explained in part as a special rule of intestate succession designed (*inter alia*) to guarantee that spurious or doubtful pregnancy will not confuse inheritance. The disposition of its property is in any case a matter of indifference to a dead fetus. Finally, the reluctance of the courts to treat the fetus as a human person in criminal-law contexts other than abortion requested by a pregnant woman[20] can be explained as reflecting an unwillingness of courts to read criminal statutes more broadly than their language requires.

Nor is it necessary that the opponent of abortion insist that abortion be treated, legally or socially, as murder. The difficult situation pregnancy often poses for a woman, and the difficulty many people feel in regarding the fetus as a human person—in particular the understandable difficulty some women have in regarding the fetus as a person separate from themselves—suffice to mitigate abortion to a moral analogue of (voluntary) manslaughter. Another analogy is the special offense of infanticide which exists in a number of jurisdictions.[21] On the other hand, while these mitigating circumstances are quite powerful when the well-being of another human being—the mother—is at stake, the opponent of abortion need have no hesitation in regarding as murder (and demanding the severest punishment for) the killing of embryos where what is at stake is only scientific curiosity—for instance when embryos conceived *in vitro* are disposed of, or when embryos are conceived *in vitro* with the intent that they should be so disposed of if they survive.

When conventional morality is ambiguous, the rational course is to resolve its ambiguities in the most coherent way possible. And the result of so doing is to ascribe a right to live to the fetus or embryo from the sixth week of gestation at the very latest, since this is the latest point at which the possibility of arousing sympathy might be said to begin. It should be added that, where there is even some probability that the life at stake in a decision is that of a human person, some morally persuasive reason, even if not so grave a one as is required to warrant what is clearly homicide, is required if that life is to be rightly taken.

• • •

I would also argue—though I cannot do so in detail here —that if unborn children are persons there is no reason why the law should not accord them protection.[22] Even if their status is a matter of reasonable doubt, the law might well prefer to be on the safe side on this issue. Protecting unborn children against killing falls squarely within the scope of the principle permitting restrictions on liberty to avert harm to others. And the argument sometimes made against anti-abortion laws—that they forbid inconspicuous conduct not clearly condemned by the prevailing moral culture—is not of sufficient strength to require us to tolerate unjustified killing.

A woman's right to control the use made of her body might, in legal contexts at least, override the unborn child's right to life in cases of rape, where one can fairly say that the woman has been forced to become pregnant. But when the risk of conception has been voluntarily assumed, such an argument has considerably less force. And there ought to be ways of helping distressed pregnant women, and of improving the lot of the poor, which do not involve the taking of human life.

There is, moreover, no objection in principle to judicial intervention to protect the unborn (as has taken place in West Germany). But judicial intervention to withdraw such protection (as has happened in the United States) is in the highest degree objectionable both from a legal and from a moral standpoint. It is a matter for bitter irony that the Supreme Court should have deferred to the judgment of the elected representatives of the people when judicial homicide was in question, but have substituted its own judgment on the side of killing when the issue was one of the protection of life.[23]

NOTES

1. Joel Feinberg, ed., *The Problem of Abortion* (Belmont, Calif., 1973), p. 4.

2. "Individual: . . . An object which is determined by properties peculiar to itself and cannot be divided into others of the same kind" (OED). Thus bicycles, embryos of more than four weeks gestation, and infants are individuals, whereas water droplets, zygotes, and amoebas are not. Nor, by a natural extension of the same idea, are pairs of sperm and egg, since they can be split and rearranged to form other pairs.

3. See Mortimer Adler, *The Difference of Man and the Difference It Makes* (New York, 1967). As Adler notices, the belief that man differs radically from brute animals would not be refuted by a discovery that dolphins (say) were not brute animals after all.

4. See Robert Morison, "Death: Process or Event?" and Leon R. Kass, "Death as an Event: A Commentary on Robert Morison," both in Richard W. Wertz, ed., *Readings on Ethical and Social Aspects of Bio-medicine* (Englewood Cliffs, N.J., 1973), pp. 105–109, 109–113.

5. If the child were under ten, G. R. Grice would presumably think he could be (*Grounds of Moral Judgement* [Cambridge, Eng., 1967], pp. 147–150).

6. There does not appear to be any information on the sentencing of those, other than their parents, who kill children, since statistics on punishment are gathered according to the characteristics of the offender rather than those of the victim.

7. This is the argument made in Morison.

8. So, following Hume, Derek Parfit, "Personal Identity," *Philosophical Review*, 80 (1971), 13–27.

9. These strategies are taken from John Perry, "Can the Self Divide?" *Journal of Philosophy*, 69 (1972), 463–488.

10. The move to which I am objecting is made by Lawrence C. Becker, "Human Being: The Boundaries of the Concept," *Philosophy & Public Affairs*, 4 (1975), esp. p. 340.

11. See Wertheimer, and Ronald Green, ''Conferred Rights and the Fetus,'' *Journal of Religious Ethics,* Spring 1974 (contrasting the sympathy-arousing circumstances in which we view new-born infants). Green sees that the situation of doctors and nurses—who are asked actually to *perform* abortions—is rather different (pp. 70ff.). His response to their problem seems to be to counsel self-deception.

12. Baruch Brody, *Abortion and the Sanctity of Human Life* (Cambridge, Mass., 1975), pp. 113–114.

13. H. Tristram Engelhardt, ''Viability, Abortion, and the Difference between a Fetus and an Infant,'' *American Journal of Obstetrics and Gynecology,* 116 (1973), 432.

14. Ralph B. Potter, Jr., ''The Abortion Debate,'' in Donald R. Cutler, ed., *Updating Life and Death* (Boston, 1969), p. 117.

15. *Jones v. Jones,* 114 N.Y.S. 2d 820 (1955).

16. See also the testimony from art and literature eloquently mustered by Noonan, *How to Argue about Abortion* (New York, 1974), pp. 17–19.

17. The suggestion is due to William T. Barker.

18. See for instance *Burns v. Alcala,* 95 S. Ct. 1180, 1187–1189 (Marshall, J. dissenting). Justice Marshall was part of the majority in the abortion decisions.

19. John Salmond, *Jurisprudence,* 11th ed., p. 355, quoted in *Problems of Abortion,* p. 7. Notice the pronouns, however.

20. *Keeler v. Superior Court,* 470 P. 2d 617 (Calif., 1970) (killing of unborn child by woman's estranged husband not murder), *State v. Dickinson,* 28 Ohio St. 65 (1970) (vehicular homicide). The *Keeler* holding has been reversed by statute, California Penal Code, sec. 187 (feticide under some circumstances murder).

21. Compare Kant's remarks on bastard infanticide in the *Metaphysical Elements of Justice,* John Ladd, tr. (New York, 1965), p. 106.

22. Next to abortion, the forms of private homicide whose legal aspects have received the most attention are suicide and euthanasia.

23. On abortion and the law, see Baruch Brody, *Abortion and the Sanctity of Human Life* (Cambridge, Mass., 1975), chs. 3, 10; and John Finnis, ''Three Schemes of Regulation,'' in John T. Noonan, Jr., ed., *The Morality of Abortion* (Cambridge, Mass., 1970). On the constitutional aspects, see John Hart Ely, ''The Wages of Crying Wolf,'' *Yale Law Journal,* 82 (1973), 923–947.

SUGGESTED READINGS FOR CHAPTER 6

Annas, George J. ''The Supreme Court and Abortion: The Irrelevance of Medical Judgment.'' *Hastings Center Report* 10 (October 1980), 23–24.

Brandt, Richard B. ''The Morality of Abortion.'' *The Monist* 36 (October 1972), 503–526.

Brody, Baruch A. ''Abortion and the Sanctity of Human Life.'' *American Philosophical Quarterly* 10 (April 1973), 133–140.

Callahan, Daniel. *Abortion: Law, Choice and Morality.* New York: Macmillan, 1970.

———. ''Abortion and Government Policy.'' *Family Planning Perspectives* 11 (September–October 1979), 275–279.

Connery, John R. *Abortion: The Development of the Roman Catholic Perspective.* Chicago: Loyola University Press, 1977.

Daniels, Charles B. ''Abortion and Potential.'' *Dialogue* 18 (June 1979), 220–223.

Ely, John Hart. ''The Wages of Crying Wolf: A Comment on Roe v. Wade.'' *Yale Law Journal* 82 (April 1973), 920–949.

Engelhardt, H. Tristram, Jr. ''The Ontology of Abortion.'' *Ethics* 84 (April 1974), 217–234.

———. ''Viability and the Use of the Fetus.'' In Beauchamp, Tom L., and Pinkard, Terry. *Ethics and Public Policy,* 2nd edition. Englewood Cliffs, N.J.: Prentice-Hall, 1982. Chap. 9.

English, Jane. ''Abortion and the Concept of a Person.'' *Canadian Journal of Philosophy* 5 (October 1975), 233–243.

Feinberg, Joel, ed. *The Problem of Abortion.* Belmont, Calif.: Wadsworth Publishing Company, 1973.

———. ''Abortion.'' In Regan, Tom, ed. *Matters of Life and Death.* New York: Random House, 1980, pp. 183–217.

Finnis, John. ''The Rights and Wrongs of Abortion: A Reply to Judith Thomson.'' *Philosophy and Public Affairs* 2 (Winter 1973), 117–145.

———. ''Abortion: Legal Aspects.'' In Reich, Warren T., ed., *Encyclopedia of Bioethics.* New York: Free Press, 1978. Vol. 1, pp. 26–32.

Foot, Philippa. ''The Problem of Abortion and the Doctrine of Double Effect.'' *The Oxford Review* 5 (1967), 59–70.

Glover, Jonathan. *Causing Death and Saving Lives.* Harmondsworth, England: Penguin Books, 1977.

Goldman, Alan H. ''Abortion and the Right to Life.'' *Personalist* 60 (October 1979), 402–406.

Hare, R. M. ''Abortion and the Golden Rule.'' *Philosophy and Public Affairs* 4 (Spring 1975), 201–222.

King, Patricia A. ''The Juridical Status of the Fetus: A Proposal for Legal Protection of the Unborn.'' *Michigan Law Review* 77 (August 1979), 1647–1687.

McCormick, Richard A. ''Past Church Teaching on Abortion.'' *Proceedings of the Catholic Theological Society of America* 23 (1968), 131–151.

Mechanic, David. ''The Supreme Court and Abortion: Sidestepping Social Realities.'' *Hastings Center Report* 10 (December 1980), 17–19.

Nicholson, Susan Teft. *Abortion and the Roman Catholic Church.* Knoxville, Tenn.: *Journal of Religious Ethics* Monographs (1978).

Noonan, John T., Jr., ed. *The Morality of Abortion: Legal and Historical Perspectives.* Cambridge, Mass.: Harvard University Press, 1970.

———. *A Private Choice: Abortion in America in the Seventies.* New York: Free Press, 1979.

———. ''The Supreme Court and Abortion: Upholding Constitutional Principles.'' *Hastings Center Report* 10 (December 1980), 14–16.

Perkins, Robert, ed. *Abortion: Pro and Con.* Cambridge, Mass.: Schenkman Publishing Company, 1974.

Ramsey, Paul. ''The Morality of Abortion.'' In Labby, Daniel H., ed. *Life or Death: Ethics and Options.* Seattle, Wash.: University of Washington Press, 1968, pp. 60–93.

Singer, Peter. *Practical Ethics.* New York: Cambridge University Press, 1979. Chap. 6.

Sterba, James P. ''Abortion, Distant Peoples and Future Generations.'' *Journal of Philosophy* 77 (July 1980), 424–440.

Sumner, L. W. *Abortion and Moral Theory.* Princeton, N.J.: Princeton University Press, 1981.

Thomson, Judith Jarvis. ''Rights and Deaths.'' *Philosophy and Public Affairs* 2 (Winter 1973), 146–155.

Tooley, Michael. ''Abortion and Infanticide.'' *Philosophy and Public Affairs* 2 (Fall 1972), 37–65.

Tribe, Laurence H. ''Toward a Model of Roles in the Due Process of Life and Law." *Harvard Law Review* 87 (November 1973), 1–53.

Veatch, Robert M. *Case Studies in Medical Ethics*. Cambridge, Mass.: Harvard University Press, 1977. Chap. 7.

Werner, Richard. "Abortion: The Ontological and Moral Status of the Unborn." In Wasserstrom, Richard A., ed. *Today's Moral Problems,* 2nd edition. New York: Macmillan, 1979, pp. 51–74.

Wertheimer, Roger. "Understanding the Abortion Argument." *Philosophy and Public Affairs* 1 (Fall 1971), 67–95.

Zaitchik, Alan. "Viability and the Morality of Abortion." *Philosophy and Public Affairs* 10 (Winter 1981), 18–26.

BIBLIOGRAPHIES

Goldstein, Doris Mueller. *Bioethics: A Guide to Information Sources*. Detroit: Gale Research Company, 1982. See under "Abortion" and "Treatment for Defective Newborns and Infanticide."

Lineback, Richard H., ed. *Philosopher's Index*. Vols. 1– . Bowling Green, Ohio: Philosophy Documentation Center, Bowling Green State University. Issued quarterly. See under "Abortion," "Dignity," "Fetus(es)," "Infanticide," "Life," "Mentally Retarded," "Persons," "Right to Life," "Sanctity of Life," and "Therapeutic Abortion."

Walters, LeRoy, ed. *Bibliography of Bioethics*. Vols. 1– . New York: Free Press. Issued annually. See under "Abortion," "Selective Abortion," and "Therapeutic Abortion." (The information contained in the annual *Bibliography of Bioethics* can also be retrieved from BIOETHICSLINE, an online data base of the National Library of Medicine.)

7.
The Definition and Determination of Death

The subject matter of this chapter has been anticipated in part by Chapter 3, which discussed the problem of personhood. The present chapter is also closely related to Chapter 6, in which several biological aspects of early human development were surveyed, and the problem of personhood further studied. Chapter 7, and Chapter 8 as well, focus on conceptual and ethical issues at the end of human life.

RECENT COMPLICATIONS IN THE DEFINITION OF DEATH

Until recently the definition of death seemed relatively clear and unambiguous. Most persons would have accepted, without question, the following definition from *Black's Law Dictionary:*

[Death is:] the cessation of life; the ceasing to exist; defined by physicians as a total stoppage of the circulation of the blood, and a cessation of the animal and vital functions consequent thereon, such as respiration, pulsation, etc.[1]

Two recent biomedical developments have complicated the definition of death. The first is the widespread and increasing use of new devices for the prolongation of life, particularly the artificial respirator. With the aid of such devices, respiration (and consequently heartbeat) can be artificially sustained, at least for a few days, even when the capacity for spontaneous respiration has been temporarily or permanently lost. Thus, a simple reliance on the traditional criteria of blood circulation and respiration may no longer be possible in cases where certain types of artificial life-support systems are employed.

A second development that has pointed up the need for a more adequate definition of death is the use of cadaver organs for transplantation. There are two potentially conflicting interests in the transplantation situation. On the one hand, patients, their families, and the society generally want to be assured that no novel definition of death will allow for the removal of organs from still-living persons. On the other hand, physicians know that the prospects for a successful transplant are improved if an organ can be removed from a cadaver immediately after death has occurred.

In response to these developments, an Ad Hoc Committee of the Harvard Medical School published in 1968 a report entitled "A Definition of Irreversible Coma." Although this document has subsequently been criticized on numerous grounds, it has been primarily responsible for setting the parameters of the current debate on the definition of death.

ANATOMICAL AND PHYSIOLOGICAL BACKGROUND

There are three primary divisions of the human brain: the cerebrum, with its outer shell called the cortex; the cerebellum; and the brainstem. The cerebrum is the center of consciousness and reasoning in human beings. Spontaneous respiration is controlled by the brainstem; in routine situations the respiratory centers in the brainstem control the rate of breathing by sending neural impulses to the muscles of the chest and to the diaphragm via the spinal cord. Before the development of the artificial respirator, any injury that destroyed or incapacitated the brainstem led within twenty minutes to the permanent cessation of spontaneous respiration and heartbeat, that is, to death (as defined by *Black's Law Dictionary* and other standard sources). However, the use of various resuscitative techniques can sometimes arrest this rapid transition from life to death, leaving the injured patient in a partially functioning status. In some cases the patient can be restored to full function. In others the deterioration process can only be delayed but not stopped, and the patient dies within a few days or weeks. In still other cases the patient remains indefinitely in a state somewhere between full function and death.

Two types of partially functioning status have provoked considerable discussion. In the first case, the brainstem is destroyed but respiration continues with the aid of a respirator. This state is only temporary, however, since heartbeat inevitably ceases within a few days or at most a few weeks in the absence of brainstem activity. Nonetheless, serious questions about the prolongation of life and about resource allocation may arise during the interval between brainstem death and the cessation of heartbeat. In the second case, the brainstem is intact but the cerebrum or the cerebral cortex has been rendered permanently functionless. This constellation of factors often leads to a chronic vegetative state in which there is spontaneous respiration and spontaneous heartbeat but no return of consciousness.

MAJOR CATEGORIES IN THE DEFINITION AND DETERMINATION OF DEATH

Three distinct categories in the discussion of death can be identified: (1) the basic philosophical concept of death; (2) physiological standards for recognizing death; and (3) methods for determining whether the physiological standards have been fulfilled in a particular case.[2]

THE BASIC PHILOSOPHICAL CONCEPT OF DEATH

This category refers to general concepts, or definitions, of death. These concepts of death are frequently based on particular theories of human personhood (see Chapter 3) and are generally not testable through the use of empirical measurements. Among the concepts of death that have been proposed in philosophical discussions are the loss of the capacity for rationality, the loss of the capacity for psychological continuity and connectedness, and the departure of the soul from the body.

PHYSIOLOGICAL STANDARDS

Unlike the basic concepts of death, these standards focus on the functioning of specific bodily systems or organs. In most cases empirical tests are available for verifying that the standards have, or have not, been fulfilled. The traditional physiological standard for recognizing death has been the (irreversible) loss of circulatory and/or respiratory function. Since the advent of artificial respirators, this standard has sometimes been limited to the (irreversible) loss of *spontaneous* circulatory and/or respiratory function. Several recently developed physiological standards focus primary attention on the central nervous system—the brain and spinal cord. Among these standards are the (irreversible) loss of the following functions: reflex activity mediated through the brain or spinal cord; electrical activity in the cerebral neocortex; and/or cerebral blood flow. Both the traditional and the more recently developed standards can be employed either individually or in combination.

METHODS FOR DETERMINING THE FULFILLMENT OF STANDARDS

This category is closely related to the second but refers to specific means for testing whether the physiological standards have been fulfilled. These testing methods frequently change in response to technological advances. In addition, it is possible in some cases to apply several alternative tests to a single standard. For example, the loss of circulatory function can be determined either by taking the patient's pulse or by recording an electrocardiogram. Testing methods that are employed to determine the fulfillment of other standards include the use of electroencephalography to measure electrical activity in the neocortex and the injection of radioactive tracers into the circulatory system for detecting cerebral blood flow.

There is obviously a close correlation between the second and third categories outlined above, the general standards and the specific testing methods. However, the relationship between the first category, basic concepts of death, and the other two categories is a matter of debate. It seems likely that there are correlations between particular concepts of death and particular physiological standards for recognizing death. A stronger and more controversial claim would be that one's concept of death either influences or determines one's choice of a physiological standard for the recognition of death.

CONFLICTING PROPOSALS FOR THE DETERMINATION OF DEATH

The report of the Harvard Ad Hoc Committee discusses three primary physiological standards for recognizing "irreversible coma," which the Committee calls "a new criterion for death"[3]: (1) unreceptivity and unresponsivity; (2) no spontaneous muscular movements or spontaneous breathing; and (3) no reflexes. A confirmatory standard is the absence of cerebral function, as indicated by a flat electroencephalogram.

The essays by Jonas and Veatch represent sharply divergent responses to the position of the Harvard Ad Hoc Committee. Jonas criticizes the Ad Hoc Committee for attempting to draw a sharp line between life and death when in fact, according to Jonas, life often shades imperceptibly into death. He also rejects the Committee's requirement of *spontaneous* respiration, arguing that artificially sustained life is nonetheless life. In addition, Jonas regards the loss of central nervous system function—even the total loss of brain function—as irrelevant to the question of *defining* death. In his view, the current emphasis on whole-brain or cerebral function is based on an unhealthy mind-body dualism. Jonas's essay thus reflects a return to traditional physiological standards for recognizing death and a refusal to adjust those standards merely because of medicine's new ability to maintain respiratory function and to measure electrical activity in the brain.

A second perspective on the Harvard Ad Hoc Committee criteria is presented by Robert Veatch, who argues that the Committee did not go far enough in the direction of brain death. In his view, the irreversible loss of functioning in the highest region of the brain—the cerebral neocortex—is the primary physiological standard for the recognition of death. Other central nervous system functions, such as the mediation of spinal or brainstem reflexes or the activation of spontaneous respiration, are on this view irrelevant to the question of life and death. Indeed, Veatch seems willing to go a step further by arguing that the bare functioning of the cerebral neocortex is an inadequate physiological standard. He notes that low-level functioning of the cerebral neocortex may lead to the mistaken conclusion that a patient is alive when in fact all capacity for both consciousness and social interaction has been lost. (Think, for example, of a case like that of Karen Quinlan—discussed in Chapter 8—in which measurable cerebral activity and irreversible coma are both present.) Veatch's viewpoint thus represents the polar opposite of Jonas's position and rejects, as well, many of the standards proposed by the Harvard Ad Hoc Committee.

As the preceding paragraphs make clear, there is a close correlation between the topics of this chapter and the succeeding chapter. Indeed, some borderline cases can be analyzed *either* as cases of determining death (Chapter 7) *or* as cases involving the prolongation of life or euthanasia (Chapter 8), depending upon the physiological standard chosen. For example, Jonas and the Harvard Ad Hoc Committee would classify as ''alive'' a spontaneously breathing individual with a continuously flat electroencephalogram. Therefore, any decision concerning appropriate medical care for the individual would be a decision about whether to prolong the life of the patient. In contrast, the physiological standard proposed by Robert Veatch—electrical activity in the cerebral neocortex—would lead to the categorization of the same individual as ''already dead.'' Thus, logically speaking, the questions of prolonging life and euthanasia could not arise.

LEGAL APPROACHES TO THE DEFINITION AND DETERMINATION OF DEATH

The issue of criteria for the determination of death has been raised in several American court cases involving organ transplantation. In one civil action a plaintiff charged that his brother's heart had been removed without the family's consent and before the patient had died.[4] In another type of case, defendants charged with murder or manslaughter have argued that surgical removal of the victim's heart for transplantation, not the injury inflicted by the defendant, was the immediate cause of the patient's death.[5] Several states have also enacted statutes that adopt rather divergent criteria for the definition or determination of death.

Capron and Kass recommend the legislative route of policy formulation as preferable to judicial responses to cases that happen to reach the courts. They criticize the earliest death statutes, enacted by Kansas and Maryland, for seeming to propose two alternative ''definitions'' of death, a respiratory-circulatory definition and a brain-oriented definition. In general, Capron and Kass argue that death legislation should seek to set physiological standards for the recognition of death rather than attempting to define death or to prescribe methods for testing whether the physiological standards have been fulfilled. The authors also propose a model statute that includes two physiological standards, a respiratory-circulatory standard for patients who are not on artificial respirators and a whole-brain-oriented standard for respirator-assisted patients.

The Capron-Kass model statute was followed, in the 1970s and early 1980s, by several additional proposals for definition-of-death statutes. In 1980 and 1981 all of these model statutes, as well as existing statutory and case law, were examined in detail by a public advisory body, the President's Commission for the Study of Ethical Problems in Medicine and Biomedical and Behavioral Research. Like Capron and Kass, the Commission developed a model statute that identifies two alternative physiological standards for determining death—a respiratory-circulatory standard and a brain-oriented standard that explicitly requires the irreversible cessation of all brainstem function.

Within the spectrum of ethical positions advocated in this chapter, the model statutes of Capron-Kass and the President's Commission seem to approximate most closely the position of the Harvard Ad Hoc Committee. These model statutes are slightly more liberal than the ethical position of Jonas but considerably more conservative than that of Veatch. Thus, this chapter raises once again the thorny question discussed in the final section of

Chapter 1, namely, how one translates ethical arguments and conclusions into appropriate public policies.

L. W.

NOTES

1. *Black's Law Dictionary,* revised 4th edition, 1968, p. 488.

2. Similar distinctions are developed by Alexander M. Capron and Leon R. Kass in the final selection of this chapter. The categories designated by Capron and Kass as ''general physiological standards'' and ''operational criteria'' have been combined under the single heading ''physiological standards.''

3. Reprinted in this chapter.

4. City of Richmond, Law and Equity Court, *Tucker's Administrator v. Lower,* No. 2831, May 25, 1972.

5. See, for example, the cases discussed by Linda Ekstrom Stanley. ''The Law of Homicide: Does It Require a Definition of Death?'' *Wake Forest Law Review* 11 (June, 1975), especially pp. 253–255.

THE AD HOC COMMITTEE[1]

A Definition of Irreversible Coma

Our primary purpose is to define irreversible coma as a new criterion for death. There are two reasons why there is need for a definition: (1) Improvements in resuscitative and supportive measures have led to increased efforts to save those who are desperately injured. Sometimes these efforts have only partial success so that the result is an individual whose heart continues to beat but whose brain is irreversibly damaged. The burden is great on patients who suffer permanent loss of intellect, on their families, on the hospitals, and on those in need of hospital beds already occupied by these comatose patients. (2) Obsolete criteria for the definition of death can lead to controversy in obtaining organs for transplantation.

Irreversible coma has many causes, but *we are concerned here only with those comatose individuals who have no discernible central nervous system activity.* If the characteristics can be defined in satisfactory terms, translatable into action—and we believe this is possible—then several problems will either disappear or will become more readily soluble.

More than medical problems are present. There are moral, ethical, religious, and legal issues. Adequate definition here will prepare the way for better insight into all of these matters as well as for better law than is currently applicable.

CHARACTERISTICS OF IRREVERSIBLE COMA

An organ, brain or other, that no longer functions and has no possibility of functioning again is for all practical purposes dead. Our first problem is to determine the characteristics of a *permanently* nonfunctioning brain.

A patient in this state appears to be in deep coma.

Reprinted by permission of the author and the publisher from "A Definition of Irreversible Coma," a report of the Ad Hoc Committee of the Harvard Medical School, *Journal of the American Medical Association,* Vol. 205, No. 6 (August 1968), pp. 337–340. Copyright 1968, American Medical Association.

The condition can be satisfactorily diagnosed by points 1, 2, and 3 to follow. The electroencephalogram (point 4) provides confirmatory data, and when available it should be utilized. In situations where for one reason or another electroencephalographic monitoring is not available, the absence of cerebral function has to be determined by purely clinical signs, to be described, or by absence of circulation as judged by standstill of blood in the retinal vessels, or by absence of cardiac activity.

1. *Unreceptivity and Unresponsitivity.* There is a total unawareness to externally applied stimuli and inner need and complete unresponsiveness—our definition of irreversible coma. Even the most intensely painful stimuli evoke no vocal or other response, not even a groan, withdrawal of a limb, or quickening of respiration.

2. *No Movements or Breathing.* Observations covering a period of at least one hour by physicians is adequate to satisfy the criteria of no spontaneous muscular movements or spontaneous respiration or response to stimuli such as pain, touch, sound, or light. After the patient is on a mechanical respirator, the total absence of spontaneous breathing may be established by turning off the respirator for three minutes and observing whether there is any effort on the part of the subject to breathe spontaneously. (The respirator may be turned off for this time provided that at the start of the trial period the patient's carbon dioxide tension is within the normal range, and provided also that the patient had been breathing room air for at least 10 minutes prior to the trial.)

3. *No Reflexes.* Irreversible coma with abolition of central nervous system activity is evidenced in part by the absence of elicitable reflexes. The pupil will be fixed and dilated and will not respond to a direct source of bright light. Since the establishment of a fixed, dilated pupil is clear-cut in clinical practice, there should be no uncertainty as to its presence.

Ocular movement (to head turning and to irrigation of the ears with ice water) and blinking are absent. There is no evidence of postural activity (decerebrate or other). Swallowing, yawning, vocalization are in abeyance. Corneal and pharyngeal reflexes are absent.

As a rule the stretch of tendon reflexes cannot be elicited; i.e., tapping the tendons of the biceps, triceps, and pronator muscles, quadriceps and gastrocnemius muscles with the reflex hammer elicits no contraction of the respective muscles. Plantar or noxious stimulation gives no response.

4. *Flat Electroencephalogram*. Of great confirmatory value is the flat or isoelectric EEG. We must assume that the electrodes have been properly applied, that the apparatus is functioning normally, and that the personnel in charge is competent. We consider it prudent to have one channel of the apparatus used for an electrocardiogram. This channel will monitor the ECG so that, if it appears in the electroencephalographic leads because of high resistance, it can be readily identified. It also establishes the presence of the active heart in the absence of the EEG. We recommend that another channel be used for a noncephalic lead. This will pick up space-borne or vibration-borne artifacts and identify them. The simplest form of such a monitoring noncephalic electrode has two leads over the dorsum of the hand, preferably the right hand, so the ECG will be minimal or absent. Since one of the requirements of this state is that there be no muscle activity, these two dorsal hand electrodes will not be bothered by muscle artifact. The apparatus should be run at standard gains 10μv/mm, 50μv/5 mm. Also it should be isoelectric at double this standard gain, which is 5μv/5 mm or 25μv/5 mm. At least ten full minutes of recording are desirable, but twice that would be better.

It is also suggested that the gains at some point be opened to their full amplitude for a brief period (5 to 100 seconds) to see what is going on. Usually in an intensive care unit artifacts will dominate the picture, but these are readily identifiable. There shall be no electroencephalographic response to noise or to pinch.

All of the above tests shall be repeated at least 24 hours later with no change.

The validity of such data as indications of irreversible cerebral damage depends on the exclusion of two conditions: hypothermia (temperature below 90 F [32.2C]) or central nervous system depressants, such as barbiturates.

OTHER PROCEDURES

The patient's condition can be determined only by a physician. When the patient is hopelessly damaged as defined above, the family and all colleagues who have participated in major decisions concerning the patient, and all nurses involved, should be so informed. Death is to be declared and *then* the respirator turned off. The decision to do this and the responsibility for it are to be taken by the physician-in-charge, in consultation with one or more physicians who have been directly involved in the case. It is unsound and undesirable to force the family to make the decision.

LEGAL COMMENTARY

The legal system of the United States is greatly in need of the kind of analysis and recommendations for medical procedures in cases of irreversible brain damage as described. At present, the law of the United States, in all 50 states and in the federal courts, treats the question of human death as a question of fact to be decided in every case. When any doubt exists, the courts seek medical expert testimony concerning the time of death of the particular individual involved. However, the law makes the assumption that the medical criteria for determining death are settled and not in doubt among physicians. Furthermore, the law assumes that the traditional method among physicians for determination of death is to ascertain the absence of all vital signs. To this extent, *Black's Law Dictionary* (fourth edition, 1951) defines death as

The cessation of life; the ceasing to exist; *defined by physicians* as a total stoppage of the circulation of the blood, and a cessation of the animal and vital functions consequent thereupon, such as respiration, pulsation, etc. [italics added].

In the few modern court decisions involving a definition of death, the courts have used the concept of the total cessation of all vital signs. Two cases are worthy of examination. Both involved the issue of which one of two persons died first.

In *Thomas v. Anderson*, (96 Cal App 2d 371, 211 P 2d 478) a California District Court of Appeal in 1950 said, "In the instant case the question as to which of the two men died first was a question of fact for the determination of the trial court . . ."

The appellate court cited and quoted in full the definition of death from *Black's Law Dictionary* and concluded, ". . . death occurs precisely when life ceases and does not occur until the heart stops beating and respiration ends. Death is not a continuous event and is an event that takes place at a precise time."

The other case is *Smith v. Smith* (229 Ark, 579, 317 SW 2d 275) decided in 1958 by the Supreme Court of Arkansas. In this case the two people were husband and wife involved in an auto accident. The husband was found dead at the scene of the accident. The wife was taken to the hospital unconscious. It is alleged that she "remained in coma due to brain injury" and died at the hospital 17 days later. The petitioner in court tried to argue that the two people died simultaneously. The judge writing the opinion said the petition contained a "quite unusual and unique allegation." It was quoted as follows:

That the said Hugh Smith and his wife, Lucy Coleman Smith, were in an automobile accident on the 19th day of April, 1957, said accident being instantly fatal to each of them at the same time, although the doctors maintained a vain hope of survival and made every effort to revive and resuscitate said Lucy Coleman Smith until May 6th, 1957, when it was finally determined by the attending physicians that their hope of resuscitation and possible restoration of human life to the said Lucy Coleman Smith was entirely vain, and

That as a matter of modern medical science, your petitioner alleges and states, and will offer the Court competent proof that the said Hugh Smith, deceased, and said Lucy Coleman Smith, deceased, lost their power to will at the same instant, and that their demise as earthly human beings occurred at the same time in said automobile accident, neither of them ever regaining any consciousness whatsoever.

The court dismissed the petition as a *matter of law*. The court quoted *Black's* definition of death and concluded

Admittedly, this condition did not exist, and as a matter of fact, it would be too much of a strain of credulity for us to believe any evidence offered to the effect that Mrs. Smith was dead, scientifically or otherwise, unless the conditions set out in the definition existed.

Later in the opinion the court said, "Likewise, we take judicial notice that one breathing, though unconscious, is not dead."

"Judicial notice" of this definition of death means that the court did not consider that definition open to serious controversy; it considered the question as settled in responsible scientific and medical circles. The judge thus makes proof of uncontroverted facts unnecessary so as to prevent prolonging the trial with unnecessary proof and also to prevent fraud being committed upon the court by quasi "scientists" being called into court to controvert settled scientific principles at a price. Here, the Arkansas Supreme Court considered the definition of death to be a settled, scientific, biological fact. It refused to consider the plaintiff's offer of evidence that "modern medical science" might say otherwise. In simplified form, the above is the state of the law in the United States concerning the definition of death.

In this report, however, we suggest that responsible medical opinion is ready to adopt new criteria for pronouncing death to have occurred in an individual sustaining irreversible coma as a result of permanent brain damage. If this position is adopted by the medical community, it can form the basis for change in the current legal concept of death. No statutory change in the law should be necessary since the law treats this question essentially as one of fact to be determined by physicians. The only circumstance in which it would be necessary that legislation be offered in the various states to define "death" by law would be in the event that great controversy were engendered surrounding the subject and physicians were unable to agree on the new medical criteria.

It is recommended as a part of these procedures that judgment of the existence of these criteria is solely a medical issue. It is suggested that the physician in charge of the patient consult with one or more other physicians directly involved in the case before the patient is declared dead on the basis of these criteria. In this way, the responsibility is shared over a wider range of medical opinion, thus providing an important degree of protection against later questions which might be raised about the particular case. It is further suggested that the decision to declare the person dead, and then to turn off the respirator, be made by physicians not involved in any later effort to transplant organs or tissue from the deceased individual. This is advisable in order to avoid any appearance of self-interest by the physicians involved.

It should be emphasized that we recommend the patient be declared dead before any effort is made to take him off a respirator, if he is then on a respirator. This declaration should not be delayed until he has been taken off the respirator and all artificially stimulated signs have ceased. The reason for this recommendation is that in our judgment it will provide a greater degree of legal protection to those involved. Otherwise, the physicians would be turning off the respirator on a person who is, under the present strict, technical application of law, still alive.

COMMENT

Irreversible coma can have various causes: cardiac arrest; asphyxia with respiratory arrest; massive brain damage; intracranial lesions, neoplastic or vascular. It can be produced by other encephalopathic states such as the metabolic derangements associated, for example, with uremia. Respiratory failure and impaired circulation underlie all of these conditions. They result in hypoxia and ischemia of the brain.

From ancient times down to the recent past it was clear that, when the respiration and heart stopped, the brain would die in a few minutes; so the obvious criterion of no heartbeat as synonymous with death was sufficiently accurate. In those times the heart was considered to be the central organ of the body; it is not surprising that its failure marked the onset of death. This is no longer valid when modern resuscitative and supportive measures are used. These improved activities can now restore "life" as judged by the ancient standards of persistent respiration and continuing heartbeat. This can be the case even when there is not the remotest possibility of an individual recovering consciousness following massive brain damage. In other situations "life" can be maintained only by means of artificial respiration and electrical stimulation of the heartbeat, or in temporarily bypassing the heart, or, in conjunction with these things, reducing with cold the body's oxygen requirement.

In an address, "The Prolongation of Life" (1957),[2] Pope Pius XII raised many questions; some conclusions stand out: (1) In a deeply unconscious individual vital functions may be maintained over a prolonged period only by extraordinary means. Verification of the moment of death can be determined, if at all, only by a physician. Some have suggested that the moment of death is the moment when irreparable and overwhelming brain damage occurs. Pius XII acknowledged that it is not "within the competence of the Church" to determine this. (2) It is incumbent on the physician to take all reasonable, ordinary means of restoring the spontaneous vital functions and consciousness, and to employ such extraordinary means

as are available to him to this end. It is not obligatory, however, to continue to use extraordinary means indefinitely in hopeless cases. "But normally one is held to use only ordinary means—according to circumstances of persons, places, times, and cultures—that is to say, means that do not involve any grave burden for oneself or another." It is the church's view that a time comes when resuscitative efforts should stop and death be unopposed.

SUMMARY

The neurological impairment to which the terms "brain death syndrome" and "irreversible coma" have become attached indicates diffuse disease. Function is abolished at cerebral, brain-stem, and often spinal levels. This should be evident in all cases from clinical examination alone. Cerebral, cortical, and thalamic involvement are indicated by a complete absence of receptivity of all forms of sensory stimulation and a lack of response to stimuli and to inner need. The term "coma" is used to designate this state of unreceptivity and unresponsivity. But there is always coincident paralysis of brain-stem and basal ganglionic mechanisms as manifested by an abolition of all postural reflexes, including induced decerebrate postures; a complete paralysis of respiration; widely dilated, fixed pupils; paralysis of ocular movements; swallowing; phonation; face and tongue muscles. Involvement of spinal cord, which is less constant, is reflected usually in loss of tendon reflex and all flexor withdrawal or nocifensive reflexes. Of the brain-stem-spinal mechanisms which are conserved for a time, the vasomotor reflexes are the most persistent, and they are responsible in part for the paradoxical state of retained cardiovascular function, which is to some extent independent of nervous control, in the face of widespread disorder of cerebrum, brain stem, and spinal cord.

Neurological assessment gains in reliability if the aforementioned neurological signs persist over a period of time, with the additional safeguards that there is no accompanying hypothermia or evidence of drug intoxication. If either of the latter two conditions exist, interpretation of the neurological state should await the return of body temperature to normal level and elimination of the intoxicating agent. Under any other circumstances, repeated examinations over a period of 24 hours or longer should be required in order to obtain evidence of the irreversibility of the condition.

NOTES

1. The Ad Hoc Committee includes Henry K. Beecher, MD, *chairman;* Raymond D. Adams, MD; A. Clifford Barger, MD;

William J. Curran, LLM, SMHyg; Derek Denny-Brown, MD; Dana L. Farnsworth, MD; Jordi Folch-Pi, MD; Everett I. Mendelsohn, PhD; John P. Merrill, MD; Joseph Murray, MD; Ralph Potter, ThD; Robert Schwab, MD; and William Sweet, MD.

2. Pius XII: The Prolongation of Life, *Pope Speaks* 4:393–398 (No. 4) 1958.

R O B E R T   M .   V E A T C H

Defining Death Anew: Technical and Ethical Problems

Four separate levels in the definition of death debate must be distinguished. First, there is the purely formal analysis of the term *death*, an analysis that gives the structure and specifies framework that must be filled in with content. Second, the *concept* of death is considered, attempting to fill the content of the formal definition. At this level the question is, What is so essentially significant about life that its loss is termed *death?* Third, there is the question of the locus of death: where in the organism ought one to look to determine whether death has occurred? Fourth, one must ask the question of the criteria of death: what technical tests must be applied at the locus to determine if an individual is living or dead?

Serious mistakes have been made in slipping from one level of the debate to another and in presuming that expertise on one level necessarily implies expertise on another. For instance, the Report of the Ad Hoc Committee of the Harvard Medical School to Examine the Definition of Brain Death is titled "A Definition of Irreversible Coma."[1] The report makes clear that the committee members are simply reporting empirical measures which are criteria for predicting an irreversible coma. (I shall explore later the possibility that they made an important mistake even at this level.) Yet the name of the committee seems to

Reprinted with permission of the publisher from *Death, Dying and the Biological Revolution: Our Last Quest for Responsibility* (New Haven: Yale University Press, 1976), pp. 24–26, 29–33, 36–51.

point more to the question of locus, where to look for measurement of death. The committee was established to examine the death of the brain. The implication is that the empirical indications of irreversible coma are also indications of "brain death." But by the first sentence of the report the committee claims that "Our primary purpose is to define irreversible coma as a new criterion for death." They have now shifted so that they are interested in "death." They must be presuming a philosophical concept of death—that a person in irreversible coma should be considered dead—but they nowhere argue this or even state it as a presumption.

Even the composition of the Harvard committee membership signals some uncertainty of purpose. If empirical criteria were their concern, the inclusion of nonscientists on the panel was strange. If the philosophical concept of death was their concern, medically trained peopole were overrepresented. As it happened, the committee did not deal at all with conceptual matters. The committee and its interpreters have confused the questions at different levels. The remainder of this [essay] will discuss the meaning of death at these four levels.

THE FORMAL DEFINITION OF DEATH

A strictly formal definition of death might be the following:

Death means a complete change in the status of a living entity

Such a definition would apply equally well to a human being, a nonhuman animal, a plant, an organ, a cell, or even metaphorically to a social phenomenon like a society or to any temporally limited entity like a research project, a sports event, or a language. To define the death of a human being, we must recognize the characteristics that are essential to humanness. It is quite inadequate to limit the discussion to the death of the heart or the brain.

Henry Beecher, the distinguished physician who chaired the Harvard committee that proposed a "definition of irreversible coma," has said that "at whatever level we *choose* . . ., it is an arbitrary decision" [italics added].[2] But he goes on, "It is *best* to choose a level where although the brain is dead, usefulness of other organs is still present" [italics added]. Now, clearly he is not making an "arbitrary decision" any longer. He recognizes that there are policy payoffs. He, like the rest of us, realizes that death already has a well-established meaning. It is the task of the current debate to clarify that meaning for a few rare and difficult cases. We use the term *death* to mean the loss of what is essentially significant to an entity—in the case of man, the loss of humanness. The direct link of a word *death* to what is "essentially significant" means that the task of defining it in this sense is first and foremost a philosophical, theological, ethical task.

•   •   •

THE CONCEPT OF DEATH

To ask what is essentially significant to a human being is a philosophical question—a question of ethical and other values. Many elements make human beings unique—their opposing thumbs, their possession of rational souls, their ability to form cultures and manipulate symbol systems, their upright postures, their being created in the image of God, and so on. Any concept of death will depend directly upon how one evaluates these qualities. Four choices seem to me to cover the most plausible approaches.

IRREVERSIBLE LOSS OF FLOW OF VITAL FLUIDS

At first it would appear that the irreversible cessation of heart and lung activity would represent a simple and straightforward statement of the traditional understanding of the concept of death in Western culture. Yet upon reflection this proves otherwise. If

patients simply lose control of their lungs and have to be permanently supported by a mechanical respirator, they are still living persons as long as they continue to get oxygen. If modern technology produces an efficient, compact heart-lung machine capable of being carried on the back or in a pocket, people using such devices would not be considered dead, even though both heart and lungs were permanently nonfunctioning. Some might consider such a technological man an affront to human dignity; some might argue that such a device should never be connected to a human; but even they would, in all likelihood, agree that such people are alive.

What the traditional concept of death centered on was not the heart and lungs as such, but the flow of vital fluids, that is, the breath and the blood. It is not without reason that these fluids are commonly referred to as "vital." The nature of man is seen as related to this vitality—or vital activity of fluid flow—which man shares with other animals. This fluidity, the movement of liquids and gases at the cellular and organismic level, is a remarkable biological fact. High school biology students are taught that the distinguishing characteristics of "living" things include respiration, circulation of fluids, movement of fluids out of the organism, and the like. According to this view the human organism, like other living organisms, dies when there is an irreversible cessation of the flow of these fluids.

IRREVERSIBLE LOSS OF THE SOUL FROM THE BODY

There is a longstanding tradition, sometimes called vitalism, that holds the essence of man to be independent of the chemical reactions and electrical forces that account for the flow of the bodily fluids. Aristotle and the Greeks spoke of the soul as the animating principle of life. The human being, according to Aristotle, differs from other living creatures in possessing a rational soul as well as vegetative and animal souls. This idea later became especially pronounced in the dualistic philosophy of gnosticism, where salvation was seen as the escape of the enslaved soul from the body. Christianity in its Pauline and later Western forms shares the view that the soul is an essential element in the living man. While Paul and some later theologian-scholars including Erasmus and Luther sometimes held a tripartite anthropology that included spirit as well as body and soul, a central element in all their thought seems to be animation of the body by a noncorporeal force. In Christianity, however, contrasting to the gnostic tradition, the body is a crucial element—not a prison from which the soul escapes, but a significant part of the person. This will become important later in this discussion. The soul remains a central element in the concept of man in most folk religion today.

The departure of the soul might be seen by believers as occurring at about the time that the fluids stop flowing. But it would be a mistake to equate these two concepts of death, as according to the first fluid stops from natural, if unexplained, causes, and death means nothing more than that stopping of the flow which is essential to life. According to the second view, the fluid stops flowing at the time the soul departs, and it stops because the soul is no longer present. Here the essential thing is the loss of the soul, not the loss of the fluid flow.

THE IRREVERSIBLE LOSS OF THE CAPACITY FOR BODILY INTEGRATION

In the debate between those who held a traditional religious notion of the animating force of the soul and those who had the more naturalistic concept of the irreversible loss of the flow of bodily fluids, the trend to secularism and empiricism made the loss of fluid flow more and more the operative concept of death in society. But man's intervention in the dying process through cardiac pacemakers, respirators, intravenous medication and feeding, and extravenous purification of the blood has forced a sharper examination of the naturalistic concept of death. It is now possible to manipulate the dying process so that some parts of the body cease to function while other parts are maintained indefinitely. This has given rise to disagreements within the naturalistic camp itself. In its report, published in 1968, the interdisciplinary Harvard Ad Hoc Committee to Examine the Definition of Brain Death gave two reasons for their undertaking. First, they argued that improvements in resuscitative and supportive measures had sometimes had only partial success, putting a great burden on "patients who suffer permanent loss of intellect, on their families, on the hospitals, and on those in need of hospital beds already occupied by these comatose patients." Second, they argued that "obsolete criteria for the definition of death can lead to controversy in obtaining organs for transplantation."

These points have proved more controversial than

they may have seemed at the time. In the first place, the only consideration of the patient among the reasons given for changing the definition of death was the suggestion that a comatose patient can feel a "great burden." If the committee is right, however, in holding that the person is in fact dead despite continued respiration and circulation, then all the benefits of the change in definition will come to other individuals or to society at large. For those who hold that the primary ethical consideration in the care of the patient should be the patient's own interest, this is cause for concern.

In the second place, the introduction of transplant concerns into the discussion has attracted particular criticism. Paul Ramsey, among others, has argued against making the issue of transplant a reason for updating the definition of death:

If no person's death should *for this purpose* be hastened, then the definition of death should not *for this purpose* be updated, or the procedures for stating that a man has died be revised as a means of affording easier access to organs.[3]

• • •

At first it would appear that the irreversible loss of brain activity is the concept of death held by those no longer satisfied with the vitalistic concept of the departure of the soul or the animalistic concept of the irreversible cessation of fluid flow. This is why the name *brain death* is frequently given to the new proposals, but the term is unfortunate for two reasons.

First, as we have seen, it is not the heart and lungs as such that are essentially significant but rather the vital functions—the flow of fluids—which we believe according to the best empirical human physiology to be associated with these organs. An "artificial brain" is not a present-day possibility but a walking, talking, thinking individual who had one would certainly be considered living. It is not the collection of physical tissues called the brain, but rather their functions—consciousness; motor control; sensory feeling; ability to reason; control over bodily functions including respiration and circulation; major integrating reflexes controlling blood pressure, ion levels, and pupil size; and so forth—which are given essential significance by those who advocate adoption of a new concept of death or clarification of the old one. In short they see the body's capacity for integrating its functions as the essentially significant indication of life.

Second, as suggested earlier, we are not interested in the death of particular cells, organs, or organ systems but in the death of the person as a whole—the point at which the person as a whole undergoes a quantum change through the loss of characteristics held to be essentially significant, the point at which "death behavior" becomes appropriate. Terms such as *brain death* or *heart death* should be avoided because they tend to obscure the fact that we are searching for the meaning of the death of the person as a whole. At the public policy level, this has very practical consequences. A statute adopted in Kansas specifically refers to "alternative definitions of death" and says that they are "to be used for all purposes in this state. . . ." According to this language, which has resulted from talking of brain and heart death, a person in Kansas may be simultaneously dead according to one definition and alive according to another. When a distinction must be made, it should be made directly on the basis of the philosophical significance of the functions mentioned above rather than on the importance of the tissue collection called the brain. For purposes of simplicity we shall use the phrase *the capacity for bodily integration* to refer to the total list of integrating mechanisms possessed by the body. The case for these mechanisms being the ones that are essential to humanness can indeed be made. Man is more than the flowing of fluids. He is a complex, integrated organism with capacities for internal regulation. With and only with these integrating mechanisms is *Homo sapiens* really a human person.

There appear to be two general aspects to this concept of what is essentially significant: first, a capacity for integrating one's internal bodily environment (which is done for the most part unconsciously through highly complex homeostatic, feedback mechanisms) and, secondly, a capacity for integrating one's self, including one's body, with the social environment through consciousness, which permits interaction with other persons. Clearly these taken together offer a more profound understanding of the nature of man than does the simple flow of bodily fluids. Whether or not it is more a profound concept of man than that which focuses simply on the presence or absence of the soul, it is clearly a very different one. The ultimate test between the two is that of meaningfulness and plausibility. For many in the modern secular society, the concept of loss of capacity for bodily integration seems much more meaningful and plausible, that is, we see it as a much more accurate description of the essential significance of man and of what is lost at the time of death. Accord-

ing to this view, when individuals lose all of these "truly vital" capacities we should call them dead and behave accordingly.

At this point the debate may just about have been won by the defenders of the neurologically oriented concept. For the most part the public sees the main dispute as being between partisans of the heart and the brain. Even court cases like the Tucker suit and the major articles in the scientific and philosophical journals have for the most part confined themselves to contrasting these two rather crudely defined positions. If these were the only alternatives, the discussion probably would be nearing an end. There are, however, some critical questions that are just beginning to be asked. This new round of discussion was provoked by the recognition that it may be possible in rare cases for a person to have the higher brain centers destroyed but still retain lower brain functions, including spontaneous respiration.[4] This has led to the question of just what brain functions are essentially significant to man's nature. A fourth major concept of death thus emerges.

THE IRREVERSIBLE LOSS OF THE CAPACITY FOR SOCIAL INTERACTION

The fourth major alternative for a concept of death draws on the characteristics of the third concept and has often been confused with it. Henry Beecher offers a summary of what he considers to be essential to man's nature:

the individual's personality, his conscious life, his uniqueness, his capacity for remembering, judging, reasoning, acting, enjoying, worrying, and so on. . . .[5]

Beecher goes on immediately to ask the anatomical question of locus. He concludes that these functions reside in the brain and that when the brain no longer functions, the individual is dead. We shall take up the locus question later in this chapter. What is remarkable is that Beecher's list, with the possible exception of "uniqueness," is composed entirely of functions explicitly related to consciousness and the capacity to relate to one's social environment through interaction with others. All the functions which give the capacity to integrate one's internal bodily environment through unconscious, complex, homeostatic reflex mechanisms—respiration, circulation, and major integrating reflexes—are omitted. In fact, when asked what was essentially significant to man's living, Beecher replied simply, "Consciousness."

Thus a fourth concept of death is the irreversible loss of the capacity for consciousness or social integration. This view of the nature of man places even more emphasis on social character. Even, given a hypothetical human being with the full capacity for integration of bodily function, if he had irreversibly lost the capacity for consciousness and social interaction, he would have lost the essential character of humanness and, according to this definition, the person would be dead.

Even if one moves to the so-called higher functions and away from the mere capacity to integrate bodily functions through reflex mechanisms, it is still not clear precisely what is ultimately valued. We must have a more careful specification of "consciousness or the capacity for social integration." Are these two capacities synonymous and, if not, what is the relationship between them? Before taking up that question, we must first make clear what is meant by capacity.

Holders of this concept of death and related concepts of the essence of man specifically do not say that individuals must be valued by others in order to be human. This would place life at the mercy of other human beings who may well be cruel or insensitive. Nor does this concept imply that the essence of man is the fact of social interaction with others, as this would also place a person at the mercy of others. The infant raised in complete isolation from other human contact would still be human, provided that the child retained the mere capacity for some form of social interaction. This view of what is essentially significant to the nature of man makes no quantitative or qualitative judgments. It need not, and for me could not, lead to the view that those who have more capacity for social integration are more human. The concepts of life and death are essentially bipolar, threshhold concepts. Either one has life or one does not. Either a particular type of death behavior is called for or it is not. One does not pronounce death half-way or read a will half-way or become elevated from the vice presidency to the presidency half-way.

One of the real dangers of shifting from the third concept of death to the fourth is that the fourth, in focusing exclusively on the capacity for consciousness or social interaction, lends itself much more readily to quantitative and qualitative considerations. When the focus is on the complete capacity for bodily integration, including the ability of the body to carry out spontaneous respiratory activity and major reflexes, it is quite easy to maintain that if any such integrating function is present the person is alive. But when the question begins to be, "What kinds of integrating capacity are really significant?" one finds oneself on the slippery slope of evaluating kinds of consciousness or social interaction. If consciousness is what counts, it might be asked if a long-term catatonic schizophrenic or a patient with extreme senile dementia really has the capacity for consciousness. To position oneself for such a slide down the slope of evaluating the degree of capacity for social interaction is extremely dangerous. It seems to me morally obligatory to stay off the slopes.

Precisely what are the functions considered to be ultimately significant to human life according to this concept? There are several possibilities.

The capacity for rationality is one candidate. *Homo sapiens* is a rational animal, as suggested by the name. The human capacity for reasoning is so unique and so important that some would suggest that it is the critical element in man's nature. But certainly infants lack any such capacity and they are considered living human beings. Nor is possession of the potential for reasoning what is important. Including potential might resolve the problem of infants, but does not explain why those who have no potential for rationality (such as the apparently permanent back ward psychotic or the senile individual) are considered to be humanly living in a real if not full sense and to be entitled to the protection of civil and moral law.

Consciousness is a second candidate that dominates much of the medical and biological literature. If the rationalist tradition is reflected in the previous notion, then the empiricalist philosophical tradition seems to be represented in the emphasis on consciousness. What may be of central significance is the capacity for experience. This would include the infant and the individual who lacks the capacity for rationality, and focuses attention on the ability for sensory activity summarized as consciousness. Yet, this is a very individualistic understanding of man's nature. It describes what is essentially significant to the human life without any reference to other human beings.

Social interaction is a third candidate. At least in the Western tradition, man is seen as an essentially social animal. Perhaps it is man's capacity or potential for social interaction that has such ultimate significance that its loss is considered death. Is this in any sense different from the capacity for experience? Certainly it is conceptually different and places a very different emphasis on man's essential role. Yet it may well be that the two functions, experience and social interaction, are completely conterminous. It is difficult to conceive a case where the two could be separated, at least if social interaction is understood in its most elementary form. While it may be important for a philosophical understanding of man's nature to distinguish between these two functions, it may not be necessary for deciding when a person has died. Thus, for our purposes we can say that the fourth concept of death is one in which the essential element that is lost is the capacity for consciousness or social interaction or both.

The concept presents one further problem. The Western tradition which emphasizes social interaction also emphasizes, as we have seen, the importance of the body. Consider the admittedly remote possibility that the electrical impulses of the brain could be transferred by recording devices onto magnetic computer tape. Would that tape together with some kind of minimum sensory device be a living human being and would erasure of the tape be considered murder? If the body is really essential to man, then we might well decide that such a creature would not be a living human being.

Where does this leave us? The alternatives are summarized in the table at the end of the [essay]. The earlier concepts of death—the irreversible loss of the soul and the irreversible stopping of the flow of vital body fluids—strike me as quite implausible. The soul as an independent nonphysical entity that is necessary and sufficient for a person to be considered alive is a relic from the era of dichotomized anthropologies. Animalistic fluid flow is simply too base a function to be the human essence. The capacity for bodily integration is more plausible, but I suspect it is attractive primarily because it includes those higher functions that we normally take to be central—consciousness, the ability to think and feel and relate to others. When the reflex networks that regulate such things as blood pressure and respiration are separated from the higher functions, I am led to conclude that it is the higher functions which are so essential that their loss ought to be taken as the death of the person. While consciousness is certainly important, man's social nature and embodiment seem to me to be the truly essential

characteristics. I therefore believe that death is most appropriately thought of as the irreversible loss of the embodied capacity for social interaction.

THE LOCUS OF DEATH

Thus far I have completely avoided dealing with anatomy. Whenever the temptation arose to formulate a concept of death by referring to organs or tissues such as the heart, lungs, brain, or cerebral cortex, I have carefully resisted. Now finally I must ask, "Where does one look if one wants to know whether a person is dead or alive?" This question at last leads into the field of anatomy and physiology. Each concept of death formulated in the previous section (by asking what is of essential significance to the nature of man) raises a corresponding question of where to look to see if death has occurred. This level of the definitional problem may be called the locus of death.

The term *locus* must be used carefully. I have stressed that we are concerned about the death of the individual as a whole, not a specific part. Nevertheless, differing concepts of death will lead us to look at different body functions and structures in order to diagnose the death of the person as a whole. This task can be undertaken only after the conceptual question is resolved, if what we really want to know is where to look to determine if a person is dead rather than where to look to determine simply if the person has irreversibly lost the capacity for vital fluid flow or bodily integration or social interaction. What then are the different loci corresponding to the different concepts?

The *loci* corresponding to the irreversible loss of vital fluid flow are clearly the heart and blood vessels, the lungs and respiratory tract. At least according to our contemporary empirical knowledge of physiology and anatomy, in which we have good reason to have confidence, these are the vital organs and organ systems to which the tests should have applied to determine if a person has died. Should a new Harvey reveal evidence to the contrary, those who hold to the concept of the irreversible loss of vital fluid flow would probably be willing to change the site of their observations in diagnosing death.

The locus, or the "seat," of the soul has not been dealt with definitively since the day of Descartes. In his essay, "The Passions of the Soul," Descartes pursues the question of the soul's dwelling place in the body. He argues that the soul is united to all the portions of the body conjointly, but, nevertheless, he concludes:

There is yet . . . a certain part in which it exercises its functions more particularly than in all the others; and it is usually believed that this part is the brain, or possibly the heart: the brain, because it is with it that the organs of sense are connected, and the heart because it is apparently in it that we experience the passions. But in examining the matter with care, it seems as though I had clearly ascertained that the part of the body in which the soul exercises its functions immediately is in no wise the heart, not the whole of the brain, but merely the most inward of all its parts, to wit, a certain very small gland which is situated in the middle of its substance. . . .[6]

Descartes is clearly asking the questions of locus. His anatomical knowledge is apparently sound, but his conclusion that the soul resides primarily and directly in the pineal body raises physiological and theological problems which most of us are unable to comprehend today. What is significant is that he seemed to hold that the irreversible loss of the soul is the critical factor in determining death, and he was asking the right kind of question about where to look to determine whether a man is dead.

The fact that the Greek term *pneuma* has the dual meaning of both breath and soul or spirit could be interpreted to imply that the presence of this animating force is closely related to (perhaps synonymous with) breath. This gives us another clue about where holders of the irreversible loss of the soul concept of death might look to determine the presence or absence of life.

The locus for loss of capacity for bodily integration is a more familiar concept today. The anatomist and physiologist would be sure that the locus of the integrating capacity is the central nervous system, as Sherrington has ingrained into the biomedical tradition. Neurophysiologists asked to find this locus might reasonably request a more specific concept, however. They are aware that the autonomic nervous system and spinal cord play a role in the integrating capacity, both as transmitters of nervous impulses and as the central analyzers for certain simple acts of integration (for example, a withdrawal reflex mediated through the spinal cord); they would have to know whether one was interested in such simple reflexes.

Beecher gives us the answer quite specifically for his personal concept of death: he says spinal reflexes are to be omitted.[7] This leaves the brain as essentially the place to look to determine whether a man is dead according to the third concept of death. The brain's highly complex circuitry provides the minimal essentials for the body's real integrating capacity. This third concept quite specifically includes unconscious homeostatic and higher reflex mechanisms such as spontaneous respiration and pupil reflexes. Thus, anatomically, according to our reading of neurophysiology, we are dealing with the whole brain, including the cerebellum, medulla, and brainstem. This is the basis for calling the third concept of death *brain death,* and we already discussed objections to this term.

Where to seek the locus for irreversible loss of the capacity for social interaction, the fourth conception of death, is quite another matter. We have eliminated unconscious reflex mechanisms. The answer is clearly not the whole brain—it is much too massive. Determining the locus of consciousness and social interaction certainly requires greater scientific understanding, but evidence points strongly to the neocortex or outer surface of the brain as the site.[8] Indeed, if this is the locus of consciousness, the presence or absence of activity in the rest of the brain will be immaterial to the holder of this view.

THE CRITERIA OF DEATH

Having determined a concept of death, which is rooted in a philosophical analysis of the nature of man, and a locus of death, which links this philosophical understanding to the anatomy and physiology of the human body, we are finally ready to ask the operational question, What tests or measurements should be applied to determine if an individual is living or dead? At this point we have moved into a more technical realm in which the answer will depend primarily on the data gathered from the biomedical sciences.

Beginning with the first concept of death, irreversible loss of vital fluid flow, what criteria can be used to measure the activity of the heart and lungs, the blood vessels and respiratory track? The methods are simple: visual observation of respiration, perhaps by the use of the classic mirror held at the nostrils; feeling the pulse; and listening for the heartbeat. More technical measures are also now available to the trained clinician: the electrocardiogram and direct measures of oxygen and carbon dioxide levels in the blood.

If Descartes' conclusion is correct that the locus of the soul is in the pineal body, the logical question would be "How does one know when the pineal body has irreversibly ceased to function?" or more precisely "How does one know when the soul has irreversibly departed from the gland?" This matter remains baffling for the modern neurophysiologist. If, however, holders of the soul-departing concept of death associate the soul with the breath, as suggested by the word *pneuma,* this might give us another clue. If respiration and specifically breath are the locus of the soul, then the techniques discussed above as applying to respiration might also be the appropriate criteria for determining the loss of the soul.

We have identified the (whole) brain as the locus associated with the third concept of death, the irreversible loss of the capacity for bodily integration. The empirical task of identifying criteria in this case is to develop accurate predictions of the complete and irreversible loss of brain activity. This search for criteria was the real task carried out by the Ad Hoc Committee to Examine the Definition of Brain Death of Harvard Medical School; the simple criteria they proposed have become the most widely recognized in the United States:

1. Unreceptivity and unresponsivity
2. No movements or breathing
3. No reflexes
4. Flat electroencephalogram

The report states that the fourth criterion is "of great confirmatory value." It also calls for the repetition of these tests twenty-four hours later. Two types of cases are specifically excluded: hypothermia (body temperature below 90° F) and the presence of central nervous system depressants such as barbiturates.[9]

Other criteria have been proposed to diagnose the condition of irreversible loss of brain function. James Toole, a neurologist at the Bowman Gray School of Medicine, has suggested that metabolic criteria such as oxygen consumption of the brain or the measure of metabolic products in the blood or cerebrospinal fluid could possibly be developed as well.[10]

European observers seem to place more emphasis on demonstrating the absence of circulation in the brain. This is measured by angiography,* radioisotopes, or sonic techniques.[11] In Europe sets of criteria analogous to the Harvard criteria have been proposed. G. P. J. Alexandre, a surgeon who heads a Belgian renal transplant department, reports that in addition to absence of reflexes as criteria of irreversible destruction of the brain, he uses lack of spontaneous respiration, a flat EEG, complete bilateral mydriasis,† and falling blood pressure necessitating increasing amounts of vasopressive‡ drugs.[12] J. P. Revillard, a Frenchman, reportedly uses these plus angiography and absence of reaction to atropine.[13] Even among those who agree on the types of measures, there may still be disagreement on the levels of measurement. This is especially true for the electroencephalogram, which can be recorded at varying sensitivities and for different time periods. The Harvard-proposed twenty-four-hour period is now being questioned as too conservative.

While these alternate sets of criteria are normally described as applicable to measuring loss of brain function (or "brain death" as in the name of the Harvard committee), it appears that many of these authors, especially the earlier ones, have not necessarily meant to distinguish them from criteria for measuring the narrower loss of cerebral function.

The criteria for irreversible loss of the capacity for social interaction are far more selective. It should be clear from the above criteria that they measure loss of all brain activity, including spontaneous respiration and higher reflexes and not simply loss of consciousness. This raises a serious problem about whether the Harvard criteria really measure "irreversible coma" as the report title indicates. Exactly what is measured is an entirely empirical matter. In any case, convincing evidence has been cited by the committee and more recently by a committee of the Institute of Society, Ethics and the Life Sciences that no one will falsely be pronounced in irreversible coma. In 128 patients who underwent autopsy, the brain was found to be "obviously destroyed" in each case.[14] Of 2,650 patients with isoelectric EEGs of twenty-four hours' duration, not one patient recovered ("excepting three who had received anesthetic doses of CNS depressants, and who were, therefore, outside the class of patients covered by the report.")[15]

What then is the relationship between the more inclusive Harvard criteria and the simple use of electrocerebral silence as measured by an isoelectric or flat electroencephalogram? The former might be ap-

*Ed. note: X-ray visualization of blood vessels.

†Ed. note: Extreme dilation of both pupils of the eyes.
‡Ed. note: Causing constriction of blood vessels and increase of blood pressure.

propriate for those who associate death with the disappearance of any neurological function of the brain. For those who hold the narrower concept based simply on consciousness or capacity for social interaction, however, the Harvard criteria may suffer from exactly the same problem as the old heart- and lung-oriented criteria. With those criteria, every patient whose circulatory and respiratory function had ceased was indeed dead, but the criteria might be too conservative, in that some patients dead according to the "loss of bodily integrating capacity" concept of death (for which the brain is the corresponding locus) would be found alive according to heart- and lung-oriented criteria. It might also happen that some patients who should be declared dead according to the irreversible loss of consciousness and social interaction concept would be found to be alive according to the Harvard criteria.[16] All discussions of the neurological criteria fail to consider that the criteria might be too inclusive, too conservative. The criteria might, therefore, give rise to classifying patients as dead according to the consciousness or social interaction conception, but as alive according to the full Harvard criteria.

A report in *Lancet* by the British physician J. B. Brierley and his colleagues, implies this may indeed be the case.[17] In two cases in which patients had undergone cardiac arrest resulting in brain damage, they report, "the electroencephalogram (strictly defined) was isoelectric throughout. Spontaneous respiration was resumed almost at once in case 2, but not until day 21 in case 1."[18] They report that the first patient did not "die" until five months later. For the second patient they report, "The Patient died on day 153." Presumably in both cases they were using the traditional heart and lung locus and correlated criteria for death as they pronounced it. They report that subsequent detailed neuropathological analysis confirmed that the "neocortex was dead while certain brainstem and spinal centers remained intact." These intact centers specifically involved the functions of spontaneous breathing and reflexes: eye-opening, yawning, and "certain reflex activities at brainstem

Table 1. Levels of the Definition of Death*

Concept of death:	Locus of death:	Criteria of death:
Philosophical or theological judgment of the essentially significant change at death.	Place to look to determine if a person has died.	Measurements physicians or other officials use to determine whether a person is dead—to be determined by scientific empirical study.
1. The irreversible stopping of the flow of "vital" body fluids, i.e., the blood and breath	Heart and lungs	1. Visual observation of respiration, perhaps with the use of a mirror 2. Feeling of the pulse, possibly supported by electrocardiogram
2. The irreversible loss of the soul from the body	The pineal body? (according to Descartes) The respiratory track?	Observation of breath?
3. The irreversible loss of the capacity for bodily integration and social interaction	The brain	1. Unreceptivity and unresponsitivity 2. No movements or breathing 3. No reflexes (except spinal reflexes) 4. Flat electroencephalogram (to be used as confirmatory evidence) —All tests to be repeated 24 hours later (excluded conditions: hypothermia and central nervous system drug depression)
4. Irreversible loss of consciousness or the capacity for social interaction	Probably the neocortex	Electroencephalogram

Formal Definition: Death means a complete change in the status of a living entity characterized by the irreversible loss of those characteristics that are essentially significant to it.

Note: The possible concepts, loci, and criteria of death are much more complex than the ones given here. These are meant to be simplified models of types of positions being taken in the current debate. It is obvious that those who believe that death means the irreversible loss of the capacity for bodily integration (3) or the irreversible loss of consciousness (4) have no reservations about pronouncing death when the heart and lungs have ceased to function. This is because they are willing to use loss of heart and lung activity as shortcut criteria for death, believing that once heart and lungs have stopped, the brain or neocortex will necessarily stop as well.

and spinal cord levels.'' As evidence that lower brain activity remained, they report that an electroretinogram (measuring electrical activity of the eye) in patient 1 was normal on day 13. After day 49 there still remained reactivity of the pupils to light in addition to spontaneous respiration.

If this evidence is sound, it strongly suggests that it is empirically as well as theoretically possible to have irreversible loss of cortical function (and therefore loss of consciousness) while lower brain functions remain intact.

This leaves us with the empirical question of the proper criteria for the irreversible loss of consciousness which is thought to have its locus in the neocortex of the cerebrum. Brierley and his colleagues suggest that the EEG alone (excluding the other three criteria of the Harvard report) measures the activity of the neocortex.[19] Presumably this test must also meet the carefully specified conditions of amplifier gain, repeat of the test after a given time period, and exclusion of the exceptional cases, if it is to be used as the criterion for death according to our fourth concept, irreversible loss of capacity for social interaction. The empirical evidence is not all in, but it would seem that the 2,650 cases of flat EEG without recovery which are cited to support the Harvard criteria would also be persuasive preliminary empirical evidence for the use of the EEG alone as empirical evidence for the irreversible loss of consciousness and social interaction which (presumably) have their locus in the neocortex. What these 2,650 cases would have to include for the data to be definitive would be a significant number of Brierley-type patients where the EEG criteria were met without the other Harvard criteria being met. This is a question for the neurophysiologists to resolve.

There is another problem with the use of electroencephalogram, angiography, or other techniques for measuring cerebral function as a criterion for the irreversible loss of consciousness. Once again we must face the problem of a false positive diagnosis of life. The old heart and lung criteria may provide a false positive diagnosis for a holder of the bodily integrating capacity concept, and the Harvard criteria may give false positive indications for a holder of the consciousness or social interaction concept. Could a person have electroencephalographic activity but still have no capacity for consciousness or social interaction? Whether this is possible empirically is difficult to say, but at least theoretically there are certainly portions of the neocortex which could be functioning and presumably be recorded on an electroencephalo-

gram without the individual having any capacity for consciousness. For instance, what if through an accident or vascular occlusion the motor cortex remained viable but the sensory cortex did not? Even the most narrow criterion of the electroencephalogram alone may still give false positive diagnoses of living for holders of the social interaction concept.

NOTES

1. Ad Hoc Committee of the Harvard Medical School to Examine the Definition of Brain Death, ''A Definition of Irreversible Coma,'' *Journal of the American Medical Association* 205 (1968), pp. 337–40. [Reprinted]

2. Henry K. Beecher, ''The New Definition of Death, Some Opposing Views,'' unpublished paper presented at the meeting of the American Association for the Advancement of Science, December 1970, p. 2.

3. Paul Ramsey, ''On Updating Procedures for Stating That a Man Has Died,'' in *The Patient as Person* (New Haven: Yale University Press, 1970), p. 103.

4. J. B. Brierley, J. A. H. Adams, D. I. Graham, and J. A. Simpson, ''Neocortical Death after Cardiac Arrest,'' *Lancet,* September 11, 1971, pp. 560–65.

5. Beecher, ''The New Definition of Death,'' p. 4.

6. René Descartes, ''The Passions of the Soul,'' in *The Philosophical Works of Descartes,* vol. 1 (Cambridge: Cambridge University Press, 1911), p. 345.

7. Beecher, ''The New Definition of Death,'' p. 2.

8. Brierley *et al.,* ''Neocortical Death.''

9. Ad Hoc Committee of the Harvard Medical School, ''A Definition of Irreversible Coma,'' pp. 337–38. See also F. Mellerio, ''Clinical and EEG Study of a Case of Acute Poisoning with Cerebral Electrical Silence, Followed by Recovery,'' *Electroencephalography Clinical Neurophysiology* 30 (1971), pp. 270–71.

10. James F. Toole, ''The Neurologist and the Concept of Brain Death,'' *Perspectives in Biology and Medicine* (Summer 1971), p. 602.

11. See, for example, A. A. Hadjidimos, M. Brock, P. Baum, and K. Schurmann, ''Cessation of Cerebral Blood Flow in Total Irreversible Loss of Brain Function,'' in *Cerebral Blood Flow,* ed. M. Brock, C. Fieschi, D. H. Ingvar, N. A. Lassen, and K. Schurmann (Berlin: Springer-Verlag, 1969), pp. 209–12; A. Beis *et al.,* ''Hemodynamic and Metabolic Studies in 'Coma Depassé,' '' ibid., pp. 213–15.

12. G. E. W. Wolstenholme and Maeve O'Connor, eds., *Ethics in Medical Progress: With Special Reference to Transplantation* (Boston: Little, Brown, 1966), p. 69.

13. Ibid., p. 71.

14. Task Force on Death and Dying of the Institute of Society, Ethics and the Life Sciences, ''Refinements in Criteria for the Determination of Death: An Appraisal.'' *Journal of the American Medical Association* 221 (1972), pp. 50–51.

15. Daniel Silverman, Richard L. Masland, Michael G. Saunders, and Robert S. Schwab, ''Irreversible Coma Associated with Electrocerebral Silence,'' *Neurology* 20 (1970), pp. 525–33.

16. The inclusion of absence of breathing and reflexes in the criteria suggests this, but does not necessarily lead to this. It might

be that, empirically, it is necessary for lower brain reflexes and breathing to be absent for twenty-four hours in order to be sure that the patient not only will never regain these functions but will never regain consciousness.

17. Brierley *et al.*, "Neocortical Death." See also Ricardo Ceballos and Samuel C. Little, "Progressive Electroencephalographic Changes in Laminar Necrosis of the Brain," *Southern Medical Journal* 64 (1971), pp. 1370–76.

18. Ibid., p. 560.

19. Brierley *et al.*, "Neocortical Death."

HANS JONAS

Against the Stream: Comments on the Definition and Redefinition of Death

The by now famous "Report of the *Ad Hoc* Committee of the Harvard Medical School to Examine the Definition of Brain Death" advocates the adoption of "irreversible coma as a new definition of death."[1] The report leaves no doubt of the practical reasons "why there is need for a definition," naming these two: relief of patient, kin, and medical resources from the burdens of indefinitely prolonged coma; and removal of controversy on obtaining organs for transplantation. On both counts, the new definition is designed to give the physician the right to terminate the treatment of a condition which not only cannot be improved by such treatment, but whose mere prolongation by it is utterly meaningless to the patient himself. The last consideration, of course, is ultimately the only valid rationale for termination (and for termination only!) and must support all the others. It does so with regard to the reasons mentioned under the first head, for the relief of the patient means automatically also that of his family, doctor, nurses, apparatus, hospital space, and so on. But the other reason—freedom for organ use—has possible implications that are not equally covered by the primary rationale, which is the patient himself. For with this primary rationale (the senselessness of mere vegetative function) the Report has strictly speaking defined not death, the ultimate state, itself, but a criterion for permitting it to take

place unopposed—e.g., by turning off the respirator. The Report, however, purports by that criterion to have defined death itself, declaring it on its evidence as already given, not merely no longer to be opposed. But if "the patient is declared dead on the basis of these criteria," i.e., if the comatose individual is not a patient at all but a corpse, then the road to other uses of the definition, urged by the second reason, has been opened in principle and will be taken in practice, unless it is blocked in good time by a special barrier. What follows is meant to reinforce what I called "my feeble attempt" to help erect such a barrier on theoretical grounds.

My original comments of 1968 on the then newly proposed "redefinition of death"[2] . . . were marginal to the discussion of "experimentation on human subjects," which has to do with the living and not the dead. They have since, however, drawn fire from within the medical profession, and precisely in connection with the second of the reasons given by the Harvard Committee why a new definition is wanted, namely, the *transplant* interest, which my kind critics felt threatened by my layman's qualms and lack of understanding. Can I take this as corroborating my initial suspicion that this *interest*, in spite of its notably muted expression in the Committee Report, was and is the major motivation behind the definitional effort? I am confirmed in this suspicion when I hear Dr. Henry K. Beecher, author of the Committee's Report (and its Chairman), ask elsewhere: "Can society afford to discard the tissues and organs of the hopelessly unconscious patient when they could be

From Hans Jonas, *Philosophical Essays: From Ancient Creed to Technological Man,* copyright 1974, pp. 132–140. Reprinted by permission of Prentice-Hall, Inc., Englewood Cliffs, New Jersey, and the author. A 1980 reedition of the *Philosophical Essays* is available from the University of Chicago Press.

used to restore the otherwise hopelessly ill, but still salvageable individual?'' In any case, the tenor and passion of the discussion which my initial polemic provoked from my medical friends left no doubt where the surgeon's interest in the definition lies. I contend that, pure as this interest, viz., to save other lives, is in itself, its intrusion into the *theoretical* attempt to define death makes the attempt impure; and the Harvard Committee should never have allowed itself to adulterate the purity of its scientific case by baiting it with the prospect of this *extraneous*—though extremely appealing—gain. But purity of theory is not my concern here. My concern is with certain practical consequences which under the urgings of that extraneous interest can be drawn from the definition and would enjoy its full sanction, once it has been officially accepted. Doctors would be less than human if certain formidable advantages of such possible consequences would not influence their judgment as to the theoretical adequacy of a definition that yields them—just as I freely admit that my shudder at one aspect of those consequences, and at the danger of others equally sanctioned by that definition, keeps my theoretical skepticism in a state of extreme alertness.

． ． ．

I had to answer three charges made à propos of the pertinent part of my *Daedalus* essay: that my reasoning regarding ''cadaver donors'' counteracts sincere life-saving efforts of physicians; that I counter precise scientific facts with vague philosophical considerations; and that I overlook the difference between death of ''the organism as a whole'' and death of ''the whole organism,'' with the related difference between spontaneous and externally induced respiratory and other movements.

I plead, of course, guilty to the first charge for the case where the cadaver status of the donor is in question, which is precisely what my argument is about. The use of the term ''cadaver donor'' here simply begs the question, to which only the third charge (see below) addresses itself.

As to the charge of vagueness, it might just be possible that it vaguely reflects the fact that mine is an argument—a precise argument, I believe—*about* vagueness, viz., the vagueness of a condition. Giving intrinsic vagueness its due is not being vague. Aristotle observed that it is the mark of a well-educated man not to insist on greater precision in knowledge than the subject admits, e.g., the same in politics as in mathematics. Reality of certain kinds—of which the life-death spectrum is perhaps one—may be imprecise in itself, or the knowledge obtainable of it may be. To acknowledge such a state of affairs is more adequate to it than a precise definition which does violence to it. I am challenging the undue precision of a definition and of its practical application to an imprecise field.

The third point—which was made by Dr. Otto Guttentag—is highly relevant and I will deal with it step by step.

a. The difference between ''organism as a whole'' and ''whole organism'' which he has in mind is perhaps brought out more clearly if for ''whole organism'' we write ''every and all parts of the organism.'' If this is the meaning, then I have been speaking throughout of ''death of the organism as a whole,'' not of ''death of the whole organism''; and any ambiguity in my formulations can be easily removed. Local subsystems—single cells or tissues—may well continue to function locally, i.e., to display biochemical activity for themselves (e.g., growth of hair and nails) for some time after death, without this affecting the definition of death by the larger criteria of the whole. But respiration and circulation do not fall into this class, since the effect of their functioning, though performed by subsystems, extends through the total system and insures the functional preservation of its other parts. Why else prolong them artificially in prospective ''cadaveric'' organ donors (e.g., ''maintain renal circulation of cadaver kidneys in situ'') except to keep those other parts ''in good shape''—viz., alive—for eventual transplantation? The comprehensive system thus sustained is even capable of continued overall metabolism when intravenously fed, and then, presumably, of diverse other (e.g. glandular) functions as well—in fact, I suppose, of pretty much everything not involving neural control. There are stories of comatose patients lingering on for months with those aids; the metaphor of the ''human vegetable'' recurring in the debate (strangely enough, sometimes in support of redefining death—as if ''vegetable'' were not an instance of life!) say as much. In short, what is here kept going by various artifices must—with the caution due in this twilight zone—be equated with ''the organism as a whole'' named in the classical definition of death—much more so, at least, than with any mere separable part of it.

b. Nor, to my knowledge, does that older definition specify that the functioning whose "irreversible cessation" constitutes death must be spontaneous and does not count for life when artificially induced and sustained (the implications for therapy would be devastating). Indeed, "irreversible" cessation can have a twofold reference: to the function itself or only to the spontaneity of it. A cessation can be irreversible with respect to spontaneity but still reversible with respect to the activity as such—in which case the reversing external agency must continuously substitute for the lost spontaneity. This is the case of the respiratory movements and heart contractions in the comatose. The distinction is not irrelevant, because if we could do for the disabled brain—let's say, the lower nerve centers only—what we can do for the heart and lungs, viz., *make* it work by the continuous input of some external agency (electrical, chemical, or whatever), we would surely do so and not be finicky about the resulting function lacking spontaneity: the functioning as such would matter. Respirator and stimulator could then be turned off, because the nerve center presiding over heart contractions (etc.) has again taken over and returned *them* to being "spontaneous"—just as systems presided over by circulation had enjoyed spontaneity of function when the circulation was only nonspontaneously active. The case is wholly hypothetical, but I doubt that a doctor would feel at liberty to pronounce the patient dead on the ground of the nonspontaneity at the cerebral source, when it can be *made* to function by an auxiliary device.

The purpose of the foregoing thought-experiment was to cast some doubt (a layman's, to be sure) on the seeming simplicity of the spontaneity criterion. With the stratification and interlocking of functions, it seems to me, organic spontaneity is distributed over many levels and loci—any superordinated level enabling its subordinates to be naturally spontaneous, be its own action natural or artificial.

c. The point with irreversible coma as defined by the Harvard group, of course, is precisely that it is a condition which precludes reactivation of any part of the brain in *every* sense. We then have an "organism as a whole" minus the brain, maintained in some partial state of life so long as the respirator and other artifices are at work. And here the question is not: has the patient died? but: how should he—still a patient—be dealt with? Now *this* question must be settled, surely not by a definition of death, but by a definition of man and of what life is human. That is to say, the question cannot be answered by decreeing that death has already occurred and the body is therefore in the domain of things; rather it is by holding, e.g., that it is humanly not justified—let alone, demanded—to artificially prolong the life of a brainless body. This is the answer I myself would advocate. On that philosophical ground, which few will contest, the physician can, indeed should, turn off the respirator and let the "definition of death" take care of itself by what then inevitably happens. (The later utilization of the corpse is a different matter I am not dealing with here, though it too resists the comfortable patness of merely utilitarian answers.) The decision to be made, I repeat, is an axiological one and not already made by clinical fact. It begins when the diagnosis of the condition has spoken: it is not diagnostic itself. Thus, as I have pointed out before, no redefinition of death is needed; only, perhaps, a redefinition of the physician's presumed duty to prolong life under all circumstances.

d. But, it might be asked, is not a definition of death made into law the simpler and more precise way than a definition of medical ethics (which is difficult to legislate) for sanctioning the same practical conclusion, while avoiding the twilight of value judgment and possible legal ambiguity? It would be, if it really sanctioned the same conclusion, and no more. But it sanctions indefinitely more: it opens the gate to a whole range of other possible conclusions, the extent of which cannot even be foreseen, but some of which are disquietingly close at hand. The point is, if the comatose patient is by definition dead, he is a patient no more but a corpse, with which can be done whatever law or custom or the deceased's will or next of kin permit and sundry interests urge doing with a corpse. This includes—why not?—the protracting of the inbetween state, for which we must find a new name ("simulated life"?) since that "life" has been preempted by the new definition of death, and extracting from it all the profit we can. There are many. So far the "redefiners" speak of no more than keeping the respirator going until the transplant organ is to be removed, then turning it off,[3] then beginning to cut into the "cadaver," this being the end of it—which sounds innocent enough. But why must it be the end? Why turn the respirator off? Once we are assured that we are dealing with a cadaver, there are no logical reasons against (and strong pragmatic reasons for) going on with the artificial "animation" and keeping the "deceased's" body on call, as a bank for life-fresh organs, possibly also as a plant for manufacturing hormones or other biochemical compounds in demand. I have no doubts that methods exist or can be perfected which allow the natural powers for the healing of surgical wounds by new tissue growth to stay "alive" in such a body. Tempting also is the idea of a self-replenishing blood bank. And that is not all. Let us not forget research. Why shouldn't the most wonderful surgical and grafting experiments be conducted on the complaisant subject-nonsubject, with no limits set to daring? Why not immunological explorations, infection with diseases old and new, trying out of drugs? We have the active cooperation of a functional organism declared to be dead; we have, that is, the advantages of the living donor without the disadvantages imposed by his rights and interests (for a corpse has none). What a boon for medical instruction, for anatomical and physiological demonstration and practicing on so much better material than the inert cadavers otherwise serving in the dissection room! What a chance for the apprentice to learn *in vivo*, as it were, how to amputate a leg, without his mistakes mattering! And so on, into the wide open field. After all, what is advocated is "the full utilization of modern means to maximize the value of cadaver organs." Well, this is it.

Come, come, the members of the profession will say, nobody is thinking of this kind of thing. Perhaps not; but I have just shown that one *can* think of them. And the point is that the proposed definition of death has removed any reasons not to think of them and, once thought of, not to do them when found desirable (and the next of kin are agreeable). We must remember that what the Harvard group offered was not a definition of irreversible coma as a rationale for breaking off sustaining action, but a definition of death by the criterion of irreversible coma as a rationale for conceptually transposing the patient's body to the class of dead things, *regardless* of whether sustaining action is kept up or broken off. It would be hypocritical to deny that the redefinition amounts to an antedating of the accomplished fact of death (compared to conventional signs that may outlast it); that it was motivated not by exclusive concern with the patient but with certain extraneous interests in mind (organ donorship mostly named so far); and that the actual use of the general license it grants is implicitly anticipated. But no matter what particular use is or is not anticipated at the moment, or even anathematized—it would be naive to think that a line can be drawn anywhere for such uses when strong enough

interests urge them, seeing that the definition (which is absolute, not graded) negates the very principle for drawing a line. (Given the ingenuity of medical science, in which I have great faith, I am convinced that the "simulated life" can eventually be made to comprise practically every extraneural activity of the human body; and I would not even bet on its never comprising *some* artificially activated neural functions as well: which would be awkward for the argument of nonsensitivity, but still under the roof of that nonspontaneity.)

e. Now my point is a very simple one. It is this. We do not know with certainty the borderline between life and death, and a definition cannot substitute for knowledge. Moreover, we have sufficient grounds for suspecting that the artificially supported condition of the comatose patient may still be one of life, however reduced—i.e., for doubting that, even with the brain function gone, he is completely dead, In this state of marginal ignorance and doubt the only course to take is to lean over backward toward the side of possible life. It follows that interventions as I described should be regarded on a par with vivisection and on no account be performed on a human body in that equivocal or threshold condition. And the definition that allows them, by stamping as unequivocal what at best is equivocal, must be rejected. But mere rejection in discourse is not enough. Given the pressure of the—very real and very worthy—medical interests, it can be predicted that the permission it implies in theory will be irresistible in practice, once the definition is installed in official authority. Its becoming so installed must therefore be resisted at all cost. It is the only thing that still can be resisted; by the time the practical conclusions beckon, it will be too late. It is a clear case of *principiis obsta*.

The foregoing argumentation was strictly on the plane of common sense and ordinary logic. Let me add, somewhat conjecturally, two philosophical observations.

I see lurking behind the proposed definition of death, apart from its obvious pragmatic motivation, a curious remnant of the old soul-body dualism. Its new apparition is the dualism of brain and body. In a certain analogy to the former it holds that the true human person rests in (or is represented by) the brain, of which the rest of the body is a mere subservient tool. Thus, when the brain dies, it is as when the soul departed: what is left are "mortal remains." Now nobody will deny that the cerebral aspect is decisive for the human quality of the life of the organism that is man's. The position I advanced acknowledges just this by recommending that with the irrecoverable total loss of brain function one should not hold up the naturally ensuing death of the rest of the organism. But it is no less an exaggeration of the cerebral aspect as it was of the conscious soul, to deny the extracerebral body its essential share in the identity of the person. The body is as uniquely the body of this brain and no other, as the brain is uniquely the brain of this body and no other. What is under the brain's central control, the bodily total, is as individual, as much "myself," as singular to my identity (fingerprints!), as noninterchangeable, as the controlling (and reciprocally controlled) brain itself. My identity is the identity of the whole organism, even if the higher functions of personhood are seated in the brain. How else could a man love a woman and not merely her brains? How else could we lose ourselves in the aspect of a face? Be touched by the delicacy of a frame? It's this person's, and no one else's. Therefore, the body of the comatose, so long as—even with the help of art—it still breathes, pulses, and functions otherwise, must still be considered a residual continuance of the subject that loved and was loved, and as such is still entitled to some of the sacrosanctity accorded to such a subject by the laws of God and men. That sacrosanctity decrees that it must not be used as a mere means.

My second observation concerns the morality of our time, to which our "redefiners" pay homage with the best of intentions, which have their own subtle sophistry. I mean the prevailing attitude toward death, whose faintheartedness they indulge in a curious blend with the toughmindedness of the scientist. The Catholic Church had the guts to say: under these circumstances let the patient die—speaking of the patient alone and not of outside interests (society's, medicine's, etc.). The cowardice of modern secular society which shrinks from death as an unmitigated evil needs the assurance (or fiction) that he is already dead when the decision is to be made. The responsibility of a value-laden decision is replaced by the mechanics of a value-free routine. Insofar as the redefiners of death—by saying "he is already dead"—seek to allay the scruples about turning the respirator off, they cater to this modern cowardice which has forgotten that death has its own fitness and dignity,

and that a man has a right to be let die. Insofar as by saying so they seek to provide an even better conscience about keeping the respirator on and freely utilizing the body thus arrested on the threshold of life and death, they serve the ruling pragmatism of our time which will let no ancient fear and trembling interfere with the relentless expanding of the realm of sheer thinghood and unrestricted utility. The "splendor and misery" of our age dwells in that irresistible tide.

POSTSCRIPT OF DECEMBER 1976

The predictions or premonitions voiced in this essay of 1970 by way of warning have meanwhile begun to come true in the glaring light of the operating theatre. On December 5, 1976, *The New York Times* brought a news report by Robert E. Tomasson under the headline "Girl is ruled dead while respirated," from which I quote the opening paragraph and the crucial statement of the act performed.

A 17-year-old Islip, L. I., schoolgirl who suffered extensive brain damage in an apparent mugging, was pronounced dead on Thursday while she was being sustained with the aid of a respirator. The death certificate was signed, with the consent of her parents, by the family doctor and by the head of the Suffolk County Medical Society. . . .

Within an hour, the girl's eyes and kidneys were removed for transplants. The respirator, which the doctors said was kept going to maintain the viability of the organs, was then disconnected and the forced respiration stopped.

It is to be noted that here the *new definition of death* was actually used for allowing to perform the organ excision *while the "donor" was still,* thanks to the respirator, *in the "equivocal or threshold condition"* (as I have called it) of the comatose. The respirator was disconnected after, not before, the removal of eyes and kidneys, and then only because no further utilization of her body, now or later, happened to be contemplated (or could be because of its non-"viability" without kidneys). But to keep it going beyond the first two surgeries would have required no further legitimation and no new decision of principle. Thus by at least one precedent the door I tried to keep shut has already been opened—and with it the road to the indefinite line of practical possibilities which my lurid imagination descried and whose election no law or qualm or principle any longer blocks. The beginning has been made; fiction cedes to enterprise, and the end is nowhere in sight. All that my essay now can still do—with little hope that it or its like will—is to help ensure that "society," this blurriest of entities, goes through that door with its eyes open and not shut. Inconsistent as man blessedly is, he may still draw the line somewhere without benefit of consistent rule.

NOTES

1. *Ed. note:* See the first essay in this chapter.

2. *Ed. note:* Jonas's essay, "Philosophical Reflections on Experimenting with Human Subjects," was originally published in *Daedalus* 98 (2): 219–247, Spring, 1969.

3. This has turned out to be too charitable an assumption—See *Postscript*.

Legal Issues

ALEXANDER M. CAPRON AND LEON R. KASS

A Statutory Definition of the Standards for Determining Human Death: An Appraisal and a Proposal

In recent years, there has been much discussion of the need to refine and update the criteria for determining that a human being has died.[1] In light of medicine's increasing ability to maintain certain signs of life artificially and to make good use of organs from newly dead bodies, new criteria of death have been proposed by medical authorities.[2] Several states have enacted or are considering legislation to establish a statutory "definition of death," at the prompting of some members of the medical profession who apparently feel that existing, judicially framed standards might expose physicians, particularly transplant surgeons, to civil or criminal liability.[3] Although the leading statute in this area[4] appears to create more problems than it resolves, some legislation may be needed for the protection of the public as well as the medical profession, and, in any event, many more states will probably be enacting such statutes in the near future.

• • •

Reprinted with permission of University of Pennsylvania Law Review and Fred B. Rothman & Company from *University of Pennsylvania Law Review,* Vol. 121, No. 1 (November 1972), pp. 87–88, 102–118.

WHAT CAN AND SHOULD BE LEGISLATED?

Arguments both for and against the desirability of legislation "defining" death often fail to distinguish among the several different subjects that might be touched on by such legislation. As a result, a mistaken impression may exist that a single statutory model is, and must be, the object of debate. An appreciation of the multiple meanings of a "definition of death" may help to refine the deliberations.

Death, in the sense the term is of interest here, can be defined purely formally as the transition, however abrupt or gradual, between the state of being alive and the state of being dead.[5] There are at least four levels of "definitions" that would give substance to this formal notion; in principle, each could be the subject of legislation: (1) the basic concept or idea; (2) general physiological standards; (3) operational criteria; and (4) specific tests or procedures.[6]

The *basic concept* of death is fundamentally a philosophical matter. Example of possible "definitions" of death at this level include "permanent cessation of the integrated functioning of the organism as a whole," "departure of the animating or vital principle,'' or ''irreversible loss of personhood.'' These abstract definitions offer little concrete help in the practical task of determining whether a person has died but they may very well influence how one goes about devising standards and criteria.

In setting forth the *general physiological standard(s)* for recognizing death, the definition moves to a level which is more medicotechnical, but not wholly so. Philosophical issues persist in the choice to define death in terms of organ systems, physiological functions, or recognizable human activities, capacities, and conditions. Examples of possible general standards include ''irreversible cessation of spontaneous respiratory and/or circulatory functions,'' ''irreversible loss of spontaneous brain functions,'' ''irreversible loss of the ability to respond or communicate,'' or some combination of these.

Operational criteria further define what is meant by the general physiological standards. The absence of cardiac contraction and lack of movement of the blood are examples of traditional criteria for ''cessation of spontaneous circulatory functions,'' whereas deep coma, the absence of reflexes, and the lack of spontaneous muscular movements and spontaneous respiration are among criteria proposed for ''cessation of spontaneous brain functions'' by the Harvard Committee.

Fourth, there are the *specific tests and procedures* to see if the criteria are fulfilled. Pulse, heartbeat, blood pressure, electrocardiogram, and examination of blood flow in the retinal vessels are among the specific tests of cardiac contraction and movement of the blood. Reaction to painful stimuli, appearance of the pupils and their responsiveness to light, and observation of movement and breathing over a specified time period are among specific tests of the ''brain function'' criteria enumerated above.

There appears to be general agreement that legislation should not seek to ''define death'' at either the most general or the most specific levels (the first and fourth). In the case of the former, differences of opinion would seem hard to resolve, and agreement, if it were possible, would provide little guidance for practice. In the case of the latter, the specific tests and procedures must be kept open to changes in medical knowledge and technology. Thus, arguments concerning the advisability and desirability of a statutory definition of death are usually confined to the two levels we have called ''standards'' and ''criteria,'' yet

often without any apparent awareness of the distinction between them. The need for flexibility in the face of medical advance would appear to be a persuasive argument for not legislating any specific operational criteria. Moreover, these are almost exclusively technical matters, best left to the judgment of physicians. Thus, the kind of ''definition'' suitable for legislation would be a definition of the general physiological standard or standards. Such a definition, while not immutable, could be expected to be useful for a long period of time and would therefore not require frequent amendment.

There are other matters that could be comprehended in legislation ''defining'' death. The statute could specify who (and how many) shall make the determination. In the absence of a compelling reason to change past practices, this may continue to be set at ''a physician,''[7] usually the doctor attending a dying patient or the one who happens to be at the scene of an accident. Moreover, the law ought probably to specify the ''time of death.'' The statute may seek to fix the precise time when death may be said to have occurred, or it may merely seek to define a time that is clearly after ''the precise moment,'' that is, a time when it is possible to say ''the patient is dead,'' rather than ''the patient has just now died.'' If the medical procedures used in determining that death has occurred call for verification of the findings after a fixed period of time (for example, the Harvard Committee's recommendation that the tests be repeated after twenty-four hours), the statute could in principle assign the ''moment of death'' to either the time when the criteria were first met or the time of verification. The former has been the practice with the traditional criteria for determining death.

Finally, legislation could speak to what follows upon the determination. The statute could be permissive or prescriptive in determining various possible subsequent events, including especially the pronouncement and recording of the death, and the use of the body for burial or other purposes.[8] It is our view that these matters are best handled outside of a statute which has as its purpose to ''define death.''

PRINCIPLES GOVERNING THE FORMULATION OF A STATUTE

In addition to carefully selecting the proper degree of specificity for legislation, there are a number of other principles we believe should guide the drafting of a statute ''defining'' death. First, the phenomenon of interest to physicians, legislators, and laymen alike is human death. Therefore, the statute should concern the death of a human being, not the death of his cells, tissues or organs, and not the ''death'' or cessation of his role as a fully functioning member of his family or community. This point merits considerable emphasis. There may be a proper place for a statutory standard for deciding when to turn off a respirator which is ventilating a patient still clearly alive, or, for that matter, to cease giving any other form of therapy. But it is crucial to distinguish this question of ''when to allow to die?'' from the question with which we are here concerned, namely, ''when to declare dead?'' Since very different issues and purposes are involved in these questions, confusing the one with the other clouds the analysis of both. The problem of determining when a person is dead is difficult enough without its being tied to the problem of whether physicians, or anyone else, may hasten the death of a terminally ill patient, with or without his consent or that of his relatives, in order to minimize his suffering or to conserve scarce medical resources. Although the same set of social and medical conditions may give rise to both problems, they must be kept separate if they are to be clearly understood.

Distinguishing the question ''is he dead?'' from the question ''should he be allowed to die?'' also assists in preserving continuity with tradition, a second important principle. By restricting itself to the ''is he dead?'' issue, a revised ''definition'' permits practices to move incrementally, not by replacing traditional cardiopulmonary standards for the determination of death but rather by supplementing them. These standards are, after all, still adequate in the majority of cases, and are the ones that both physicians and the public are in the habit of employing and relying on. The supplementary standards are needed primarily for those cases in which artificial means of support of comatose patients render the traditional standards unreliable.

Third, this incremental approach is useful for the additional and perhaps most central reason that any new means for judging death should be seen as just that and nothing more—a change in method dictated by advances in medical practice, but not an alteration of the meaning of ''life'' and ''death.'' By indicating that the various standards for measuring death relate to a single phenomenon, legislation can serve to reduce a primary source of public uneasiness on this subject. Once it has been established that certain consequences—for example, burial, autopsy, transfer of property to the heirs, and so forth—follow from a

determination of death, definite problems would arise if there were a number of ''definitions'' according to which some people could be said to be ''more dead'' than others.

There are, of course, many instances in which the law has established differing definitions of a term, each framed to serve a particular purpose. One wonders, however, whether it does not appear somewhat foolish for the law to offer a number of arbitrary definitions of a natural phenomenon such as death. Nevertheless, legislators might seek to identify a series of points during the process of dying, each of which might be labelled ''death'' for certain purposes. Yet so far as we know, no arguments have been presented for special-purpose standards except in the area of organ transplantation. Such a separate ''definition of death,'' aimed at increasing the supply of viable organs, would permit physicians to declare a patient dead before his condition met the generally applicable standards for determining death if his organs are of potential use in transplantation. The adoption of a special standard risks abuse and confusion, however. The status of prospective organ donor is an arbitrary one to which a person can be assigned by relatives[9] or physicians and is unrelated to anything about the extent to which his body's functioning has deteriorated. A special ''definition'' of death for transplantation purposes would thus need to be surrounded by a set of procedural safeguards that would govern not only the method by which a person is to be declared dead but also those by which he is to be classified as an organ donor. Even more troublesome is the confusion over the meaning of death that would probably be engendered by multiple ''definitions.'' Consequently, it would be highly desirable if a statute on death could avoid the problems with a special ''definition.'' Should the statute happen to facilitate organ transplantation, either by making more organs available or by making prospective donors and transplant surgeons more secure in knowing what the law would permit, so much the better.

If, however, more organs are needed for transplantation than can be legally obtained, the question whether the benefits conferred by transplantation justify the risks associated with a broader ''definition'' of death should be addressed directly rather than by attempting to subsume it under the question ''what is death?'' Such a direct confrontation with the issue could lead to a discussion about the standards and procedures under which organs might be taken from persons near death, or even those still quite alive, at their own option[10] or that of relatives, physicians, or representatives of the state. The major advantage of keeping the issues separate is not, of course, that this will facilitate transplantation, but that it will remove a present source of concern: it is unsettling to contemplate that as you lie slowly dying physicians are free to use a more "lenient" standard to declare you dead if they want to remove your organs for transplantation into other patients.

Fourth, the standards for determining death ought not only to relate to a single phenomenon but should also be applied uniformly to all persons. A person's wealth or his "social utility" as an organ donor should not affect the way in which the moment of his death is determined.

Finally, while there is a need for uniformity of application at any one time, the fact that changes in medical technology brought about the present need for "redefinition" argues that the new formulation should be flexible. As suggested in the previous section, such flexibility is most easily accomplished if the new "definition" confines itself to the general standards by which death is to be determined and leaves to the continuing exercise of judgment by physicians the establishment and application of appropriate criteria and specific tests for determining that the standards have been met.

THE KANSAS STATUTE

The first attempt at a legislative resolution of the problems discussed here was made in 1970 when the State of Kansas adopted "An Act relating to and defining death."[11] The Kansas statute has received a good deal of attention; similar legislation was enacted in the spring of 1972 in Maryland and is presently under consideration in a number of other jurisdictions.[12] The Kansas legislation, which was drafted in response to developments in organ transplantation and medical support of dying patients, provides "alternative definitions of death,"[13] set forth in two paragraphs. Under the first, a person is considered "medically and legally dead" if a physician determines "there is the absence of spontaneous respiratory and cardiac function and . . . attempts at resuscitation are considered hopeless."[14] In the second "definition," death turns on the absence of spontaneous brain function if during "reasonable at-

tempts" either to "maintain or restore spontaneous circulatory or respiratory function," it appears that "further attempts at resuscitation or supportive maintenance will not succeed."[15] The purpose of the latter "definition" is made clear by the final sentence paragraph:

Death is to be pronounced before artificial means of supporting respiratory and circulatory function are terminated and *before any vital organ is removed for the purpose of transplantation.*[16]

The primary fault with this legislation is that it appears to be based on, or at least gives voice to, the misconception that there are two separate phenomena of death. This dichotomy is particularly unfortunate because it seems to have been inspired by a desire to establish a special definition for organ transplantation, a definition which physicians would not, however, have to apply, in the draftsman's words, "to prove the irrelevant deaths of most persons."[17] Although there is nothing in the Act itself to indicate that physicians will be less concerned with safeguarding the health of potential organ donors, the purposes for which the Act was passed are not hard to decipher, and they do little to inspire the average patient with confidence that his welfare (including his not being prematurely declared dead) is of as great concern to medicine and the State of Kansas as is the facilitation of organ transplantation.[18] As Professor Kennedy cogently observes, "public disquiet [over transplantation] is in no way allayed by the existence in legislative form of what appear to be alternative definitions of death."[19] One hopes that the form the statute takes does not reflect a conclusion on the part of the Kansas legislature that death occurs at two distinct points during the process of dying.[20] Yet this inference can be derived from the Act, leaving open the prospect "that X at a certain stage in the process of dying can be pronounced dead, whereas Y, having arrived at the same point, is not said to be dead."[21]

The Kansas statute appears also to have attempted more than the "definition" of death, or rather, to have tried to resolve related questions by erroneously treating them as matters of "definition." One supporter of the statute praises it, we think mistakenly, for this reason: "Intentionally, the statute extends to these questions: When can a physician avoid attempting resuscitation? When can he terminate resuscitative efforts? When can he discontinue artificial maintenance?"[22] To be sure, "when the patient is dead'' is one obvious answer to these questions, but by no means the only one. As indicated above, we believe that the question ''when is the patient dead?'' needs to be distinguished and treated separately from the questions ''when may the doctor turn off the respirator?'' or ''when may a patient—dying yet still alive—be allowed to die?''

A STATUTORY PROPOSAL

As an alternative to the Kansas statute we propose the following:

A person will be considered dead if in the announced opinion of a physician, based on ordinary standards of medical practice, he has experienced an irreversible cessation of spontaneous respiratory and circulatory functions. In the event that artificial means of support preclude a determination that these functions have ceased, a person will be considered dead if in the announced opinion of a physician, based on ordinary standards of medical practice, he has experienced an irreversible cessation of spontaneous brain functions. Death will have occurred at the time when the relevant functions ceased.

This proposed statute provides a ''definition'' of death confined to the level of *general physiological standards,* and it has been drafted in accord with the five principles set forth above. . . . First, the proposal speaks in terms of the *death* of a *person.* The determination that a person has died is to be based on an evaluation of certain vital bodily functions, the permanent absence of which indicates that he is no longer a living human being. By concentrating on the death of a human being as a whole, the statute rightly disregards the fact that some cells or organs may continue to ''live'' after this point, just as others may have ceased functioning long before the determination of death. This statute would leave for resolution by other means the question of when the absence or deterioration of certain capacities, such as the ability to communicate, or functions, such as the cerebral, indicates that a person may or should be allowed to die without further medical intervention.

Second, the proposed legislation is predicated upon the single phenomenon of death. Moreover, it applies uniformly to all persons,[23] by specifying the circumstances under which each of the standards is to be used rather than leaving this to the unguided discretion of physicians. Unlike the Kansas law, the model statute does not leave to arbitrary decision a choice between two apparently equal yet different ''alternative definitions of death.''[24] Rather, its sec-ond standard is applicable only when ''artificial means of support preclude'' use of the first. It does not establish a separate kind of death, called ''brain death.'' In other words, the proposed law would provide two standards gauged by different functions, for measuring different manifestations of the same phenomenon. If cardiac and pulmonary functions have ceased, brain functions cannot continue; if there is no brain activity and respiration has to be maintained artificially, the same state (*i.e.,* death) exists. Some people might prefer a single standard, one based either on cardiopulmonary or brain functions. This would have the advantage of removing the last trace of the ''two deaths'' image, which any reference to alternative standards may still leave. Respiratory and circulatory indicators, once the only touchstone, are no longer adequate in some situations. It would be possible, however, to adopt the alternative, namely that death is *always* to be established by assessing spontaneous brain functions. Reliance only on brain activity, however, would represent a sharp and unnecessary break with tradition. Departing from continuity with tradition is not only theoretically unfortunate in that it violates another principle of good legislation . . . but also practically very difficult, since most physicians customarily employ cardiopulmonary tests for death and would be slow to change, especially when the old tests are easier to perform, more accessible and acceptable to the lay public, and perfectly adequate for determining death in most instances.

Finally, by adopting standards for death in terms of the cessation of certain vital bodily functions but not in terms of the specific criteria or tests by which these functions are to be measured, the statute does not prevent physicians from adapting their procedures to changes in medical technology.

A basic substantive issue remains: what are the merits of the proposed standards? For ordinary situations, the appropriateness of the traditional standard, ''an irreversible cessation of spontaneous respiratory and circulatory functions,'' does not require elaboration. Indeed, examination by a physician may be more a formal than a real requirement in determining that most people have died. In addition to any obvious injuries, elementary signs of death such as absence of heartbeat and breathing, cold skin, fixed pupils, and so forth, are usually sufficient to indicate even to a layman that the accident victim, the elderly person who passes away quietly in the night, or the patient stricken with a sudden infarct has died. The difficulties arise when modern medicine intervenes to sustain a patient's respiration and circulation. . . . The indicators of brain damage appear reliable, in that studies have shown that patients who fit the Harvard criteria have suffered such extensive damage that they do not recover. Of course, the task of the neurosurgeon or physician is simplified in the common case where an accident victim has suffered such gross, apparent injuries to the head that it is not necessary to apply the Harvard criteria in order to establish cessation of brain functioning.

The statutory standard, "irreversible cessation of spontaneous brain functions," is intended to encompass both higher brain activities and those of the brainstem. There must, of course, also be no spontaneous respiration; the second standard is applied only when breathing is being artificially maintained. The major emphasis placed on brain functioning, although generally consistent with the common view of what makes man distinctive as a living creature, brings to the fore a basic issue: What aspects of brain function should be decisive? The question has been reframed by some clinicians in light of their experience with patients who have undergone what they term "neocortical death" (that is, complete destruction of higher brain capacity, demonstrated by a flat EEG). "Once neocortical death has been unequivocally established and the possibility of any recovery of consciousness and intellectual activity [is] thereby excluded, . . . although [the] patient breathes spontaneously, is he or she alive?"[25] While patients with irreversible brain damage from cardiac arrest seldom survive more than a few days, cases have recently been reported of survival for up to two and one-quarter years.[26] Nevertheless, though existence in this state falls far short of a full human life, the very fact of spontaneous respiration, as well as coordinated movements and reflex activities at the brainstem and spinal cord levels, would exclude these patients from the scope of the statutory standards.[27] The condition of "neocortical death" may well be a proper justification for interrupting all forms of treatment and allowing these patients to die, but this moral and legal problem cannot and should not be settled by "defining" these people "dead."

The legislation suggested here departs from the Kansas statute in its basic approach to the problem of "defining" death: the proposed statute does not set about to establish a special category of "brain death" to be used by transplanters. Further, there are a number of particular points of difference between them. For example, the proposed statute does not speak of persons being "medically and legally dead," thus avoiding redundancy and, more importantly, the mistaken implication that the "medical" and "legal" definitions could differ. Also, the proposed legislation does not include the provision that "death is to be pronounced before" the machine is turned off or any organs removed. Such a *modus operandi,* which was incorporated by Kansas from the Harvard Committee's report, may be advisable for physicians on public relations grounds, but it has no place in a statute "defining" death. The proposed statute already provides that "Death will have occurred at the time when the relevant functions ceased." If supportive aids, or organs, are withdrawn after this time, such acts cannot be implicated as having caused death. The manner in which, or exact time at which, the physician should articulate his finding is a matter best left to the exigencies of the situation, to local medical customs or hospital rules, or to statutes on the procedures for certifying death or on transplantation if the latter is the procedure which raises the greatest concern of medical impropriety. The real safeguard against doctors killing patients is not to be found in a statute "defining" death. Rather, it inheres in physicians' ethical and religious beliefs, which are also embodied in the fundamental professional ethic of *primum non nocere* and are reinforced by homicide and "wrongful death" laws and the rules governing medical negligence applicable in license revocation proceedings or in private actions for damages.

•   •   •

CONCLUSION

Changes in medical knowledge and procedures have created an apparent need for a clear and acceptable revision of the standards for determining that a person has died. Some commentators have argued that the formulation of such standards should be left to physicians. The reasons for rejecting this argument seem compelling: the "definition of death" is not merely a matter for technical expertise, the uncertainty of the present law is unhealthy for society and physicians alike, there is a great potential for mischief and harm through the possibility of conflict between the standards applied by some physicians and those assumed to be applicable by the community at large and its legal system, and patients and their relatives are made uneasy by physicians apparently being free to shift around the meaning of death without any societal guidance. Accordingly, we conclude the public has a legitimate role to play in the formulation and adoption of such standards. This article has proposed a model statute which bases a determination of death primarily on the traditional standard of final respiratory and circulatory cessation; where the artificial maintenance of these functions precludes the use of such a standard, the statute authorizes that death be determined on the basis of irreversible cessation of spontaneous brain functions. We believe the legislation proposed would dispel public confusion and concern and protect physicians and patients, while avoiding the creation of "two types of death," for which the statute on this subject first adopted in Kansas has been justly criticized. The proposal is offered not as the ultimate solution to the problem, but as a catalyst for what we hope will be a robust and well-informed public debate over a new "definition." Finally, the proposed statute leaves for future resolution the even more difficult problems concerning the conditions and procedures under which a decision may be reached to cease treating a terminal patient who does not meet the standards set forth in the statutory "definition of death."

NOTES

1. *See, e.g.,* P. Ramsey, The Patient as Person 59–119 (1970); Louisell, *Transplantation; Existing Legal Constraints,* in Ethics in Medical Progress: With Special Reference to Transplantation 91–92 (G. Wolstenholme & M. O'Connor eds. 1966) [hereinafter cited as Medical Progress]: *Discussion* of Murray, *Organic Transplantation: The Practical Possibilities,* in *id.* 68 (comments of Dr. G. E. Schreiner), 71 (comments of Dr. M. F. A. Woodruff); Wasmuth & Stewart, *Medical and Legal Aspects of Human Organ Transplantation,* 14 Clev.-Mar. L. Rev 442 (1965); Beecher, *Ethical Problems Created by the Hopelessly Unconscious Patient,* 278 New Eng. J. Med 1425 (1968); Wasmuth, *The Concept of Death,* 30 Ohio St. L. J. 32 (1969); Note, *The Need for a Redefinition of "Death,"* 45 Chi.-Kent L. Rev. 202 (1969).

2. *See, e.g.,* Ad Hoc Committee of the Harvard Medical School to Examine the Definition of Brain Death, *A Definition of Irreversible Coma,* 205 J.A.M.A. 337 (1968) [hereinafter cited as *Irreversible Coma*]; *Discussion* of Murray, *Organ Transplantation: The Practical Possibilities,* in Medical Progress, *supra* note 1, at 69–74 (remarks of Drs. G. P. J. Alexandre, R. Y. Calne, J. Hamburger, J. E. Murray, J. P. Revillard & G. E. Schreiner); *When Is a Patient Dead?,* 204 J.A.M.A. 1000 (1968) (editorial); *Updating the Definition of Death,* Med. World News, Apr. 28, 1967, at 47. . . .

3. *See, e.g.,* Taylor, *A Statutory Definition of Death in Kansas,* 215 J.A.M.A. 296 (1971) (letter to the editor), in which the principal draftsman of the Kansas statute states that the law was believed necessary to protect transplant surgeons against the risk of "a criminal charge, for the existence of a resuscitated heart in another body should be excellent evidence that the donor was not dead

[under the "definition" of death then existing in Kansas] until the operator excised the heart." . . . The specter of civil liability was raised in *Tucker v. Lower,* a recent action brought by the brother of a heart donor against the transplantation team at the Medical College of Virginia. . . .

4. Kan. Stat. Ann. § 77–202 (Supp. 1971); see notes 11–24 *infra* & accompanying text for a discussion of this statute.

5. For a debate on the underlying issues see Morison, *Death: Process or Event?* 173 Science 694 (1970); Kass, *Death as an Event: A Commentary on Robert Morison,* 173 Science 698 (1971).

6. To our knowledge, this delineation of four levels has not been made elsewhere in the existing literature on this subject. Therefore, the terms "concept," "standard," "criteria," and "tests and procedures" as used here bear no necessary connection to the ways in which others may use these same terms, and in fact we recognize that in some areas of discourse, the term "standards" is more, rather than less, operational and concrete than "criteria"—just the reverse of our ordering. Our terminology was selected so that the category we call "criteria" would correspond to the level of specificity at which the Ad Hoc Harvard Committee framed its proposals, which it called and which are widely referred to as the *"new criteria"* for determining death. We have attempted to be consistent in our use of these terms throughout this Article. Nevertheless, our major purpose here is not to achieve public acceptance of our terms, but to promote awareness of the four different levels of a "definition" of death to which the terms refer.

7. Cf. Uniform Anatomical Gift Act § 7(b).

8. If . . . sound procedures for stating death are agreed to and carried out, then theologians and moralists and every other thoughtful person should agree with the physicians who hold that it is *then* permissible to maintain circulation of blood and supply of oxygen in the corpse of a donor to preserve an *organ* until it can be used in transplantation. Whether one gives the body over for decent burial, performs an autopsy, gives the cadaver for use in medical education, or uses it as a "vital organ bank" are all alike procedures governed by decent respect for the bodies of deceased men and specific regulations that ensure this. The ventilation and circulation of organs for transplant raises no question not already raised by these standard procedures. None are life-and-death matters. P. Ramsey, The Patient as Person 72 (1970).

9. Uniform Anatomical Gift Act § 2(c). For example, if a special standard were adopted for determining death in potential organ donors, relatives of a dying patient with limited financial means might feel substantial pressure to give permission for his organs to be removed in order to bring to a speedier end the care given the patient.

10. *See, e.g.,* Blachly, *Can Organ Transplantation Provide an Altruistic-Expiatory Alternative to Suicide?,* 1 Life-Threatening Behavior 6 (1971); Scribner, *Ethical Problems of Using Artificial Organs to Sustain Human Life,* 10 Trans. Am. Soc. Artif. Internal Organs 209, 211 (1964) (advocating legal guidelines to permit voluntary euthanasia for purpose of donating organs for transplantation).

11. Law of Mar. 17, 1970, ch. 378 [1970] Kan. Laws 994 [codified at Kan. Stat. Ann. § 77–202 (Supp. 1971)]. It provides in full:

A person will be considered medically and legally dead if, in the opinion of a physician, based on ordinary standards of medical practice, there is the absence of spontaneous brain function; and if based on ordinary standards of medical practice, during reasonable attempts to either maintain or restore spontaneous circulatory or respiratory function in the absence of aforesaid brain function, it appears that further attempts at resuscitation or supportive maintenance will not succeed, death will have occurred at the time when these conditions first coincide. Death is to be pronounced before artificial means of supporting respiratory and circulatory function are terminated and before any vital organ is removed for purposes of transplantation.

These alternative definitions of death are to be utilized for all purposes in this state, including the trials of civil and criminal cases, any laws to the contrary notwithstanding.

12. . . . In the Maryland law, which is nearly identical to its Kansas progenitor, the phrase "in the opinion of a physician" was deleted from the first paragraph, and the phrase "and because of a known disease or condition" was added to the second paragraph following "ordinary standards of medical practice." Maryland Sessions Laws ch. 693 (1972). Interestingly, Kansas and Maryland were also among the first states to adopt the Uniform Anatomical Gift Act in 1968, even prior to its official revision and approval by the National Conference of Commissioners on Uniform State Laws.

13. Note 11 *supra*.

14. *Id*. In using the term "hopeless," the Kansas legislature apparently intended to indicate that the "absence of spontaneous respiratory and cardiac function" must be irreversible before death is pronounced. In addition to being rather roundabout, this formulation is also confusing in that it might be taken to address the "when to allow to die?" question as well as the "is he dead?" question. *See* note 22 *infra* and accompanying text.

15. Note 11 *supra*.

16. *Id*. (emphasis added).

17. Taylor, *supra* note 3 at 296.

18. Cf. Kass, *A Caveat on Transplants*, The Washington Post, Jan. 14, 1968, § B, at 1, col. 1.

19. Kennedy, *The Kansas Statute on Death: An Appraisal*, 285 New Eng. J. Med. 947 (1971).

20. General use of the term "resuscitation" might suggest the existence of a common notion that a person can die once, be revived (given life again), and then die again at a later time—in the other words, that death can occur at two or more distinct points in time. But resuscitation only restores life "from *apparent* death or unconsciousness." Webster's Third New International Dictionary 1937 (1966) (emphasis added). The proposed statute, text accompanying note 24 infra, takes account of the possibility of resuscitation by providing that death occurs only when there has been an *irreversible* cessation of the relevant vital bodily functions. Cf. 3 M. Houts & I. H. Haut, Courtroom Medicine § 1.01 (3)(d) (1971):

"The ability to resuscitate patients after apparent death, coupled with observations that in many cases the restoration was not to a state of consciousness, understanding and intellectual functioning, but merely to a decerebrate, vegetative existence, and with advances in neurology that have brought greater, though far from complete, understanding of the functions of the nervous system,

has drawn attention to the role of the nervous system in maintaining life."

21. Kennedy, *op. cit.*

22. Mills, *The Kansas Death Statute: Bold and Innovative,* 285 New Eng. J. Med. 968 (1971).

23. Differences in the exact mode of diagnosing death will naturally occur as a result of differing circumstances under which the physician's examination is made. Thus the techniques employed with an automobile accident victim lying on the roadside at night may be less sophisticated than those used with a patient who has been receiving treatment in a well-equipped hospital.

24. Kan. Stat. Ann. § 77–202 (Supp. 1971).

25. Brierley, Adams, Graham & Simpson, *Neocortical Death After Cardiac Arrest,* 2 Lancet 560, 565 (1971) [hereinafter cited as Brierley]. In addition to a flat (isoelectric) electroencephalogram, a "neuropathological examination of a biopsy specimen . . . from the posterior half of a cerebral hemisphere" provides further confirmation. *Id*. The editors of a leading medical journal question "whether a state of cortical death can be diagnosed clinically." Editorial, *Death of a Human Being,* 2 Lancet 590 (1971). Cf. note 14 *supra* [original text].

26. Brierley and his colleagues report two cases of their own in which the patients each survived in a comatose condition for five months after suffering cardiac arrest before dying of pulmonary complications. They also mention two unreported cases of a Doctor Lewis, in one of which the patient survived for 2¼ years. Brierley, *supra* note 25, at 565.

27. The exclusion of patients without neocortical function from the category of death may appear somewhat arbitrary in light of our disinclination to engage in a philosophical discussion of the basic concepts of human "life" and "death." *See* text accompanying notes 5–6 *supra*. Were the "definition" contained in the proposed statute a departure from what has traditionally been meant by "death," such a conceptual discussion would clearly be in order. But, as this Article has tried to demonstrate, our intention has been more modest: to provide a clear restatement of the traditional understanding in terms which are useful in light of modern medical capabilities and practices. . . .

A philosophical examination of the essential attributes of being "human" might lead one to conclude that persons who, for example, lack the mental capacity to communicate in any meaningful way, should be regarded as "not human" or "dead." It would nevertheless probably be necessary and prudent to treat the determination of that kind of "death" under special procedures until such time as medicine is able routinely to diagnose the extent and irreversibility of the loss of the "central human capacities" (however defined) with the same degree of assurance now possible in determining that death has occurred. Consequently, even at the conceptual level, we are inclined to think that it is best to distinguish the question "is he dead?" from such questions as "should he be allowed to die?" and "should his death be actively promoted?"

PRESIDENT'S COMMISSION FOR THE STUDY OF ETHICAL PROBLEMS IN MEDICINE AND BIOMEDICAL AND BEHAVIORAL RESEARCH

A Proposed Uniform Determination of Death Act

Editor's note. Between 1972, when Capron and Kass proposed their model statute, and 1981, when the President's Commission completed its report, three major model definition-of-death statutes were proposed in the United States.

1. American Bar Association (1975):

For all legal purposes, a human body, with irreversible cessation of total brain function, according to usual and customary standards of medical practice, shall be considered dead.

2. National Conference of Commissioners on Uniform State Laws, "The Uniform Brain Death Act" (1978):

For legal and medical purposes, an individual who has sustained irreversible cessation of all functioning of the brain, including the brain stem, is dead. A determination under this section must be made in accordance with reasonable medical standards.

3. American Medical Association (1979):

Section 1. An individual who has sustained either (1) irreversible cessation of circulatory and respiratory functions, or (2) irreversible cessation of all functions of the entire brain, shall be considered dead. A determination of death shall be made in accordance with accepted medical standards.

Section 2. A physician or any other person authorized by law to determine death who makes such determination in accordance with Section 1 is not liable for damages in any civil action or subject to prosecution in any criminal proceeding for his acts or the acts of others based on that determination. . . .

From the Commission's July 1981 final report entitled: *"Defining Death": A Report on the Medical, Legal and Ethical Issues in the Determination of Death.*

Variations of these model statutes, the Capron-Kass proposal, and the 1970 Kansas law have been adopted in twenty-two of the fifty states.

In 1981 the Law Reform Commission of Canada published an additional model statute on the determination of death:

For all purposes within the jurisdiction of the Parliament of Canada,
(1) a person is dead when an irreversible cessation of all that person's brain functions has occurred.
(2) the irreversible cessation of brain functions can be determined by the prolonged absence of spontaneous circulatory and respiratory functions.
(3) when the determination of the prolonged absence of spontaneous circulatory and respiratory functions is made impossible by the use of artificial means of support, the irreversible cessation of brain functions can be determined by any means recognized by the ordinary standards of current medical practice.

—L.W.

THE LANGUAGE AND ITS HISTORY

The array of "model laws" and state variations reveals two major problems: first, their diversity, and second, the overly complex or inexact wording that characterizes many of them. Diversity is a problem for several reasons. In the case of enacted statutes, diversity means nonuniformity among jurisdictions. In most areas of the law, provisions that diverge from one state to the next create, at worst, inconvenience and the occasional failure of a finely honed business or personal plan to achieve its intended result. But on the subject of death, nonuniformity has a jarring effect. Of course, the diversity is really only superficial; all the enacted statutes appear to have the same intent.

Yet even small differences raise the question: if the statutes all mean the same thing, why are they so varied? And it is possible to think of medical situations—and, even more freely, of legal cases that would be unlikely but not bizarre—in which the differences in statutory language *could* lead to different outcomes.

More fundamental is the obstacle that diversity presents for the process of statutory enactment. Legislators, presented with a variety of proposals and no clear explanation of the significance of their differences, are (not surprisingly) wary of *all* the choices. Proponents of each of the models (and other critics) compounded this difficulty by objecting to the language of the other statutes. . . .

A uniform proposal that is broadly acceptable would significantly ease the enactment of good law on death throughout the United States. To that end, the Commission's Executive Director met in May 1980 with representatives of the American Bar Association, the American Medical Association, and the National Conference of Commissioners on Uniform State Laws. Through a comparison of the then existing "models" with the objectives that a statute ought to serve, they arrived at a proposed Uniform Determination of Death Act:

1. [*Determination of Death.*] An individual who has sustained either (1) irreversible cessation of circulatory and respiratory functions, or (2) irreversible cessation of all functions of the entire brain, including the brainstem, is dead. A determination of death must be made in accordance with accepted medical standards.

2. [*Uniformity of Construction and Application.*] This act shall be applied and construed to effectuate its general purpose to make uniform the law with respect to the subject of this Act among states enacting it.

This model law has now been approved by the Uniform Law Commissioners, the ABA, and the AMA as a substitute for their previous proposals. It has also been endorsed by the American Academy of Neurology and the American Electroencephalographic Society.

CONSTRUCTION OF THE STATUTE

The proposed statute addresses the matter of "defining" death at the level of general physiological standards rather than at the level of more abstract concepts or the level of more precise criteria and tests.

The proposed statute articulates alternative standards, since in the vast majority of cases irreversible circulatory and respiratory cessation will be the obvious and sufficient basis for diagnosing death. When a patient is not supported on a respirator, the need to evaluate brain functions does not arise. The basic statute in this area should acknowledge that fact by setting forth the basis on which death *is* determined in such cases (namely, that breathing and blood flow have ceased and cannot be restored or replaced).

It would be possible, as in the statute drafted by the Law Reform Commission of Canada, to propound the irreversible cessation of brain functions as *the* "definition" and then to permit that standard to be met not only by direct measures of brain activity but also "by the prolonged absence of spontaneous cardiac and respiratory functions."[1] Although conceptually acceptable (and vastly superior to the adoption of brain cessation as a primary standard conjoined with a nonspecific reference to other, apparently unrelated "usual and customary procedures"[2]), the Canadian proposal breaks with tradition in a manner that appears to be unnecessary. For most lay people—and in all probability for most physicians as well—the permanent loss of heart and lung function (for example, in an elderly person who has died in his or her sleep) clearly manifests death. Biomedical scientists can explain the brain's particularly important—and vulnerable—role in the organism as a whole and show how temporary loss of blood flow (ischemia) becomes permanent cessation because of the damage it inflicts on the brain. Nonetheless, most of the time people do not, and need not, go through this two-step process. Irreversible loss of circulation is recognized as death because—setting aside any mythical connotations of the heart—a person without blood flow simply cannot live. Thus, the Commission prefers to employ language which would reflect the continuity of the traditional standard and the newer, brain-based standard.

"INDIVIDUAL"

Other aspects of the statutory language, as well as several phrases that were intentionally omitted, deserve special mention. First, the word "individual" is employed here to conform to the standard designation of a human being in the language of the uniform acts. The term "person" was not used here because it is sometimes used by the law to include a corporation. Although that particular confusion would be unlikely to arise here, the narrower term "individual" is more precise and thus avoids the possibility of confusion.

Second, the statute emphasizes the degree of damage to the brain required for a determination of death by stating "*all* functions of the *entire* brain, *including the brainstem*" (emphasis added). This may be thought doubly redundant, but at least it should make plain the intent to *exclude* from application under the "definition" any patient who has lost only "higher" brain functions or, conversely, who maintains those functions but has suffered solely a direct injury to the brainstem which interferes with the vegetative functions of the body.

The phrase "cessation of *functions*" reflects an important choice. It stands in contrast to two other terms that have been discussed in this field: (a) "loss of activity" and (b) "destruction of the organ."

Bodily parts, and the subparts that make them up, are important for the functions they perform. Thus, detecting a loss of the ability to function is the central aim of diagnosis in this field. After an organ has lost the ability to *function* within the organism, electrical and metabolic *activity* at the level of individual cells or even groups of cells may continue for a period of time. Unless this cellular activity is integrated, however, it cannot contribute to the operation of the organism as a whole. Thus, cellular activity alone is irrelevant in judging whether the organism, as opposed to its components, is "dead."

At the other pole, several commentators have argued that organic *destruction* rather than cessation of functions should be the basis for declaring death.[3] They assert that until an organ has been destroyed there is always the *possibility* that it might resume functioning. The Commission has rejected this position for several reasons. Once brain cells have permanently ceased metabolizing, the body cannot regenerate them. The loss of the brain's functions precedes the destruction of the cells and liquefaction of the tissues.

Theoretically, even *destruction* of an organ does not prevent its functions from being restored. Any decision to recognize "the end" is inevitably restricted by the limits of available medical knowledge and techniques.[4] Since "irreversibility" adjusts to the times, the proposed statute can incorporate new clinical capabilities. Many patients declared dead fifty years ago because of heart failure would not have experienced an "*irreversible* cessation of circulatory and respiratory functions" in the hands of a modern hospital.

Finally, the argument for using "brain destruction" echoes the proposal about "putrefaction" made two centuries ago and overcome by advances in diagnostic techniques. The traditional cardiopulmonary standard relies on the vital signs as a measure of heart-lung function; the declaration of death does not await evidence of destruction. Since the evidence reviewed by the Commission indicates that brain criteria, properly applied, diagnose death as reliably as cardiopulmonary criteria, the Commission sees no reason not to use the same standards of cessation for both. The requirement of "irreversible cessation of functions" should apply to both cardiopulmonary and brain-based determinations.

"IS DEAD"

Most of the model statutes previously proposed state that a person meeting the statutory standards "will [or shall] be considered dead." This formulation, although probably effective in achieving the desired clarification of the place of "brain death" in the law, is somewhat disconcerting since it might be read to indicate that the law will *consider* someone dead who by some other, perhaps wiser, standard *is not* dead. The President's Commission does not endorse this view. It favors stating more directly (as had the Uniform State Law Commissioners in their 1978 proposal) that a person "is dead" when he or she meets one of the standards set forth in the statute.

In declaring that an individual "is dead," physicians imply that at some moment prior to the diagnosis the individual moved from the status of "being alive" to "being dead." The Commission concurs in the view that "death should be viewed not as a process but as the event that separates the process of dying from the process of distintegration."[5] Although it assumes that each dead person became dead at some moment prior to the time of diagnosis, the statute does not specify that moment. Rather, this calculation is left to "accepted medical practices" and the law of each jurisdiction.

Determining the time of passage from living to dead can be troublesome in certain situations; like all aspects of assessing whether a body is dead, it relies heavily on the clinical skills and judgment of the person making the determination. In most cases, it appears to be the custom simply to record the time when a diagnosis of death is made as the time of death. When precision is important for legal purposes, the scientific basis for determining the time of death may be reexamined and resolved through legal proceedings.

A determination of death immediately changes the attitudes and behavior of the living toward the body that has gone from being a person to being a corpse. Discontinuation of medical care, mourning, and burial are examples of customary behavior; people usually provide intimate care for living patients and identify with them, while withdrawing from contact with the dead. In ordinary circumstances, the time at which medical diagnosis causes a change in legal status should be synchronous with the time that social behaviors naturally change.

In some cases of death determined by neurologic criteria, however, it is necessary to allow for repeated testing, observation, or metabolism of drugs. This may interpose hours or even days between the actual time of death and its confirmation. Procedures for certifying time of death, like those for determining the status of being dead, will be a matter for locally "accepted medical standards," hospital rules and custom, community mores and state death certificate law. Present practice in most localities now parallels the determination of death by cardiopulmonary criteria: death by brain criteria is certified at the time that the fact of death is established, that is, after all tests and confirmatory observation periods are complete.

When the time of "brain death" has legal importance, a best medical estimate of the actual time when all brain functions irreversibly ceased will probably be appropriate. Where this is a matter of controversy, it becomes a point to be resolved by the law of the jurisdiction. Typically, judges decide this on the basis of expert testimony—as they do with a contested determination of unwitnessed cessation of cardiopulmonary functions.

"ACCEPTED MEDICAL STANDARDS"

The proposed statutes variously describe the basis on which the criteria and tests actually used to diagnose death may be selected. The variations were:

Capron-Kass (1972):   "based on ordinary standards of medical practice"

ABA (1975):   "according to usual and customary standards of medical practice"

NCCUSL (1978):   "in accordance with reasonable medical standards"

AMA (1979):   "in accordance with accepted medical standards"

Despite their linguistic differences, the Capron-Kass, ABA, and AMA models apparently intend the same result: to require the use of diagnostic measures and procedures that have the normal test of scrutiny and adoption by the biomedical community. In contrast, the 1978 Uniform proposal sounded a different note by proposing "reasonableness" as the standard. The problem is: whose reasonableness? Might lay jurors conclude that a medical practice, although generally adopted, was "unreasonable"? It would be unfair to subject a physician (and others acting pursuant to his or her instructions) to liability on the basis of an after-the-fact determination of standards if he or she had been acting in good faith and according to the norms of professional practice and belief. Even the prospect of this liability would unnecessarily disrupt orderly decision-making in this field.

The process by which a norm of medical practice becomes "accepted" varies according to the field and the type of procedure at issue. The statutory language should eliminate wholly idiosyncratic standards or the use of experimental means of diagnosis (except in conjunction with adequate customary procedures). On the other hand, the statute does not require a procedure to be universally adopted; it is enough if, like any medical practice which is later challenged, it has been accepted by a substantial and reputable body of medical men and women as safe and efficacious for the purpose for which it is being employed.[6]

The Commission has also concluded that the statute need not elaborate the legal consequences of following accepted practices. The model statute proposed earlier by the AMA contained separate sections precluding criminal and civil prosecution or liability for determinations of death made in accordance with the statute or actions taken "in good faith in reliance on a determination of death."[7] It is not necessary to address this issue in a statute because the existing common law already eliminates such liability.

• • •

PERSONAL BELIEFS

Should a statute include a "conscience clause" permitting an individual (or family members, where the individual is incompetent) to specify the standard to be used for determining his or her death based upon personal or religious beliefs?[8] While sympathetic to the concerns and values that prompt this suggestion, the Commission has concluded that such a provision has no place in a statute on the determination of death. Were a nonuniform standard permitted, unfortunate and mischievous results are easily imaginable.[9]

If the question were what actions (e.g., termination of treatment, autopsy, removal of organs, etc.) could be taken, there might be room for such a conscience clause. Yet, as the question is one of legal *status,* on which turn the rights and interests not only of the one individual but also of other people and of the state itself, the subject is not one for personal (or familial) self-determination.

The statute specifies that death has occurred if *either* cardiopulmonary or brain criteria are met. Although, as a legal matter, there is no personal discretion as to the *fact* of death when either criterion is met, room remains for reasonable accommodation of personal beliefs regarding the actions to be taken once a determination of death has been made. Such actions, whether medical (e.g., maintaining a deady body on a respirator until organs are removed for transplantation) or religious (e.g., withholding religious pronouncement of death until the blood has ceased flowing), can very with the circumstances. Some subjects in the Commission's hospital survey, for example, were maintained on ventilators for several hours after they were dead, in deference to family wishes or in order for the family to decide whether to donate the deceased's organs.

· · ·

NOTES

1. Law Reform Commission of Canada. *Criteria for the Determination of Death* (Report, No. 15), Minister of Supply and Service, Canada (1981) at 7–20.

2. See, e.g., Cal. Health and Safety Code §7180 (West 1975).

3. Paul A. Byrne, Sean O'Reilly, and Paul M. Quay, "Brain Death: An Opposing Viewpoint," 242 *J.A.M.A.* 1985 (1979).

4. Already, a hand "destroyed" in an accident can be reconstructed using advanced surgical methods. The functions of the kidney can be artificially restored through extracorporeal devices; an implantable artificial heart has been tested in animals and is now proposed for human trials. It is impossible to predict what other "miracles" biomedical science may some day produce in the restoration of natural functions or their substitution through artificial means.

5. James L. Bernat, Charles M. Culver, and Bernard Gert, "On the Definition and Criterion of Death," 94 *Ann. Int. Med.* 389 (1981): "If we regard death as a process then either the process starts when the person is still living, which confuses the 'process of death' with the process of dying, for we all regard someone who is dying as not yet dead, or the 'process of death' starts when the

person is no longer alive, which confuses death with the process of disintegration." *Id.*

6. Edwards v. United States, 519 F.2d 1137 (5th Cir. 1975); Price v. Neyland, 320 F.2d 674 (D.C. Cir. 1963).

7. 243 *J.A.M.A.* 420 (1980) (editorial).

8. Robert M. Veatch, *Death, Dying and the Biological Revolution: Our Last Quest for Responsibility,* Yale University Press, New Haven, Connecticut (1977) at 72–76; Michael T. Sullivan, "The Dying Person—His Plight and His Right," 216 *New Eng. L. Rev.* 1978 (1973).

9. Alexander M. Capron, "Legal Definition of Death," 315 *Ann. N.Y. Acad. Sci.* 349, 356–357 (1978).

SUGGESTED READINGS FOR CHAPTER 7

Beauchamp, Tom L., and Perlin, Seymour, eds. *Ethical Issues in Death and Dying.* Englewood Cliffs, N.J.: Prentice-Hall, 1978. Chap. 1.

Beecher, Henry K. "After the 'Definition of Irreversible Coma'." *New England Journal of Medicine* 281 (November 6, 1969), 1070–1071.

———. "Ethical Problems Created by the Hopelessly Unconscious Patient." *New England Journal of Medicine* 278 (June 27, 1968), 1425–1430.

Bernat, James L., *et al.* "On the Definition and Criterion of Death." *Annals of Internal Medicine* 94 (March 1981), 389–394.

Black, Peter M. "Brain Death." *New England Journal of Medicine* 299 (August 17 and 24, 1978), 338–344, 393–401.

———. "Three Definitions of Death." *Monist* 60 (January 1977), 136–146.

Brierley, J. B., *et al.* "Neocortical Death after Cardiac Arrest." *Lancet* 2 (September 11, 1971), 560–565.

Byrne, Paul A., *et al.* "Brain Death—An Opposing Viewpoint." *Journal of the American Medical Association* 242 (November 2, 1979), 1985–1990.

Canada, Law Reform Commission. *Criteria for the Determination of Death.* Ottawa: Law Reform Commission of Canada, 1979.

Capron, Alexander M. "Death, Definition and Determination of: Legal Aspects of Pronouncing Death." In Reich, Warren T., ed. *Encyclopedia of Bioethics.* New York: Free Press, 1978. Vol. 1, pp. 296–301.

Conference of Medical Royal Colleges and Faculties of the United Kingdom. "Diagnosis of Brain Death." *Lancet* 2 (November 13, 1976), 1069–1070.

Engelhardt, H. Tristram. "Definition of Death: Where to Draw the Lines and Why." In McMullin, Ernan, ed. *Death and Decision.* Boulder, Colo.: Westview Press, 1978, pp. 15–34.

Gaylin, Willard. "Harvesting the Dead." *Harper's* 249 (September 1974), 23–28+.

Green, Michael B., and Wikler, Daniel. "Brain Death and Personal Identity." *Philosophy and Public Affairs* 9 (Winter 1980), 105–133.

High, Dallas M. "Death, Definition and Determination of: Philosophical and Theological Foundations." In Reich, Warren T., ed. *Encyclopedia of Bioethics.* New York: Free Press, 1978. Vol. 1, pp. 301–307.

Institute of Society, Ethics and the Life Sciences, Task Force on Death and Dying. "Refinements in Criteria for the Determination of Death." *Journal of the American Medical Association* 221 (July 3, 1972), 48–53.

Jennett, Bryan, *et al.* "Brain Death in Three Neurosurgical Units." *British Medical Journal* 282 (February 14, 1981), 533–539.

Korein, Julius, ed. "Brain Death: Interrelated Medical and Social Issues." *Annals of the New York Academy of Sciences* 315 (1978), 1–454.

Margolis, Joseph. *Negativities.* Columbus, Ohio: Charles E. Merrill Co., 1975. Chap. 1.

Molinari, Gaetano F. "Death, Definition and Determination of: Criteria for Death." In Reich, Warren T., ed. *Encyclopedia of Bioethics.* New York: Free Press, 1978. Vol. 1, pp. 292–296.

Morrison, Robert, and Kass, Leon. "Death—Process or Event?" *Science* 173 (August 20, 1971), 694–702.

United States, President's Commission for the Study of Ethical Problems in Medicine and Biomedical and Behavioral Research. "Defining Death": A Report on the Medical, Legal and Ethical Issues in the Determination of Death. Washington, D.C.: President's Commission, July 1981.

Van Till, H. A. H. "Diagnosis of Death in Comatose Patients under Resuscitation Treatment: A Critical Review of the Harvard Report." *American Journal of Law and Medicine* 2 (Summer 1976), 1–40.

Veatch, Robert M. *Death, Dying and the Biological Revolution: Our Last Quest for Responsibility.* New Haven: Yale University Press, 1976. Chap. 2.

Veith, Frank J., *et al.* "Brain Death." *Journal of the American Medical Association* 238 (October 10 and 17, 1977), 1651–1655, 1744–1748.

BIBLIOGRAPHIES

Goldstein, Doris Mueller. *Bioethics: A Guide to Information Sources.* Detroit: Gale Research Company, 1982. See under "Definition and Determination of Death."

Lineback, Richard H., ed. *Philosopher's Index.* Vols. 1– . Bowling Green, Ohio: Philosophy Documentation Center, Bowling Green State University. Issued quarterly. See under "Brain Death," "Death," and "Life."

Walters, LeRoy, ed. *Bibliography of Bioethics.* Vols. 1– . New York: Free Press. Issued annually. See under "Brain Death" and "Determination of Death." (The information contained in the annual *Bibliography of Bioethics* can also be retrieved from BIOETHICSLINE, an online data base of the National Library of Medicine.)

8.
Euthanasia and the Prolongation of Life

The previous chapter examined concepts of death and the standards for recognizing when death has occurred. The present chapter considers ethical issues in the treatment of living persons who are seriously or terminally ill. In the discussion of these issues a variety of words and phrases have been employed, including "death with dignity," "euthanasia," "the prolongation of life," "allowing to die," and even "mercy killing." As we shall see, alternative ways of conceptualizing the topic of this chapter are sometimes correlated with divergent ethical perspectives.

GENERAL CONCEPTUAL AND ETHICAL QUESTIONS

Three major conceptual issues frequently arise in discussions of euthanasia and the prolongation of life: (1) the distinction between killing and allowing to die; (2) the distinction between "voluntary" and "involuntary" decisions concerning death; and (3) the proper usage of the term "euthanasia."

The killing/allowing to die debate includes two distinct subquestions: Is it possible to draw a clear logical distinction between actions and omissions? And, even if such a distinction can be drawn, is it morally relevant? Several commentators, among them John Lorber and the American Medical Association (AMA), assert that a meaningful logical distinction can be drawn between killing and allowing to die. Two major arguments are commonly adduced in support of this distinction:

1. Ordinary language—Speakers of English regularly distinguish without difficulty between "causing harm or death" and "permitting harm or death to occur." Most English-speakers would classify allowing to die as an instance of the latter category, killing, of the former.
2. Causation—In cases where a terminally ill or seriously injured patient dies following nontreatment, the proximate cause of death is the patient's disease or injury, not nontreatment, a principle traditionally recognized in the law.

James Rachels, on the other hand, argues that the cessation of treatment in terminal cases is "the intentional termination of the life of one human being by another" and, more generally, that letting a patient die is an action, not merely an omission. He therefore questions whether any clear conceptual distinction between killing and allowing to die can be sustained. (R. B. Zachary also notes how, in practice, allowing to die can shade gradually into killing.)

On the second subquestion, the moral relevance of the killing/allowing-to-die distinction, Rachels holds that if it is morally permissible to intend that a patient die, then acting directly to terminate a patient's life is justified if it causes less suffering to the patient than simply allowing him or her to die. By contrast, Tom Beauchamp argues that active or direct killing may not be justified in a *particular* case even if it causes less suffering for the patient, on grounds that seriously harmful consequences might occur if the active/passive distinction were generally viewed as morally irrelevant.

On this subquestion, however, there is some measure of agreement between Rachels and his opponents. Neither side accepts a simple correlation between the killing/letting die distinction and the wrong/right distinction. For example, Rachels and Beauchamp agree that certain omissions that allow another to die are morally or legally blameworthy. Even the AMA statement (cited by Rachels) implicitly recognizes the moral accountability of physicians for some types of omissions by carefully circumscribing the conditions in which the cessation of treatment is considered to be justified: only "extraordinary" means may be withheld and then only in cases in which there is "irrefutable evidence" that biological death is imminent. On the other hand, the AMA statement seems to regard the killing of a patient, even for humane reasons, as morally wrong; thus, in its view there is a close connection between killing (a patient) and morally wrong action. Rachels obviously disagrees. Beauchamp adopts an intermediate position, arguing that there are rule-utilitarian reasons for preserving the killing/letting die distinction; however, he does not regard killing for humane reasons as necessarily correlated with morally wrong action.

The conceptual distinction between "voluntary" and "involuntary" decisions about death is less controversial; however, the term "involuntary" is ambiguous. Voluntary decisions about death are those in which a competent patient requests or gives informed consent to a particular course of treatment or nontreatment. The term "involuntary," however, is not generally applied to situations in which the expressed will of a competent patient is overridden but rather to cases in which the patient—because of age, mental impairment, or unconsciousness—is not competent to give informed consent to life-death decisions. In such cases, where decisions must be made by others on the patient's behalf, the term "nonvoluntary" might be more appropriate, since it lacks the coercive overtones of "involuntary." However, the term "involuntary" is well established in the discussion of life-and-death questions and will therefore be employed in its noncoercive sense in the remainder of this introduction.

The third issue identified above is perhaps the most difficult: What is the proper usage of the term "euthanasia"? The answer to this question is complicated by the fact that the *descriptive definition* (see Chapter 2) of the term may be in transition. Originally, euthanasia was derived from two Greek roots meaning simply "good death." In *Webster's Third New International Dictionary (Unabridged),* originally published in 1961, the definition of euthanasia was further specified as (1) "an easy death or means of inducing one" and (2) "the act or practice of painlessly putting to death persons suffering from incurable conditions or diseases." Two features of these definitions may be noted: both seem to employ the language of acting rather than omitting to act, or killing rather than allowing to die; and the second definition suggests that the action is performed by a party other than the patient. By contrast, a 1975 reference work, the *New Columbia Encyclopedia,* defines euthanasia as "either painlessly putting to death or failing to prevent death from natural causes in cases of terminal illness." The euthanasia entry continues:

The term formerly referred only to the act of painlessly putting incurably ill patients to death. However, technological advances in medicine, which have made it possible to prolong the lives of patients who have no hope of recovery, have led to the use of the term *negative euthanasia,* i.e., the withdrawing of extraordinary means used to preserve life.[1]

If Webster's definition is accepted, then the paradigm case of euthanasia is the (active) termination of a suffering patient's life by a second party. If the termination is requested or consented to by the patient, then the action is called "voluntary euthanasia." In cases where the patient is not mentally competent to give consent, the action is called "involuntary euthanasia." If, however, one accepts the definition proposed by the *New Columbia Encyclopedia,* two discrete subtypes of euthanasia are distinguishable, active (or positive) euthanasia and passive (or negative) euthanasia. On this view, the paradigm case of euthanasia just described is an instance of active euthanasia. The combination of the voluntary/involuntary distinction with the *New Columbia Encyclopedia* definition of euthanasia would thus yield four subtypes of euthanasia, which can be represented schematically as follows:

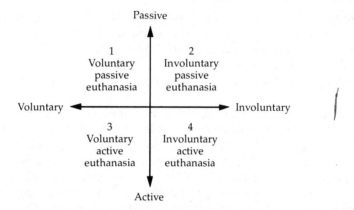

Adherents of Webster's definition, however, would insist on a sharp conceptual distinction between euthanasia and allowing to die and would probably deny that both concepts can be included on a single graph.

In the present chapter, Rachels and H. Tristram Engelhardt apply the term euthanasia both to cases of killing and to cases of allowing to die. By contrast, the California Natural Death Act and John Lorber draw a sharp distinction between euthanasia and either refusing treatment or allowing to die. A similar distinction seems to be presupposed by the British Voluntary Euthanasia Bill, which confines its attention to the "painless inducement of death," and by the essays of Yale Kamisar and Glanville Williams, which discuss only issues related to mercy-killing.

DECISIONS BY COMPETENT ADULTS

This section focuses on voluntary decisions by patients and carries forward the discussion of the professional-patient relationship (Chapter 4) and informed consent (Chapter 5). It is also related to the analyses of autonomy, liberty, and paternalism in Chapter 1.

Life and death decisions, even when they involve competent patients, are frequently presented as dilemmas for health professionals: What are the obligations of the physician or nurse to the dying patient? But it is also possible to approach such decisions from the standpoint of the patient and to ask: Under what circumstances does the patient have a moral right to refuse treatment or to request the termination of life? and, Do patients have a moral obligation to accept low-risk, life-saving treatments that offer a high probability of success?

Tangible ways for patients to express their wishes concerning terminal care are presented by the British Voluntary Euthanasia Act, the Living Will developed by the Euthanasia Educational Council,[2] and the California Natural Death Act. The British bill, which was never adopted by Parliament, would have made legal provision for the active termination of life, but only in the case of patients suffering from what the bill calls "irremediable conditions." The general form of the declaration included in the Voluntary

Euthanasia Act is preserved in the Living Will, but there are important differences. Since it is not a legal document, the Living Will is technically a declaration of intention rather than a will. The signer of the Living Will requests that in case of apparently irreversible illness no "artificial means" or heroic measures be employed to prolong his or her life. Although this document focuses primary attention on the patient's right to refuse treatment, its allusion to pain-killing medication (e.g., morphine) that may also "hasten the moment of death" indicates one of the practical difficulties in maintaining a clear distinction between killing and allowing to die.

Like the British act, the California Natural Death Act provides legal authorization for a patient to make a formal declaration of intention in case of terminal illness. However, the California law, which was enacted in 1976, specifically does not apply to requests for the active termination of life. Robert Veatch assesses the comparative merits of the approaches represented in these three documents and of alternative public-policy options, as well.

In the essays of Yale Kamisar and Glanville Williams one is clearly confronted with the issue of mercy-killing. Williams argues that the case for the voluntary inducement of death in the terminal stages of painful diseases is based on two values. The first is liberty; that is, like the California Natural Death Act, Williams accords a central role to patient autonomy but, unlike the Act, extends the sphere of patient self-determination to include the right to have one's life directly terminated. The second value espoused by Williams is the prevention of cruelty, which is closely related to the principle of beneficence discussed in Chapter 1.

Kamisar raises three primary objections to voluntary mercy-killing: (1) the diagnosis that a patient's disease is "incurable" may be mistaken, or a cure for the disease may be discovered; (2) the "voluntary" character of decisions by seriously ill patients is open to question; and (3) programs of voluntary mercy-killing are likely to be the opening wedge for proposed programs of involuntary mercy-killing. Kamisar is prepared to concede that in individual, extreme cases the voluntary inducement of death could be morally justified. His essay can therefore be interpreted as a rule-utilitarian argument against both the general practice of mercy-killing and the legalization of the practice. (The discussion of rule-utilitarianism in Beauchamp's essay reaches similar conclusions.)

It is at least conceivable that some of Kamisar's objections to mercy-killing could also be raised against the refusal of life-saving treatment. Medical diagnoses could be equally mistaken in treatment-refusal cases. Similarly, the voluntary character of a seriously ill patient's decision to refuse treatment might be open to question, particularly if the patient were pressured by family or society to assert his or her "right to die." Thus, one might find oneself driven to the view that the morally safest policy is to request (or provide) maximal treatment in every case of life-threatening illness. However, this "safe" policy might raise ethical problems of its own, particularly with respect to patient autonomy, the suffering of patients, and the allocation of scarce biomedical resources.

DECISIONS ABOUT INFANTS AND OTHER INCOMPETENT INDIVIDUALS

In recent years the question of appropriate treatment for handicapped newborn infants and seriously ill, comatose patients has become a matter of intense public concern. Interest in this question has been stimulated in part by a series of dramatic cases, including the "Quinlan case," the "Saikewicz case," and the "Johns Hopkins case." In the latter case an infant born with Down's Syndrome (mongolism) and an intestinal blockage was denied corrective surgery and allowed to die at the parents' request.

Decisions about the treatment of infants and comatose patients are of necessity made by parties other than the patients themselves. They are thus *involuntary* decisions in the sense proposed above. Until now, the public debate has centered primarily on the issue of allowing patients to die rather than on the active termination of life, although several authors in this chapter, most notably Engelhardt, devote attention to the latter issue, as well.

Three major ethical positions on the treatment of handicapped infants and comatose patients can be distinguished. The first position would argue that the life of every infant and incompetent patient should be saved, if medically possible. As Lorber points out, a policy of maximal treatment was, in fact, followed during the 1960s for newborns suffering from an often severe defect of the spinal column (meningomyelocele). This position excludes both killing and allowing to die. The primary justifications for this position are, negatively, that no one should be authorized to make life-death decisions on behalf of another and, positively, that every patient, regardless of his or her condition, has an overriding right to life.

A second position would make the decision about treatment on the basis of the patient's projected long-term welfare. In this case a proxy for the patient seeks to make an anticipatory judgment concerning the quality of life that the patient is likely to experience as balanced against the suffering that the patient is likely to endure. Several selections in this chapter espouse this patient-oriented standard. R. B. Zachary, for example, asks his readers to envision the positive qualities of life with spina bifida. The New Jersey Supreme Court considers what Karen Quinlan would have decided about her own treatment had she enjoyed a brief "lucid interval." And the Supreme Judicial Court of Massachusetts displays sensitivity to the effects that a rigorous course of therapy might have on a profoundly retarded patient.

A third position would allow decisions concerning the treatment of infants and the incompetent to be determined, or at least strongly influenced, by familial and broader social considerations. If the patient's continued existence would be likely to undermine a marriage, adversely affect other family members, or claim an undue share of society's scarce resources, then a decision to allow the patient to die would be morally approved. A benefit-harm calculus underlies this third position, as it did the second. However, factors other than patient benefit are also included in the calculus. Without explicitly opting for this third position, Engelhardt argues that parents, in addition to anticipating the future suffering of a severely handicapped child, may also include familial considerations, such as excessive cost or inconvenience, in their decisions about appropriate treatment for their child.

The presence of two court decisions in this chapter serves as a reminder that public policy in the arena of death and dying can be formulated by the judicial as well as by the legislative branch. Both decisions raise the difficult question of the appropriate role for family members, appointed guardians, health professionals, ethics committees, and judges in life-death situations involving incompetent individuals. The Quinlan court seems reluctant to entrust sole decision-making authority to the patient's family or physician. It therefore recommends consultation by the physician with other individuals and groups, including, for example, discussion of difficult cases with interprofessional hospital-based ethics committees. According to the court, such broad-based local review would protect physicians as well as patients and their families and would, in most cases, obviate the need for formal judicial review. The perspective adopted by the Saikewicz court is different in the sense that the court itself is the primary decision-maker. However, both the Quinlan and the Saikewicz decisions fit consistently into a framework in which the judgment of one party is legitimately substituted for that of another (thus forming a mechanism of consent) and in which the legal right to privacy of incompetent individuals is accepted as a fundamental and overriding right.

L.W.

NOTES

1. William H. Harris and Judith S. Levey, eds. *The New Columbia Encyclopedia* (New York: Columbia University Press, 1975), p. 904.

2. Subsequent to 1974, the Euthanasia Educational Council divided into two successor groups: the Society for the Right to Die, which actively supports the reform of laws relating to voluntary death and the refusal of treatment, and Concern for Dying, whose primary focus is education rather than legal reform.

JAMES RACHELS

Active and Passive Euthanasia

The distinction between active and passive euthanasia is thought to be crucial for medical ethics. The idea is that it is permissible, at least in some cases, to withhold treatment and allow a patient to die, but it is never permissible to take any direct action designed to kill the patient. This doctrine seems to be accepted by most doctors, and it was endorsed in a statement adopted by the House of Delegates of the American Medical Association on December 4, 1973:

The intentional termination of the life of one human being by another—mercy killing—is contrary to that for which the medical profession stands and is contrary to the policy of the American Medical Association.

The cessation of the employment of extraordinary means to prolong the life of the body when there is irrefutable evidence that biological death is imminent is the decision of the patient and/or his immediate family. The advice and judgment of the physician should be freely available to the patient and/or his immediate family.

However, a strong case can be made against this doctrine. In what follows I will set out some of the relevant arguments, and urge doctors to reconsider their views on this matter.

To begin with a familiar type of situation, a patient who is dying of incurable cancer of the throat is in terrible pain, which can no longer be satisfactorily alleviated. He is certain to die within a few days, even if present treatment is continued, but he does not want to go on living for those days since the pain is unbearable. So he asks the doctor for an end to it, and his family joins in the request.

Suppose the doctor agrees to withhold treatment, as the conventional doctrine says he may. The justification for his doing so is that the patient is in terrible agony, and since he is going to die anyway, it would

be wrong to prolong his suffering needlessly. But now notice this. If one simply withholds treatment, it may take the patient longer to die, and so he may suffer more than he would if more direct action were taken and a lethal injection given. This fact provides strong reason for thinking that, once the initial decision not to prolong his agony has been made, active euthanasia is actually preferable to passive euthanasia, rather than the reverse. To say otherwise is to endorse the option that leads to more suffering rather than less, and is contrary to the humanitarian impulse that prompts the decision not to prolong his life in the first place.

Part of my point is that the process of being "allowed to die" can be relatively slow and painful, whereas being given a lethal injection is relatively quick and painless. Let me give a different sort of example. In the United States about one in 600 babies is born with Down's syndrome. Most of these babies are otherwise healthy—that is, with only the usual pediatric care, they will proceed to an otherwise normal infancy. Some, however, are born with congenital defects such as intestinal obstructions that require operations if they are to live. Sometimes, the parents and the doctor will decide not to operate, and let the infant die. Anthony Shaw describes what happens then.

. . . When surgery is denied [the doctor] must try to keep the infant from suffering while natural forces sap the baby's life away. As a surgeon whose natural inclination is to use the scalpel to fight off death, standing by and watching a salvageable baby die is the most emotionally exhausing experience I know. It is easy at a conference, in a theoretical discussion, to decide that such infants should be allowed to die. It is altogether different to stand by in the nursery and watch as dehydration and infection wither a tiny being over hours and days. This is a terrible ordeal for me and the hospital staff—much more so than for the parents who never set foot in the nursery.[1]

Reprinted with permission from *The New England Journal of Medicine*, Vol. 292, No. 2 (Jan. 9, 1975), pp. 78–80.

I can understand why some people are opposed to all euthanasia, and insist that such infants must be allowed to live. I think I can also understand why other people favor destroying these babies quickly and painlessly. But why should anyone favor letting "dehydration and infection wither a tiny being over hours and days?" The doctrine that says that a baby may be allowed to dehydrate and wither, but may not be given an injection that would end its life without suffering, seems so patently cruel as to require no further refutation. The strong language is not intended to offend, but only to put the point in the clearest possible way.

My second argument is that the conventional doctrine leads to decisions concerning life and death made on irrelevant grounds.

Consider again the case of the infants with Down's syndrome who need operations for congenital defects unrelated to the syndrome to live. Sometimes there is no operation, and the baby dies, but when there is no such defect, the baby lives on. Now, an operation such as that to remove an intestinal obstruction is not prohibitively difficult. The reason why such operations are not performed in these cases is, clearly, that the child has Down's syndrome and the parents and doctor judge that because of that fact it is better for the child to die.

But notice that this situation is absurd, no matter what view one takes of the lives and potentials of such babies. If the life of such an infant is worth preserving, what does it matter if it needs a simple operation? Or, if one thinks it better that such a baby should not live on, what difference does it make that it happens to have an unobstructed intestinal tract? In either case, the matter of life and death is being decided on irrelevant grounds. It is the Down's syndrome, and not the intestines, that is the issue. The matter should be decided, if at all, on that basis, and not be allowed to depend on the essentially irrelevant question of whether the intestinal tract is blocked.

What makes this situation possible, of course, is the idea that when there is an intestinal blockage, one can "let the baby die," but when there is no such defect there is nothing that can be done, for one must not "kill" it. The fact that this idea leads to such results as deciding life or death on irrelevant grounds is another good reason why the doctrine should be rejected.

One reason why so many people think that there is an important moral difference between active and passive euthanasia is that they think killing someone is morally worse than letting someone die. But is it? Is killing, in itself, worse than letting die? To investigate this issue, two cases may be considered that are exactly alike except that one involves killing whereas the other involves letting someone die. Then, it can be asked whether this difference makes any difference to the moral assessments. It is important that the cases be exactly alike, except for this one difference, since otherwise one cannot be confident that it is this difference and not some other that accounts for any variation in the assessments of the two cases. So, let us consider this pair of cases:

In the first, Smith stands to gain a large inheritance if anything should happen to his six-year-old cousin. One evening while the child is taking his bath, Smith sneaks into the bathroom and drowns the child, and then arranges things so that it will look like an accident.

In the second, Jones also stands to gain if anything should happen to his six-year-old cousin. Like Smith, Jones sneaks in planning to drown the child in his bath. However, just as he enters the bathroom Jones sees the child slip and hit his head, and fall face down in the water. Jones is delighted; he stands by, ready to push the child's head back under if it is necessary, but it is not necessary. With only a little thrashing about, the child drowns all by himself, "accidentally," as Jones watches and does nothing.

Now Smith killed the child, whereas Jones "merely" let the child die. That is the only difference between them. Did either man behave better, from a moral point of view? If the difference between killing and letting die were in itself a morally important matter, one should say that Jones's behavior was less reprehensible than Smith's. But does one really want to say that? I think not. In the first place, both men acted from the same motive, personal gain, and both had exactly the same end in view when they acted. It may be inferred from Smith's conduct that he is a bad man, although that judgment may be withdrawn or modified if certain further facts are learned about him—for example, that he is mentally deranged. But would not the very same thing be inferred about Jones from his conduct? And would not the same further considerations also be relevant to any modification of this judgment? Moreover, suppose Jones pleaded, in his own defense, "After all, I didn't do anything except just stand there and watch the child drown. I didn't kill him; I only let him die." Again, if letting die were in itself less bad than killing, this defense should have at least some weight. But it does not. Such a "defense" can only be regarded as a grotesque perversion of moral reasoning. Morally speaking, it is no defense at all.

Now it may be pointed out, quite properly, that the cases of euthanasia with which doctors are concerned are not like this at all. They do not involve personal gain or the destruction of normal healthy children. Doctors are concerned only with cases in which the patient's life is of no further use to him, or in which the patient's life has become or will soon become a terrible burden. However, the point is the same in these cases: the bare difference between killing and letting die does not, in itself, make a moral difference. If a doctor lets a patient die, for humane reasons, he is in the same moral position as if he had given the patient a lethal injection for humane reasons. If his decision was wrong—if, for example, the patient's illness was in fact curable—the decision would be equally regrettable no matter which method was used to carry it out. And if the doctor's decision was the right one, the method used is not in itself important.

The AMA policy statement isolates the crucial issue very well; the crucial issue is "the intentional termination of the life of one human being by another." But after identifying this issue, and forbidding "mercy killing," the statement goes on to deny that the cessation of treatment is the intentional termination of a life. This is where the mistake comes in, for what is the cessation of treatment, in these circumstances, if it is not "the intentional termination of the life of one human being by another?" Of course it is exactly that, and if it were not, there would be no point to it.

Many people will find this judgment hard to accept. One reason, I think, is that it is very easy to conflate the question of whether killing is, in itself, worse than letting die, with the very different question of whether most actual cases of killing are more reprehensible than most actual cases of letting die. Most actual cases of killing are clearly terrible (think, for example, of all the murders reported in the newspapers), and one hears of such cases every day. On the other hand, one hardly ever hears of a case of letting die, except for the actions of doctors who are motivated by humanitarian reasons. So one learns to think of killing in a much worse light than of letting die. But this does not mean that there is something about killing that makes it in itself worse than letting die, for it is not the bare difference between killing and letting die that makes the difference in these cases. Rather, the other factors—the murderer's motive of personal gain, for example, contrasted with the doctor's humanitarian motivation—account for different reactions to the different cases.

I have argued that killing is not in itself any worse than letting die; if my contention is right, it follows that active euthanasia is not any worse than passive euthanasia. What arguments can be given on the other side? The most common, I believe, is the following:

"The important difference between active and passive euthanasia is that, in passive euthanasia, the doctor does not do anything to bring about the patient's death. The doctor does nothing, and the patient dies of whatever ills already afflict him. In active euthanasia, however, the doctor does something to bring about the patient's death: he kills him. The doctor who gives the patient with cancer a lethal injection has himself caused his patient's death; whereas if he merely ceases treatment, the cancer is the cause of the death."

A number of points need to be made here. The first is that it is not exactly correct to say that in passive euthanasia the doctor does nothing, for he does do one thing that is very important: he lets the patient die. "Letting someone die" is certainly different, in some respects, from other types of action—mainly in that it is a kind of action that one may perform by way of not performing certain other actions. For example, one may let a patient die by way of not giving medication, just as one may insult someone by way of not shaking his hand. But for any purpose of moral assessment, it is a type of action nonetheless. The decision to let a patient die is subject to moral appraisal in the same way that a decision to kill him would be subject to moral appraisal: it may be assessed as wise or unwise, compassionate or sadistic, right or wrong. If a doctor deliberately let a patient die who was suffering from a routinely curable illness, the doctor would certainly be to blame for what he had done, just as he would be to blame if he had needlessly killed the patient. Charges against him would then be appropriate. If so, it would be no defense at all for him to insist that he didn't "do anything." He would have done something very serious indeed, for he let his patient die.

Fixing the cause of death may be very important from a legal point of view, for it may determine whether criminal charges are brought against the doctor. But I do not think that this notion can be used to show a moral difference between active and passive euthanasia. The reason why it is considered bad to be the cause of someone's death is that death is regarded as a great evil—and so it is. However, if it has been decided that euthanasia—even passive euthanasia—is desirable in a given case, it has also been decided that in this instance death is no greater an evil than the patient's continued existence. And if this is true, the usual reason for not wanting to be the cause of someone's death simply does not apply.

Finally, doctors may think that all of this is only of academic interest—the sort of thing that philosophers may worry about but that has no practical bearing on their own work. After all, doctors must be concerned about the legal consequences of what they do, and active euthanasia is clearly forbidden by the law. But even so, doctors should also be concerned with the fact that the law is forcing upon them a moral doctrine that may well be indefensible, and has a considerable effect on their practices. Of course, most doctors are not now in the position of being coerced in this matter, for they do not regard themselves as merely going along with what the law requires. Rather, in statements such as the AMA policy statement that I have quoted, they are endorsing this doctrine as a central point of medical ethics. In that statement, active euthanasia is condemned not merely as illegal but as "contrary to that for which the medical profession stands," whereas passive euthanasia is approved. However, the preceding considerations suggest that there is really no moral difference between the two, considered in themselves (there may be important moral differences in some cases in their *consequences,* but, as I pointed out, these differences may make active euthanasia, and not passive euthanasia, the morally preferable option). So, whereas doctors may have to discriminate between active and passive euthanasia to satisfy the law, they should not do any more than that. In particular, they should not give the distinction any added authority and weight by writing it into official statements of medical ethics.

NOTES

1. A. Shaw, "Doctor, Do We Have a Choice?" *The New York Times Magazine,* January 30, 1972, p.54.

TOM L. BEAUCHAMP

A Reply to Rachels on Active and Passive Euthanasia

James Rachels has recently argued that the distinction between active and passive euthanasia is neither appropriately used by the American Medical Association nor generally useful for the resolution of moral problems of euthanasia.[1] Indeed he believes this distinction—which he equates with the killing/letting die distinction—does not in itself have any moral importance. The chief object of his attack is the following statement adopted by the House of Delegates of the American Medical Association in 1973:

From Tom L. Beauchamp and Seymour Perlin, eds., *Ethical Issues in Death and Dying* (Englewood Cliffs, N.J.: Prentice-Hall, 1978), pp. 246–258. This is a heavily revised version of an article by the same title first published in Thomas Mappes and Jane Zembaty, eds. *Social Ethics,* (New York: McGraw-Hill, 1976).

The intentional termination of the life of one human being by another—mercy killing—is contrary to that for which the medical profession stands and is contrary to the policy of the American Medical Association.

The cessation of the employment of extraordinary means to prolong the life of the body when there is irrefutable evidence that biological death is imminent is the decision of the patient and/or his immediate family. The advice and judgment of the physician should be freely available to the patient and/or his immediate family (p. 313).

Rachels constructs a powerful and interesting set of arguments against this statement. In this paper I attempt the following: (1) to challenge his views on the grounds that he does not appreciate the moral reasons which give weight to the active/passive distinction;

(2) to provide a constructive account of the moral relevance of the active/passive distinction; and (3) to offer reasons showing that Rachels may nonetheless be correct in urging that we *ought* to abandon the active/passive distinction for purposes of moral reasoning.

I

I would concede that the active/passive distinction is *sometimes* morally irrelevant. Of this Rachels convinces me. But it does not follow that it is *always* morally irrelevant. What we need, then, is a case where the distinction is a morally relevant one and an explanation why it is so. Rachels himself uses the method of examining two cases which are exactly alike except that "one involves killing whereas the other involves letting die" (p. 314). We may profitably begin by comparing the kinds of cases governed by the AMA's doctrine with the kinds of cases adduced by Rachels in order to assess the adequacy and fairness of his cases.

The second paragraph of the AMA statement is confined to a narrowly restricted range of passive euthanasia cases, viz., those (a) where the patients are on extraordinary means, (b) where irrefutable evidence of imminent death is available, and (c) where patient or family consent is available. Rachels' two cases involve conditions notably different from these:

In the first, Smith stands to gain a large inheritance if anything should happen to his six-year-old cousin. One evening while the child is taking his bath, Smith sneaks into the bathroom and drowns the child, and then arranges things so that it will look like an accident.

In the second, Jones also stands to gain if anything should happen to his six-year-old cousin. Like Smith, Jones sneaks in planning to drown the child in his bath. However, just as he enters the bathroom Jones sees the child slip and hit his head, and fall face down in the water. Jones is delighted; he stands by, ready to push the child's head back under if it is necessary, but it is not necessary. With only a little thrashing about, the child drowns all by himself, "accidentally," as Jones watches and does nothing.

Now Smith killed the child, whereas Jones "merely" let the child die. That is the only difference between them (p. 314).

Rachels says there is no moral difference between the cases in terms of our moral assessments of Smith and Jones' behavior. This assessment seems fair enough, but what can Rachels' cases be said to prove, as they are so markedly disanalogous to the sorts of cases envisioned by the AMA proposal? Rachels concedes important disanalogies, but thinks them irrelevant:

The point is the same in these cases: the bare difference between killing and letting die does not, in itself, make a moral difference. If a doctor lets a patient die, for humane reasons, he is in the same moral position as if he had given the patient a lethal injection for humane reasons (p. 315).

Three observations are immediately in order. First, Rachels seems to infer that from such cases we can conclude that the distinction between killing and letting die is *always* morally irrelevant. This conclusion is fallaciously derived. What the argument in fact shows, being an analogical argument, is only that in all *relevantly similar* cases the distinction does not in itself make a moral difference. Since Rachels concedes that other cases are disanalogous, he seems thereby to concede that his argument is as weak as the analogy itself. Second, Rachels' cases involve two *unjustified* actions, one of killing and the other of letting die. The AMA statement distinguishes one set of cases of unjustified killing and another of *justified* cases of allowing to die. Nowhere is it claimed by the AMA that what makes the difference in these cases is the active/passive distinction itself. It is only implied that one set of cases, the justified set, *involves* (passive) letting die while the unjustified set *involves* (active) killing. While it is said that justified euthanasia cases are passive ones and unjustified ones active, it is not said either that what makes some acts justified is the fact of their being passive or that what makes others unjustified is the fact of their being active. This fact will prove to be of vital importance.

The third point is that in both of Rachels' cases the respective moral agents—Smith and Jones—are morally responsible for the death of the child and are morally blameworthy—even though Jones is presumably not causally responsible. In the first case death is caused by the agent, while in the second it is not; yet the second agent is no less morally responsible. While the law might find only the first homicidal, morality condemns the motives in each case as equally wrong, and it holds that the duty to save life in such cases is as compelling as the duty not to take life. I suggest that it is largely because of this equal degree of moral responsibility that there is no morally relevant difference in Rachels' cases. In the cases envisioned by the AMA, however, an agent is held to be responsible for taking life by actively killing but is not held to be morally required to preserve life, and so not responsible for death, when removing the patient from extraordinary means (under conditions a–c above). I shall elaborate this latter point momentarily. My only conclusion thus far is the negative one that Rachels' arguments rest on weak foundations. His cases are not relevantly similar to euthanasia cases and do not support his apparent conclusion that the active/passive distinction is *always* morally irrelevant.

II

I wish first to consider an argument that I believe has powerful intuitive appeal and probably is widely accepted as stating the main reason for rejecting Rachels' views. I will maintain that this argument fails, and so leaves Rachels' contentions untouched.

I begin with an actual case, the celebrated Quinlan case.[2] Karen Quinlan was in a coma, and was on a mechanical respirator which artifically sustained her vital processes and which her parents wished to cease. At least some physicians believed there was irrefutable evidence that biological death was imminent and the coma irreversible. This case, under this description, closely conforms to the passive cases envisioned by the AMA. During an interview the father, Mr. Quinlan, asserted that he did not wish to kill his daughter, but only to remove her from the machines in order to see whether she would live or would die a natural death.[3] Suppose he had said—to envision now a second and hypothetical, but parallel case—that he wished only to see her die painlessly and therefore wished that the doctor could induce death by an overdose of morphine. Most of us would think the second act, which involves active killing, morally unjustified in these circumstances, while many of us would think the first act morally justified. (This is not the place to consider whether in fact it is justified, and if so under what conditions.) What accounts for the apparent morally relevant difference?

I have considered these two cases together in order to follow Rachels' method of entertaining parallel cases where the only difference is that the one case involves killing and the other letting die. However, there is a further difference, which crops up in the euthanasia context. The difference rests in our judgments of medical fallibility and moral responsibility. Mr. Quinlan seems to think that, after all, the doctors might be wrong. There is a remote possibility that she

might live without the aid of a machine. But whether or not the medical prediction of death turns out to be accurate, if she dies then no one is morally responsible for directly bringing about or causing her death, as they would be if they caused her death by killing her. Rachels finds explanations which appeal to causal conditions unsatisfactory; but perhaps this is only because he fails to see the nature of the causal link. To bring about her death is by that act to preempt the possibility of life. To "allow her to die" by removing artificial equipment is to allow for the possibility of wrong diagnosis or incorrect prediction and hence to absolve oneself of moral responsibility for the taking of life under false assumptions. There may, of course, be utterly no empirical possibility of recovery in some cases since recovery would violate a law of nature. However, judgments of empirical impossibility in medicine are notoriously problematic—the reason for emphasizing medical fallibility. And in all the hard cases we do not *know* that recovery is empirically impossible, even if good *evidence* is available.

The above reason for invoking the active/passive distinction can now be generalized: Active termination of life removes all possibility of life for the patient, while passively ceasing extraordinary means may not. This is not trivial since patients have survived in several celebrated cases where, in knowledgeable physicians' judgments, there was "irrefutable" evidence that death was imminent.[4]

One may, of course, be entirely responsible and culpable for another's death either by killing him or by letting him die. In such cases, of which Rachels' are examples, there is no morally significant difference between killing and letting die precisely because whatever one does, omits, or refrains from doing does not absolve one of responsibility. Either active or passive involvement renders one responsible for the death of another, and both involvements are equally wrong for the same principled moral reason: it is (prima facie) morally wrong to bring about the death of an innocent person capable of living whenever the causal intervention or negligence is intentional. (I use causal terms here because causal involvement need not be active, as when by one's negligence one is nonetheless causally responsible.) But not all cases of killing and letting die fall under this same moral principle. One is sometimes culpable for killing, because morally responsible as the agent for death, as when one pulls the plug on a respirator sustaining a recovering patient (a murder). But one is sometimes not culpable for letting die because not morally responsible as agent, as when one pulls the plug on a respirator sustaining an irreversibly comatose and unrecoverable patient (a routine procedure, where one is *merely* causally responsible).[5] Different degrees and means of involvement assess different degrees of responsibility, and our assessments of culpability can become intricately complex. The only point which now concerns us, however, is that because different moral principles may govern very similar circumstances, we are sometimes morally culpable for killing but not for letting die. And to many people it will seem that in passive cases we are not morally responsible for causing death, though we are responsible in active cases.

This argument is powerfully attractive. Although I was once inclined to accept it in virtually the identical form just developed,[6] I now think that, despite its intuitive appeal, it cannot be correct. It is true that different degrees and means of involvement entail different degrees of responsibility, but it does not follow that we are *not* responsible and therefore are absolved of possible culpability in *any* case of intentionally allowing to die. We are responsible and *perhaps* culpable in either active or passive cases. Here Rachels' argument is entirely to the point: It is not primarily a question of greater or lesser responsibility by an active or a passive means that should determine culpability. Rather, the question of culpability is decided by the moral *justification* for choosing either a passive or an active means. What the argument in the previous paragraph overlooks is that one might be unjustified in using an active means or unjustified in using a passive means, and hence be culpable in the use of either; yet one might be justified in using an active means or justified in using a passive means, and hence not be culpable in using either. Fallibility might just as well be present in a judgment to use one means as in a judgment to use another. (A judgment to allow to die is just as subject to being based on *knowledge which is fallible* as a judgment to kill.) Moreover, in either case, it is a matter of what one knows and believes, and not a matter of a particular kind of causal connection or causal chain. If we kill the patient, then we are certainly causally responsible for his death. But, similarly, if we cease treatment, and the patient dies, the patient might have recovered if treatment had been continued. The patient might have been saved in either case, and hence there is no morally relevant difference between the two cases. It is, therefore, simply beside the point that "one is sometimes culpable for killing . . . but one is sometimes not culpable for letting die"—as the above argument concludes.

Accordingly, despite its great intuitive appeal and frequent mention, this argument from responsibility fails.

III

There may, however, be more compelling arguments against Rachels, and I wish now to provide what I believe is the most significant argument that can be adduced in defense of the active/passive distinction. I shall develop this argument by combining (1) so-called wedge or slippery slope arguments with (2) recent arguments in defense of rule utilitarianism. I shall explain each in turn and show how in combination they may be used to defend the active-passive distinction.

(1) *Wedge arguments* proceed as follows: if killing were allowed, even under the guise of a merciful extinction of life, a dangerous wedge would be introduced which places all "undesirable" or "unworthy" human life in a precarious condition. Proponents of wedge arguments believe the initial wedge places us on a slippery slope for at least one of two reasons: (i) It is said that our justifying principles leave us with no principled way to avoid the slide into saying that all sorts of killings would be justified under similar conditions. Here it is thought that once killing is allowed, a firm line between justified and unjustified killings cannot be securely drawn. It is thought best not to redraw the line in the first place, for redrawing it will inevitably lead to a downhill slide. It is then often pointed out that as a matter of historical record this is precisely what has occurred in the darker regions of human history, including the Nazi era, where euthanasia began with the best intentions for horribly ill, non-Jewish Germans and gradually spread to anyone deemed an enemy of the people. (ii) Second, it is said that our basic principles against killing will be gradually eroded once some form of killing is legitimated. For example, it is said that permitting voluntary euthanasia will lead to permitting involuntary euthanasia, which will in turn lead to permitting euthanasia for those who are a nuisance to society (idiots, recidivist criminals, defective newborns, and the insane, e.g.). Gradually other principles which instill respect for human life will be eroded or abandoned in the process.

I am not inclined to accept the first reason (i).[7] If

our justifying principles are themselves justified, then any action they warrant would be justified. Accordingly, I shall only be concerned with the second approach (ii).

(2) *Rule utilitarianism* is the position that a society ought to adopt a rule if its acceptance would have better consequences for the common good (greater social utility) than any comparable rule could have in that society. Any action is right if it conforms to a valid rule and wrong if it violates the rule. Sometimes it is said that alternative rules should be measured against one another, while it has also been suggested that whole moral *codes* (complete sets of rules) rather than individual rules should be compared. While I prefer the latter formulation (Brandt's), this internal dispute need not detain us here. The important point is that a particular rule or a particular code of rules is morally justified if and only if there is no other competing rule or moral code whose acceptance would have a higher utility value for society, and where a rule's acceptability is contingent upon the consequences which would result if the rule were made current.

Wedge arguments, when conjoined with rule utilitarian arguments, may be applied to euthanasia issues in the following way. We presently subscribe to a no-active-euthanasia rule (which the AMA suggests we retain). Imagine now that in our society we make current a restricted-active-euthanasia rule (as Rachels seems to urge). Which of these two moral rules would, if enacted, have the consequence of maximizing social utility? Clearly a restricted-active-euthanasia rule would have *some* utility value, as Rachels notes, since some intense and uncontrollable suffering would be eliminated. However, it may not have the highest utility value in the structure of our present code or in any imaginable code which could be made current, and therefore may not be a component in the ideal code for our society. If wedge arguments raise any serious questions at all, as I think they do, they rest in this area of whether a code would be weakened or strengthened by the addition of active euthanasia principles. For the disutility of introducing legitimate killing into one's moral code (in the form of active euthanasia rules) may, in the long run, outweigh the utility of doing so, as a result of the eroding effect such a relaxation would have on rules in the code which demand respect for human life. If, for example, rules permitting active killing were intro-

duced, it is not implausible to suppose that destroying defective newborns (a form of involuntary euthanasia) would become an accepted and common practice, that as population increases occur the aged will be even more neglectable and neglected than they now are, that capital punishment for a wide variety of crimes would be increasingly tempting, that some doctors would have appreciably reduced fears of actively injecting fatal doses whenever it seemed to them propitious to do so, and that laws of war against killing civilians would erode in efficacy even beyond their already abysmal level.

A hundred such possible consequences might easily be imagined. But these few are sufficient to make the larger point that such rules permitting killing could lead to a general reduction of respect for human life. Rules against killing in a moral code are not *isolated* moral principles; they are pieces of a web of rules against killing which forms the code. The more threads one removes, the weaker the fabric becomes. And if, as I believe, moral principles against active killing have the deep and continuously civilizing effect of promoting respect for life, and if principles which allow passively letting die (as envisioned in the AMA statement) do not themselves cut against this effect, then this seems an important reason for the maintenance of the active/passive distinction. (By the logic of the above argument, passively letting die would also have to be prohibited if a rule permitting it had the serious adverse consequence of eroding acceptance or rules protective of respect for life. While this prospect seems to me improbable, I can hardly claim to have refuted those conservatives who would claim that even rules that sanction letting die place us on a precarious slippery slope.)

A troublesome problem, however, confronts my use of utilitarian and wedge arguments. Most all of us would agree that both killing and letting die are justified under some conditions. Killings in self-defense and in "just" wars are widely accepted as justified because the conditions excuse the killing. If society can withstand these exceptions to moral rules prohibiting killing, then why is it not plausible to suppose society can accept another excusing exception in the form of justified active euthanasia? This is an important and worthy objection, but not a decisive one. The defenseless and the dying are significantly different classes of persons from aggressors who attack individuals and/or nations. In the case of aggressors, one does not confront the question whether their lives are no longer *worth living*. Rather, we reach the judgment that the aggressors' morally blameworthy actions justify counteractions. But in the case of the dying and the otherwise ill, there is no morally blameworthy action to justify our own. Here we are required to accept the judgment that their lives are no longer *worth living* in order to believe that the termination of their lives is justified. It is the latter sort of judgment which is feared by those who take the wedge argument seriously. We do not now permit and never have permitted the taking of morally blameless lives. I think this is the key to understanding why recent cases of intentionally allowing the death of defective newborns (as in the now famous case at the Johns Hopkins Hospital) have generated such protracted controversy. Even if such newborns could not have led meaningful lives (a matter of some controversy), it is the wedged foot in the door which creates the most intense worries. For if we once take a decision to allow a restricted infanticide justification or any justification at all on grounds that a life is not meaningful or not worth living, we have qualified our moral rules against killing. That this qualification is a matter of the utmost seriousness needs no argument. I mention it here only to show why the wedge argument may have moral force even though we *already* allow some very different conditions to justify intentional killing.

There is one final utilitarian reason favoring the preservation of the active/passive distinction.[8] Suppose we distinguish the following two types of cases of wrongly diagnosed patients:

1. Patients wrongly diagnosed as hopeless, and who will survive even if a treatment *is* ceased (in order to allow a natural death).
2. Patients wrongly diagnosed as hopeless, and who will survive only if the treatment is *not ceased* (in order to allow a natural death).

If a social rule permitting only passive euthanasia were in effect, then doctors and families who "allowed death" would lose only patients in class 2, not those in class 1; whereas if active euthanasia were permitted, at least some patients in class 1 would be needlessly lost. Thus, the consequence of a no-active-euthanasia rule would be to save some lives which could not be saved if both forms of euthanasia were allowed. This reason is not a *decisive* reason for favoring a policy of passive euthanasia, since these classes (1 and 2) are likely to be very small and since there might be counterbalancing reasons (extreme pain, autonomous expression of the patient, etc.) in

favor of active euthanasia. But certainly it is *a* reason favoring only passive euthanasia and one which is morally relevant and ought to be considered along with other moral reasons.

IV

It may still be insisted that my case has not touched Rachels' leading claim, for I have not shown, as Rachels puts it, that it is "the bare difference between killing and letting die that makes the difference in these cases" (p. 315). True, I have not shown this and in my judgment it cannot be shown. But this concession does not require capitulation to Rachels' argument. I adduced a case which is at the center of our moral intuition that killing is morally different (in at least some cases) from letting die; and I then attempted to account for at least part of the grounds for this belief. The grounds turn out to be other than the *bare* difference, but nevertheless *make* the distinction morally relevant. The identical point can be made regarding the voluntary/involuntary distinction, as it is commonly applied to euthanasia. It is not the bare difference between voluntary euthanasia (i.e., euthanasia with patient consent) and involuntary euthanasia (i.e., without patient consent) that makes one justifiable and one not. Independent moral grounds based on, for example, respect for autonomy or beneficence, or perhaps justice will alone make the moral difference.

In order to illustrate this general claim, let us presume that it is sometimes justified to kill another person and sometimes justified to allow another to die. Suppose, for example, that one may kill in self-defense and may allow to die when a promise has been made to someone that he would be allowed to die. Here conditions of self-defense and promising justify actions. But suppose now that someone *A* promises in exactly similar circumstances to kill someone *B* at *B*'s request, and also that someone *C* allows someone *D* to die in an act of self-defense. Surely *A* is obliged equally to kill or to let die if he promised; and surely *C* is permitted to let *D* die if it is a matter of defending *C*'s life. If this analysis is correct, then it follows that killing is sometimes right, sometimes wrong, depending on the circumstances, and the same is true of letting die. It is the justifying reasons which make the difference whether an action is right, not merely the kind of action it is.

Now, *if* letting die led to disastrous conclusions but

killing did not, then letting die but not killing would be wrong. Consider, for example, a possible world in which dying would be indefinitely prolongable even if all extraordinary therapy were removed and the patient were allowed to die. Suppose that it costs over one million dollars to let each patient die, that nurses consistently commit suicide from caring for those being "allowed to die," that physicians are constantly being successfully sued for malpractice for allowing death by cruel and wrongful means, and that hospitals are uncontrollably overcrowded and their wards filled with communicable diseases which afflict only the dying. Now suppose further that killing in this possible world is quick, painless, and easily monitored. I submit that in this world we would believe that *killing is morally acceptable but that allowing to die is morally unacceptable*. The point of this example is again that it is the circumstances that make the difference, not the bare difference between killing and letting die.

It is, however, worth noticing that there is nothing in the AMA statement which says that the bare difference between killing and letting die itself and alone makes the difference in our differing moral assessments of rightness and wrongness. Rachels forces this interpretation on the statement. Some philosophers may have thought bare difference makes the difference, but there is scant evidence that the AMA or any thoughtful ethicist *must* believe it in order to defend the relevance and importance of the active/passive distinction. When this conclusion is coupled with my earlier argument that from Rachels' paradigm cases it follows only that the active/passive distinction is sometimes, but not always, morally irrelevant, it would seem that his case against the AMA is rendered highly questionable.

V

There remains, however, the important question as to whether we *ought* to accept the distinction between active and passive euthanasia, now that we are clear about (at least one way of drawing) the moral grounds for its invocation. That is, should we employ the distinction in order to judge some acts of euthanasia justified and others not justified? Here, as the hesitant previous paragraph indicates, I am uncertain. This problem is a substantive moral issue—not merely a conceptual one—and would require at a minimum a lengthy assessment of wedge arguments and related

utilitarian considerations. In important respects empirical questions are involved in this assessment. We should like to know, and yet have hardly any evidence to indicate, what the consequences would be for our society if we were to allow the use of active means to produce death. The best hope for making such an assessment has seemed to some to rest in analogies to suicide and capital punishment statutes. Here it may reasonably be asked whether recent liberalizations of laws limiting these forms of killing have served as the thin end of a wedge leading to a breakdown of principles protecting life or to widespread violations of moral principles. Nonetheless, such analogies do not seem to me promising, since they are still fairly remote from the pertinent issue of the consequences of allowing active humanitarian killing of one person by another.

It is interesting to notice the outcome of the Kamisar-Williams debate on euthanasia—which is almost exclusively cast by both writers in a consequential, utilitarian framework.[9] At one crucial point in the debate, where possible consequences of laws permitting euthanasia are under discussion, they exchange "perhaps" judgments:

I [Williams] will return Kamisar the compliment and say: "Perhaps." We are certainly in an area where no solution is going to make things quite easy and happy for everybody, and all sorts of embarrassments may be conjectured. But these embarrassments are not avoided by keeping to the present law: we suffer from them already.[10]

Because of the grave difficulties which stand in the way of making accurate predictions about the impact of liberalized euthanasia laws—especially those that would permit active killing—it is not surprising that those who debate the subject would reach a point of exchanging such "perhaps" judgments. And that is why, so it seems to me, we are uncertain whether to perpetuate or to abandon the active-passive distinction in our moral thinking about euthanasia. I think we *do* perpetuate it in medicine, law, and ethics because we are still somewhat uncertain about the conditions under which *passive* euthanasia should be permitted by law (which is one form of social *rule*). We are unsure about what the consequences will be of the California "Natural Death Act" and all those similar acts passed by other states which have followed in its path. If no untoward results occur, and the balance of the results seems favorable, then we will perhaps be less concerned about further liberalizations of euthanasia laws. If untoward results do occur (on a wide-spread scale), then we would be most reluctant to accept further liberalizations and might even abolish natural death acts.

In short, I have argued in this section that euthanasia in its active and its passive forms presents us with a dilemma which can be developed by using powerful consequentialist arguments on each side, yet there is little clarity concerning the proper resolution of the dilemma precisely because of our uncertainty regarding proclaimed consequences.

VI

I reach two conclusions at the end of these several arguments. First, I think Rachels is incorrect in arguing that the distinction between active and passive is (always) morally irrelevant. It may well be relevant, and for moral reasons—the reasons adduced in section III above. Second, I think nonetheless that Rachels may ultimately be shown correct in his contention that we ought to dispense with the active-passive distinction—for reasons adduced in sections IV–V. But if he is ultimately judged correct, it will be because we have come to see that some forms of active killing have generally acceptable social consequences, and not primarily because of the arguments he adduces in his paper—even though *something* may be said for each of these arguments. Of course, in one respect I have conceded a great deal to Rachels. The bare difference argument is vital to his position, and I have fully agreed to it. On the other hand, I do not see that the bare difference argument does play or need play a major role in our moral thinking—or in that of the AMA.

NOTES

1. "Active and Passive Euthanasia," *New England Journal of Medicine* 292 (January 9, 1975), 78–80. [All page references in parentheses refer to Rachels' article as reprinted in this chapter.]

2. As recorded in the Opinion of Judge Robert Muir, Jr., Docket No. C-201-75 of the Superior Court of New Jersey, Chancery Division, Morris County (November 10, 1975).

3. See Judge Muir's Opinion, p. 18—a slightly different statement but on the subject.

4. This problem of the strength of evidence also emerged in the Quinlan trial, as physicians disagreed whether the evidence was "irrefutable." Such disagreement, when added to the problems of medical fallibility and causal responsibility just outlined, provides in the eyes of some one important argument against the *legalization* of active euthanasia, as perhaps the AMA would agree. Cf. Kamisar's arguments in this chapter.

5. Among the moral reasons why one is held to be responsible in the first sort of case and not responsible in the second sort are, I believe, the moral grounds for the active/passive distinction under discussion in this section.

6. In *Social Ethics,* as cited in the permission note to this article.

7. An argument of this form, which I find unacceptable for reasons given below, is Arthur Dyck, "Beneficent Euthanasia and Benemortasia: Alternative Views of Mercy," in M. Kohl, ed., *Beneficent Euthanasia* (Buffalo: Prometheus Books, 1975), pp. 121f.

8. I owe most of this argument to James Rachels, whose comments on an earlier draft of this paper led to several significant alterations.

9. Williams bases his pro-euthanasia argument on the prevention of two consequences: (1) loss of liberty and (2) cruelty. Kamisar bases his anti-euthanasia position on three projected consequences of euthanasia laws: (1) mistaken diagnosis, (2) pressured decisions by seriously ill patients, and (3) the wedge of the laws will lead to legalized involuntary euthanasia. Kamisar admits that individual acts of euthanasia are sometimes justified. It is the rule that he opposes. He is thus clearly a rule-utilitarian, and I believe Williams is as well (cf. his views on children and the senile). Their assessments of wedge arguments are, however, radically different.

10. Glanville Williams, "Mercy-Killing Legislation—A Rejoinder," *Minnesota Law Review,* 43, no. 1 (1958), 5.

YALE KAMISAR

Some Nonreligious Views Against Proposed "Mercy-Killing" Legislation

A recent book, Glanville Williams' *The Sanctity of Life and the Criminal Law,* once again brings to the fore the controversial topic of euthanasia, more popularly known as "mercy killing." In keeping with the trend of the euthanasia movement over the past generation, Williams concentrates his efforts for reform on the *voluntary* type of euthanasia, for example, the cancer victim begging for death; as opposed to the *involuntary variety,* that is the case of the congenital idiot, the permanently insane or the senile. . . .

The Law On The Books condemns all mercy-killings.[1] That this has a substantial deterrent effect, even its harshest critics admit. Of course, it does not stamp out all mercy-killings, just as murder and rape provisions do not stamp out all murder and rape, but presumably it does impose a substantially greater responsibility on physicians and relatives in a euthanasia situation and turns them away from significantly more doubtful cases than would otherwise be the practice under any proposed euthanasia legislation to date. When a mercy-killing occurs, however, The Law In Action is as malleable as The Law On The Books is uncompromising. The high incidence of failures to indict, acquittals, suspended sentences and reprieves lend considerable support to the view that:

If the circumstances are so compelling that the defendant ought to violate the law, then they are compelling enough for the jury to violate their oaths. The law does well to declare these homicides unlawful. It does equally well to put no more than the sanction of an oath in the way of an acquittal.[2]

The complaint has been registered that "the prospect of a sentimental acquittal cannot be reckoned as a

certainty."[3] Of course not. The defendant is not always *entitled* to a sentimental acquittal. The few American convictions cited for the proposition that the present state of affairs breeds "inequality" in application may be cited as well for the proposition that it is characterized by elasticity and flexibility. In any event, if inequality of application suffices to damn a particular provision of the criminal law, we might as well tear up all our codes—beginning with the section on chicken-stealing. . . .

The existing law on euthanasia is hardly perfect. But if it is not too good, neither, as I have suggested, is it much worse than the rest of the criminal law. At any rate, the imperfections of the existing law are not cured by Williams' proposal. Indeed, I believe adoption of his views would add more difficulties than it would remove.

Williams strongly suggests that "euthanasia can be condemned only according to a religious opinion."[4] He tends to view the opposing camps as Roman Catholics versus Liberals. Although this has a certain initial appeal to me, a non-Catholic and a self-styled liberal, I deny that this is the only way the battle lines can, or should, be drawn. I leave the religious arguments to the theologians. I share the view that "those who hold the faith may follow its precepts without requiring those who do not hold it to act as if they did."[5] But I do find substantial utilitarian obstacles on the high road to euthanasia.

As an ultimate philosophical proposition, the case for voluntary euthanasia is strong. Whatever may be said for and against suicide generally, the appeal of death is immeasurably greater when it is sought not for a poor reason or just any reason, but for "good cause," so to speak; when it is invoked not on behalf of a "socially useful" person, but on behalf of, for example, the pain-racked "hopelessly incurable"

Reprinted with permission of the author and the publisher from *Minnesota Law Review,* Vol. 42, No. 6 (May 1958).

cancer victim. *If* a person is *in fact* (1) presently incurable, (2) beyond the aid of any respite which may come along in his life expectancy, suffering (3) intolerable and (4) unmitigable pain and of a (5) fixed and (6) rational desire to die, I would hate to have to argue that the hand of death should be stayed. But abstract propositions and carefully formed hypotheticals are one thing; specific proposals designed to cover everyday situations are something else again.

In essence, Williams' specific proposal is that death be authorized for a person in the above situation "by giving the medical practitioner a wide discretion and trusting to his good sense."[6] This, I submit, raises too great a risk of abuse and mistake to warrant a change in the existing law. That a proposal entails risk of mistake is hardly a conclusive reason against it. But neither is it irrelevant. Under any euthanasia program the consequences of mistake, of course, are always fatal. As I shall endeavor to show, the incidence of mistake of any kind or another is likely to be quite appreciable. If this indeed be the case, unless the need for the authorized conduct is compelling enough to override it, I take it the risk of mistake *is* a conclusive reason against such authorization. I submit, too, that the possible radiations from the proposed legislation, *e.g.,* involuntary euthanasia of idiots and imbeciles (the typical "mercy-killings" reported by the press) and the emergence of the legal precedent that there are lives not "worth living," give additional cause to pause.

I see the issue, then, as the need for voluntary euthanasia versus (1) the incidence of mistake and abuse; and (2) the danger that legal machinery initially designed to kill those who are a nuisance to themselves may someday engulf those who are a nuisance to others.

The "freedom to choose a merciful death by euthanasia " may well be regarded . . . "as a special area of civil liberties." . . . The civil liberties angle is definitely a part of Professor Williams' approach:

> If the law were to remove its ban on euthanasia, the effect would merely be to leave this subject to the individual conscience. This proposal would . . . be easy to defend, as restoring personal liberty in a field in which men differ on the question of conscience. . . .
> On a question like this there is surely everything to be said for the liberty of the individual.[7]

I am perfectly willing to accept civil liberties as the battlefield, but issues of "liberty" and "freedom" mean little until we begin to pin down *whose* "liberty" and "freedom" and for *what* need and at *what* price. . . .

I am more concerned about the life and liberty of those who would needlessly be killed in the process or who would irrationally choose to partake of the process. Williams' price on behalf of those who are *in fact* "hopeless incurables" and *in fact* of a fixed and rational desire to die is the sacrifice of (1) some few, who, though they know it not, because their physicians know it not, need not and should not die; (2) others, probably not so few, who, though they go through the motions of "volunteering," are casualties of strain, pain or narcotics to such an extent that they really know not what they do. My price on behalf of those who, despite appearances to the contrary, have some relatively normal and reasonably useful life left in them, or who are incapable of making the choice, is the lingering on for a while of those who, if you will, *in fact* have no desire and no reason to linger on. . . .

THE "CHOICE"

Under current proposals to establish legal machinery, elaborate or otherwise, for the administration of a quick and easy death, it is not enough that those authorized to pass on the question decide that the patient, in effect, is "better off dead." The patient must concur in this opinion. Much of the appeal in the current proposal lies in this so-called "voluntary" attribute.

But is the adult patient really in a position to concur? Is he truly able to make euthanasia a "voluntary" act? There is a good deal to be said, is there not, for Dr. Frohman's pithy comment that the "voluntary" plan is supposed to be carried out "only if the victim is both sane and crazed by pain."[8]

By hypothesis, voluntary euthanasia is not to be resorted to until narcotics have long since been administered and the patient has developed a tolerance to them. *When,* then, does the patient make the choice? While heavily drugged? Or is narcotic relief to be withdrawn for the time of decision? But if heavy dosage no longer deadens pain, indeed, no longer makes it bearable, how overwhelming is it when whatever relief narcotics offer is taken away, too?

"Hypersensitivity to pain after the analgesia has worn off is nearly always noted."[9] Moreover, "the mental side-effects of narcotics, unfortunately for anyone wishing to suspend them temporarily without unduly tormenting the patient, appear to outlast the analgesic effect'' and ''by many hours.''[10] The situation is further complicated by the fact that ''a person in terminal stages of cancer who had been given morphine steadily for a matter of weeks would certainly be dependent upon it physically and would probably be addicted to it and react with the addict's response.''[11]

The narcotics problem aside, Dr. Benjamin Miller, who probably has personally experienced more pain than any other commentator on the euthanasia scene, observes:

Anyone who has been severely ill knows how distorted his judgment became during the worst moments of the illness. Pain and the toxic effect of disease, or the violent reaction to certain surgical procedures may change our capacity for rational and courageous thought.[12]

If, say, a man in this plight were a criminal defendant and he were to decline the assistance of counsel, would the courts hold that he had ''intelligently and understandingly waived the benefit of counsel?''[13]

Undoubtedly, some euthanasia candidates will have their lucid moments. How they are to be distinguished from fellow-sufferers who do not, or how these instances are to be distinguished from others when the patient is exercising an irrational judgment is not an easy matter. Particularly is this so under Williams' proposal, where no specially qualified persons, psychiatrically trained or otherwise, are to assist in the process.

Assuming, for purposes of argument, that the occasion when a euthanasia candidate possesses a sufficiently clear mind can be ascertained and that a request for euthanasia is then made, there remain other problems. The mind of the pain-racked may occasionally be clear, but is it not also likely to be uncertain and variable? This point was pressed hard by the great physician, Lord Horder, in the House of Lords debates:

During the morning depression he [the patient] will be found to favour the application under this Bill; later in the day he will think quite differently, or will have forgotten all about it. The mental clarity with which noble Lords who present this Bill are able to think and to speak must not be thought to have any counterpart in the alternating moods and confused judgments of the sick man.[14]

The concept of ''voluntary'' in voluntary euthanasia would have a great deal more substance to it if, as is the case with voluntary admission statutes for the mentally ill, the patient retained the right to reverse the process within a specified number of days after he gives written notice of his desire to do so—but unfortunately this cannot be. The choice here, of course, is an irrevocable one.

The likelihood of confusion, distortion or vacillation would appear to be serious drawbacks to any voluntary plan. Moreover, Williams' proposal is particularly vulnerable in this regard, since, as he admits, by eliminating the fairly elaborate procedure of the American and English Societies' plans, he also eliminates a time period which would furnish substantial evidence of the patient's settled intention to avail himself of euthanasia.[15] But if Williams does not always choose to slug it out, he can box neatly and parry gingerly:

[T]he problem can be exaggerated. Every law has to face difficulties in application, and these difficulties are not a conclusive argument against a law if it has a beneficial operation. The measure here proposed is designed to meet the situation where the patient's consent to euthanasia is clear and incontrovertible. The physician, conscious of the need to protect himself against malicious accusations, can devise his own safeguards appropriate to the circumstances; he would normally be well advised to get the patient's consent in writing, just as is now the practice before operations. Sometimes, the patient's consent will be particularly clear because he will have expressed a desire for ultimate euthanasia while he is still clear-headed and before he comes to be racked by pain; if the expression of desire is never revoked, but rather is reaffirmed under the pain, there is the best possible proof of full consent. If, on the other hand, there is no such settled frame of mind, and if the physician chooses to administer euthanasia when the patient's mind is in a variable state, he will be walking in the margin of the law and may find himself unprotected.[16]

If consent is given at a time when the patient's condition has so degenerated that he has become a fit candidate for euthanasia, when, if ever, will it be ''clear and incontrovertible?'' Is the suggested alternative of consent in advance a satisfactory solution? Can such a consent be deemed an informed one? Is this much different from holding a man to a prior statement of intent that if such and such an employment opportunity would present itself he would accept it, or if such and such a young woman were to come along he would marry her? Need one marshal authority for the proposition that many an "iffy" inclination is disregarded when the actual facts are at hand?

Professor Williams states that where a pre-pain desire for "ultimate euthanasia" is "reaffirmed" under pain, "there is the best possible proof of full consent." Perhaps. But what if it is alternately renounced and reaffirmed under pain? What if it is neither affirmed or renounced? What if it is only renounced? Will a physician be free to go ahead on the ground that the prior desire was "rational," but the present desire "irrational"? Under Williams' plan, will not the physician frequently "be walking in the margin of the law"—just as he is now? Do we really accomplish much more under this proposal than to put the euthanasia principle on the books?

Even if the patient's choice could be said to be "clear and incontrovertible," do not other difficulties remain? Is this the kind of choice, assuming that it can be made in a fixed and rational manner, that we want to offer a gravely ill person? Will we not sweep up, in the process, some who are not really tired of life but think others are tired of them; some who do not really want to die but who feel they should not live on, because to do so when there looms the legal alternative of euthanasia is to do a selfish or a cowardly act? Will not some feel an obligation to have themselves "eliminated" in order that funds allocated for their terminal care might be better used by their families, or, financial worries aside, in order to relieve their families of the emotional strain involved?

It would not be surprising for the gravely ill person to seek to inquire of those close to him whether he should avail himself of the legal alternative of euthanasia. Certainly, he is likely to wonder about their attitude in the matter. It is quite possible, is it not, that he will not exactly be gratified by any inclination on their part—however noble their motives may be in fact—that he resort to the new procedure? At this stage, the patient-family relationship may well be a good deal less than it ought to be. . . .

And what of the relatives? If their views will not always influence the patient, will they not at least influence the attending physician? Will a physician assume the risks to his reputation, if not his pocketbook, by administering the *coup de grace* over the objection—however irrational—of a close relative? Do not the relatives, then, also have a "choice?" Is not the decision on their part to do nothing and say nothing *itself* a "choice?" In many families there will be some, will there not, who will consider a stand

against euthanasia the only proof of love, devotion and gratitude for past events? What of the stress and strife if close relatives differ—as they did in the famous *Sander* case—over the desirability of euthanatizing the patient?

• • •

At such a time, members of the family are not likely to be in the best state of mind, either, to make this kind of decision. Financial stress and conscious or unconscious competition for the family's estate aside:

The chronic illness and persistent pain in terminal carcinoma may place strong and excessive stresses upon the family's emotional ties with the patient. The family members who have strong emotional attachment to start with are most likely to take the patient's fears, pains and fate personally. Panic often strikes them. Whatever guilt feelings they may have toward the patient emerge to plague them.

If the patient is maintained at home, many frustrations and physical demands may be imposed on the family by the advanced illness. There may develop extreme weakness, incontinence and bad odors. The pressure of caring for the individual under these circumstances is likely to arouse a resentment and, in turn, guilt feelings on the part of those who have to do the nursing.[17]

Nor should it be overlooked that while Professor Williams would remove the various procedural steps and the various personnel contemplated in the American and English Bills and bank his all on the "good sense" of the general practitioner, no man is immune to the fear, anxieties and frustrations engendered by the apparently helpless, hopeless patient. Not even the general practitioner:

Working with a patient suffering from a malignancy causes special problems for the physician. First of all, the patient with a malignancy is most likely to engender anxiety concerning death, even in the doctor. And at the same time, this type of patient constitutes a serious threat or frustration to medical ambition. As a result, a doctor may react more emotionally and less objectively than in any other area of medical practice. . . . His deep concern may make him more pessimistic than is necessary. As a result of the feeling of frustration in his wish to help, the doctor may have moments of annoyance with the patient. He may even feel almost included to want to avoid this type of patient.[18]

• • •

Putting aside the problem of whether the good sense of the general practitioner warrants dispensing with other personnel, there still remain the problems posed by *any* voluntary euthanasia program: the aforementioned considerable pressures on the patient and his family. Are these the kind of pressures we want to inflict on any person, let alone a very sick person? Are these the kind of pressures we want to impose on any family, let alone an emotionally shattered family? And if so, why are they not also proper considerations for the crippled, the paralyzed, the quadruple amputee, the iron lung occupant and their families?

Might it not be said of the existing ban on euthanasia, as Professor Herbert Wechsler has said of the criminal law in another connection:

It also operates, and perhaps more significantly, at anterior stages in the patterns of conduct, the dark shadow of organized disapproval eliminating from the ambit of consideration alternatives that might otherwise present themselves in the final competition of choice.[19]

THE "HOPELESSLY INCURABLE" PATIENT AND THE FALLIBLE DOCTOR

Professor Williams notes as "standard argument" the plea that "no sufferer from an apparently fatal illness should be deprived of his life because there is always the possibility that the diagnosis is wrong, or else that some remarkable cure will be discovered in time."[20]

Until the euthanasia societies of England and America had been organized and a party decision reached, shall we say, to advocate euthanasia only for incurables on their request, Dr. Abraham L. Wolbarst, one of the most ardent supporters of the movement, was less troubled about putting away "insane or defective people [who] have suffered mental incapacity and tortures of the mind for many years" than he was about the "incurables."[21] He recognized the "difficulty involved in the decision as to the incurability" as one of the "doubtful aspects of euthanasia."

Doctors are only human beings, with few if any supermen among them. They make honest mistakes, like other men, because of the limitations of the human mind.[22]

He noted further that "it goes without saying that, in recently developed cases with a possibility of cure, euthanasia should not even be considered," that "the law might establish a limit of, say, ten years in which there is a chance of the patient's recovery."[23]

Dr. Benjamin Miller [has a more personal interest in the problem of euthanasia.] He himself was left to die the death of a "hopeless" tuberculosis victim only to discover that he was suffering from a rare malady which affects the lungs in much the same manner but seldom kills. Five years and sixteen hospitalizations later, Dr. Miller dramatized his point by recalling the last diagnostic clinic of the brilliant Richard Cabot, on the occasion of his official retirement:

He was given the case records [complete medical histories and results of careful examinations] of two patients and asked to diagnose their illnesses. . . . The patients had died and only the hospital pathologist knew the exact diagnosis beyond doubt, for he had seen the descriptions of the postmortem findings. Dr. Cabot, usually very accurate in his diagnosis, that day missed both.

The chief pathologist who had selected the cases was a wise person. He had purposely chosen two of the most deceptive to remind the medical students and young physicians that even at the end of a long and rich experience one of the greatest diagnosticians of our time was still not infallible.[24]

Richard Cabot was the John W. Davis, the John Lord O'Brian, of his profession. When one reads the account of his last clinic, one cannot help but think of how fallible the *average* general practitioner must be, how fallible the *young doctor just starting practice* must be—and this, of course, is all that some small communities have in the way of medical care—how fallible the *worst* practitioner, young or old, must be. If the range of skill and judgment among licensed physicians approaches the wide gap between the very best and the very worst members of the bar—and I have no reason to think it does not—then the minimally competent physician is hardly the man to be given the responsibility for ending another's life. Yet, under Williams' proposal at least, the marginal physician, as well as his more distinguished brethren, would have legal authorization to make just such decisions. Under Williams' proposal, euthanatizing a patient or two would all be part of the routine day's work.

.   .   .

Faulty diagnosis is only one ground for error. Even if the diagnosis is correct, a second ground for error lies in the possibility that some measure of relief, if not a full cure, may come to the fore within the life expectancy of the patient. Since Glanville Williams does not deign this objection to euthanasia worth more than a passing reference,[25] it is necessary to turn elsewhere to ascertain how it has been met.

One answer is:

It must be little comfort to a man slowly coming apart from multiple sclerosis to think that, fifteen years from now, death might not be his only hope.[26]

To state the problem this way is of course, to avoid it entirely. How do we know that fifteen *days* or fifteen *hours* from now, "death might not be [the incurable's] only hope?"

A second answer is:

[N]o cure for cancer which might be found "tomorrow" would be of any value to a man or woman "so far advanced in cancerous toxemia as to be an applicant for euthanasia."[27]

As I shall endeavor to show, this approach is a good deal easier to formulate than it is to apply. For one thing, it presumes that we know today *what* cures will be found tomorrow. For another, it overlooks that if such cases can be said to exist, the patient is likely to be *so far* advanced in cancerous toxemia as to be no longer capable of understanding the step he is taking and hence *beyond* the stage when euthanasia ought to be administered.

A generation ago, Dr. Haven Emerson, then President of the American Public Health Association, made the point that "no one can say today what will be incurable tomorrow. No one can predict what disease will be fatal or premanently incurable until medicine becomes stationary and sterile." Dr. Emerson went so far as to say that "to be at all accurate we must drop altogether the term 'incurables' and substitute for it some such term as 'chronic illness'."[28]

That was a generation ago. Dr. Emerson did not have to go back more than a decade to document his contention. Before Banting and Best's insulin discovery, many a diabetic had been doomed. Before the Whipple-Minot-Murphy liver treatment made it a relatively minor malady, many a pernicious anemia sufferer had been branded "hopeless." Before the uses of sulfanilimide were disclosed, a patient with widespread streptococcal blood poisoning was a condemned man.[29]

Today, we may take even that most resolute disease, cancer, and we need to look back no further than the last decade of research in this field to document the same contention.

•   •   •

True, many types of cancer still run their course virtually unhampered by man's arduous efforts to inhibit them. But the number of cancers coming under some control is ever increasing. With medicine attacking on so many fronts with so many weapons who would bet a man's life on when and how the next type of cancer will yield, if only just a bit?

•   •   •

VOLUNTARY V. INVOLUNTARY EUTHANASIA

Ever since the 1870s, when what was probably the first euthanasia debate of the modern era took place, most proponents of the movement—at least when they are pressed—have taken considerable pains to restrict the question to the plight of the unbearably suffering incurable who *voluntarily seeks* death, while most of their opponents have striven equally hard to frame the issue in terms which would encompass certain involuntary situations as well, *e.g.*, the "congenital idiots," the "permanently insane," and the senile.

Glanville Williams reflects the outward mood of many euthanasiasts when he scores those who insist on considering the question from a broader angle:

The [English Society's] bill [debated in the House of Lords in 1936 and 1950] excluded any question of compulsory euthanasia, even for hopelessly defective infants. Unfortunately, a legislative proposal is not assured of success merely because it is worded in a studiously moderate and restrictive form. The method of attack, by those who dislike the proposal, is to use the "thin edge of the wedge" argument. . . . There is no proposal for reform on any topic, however conciliatory and moderate, that cannot be opposed by this dialectic.[30]

Why was the bill "worded in a studiously moderate and restrictive form?" If it were done as a matter of principle, if it were done in recognition of the ethico-moral-legal "wall of separation" which stands between voluntary and compulsory "mercy-killings," much can be said for the euthanasiasts' lament about the methods employed by the opposition. But if it were done as a matter of political expediency—with great hopes and expectations of pushing through a second and somewhat less restrictive bill as soon as the first one had sufficiently ''educated'' public opinion and next a third still less restrictive bill—what standing do the euthanasiasts then have to attack the methods of the opposition? No cry of righteous indignation could ring more hollow, I would think, than the protest from those utilizing the ''wedge'' principle themselves that their opponents are making the wedge objection.

• • •

The boldness and daring which characterizes most of Glanville Williams' book dims perceptibly when he comes to involuntary euthanasia proposals. As to the senile, he states:

At present the problem has certainly not reached the degree of seriousness that would warrant an effort being made to change traditional attitudes toward the sanctity of life of the aged. Only the grimmest necessity could bring about a change that, however cautious in its approach, would probably cause apprehension and deep distress to many people, and inflict a traumatic injury upon the accepted code of behaviour built up by two thousand years of the Christian religion. It may be however, that as the problem becomes more acute it will itself cause a reversal of generally accepted values.[31]

To me, this passage is the most startling one in the book. On page 348 Williams invokes ''traditional attitudes towards the sanctity of life'' and ''the accepted code of behaviour built up by two thousand years of the Christian religion'' to check the extension of euthanasia to the senile, but for 347 pages he had been merrily rolling along debunking both. Substitute ''cancer victim'' for ''the aged'' and Williams' passage is essentially the argument of many of his *opponents* on the voluntary euthanasia question.

The unsupported comment that ''the problem [of senility] has certainly not reached the degree of seriousness'' to warrant euthanasia is also rather puzzling, particularly coming as it does after an observation by Williams on the immediately preceding page that ''it is increasingly common for men and women to reach an age of 'second childishness and mere oblivion,' with a loss of almost all adult faculties except that of digestion.'[32]

How ''serious'' does a problem have to be to warrant a change in these ''traditional attitudes''? If, as the statement seems to indicate, ''seriousness'' of a problem is to be determined numerically, the problem of the cancer victim does not appear to be as substantial as the problem of the senile. For example, taking just the 95,837 first admissions to ''public prolonged-care hospitals'' for mental diseases in the United States in 1955, 23,561—or one-fourth—were cerebral arteriosclerosis or senile brain disease cases.[33] I am not at all sure that there are 20,000 cancer victims per year who die *unbearably painful* deaths. Even if there were, I cannot believe that among their ranks are some 20,000 per year who, when still in a rational state, so long for a quick and easy death that they would avail themselves of legal machinery for euthanasia.

If the problem of the incurable cancer victim ''has reached the degree of seriousness that would warrant an effort being made to change traditional attitudes toward the sanctity of life,'' as Williams obviously thinks it has, then so has the problem of senility. In any event, the senility problem will undoubtedly soon reach even Williams' requisite degree of seriousness:

A decision concerning the senile may have to be taken within the next twenty years. The number of old people are increasing by leaps and bounds. Pneumonia, ''the old man's friend,'' is now checked by antibiotics. The effects of hardship, exposure, starvation and accident are now minimized. Where is this leading us? . . . What of the drooling, helpless, disorientated old man or the doubly incontinent old woman lying log-like in bed? Is it here that the real need for euthanasia exists?[34]

If, as Williams indicates ''seriousness'' of the problem is a major criterion for euthanatizing a category of unfortunates, the sum total of mentally deficient persons would appear to warrant high priority, indeed.

When Williams turns to the plight of the ''hopelessly defective infants,'' his characteristic vim and vigor are, as in the senility discussion, conspicuously absent:

While the Euthanasia Society of England has never advocated this, the Euthanasia Society of America did include it in its original program. The proposal certainly escapes the chief objection to the similar proposal for senile dementia: it does not create a sense of insecurity in society, because infants cannot, like adults, feel anticipatory dread of being done to death if their condition should worsen. Moreover, the proposal receives some support on eugenic grounds, and more importantly on humanitarian grounds—both on account of the parents, to whom the child will be a burden all their lives, and on account of the handicapped child itself.

(It is not, however, proposed that any child should be destroyed against the wishes of its parents.) Finally, the legalization of euthanasia for handicapped children would bring the law into closer relation to its practical administration, because juries do not regard parental mercy-killing as murder. For these various reasons the proposal to legalize humanitarian infanticide is put forward from time to time by individuals. They remain in a very small minority, and the proposal may at present be dismissed as politically insignificant.[35]

It is understandable for a reformer to limit his present proposals for change to those with a real prospect of success. But it is hardly reasuring for Williams to cite the fact that only "a very small minority" has urged euthanasia for "hopelessly defective infants" as the *only* reason for not pressing for such legislation now. If, as Williams sees it, the only advantage voluntary euthanasia has over the involuntary variety lies in the organized movements on its behalf, that advantage can readily be wiped out.

In any event, I do not think that such "a very small minority" has advocated "humanitarian infanticide." Until the organization of the English and American societies led to a concentration on the voluntary type, and until the by-products of the Nazi euthanasia program somewhat embarrassed, if only temporarily, most proponents of involuntary euthanasia, about as many writers urged one type as another. Indeed, some euthanasiasts have taken considerable pains to demonstrate the superiority of defective infant euthanasia over incurably ill euthanasia.

As for dismissing euthanasia of defective infants as "politically insignificant," the only poll that I know of which measured the public response to both types of euthanasia revealed that *45 percent favored euthanasia for defective infants under certain conditions while only 37.3 percent approved euthanasia for the incurably and painfully ill under any conditions.*[36] Furthermore, of those who favored the mercy-killing cure for incurable adults, some 40 percent would require only family permission or medical board approval, but not the patient's permission.[37]

Nor do I think it irrelevant that while public resistance caused Hitler to yield on the adult euthanasia front, the killing of malformed and idiot children continued unhindered to the end of the war, the definition of "children" expanding all the while.[38] Is it the embarrassing experience of the Nazi euthanasia program which has rendered destruction of defective infants presently "politically insignificant"? If so, is it any more of a jump from the incurably and painfully

ill to the unorthodox political thinker than it is from the hopelessly defective infant to the same "unsavory character?" Or is it not so much that the euthanasiasts are troubled by the Nazi experience as it is that they are troubled that the public is troubled by the Nazi experience?

I read Williams' comments on defective infants [as arguments] for the proposition that there are some very good reasons for euthanatizing defective infants, but the time is not yet ripe. When will it be? When will the proposal become politically significant? After a voluntary euthanasia law is on the books and public opinion is sufficiently "educated?"

Williams' reasons for not extending euthanasia— once we legalize it in the narrow "voluntary" area—to the senile and the defective are much less forceful and much less persuasive than his arguments for legalizing voluntary euthanasia in the first place. I regard this as another reason for not legalizing voluntary euthanasia in the first place.

. . .

A FINAL REFLECTION

There have been and there will continue to be compelling circumstances when a doctor or relative or friend will violate The Law On The Books and, more often than not, receive protection from The Law In Action. But this is not to deny that there are other occasions when The Law On The Books operates to stay the hand of all concerned, among them situations where the patient is in fact (1) presently incurable, (2) beyond the aid of any respite which may come along in his life expectancy, suffering (3) intolerable and (4) unmitigable pain and of a (5) fixed and (6) rational desire to die. That any euthanasia program may only be the opening wedge for far more objectionable practices, and that even within the bounds of a "voluntary" plan such as Williams' the incidence of mistake or abuse is likely to be substantial, is not much solace to one in the above plight.

It may be conceded that in a narrow sense it is an "evil" for such a patient to have to continue to suffer—if only for a little while. But in a narrow sense, long-term sentences and capital punishment are "evils," too.[39] If we can justify the infliction of imprisonment and death by the state "on the ground of the social interests to be protected,"[40] then surely we can similarly justify the postponement of death by the state. The objection that the individual is thereby treated not as an "end" in himself but only as a "means" to further the common good was, I think, aptly disposed of by Holmes long ago. "If a man lives in society, he is likely to find himself so treated."[41]

NOTES

1. In Anglo-American jurisprudence a "mercy-killing" is murder. In theory, neither good motive nor consent of the victim is relevant. See, *e.g.*, 2 Burdick, Law of Crimes §§ 422, 447 (1946); Miller, Criminal Law 55, 172 (1934); Perkins, Criminal Law 721 (1957); 1 Wharton, Criminal Law and Procedure § 194 (Anderson 1957); Orth, *Legal Aspects Relating to Euthanasia*, 2 Md. Med. J. 120 (1953) (symposium on euthanasia); 48 Mich. L. Rev. 1199 (1950); Anno., 25 A.L.R. 1007 (1923).

In a number of countries, *e.g.*, Germany, Norway, Switzerland, a compassionate motive and/or "homicide upon request" operate to reduce the penalty. See generally Helen Silving's valuable comparative study, *supra* note 7 [in original text]. However, apparently only Uruguayan law completely immunizes a homicide characterized by both of the above factors. *Id.* at 369 and n. 21. The Silving article only contains an interesting and fairly extensive comparative study of assisted suicide and the degree to which it is treated differently from a direct "mercy-killing." In this regard see also Friedman, *Suicide, Euthanasia and the Law,* 85 Med. Times 681 (1957).

2. Curtis, It's Your Law 95 (1954).

3. Williams, The Sanctity of Life and the Criminal Law (1957), p. 328.

4. *Id.* at 312.

5. Wechsler and Michael, *A Rationale of the Law of Homicide: I,* 37 Columbia L. Rev. 740 (1937).

6. Williams, p. 339.

7. *Id.* at 341, 346.

8. Frohman, *Vexing Problems in Forensic Medicine: A Physician's View,* 31 N.Y.U.L. Rev. 1215, 1222 (1956).

9. Goodman and Gilman, The Pharmacological Basis of Therapeutics 235 (2d ed. 1955).

10. Sharpe, *Medication As a Threat to Testamentary Capacity,* 35 N.C.L. Rev. 380, 392 (1957) and medical authorities cited therein.

11. *Id.* at 384.

12. Miller, *Why I Oppose Mercy Killings,* Woman's Home Companion, June 1950, pp. 38, 103.

13. Moore v. Michigan, 355 U.S. 155, 161 (1957).

14. 103 House of Lords Debates (5th ser.) 466, 492–93 (1936).

15. Williams, pp. 343–44.

16. *Id.* at 344.

17. Zarling, *Psychological Aspects of Pain in Terminal Malignancies,* in Management of Pain in Cancer, 211–12 (Schiffrin, ed., 1956).

18. *Id.* at 213–14.

19. Wechsler, *The Issues of the Nuremberg Trial,* 62 Pol. Sci. Q. 11, 16 (1947).

20. Williams, p. 318.

21. Wolbarst, *Legalize Euthanasia!,* 94 The Forum 330, 332 (1935). *But see* Wolbarst, *The Doctor Looks at Euthanasia,* 149 Medical Record, 354 (1939).

22. Wolbarst, *Legalize Euthanasia!,* 94 The Forum 330, 331 (1935).

23. *Id.* at 332.

24. Miller, *supra* note 12, at 39.

25. See Williams, p. 318.

26. *Pro & Con: Shall We Legalize "Mercy Killing"?,* Readers Digest, Nov. 1938, pp. 94, 96.

27. James, *Euthanasia—Right or Wrong?* Survey Graphic, May, 1948, pp. 241, 243; Wolbarst, *The Doctor Looks at Euthanasia,* 149 Medical Record, 354, 355 (1939).

28. Emerson, *Who Is Incurable? A Query and Reply,* N.Y. Times, Oct. 22, 1933, § 8, p. 5, col. 1.

29. *Ibid.,* Miller, *supra* note 12, at 39.

30. Williams, pp. 333–34.

31. *Id.* at 348.

32. *Id.* at 347.

33. U.S. Dep't of Health, Education and Welfare, Patients in Mental Institutions 1955, Part II, Public Hospitals for the Mentally Ill 21. Some 13,972 were cerebral arteriosclerosis cases; 9,589 had senile brain diseases.

34. Banks, *Euthanasia,* 26 Bull. N.Y. Acad. Med. 297, 305 (1950).

35. Williams, pp. 349–50.

36. *The Fortune Quarterly Survey:* IX, Fortune, July 1937, pp. 96, 106.

37. *Id.* at 106.

38. Mitscherlich and Mielke, Doctors of Infamy 114 (1949).

39. Perhaps this would not be true if the only purpose of punishment was to reform the criminal. But whatever *ought to be* the case, this obviously *is not.* "If it were, every prisoner should be released as soon as it appears clear that he will never repeat his offence, and if he is incurable he should not be punished at all." Holmes, The Common Law 42 (1881).

40. Michael and Adler, Crime, Law and Social Science 351 (1933).

41. Holmes, The Common Law 44 (1881).

GLANVILLE WILLIAMS

"Mercy-Killing" Legislation—A Rejoinder

I welcome Professor Kamisar's reply to my argument for voluntary euthanasia, because it is on the whole a careful, scholarly work, keeping to knowable facts and accepted human values. It is, therefore, the sort of reply that can be rationally considered and dealt with. In this short rejoinder I shall accept most of Professor Kamisar's valuable footnotes, and merely submit that they do not bear out his conclusion.

The argument in favour of voluntary euthanasia in the terminal stages of painful diseases is quite a simple one, and is an application of two values that are widely recognized. The first value is the prevention of cruelty. Much as men differ in their ethical assessments, all agree that cruelty is an evil—the only difference of opinion residing in what is meant by cruelty. Those who plead for the legalization of euthanasia think that it is cruel to allow a human being to linger for months in the last stages of agony, weakness and decay, and to refuse him his demand for merciful release. There is also a second cruelty involved—not perhaps quite so compelling, but still worth consideration: the agony of the relatives in seeing their loved one in his desparate plight. Opponents of euthanasia are apt to take a cynical view of the desires of relatives, and this may sometimes be justified. But it cannot be denied that a wife who has to nurse her husband through the last stages of some terrible disease may herself be so deeply affected by the experience that her health is ruined, either mentally or physically. Whether the situation can be eased for such a person by voluntary euthanasia I do not know; probably it depends very much on the individuals concerned, which is as much as to say that no solution in terms of a general regulatory law can be satisfactory. The conclusions should be in favour of individual discretion.

Reprinted with permission of the author and the publisher from *Minnesota Law Review*, Vol. 43, No. 1 (1958).

The second value involved is that of liberty. The criminal law should not be invoked to repress conduct unless this is demonstrably necessary on social grounds. What social interest is there in preventing the sufferer from choosing to accelerate his death by a few months? What positive value does his life still possess for society, that he is to be retained in it by the terrors of the criminal law?

And, of course, the liberty involved is that of the doctor as well as that of the patient. It is the doctor's responsibility to do all he can to prolong worth-while life, or, in the last resort, to ease his patient's passage. If the doctor honestly and sincerely believes that the best service he can perform for his suffering patient is to accede to his request for euthanasia, it is a grave thing that the law should forbid him to do so.

This is the short and simple case for voluntary euthanasia, and, as Kamisar admits, it cannot be attacked directly on utilitarian grounds. Such an attack can only be by finding possible evils of an indirect nature. These evils, in the view of Professor Kamisar, are (1) the difficulty of ascertaining consent, and arising out of that the danger of abuse; (2) the risk of an incorrect diagnosis; (3) the risk of administering euthanasia to a person who could later have been cured by developments in medical knowledge; (4) the "wedge" argument.

Before considering these matters, one preliminary comment may be made. In some parts of his Article Kamisar hints at recognition of the fact that a practice of mercy-killing exists among the most reputable of medical practitioners. Some of the evidence for this will be found in my book. [The Sanctity of Life and the Criminal Law 334–39 (1957).] In the first debate in the House of Lords, Lord Dawson admitted the fact, and claimed that it did away with the need for legislation. In other words, the attitude of conservatives is this: let medical men do mercy-killing, but let it continue to be called murder, and be treated as such if the legal machinery is by some unlucky mischance made to work; let us, in other words, take no steps to translate the new morality into the concepts of the law. I find this attitude equally incomprehensible in a doctor, as Lord Dawson was, and in a lawyer, as Professor Kamisar is. Still more baffling does it become when Professor Kamisar seems to claim as a virture of the system that the jury can give a merciful acquittal in breach of their oaths. The result is that the law frightens some doctors from interposing, while not frightening others—though subjecting the braver group to the risk of prosecution and possible loss of liberty and livelihood. Apparently, in Kamisar's view, it is a good thing if the law is broken in a proper case, because that relieves suffering, but also a good thing that the law is there as a threat in order to prevent too much mercy being administered; thus, whichever result the law has is perfectly right and proper. It is hard to understand on what moral principle this type of ethical ambivalence is to be maintained. If Kamisar does approve of doctors administering euthanasia in some clear cases, and of juries acquitting them if they are prosecuted for murder, how does he maintain that it is an insuperable objection to euthanasia that diagnosis may be wrong and medical knowledge subsequently extended?

However, the references to merciful acquittals disappear after the first few pages of the article, and thenceforward the argument develops as a straight attack on euthanasia. So although at the beginning Kamisar says that he would hate to have to argue against mercy-killing in a clear case, in fact he does proceed to argue against it with some zest.

. . .

Kamisar's first objection, under the heading of "The Choice," is that there can be no such thing as truly volunatry euthanasia in painful and killing diseases. He seeks to impale the advocates of euthanasia on an old dilemma. Either the victim is not yet suffering pain, in which case his consent is merely an uninformed and anticipatory one—and he cannot bind himself by contract to be killed in the future—or he is crazed by pain and stupefied by drugs, in which case he is not of sound mind. I have dealt with this problem in my book; Kamisar has quoted generously from it, and I leave the reader to decide. As I understand Kamisar's position, he does not really persist in the objection. With the laconic "Perhaps," he seems to grant me, though unwillingly, that there are cases

where one can be sure of the patient's consent. But having thus abandoned his own point, he then goes off to a different horror, that the patient may give his consent only in order to relieve his relatives of the trouble of looking after him.

On this new issue, I will return Kamisar the compliment and say: "Perhaps." We are certainly in an area where no solution is going to make things quite easy and happy for everybody, and all sorts of embarrassments may be conjectured. But these embarrassments are not avoided by keeping to the present law: we suffer from them already. If a patient, suffering pain in a terminal illness, wishes for euthanasia partly because of this pain and partly because he sees his beloved ones breaking under the strain of caring for him, I do not see how this decision on his part, agonizing though it may be, is necessarily a matter of discredit either to the patient himself or to his relatives. The fact is that, whether we are considering the patient or his relatives, there are limits to human endurance.

The author's next objection rests on the possibility of mistaken diagnosis. . . . I agree with him that, before deciding on euthanasia in any particular case, the risk of mistaken diagnosis would have to be considered. Everything that is said in the article would, therefore, be most relevant when the two doctors whom I propose in my suggested measure come to consult on the question of euthanasia; and the possibility of mistake might most forcefully be brought before the patient himself. But have these medical questions any real relevance to the legal discussion?

Kamisar, I take it, notwithstanding his wide reading in medical literature, is by training a lawyer. He has consulted much medical opinion in order to find arguments against changing the law. I ought not to object to this, since I have consulted the same opinion for the opposite purpose. But what we may well ask ourselves is this: is it not a trifle bizarre that we should be doing it at all? Our profession is the law, not medicine; how does it come about that lawyers have to examine medical literature to assess the advantages and disadvantages of a medical practice?

If the import of this question is not immediately clear, let me return to my imaginary State of Ruritania. Many years ago, in Ruritania as elsewhere, surgical operations were attended with great risk. Pasteur had not made his discoveries, and surgeons killed as often as they cured. In this state of things, the legislature of Ruritania passed a law declaring all surgical operations to be unlawful in principle but providing that each specific type of operation might be legalized by a statute specially passed for the purpose. The result is that, in Ruritania, as expert medical opinion sees the possibility of some new medical advance, a pressure group has to be formed in order to obtain legislative approval for it. Since there is little public interest in these technical questions, and since, moreover, surgical operations are thought in general to be inimical to the established religion, the pressure group has to work for many years before it gets a hearing. When at last a proposal for legalization is seriously mooted, the lawyers and politicians get to work upon it, considering what possible dangers are inherent in the new operation. Lawyers and politicians are careful people, and they are perhaps more prone to see the dangers than the advantages in a new departure. Naturally they find allies among some of the more timid or traditional or less knowledgeable members of the medical profession, as well as among the priesthood and the faithful. Thus it is small wonder that whereas appendicectomy has been practised in civilised countries since the beginning of the present century, a proposal to legalize it has still not passed the legislative assembly of Ruritania.

It must be confessed that on this particular matter the legal prohibition has not been an unmixed evil for the Ruritanians. During the great popularity of the appendix operation in much of the civilised world during the twenties and thirties of this century, large numbers of these organs were removed without adequate cause, and the citizens of Ruritania have been spared this inconvenience. On the other hand, many citizens of that country have died of appendicitis who would have been saved if they had lived elsewhere. And whereas in other countries the medical profession has now learned enough to be able to perform this operation with wisdom and restraint, in Ruritania it is still not being performed at all. Moreover, the law has destroyed scientific inventiveness in that country in the forbidden fields.

Now, in the United States and England we have no such absurd general law on the subject of surgical operations as they have in Ruritania. In principle, medical men are left free to exercise their best judgement, and the result has been a brilliant advance in knowledge and technique. But there are just two—or possibly three—operations which are subject to the Ruritanian principle. These are abortion, euthanasia, and possibly sterilization of convenience. In these fields we, too, must have pressure groups, with lawyers and politicians warning us of the possibility

of inexpert practitioners and mistaken diagnosis, and canvassing medical opinion on the risk of an operation not yielding the expected results in terms of human happiness and the health of the body politic. In these fields we, too, are forbidden to experiment to see if the foretold dangers actually come to pass. Instead of that, we are required to make a social judgment on the probabilities of good and evil before the medical profession is allowed to start on its empirical tests.

This anomaly is perhaps more obvious with abortion than it is with euthanasia. Indeed, I am prepared for ridicule when I describe euthanasia as a medical operation. Regarded as surgery it is unique, since its object is not to save or prolong life but the reverse. But euthanasia has another object which it shares with many surgical operations—the saving of pain. And it is now widely recognised, as Lord Dawson said in the debate in the House of Lords, that the saving of pain is a legitimate aim of medical practice. The question whether euthanasia will effect a net saving of pain and distress is, perhaps, one that can be only finally answered by trying it. But it is obscurantist to forbid the experiment on the ground that until it is performed we cannot certainly know its results. Such an attitude, in any other field of medical endeavor, would have inhibited progress.

The argument based on mistaken diagnosis leads into the argument based on the possibility of dramatic medical discoveries. Of course, a new medical discovery which gives the opportunity of remission or cure will almost at once put an end to mercy-killings in the particular group of cases for which the discovery is made. On the other hand, the discovery cannot affect patients who have already died from their disease. The argument based on mistaken diagnosis is therefore concerned only with those patients who have been mercifully killed just before the discovery becomes available for use. The argument is that such persons may turn out to have been "mercy–killed" unnecessarily, because if the physician had waited a bit longer they would have been cured. Because of this risk for this tiny fraction of the total number of patients, patients who are dying in pain must be left to do so, year after year, against their entreaty to have it ended.

Just how real is the risk? When a new medical discovery is claimed, some time commonly elapses before it becomes tested sufficiently to justify large-scale production of the drug, or training in the techniques involved. This is a warning period when euthanasia in the particular class of case would probable be halted anyway. Thus it is quite probable that when the new discovery becomes available, the euthanasia process would not in fact show any mistakes in this regard.

Kamisar says that in my book I ''did not deign this objection to euthanasia more than a passing reference.'' I still do not think it is worth any more than that.

The author advances the familiar but hardly convincing argument that the quantitative need for euthanasia is not large. As one reason for this argument, he suggests that not many patients would wish to benefit from euthanasia, even if it were allowed. I am not impressed by the argument. It may be true, but it is irrelevant. So long as there are *any* persons dying in weakness and grief who are refused their request for a speeding of their end, the argument for legalizing euthanasia remains. Next, the Article suggests that there is no great need for euthanasia because of the advances made with pain-killing drugs. . . . In my book, recognising that medical science does manage to save many dying patients from the extreme of physical pain, I pointed out that it often fails to save them from an artificial, twilight existence, with nausea, giddiness, and extreme restlessness, as well as the long hours of consciousness of a hopeless condition. A dear friend of mine, who died of cancer of the bowel, spent his last months in just this state, under the influence of morphine, which deadened pain, but vomiting incessantly, day in and day out. The question that we have to face is whether the unintelligent brutality of such an existence is to be imposed on one who wished to end it.

. . .

The last part of the Article is devoted to the ancient ''wedge'' argument which I have already examined in my book. It is the trump card of the traditionalist, because no proposal for reform, however strong the arguments in favour, is immune from the wedge objection. In fact, the stronger the arguments in favour of a reform, the more likely it is that the traditionalist will take the wedge objection—it is then the only one he has. C. M. Cornford put the argument in its proper place when he said that the wedge objection means

this, that you should not act justly today, for fear that you may be asked to act still more justly tomorrow.

We heard a great deal of this type of argument in England in the nineteenth century, when it was used to resist almost every social and economic change. In the present century we have had less of it, but (if I may claim the hospitality of these columns to say so) it seems still to be accorded an exaggerated importance in American thought. When lecturing on the law of torts in an American university a few years ago, I suggested that just as compulsory liability insurance for automobiles had spread practically through the civilised world, so we should in time see the law of tort superseded in this field by a system of state insurance for traffic accidents, administered independently of proof of fault. The suggestion was immediately met by one student with a horrified reference to ''creeping socialism.'' That is the standard objection made by many people to any proposal for a new department of state activity. The implication is that you must resist every proposal, however admirable in itself, because otherwise you will never be able to draw the line. On the particular question of socialism, the fear is belied by the experience of a number of countries which have extended state control of the economy without going the whole way to socialistic state regimentation.

Kamisar's particular bogey, the racial laws of Nazi Germany, is an effective one in the democratic countries. Any reference to the Nazis is a powerful weapon to prevent change in the traditional taboo on sterilization as well as euthanasia. The case of sterilization is particularly interesting on this; I dealt with it at length in my book, though Kamisar does not mention its bearing on the argument. When proposals are made for promoting voluntary sterilization on eugenic and other grounds, they are immediately condemned by most people as the thin end of a wedge leading to involuntary sterilization; and then they point to the practices of the Nazis. Yet a more persuasive argument pointing in the other direction can easily be found. Several American states have sterilization laws, which for the most part were originally drafted in very wide terms, to cover desexualisation as well as sterilization, and authorizing involuntary as well as voluntary operations. This legislation goes back long before the Nazis; the earliest statute was in Indiana in 1907. What has been its practical effect? In several states it has hardly been used. A few have used it, but in practice they have progressively restricted it until now it is virtually confined to voluntary sterilization. This is so, at least, in North Carolina, as Mrs. Woodside's study strikingly shows. In my book I summed up the position as follows:

The American experience is of great interest because it shows how remote from reality in a democratic community is the fear—frequently voiced by Americans themselves—that voluntary sterilization may be the "thin end of the wedge," leading to a large-scale violation of human rights as happened in Nazi Germany. In fact, the American experience is the precise opposite—starting with compulsory sterilization, administrative practice has come to put the operation on a voluntary footing.

But it is insufficient to answer the "wedge" objection in general terms; we must consider the particular fears to which it gives rise. Kamisar professes to fear certain other measures that the euthanasia societies may bring up if their present measure is conceded to them. Surely, these other measures, if any, will be debated on their merits? Does he seriously fear that anyone in the United States is going to propose the extermination of people of a minority race or religion? Let us put aside such ridiculous fancies and discuss practical politics.

The author is quite right in thinking that a body of opinion would favour the legalization of the involuntary euthanasia of hopelessly defective infants, and some day a proposal of this kind may be put forward. The proposal would have distinct limits, just as the proposal for voluntary euthanasia of incurable sufferers has limits. I do not think that any responsible body of opinion would now propose the euthanasia of insane adults, for the perfectly clear reason that any such practice would greatly increase the sense of insecurity felt by the borderline insane and by the large number of insane persons who have sufficient understanding on this particular matter.

Kamisar expresses distress at a concluding remark in my book in which I advert to the possibility of old people becoming an overwhelming burden on mankind. I share his feeling that there are profoundly disturbing possibilities here; and if I had been merely a propagandist, intent upon securing agreement for a specific measure of law reform, I should have done wisely to have omitted all reference to this subject. Since, however, I am merely an academic writer, trying to bring such intelligence as I have to bear on moral and social issues, I deemed the topic too important and threatening to leave without a word. I think I have made it clear, in the passages cited, that I am not for one moment proposing any euthanasia of the aged in present society; such an idea would shock me as much as it shocks Kamisar and would shock everybody else. Still, the fact that we may one day have to face is that medical science is more successful in preserving the body than in preserving the mind. It is not impossible that, in the foreseeable future, medical men will be able to preserve the mindless body until the age, say, of 1000, while the mind itself will have lasted only a tenth of that time. What will mankind do then? It is hardly possible to imagine that we shall establish huge hospital-mausolea where the aged are kept in a kind of living death. Even if it is desired to do this, the cost of the undertaking may make it impossible.

This is not an immediately practical problem, and we need not yet face it. The problem of maintaining persons afflicted with senile dementia is well within our economic resources as the matter stands at present. Perhaps some barrier will be found to medical advance which will prevent the problem becoming more acute. Perhaps, as time goes on, and as the alternatives become more clearly realised, men will become more resigned to human control over the mode of termination of life. Or the solution may be that after the individual has reached a certain age, or a certain degree of decay, medical science will hold its hand, and allow him to be carried off by natural causes. But what if these natural causes are themselves painful? Would it not be better kindness to substitute human agency?

In general, it is enough to say that we do not have to know the solutions to these problems. The only doubtful moral question on which we have to make an immediate decision in relation to involuntary euthanasia is whether we owe a moral duty to terminate the life of an insane person who is suffering from a painful and incurable disease. Such a person is left unprovided for under the legislative proposal formulated in my book. The objection to any system of involuntary euthanasia of the insane is that it may cause a sense of insecurity. It is because I think that the risk of this fear is a serious one that a proposal for the reform of the law must leave the insane out.

GREAT BRITAIN, PARLIAMENT, HOUSE OF LORDS

Voluntary Euthanasia Bill*

An act to provide in certain circumstances for the administration of euthanasia to persons who request it and who are suffering from an irremediable condition, and to enable persons to request in advance the administration of euthanasia in the event of their suffering from such a condition at a future date.

Be it enacted by the Queen's most Excellent Majesty, by and with the consent of the Lords Spiritual and Temporal, and Commons, in this present Parliament assembled, and by the authority of the same, as follows:—

1. Authorization of euthanasia

(1) Subject to the provisions of this Act, it shall be lawful for a physician to administer euthanasia to a qualified patient who has made a declaration that is for the time being in force.

(2) For the purposes of this Act:

'physician' means a registered medical practitioner;

'euthanasia' means the painless inducement of death;

'qualified patient' means a patient over the age of majority in respect of whom two physicians (one being of consultant status) have certified in writing that the patient appears to them to be suffering from an irremediable condition;

'irremediable condition' means a serious physical illness or impairment reasonably thought in the patient's case to be incurable and expected to cause him severe distress or render him incapable of rational existence;

'declaration' means a witnessed declaration in writing made substantially in the form set out in the schedule to this Act.

2. Declaration made in advance

(1) Subject to the provisions of this section, a declaration shall come into force 30 days after being made and shall remain in force (unless revoked) for 3 years.

(2) A declaration re-executed within the 12 months preceding its expiry date shall remain in force (unless revoked) during the lifetime of the declarant.

3. Mode of revocation

A declaration may be revoked at any time by destruction or by notice of cancellation shown on its face, effected (in either case) by the declarant or to his order.

4. Duties and rights of physicians and nurses

(1) Before causing euthanasia to be administered to a mentally responsible patient the physician in charge shall ascertain to his reasonable satisfaction that the declaration and all steps proposed to be taken under it accord with the patient's wishes.

(2) Euthanasia shall be deemed to be administered by a physician if treatment prescribed by a physician is given to the patient by a state registered or state enrolled nurse.

(3) No person shall be under any duty, whether by contract or by any statutory or other legal requirement, to participate in any treatment authorized by this Act to which he has a conscientious objection.

5. Protection for physicians and nurses

(1) A physician or nurse who, acting in good faith, causes euthanasia to be administered to a qualified patient in accordance with what the person so acting believes to be the patient's declaration and wishes shall not be guilty of any offence.

(2) Physicians and nurses who have taken part in the administration of euthanasia shall be deemed

*Ed. note: This bill was introduced by Lord Raglan; it was debated and defeated on its second reading. See House of Lords Official Report, *Parliamentary Debates* (Hansard), Vol. 300, No. 50 (March 25, 1969), cols. 1143–1254.

not to be in breach of any professional oath or affirmation.

6. Offenses

(1) It shall be an offence punishable on indictment by a sentence of life imprisonment wilfully to conceal, destroy, falsify or forge a declaration with intent to create a false impression of another person's wishes with regard to euthanasia.

(2) A person signing a declaration by way of attestation who wilfully puts his signature to a statement he knows to be false shall be deemed to have committed an offence under section 2 of the Perjury Act 1911.

7. Insurance policies

No policy of insurance that has been in force for 12 months shall be vitiated by the administration of euthanasia to the insured.

8. Administration of drugs to patients suffering severe distress

For the removal of doubt it is declared that a patient suffering from an irremediable condition reasonably thought in his case to be terminal shall be entitled to the administration of whatever quantity of drugs may be required to keep him free from pain, and such a patient in whose case severe distress cannot be otherwise relieved shall, if he so requests, be entitled to drugs rendering him continuously unconscious.

9. Power to make regulations

(1) The Secretary of State for Social Services shall make regulations under this Act by statutory instrument for determining classes of persons who may or may not sign a declaration by way of attestation, for regulating the custody of declarations, for appointing (with their consent) hospital physicians having responsibility in relation to patients who have made or wish to make a declaration, and for the prescribing of any matters he may think fit to prescribe for the purposes of this Act.

(2) Any statutory instrument made under this Act shall be subject to annulment in pursuance of a resolution of either House of Parliament.

10. Short title and extent

(1) This Act may be cited as the Voluntary Euthanasia Act 1969.

(2) This Act does not extend to Northern Ireland.

SCHEDULE

FORM OF DECLARATION UNDER THE VOLUNTARY EUTHANASIA ACT 1969

Declaration made   19 [and re-executed

                                  19   ]

    by

    of

I DECLARE that I subscribe to the code set out under the following articles:—

A. If I should at any time suffer from a serious physical illness or impairment reasonably thought in my case to be incurable and expected to cause me severe distress or render me incapable of rational existence, I request the administration of euthanasia at a time or in circumstances to be indicated or specified by me or, if it is apparent that I have become incapable of giving directions, at the discretion of the physician in charge of my case.

B. In the event of my suffering from any of the conditions specified above, I request that no active steps should be taken, and in particular that no resuscitatory techniques should be used, to prolong my life or restore me to consciousness.

C. This declaration is to remain in force unless I revoke it, which I may do at any time, and any request I may make concerning action to be taken or withheld in connection with this declaration will be made without further formalities.

I WISH it to be understood that I have confidence in the good faith of my relatives and physicians, and fear degeneration and indignity far more than I fear premature death. I ask and authorize the physician in charge of my case to bear these statements in mind when considering what my wishes would be in any uncertain situation.

SIGNED

[SIGNED ON RE-EXECUTION]

WE TESTIFY that the above-named declarant *[signed] *[was unable to write but assented to] this declaration in our presence, and appeared to appreciate its significance. We do not know of any pressure being brought on him to make a declaration, and we believe it is made by his own wish. So far as we are aware, we are entitled to attest this declaration and do not stand to benefit by the death of the declarant.

Signed by	Signed by
of	of
[Signed by	[Signed by
of	of
on re-execution]	on re-execution]

*Strike out whichever words do not apply.

EUTHANASIA EDUCATIONAL COUNCIL

A Living Will

TO MY FAMILY, MY PHYSICIAN, MY LAWYER, MY
CLERGYMAN; TO ANY MEDICAL FACULTY IN
WHOSE CARE I HAPPEN TO BE; TO ANY
INDIVIDUAL WHO MAY BECOME RESPONSIBLE
FOR MY HEALTH, WELFARE OR AFFAIRS

Death is as much a reality as birth, growth, maturity and old age—it is the one certainty of life. If the time comes when I, _____ _____can no longer take part in decisions for my own future, let this statement stand as an expression of my wishes, while I am still of sound mind.

If the situation should arise in which there is no reasonable expectation of my recovery from physical or mental disability, I request that I be allowed to die and not be kept alive by artificial means or "heroic measures." I do not fear death itself as much as the indignities of deterioration, dependence and hopeless pain. I, therefore, ask that medication be mercifully administered to me to alleviate suffering even though this may hasten the moment of death.

This request is made after careful consideration. I hope you who care for me will feel morally bound to follow its mandate. I recognize that this appears to place a heavy responsibility upon you, but it is with the intention of relieving you of such responsibility and of placing it upon myself in accordance with my strong convictions, that this statement is made.

Signed _____

Date _____

Witness _____

Witness _____

Copies of this request have been given to _____

_____

_____

_____

Published April 1974 and reprinted with permission of the Euthanasia Educational Council, New York.

THE STATE OF CALIFORNIA

Natural Death Act

LEGISLATIVE COUNSEL'S DIGEST

AB 3060, Keene. Cessation of medical care for terminal patients.

No existing statute prescribes a procedure whereby a person may provide in advance for the withholding or withdrawal of medical care in the event the person should suffer a terminal illness or mortal injury.

This bill would expressly authorize the withholding or withdrawal of life-sustaining procedures, as defined, from adult patients afflicted with a terminal condition, as defined, where the patient has executed a directive in the form and manner prescribed by the bill. Such a directive would generally be effective for 5 years from the date of execution unless sooner revoked in a specified manner. This bill would relieve physicians, licensed health professionals acting under the direction of a physician, and health facilities from civil liability, and would relieve physicians and licensed health professionals acting under the direction of a physician from criminal prosecution or charges of unprofessional conduct, for withholding or withdrawing life-sustaining procedures in accordance with the provisions of the bill.

The bill would provide that such a withholding or withdrawal of life-sustaining procedures shall not constitute a suicide nor impair or invalidate life insurance, and the bill would specify that the making of such a directive shall not restrict, inhibit, or impair the sale, procurement, or issuance of life insurance or modify existing life insurance. The bill would provide that health insurance carriers, as prescribed, could not require execution of a directive as a condition for being insured for, or receiving, health care services.

The bill would make it a misdemeanor to willfully conceal, cancel, deface, obliterate, or damage the directive of another without the declarant's consent. Any person, not justified or excused by law, who

From *California Health and Safety Code,* Part I, Division 7, Chapter 3.9, Sections 7185-7195. Approved by the Governor on the 30th of September, 1976.

falsifies or forges the directive of another or willfully conceals or withholds personal knowledge of a prescribed revocation with the intent to cause a withholding or withdrawal of life-sustaining procedures contrary to the wishes of the declarant and thereby causes life-sustaining procedures to be withheld or withdrawn, and death to thereby be hastened, would be subject to prosecution for unlawful homicide.

• • •

The people of the State of California do enact as follows:

. . . Chapter 3.9 (commencing with Section 7185) is added to Part 1 of Division 7 of the Health and Safety Code, to read:

CHAPTER 3.9. NATURAL DEATH ACT

7185. This act shall be known and may be cited as the Natural Death Act.

7186. The Legislature finds that adult persons have the fundamental right to control the decisions relating to the rendering of their own medical care, including the decision to have life-sustaining procedures withheld or withdrawn in instances of a terminal condition.

The Legislature further finds that modern medical technology has made possible the artificial prolongation of human life beyond natural limits.

The Legislature further finds that, in the interest of protecting individual autonomy, such prolongation of life for persons with a terminal condition may cause loss of patient dignity and unnecessary pain and suffering, while providing nothing medically necessary or beneficial to the patient.

The Legislature further finds that there exists considerable uncertainty in the medical and legal professions as to the legality of terminating the use or application of life-sustaining procedures where the patient has voluntarily and in sound mind evidenced a desire that such procedures be withheld or withdrawn.

In recognition of the dignity and privacy which patients have a right to expect, the Legislature hereby declares that the laws of the State of California shall recognize the right of an adult person to make a written directive instructing his physician to withhold or withdraw life-sustaining procedures in the event of a terminal condition.

7187. The following definitions shall govern the construction of this chapter:

(a) "Attending physician" means the physician selected by, or assigned to, the patient who has primary responsibility for the treatment and care of the patient.

(b) "Directive" means a written document voluntarily executed by the declarant in accordance with the requirements of Section 7188. The directive, or a copy of the directive, shall be made part of the patient's medical records.

(c) "Life-sustaining procedure" means any medical procedure or intervention which utilizes mechanical or other artificial means to sustain, restore, or supplant a vital function, which, when applied to a qualified patient, would serve only to artificially prolong the moment of death and where, in the judgment of the attending physician, death is imminent whether or not such procedures are utilized. "Life-sustaining procedure" shall not include the administration of medication or the performance of any medical procedure deemed necessary to alleviate pain.

(d) "Physician" means a physician and surgeon licensed by the Board of Medical Quality Assurance or the Board of Osteopathic Examiners.

(e) "Qualified patient" means a patient diagnosed and certified in writing to be afflicted with a terminal condition by two physicians, one of whom shall be the attending physician, who have personally examined the patient.

(f) "Terminal condition" means an incurable condition caused by injury, disease, or illness, which, regardless of the application of life-sustaining procedures, would, within reasonable medical judgment, produce death, and where the application of life-sustaining procedures serve only to postpone the moment of death of the patient.

7188. Any adult person may execute a directive directing the withholding or withdrawal of life-sustaining procedures in a terminal condition. The directive shall be signed by the declarant in the presence of two witnesses not related to the declarant by blood or marriage and who would not be entitled to any portion of the estate of the declarant upon his decease under any will of the declarant or codicil thereto then existing or, at the time of the directive, by operation of law then existing. In addition, a witness to a directive shall not be the attending physician, an employee of the attending physician or a health facility in which the declarant is a patient, or any person who has a claim against any portion of the estate of the declarant upon his decease at the time of the execution of the directive. The directive shall be in the following form:

DIRECTIVE TO PHYSICIANS

Directive made this _____ day of _____ (month, year).

I _____, being of sound mind, willfully, and voluntarily make known my desire that my life shall not be artificially prolonged under the circumstances set forth below, do hereby declare:

1. If at any time I should have an incurable injury, disease, or illness certified to be a terminal condition by two physicians, and where the application of life-sustaining procedures would serve only to artificially prolong the moment of my death and where my physician determines that my death is imminent whether or not life-sustaining procedures are utilized, I direct that such procedures be withheld or withdrawn, and that I be permitted to die naturally.

2. In the absence of my ability to give directions regarding the use of such life-sustaining procedures, it is my intention that this directive shall be honored by my family and physician(s) as the final expression of my legal right to refuse medical or surgical treatment and accept the consequences from such refusal.

3. If I have been diagnosed as pregnant and that diagnosis is known to my physician, this directive shall have no force or effect during the course of my pregnancy.

4. I have been diagnosed and notified at least 14 days ago as having a terminal condition by _____ M.D., whose address is _____, and whose telephone number is _____. I understand that if I have not filled in the physician's name and address, it shall be presumed that I did not have a terminal condition when I made out this directive.

5. This directive shall have no force or effect five years from the date filled in above.

6. I understand the full import of this directive and

I am emotionally and mentally competent to make this directive.

Signed _____

City, County and State of Residence _____

The declarant has been personally known to me and I believe him or her to be of sound mind.

Witness _____

Witness _____

7188.5. A directive shall have no force or effect if the declarant is a patient in a skilled nursing facility as defined in subdivision (c) of Section 1250 at the time the directive is executed unless one of the two witnesses to the directive is a patient advocate or ombudsman as may be designated by the State Department of Aging for this purpose pursuant to any other applicable provision of law. The patient advocate or ombudsman shall have the same qualifications as a witness under Section 7188.

The intent of this section is to recognize that some patients in skilled nursing facilities may be so insulated from a voluntary decisionmaking role, by virtue of the custodial nature of their care, as to require special assurance that they are capable of willfully and voluntarily executing a directive.

7189. (a) A directive may be revoked at any time by the declarant, without regard to his mental state or competency, by any of the following methods:

(1) By being canceled, defaced, obliterated, or burnt, torn, or otherwise destroyed by the declarant or by some person in his presence and by his direction.

(2) By a written revocation of the declarant expressing his intent to revoke, signed and dated by the declarant. Such revocation shall become effective only upon communication to the attending physician by the declarant or by a person acting on behalf of the declarant. The attending physician shall record in the patient's medical record the time and date when he received notification of the written revocation.

(3) By a verbal expression by the declarant of his intent to revoke the directive. Such revocation shall become effective only upon communication to the attending physician by the declarant or by a person acting on behalf of the declarant. The attending physician shall record in the patient's medical record the time, date, and place of the revocation and the time, date, and place, if different, of when he received notification of the revocation.

(b) There shall be no criminal or civil liability on the part of any person for failure to act upon a revocation made pursuant to this section unless that person has actual knowledge of the revocation.

7189.5. A directive shall be effective for five years from the date of execution thereof unless sooner revoked in a manner prescribed in Section 7189. Nothing in this chapter shall be construed to prevent a declarant from reexecuting a directive at any time in accordance with the formalities of Section 7188, including reexecution subsequent to a diagnosis of a terminal condition. If the declarant has executed more than one directive, such time shall be determined from the date of execution of the last directive known to the attending physician. If the declarant becomes comatose or is rendered incapable of communicating with the attending physician, the directive shall remain in effect for the duration of the comatose condition or until such time as the declarant's condition renders him or her able to communicate with the attending physician.

7190. No physician or health facility which, acting in accordance with the requirements of this chapter, causes the withholding or withdrawal of life-sustaining procedures from a qualified patient, shall be subject to civil liability therefrom. No licensed health professional, acting under the direction of a physician, who participates in the withholding or withdrawal of life-sustaining procedures in accordance with the provisions of this chapter shall be subject to any civil liability. No physician, or licensed health professional acting under the direction of a physician, who participates in the withholding or withdrawal of life-sustaining procedures in accordance with the provisions of this chapter shall be guilty of any criminal act or of unprofessional conduct.

7191. (a) Prior to effecting a withholding or withdrawal of life-sustaining procedures from a qualified patient pursuant to the directive, the attending physician shall determine that the directive complies with Section 7188, and, if the patient is mentally competent, that the directive and all steps proposed by the attending physician to be undertaken are in accord with the desires of the qualified patient.

(b) If the declarant was a qualified patient at least 14 days prior to executing or reexecuting the directive, the directive shall be conclusively presumed, unless revoked, to be the directions of the patient regarding the withholding or withdrawal of life-sustaining procedures. No physician, and no licensed health professional acting under the direction of a physician, shall be criminally or civilly liable for failing to effectuate the directive of the qualified patient pursuant to this subdivision. A failure by a physician to effectuate the directive of a qualified patient pursuant to this division shall constitute unprofessional conduct if the physician refuses to make the necessary arrangements, or fails to take the necessary steps, to effect the transfer of the qualified patient to another physician who will effectuate the directive of the qualified patient.

(c) If the declarant becomes a qualified patient subsequent to executing the directive, and has not subsequently reexecuted the directive, the attending physician may give weight to the directive as evidence of the patient's directions regarding the withholding or withdrawal of life-sustaining procedures and may consider other factors, such as information from the affected family or the nature of the patient's illness, injury, or disease, in determining whether the totality of circumstances known to the attending physician justify effectuating the directive. No physician, and no licensed health professional acting under the direction of a physician, shall be criminally or civilly liable for failing to effectuate the directive of the qualified patient pursuant to this subdivision.

7192. (a) The withholding or withdrawal of life-sustaining procedures from a qualified patient in accordance with the provisions of this chapter shall not, for any purpose, constitute a suicide.

(b) The making of a directive pursuant to Section 7188 shall not restrict, inhibit, or impair in any manner the sale, procurement, or issuance of any policy of life insurance, nor shall it be deemed to modify the terms of an existing policy of life insurance. No policy of life insurance shall be legally impaired or invalidated in any manner by the withholding or withdrawal of life-sustaining procedures from an insured

qualified patient, notwithstanding any term of the policy to the contrary.

(c) No physician, health facility, or other provider, and no health care service plan, insurer issuing disability insurance, self-insured employee welfare benefit plan, or nonprofit hospital service plan, shall require any person to execute a directive as a condition for being insured for, or receiving, health care services.

7193. Nothing in this chapter shall impair or supersede any legal right or legal responsibility which any person may have to effect the withholding or withdrawal of life-sustaining procedures in any lawful manner. In such respect the provisions of this chapter are cumulative.

7194. Any person who willfully conceals, cancels, defaces, obliterates, or damages the directive of another without such declarant's consent shall be guilty of a misdemeanor. Any person who, except where justified or excused by law, falsifies or forges the directive of another, or willfully conceals or withholds personal knowledge of a revocation as provided in Section 7189, with the intent to cause a withholding or withdrawal of life-sustaining procedures contrary to the wishes of the declarant, and thereby, because of any such act, directly causes life-sustaining procedures to be withheld or withdrawn and death to thereby be hastened, shall be subject to prosecution for unlawful homicide as provided in Chapter 1 (commencing with Section 187) of Title 8 of Part 1 of the Penal Code.

7195. Nothing in this chapter shall be construed to condone, authorize, or approve mercy killing, or to permit any affirmative or deliberate act or omission to end life other than to permit the natural process of dying as provided in this chapter.

ROBERT M. VEATCH

Death and Dying: The Legislative Options

A man in his eighties, without any relatives, was admitted to the hospital in respiratory distress from pneumonia. He had metastisized cancer and was convinced that he would eventually die from it. By the next morning he was dead. Acting on benevolent and humane motives, the medical staff had decided to let the patient die of pneumonia now rather than of cancer later. They had heard the "death-with-dignity" message. But they had not bothered to ask the patient how he felt about dying in this way.

The case illustrates the confusion that has followed upon the increasingly vigorous calls for the right to die with dignity. It also illustrates why many people, including those who are strongly committed to right-to-life positions and to continued medical treatment for the terminally ill, are beginning to explore legislative options to clarify the individual's rights to control decisions about terminal care.

A combination of several factors has apparently led to this recent round of legislative effort. Many of the state legislators who have introduced bills say they were motivated by unnecessarily tragic deaths in their own families. Underlying these personal experiences, however, is a shift in the cultural mood, a reaction against the excessive technologizing of the dying process and its control by the professional rather than the family.

I have examined eighty-five pieces of draft legislation which address this problem. In 1977 alone bills have been introduced into forty state legislatures; eight states have passed legislation: Arkansas, California, Idaho, Nevada, New Mexico, North Carolina, Oregon, and Texas. The others are at various stages in the legislative process.[1] Some of the bills seem to provide needed clarification, making relatively minor adjustments in our present public policy. Others seem

to be extremely dangerous and confusing, perhaps depriving individuals of rights and responsibilities they now possess and would not want to surrender. The brief history of legislative research and development may explain why some of the bills are so inadequate.

The merits of the bills notwithstanding, it is no longer possible to take the position that there should be no policy at all. In an older and simpler day, an informal policy could suffice. The physician could decide what treatments were appropriate and when to stop treatment. We thought he was making a technical judgment. Certainly this is not the case today. There is such an obvious variation in views about what treatment is appropriate for a terminally ill patient that informal consensus is no longer adequate. Physicians, like the general public, have views ranging from "treatment at all costs to the very end," to "let the patient die even if the patient is not ready to die."

Policies regarding decisions to treat or not treat the terminally ill should be clarified publicly. The eighty-five bills I have examined fall into three basic types: (1) bills that would apparently legalize active killing, (2) bills that would clarify the rights of competent patients to accept or refuse treatment, and (3) bills that would clarify who should make medical decisions in cases where the patient is incompetent.

BILLS APPARENTLY LEGALIZING ACTIVE KILLING

At least seven bills that would apparently legalize active killing have been introduced into legislative bodies. The movement began in 1936 in Britain with the introduction of the voluntary euthanasia bill, which was defeated in the House of Lords. Two years later, a similar bill was introduced in Nebraska. In 1947 such a bill was introduced in New York. More recently, still following the British pattern, bills that would apparently legalize active killings on grounds of mercy were introduced into Idaho in 1969, and

From *Hastings Center Report* 7 (October 1977), 5–8. Reprinted with permission of the Hastings Center: ©Institute of Society, Ethics, and the Life Sciences, 360 Broadway, Hastings-on-Hudson, N.Y. 10706.

Montana and Oregon in 1973. The authors of these older bills were apparently not adequately aware of the distinction between active killing and letting die. They refer to "the administration of euthanasia," seeming to authorize active killing.

Active killing on grounds of mercy remains illegal both in Britain and in the United States. At least thirteen such cases have gone to trial, resulting in four convictions and nine acquittals. All the acquittals, however, were either on grounds of insanity or inability to prove the cause of death. Thus, if active killing were to become public policy, legislation legalizing it would be required.

Both moral and practical reasons can be raised against such legalization. Many believe active killing is morally unacceptable because a human agent causes the death rather than simply decides that an omission is acceptable. Or, they believe that active killing in the exceptional case on grounds of mercy would lead to active killings on other, less acceptable grounds. The practical arguments against legalization of active killings include the claim that pain can be adequately controlled with proper medication and that there is apparently a high error rate in making decisions to kill actively. It would be extremely difficult to identify a killing that resulted from maliciousness or an error in prognosis. In cases of omission, it is argued, there is more of a chance for judicial review. In addition, since a majority of both professionals and lay people are clearly opposed to the legalization of active killing, it seems politically unfeasible; on the other hand, public opinion apparently favors the refusal of medical treatment in some circumstances. Thus, clarification of policy regarding those refusals should not be delayed by needless debate over the morality of active killing.

Two real problems need resolution today. First, people need to be assured that high-technology resuscitation will be stopped at an appropriate time after they are not fully competent to refuse treatment or execute a request that treatment be stopped. Second, the decision-making process for the incompetent patient should be clarified. Legislative proposals to legalize active killing upon the request of the patient deal with neither of these problems.

BILLS CLARIFYING THE RIGHTS OF COMPETENT PATIENTS.

A second kind of legislation began with the introduction of a bill into the Wisconsin legislature in 1971. It gained momentum in 1973 when a bill was introduced into the Florida legislature by a physician-representative, Walter Sackett. His bill would have clarified the right of competent persons to execute a document indicating that they do not desire certain kinds of intervention if and when they become terminally ill. The effects of that legislative proposal are still being felt. Proposals following this pattern have been introduced in many other states, including Delaware, Washington, and Illinois in 1973 and Massachusetts in 1974. Some of the early bills had serious drawbacks. They did not make clear whether the documents to be executed were legally binding, and there were no penalties for ignoring the instruction— not even penalties for forging such documents. Many of the definitions were poor, and some of the bills provided no minimum age.

The real breakthrough came in 1976, when California passed the Natural Death Act, the first piece of legislation of this kind in the United States. The California law meets one very narrow but important need. It makes clear that instructions written while competent but after one is certifiably terminally ill remain in effect after one lapses into incompetency.

There are several problems, however, First, the California Natural Death Act does not provide assurance that if a person writes something *now* his wishes will be followed should he become terminally ill. California law states: "If the declarant becomes a qualified patient subsequent to executing the directive, and has not subsequently reexecuted the directive, the attending physician *may give weight* (but) . . . may consider other factors such as information from the affected family or the nature of the patient's illness, injury or disease, in determining whether the totality of circumstances known to the attending physician justify effectuating the directive."

Under that law, Karen Quinlan's respirator treatment could not be stopped even if she had filled out the directive in accordance with the law. It would give no assurance to anyone who fears being maintained after an accident or stroke. In fact, it may even deprive individuals of certain already existing rights to refuse medical treatment; but to make matters more confusing, the law says that "nothing in this chapter shall impair or supersede any legal right or legal responsibility which any person may have to effect the withholding or withdrawal of life sustaining procedures. . . ."

Before this law was passed, it might have been

possible to write ahead of time a legally binding Living Will that would require stopping treatment, although the legality of such documents was unclear. Now in California there is clearly no confusion: one does not have any assurance that treatment will be stopped even if one has filled out a document.

A second problem is that the California law defines terminal illness in a hopelessly narrow way. A terminal condition is an "incurable condition caused by injury, disease, or illness which, regardless of the application of life-sustaining procedures, would, within reasonable medical judgment, produce death, and where the application of life-sustaining procedures serves only to postpone the moment of death of the patient." This excludes many situations where treatment refusal is normally acceptable; for example, a man in chronic kidney failure receiving agonizing hemodialysis probably should not be able to make use of the law's provisions to assure that treatment would be stopped, because he would not meet the definition of being terminally ill. Furthermore, the directive only takes effect when "my death is imminent." Thus many patients would not be permitted to have treatment stopped at a time when they are declining and treatment has become burdensome, useless, or both, but when death is still not imminent.

Another bill that would clarify the rights of the competent patient was introduced in Alabama in 1976. It provides that certain individuals "have the right to self-determination regarding the acceptance, continuance, rejection or refusal of medical treatment." It makes clear that the moral basis of the bill is the individual's right of privacy and self-determination. In contrast, the California bill, in spite of the fact that it claims to focus on self-determination, really abandons patient autonomy, at least for patients who are not terminally ill or for whom death is not imminent. The Alabama bill, in contrast, is not limited to terminally ill patients. Any individual over the age of nineteen would have the right to "make a declaration instructing any physician . . . to cease or refrain from medical or surgical treatment during possible prestated future states of incompetency as long as such demands do not result in undue harm to society as judged by court decision." This permits a person to specify conditions fitting his own moral and religious belief. It does not limit the application to conditions where the patient will die regard-less of treatment. It deals realistically with a wide variety of moral positions on a set of complicated issues.

None of these bills deals with the most serious problem: the patient who arrives at the emergency room comatose without having filled out a Living Will; or the patient who was never competent, the child, the retarded person, or others never having had the competency to fill out treatment refusal or acceptance instructions.

BILL CLARIFYING CASES OF INCOMPETENT PATIENTS

Even if there were laws permitting individuals to write binding instructions about their care should they become incompetent and terminally ill, realistically many people will not fill out such documents, and many others, especially children, will never have had the opportunity to do so. At least twelve bills have been introduced to try to clarify who has the authority to make decisions in such cases. All these bills begin with a section providing the right of the competent patient to execute a document, much as the previously discussed bills do. However, they differ in providing mechanisms for decision making. It is clear that someone must have the authority to decide what constitutes appropriate treatment for such patients. There are many possible candidates: the physician, the nurse, the combined medical staff, the patient's next of kin, all of the relatives acting together, a judge, or a guardian appointed by the courts.

Two of the bills give decision-making authority to physicians. A bill introduced in Virginia in 1976 provided that "in the absence of the patient having so communicated his or her wishes to the physician, the physician may seek the advice of the patient's immediate family, but not be bound thereby." The Quinlan case is the prime example of the problems such a provision would create.

A similar bill was introduced in the New York Assembly in 1977. That bill stated "if the person is not already receiving extraordinary treatment, the decision to commence such treatment shall be left to the attending physician in consultation with the patient's guardian or next of kin." Again the guardian or family of the patient is granted only weak authority. To my knowledge the New York draft bill is the only one that uses the distinction between stopping treatment and not starting treatment in the first place. The New York bill would only permit physicians to make decisions not to start so-called extraordinary treatments. It would not authorize treatment stoppages, even if the treatment is considered extraordinary.

Some see serious problems with bills giving physicians such authority. If there is a wide range of acceptable views on what constitutes appropriate treatment, it seems unreasonable that a patient should be subjected randomly to the personal values of the physician. A patient who has long opposed so-called heroic measures might be treated by a physician who believes his duty is to prolong life. On the other hand, a patient with long membership in a right-to-life movement may be treated by a physician who believes he should provide immediate "death with dignity." It seems more reasonable that the person who best knows the values of the patient should be given the guardianship authority. The question is not one of lack of trust in physicians; it is simply that normally the physician is not the person most likely to know the long-held values and religious beliefs of the patient upon which such judgments might be based.

All the other legislative proposals in this category give authority to someone selected because the person is likely to know best those values. The first bill in the current round of legislative proposals was a Florida bill introduced by Representative Sackett in 1970. It would have given authority to the spouse or next of kin, focusing on the integrity, privacy, and responsibility of the family in making such decisions. A number of criticisms were offered at the time. Some relatives would greedily try to kill off a rich old uncle, it was said, or would unreasonably use deviant religious convictions to refuse treatments on patients for whom treatment should not be stopped. Or, in some cases, family members would simply be unable psychologically to handle the difficulty of such decisions.

Similar problems are faced currently by courts when parents make apparently malicious or foolish decisions about refusing to consent to medical care for their children. The courts routinely review such cases, and, in situations where the parents' judgment is so unreasonable that it cannot be tolerated, a new guardian is appointed. Presumably such provisions would still be available in a state where a bill such as that proposed in Florida would be passed.

On March 30, 1977, Arkansas passed a law adopting almost verbatim the Florida provisions. In April, New Mexico passed a similar law, but it limited guardian refusal to cases where the patient is a minor. Apparently other incompetents are given no

similar legal protections. Both the New Mexico and Arkansas laws apply only to terminally ill patients.

A number of variants are being considered on the proposal to give guardianship for purposes of treatment acceptance or refusal to the next of kin. I have suggested in *Death, Dying, and the Biological Revolution* that the most reasonable first line of authority would be someone the patient himself might have designated while competent. Under such a provision one might designate some other relative, a personal friend, a clergyman, or even a physician as an agent for purposes of making treatment acceptance or refusal decisions. This provision has been incorporated into a law in draft form to be introduced in Michigan. The Michigan proposal does not deal with the question of who shall have the authority to make treatment decisions in cases where someone has not been designated by the patient while competent.

Other proposals would then give authority to the next of kin until such time as the next-of-kin's decision is judged so unreasonable that society must intervene and appoint a new guardian. The objective of legislative proposals of this type is to facilitate patient and familial integrity and self-determination. They attempt to clarify the proper authority. There is a potential conflict among family members in deciding treatment on the basis of the values held by the next of kin, or the values believed to be held by the patient himself. It would seem in the case of once-competent patients that the family's task is to be an agent for the patient, representing to the best of their ability the views held by the patient; but in cases where the patient has never been competent, we have traditionally given the family wide latitude in making such judgments.

The legislative proposals are attempts to clarify which decisions are legally to be accepted by our society and who would have the authority to make such decisions. No bill has yet succeeded in doing this. If there is to be a legislative solution, what factors need to be taken into consideration?

ELEMENTS OF A MODEL BILL

A model bill should do several things. First, it should make clear that wishes expressed while competent and never disavowed should remain valid when individuals are not able to express themselves. Mechanisms for disavowal should be spelled out. Since all competent persons have the right to refuse medical treatment even if it will lead to death, it seems reasonable that their wishes should remain valid when they become incompetent. The right to have one's instructions followed should not be limited to the terminally ill no matter how defined.

A good bill will also specify the penalty for failure to follow such instructions and for forging a document. Probably the penalty for falsely making it appear someone wants treatment stopped should be different from falsely making it appear someone wants treatment to go on.

The rights of medical personnel to withdraw from a case, as long as other suitable professional support is provided, when the patient's instructions violate the professional's conscience should be spelled out, as well as the right of patients to be informed of the right to accept or refuse treatment.

The bill should clearly state that deaths resulting from treatment refusal are not suicide for legal and insurance purposes, and that medical professionals are not guilty of homicide for following such instructions.

If these guidelines are followed, ambiguous terms such as "extraordinary means" and "terminal patient" will not have to be included, but, if such terms are used they should be defined.

A minimum age for execution of a treatment acceptance or refusal document should be stated, probably the age of majority in the state for purposes of legally accepting or refusing medical treatments in general and for executing other critical documents.

The bill should also address the problem of who should make decisions in cases where the patient is incompetent because of age or other reasons. For formerly competent patients, a person designated by the individual while competent is a reasonable first authority. For the never-competent, the next of kin is currently presumed to have the authority to consent to medical treatment. Logically the right to refuse consent is implied, but this right should be made explicit. A full statute would permit agents delegated by the individual to make treatment acceptance or refusal decisions and would make clear who has that authority in cases where no one has been so designated.

The movement to legislate "death with dignity" has gained momentum, fueled by public opinion and rising emotion. Careful analysis and attention to the consequences are essential to assure that these laws achieve their goals rather than obscuring or hindering them.

NOTES

1. For an account of the evolution of the California Natural Death Act, see Michael Garland, "Politics, Legislation, and Natural Death," *Hastings Center Report,* October, 1976, pp. 5–6.

JOHN LORBER

Early Results of Selective Treatment of Spina Bifida Cystica

INTRODUCTION

Two major revolutions have occurred in the past 15 years in the treatment of myelomeningocele.* The first was the enthusiasm or moral compulsion to treat all infants, irrespective of the degree of their handicap—largely the result of the insistence of the Sheffield team[1,2] The main reason for this enthusiasm was the introduction of the ventriculoatrial shunt* in 1958. This procedure was able to control hydrocephalus* effectively for the first time.

The second event was the disillusionment which occurred because the technical advances, especially the use of unidirectional valve systems to control the associated hydrocephalus, led to hopes that were unfortunately not fulfilled. Analysis of the results[3,4] have shown that treating all infants still resulted in a high mortality rate in those cases severely affected at birth and yet led to the prolonged survival of many severely handicapped children, with gross paralysis, multiple deformities of the legs, fractures, kyphosis,* scoliosis,* and incontinence of urine and faeces with frequent secondary effects of hydronephrosis, chronic pyelonephritis, and arterial hypertension. Hydrocephalus was usually well controlled with shunt therapy—in those who needed the operation—but the complications of shunt therapy are extremely common, requiring repeated operations. The mortality rate from these complications alone was 20% within seven years of the first shunt operation in a large group of children. Over half of the shunt-treated survivors were mentally handicapped and very few had an I.Q. over 100. At best not more than 10% of all the survivors (with and without hydrocephalus) were likely to have a chance of earning a living in competitive employment.

The survival of so many severely handicapped children gave rise to progressively greater anxiety among doctors, nurses, parents, teachers, and the general public. This became evident with the rising tide of comments on television, radio, in newspapers, and other media. The ethical validity of prolongation of profoundly handicapped lives, consisting of frequent operations, hospital admissions, and absence from home and school and with no prospect of marriage or employment, became less and less tenable. The cost of maintaining each such child is now about £3,000 a year. A change in policy was bound to come.

Though most infants were offered active treatment during the 1960s this practice was not universal, but those who did not treat all patients or were reluctant to do so did not report their views or results until recently. Nevertheless, in Oxford[5] and in Edinburgh[6] a policy of selection was carried out and, though exact criteria were not laid down where the line should be drawn, very few selectively untreated infants survived to two years of age and the condition of these survivors was probably no worse than if they had been treated. In Stark and Drummond's[6] treated patients the condition of the survivors was more favourable than in those series in which all patients were treated without selection. A policy of selection was also practised in the large spina bifida clinic in Melbourne,[7] where a complex system of criteria were laid down and which were similar to those proposed in England in the past two years.[3]

From *British Medical Journal* 4 (October 27, 1973), 201–204. Reprinted with permission of the author and the *British Medical Journal*.

Ed. Note: Myelomeningocele: protrusion of the spinal cord and its covering through a defect in the spinal column. The protrusion often forms a sac that is filled with cerebrospinal fluid.

Ventriculoatrial shunt: a draining system that allows excess fluid to flow from the ventricles, or cavities, of the brain to the atrium, one of the chambers of the heart.

Hydrocephalus: an excess of fluid in the ventricles of the brain, which may, if untreated, lead to the swelling of the head and damage to the brain.

Kyphosis: abnormal backward curvature of the spine, which produces a hunchbacked appearance.

Scoliosis: abnormal lateral curvature of the spine.

In my experience a detailed correlation between the physical findings soon after birth and the results of therapy has clearly indicated that it is possible to define a line of division as criteria for treatment. No infant among 400 consecutive cases treated from the first day of life who had any one or any combination of the adverse features shown in the appendix survived with less than very severe combined handicaps, while in the absence of these criteria many children survived with only "moderate" handicaps. Only half of the latter were treated with a shunt, their average intelligence was normal, and they had far fewer operations. Only 16% without adverse criteria died by 7 years compared with 59% of those with adverse criteria. In view of the predictability of the minimal likely handicap, I proposed . . . that these criteria should be adopted for selection. The publication of these results[3,4] led to the second revolution in the management of myelomeningocele—namely, an almost universal acceptance of selection[8] which has been officially recognized as legitimate practice.[9] Selection is now being practised in some of the largest units—for example, at the Queen Mary's Hospital, Carshalton,[10] and at the Hospital for Sick Children.[11] There has been no difficulty with the nursing staff, who fully understand the humane purpose and the need for such practice, so long as they are taken into the confidence of the medical staff.

PRESENT INVESTIGATION

This study describes the experiences and results of a policy of selection based on the proposed line of division (see appendix) and examines the validity of this dividing line. In the current investigation it was necessary only to use the criteria for selection which were present at birth.

PATIENTS AND METHODS

Between May, 1971, when my policy of "selection" was put into practice, and 31 January 1973, 37 newborn infants born with spina bifida cystica were referred to the medical paediatric unit for assessment, and for treatment if thought appropriate. The infants were born either in the Jessop Hospital, in our own maternity unit (seven cases), or were referred by consultant paediatricians in the region who used to refer cases of spina bifida to the Combined Clinic of the Children's Hospital in the past (30 cases).

All the infants were assessed fully from every point of view. This included a full orthopaedic assessment by Mr. W. J. W. Sharrard or members of his staff. The decision whether to treat or not was entirely that of the paediatric team. If any infant had one or more of the "adverse criteria" (see appendix) as described earlier,[4] the father or both parents were interviewed by me (or in my absence by my senior assistant) in the presence of a member of the junior medical staff and a member of the nursing staff.

The infant's condition was fully explained and the facts were repeated, so as to leave no doubt in the parents' minds. The many possible therapeutic actions were described to them and a prognosis was given as to the *likely minimal handicap* their child might have if he was offered total treatment and *if everything went well*. The risks and possible complications were also explained without bias. Finally, a recommendation was made together with an offer for a second opinion. The interview took up to two hours and, if necessary, was repeated later.

No parent was asked to sign a consent form for operation without fully understanding what it would mean to the infant and the family. All but one couple accepted the doctor's recommendation. In one instance where the infant's condition was near the borderline, treatment was advised, but the parents refused to give permission. The infant died shortly afterwards.

Several paediatricians in the region accepted the principle of selection and did not send those infants who had adverse criteria to the Children's Hospital. These included eight born in Sheffield, all of whom died very quickly. Partly as a result of this new policy a substantially smaller number of infants was referred to the hospital, and not all who were referred were treated.

RESULTS

Active treatment was recommended for and accepted by the parents of 12 infants. Twenty-five were not treated.

Treated Infants. Of the 12 treated infants 11 had no adverse criteria on admission, but one had a large thoracolumbosacral* lesion. [Despite early surgical treatment, the infant with the large thoracolumbosacral lesion developed severe complications, including paralysis of the legs, incontinence, curvature of the spine, and progressive hydrocephalus.]

Ed. Note: Thoracolumbosacral: affecting the upper, middle, and lower parts of the spinal column.

There was progressive deterioration in [this patient's] renal* conditon and function studies showed little renal reserve. Thus the size and site of her spina bifida was an accurate prognostic sign, yet had she not been operated on at an early stage the gross loss of muscle function and her other problems might well have been attributed to failure of treatment.

The remaining 11 patients' spina bifida was upper thoracic*(1), lumbar (1), low lumbosacral (6), and sacral (3).* One treated infant died on the surgical ward from respiratory arrest on the second day of life. . . . All the remaining 10 infants are alive and are between 5 and 18 months of age at the time of writing. None have severe sequelae[3] (Table I). Three are fully normal. Seven have slight paraplegia but four of these pass a normal stream of urine and have good anal tone. Three have dribbling incontinence and patulous* anus as well as having mild paraplegia.

Table I. Condition of 12 Treated Infants

	No. of Patients
Alive	11
Fully normal	3
Slight paralysis, continent	3
Slight paralysis, continent, shunt	1
Slight paralysis, incontinent	1
Slight paralysis, incontinent, shunt	2
Severe paralysis, incontinent, hydronephrosis,* scoliosis, hydrocephalus (no shunt)	1[a]
Died (aged 2 days)	1

[a]The only child who had adverse criteria (thoracolumbosacral lesion) at birth.

Four of the 11 survivors have no hydrocephalus, two had moderate hydrocephalus which required no treatment, two other infants' moderate hydrocephalus was fully controlled with isosorbide, and the remaining three have shunt-treated hydrocephalus (Table II). None has an abnormally large head. None has required a revision of shunt treatment, so far. All have normal milestones of development.

The 12 treated infants had 16 operations, including the primary closure, three shunt operations, and one foot correction during a total of 160 months of observation.

Ed. Note: Renal: pertaining to the kidney.

Thoracic lesions are at the level of the chest, or thorax; lumbar lesions are at the level of the upper part of the hip; sacral lesions are at the level of the lower part of the hip.

Patulous: open.

Hydronephrosis: swelling and distension of the kidney caused by a blockage in the urinary tract.

Table II. Incidence of Hydrocephalus in 11 Surviving Treated Infants

	No. of Patients
No hydrocephalus	4
Moderate hydrocephalus, no treatment	2
Moderate hydrocephalus, controlled with isosorbide	2
Moderate hydrocephalus, isosorbide followed by shunt	2
Severe hydrocephalus, shunt	1

Untreated Infants. One infant had no adverse criteria, though she had moderately severe asymmetrical paraplegia, was incontinent, and had hydrocephalus. After much discussion with both parents they decided against treatment and the infant died at home under 1 month of age. The parents later wrote a thoughtful and appreciative letter to *The Times*[12]. Most patients (21 out of 25) had two or more adverse criteria (Table III). These consisted mostly of gross paralysis (24) and thoracolumbosacral lesions (20), but clinical kyphosis or scoliosis was also very common (13) (Table IV) . . . .

Once a decision was made not to treat these infants they were looked after as normal babies, given normal nursing-care, and were fed on demand. Analgesics

Table III. Number of "Adverse Criteria" on Admission in 25 Untreated Patients

	No. of Patients
No adverse criterion†	1
Only one adverse criterion	3
Two adverse criteria	6
Three adverse criteria	10
Four adverse criteria	5

†Parents refused treatment.

Table IV. "Adverse Criteria" on Admission in 25 Untreated Patients

	No. of Patients
Gross paralysis	24
Thoracolumbosacral lesion	20
Kyphosis (with or without scoliosis)	13
Cerebral birth injury or multiple congenital defects	5
Grossly enlarged head	4

were given as required, but no other treatment was offered: no oxygen, tube feeding, antibiotic drugs, or resuscitation. No painful investigations were carried out: no ventriculography,* blood tests, etc. The parents could take the infant home (including for weekends), but they were not expected to do so. Infants born in Sheffield were kept on the ward. The others were returned to their base unit under their own paediatrician's care. (This was invariably agreed to before the infant's transfer to Sheffield.)

Death occurred within nine months in all 25 (Table V): three died within a week and 18 (72%) by 3 months of age. Three infants lived for six months or longer. Two went home from the local hospital, and the third was unfortunately being tube-fed for months before dying of esophageal ulceration and aspirated vomit.

Table V. Age at Death in 25 Untreated Infants

	No. of Patients
Alive at:	
1 Day	25
1 Week	22
1 Month	14
3 Months	7
6 Months	2
9 Months	0

DISCUSSION

The fear that some untreated severe cases of myelomeningocele might survive for long has not been substantiated, and so far the strict criteria for selection have proved reliable. The parents were invariably appreciative of the painless and humane nursing of their untreated infants. Everyone realizes that the solution offered by "selection" is not a good one. There is no "good solution" to a desperate, insoluble problem, merely a "least bad solution," which is being offered.

Selection has also led to an undoubtedly better quality of the survivors than was the case for the less severely affected infants in the past. None has "severe handicaps" so far, except the one treated infant who did have adverse criteria (thoracolumbosacral le-

sion) at birth. This shows the need for the utmost strictness in applying the criteria for selection.

The results in the untreated infants are similar to the larger series reported from Oxford, but where the decision not to treat was not based on exact criteria[5] and the subsequent management of the infants was not necessarily uniform. This may explain why 4% of the patients survived to two years of age.

One of the advantages of the proposed criteria for selection is that the infants are so severely affected at birth that no appreciable functional loss can result from failure to treat on the first day. On the contrary, at least their hydrocephalus is less likely to be rapidly progressive. If an occasional infant were to survive in good general condition for over six months and seemed likely to live, then he could be "brought back into the fold" and be treated for his hydrocephalus and for his renal, orthopaedic, and other problems as necessary.

If it is the open objective of "no treatment" that the infant should die soon and painlessly, then why cannot euthanasia be carried out?[13] I wholly disagree with euthanasia. Though it is fully logical, and in expert and conscientious hands it could be the most humane way of dealing with such a situation, legalizing euthanasia would be a most dangerous weapon in the hands of the State or ignorant or unscrupulous individuals. One does not have to go far back in history to know what crimes can be committed if euthanasia were legalized. The best hope for the future is to discover the cause or causes of spina bifida and to prevent its occurrence. Already there is a chink of hope on the horizon, and the recent dramatic decline in the incidence of spina bifida in Sheffield (J. Lorber, unpublished data, 1973) gives us the hope that one day it will not be such a major problem for our children and their families.

I am grateful for the whole-hearted co-operation in this study to the numerous colleagues who referred cases under their care, to my own junior medical staff and my nurses who uphold and practice this policy, and especially to the parents whose active co-operation makes selection less difficult, though a far from easy task.

APPENDIX—*Contraindications to Active Therapy*

At birth:

(a) Gross paralysis of the legs. . . .

(b) Thoracolumbar or thoracolumbosacral lesions related to vertebral levels.

(c) Kyphosis or scoliosis.

*Ed. note: Ventriculography: X-ray of the head following removal of the fluid from the ventricles of the brain and replacement of the fluid with air or a radiopaque substance.

(d) Grossly enlarged head, with maximal circumference of 2 cm or more above the 90th percentile related to birth weight.

(e) Intracerebral birth injury.

(f) Other gross congenital defects—for example, cyanotic heart disease, ectopia of bladder, and mongolism.

After closure, in the newborn period:

Meningitis or ventriculitis* in an infant who already has serious neurological handicap and hydrocephalus.

Later:

In any life-threatening episode in a child who is severely handicapped by gross mental and neurological defects.

NOTES

1. Sharrard, W. J. W., Zachary, R. B., Lorber, J., and Bruce, A. M. (1963). *Archives of Disease in Childhood*, 38, 18.

2. Zachary, R. B. (1968). *Lancet*, 2, 274.

Ed. note: Ventriculitis: inflammation of the ventricles in the brain.

3. Lorber, J. (1971). *Developmental Medicine and Child Neurology*, 13, 279.

4. Lorber, J. (1972). *Archives of Disease in Childhood*, 47, 854.

5. Hide, D. W., Williams, H. P., and Ellis, H. L. (1972). *Developmental Medicine and Child Neurology*, 14, 304.

6. Stark, G. D., and Drummond, M. (1973). *Archives of Diseases in Childhood*, 48, 676.

7. *Medical Journal of Australia*, 1971, 2, 1151.

8. Personal communications from most paediatricians and paediatric surgeons in Britain.

9. Department of Health and Social Security (1973). *Care of the Child with Spina Bifida*. London, D.H.S.S.

10. Collis, V. R. (1972). *Developmental Medicine and Child Neurology*, 14, Suppl. no. 27, p. 34.

11. Eckstein, H. B. (1973). *British Medical Journal*, 2, 284.

12. *The Times*, 21 August 1972, p. 11.

13. Freeman, J. M. (1972), *Journal of Pediatrics*, 80, 904.

R. B. ZACHARY

Life with Spina Bifida

Spina bifida is a broad term that includes minimal lesions such as spina bifida occulta* and cystic swellings not containing any neural tissue (spina bifida with meningocele). Our main concern, however, is spina bifida with open myelomeningocele, in which the neural tissue is exposed on the surface of the cystic swelling.

The neural tissue in this exposed plaque is abnormal and defective, so that the muscles innervated by it, and indeed distal to the plaque, may be partly or completely paralysed. Naturally, innervation of the bladder and bowels is almost always defective.

In addition, about 90 percent of the children with open myelomeningocele have hydrocephalus,* but

From *British Medical Journal* 2 (December 3, 1977), 1460–1462. Reprinted with permission of the author and the *British Medical Journal*.

Ed. note: Spina bifida occulta: a mild form of spina bifida in which there is a defect in the spine but little or no protrusion of the spinal cord or its covering.

Hydrocephalus: an excess of fluid in the ventricles of the brain, which, if untreated, leads to a swelling of the head and damage to the brain.

the degree of ventricular dilatation and intracranial tension varies and is not directly related to the appearance of the back lesion. If an infant had an operation to close the back wound in the neonatal period he might require a valve for the hydrocephalus within the first six to eight weeks. Complete paralysis of the legs may lead to no deformity whatever, but partial paralysis may lead to dislocation of the hip and to foot deformities. If it is decided to encourage the child to walk with appliances several operations may be needed on the feet and also a muscle transplant at the hip to keep the hip in joint after reduction. The other serious orthopaedic problem is the spinal deformity caused by unopposed action of certain muscles, which leads to kyphosis or kyphoscoliosis* and which may require major surgery for partial correction.

In treating the hydrocephalus the excess ventricular fluid can be shunted through the Holter valve back into the bloodstream, and although some patients re-

Ed. note: Kyphosis is an abnormal backward curvature of the spine, which produces a hunchback appearance. Kyphoscoliosis is a combination of backward and lateral curvature of the spine.

quire revision of the valve several times in the first ten years, the hydrocephalus can be reasonably well controlled. We are learning in Sheffield how to prevent, and also recognise and treat, infection of the valve system; but as with any foreign body, the risk of infection remains.

Defective bladder emptying may lead to stasis of urine within the renal tract and a tendency to infection, and in certain cases may lead to high pressures that cause the upper tract to dilate. Careful and frequent monitoring of the renal tract has enabled us to detect the early signs of trouble and give appropriate treatment, and there is no doubt that young children under treatment now have better kidneys than did children ten years ago. Even so, a ten-year review of survivors of an unselected series showed that nearly a quarter of them had normal or nearly normal bladder control.

Expression of the bladder every two hours may enable the incontinent to be socially dry; but, if not, a penile appliance will help the boys, and an indwelling Foley catheter* has been a tremendous boon in many girls. We still, however, have to undertake a urinary diversion in many of these patients.

A typical 10-year-old with severe spina bifida will therefore spend most of his time in a wheelchair but can make some progress in long calipers;* his hydrocephalus is controlled with a valve that may have needed two or three revisions during the growth period. Most children have an IQ within the normal range but below the mean; intellectual attainment will depend on the degree of hydrocephalus at the time when treatment was started, whether there has been infection, the speed with which obstruction has been relieved, and the opportunities for intellectual stimulation. I noticed a remarkable change in the children when the spina bifida school was first opened in Sheffield, because many were receiving stimulation that had not been possible before. A boy will probably have a good upper renal tract and may be wearing a penile appliance if he cannot be kept dry by expression of the bladder. A girl may have an indwelling Foley catheter or may have needed an ileal conduit.*

Ed note: Foley catheter: a device for draining urine from the bladder.

Calipers: braces for the legs.

Ileal conduit: a segment of the small intestine that is surgically removed and connected to the urinary tract, to facilitate the passage of fluid from the kidneys to the bladder.

This is not an unusual picture of the young person with spina bifida and hydrocephalus. I would emphasize that this is a *person* who has spina bifida, and it is very important that we always refer to them and treat them as persons. The picture at 15 or 20 years is unlikely to change significantly, unless there is an untreated obstruction of the valve system or an uncorrected stasis and back pressure in the renal tract.

SHOULD THEY BE ALLOWED TO DIE?

At the end of the 1960s my medical colleague Dr. John Lorber became very concerned about the degree of handicap of these young people and the morbidity and hospital admissions that resulted.† His extensive study showed that those who have a gross lesion at birth are likely to be severely handicapped when they grow up. He came to the view that the degree of handicap could be forecast at birth, and became strongly opposed to any treatment at all of severely affected babies in the newborn period. He proposed certain criteria for selecting those infants who should be allowed to die, and these were widely accepted— partly because of the human appeal of the view that these children should not allowed to suffer, and that their parents should not have the burden of looking after them. It was also attractive to administrative authorities because the burden of the financial support needed to treat and care for children with spina bifida would be greatly reduced.

The cardinal error in these proposals is the expression, they should be allowed to die. Thirty years ago I was concerned with the care of many patients with spina bifida at the Children's Hospital in Boston, Mass., under Dr. Franc Ingraham. The policy was that *none* of these children should have a neonatal operation. The lesion was covered by a simple dressing and protected by a ring; and after about a week or ten days the children went home to be looked after by their parents and the local paediatrician, with monthly visits to the neurosurgical and orthopaedic clinics. I have seen many children with severe lesions that epithelialised* spontaneously, who then had the operation to close the back wound at about 18 months. Several of the very severely affected ones died at home, but I myself have handled many survivors with serious lesions. I thought it was an unduly heavy burden for the mother to have to look after the swelling on the back, and when I first came to Sheffield I

---

†*Ed. note:* J. Lorber, *Developmental Medicine and Child Neurology,* 1971, *13,* 279.

Epithelialized: became covered with skin.

decided to remove the swelling in the neonatal period if possible. Even so, for several years I continued to see children with quite obvious severe lesions who had not undergone any operation immediately after birth.

There is a widespread myth that if you operate on a child with spina bifida the child will live, and if you do not operate he will die. This is nonsense. They will not all die spontaneously.

"NO TREATMENT" METHODS

How is it then that those who write about the value of selection can point to a high mortality, usually 100 percent, in those that they have selected out? I am sure it has nothing to do with the administration of antibiotics, because those young patients in Boston had no antibiotics 30 years ago. We must look at the exact method of management of those who have no treatment.

One paediatrician has said that they receive the same care and attention as any other baby, being fed and picked up and loved, and even taken out into the sunshine in a pram. Yet these babies are receiving 60 mg/kg body weight of chloral hydrate*, not once but four times a day. This is eight times the sedative dose of chloral hydrate recommended in the most recent volume of *Nelson's Paediatrics* and four times the hypnotic dose, and it is being administered four times every day. No wonder these babies are sleepy and demand no feed, and with this regimen most of them will die within a few weeks, many within the first week.

It is sometimes said that the chloral hydrate is being administered for pain, either in the back or due to the hydrocephalus, but I personally have seen little evidence that the babies have pain in the newborn period, nor have I found them unable to sleep. And if chloral hydrate is such a good drug, why is it not given to those who are intended to survive?

There is nothing secret or confidential about this method of management, for the paediatrician has stated that he has published the details of management for all to see. At a meeting of doctors, social workers, and theologians another paediatrician explained his method of asking the registrar* to administer morphine. He claimed that the parents were taken fully into his confidence and were 100 percent behind him.

When closely questioned he admitted that he did not tell them that the child would receive morphine—merely that the child would die.

In another centre only one out of 24 patients was operated on—all the others died. When asked, "Did they fall or were they pushed"—into death—the reply was, "They were pushed of course." At another meeting I attended a paediatrician was asked by a medical student what was his method of management, and the reply was, "We don't feed them."

I have mentioned the various problems that a person with a moderately severe spina bifida might have in his life, and emphasised that the duration of life would depend on the attitude of the doctor in charge. Some have been prepared to say in public that they would administer drugs, whose direct purpose and effect is the death of the child in a relatively short time. I think there are some paediatricians who have misunderstood the likely consequences of simply withholding surgery, and I have had to deal with children at 6 months of age in whom the total drug treatment part of the regimen had been omitted. I have indeed treated some who have had chloral hydrate, later phenobarbitone, and later morphine and have still survived to require operation. Such doctors are entitled to their view that their actions are best for the child and family, but there should not be any pretence that all these babies are dying spontaneously. Indeed, one must ask, "Are not these actions outside the law?"

I think it is extremely important from a strictly scientific point of view that we cannot regard the non-operative mortality figures as indicating accurately how many babies who are selected for no treatment will die spontaneously—there is, so to speak, an inbuilt insurance policy. There is one further worrying aspect. The editors of medical journals are conscious of their responsibility not to publish papers that are clearly unethical—for example, reporting research that required unnecessary operation or any appreciable risk. How much more carefully should they look at contributions based on studies that include the administration of drugs to accomplish the death of a child?

CRITERIA FOR OPERATION

It may be asked whether I would advocate operation on every baby with spina bifida. Of course not. As with every aspect of surgery, there are criteria for

---

Ed. note: Chloral hydrate is a hypnotic drug, often used by adults for the relief of insomnia.

A registrar, in British hospitals, is a resident specialist who assists the patient's physician.

selection, which should be based on sound medical and surgical principles and a knowledge of the prospects with and without surgery. My scheme for selection for operation in open myelomeningocele is as follows, babies in categories 1 and 2 having no operation.

CATEGORY 1

This category includes those patients who are judged likely to die within a few days or a week or so—for example, babies with severe intracranial haemorrhage or another major life-threatening anomaly. There will be no operation on the back in these children because it could have no bearing at all on whether they lived or died.

CATEGORY 2

Some of the children who seem unlikely to die spontaneously in a short time will have a serious lesion of the back—for example, a very wide lesion or one producing a severe kyphosis, in which the chances of primary healing after surgery would be small: there would be a risk of wound breakdown, which would be far worse than no operation at all. Epithelium is likely to grow over the exposed plaque with simple protection of the wound, and this would be the method of treatment.

CATEGORY 3

Other babies are judged to have a good chance of primary wound healing after operation, and these are placed in three grades of severity.

Grade 1—Active movement of the legs has been observed after birth. These babies need urgent operation because otherwise some of that active movement may be lost.

Grade 2—Babies in the intermediate group have certain active muscles such as hip flexors and adductors, and perhaps quadriceps.* I think these are important muscles to preserve for the orthopaedic surgeon to use, and I would advocate urgent surgery.

Grade 3—At the other extreme there are babies who make no observed leg movements after birth; in these infants operation on the back will have no effect upon the muscular power in the legs. They can be treated either by a non-urgent operation (but within 24

Ed. note: The quadriceps is the large muscle of the front of the thigh.

to 48 hours to minimise infection) or by conservative means such as simple dressings.

The survivors, whether they have been operated on or not, will be offered surgery for hydrocephalus or for renal tract or orthopaedic problems to improve the quality of life or prevent deterioration.

Under no circumstances would I administer drugs to cause the death of the child. There is no doubt that those who are severely affected at birth will continue to be severely handicapped. But I conceive it to be my duty to overcome that handicap as much as possible and to achieve the maximum development of their potential in as many aspects of life as possible— physical, emotional, recreational, and vocational— and I find them very nice people. If in the *neonatal* period you are looking for opportunities to make sure they will die, I am sure this attitude is likely to persist even when they are older. Some have been regarded as living completely miserable and unhappy lives. Yet when I see them I find them happy people who can respond to concern for their personal welfare.

One final point. It has often been said by those who oppose abortion that the disregard for the life of a child within the uterus would spill over into postnatal life. This suggestion has been ''pooh-poohed,'' yet in spina bifida there is a clear example of this. The equanimity with which the life of a 17-week-gestation spina bifida infant is terminated after the finding of a high level of α-fetoprotein* in the amniotic fluid has, I think, spilled over to a similar disregard for the life of the child with spina bifida after birth.

Much of my surgical life over the past 30 years has been devoted to improving the quality of life of those who have been born with spina bifida. The attitude of mind that would eliminate all the severely handicapped reminds me of the poster issued by Christian Aid some years ago, which said ''Ignore the hungry and they will go away''—to their graves. If we eliminate all the severely affected children with spina bifida there will be no more problem; but why stop at spina bifida, why not all the severely affected spastics, all those with muscular dystrophy, and all those with Down's syndrome? Why stop at the neonatal period? Our aim should be that life with spina bifida is the best possible life for that person in the family and in the community.

Ed. note: Alpha-fetoprotein is an enzyme detectable during pregnancy in a woman's blood and in the amniotic fluid surrounding the fetus. Elevated alpha-fetoprotein levels in the amniotic fluid are almost always indicative of either anencephaly (malformed brain and skull) or open spina bifida in the fetus.

H. TRISTRAM ENGELHARDT

Ethical Issues in Aiding the Death of Young Children

Euthanasia in the pediatric age group involves a constellation of issues that are materially different from those of adult euthanasia.[1] The difference lies in the somewhat obvious fact that infants and young children are not able to decide about their own futures and thus are not persons in the same sense that normal adults are. While adults usually decide their own fate, others decide on behalf of young children. Although one can argue that euthanasia is or should be a personal right, the sense of such an argument is obscure with respect to children. Young children do not have any personal rights, at least none that they can exercise on their own behalf with regard to the manner of their life and death. As a result, euthanasia of young children raises special questions concerning the standing of the rights of children, the status of parental rights, the obligations of adults to prevent the suffering of children, and the possible effects on society of allowing or expediting the death of seriously defective infants.

What I will refer to as the euthanasia of infants and young children might be termed by others infanticide, while some cases might be termed the withholding of extraordinary life-prolonging treatment.[2] One needs a term that will encompass both death that results from active intervention and death that ensues when one simply ceases further therapy.[3] In using such a term, one must recognize that death is often not directly but only obliquely intended. That is, one often intends only to treat no further, not actually to have death follow, even though one knows death will follow.[4]

Finally, one must realize that deaths as the result of withholding treatment constitute a significant proportion of neonatal deaths. For example, as high as 14 percent of children in one hospital have been identified as dying after a decision was made not to treat

From Marvin Kohl, ed., *Beneficent Euthanasia* (Buffalo, N.Y.: Prometheus Books, 1975), pp. 180–192. Reprinted with permission of the publisher.

further, the presumption being that the children would have lived longer had treatment been offered.[5]

Even popular magazines have presented accounts of parental decisions not to pursue treatment.[6] These decisions often involve a choice between expensive treatment with little chance of achieving a full, normal life for the child and "letting nature take its course," with the child dying as a result of its defects. As this suggests, many of these problems are products of medical progress. Such children in the past would have died. The quandaries are in a sense an embarrassment of riches; now that one *can* treat such defective children, *must* one treat them? And, if one need not treat such defective children, may one expedite their death?

I will here briefly examine some of these issues. First, I will review differences that contrast the euthanasia of adults to euthanasia of children. Second, I will review the issue of the rights of parents and the status of children. Third, I will suggest a new notion, the concept of the "injury of continued existence," and draw out some of its implications with respect to a duty to prevent suffering. Finally, I will outline some important questions that remain unanswered even if the foregoing issues can be settled. In all, I hope more to display the issues involved in a difficult question than to advance a particular set of answers to particular dilemmas.

For the purpose of this paper, I will presume that adult euthanasia can be justified by an appeal to freedom. In the face of imminent death, one is usually choosing between a more painful and more protracted dying and a less painful or less protracted dying, in circumstances where either choice makes little difference with regard to the discharge of social duties and responsibilities. In the case of suicide, we might argue that, in general, social duties (for example, the duty to support one's family) restrain one from taking one's own life. But in the face of imminent death and in the presence of the pain and deterioration of a fatal disease, such duties are usually impossible to discharge and are thus rendered moot. One can, for example, picture an extreme case of an adult with a widely disseminated carcinoma, including metastases to the brain, who because of severe pain and debilitation is no longer capable of discharging any social duties. In these and similar circumstances, euthanasia becomes the issue of the right to control one's own body, even to the point of seeking assistance in suicide. Euthanasia is, as such, the issue of assisted suicide, the universalization of a maxim that all persons should be free, *in extremis,* to decide with regard to the circumstances of their death.

Further, the choice of positive euthanasia could be defended as the more rational choice: the choice of a less painful death and the affirmation of the value of a rational life. In so choosing, one would be acting to set limits to one's life in order not to live when pain and physical and mental deterioration make further rational life impossible. The choice to end one's life can be understood as a noncontradictory willing of a smaller set of states of existence for oneself, a set that would not include a painful death. As such, it would not involve a desire to destroy oneself. That is, adult euthanasia can be construed as an affirmation of the rationality and autonomy of the self.[7]

The remarks above focus on the active or positive euthanasia of adults. But they hold as well concerning what is often called passive or negative euthanasia, the refusal of life-prolonging therapy. In such cases, the patient's refusal of life-prolonging therapy is seen to be a right that derives from personal freedom, or at least from a zone of privacy into which there are no good grounds for social intervention.[8]

Again, none of these considerations applies directly to the euthanasia of young children, because they cannot participate in such decisions. Whatever else pediatric, in particular neonatal, euthanasia involves, it surely involves issues different from those of adult euthanasia. Since infants and small children cannot commit suicide, their right to assisted suicide is difficult to pose. The difference between the euthanasia of young children and that of adults resides in the difference between children and adults. The difference, in fact, raises the troublesome question of whether young children are persons, or at least whether they are persons in the sense in which adults are. Answering that question will resolve in part at least the right of others to decide whether a young child should live or die and whether he should receive life-prolonging treatment.

THE STATUS OF CHILDREN

Adults belong to themselves in the sense that they are rational and free and therefore responsible for their actions. Adults are *sui juris*. Young children, though, are neither self-possessed nor responsible. While adults exist in and for themselves, as self-directive and self-conscious beings, young children, especially newborn infants, exist for their families and those who love them. They are not, nor can they in any sense be, responsible for themselves. If being a person is to be a responsible agent, a bearer of rights and duties, children are not persons in a strict sense. They are, rather, persons in a social sense: others must act on their behalf and bear responsibility for them. They are, as it were, entities defined by their place in social roles (for example, mother-child, family-child) rather than beings that define themselves as persons, that is, in and through themselves. Young children live as persons in and through the care of those who are responsible for them, and those responsible for them exercise the children's rights on their behalf. In this sense children belong to families in ways that most adults do not. They exist in and through their family and society.

Treating young children with respect has, then, a sense different from treating adults with respect. One can respect neither a newborn infant's or very young child's wishes nor its freedom. In fact, a newborn infant or young child is more an entity that is valued highly because it will grow to be a person and because it plays a social role as if it were a person.[9] That is, a small child is treated as if it were a person in social roles such as mother-child and family-child relationships, though strictly speaking the child is in no way capable of claiming or being responsible for the rights imputed to it. All the rights and duties of the child are exercised and "held in trust" by others for a future time and for a person yet to develop.

Medical decisions to treat or not to treat a neonate or small child often turn on the probability and cost of achieving that future status—a developed personal life. The usual practice of letting anencephalic children (who congenitally lack all or most of the brain) die can be understood as a decision based on the absence of the possibility of achieving a personal life. The practice of refusing treatment to at least some children born with meningomyelocele can be justified through a similar, but more utilitarian, calculus. In the case of anencephalic children one might argue that care for them as persons is futile since they will never be persons. In the case of a child with meningomyelocele, one might argue that when the cost of cure would likely be very high and the probable lifestyle open to attainment very truncated, there is not a positive duty to make a large investment of money and suffering. One should note that the cost here must include not only financial costs but also the anxiety and suffering that prolonged and uncertain treatment of the child would cause the parents.

This further raises the issue of the scope of positive duties not only when there is no person present in a strict sense, but when the likelihood of a full human life is also very uncertain. Clinical and parental judgment may and should be guided by the expected lifestyle and the cost (in parental and societal pain and money) of its attainment. The decision about treatment, however, belongs properly to the parents because the child belongs to them in a sense that it does not belong to anyone else, even to itself. The care and raising of the child falls to the parents, and when considerable cost and little prospect of reasonable success are present, the parents may properly decide against life-prolonging treatment.

The physician's role is to present sufficient information in a usable form to the parents to aid them in making a decision. The accent is on the absence of a positive duty to treat in the presence of severe inconvenience (costs) to the parents; treatment that is very costly is not obligatory. What is suggested here is a general notion that there is never a duty to engage in extraordinary treatment and that "extraordinary" can be defined in terms of costs. This argument concerns children (1) whose future quality of life is likely to be seriously compromised and (2) whose present treatment would be very costly. The issue is that of the circumstances under which parents would not be obliged to take on severe burdens on behalf of their children or those circumstances under which society would not be so obliged. The argument should hold as well for those cases where the expected future life would surely be of normal quality, though its attainment would be extremely costly. The fact of little likelihood of success in attaining a normal life for the child makes decisions to do without treatment more plausible because the hope of success is even more remote and therefore the burden borne by parents or society becomes in that sense more extraordinary. But very high costs themselves could be a sufficient

criterion, though in actual cases judgments in that regard would be very difficult when a normal life could be expected.[10]

The decisions in these matters correctly lie in the hands of the parents, because it is primarily in terms of the family that children exist and develop—until children become persons strictly, they are persons in virtue of their social roles. As long as parents do not unjustifiably neglect the humans in those roles so that the value and purpose of that role (that is, child) stands to be eroded (thus endangering other children), society need not intervene. In short, parents may decide for or against the treatment of their severely deformed children.

However, society has a right to intervene and protect children for whom parents refuse care (including treatment) when such care does not constitute a severe burden and when it is likely that the child could be brought to a good quality of life. Obviously, "severe burden" and "good quality of life" will be difficult to define and their meanings will vary, just as it is always difficult to say when grains of sand dropped on a table constitute a heap. At most, though, society need only intervene when the grains clearly do not constitute a heap, that is, when it is clear that the burden is light and the chance of a good quality of life for the child is high. A small child's dependence on his parents is so essential that society need intervene only when the absence of intervention would lead to the role "child" being undermined. Society must value mother-child and family-child relationships and should intervene only in cases where (1) neglect is unreasonable and therefore would undermine respect and care for children, or (2) where societal intervention would prevent children from suffering unnecessary pain.[11]

THE INJURY OF CONTINUED EXISTENCE

But there is another viewpoint that must be considered: that of the child or even the person that the child might become. It might be argued that the child has a right not to have its life prolonged. The idea that forcing existence on a child could be wrong is a difficult notion, which, if true, would serve to amplify the foregoing argument. Such an argument would allow the construal of the issue in terms of the perspective of the child, that is, in terms of a duty not to treat in circumstances where treatment would only prolong suffering. In particular, it would at least give a framework for a decision to stop treatment in cases where, though the costs of treatment are not high, the child's existence would be characterized by severe pain and deprivation.

A basis for speaking of continuing existence as an injury to the child is suggested by the proposed legal concept of "wrongful life." A number of suits have been initiated in the United States and in other countries on the grounds that life or existence itself is, under certain circumstances, a tort or injury to the living person.[12] Although thus far all such suits have ultimately failed, some have succeeded in their initial stages. Two examples may be instructive. In each case the ability to receive recompense for the injury (the tort) presupposed the existence of the individual, whose existence was itself the injury. In one case a suit was initiated on behalf of a child against his father alleging that his father's siring him out of wedlock was an injury to the child.[13] In another case a suit on behalf of a child born of an inmate of a state mental hospital impregnated by rape in that institution was brought against the state of New York.[14] The suit was brought on the grounds that being born with such historical antecedents was itself an injury for which recovery was due. Both cases presupposed that nonexistence would have been preferable to the conditions under which the person born was forced to live.

The suits for tort for wrongful life raise the issue not only of when it would be preferable not to have been born but also of when it would be *wrong* to cause a person to be born. This implies that someone should have judged that it would have been preferable for the child never to have had existence, never to have been in the position to judge that the particular circumstances of life were intolerable.[15] Further, it implies that the person's existence under those circumstances should have been prevented and that, not having been prevented, life was not a gift but an injury. The concept of tort for wrongful life raises an issue concerning the responsibility for giving another person existence, namely, the notion that giving life is not always necessarily a good and justifiable action. Instead, in certain circumstances, so it has been argued, one may have a duty *not* to give existence to another person. This concept involves the claim that certain qualities of life have a negative value, making life an injury, not a gift; it involves, in short, a concept of human accountability and responsibility for human life. It contrasts with the notion that life is a gift of God and

thus similar to other "acts of God" (that is, events for which no man is accountable). The concept thus signals the fact that humans can now control reproduction and that where rational control is possible humans are accountable. That is, the expansion of human capabilities has resulted in an expansion of human responsibilities such that one must now decide when and under what circumstances persons will come into existence.

The concept of tort for wrongful life is transferable in part to the painfully compromised existence of children who can only have their life prolonged for a short, painful, and marginal existence. The concept suggests that allowing life to be prolonged under such circumstances would itself be an injury of the person whose painful and severely compromised existence would be made to continue. In fact, it suggests that there is a duty not to prolong life if it can be determined to have a substantial negative value for the person involved.[16] Such issues are moot in the case of adults, who can and should decide for themselves. But small children cannot make such a choice. For them it is an issue of justifying prolonging life under circumstances of painful and compromised existence. Or, put differently, such cases indicate the need to develop social canons to allow a decent death for children for whom the only possibility is protracted, painful suffering.

I do not mean to imply that one should develop a new basis for civil damages. In the field of medicine, the need is to recognize an ethical category, a concept of wrongful continuance of existence, not a new legal right. The concept of injury for continuance of existence, the proposed analogue of the concept of tort for wrongful life, presupposes that life can be of a negative value such that the medical maxim *primum non nocere* ("first do no harm") would require not sustaining life.[17]

The idea of responsibility for acts that sustain or prolong life is cardinal to the notion that one should not under certain circumstances further prolong the life of a child. Unlike adults, children cannot decide with regard to euthanasia (positive or negative), and if more than a utilitarian justification is sought, it must be sought in a duty not to inflict life on another person in circumstances where that life would be painful and futile. This position must rest on the facts that (1) medicine now can cause the prolongation of the life of seriously deformed children who in the past would have died young and that (2) it is not clear that life so prolonged is a good for the child. Further, the choice is made not on the basis of costs to the parents or to society but on the basis of the child's suffering and compromised existence.

The difficulty lies in determining what makes life not worth living for a child. Answers could never be clear. It seems reasonable, however, that the life of children with diseases that involve pain and no hope of survival should not be prolonged. In the case of Tay-Sachs disease (a disease marked by a progressive increase in spasticity and dementia usually leading to death at age three or four), one can hardly imagine that the terminal stages of spastic reaction to stimuli and great difficulty in swallowing are at all pleasant to the child (even insofar as it can only minimally perceive its circumstances). If such a child develops aspiration pneumonia and is treated, it can reasonably be said that to prolong its life is to inflict suffering. Other diseases give fairly clear portraits of lives not worth living: for example, Lesch-Nyhan disease, which is marked by mental retardation and compulsive self-mutilation.

The issue is more difficult in the case of children with diseases for whom the prospects for normal intelligence and a fair lifestyle do exist, but where these chances are remote and their realization expensive. Children born with meningomyelocele present this dilemma. Imagine, for example, a child that falls within Lorber's fifth category (an IQ of sixty or less, sometimes blind, subject to fits, and always incontinent). Such a child has little prospect of anything approaching a normal life, and there is a good chance of its dying even with treatment.[18] But such judgments are statistical. And if one does not treat such children, some will still survive and, as John Freeman indicates, be worse off if not treated.[19] In such cases one is in a dilemma. If one always treats, one must justify extending the life of those who will ultimately die anyway and in the process subjecting them to the morbidity of multiple surgical procedures. How remote does the prospect of a good life have to be in order not to be worth great pain and expense?[20] It is probably best to decide, in the absence of a positive duty to treat, on the basis of the cost and suffering to parents and society. But, as Freeman argues, the prospect of prolonged or even increased suffering raises the issue of active euthanasia.[21]

If the child is not a person strictly, and if death is inevitable and expediting it would diminish the child's pain prior to death, then it would seem to follow that, all else being equal, a decision for active euthanasia would be permissible, even obligatory.[22]

The difficulty lies with "all else being equal," for it is doubtful that active euthanasia could be established as a practice without eroding and endangering children generally, since, as John Lorber has pointed out, children cannot speak in their own behalf.[23] Thus, although there is no argument in principle against the active euthanasia of small children, there could be an argument against such practices based on questions of prudence. To put it another way, even though one might have a duty to hasten the death of a particular child, one's duty to protect children in general could override that first duty. The issue of active euthanasia turns in the end on whether it would have social consequences that refraining would not, on whether (1) it is possible to establish procedural safeguards for limited active euthanasia and (2) whether such practices would have a significant adverse effect on the treatment of small children in general. But since these are procedural issues dependent on sociological facts, they are not open to an answer within the confines of this article. In any event, the concept of the injury of continued existence provides a basis for the justification of the passive euthanasia of small children—a practice already widespread and somewhat established in our society—beyond the mere absence of a positive duty to treat.[24]

CONCLUSION

Though the lack of certainty concerning questions such as the prognosis of particular patients and the social consequence of active euthanasia of children prevents a clear answer to all the issues raised by the euthanasia of infants, it would seem that this much can be maintained: (1) Since children are not persons strictly but exist in and through their families, parents are the appropriate ones to decide whether or not to treat a deformed child when (a) there is not only little likelihood of full human life but also great likelihood of suffering if the life is prolonged, or (b) when the cost of prolonging life is very great. Such decisions must be made in consort with a physician who can accurately give estimates of cost and prognosis and who will be able to help the parents with the consequences of their decision. (2) It is reasonable to speak of a duty not to treat a small child when such treatment will only prolong a painful life or would in any event lead to a painful death. Though this does not by any means answer all the questions, it does point out an important fact—that medicine's duty is not always to prolong life doggedly but sometimes is quite the contrary.

NOTES

1. I am grateful to Laurence B. McCullough and James P. Morris for their critical discussion of this paper. They may be responsible for its virtues, but not for its shortcomings.

2. The concept of extraordinary treatment as it has been developed in Catholic moral theology is useful: treatment is extraordinary and therefore not obligatory if it involves great costs, pain, or inconvenience, and is a grave burden to oneself or others without a reasonable expectation that such treatment would be successful. See Gerald Kelly, S. J., *Medico-Moral Problems* (St. Louis: The Catholic Hospital Association Press, 1958), pp. 128–141. Difficulties are hidden in terms such as "great costs" and "reasonable expectation," as well as in terms such as "successful." Such ambiguity reflects the fact that precise operational definitions are not available. That is, the precise meanings of "great," "reasonable," and "successful" are inextricably bound to particular circumstances, especially particular societies.

3. I will use the term euthanasia in a broad sense to indicate a deliberately chosen course of action or inaction that is known at the time of decision to be such as will expedite death. This use of euthanasia will encompass not only positive or active euthanasia (acting in order to expedite death) and negative or passive euthanasia (refraining from action in order to expedite death), but acting and refraining in the absence of a direct intention that death occur more quickly (that is, those cases that fall under the concept of double effect). See note 4.

4. But, both active and passive euthanasia can be appreciated in terms of the Catholic moral notion of double effect. When the doctrine of double effect is invoked, one is strictly not intending euthanasia, but rather one intends something else. That concept allows actions or omissions that lead to death (1) because it is licit not to prolong life *in extremis* (allowing death is not an intrinsic evil), (2) if death is not actually willed or actively sought (that is, the evil is not directly willed), (3) if that which is willed is a major good (for example, avoiding useless major expenditure of resources or serious pain), and (4) if the good is not achieved by means of the evil (for example, one does not will to save resources or diminish pain *by* the death). With regard to euthanasia the doctrine of double effect means that one need not expend major resources in an endeavor that will not bring health but only prolong dying and that one may use drugs that decrease pain but hasten death. See Richard McCormick, *Ambiguity in Moral Choice* (Milwaukee: Marquette University Press, 1973). I exclude the issue of double effect from my discussion because I am interested in those cases in which the good may follow directly from the evil—the death of the child. In part, though, the second section of this paper is concerned with the concept of proportionate good.

5. Raymond S. Duff and A. G. M. Campbell, "Moral and Ethical Dilemmas in the Special-Care Nursery," *The New England Journal of Medicine,* 289 (Oct. 25, 1973), pp. 890–894.

6. Roger Pell, "The Agonizing Decision of Joanne and Roger Pell," *Good Housekeeping* (January 1972), pp. 76–77, 131–135.

7. This somewhat Kantian argument is obviously made in opposition to Kant's position that suicide involves a default of one's duty to oneself ". . . to preserve his life simply because he is a person and must therefore recognize a duty to himself (and a strict one at that)," as well as a contradictory volition: "that man ought to have the authorization to withdraw himself from all obligation, that is, to be free to act as if no authorization at all were required for

this withdrawal, involves a contradiction. To destroy the subject of morality in his own person is tantamount to obliterating from the world. . ." Immanuel Kant, *The Metaphysical Principles of Virtue: Part II of the Metaphysics of Morals,* trans. James Ellington (Indianapolis: Bobbs-Merrill, 1964), p. 83; Akademie Edition, VI, 422–423.

8. Norman L. Cantor, "A Patient's Decision To Decline Life-Saving Medical Treatment: Bodily Integrity Versus the Preservation of Life," *Rutgers Law Review,* 26 (Winter 1972), p. 239.

9. By "young child" I mean either an infant or child so young as not yet to be able to participate, in any sense, in a decision. A precise operational definition of "young child" would clearly be difficult to develop. It is also not clear how one would bring older children into such decisions. See, for example, Milton Viederman, "Saying 'No' to Hemodialysis: Exploring Adaptation," and Daniel Burke, "Saying 'No' to Hemodialysis: An Acceptable Decision," both in *The Hastings Center Report,* 4 (September 1974), pp. 8–10, and John E. Schowalter, Julian B. Ferholt, and Nancy M. Mann, "The Adolescent Patient's Decision To Die," *Pediatrics,* 51 (January 1973), pp. 97–103.

10. An appeal to high costs alone is probably hidden in judgments based on statistics: even though there is a chance for a normal life for certain children with apparently severe cases of meningomyelocele, one is not obliged to treat since that chance is small, and the pursuit of that chance is very expensive. Cases of the costs being low but the expected suffering of the child being high will be discussed under the concept of the injury of continued existence. It should be noted that none of the arguments in this paper bear on cases where neither the cost nor the suffering of the child is considerable. Cases in this last category probably include, for example, children born with mongolism complicated only by duodenal atresia.

11. I have in mind here the issue of physicians, hospital administrators, or others being morally compelled to seek an injunction to force treatment of the child in the absence of parental consent. In these circumstances, the physician, who is usually best acquainted with the facts of the case, is the natural advocate of the child.

12. G. Tedeschi, "On Tort Liability for 'Wrongful Life,' " *Israel Law Review,* 1 (1966), p. 513.

13. Zepeda v. Zepeda: 41 Ill. App. 2d 240, 190 N.E. 2d 849 (1963).

14. Williams v. State of New York: 46 Misc. 2d 824, 260 N.Y.S. 2d 953 (Ct. Cl., 1965).

15. Torts: "Illegitimate Child Denied Recovery Against Father for 'Wrongful Life,' " *Iowa Law Review,* 49 (1969), p. 1009.

16. It is one thing to have a conceptual definition of the injury of continued existence (for example, causing a person to continue to live under circumstances of severe pain and deprivation when there are no alternatives but death) and another to have an operational definition of that concept (that is, deciding what counts as such severe pain and deprivation). This article has focused on the first, not the second, issue.

17. H. Tristram Engelhardt, Jr., "Euthanasia and Children: The Injury of Continued Existence," *The Journal of Pediatrics,* 83 (July 1973), pp. 170–171.

18. John Lorber, "Results of Treatment of Myelomeningocele," *Developmental Medicine and Child Neurology,* 13 (1971), p. 286.

19. John M. Freeman, "The Shortsighted Treatment of Myelomeningocele: A Long-Term Case Report," *Pediatrics,* 53 (March 1974), pp. 311–313.

20. John M. Freeman, "To Treat or Not To Treat," *Practical Management of Meningomyelocele,* ed. John Freeman (Baltimore: University Park Press, 1974), p. 21.

21. John Lorber, "Selective Treatment of Myelomeningocele: To Treat or Not To Treat, *Pediatrics,* 53 (March 1974), pp. 307–308.

22. I am presupposing that no intrinsic moral distinctions exist in cases such as these, between acting and refraining, between omitting care in the hope that death will ensue (that is, rather than the child living to be even more defective) and acting to ensure that death will ensue rather than having the child live under painful and seriously compromised circumstances. For a good discussion of the distinction between acting and refraining, see Jonathan Bennett, "Whatever the Consequences," *Analysis,* 26 (January 1966), pp. 83–102; P. J. Fitzgerald, "Acting and Refraining," *Analysis,* 27 (March 1967), pp. 133–139; Daniel Dinello, "On Killing and Letting Die," *Analysis,* 31 (April 1971), pp. 83–86.

23. Lorber, "Selective Treatment of Myelomeningocele," p. 308.

24. Positive duties involve a greater constraint than negative duties. Hence it is often easier to establish a duty not to do something (not to treat further) than a duty to do something (to actively hasten death). Even allowing a new practice to be permitted (for example, active euthanasia) requires a greater attention to consequences than does establishing the absence of a positive duty. For example, at common law there is no basis for action against a person who watches another drown without giving aid; this reflects the difficulty of establishing a positive duty.

NEW JERSEY SUPREME COURT

In the Matter of Karen Quinlan, an Alleged Incompetent

[The opinion of the Court was delivered by Hughes, Chief Justice.]

The central figure in this tragic case is Karen Ann Quinlan, a New Jersey resident. At the age of 22, she lies in a debilitated and allegedly moribund state at Saint Clare's Hospital in Denville, New Jersey. The litigation has to do, in final analysis, with her life— its continuance or cessation—and the responsibilities, rights, and duties, with regard to any fateful decision concerning it, of her family, her guardian, her doctors, the hospital, the State through its law enforcement authorities, and finally the courts of justice. . . .

The matter is of transcendent importance, involving questions related to the definition and existence of death; the prolongation of life through artificial means developed by medical technology undreamed of in past generations of the practice of the healing arts; the impact of such durationally indeterminate and artificial life prolongation on the rights of the incompetent, her family and society in general; the bearing of constitutional right and the scope of judicial responsibility, as to the appropriate response of an equity court of justice to the extraordinary prayer for relief of the plaintiff. Involved as well is the right of the plaintiff,

Reprinted from 70 *New Jersey Reports* 10. Decided March 31, 1976.

Joseph Quinlan, to guardianship of the person of his daughter.

• • •

THE FACTUAL BASE

An understanding of the issues in their basic perspective suggests a brief review of the factual base developed in the testimony and documented in greater detail in the opinion of the trial judge. *In re Quinlan,* 137 *N.J. Super.* 227 (Ch. Div. 1975).

On the night of April 15, 1975, for reasons still unclear, Karen Quinlan ceased breathing for at least two 15-minute periods. She received some ineffectual mouth-to-mouth resuscitation from friends. She was taken by ambulance to Newton Memorial Hospital. There she had a temperature of 100 degrees, her pupils were unreactive and she was unresponsive even to deep pain. The history at the time of her admission to that hospital was essentially incomplete and uninformative.

Three days later, Dr. Morse examined Karen at the request of the Newton admitting physician, Dr. McGee. He found her comatose with evidence of decortication, a condition relating to derangement of the cortex of the brain causing a physical posture in which the upper extremities are flexed and the lower extremities are extended. She required a respirator to assist her breathing. Dr. Morse was unable to obtain an adequate account of the circumstances and events leading up to Karen's admission to the Newton Hospital. Such initial history or etiology is crucial in neurological diagnosis. Relying as he did upon the Newton Memorial records and his own examination, he concluded that prolonged lack of oxygen in the bloodstream, anoxia, was identified with her condition as he saw it upon first observation. When she was later transferred to Saint Clare's Hospital she was still unconscious, still on a respirator and a tracheotomy had been performed. On her arrival Dr. Morse conducted extensive and detailed examinations. An electroencephalogram (EEG) measuring electrical rhythm of the brain was performed and Dr. Morse characterized the result as "abnormal but it showed some activity and was consistent with her clinical state." Other significant neurological tests, including a brain scan, an angiogram, and a lumbar puncture were normal in result. Dr. Morse testified that Karen has been in a state of coma, lack of consciousness, since he began treating her. He explained that there are basically two types of coma, sleep-like unresponsiveness and awake unresponsiveness. Karen was originally in a sleep-like unresponsive condition but soon developed "sleep-wake" cycles, apparently a normal improvement for comatose patients occurring within three to four weeks. In the awake cycle she blinks, cries out and does things of that sort but is still totally unaware of anyone or anything around her.

Dr. Morse and other expert physicians who examined her characterized Karen as being in a "chronic persistent vegetative state." Dr. Fred Plum, one of such expert witnesses, defined this as a "subject who remains with the capacity to maintain the vegetative parts of neurological function but who . . . no longer has any cognitive function."

Dr. Morse, as well as the several other medical and neurological experts who testified in this case, believed with certainty that Karen Quinlan is not "brain dead." They identified the Ad Hoc Committee of Harvard Medical School report . . . as the ordinary medical standard for determining brain death, and all of them were satisfied that Karen met none of the criteria specified in that report and was therefore not "brain dead" within its contemplation.

· · · ·

Because Karen's neurological condition affects her

respiratory ability (the respiratory system being a brainstem function) she requires a respirator to assist her breathing. From the time of her admission to Saint Clare's Hospital Karen has been assisted by an MA-1 respirator, a sophisticated machine which delivers a given volume of air at a certain rate and periodically provides a "sigh" volume, a relatively large measured volume of air designed to purge the lungs of excretions. Attempts to "wean" her from the respirator were unsuccessful and have been abandoned.

The experts believe that Karen cannot now survive without the assistance of the respirator; that exactly how long she would live without it is unknown; that the strong likelihood is that death would follow soon after its removal, and that removal would also risk further brain damage and would curtail the assistance the respirator presently provides in warding off infection.

It seemed to be the consensus not only of the treating physicians but also of the several qualified experts who testified in the case, that removal from the respirator would not conform to medical practices, standards and traditions.

The further medical consensus was that Karen in addition to being comatose is in a chronic and persistent "vegetative" state, having no awareness of anything or anyone around her and existing at a primitive reflex level. Although she does have some brainstem function (ineffective for respiration) and has other reactions one normally associates with being alive, such as moving, reacting to light, sound and noxious stimuli, blinking her eyes, and the like, the quality of her feeling impulses is unknown. She grimaces, makes stereotyped cries and sounds and has chewing motions. Her blood pressure is normal.

Karen remains in the intensive care unit at Saint Clare's Hospital, receiving 24-hour care by a team of four nurses characterized, as was the medical attention, as "excellent." She is nourished by feeding by way of a nasal-gastro tube and is routinely examined for infection, which under these circumstances, is a serious life threat. The result is that her condition is considered remarkable under the unhappy circumstances involved.

Karen is described as emaciated, having suffered a weight loss of at least 40 pounds, and undergoing a continuing deteriorative process. Her posture is described as fetal-like and grotesque; there is extreme flexion-rigidity of the arms, legs and related muscles and her joints are severely rigid and deformed.

From all of this evidence, and including the whole

testimonial record, several basic findings in the physical area are mandated. Severe brain and associated damage, albeit of uncertain etiology, has left Karen in a chronic and persistent vegetative state. No form of treatment which can cure or improve that condition is known or available. As nearly as may be determined, considering the guarded area of remote uncertainties characteristic of most medical science predictions, she can *never* be restored to cognitive or sapient life. Even with regard to the vegetative level and improvement therein (if such it may be called) the prognosis is extremely poor and the extent unknown if it should in fact occur.

She is debilitated and moribund and although fairly stable at the time of argument before us (no new information having been filed in the meanwhile in expansion of the record), no physician risked the opinion that she could live more than a year and indeed she may die much earlier. Excellent medical and nursing care so far has been able to ward off the constant threat of infection, to which she is peculiarly susceptible because of the respirator, the tracheal tube and other incidents of care in her vulnerable condition. Her life accordingly is sustained by the respirator and tubal feeding, and removal from the respirator would cause her death soon, although the time cannot be stated with more precision.

· · ·

We have adverted to the "brain death" concept and Karen's disassociation with any of its criteria, to emphasize the basis of the medical decision made by Dr. Morse. When plaintiff and his family, finally reconciled to the certainty of Karen's impending death, requested the withdrawal of life support mechanisms, he demurred. His refusal was based upon his conception of medical standards, practice and ethics described in the medical testimony, such as in the evidence given by another neurologist, Dr. Sidney Diamond, a witness for the State. Dr. Diamond asserted that no physician would have failed to provide respirator support at the outset, and none would interrupt its life-saving course thereafter, except in the case of cerebral death. In the latter case, he thought the respirator would in effect be disconnected from one already dead, entitling the physician under medical standards and, he thought, legal concepts, to terminate the supportive measures. We note Dr. Diamond's distinction of major surgical or transfusion procedures in a terminal case not involving cerebral death, such as here:

The subject has lost human qualities. It would be incredible, and I think unlikely, that any physician would respond to a sudden hemorrhage, massive hemorrhage or a loss of all her defensive blood cells, by giving her large quantities of blood. I think that . . . major surgical procedures would be out of the question even if they were known to be essential for continued physical existence.

This distinction is adverted to also in the testimony of Dr. Julius Korein, a neurologist called by plaintiff. Dr. Korein described a medical practice concept of "judicious neglect" under which the physician will say:

Don't treat this patient any more, . . . it does not serve either the patient, the family, or society in any meaningful way to continue treatment with this patient.

Dr. Korein also told of the unwritten and unspoken standard of medical practice implied in the foreboding initials DNR (do not resuscitate), as applied to the extraordinary terminal case:

Cancer, metastatic cancer, involving the lungs, the liver, the brain, multiple involvements, the physician may or may not write: Do not resuscitate. . . . [I]t could be said to the nurse: if this man stops breathing don't resuscitate him. . . . No physician that I know personally is going to try and resuscitate a man riddled with cancer and in agony and he stops breathing. They are not going to put him on a respirator. . . . I think that would be the height of misuse of technology.

While the thread of logic in such distinctions may be elusive to the non-medical lay mind, in relation to the supposed imperative to sustain life at all costs, they nevertheless relate to medical decisions, such as the decision of Dr. Morse in the present case. We agree with the trial court that that decision was in accord with Dr. Morse's conception of medical standards and practice.

· · ·

CONSTITUTIONAL AND LEGAL ISSUES

THE RIGHT OF PRIVACY[1]

It is the issue of the constitutional right of privacy that has given us most concern, in the exceptional circumstances of this case. Here a loving parent, *qua* parent and raising the rights of his incompetent and profoundly damaged daughter, probably irreversibly doomed to no more than a biologically vegetative remnant of life, is before the court. He seeks authorization to abandon specialized technological procedures which can only maintain for a time a body having no potential for resumption or continuance of other than a "vegetative" existence.

We have no doubt, in these unhappy circumstances, that if Karen were herself miraculously lucid for an interval (not altering the existing prognosis of the condition to which she would soon return) and perceptive of her irreversible condition, she could effectively decide upon discontinuance of the life-support apparatus, even if it meant the prospect of natural death. To this extent we may distinguish [*John F. Kennedy Memorial Hosp. v. Heston*], . . . which concerned a severely injured young woman (Delores Heston), whose life depended on surgery and blood transfusion; and who was in such extreme shock that she was unable to express an informed choice (although the Court apparently considered the case as if the patient's own religious decision to resist transfusion were at stake), but most importantly a patient apparently salvable to long life and vibrant health;—a situation not at all like the present case.

We have no hesitancy in deciding, in the instant diametrically opposite case, that no external compelling interest of the State could compel Karen to endure the unendurable, only to vegetate a few measurable months with no realistic possibility of returning to any semblance of cognitive or sapient life. We perceive no thread of logic distinguishing between such a choice on Karen's part and a similar choice which, under the evidence in this case, could be made by a competent patient terminally ill, riddled by cancer and suffering great pain; such a patient would not be resuscitated or put on a respirator in the example described by Dr. Korein, and *a fortiori* would not be kept *against his will* on a respirator.

·   ·   ·

The claimed interests of the State in this case are essentially the preservation and sanctity of human life and defense of the right of the physician to administer medical treatment according to his best judgment. In this case the doctors say that removing Karen from the respirator will conflict with their professional judgment. The plaintiff answers that Karen's present treatment serves only a maintenance function; that the respirator cannot cure or improve her condition but at best can only prolong her inevitable slow deterioration and death; and that the interests of the patient, as seen by her surrogate, the guardian, must be evaluated by the court as predominant, even in the face of an opinion *contra* by the present attending physicians. Plaintiff's distinction is significant. The nature of Karen's care and the realistic chances of her recovery are quite unlike those of the patients discussed in many of the cases where treatments were ordered. In many of those cases the medical procedure required (usually a transfusion) constituted a minimal bodily invasion, and the chances of recovery and return to functioning life were very good. We think that the State's interest *contra* weakens and the individual's right to privacy grows as the degree of bodily invasion increases and the prognosis dims. Ultimately there comes a point at which the individual's rights overcome the State interest. It is for that reason that we believe Karen's choice, if she were competent to make it, would be vindicated by the law. Her prognosis is extremely poor—she will never resume cognitive life. And the bodily invasion is very great—she requires 24 hour intensive nursing care, antibiotics, the assistance of a respirator, a catheter and feeding tube.

Our affirmation of Karen's independent right of choice, however, would ordinarily be based upon her competency to assert it. The sad truth, however, is that she is grossly incompetent and we cannot discern her supposed choice based on the testimony of her previous conversations with friends, where such testimony is without sufficient probative weight. 137 *N.J. Super.* at 260. Nevertheless we have concluded that Karen's right of privacy may be asserted on her behalf by her guardian under the peculiar circumstances here present.

If a putative decision by Karen to permit this noncognitive, vegetative existence to terminate by natural forces is regarded as a valuable incident of her right of privacy, as we believe it to be, then it should not be discarded solely on the basis that her condition prevents her conscious exercise of the choice. The only practical way to prevent destruction of the right is to permit the guardian and family of Karen to render their best judgment, subject to the qualifications hereinafter stated, as to whether she would exercise it in these circumstances. If their conclusion is in the affirmative, this decision should be accepted by a society the overwhelming majority of whose members would, we think, in similar circumstances, exercise such a choice in the same way for themselves or for those closest to them. It is for this reason that we determine that Karen's right of privacy may be asserted in her behalf, in this respect, by her guardian and family under the particular circumstances presented by this record.

· · ·

THE MEDICAL FACTOR

Having declared the substantive legal basis upon which plaintiff's rights as representative of Karen must be deemed predicated, we face and respond to the assertion on behalf of defendants that our premise unwarrantably offends prevailing medical standards. We thus turn to consideration of the medical decision supporting the determination made below, conscious of the paucity of pre-existing legislative and judicial guidance as to the rights and liabilities therein involved.

A significant problem in any discussion of sensitive medical-legal issues is the marked, perhaps unconscious, tendency of many to distort what the law is, in pursuit of an exposition of what they would like the law to be. Nowhere is this barrier to the intelligent resolution of legal controversies more obstructive than in the debate over patient rights at the end of life. Judicial refusals to order lifesaving treatment in the face of contrary claims of bodily self-determination or free religious exercise are too often cited in support of a preconceived ''right to die,'' even though the patients, wanting to live, have claimed no such right. Conversely, the assertion of a religious or other objection to lifesaving treatment is at times condemned as attempted suicide, even though suicide means something quite different in the law. [Byrn, ''Compulsory Lifesaving Treatment for the Competent Adult,'' 44 *Fordham L. Rev.* 1 (1975)].

Perhaps the confusion there adverted to stems from mention by some courts of statutory or common law condemnation of suicide as demonstrating the state's interest in the preservation of life. We would see, however, a real distinction between the self-infliction of deadly harm and a self-determination against artificial life support or radical surgery, for instance, in the face of irreversible, painful and certain imminent death. The contrasting situations mentioned are analogous to those continually faced by the medical profession. When does the institution of life-sustaining procedures, ordinarily mandatory, become the subject of medical discretion in the context of administration to persons *in extremis?* And when does the withdrawal of such procedures, from such persons already supported by them, come within the orbit of medical discretion? When does a determination as to either of the foregoing contingencies court the hazard of civil or criminal liability on the part of the physician or institution involved?

The existence and nature of the medical dilemma need hardly be discussed at length, portrayed as it is in the present case and complicated as it has recently come to be in view of the dramatic advance of medical technology. The dilemma is there, it is real, it is constantly resolved in accepted medical practice without attention in the courts, it pervades the issues in the very case we here examine. The branch of the dilemma involving the doctor's responsibility and the relationship of the court's duty was thus conceived by Judge Muir:

Doctors . . . to treat a patient, must deal with medical tradition and past case histories. They must be guided by what they do know. The extent of their training, their experience, consultation with other physicians, must guide their decision-making processes in providing care to their patient. The nature, extent and duration of care by societal standards is the responsibility of a physician. The morality and conscience of our society places this responsibility in the hands of the physician. What justification is there to remove it from control of the medical profession and place it in the hands of the courts? [137 *N.J. Super.* at 259].

Such notions as to the distribution of responsibility, heretofore generally entertained, should, however neither impede this Court in deciding matters clearly justiciable nor preclude a re-examination by the Court as to underlying human values and rights. Determinations as to these must, in the ultimate, be responsive not only to the concepts of medicine but also to the common moral judgment of the community at large. In the latter respect the Court has a non-delegable judicial responsibility.

Put in another way, the law, equity and justice must not themselves quail and be helpless in the face of modern technological marvels presenting questions hitherto unthought of. Where a Karen Quinlan, or a parent, or a doctor, or a hospital, or a State seeks the process and response of a court, it must answer with its most informed conception of justice in the previously unexplored circumstances presented to it. That is its obligation and we are here fulfilling it, for the actors and those having an interest in the matter should not go without remedy.

· · ·

The medical obligation is related to standards and practice prevailing in the profession. The physicians in charge of the case, as noted above, declined to withdraw the respirator. That decision was consistent with the proofs . . . [in the lower court] as to the then existing medical standards and practices. Under the law as it then stood, Judge Muir was correct in declining to authorize withdrawal of the respirator.

However, in relation to the matter of the declaratory relief sought by plaintiff as representative of Karen's interests, we are required to reevaluate the applicability of the medical standards projected in the court below. The question is whether there is such internal consistency and rationality in the application of such standards as should warrant their constituting an ineluctable bar to the effectuation of substantive relief for plaintiff at the hands of the court. We have concluded not.

In regard to the foregoing it is pertinent that we consider the impact on the standards both of the civil and criminal law as to medical liability and the new technological means of sustaining life irreversibly damaged.

The modern proliferation of substantial malpractice litigation and the less frequent but even more unnerving possibility of criminal sanctions would seem, for it is beyond human nature to suppose otherwise, to have bearing on the practice and standards as they exist. The brooding presence of such possible liability, it was testified here, had no part in the decision of the treating physicians. As did Judge Muir, we afford this testimony full credence. But we cannot believe that the stated factor has not had a strong influence on the standards, as the literature on the subject plainly reveals. (See footnote 2, *infra*). Moreover our attention is drawn not so much to the recognition by Drs. Morse and Javed of the extant practice and standards but to the widening ambiguity of those standards themselves in their application to the medical problems we are discussing.

The agitation of the medical community in the face of modern life prolongation technology and its search for definitive policy are demonstrated in the large volume of relevant professional commentary.[2]

The wide debate thus reflected contrasts with the relative paucity of legislative and judicial guides and standards in the same field. The medical profession has sought to devise guidelines such as the "brain death" concept of the Harvard Ad Hoc Committee mentioned above. But it is perfectly apparent from the testimony we have quoted of Dr. Korein, and indeed so clear as almost to be judicially noticeable, that humane decisions against resuscitative or maintenance therapy are frequently a recognized *de facto* response in the medical world to the irreversible, terminal, pain-ridden patient, especially with familial consent. And these cases, of course, are far short of "brain death."

We glean from the record here that physicians distinguish between curing the ill and comforting and easing the dying; that they refuse to treat the curable as if they were dying or ought to die, and that they have sometimes refused to treat the hopeless and dying as if they were curable. In this sense, as we were reminded by the testimony of Drs. Korein and Diamond, many of them have refused to inflict an undesired prolongation of the process of dying on a patient in irreversible condition when it is clear that such "therapy" offers neither human nor humane benefit. We think these attitudes represent a balanced implementation of a profoundly realistic perspective on the meaning of life and death and that they respect the whole Judeo-Christian tradition of regard for human life. No less would they seem consistent with the moral matrix of medicine, "to heal," very much in the sense of the endless mission of the law, "to do justice."

Yet this balance, we feel, is particularly difficult to perceive and apply in the context of the development by advanced technology of sophisticated and artificial life-sustaining devices. For those possibly curable, such devices are of great value, and, as ordinary medical procedures, are essential. Consequently, as pointed out by Dr. Diamond, they are necessary because of the ethic of medical practice. But in light of the situation in the present case (while the record here is somewhat hazy in distinguishing between "ordinary" and "extraordinary" measures), one would have to think that the use of the same respirator or like support could be considered "ordinary" in the context of the possibly curable patient but "extraordinary" in the context of the forced sustaining by cardio-respiratory processes of an irreversibly doomed patient. And this dilemma is sharpened in the face of the malpractice and criminal action threat which we have mentioned.

.   .   .

There must be a way to free physicians, in the pursuit of their healing vocation, from possible contamination by self-interest or self-protection concerns which would inhibit their independent medical judgments for the well-being of their dying patients. We would hope that this opinion might be serviceable to some degree in ameliorating the professional problems under discussion.

A technique aimed at the underlying difficulty (though in a somewhat broader context) is described by Dr. Karen Teel, a pediatrician and a director of pediatric education, who writes in the *Baylor Law Review* under the title "The Physician's Dilemma: A Doctor's View: What The Law Should Be." Dr. Teel recalls:

Physicians, by virtue of their responsibility for medical judgments are, partly by choice and partly by default, charged with the responsibility of making ethical judgments which we are sometimes ill-equipped to make. We are not always morally and legally authorized to make them. The physician is thereby assuming a civil and criminal liability that, as often as not, he does not even realize as a factor in his decision. There is little or no dialogue in this whole process. The physician assumes that his judgment is called for and, in good faith, he acts. Someone must and it has been the physician who has assumed the responsibility and the risk.

I suggest that it would be more appropriate to provide a regular forum for more input and dialogue in individual situations and to allow the responsibility of these judgments to be shared. Many hospitals have established an Ethics Committee composed of physicians, social workers, attorneys, and theologians, . . . which serves to review the individual circumstances of ethical dilemmas, and which has provided much in the way of assistance and safeguards for patients and their medical caretakers. Generally, the authority of these committees is primarily restricted to the hospital setting and their official status is more that of an advisory body than of an enforcing body.

The concept of an Ethics Committee which has this kind of organization and is readily accessible to those persons rendering medical care to patients, would be, I think, the most promising direction for further study at this point. . . .

[This would allow] some much-needed dialogue regarding these issues and [force] the point of exploring all of the options for a particular patient. It diffuses the responsibility for making these judgments. Many physicians, in many circumstances, would welcome this sharing of responsibility. I believe that such an entity could lend itself well to an assumption of a legal status which would allow courses of action not now undertaken because of the concern for liability. [27 *Baylor L. Rev.* 6, 8–9 (1975)].

The most appealing factor in the technique suggested by Dr. Teel seems to us to be the diffusion of professional responsibility for decision, comparable in a way to the value of multi-judge courts in finally resolving on appeal difficult questions of law. Moreover, such a system would be protective to the hospital as well as the doctor in screening out, so to speak, a case which might be contaminated by less than worthy motivations of family or physician. In the real world and in relationship to the momentous decision contemplated, the value of additional views and diverse knowledge is apparent.

· · ·

And although the deliberations and decisions which we describe would be professional in nature they should obviously include at some stage the feelings of the family of an incompetent relative. Decision-making within health care if it is considered as an expression of a primary obligation of the physician, *primum non nocere,* should be controlled primarily within the patient-doctor-family relationship, as indeed was recognized by Judge Muir in his supplemental opinion of November 12, 1975.

If there could be created not necessarily this particular system but some reasonable counterpart, we would have no doubt that such decisions, thus determined to be in accordance with medical practice and prevailing standards, would be accepted by society and by the courts, at least in cases comparable to that of Karen Quinlan.

The evidence in this case convinces us that the focal point of decision should be the prognosis as to the reasonable possibility of return to cognitive and sapient life, as distinguished from the forced continuance of that biological vegetative existence to which Karen seems to be doomed.

In summary of the present Point of this opinion, we conclude that the state of the pertinent medical standards and practices which guided the attending physicians in this matter is not such as would justify this Court in deeming itself bound or controlled thereby in responding to the case for declaratory relief established by the parties on the record before us.

ALLEGED CRIMINAL LIABILITY

Having concluded that there is a right of privacy that might permit termination of treatment in the circumstances of this case, we turn to consider the relationship of the exercise of that right to the criminal law. We are aware that such termination of treatment would accelerate Karen's death. The County Prosecutor and the Attorney General stoutly maintain that there would be criminal liability for such acceleration. Under the statutes of this State, the unlawful killing of another human being is criminal homicide. *N.J.S.A.* 2A:113–1, 2, 5. We conclude that there would be no criminal homicide in the circumstances of this case. We believe, first, that the ensuing death would not be homicide but rather expiration from existing natural causes. Secondly, even if it were to be regarded as homicide, it would not be unlawful.

These conclusions rest upon definitional and constitutional bases. The termination of treatment pursuant to the right of privacy is, within the limitations of this case, *ipso facto* lawful. Thus, a death resulting from such an act would not come within the scope of the homicide statutes proscribing only the unlawful killing of another. There is a real and in this case determinative distinction between the unlawful taking of the life of another and the ending of artificial life-support systems as a matter of self-determination.

$$\bullet \quad \bullet \quad \bullet$$

DECLARATORY RELIEF

We thus arrive at the formulation of the declaratory relief which we have concluded is appropriate to this case. Some time has passed since Karen's physical and mental condition was described to the Court. At that time her continuing deterioration was plainly projected. Since the record has not been expanded we assume that she is now even more fragile and nearer to death than she was then. Since her present treating physicians may give reconsideration to her present posture in the light of this opinion, and since we are transferring to the plaintiff as guardian the choice of the attending physician and therefore other physicians may be in charge of the case who may take a different view from that of the present attending physicians, we herewith declare the following affirmative relief on behalf of the plaintiff. Upon the concurrence of the

guardian and family of Karen, should the responsible attending physicians conclude that there is no reasonable possibility of Karen's ever emerging from her present comatose condition to a cognitive, sapient state and that the life-support apparatus now being administered to Karen should be discontinued, they shall consult with the hospital "Ethics Committee" or like body of the institution in which Karen is then hospitalized. If that consultative body agrees that there is no reasonable possibility of Karen's ever emerging from her present comatose condition to a cognitive, sapient state, the present life-support system may be withdrawn and said action shall be without any civil or criminal liability therefor on the part of any participant, whether guardian, physician, hospital or others. We herewith specifically so hold.

NOTES

1. The right we here discuss is included within the class of what have been called rights of "personality." *See* Pound, "Equitable Relief against Defamation and Injuries to Personality," 29 *Harv. L. Rev.* 640, 668–76 (1916). Equitable jurisdiction with respect to the recognition and enforcement of such rights has long been recognized in New Jersey. *See, e.g.,* Vanderbilt v. Mitchell, 72 *N.J. Eq.* 910, 919–20 (E. & A. 1907).

2. *See, e.g.,* Downing, *Euthanasia and the Right to Death* (1969); St. John-Stevas, *Life, Death and the Law* (1961); Williams, *The Sanctity of Human Life and the Criminal Law* (1957); Appel, "Ethical and Legal Questions Posed by Recent Advances in Medicine," 205 *J.A.M.A.* 513 (1968); Cantor, "A Patient's Decision To Decline Life-Saving Medical Treatment: Bodily Integrity Versus The Preservation Of Life." 26 *Rutgers L. Rev.* 228 (1973); Claypool, "The Family Deals with Death," 27 *Baylor L. Rev.* 34 (1975); Elkinton, "The Dying Patient, The Doctor and The Law," 13 *Vill. L. Rev.* 740 (1968); Fletcher, "Legal Aspects of the Decision Not to Prolong Life," 203 *J.A.M.A.* 65 (1968); Foreman, "The Physician's Criminal Liability for the Practice of Euthanasia," 27 *Baylor L. Rev.* 54 (1975); Gurney, "Is There A Right To Die?—A Study of the Law of Euthanasia," 3 *Cumb.-Sam. L. Rev.* 235 (1972); Mannes, "Euthanasia vs. The Right To Life," 27 *Baylor L. Rev.* 68 (1975); Sharp & Crofts, "Death with Dignity and the Physician's Civil Liability," 27 *Baylor L. Rev.* 86 (1975); Sharpe & Hargest, "Lifesaving Treatment for Unwilling Patients," 36 *Fordham L. Rev.* 695 (1968); Skegg, "Irreversibly Comatose Individuals: 'Alive' or 'Dead'?" 33 *Camb. L.J.* 130 (1974); Comment, "The Right to Die," 7 *Houston L. Rev.* 654 (1970); Note, "The Time Of Death—A Legal, Ethical and Medical Dilemma," 18 *Catholic Law.* 243 (1972); Note, "Compulsory Medical Treatment: The State's Interest Re-evaluated," 51 *Minn. L. Rev.* 293 (1966).

SUPREME JUDICIAL COURT OF MASSACHUSETTS, HAMPSHIRE

Superintendent of Belchertown State School v. Saikewicz

LIACOS, Justice.

On April 26, 1976, William E. Jones, superintendent of the Belchertown State School (a facility of the Massachusetts Department of Mental Health), and Paul R. Rogers, a staff attorney at the school, petitioned the Probate Court for Hampshire County for the appointment of a guardian of Joseph Saikewicz, a resident of the State school. Simultaneously they filed a motion for the immediate appointment of a guardian *ad litem*, with authority to make the necessary decisions concerning the care and treatment of Saikewicz, who was suffering with acute myeloblastic monocytic leukemia. The petition alleged that Saikewicz was a mentally retarded person in urgent need of medical treatment and that he was a person with disability incapable of giving informed consent for such treatment.

On May 5, 1976, the probate judge appointed a guardian *ad litem*. On May 6, 1976, the guardian *ad litem* filed a report with the court. The guardian *ad litem*'s report indicated that Saikewicz's illness was an incurable one, and that although chemotherapy was the medically indicated course of treatment it would cause Saikewicz significant adverse side effects and discomfort. The guardian *ad litem* concluded that these factors, as well as the inability of the ward to understand the treatment to which he would be subjected and the fear and pain he would suffer as a result, outweighed the limited prospect of any benefit from such treatment, namely, the possibility of some uncertain but limited extension of life. He therefore recommended "that not treating Mr. Saikewicz would be in his best interests."

A hearing on the report was held on May 13, 1976. Present were the petitioners and the guardian *ad litem*. . . . After hearing the evidence, the judge en-

From 370 *North Eastern Reporter, 2d Series* 417, pp. 420–423, 428–432, and 435. Decided November 28, 1977.

tered findings of fact and an order that in essence agreed with the recommendation of the guardian *ad litem*. The decision of the judge appears to be based in part on the testimony of Saikewicz's two attending physicians who recommended against chemotherapy. The judge then reported to the Appeals Court the two questions set forth in the margin.* An application for direct appellate review was allowed by this court. On July 9, 1976, this court issued an order answering the questions reported in the affirmative with the notation "rescript and opinion . . . will follow."† We now issue that opinion.

I

The judge below found that Joseph Saikewicz, at the time the matter arose, was sixty-seven years old, with an I.Q. of ten and a mental age of approximately two years and eight months. He was profoundly mentally retarded. The record discloses that, apart from his leukemic condition, Saikewicz enjoyed generally good health. He was physically strong and well built, nutritionally nourished, and ambulatory. He was not, however, able to communicate verbally—

*"(1) Does the Probate Court under its general or any special jurisdiction have the authority to order, in circumstances it deems appropriate, the withholding of medical treatment from a person even though such withholding of treatment might contribute to a shortening of the life of such person?

"(2) On the facts reported in this case, is the Court correct in ordering that no treatment be administered to said JOSEPH SAIKEWICZ now or at any time for his condition of acute myeloblastic monocytic leukemia except by further order of the Court?"

†After briefly reviewing the facts of the case, we stated in that order: "Upon consideration, based upon the findings of the probate judge, we answer the first question in the affirmative, and a majority of the Court answer the second question in the affirmative. However, we emphasize that upon receiving evidence of a significant change either in the medical condition of Saikewicz or in the medical treatment available to him for successful treatment of his condition, the probate judge may issue a further order."

resorting to gestures and grunts to make his wishes known to others and responding only to gestures or physical contacts. In the course of treatment for various medical conditions arising during Saikewicz's residency at the school, he had been unable to respond intelligibly to inquiries such as whether he was experiencing pain. It was the opinion of a consulting psychologist, not contested by the other experts relied on by the judge below, that Saikewicz was not aware of dangers and was disoriented outside his immediate environment. As a result of his condition, Saikewicz had lived in State institutions since 1923 and had resided at the Belchertown State School since 1928. Two of his sisters, the only members of his family who could be located, were notified of his condition and of the hearing, but they preferred not to attend or otherwise become involved.

On April 19, 1976, Saikewicz was diagnosed as suffering from acute myeloblastic monocytic leukemia. Leukemia is a disease of the blood. It arises when organs of the body produce an excessive number of white blood cells as well as other abornmal cellular structures, in particular undeveloped and immature white cells. Along with these symptoms in the composition of the blood the disease is accompanied by enlargement of the organs which produce the cells, e.g., the spleen, lymph glands, and bone marrow. The disease tends to cause internal bleeding and weakness, and, in the acute form, severe anemia and high susceptibility to infection. The particular form of the disease present in this case, acute myeloblastic monocytic leukemia, is so defined because the particular cells which increase are the myeloblasts, the youngest form of a cell which at maturity is known as the granulocyte. The disease is invariably fatal.

Chemotherapy, as was testified to at the hearing in the Probate Court, involves the administration of drugs over several weeks, the purpose of which is to kill the leukemia cells. This treatment unfortunately affects normal cells as well. One expert testified that the end result, in effect, is to destroy the living vitality of the bone marrow. Because of this effect, the patient becomes very anemic and may bleed or suffer infections—a condition which requires a number of blood transfusions. In this sense, the patient immediately becomes much "sicker" with the commencement of chemotherapy, and there is a possibility that infections during the initial period of severe anemia will prove fatal. Moreover, while most patients survive

chemotherapy, remission of the leukemia is achieved in only thirty to fifty per cent of the cases. Remission is meant here as a temporary return to normal as measured by clinical and laboratory means. If remission does occur, it typically lasts for between two and thirteen months although longer periods of remission are possible. Estimates of the effectiveness of chemotherapy are complicated in cases, such as the one presented here, in which the patient's age becomes a factor. According to the medical testimony before the court below, persons over age sixty have more difficulty tolerating chemotherapy, and the treatment is likely to be less successful than in younger patients. This prognosis may be compared with the doctors' estimates that, left untreated, a patient in Saikewicz's condition would live for a matter of weeks or, perhaps, several months. According to the testimony, a decision to allow the disease to run its natural course would not result in pain for the patient, and death would probably come without discomfort.

An important facet of the chemotherapy process, to which the judge below directed careful attention, is the problem of serious adverse side effects caused by the treating drugs. Among these side effects are severe nausea, bladder irritation, numbness and tingling of the extremities, and loss of hair. The bladder irritation can be avoided, however, if the patient drinks fluids, and the nausea can be treated by drugs. It was the opinion of the guardian *ad litem,* as well as the doctors who testified before the probate judge, that most people elect to suffer the side effects of chemotherapy rather than to allow their leukemia to run its natural course.

Drawing on the evidence before him, including the testimony of the medical experts, and the report of the guardian *ad litem,* the probate judge issued detailed findings with regard to the costs and benefits of allowing Saikewicz to undergo chemotherapy. The judge's findings are reproduced in part here because of the importance of clearly delimiting the issues presented in this case. The judge below found:

5. That the majority of persons suffering from leukemia who are faced with a choice of receiving or forgoing such chemotherapy, and who are able to make an informed judgment thereon, choose to receive treatment in spite of its toxic side effects and risks of failure.

6. That such toxic side effects of chemotherapy include pain and discomfort, depressed bone marrow, pronounced anemia, increased chance of infection, possible bladder irritation, and possible loss of hair.

7. That administration of such chemotherapy requires cooperation from the patient over several weeks of time, which cooperation said JOSEPH SAIKEWICZ is unable to give due to his profound retardation.

8. That, considering the age and general state of health of said JOSEPH SAIKEWICZ, there is only a 30–40 percent chance that chemotherapy will produce a remission of said leukemia, which remission would probably be for a period of time of from 2 to 13 months, but that said chemotherapy will certainly not completely cure such leukemia.

9. That if such chemotherapy is to be administered at all it should be administered immediately, inasmuch as the risks involved will increase and the chances of successfully bringing about remission will decrease as time goes by.

10. That, at present, said JOSEPH SAIKEWICZ's leukemia condition is stable and is not deteriorating.

11. That said JOSEPH SAIKEWICZ is not now in pain and will probably die within a matter of weeks or months a relatively painless death due to the leukemia unless other factors should intervene to themselves cause death.

12. That it is impossible to predict how long said JOSEPH SAIKEWICZ will probably live without chemotherapy or how long he will probably live with chemotherapy, but it is to a very high degree medically likely that he will die sooner without treatment than with it.

Balancing these various factors, the judge concluded that the following considerations weighed *against* administering chemotherapy to Saikewicz: "(1) his age, (2) his inability to cooperate with the treatment, (3) probable adverse side effects of treatment, (4) low chance of producing remission, (5) the certainty that treatment will cause immediate suffering, and (6) the quality of life possible for him even if the treatment does bring about remission."

The following considerations were determined to weigh in *favor* of chemotherapy: "(1) the chance that his life may be lengthened thereby, and (2) the fact that most people in his situation when given a chance to do so elect to take the gamble of treatment."

Concluding that, in this case, the negative factors of treatment exceeded the benefits, the probate judge ordered on May 13, 1976, that no treatment be administered to Saikewicz for his condition of acute myeloblastic monocytic leukemia except by further order of the court. The judge further ordered that all reasonable and necessary supportive measures be taken, medical or otherwise, to safeguard the well-being of Saikewicz in all other respects and to reduce as far as possible any suffering or discomfort which he might experience.

Saikewicz died on September 4, 1976, at the Belchertown State School hospital. Death was due to

bronchial pneumonia, a complication of the leukemia. Saikewicz died without pain or discomfort.

•   •   •

II

The question what legal standards govern the decision whether to administer potentially life-prolonging treatment to an incompetent person encompasses two distinct and important subissues. First, does a choice exist? That is, is it the unvarying responsibility of the State to order medical treatment in all circumstances involving the care of an incompetent person? Second, if a choice does exist under certain conditions, what considerations enter into the decision-making process?

We think that principles of equality and respect for all individuals require the conclusion that a choice exists. . . . We recognize a general right in all persons to refuse medical treatment in appropriate circumstances. The recognition of that right must extend to the case of an incompetent, as well as a competent, patient because the value of human dignity extends to both.

This is not to deny that the State has a traditional power and responsibility, under the doctrine of *parens patriae,* to care for and protect the "best interests" of the incompetent person. Indeed, the existence of this power and responsibility has impelled a number of courts to hold that the "best interests" of such a person mandate an unvarying responsibility by the courts to order necessary medical treatment for an incompetent person facing an immediate and severe danger to life. Whatever the merits of such a policy where life-saving treatment is available—a situation unfortunately not presented by this case—a more flexible view of the "best interests" of the incompetent patient is not precluded under other conditions. For example, other courts have refused to take it on themselves to order certain forms of treatment or therapy which are not immediately required although concededly beneficial to the innocent person. While some of these cases involved children who might eventually be competent to make the necessary decisions without judicial interference, it is also clear that the additional period of waiting might make the task of correction more difficult. These cases stand for the proposition that, even in the exercise of the *parens patriae* power, there must be respect for the bodily integrity of the child or respect for the rational decision of those parties, usually the parents, who for one reason or another are seeking to protect the bodily integrity or other personal interest of the child.

The "best interests" of an incompetent person are not necessarily served by imposing on such persons results not mandated as to competent persons similarly situated. It does not advance the interest of the State or the ward to treat the ward as a person of lesser status or dignity than others. To protect the incompetent person within its power, the State must recognize the dignity and worth of such a person and afford to that person the same panoply of rights and choices it recognizes in competent persons. If a competent person faced with death may choose to decline treatment which not only will not cure the person but which substantially may increase suffering in exchange for a possible yet brief prolongation of life, then it cannot be said that it is always in the "best interests" of the ward to require submission to such treatment. Nor do statistical factors indicating that a majority of competent persons similarly situated choose treatment resolve the issue. The significant decisions of life are more complex than statistical determinations. Individual choice is determined not by the vote of the majority but by the complexities of the singular situation viewed from the unique perspective of the person called on to make the decision. To presume that the incompetent person must always be subjected to what many rational and intelligent persons may decline is to downgrade the status of the incompetent person by placing a lesser value on his intrinsic human worth and vitality.

The trend in the law has been to give incompetent persons the same rights as other individuals. Recognition of this principle of equality requires understanding that in certain circumstances it may be appropriate for a court to consent to the withholding of treatment from an incompetent individual. This leads us to the question of how the right of an incompetent person to decline treatment might best be exercised so as to give the fullest possible expression to the character and circumstances of that individual.

The problem of decision-making presented in this case is one of first impression before this court, and we know of no decision in other jurisdictions squarely on point. The well publicized decision of the New Jersey Supreme Court in *In re Quinlan* provides a helpful starting point for analysis, however.

. . .

The Supreme Court of New Jersey, in a unanimous opinion authored by Chief Justice Hughes, held that the father, as guardian, could, subject to certain qualifications, exercise his daughter's right to privacy by authorizing removal of the artificial life-support systems. The court thus recognized that the preservation of the personal right to privacy against bodily intrusions, not exercisable directly due to the incompetence of the right-holder, depended on its indirect exercise by one acting on behalf of the incompetent person. The exposition by the New Jersey court of the principle of substituted judgment, and of the legal standards that were to be applied by the guardian in making this decision, bears repetition here.

If a putative decision by Karen to permit this non-cognitive, vegetative existence to terminate by natural forces is regarded as a valuable incident of her right of privacy, as we believe it to be, then it should not be discarded solely on the basis that her condition prevents her conscious exercise of the choice. The only practical way to prevent destruction of the right is to *permit the guardian and family of Karen to render their best judgment,* subject to the qualifications [regarding consultation with attending physicians and hospital 'Ethics Committee'] hereinafter stated, *as to whether she would exercise it in these circumstances.* If their conclusion is in the affirmative this decision should be accepted by a society the overwhelming majority of whose members would, we think, in similar circumstances, exercise such a choice in the same way for themselves or for those closest to them. It is for this reason that we determine that Karen's right of privacy may be asserted in her behalf, in this respect, by her guardian and family under the particular circumstances presented by this record (emphasis supplied).

The court's observation that most people in like circumstances would choose a natural death does not, we believe, detract from or modify the central concern that the guardian's decision conform, to the extent possible, to the decision that would have been made by Karen Quinlan herself. Evidence that most people would or would not act in a certain way is certainly an important consideration in attempting to ascertain the predilections of any individual, but care must be taken, as in any analogy, to ensure that operative factors are similar or at least to take notice of the dissimilarities. With this in mind, it is profitable to compare the situations presented in the *Quinlan* case and the case presently before us. Karen Quinlan, subsequent to her accident, was totally incapable of knowing or appreciating life, was physically debilitated, and was pathetically reliant on sophisticated machinery to nourish and clean her body. Any other person suffering from similar massive brain damage would be in a similar state of total incapacity, and thus it is not unreasonable to give weight to a supposed general, and widespread, response to the situation.

Karen Quinlan's situation, however, must be distinguished from that of Joseph Saikewicz. Saikewicz was profoundly mentally retarded. His mental state was a cognitive one but limited in his capacity to comprehend and communicate. Evidence that most people choose to accept the rigors of chemotherapy has no direct bearing on the likely choice that Joseph Saikewicz would have made. Unlike most people, Saikewicz had no capacity to understand his present situation or his prognosis. The guardian *ad litem* gave expression to this important distinction in coming to grips with this "most troubling aspect" of withholding treatment from Saikewicz: "If he is treated with toxic drugs he will be involuntarily immersed in a state of painful suffering, the reason for which he will never understand. Patients who request treatment know the risks involved and can appreciate the painful side-effects when they arrive. They know the reason for the pain and their hope makes it tolerable." To make a worthwhile comparison, one would have to ask whether a a majority of people would choose chemotherapy if they were told merely that something outside of their previous experience was going to be done to them, that this something would cause them pain and discomfort, that they would be removed to strange surroundings and possibly restrained for extended periods of time, and that the advantages of this course of action were measured by concepts of time and mortality beyond their ability to comprehend.

To put the above discussion in proper perspective, we realize that an inquiry into what a majority of people would do in circumstances that truly were similar assumes an objective viewpoint not far removed from a "reasonable person" inquiry. While we recognize the value of this kind of indirect evidence, we should make it plain that the primary test is subjective in nature—that is, the goal is to determine with as much accuracy as possible the wants and needs of the individual involved. This may or may not conform to what is thought wise or prudent by most people. The problems of arriving at an accurate substituted judgment in matters of life and death vary greatly in degree, if not in kind, in different circumstances. For example, the responsibility of Karen Quinlan's father to act as she would have wanted could be discharged by drawing on many years of what was apparently an affectionate and close relationship. In contrast, Joseph Saikewicz was profoundly retarded and noncommunicative his entire life, which was spent largely in the highly restrictive atmosphere of an institution. While it may thus be necessary to rely to a greater degree on objective criteria, such as the supposed inability of profoundly retarded persons to conceptualize or fear death, the effort to bring the substituted judgment into step with the values and desires of the affected individual must not, and need not, be abandoned.

The "substituted judgment" standard which we have described commends itself simply because of its straightforward respect for the integrity and autonomy of the individual. We need not, however, ignore the substantial pedigree that accompanies this phrase. The doctrine of substituted judgment had its origin over 150 years ago in the area of the administration of the estate of an incompetent person. *Ex parte Whitbread in re Hinde, a Lunatic* (1816). The doctrine was utilized to authorize a gift from the estate of an incompetent person to an individual when the incompetent owed no duty of support. The English court accomplished this purpose by substituting itself as nearly as possible for the incompetent, and acting on the same motives and considerations as would have moved him.

In modern times the doctrine of substituted judgment has been applied as a vehicle of decision in cases more analogous to the situation presented in this case. In a leading decision on this point, *Strunk v. Strunk* (Ky.Ct.App.1969), the court held: that a court of equity had the power to permit removal of a kidney from an incompetent donor for purposes of effectuating a transplant. The court concluded that, due to the nature of their relationship, both parties would benefit from the completion of the procedure, and hence the court could presume that the prospective donor would, if competent, assent to the procedure.

With this historical perspective, we now reiterate the substituted judgment doctrine as we apply it in the instant case. We believe that both the guardian *ad litem* in his recommendation and the judge in his decision should have attempted (as they did) to ascertain the incompetent person's actual interests and preferences. In short, the decision in cases such as this should be that which would be made by the incompetent person, if that person were competent, but taking into account the present and future incompetency of the individual as one of the factors which would necessarily enter into the decision-making process of the competent person. Having recognized the right of a competent person to make for himself the same decision as the court made in this case, the question is, do the facts on the record support the proposition that Saikewicz himself would have made the decision under the standard set forth. We believe they do.

The two factors considered by the probate judge to weigh in favor of administering chemotherapy were: (1) the fact that most people elect chemotherapy and (2) the chance of a longer life. Both are appropriate indicators of what Saikewicz himself would have wanted, provided that due allowance is taken for this individual's present and future incompetency. We have already discussed the perspective this brings to the fact that most people choose to undergo chemotherapy. With regard to the second factor, the chance of a longer life carries the same weight for Saikewicz as for any other person, the value of life under the law having no relation to intelligence or social position. Intertwined with this consideration is the hope that a cure, temporary or permanent, will be discovered during the period of extra weeks or months potentially made available by chemotherapy. The guardian *ad litem* investigated this possibility and found no reason to hope for a dramatic breakthrough in the time frame relevant to the decision.

The probate judge identified six factors weighing against administration of chemotherapy. Four of these—Saikewicz's age, the probable side effects of treatment, the low chance of producing remission, and the certainty that treatment will cause immediate suffering—were clearly established by the medical testimony to be considerations that any individual would weigh carefully. A fifth factor—Saikewicz's inability to cooperate with the treatment—introduces those considerations that are unique to this individual and which therefore are essential to the proper exercise of substituted judgment. The judge heard testimony that Saikewicz would have no comprehension of the reasons for the severe disruption of his formerly secure and stable environment occasioned by the chemotherapy. He therefore would experience fear without the understanding from which other patients draw strength. The inability to anticipate and prepare for the severe side effects of the drugs leaves room only for confusion and disorientation. The possibility

that such a naturally uncooperative patient would have to be physically restrained to allow the slow intravenous administration of drugs could only compound his pain and fear, as well as possibly jeopardize the ability of his body to withstand the toxic effects of the drugs.

The sixth factor identified by the judge as weighing against chemotherapy was "the quality of life possible for him even if the treatment does bring about remission." To the extent that this formulation equates the value of life with any measure of the quality of life, we firmly reject it. A reading of the entire record clearly reveals, however, the judge's concern that special care be taken to respect the dignity and worth of Saikewicz's life precisely because of his vulnerable position. The judge, as well as all the parties, were keenly aware that the supposed ability of Saikewicz, by virtue of his mental retardation, to appreciate or experience life had no place in the decision before them. Rather than reading the judge's formulation in a manner that demeans the value of the life of one who is mentally retarded, the vague, and perhaps ill-chosen, term "quality of life" should be understood as a reference to the continuing state of pain and disorientation precipitated by the chemotherapy treatment. Viewing the term in this manner, together with the other factors properly considered by the judge, we are satisfied that the decision to withhold treatment from Saikewicz was based on a regard for his actual interests and preferences and that the facts supported this decision.

•   •   •

III

Finding no State interest sufficient to counterbalance a patient's decision to decline life-prolonging medical treatment in the circumstances of this case, we conclude that the patient's right to privacy and self-determination is entitled to enforcement. Because of this conclusion, and in view of the position of equality of an incompetent person in Joseph Saikewicz's position, we conclude that the probate judge acted appropriately in this case. For these reasons we issued our order of July 9, 1976, and responded as we did to the questions of the probate judge.

SUGGESTED READINGS FOR CHAPTER 8

Bayles, Michael D., and High, Dallas M., eds. *Medical Treatment of the Dying: Moral Issues.* Cambridge, Mass.: Schenkman, 1978.

Beauchamp, Tom L. "The Moral Justification for Withholding Heroic Procedures." In Bell, Nora K., ed. *Who Decides? Conflicts of Rights in Health Care.* Clifton, N.J.: Humana Press, 1982.

———, and Childress, James F. *Principles of Biomedical Ethics.* New York: Oxford University Press, 1979. Chaps. 4, 7.

———, and Davidson, Arnold I. "The Definition of Euthanasia." *Journal of Medicine and Philosophy* 4 (September 1979), 294–312.

———, and Perlin, Seymour, eds. *Ethical Issues in Death and Dying.* Englewood Cliffs, N.J.: Prentice-Hall, 1978.

Behnke, John A., and Bok, Sissela, eds. *The Dilemma of Euthanasia.* Garden City, N.Y.: Doubleday Anchor, 1975.

Benjamin, Martin. "Moral Agency and Negative Acts in Medicine." In Robison, Wade L., and Pritchard, Michael S., eds. *Medical Responsibility: Paternalism, Informed Consent, and Euthanasia.* Clifton, N.J.: Humana Press, 1979, pp 169–180.

Bok, Sissela. "Death and Dying: Euthanasia and Sustaining Life: Ethical Views." In Reich, Warren T., ed. *Encyclopedia of Bioethics.* New York: Free Press, Macmillan, 1978. Vol. 1, pp. 268–278.

———. "Personal Directions for Care at the End of Life." *New England Journal of Medicine* 295 (August 12, 1976), 367–369.

Cantor, Norman. "A Patient's Decision to Decline Life-Saving Medical Treatment: Bodily Integrity versus the Preservation of Life." *Rutgers Law Review* 26 (Winter 1972), 228–264.

A Children's Physician. "Non-Treatment of Defective Newborn Babies." *Lancet* 2 (November 24, 1979), 1123–1124.

Childress, James F. "To Live or Let Die," in his *Priorities in Biomedical Ethics.* Philadelphia: Westminster Press, 1981, pp. 34–50.

Coburn, Robert C. "Morality and the Defective Newborn." *Journal of Medicine and Philosophy* 5 (December 1980), 340–357.

Devine, Philip E. *The Ethics of Homicide.* Ithaca, N.Y.: Cornell University Press, 1978.

Downing, A. B., ed. *Euthanasia and the Right to Die.* New York: Humanities Press, 1970.

Duff, Raymond S., and Campbell, A. G. M. "Moral and Ethical Dilemmas in the Special-Care Nursery." *New England Journal of Medicine* 289 (October 25, 1973), 890–894.

Dyck, Arthur. "An Alternative to the Ethic of Euthanasia." In Williams, Robert H., ed. *To Live and To Die: When, Why, and How.* New York: Springer-Verlag, 1973, pp. 98–112.

Feinberg, Joel. "Voluntary Euthanasia and the Inalienable Right to Life," *Philosophy and Public Affairs* 7 (Winter 1978), 93–123.

Fletcher, George P. "Prolonging Life: Some Legal Considerations." *Washington Law Review* 42 (1967), 999–1016.

Fletcher, Joseph. "Ethics and Euthanasia." In Williams, Robert H., ed. *To Live and To Die: When, Why, and How.* New York: Springer, Verlag, 1973, pp. 113–122.

Foot, Philippa. "Euthanasia." *Philosophy and Public Affairs* 6 (Winter 1977), 85–112.

Glover, Jonathan. *Causing Death and Saving Lives.* New York: Penguin Books, 1977.

Grisez, Germain, and Boyle, Joseph M. *Life and Death with Liberty and Justice: A Contribution to the Euthanasia Debate.* Notre Dame, Ind.: University of Notre Dame Press, 1979.

Gustafson, James M. "Mongolism, Parental Desires, and the Right to Life." *Perspectives in Biology and Medicine* 16 (Summer 1973), 529–557.

Hare, R. M. "Euthanasia: A Christian View." *Philosophic Exchange* 2 (Summer 1975), 43–52.

Horan, Dennis J., and Mall, David, eds. *Death, Dying, and Euthanasia.* Washington, D.C.: University Publications of America, 1977.

Jonsen, Albert R. "Dying *Right* in California: The Natural Death Act." *Clinical Research* 26 (February 1978), 55–60.

Kluge, Eike-Henner W. *The Practice of Death.* New Haven: Yale University Press, 1975.

Kohl, Marvin, ed. *Beneficent Euthanasia.* Buffalo: Prometheus Books, 1975.

———, ed. *Infanticide and the Value of Life.* Buffalo, N.Y.: Prometheus Books, 1978.

Jonsen, Albert R., and Garland, Michael J., eds. *Ethics of Newborn Intensive Care.* Berkeley: University of California, Institute of Governmental Studies, 1976.

Ladd, John, ed. *Ethical Issues Relating to Life and Death.* New York: Oxford University Press, 1979.

McCormick, Richard A. "To Save or Let Die: The Dilemma of Modern Medicine." *Journal of the American Medical Association* 229 (July 8, 1974), 172–176.

Menzel, Paul T. "Are Killing and Letting Die Morally Different in Medical Contexts?" *Journal of Medicine and Philosophy* 4 (September 1979), 269–293.

Rachels, James. "Euthanasia." In Regan, Tom, ed. *Matters of Life and Death.* New York: Random House, 1980, pp. 28–66.

———. "Killing and Starving to Death." *Philosophy* 54 (April 1979), 159–171.

Ramsey, Paul. *Ethics at the Edges of Life: Medical and Legal Intersections.* New Haven: Yale University Press, 1978.

———. *The Patient as Person.* New Haven: Yale University Press, 1970. Chapter 3.

Redleaf, Diane L., et al. "The California Natural Death Act: An Empirical Study of Physicians' Practices." *Stanford Law Review* 31 (May 1979), 913–945.

Robertson, John A., and Fost, Norman. "Passive Euthanasia of Defective Newborn Infants: Legal Considerations." *Journal of Pediatrics* 88 (May 1976), 883–889.

Singer, Peter. "Taking Life: Euthanasia." In his *Practical Ethics.* Cambridge: Cambridge University Press, 1979, pp. 127–157.

Strong, Carson. "Euthanasia: Is the Concept Really Nonevaluative?" *Journal of Medicine and Philosophy* 5 (December 1980), 313–325.

Suckiel, Ellen K. "Death and Benefit in the Permanently Unconscious Patient: A Justification of Euthanasia." *Journal of Medicine and Philosophy* 3 (March 1978), 38–52.

Swinyard, Chester A., ed. *Decision Making and the Defective Newborn.* Springfield, Ill.: Charles C Thomas, 1978.

Tooley, Michael. "Infants: Infanticide: A Philosophical Perspective." In Reich, Warren T., ed. *Encyclopedia of Bioethics.* New York: Free Press, 1978. Vol. 2, pp. 742–751.

Trammell, Richard L. "The Presumption Against Taking Life." *Journal of Medicine and Philosophy* 3 (March 1978), 53–67.

Veatch, Robert M. *Death, Dying and the Biological Revolution: Our Last Quest for Responsibility.* New Haven: Yale University Press, 1976.

Weir, Robert F., ed. *Ethical Issues in Death and Dying.* New York: Columbia Univesity Press, 1977.

Williams, Peter C. "Rights and the Alleged Right of Innocents to Be Killed." *Ethics* 87 (July 1977), 383–394.

BIBLIOGRAPHIES

Goldstein, Doris Mueller. *Bioethics: A Guide to Information Sources*. Detroit: Gale Research Company, 1982. See under "Death and Dying."

Lineback, Richard H., ed. *Philosopher's Index*. Vols. 1– . Bowling Green, Ohio: Bowling Green State University, Philosophy Documentation Center. Issued quarterly. See under "Active Euthanasia," "Death," "Dying," "Euthanasia," "Killing," and "Letting Die."

Walters, LeRoy, ed. *Bibliography of Bioethics*. Vols. 1– . New York: Free Press. Issued annually. See under "Allowing to Die," "Euthanasia," "Infanticide," "Killing," and "Terminal Care." (The information contained in the annual *Bibliography of Bioethics* can also be retrieved from BIOETHICS-LINE, an online data base of the National Library of Medicine.)

9.

The Allocation of Medical Resources

As medicine has expanded its services, a problem has accompanied this expansion: scarce resources have often become even scarcer. This scarcity is not simply one of expensive equipment and medicine. Highly specialized practitioners, artificial organs, blood for the treatment of hemophilia, donors for organ transplant operations, and research facilities are all in scarce supply. The basic *economic problem* is how these scarce resources can be most efficiently allocated, in the light of economic facts and predictions, in order to satisfy human needs and desires. The basic *ethical problem* is one of distributive justice: by what policies can we ensure justice in the distribution of available resources? These are not two entirely separate problems, of course. Rather, we should say that there is both an economic dimension and an ethical dimension to the problem of allocation.

The problem is further divisible into two levels, macroallocation and microallocation. At the macroallocation level, decisions are made concerning how much shall be expended for medical resources in society, as well as how it is to be distributed. Such decisions are taken by Congress, state legislatures, health organizations, private foundations, and health insurance companies. At the microallocation level, decisions are taken by particular hospital staffs or doctors concerning who shall obtain whatever resources are available. The problem of macroallocation is emphasized in this chapter, together with related considerations about the right to health care.

THE PROBLEM OF MACROALLOCATION

Macroallocation decisions have recently assumed an increasing significance for the distribution of health resources, largely because federal funds and foundation grants now support the bulk of ongoing medical research and specialized treatment. Local and national health planning has also taken on added significance. There are two dimensions to such planning: (1) How much in the way of the total available money and resources should be allotted to biomedical research and clinical practice? (2) Of the amount allotted to biomedicine, how much should go to which specific projects (e.g., how much to cancer research, how much to preventive medicine, and how much to the production of expensive machines used in treatment facilities)? In considering such questions, one must take account both of competing medical needs and of competing nonmedical domestic needs (such as expenditures for food, housing, education, and welfare), as well as considering the needs of persons in other countries (such as the need of hundreds of thousands of food-starved people in other nations). These problems as applied to the particular case of justifiable allocations for the treatment of hypertension are explored in this chapter by Milton Weinstein and William Stason. They are concerned to show the most cost-effective and morally acceptable way to handle the public health problems of controlling hypertension. James Childress also treats these issues, but through a more general approach.

Ethical questions of distributive justice arise at every point in such deliberations. Consider the following examples. That there is an unequal distribution of economic resources among individual nations and among persons within these nations is a fact none would deny. But what, if anything, should be done about this inequality of distribution? Do the richer nations of the world have a moral obligation to provide more medical resources to other nations than they now provide? Should more of our own tax dollars be spent for medical purposes, and if so on what medical items? Should we distribute these medical benefits in a different way than we now distribute them? Do disadvantaged or especially needy persons have a "right" to a disproportionate amount of the available resources? The latter problem especially concerns Weinstein and Stason because some of their own public policy recommendations would leave the poorest sector of society unaffected by public financing schemes. The essay by Robert Veatch also treats this key issue.

In order to answer such questions, we need to determine what constitutes an economically just system of distribution. Since there are competing systems of distribution, we must decide which are the fairest. Here practical considerations such as whether the poor should receive more medical resources than they now do, whether more hospitals should be located in rural regions, and whether all citizens should have an equal amount of money expended on them each year regardless of need are all involved.

If these questions are to be answered in a principled rather than an arbitrary way, principles of distributive justice seem required. Most societies use different principles of distribution in different contexts. In the United States, for example, unemployment and welfare payments are distributed on the basis of *need* (and to some extent on the basis of previous length of employment); jobs and promotions are in many sectors awarded (distributed) on the basis of demonstrated *achievement and merit;* the higher incomes of wealthy professionals are allowed (distributed) on the grounds of superior *effort or merit or social contribution* (or perhaps all three); and, at least theoretically, the opportunity for elementary and secondary education is distributed *equally to all* citizens.

The different ways of distributing resources—of which the above are instances—may be concisely stated as principles of distributive justice:

1. To each person an equal share.
2. To each person according to individual need.
3. To each person according to individual effort.
4. To each person according to societal contribution.
5. To each person according to merit (individual ability).

The ethical problems of macroallocation are largely those of deciding which of these principles, if any, are the proper ones to use in distributing medical goods and services, and under what conditions they should be employed. The selections by Daniels and Veatch in this chapter are concerned with precisely this issue.

It is noteworthy that this list is not a complete one for purposes of macroallocation. The five principles pertain largely to individuals rather than to institutions or branches of government. The principle of utility—to take one obvious example—is more frequently used for purposes of allocations to institutions. Consider a community hospital as illustrative of this point. The hospital must compete with other community institutions for tax dollars, but once that allocation has been made (perhaps using the principle of utility), hospital supplies and space may be allocated to individuals (perhaps on the basis of need).

A different, but especially urgent, issue is whether allocation for *preventive* medicine should take priority over allocation for *crisis* medicine. From one perspective, the prevention of disease by the alteration of unsanitary environments, by screening programs, and by the provision of health information is cheaper and more efficient in raising health levels and saving lives than is crisis medicine (in the form of surgery, kidney dialysis, intensive care units, etc.). But from another perspective, a concentrated preventive approach is morally unsatisfactory if it would lead to the neglect of needy persons who could directly benefit from the resources of crisis medicine—even if the preventive approach is more efficient in the long run in preventing disease and maintaining health. At least two aspects of this problem are apparent here. First, there is the problem of weighing maximum cost-efficiency against the costly needs of individuals. Second, there is the problem of allocation priorities when some choice must be made between preventive medicine and crisis medicine.

James Childress explores these issues in general in the present chapter, while Weinstein and Stason are concerned to explore how effectively preventive programs (especially public screening and informational programs) have functioned and can be expected to function in the case of hypertension.

THE RIGHT TO HEALTH CARE

The question of a right to a certain level of health care is at least loosely connected to these problems of distributive justice, since it is one aspect of the moral problem of how health care should be distributed.[1] In this context a "right" is understood as an *entitlement* to some measure of health care, and not simply as a *benefit*. This usage follows traditions in political philosophy, where rights have been understood as entitlements a person possesses to some good, service, or liberty. As entitlements, rights are to be contrasted with mere privileges, ideals, and acts of charity. Rights to Medicaid or to Medicare, for example, are analogous to rights to receive an insurance benefit when required premiums have been paid: anyone eligible is entitled to receive all services and goods established by the rules of the program.

As noted in Chapter 1, *legal* rights are entitlements supportable by moral systems of rules. In many nations there is a firmly established legal right to health care goods and services for all citizens. The prevailing legal view in the United States, however, seems to be that even if there are solid moral reasons for and no constitutional constraints against enactment of a right to health care, there is no *constitutional* right to health care, although there is also no constitutional obstacle to the Congress's providing some types of health care to citizens. Whether there is or ought to be a *moral* right to health care is a far more open question.

Rights claims, whether legal or moral, are commonly divided into two types: negative and positive. This distinction is based on the difference between the right to be free to do something (a right to noninterference) and the right to be provided by others with something (a right to benefits). A negative right is a right to be free to pursue a course of action or to enjoy a state of affairs, whereas a positive right is a right to obtain a good, opportunity, or service. The rights proclaimed in major political documents such as the American Bill of Rights (1776) and the French Declaration of the Rights of Man (1789) have been negative rights. These include rights to life, liberty, property, and safety. Rights to health care, by contrast, are commonly interpreted as positive rights, because they are rights to other persons' positive actions or to social goods and services. In this chapter, Robert Sade vigorously protests the idea that there is such a positive right to health care. Other writers in the chapter tend to disagree with him, and some (e.g., Beauchamp and Faden) find the positive/negative distinction itself problematic.

Many liberty rights normally classified as negative rights do at least suggest a need for active intervention, and this complexity tends to obscure any neat positive/negative distinction. For example, to assert a right to health (not health *care*) is to claim more than mere freedom from interferences that negatively affect health. It asserts that the state is obliged to enforce the rights of citizens by actively protecting them against dangerous chemicals, emissions, polluted waterways, the spread of disease, etc. A claim that some rights are rights both to freedom *and* to protection is perhaps best understood, then, as a dual claim to a negative right to freedom and to a positive right to active protection by the state. In this way, such rights can be treated as complex, containing both negative rights and positive rights within their broad scope.

It is often maintained that rights of all types are "logically correlative" to obligations: One person's right entails an obligation on another's part (either to abstain from interference or to provide something), and all obligations similarly entail rights. This correlativity thesis has been challenged on grounds that several classes of obligations do not entail rights. Duties of charity, love, and conscience, for example, often function more as services one requires of oneself than as universal moral requirements. Such a "duty" or "obligation"—as something self-required—specifies the only grounds acceptable to Sade for providing persons with state-supported health goals and services. Again, however, several authors in this chapter disagree: Though they use different approaches, Fried, Veatch, Daniels, and Beauchamp and Faden all tend to support at least a limited *obligation* to provide some health care goods and services. The correlativity thesis thus requires them—unlike Sade—to support some program (however limited) of a *right* to health care. Many points in the debates over a right to health and to health care turn on what constitutes the basis of the "obligation" to provide health care goods and services.[2]

It is sometimes assumed that we have such rights as those to life and health irrespective of competing claims or social conditions. At most, however, morality posits a right not to have one's life taken or health placed at risk *without sufficient justification*. In the language introduced in Chapter 1 of this volume, rights are *prima facie* rather than absolute—that is, they are presumptively valid standing claims that may be overridden by more stringent competing claims. Inevitably, questions of macroallocation have direct bearing on all considerations about rights to goods and services. As we shall see, many discussions about a right to health or health care involve a *balancing* of the public interest and individual rights.

JUSTICE AND HEALTH CARE

There are, of course, many different general approaches to the questions of distribution and rights raised in this chapter. One idea is that there is a right to *equal access* to health care—the view Robert Veatch seems to reach by examining various possible distributive schemes. This approach makes a direct appeal to the first and second principles (equality; need) in the preceding list for its justification. On the other hand, one might reject any broad program of equal access, as Charles Fried does, while favoring the notion of a right to a *decent minimum* of health care. (Fried's proposal is not to be understood as a right to the best possible care, since the best available treatments are often prohibitively expensive and sometimes are luxuries rather than necessities.) This decent minimum proposal cannot be directly derived from any single one of the above distributive principles. This may be because, when fully elaborated, any such proposal will make an appeal to several of the principles, or it may be because the right to health care is independent of any such scheme of principles.

The decent minimum proposal is especially interesting because—as Beauchamp and Faden observe in their essay—it raises the theoretical and practical problem of whether one can consistently, fairly, and unambiguously structure a public policy that recognizes a right to have primary human needs for health care met but without thereby incorporating a right to exotic and expensive forms of treatment. The problem of justifying expense is also prominent in the final two essays in the chapter, those by Weinstein and Stason and Rashi

Fein. These essays explore the relationships between economic analysis and distributive justice.

These problems of macroallocation and rights make the urgency of moral decision apparent. These moral dilemmas cannot be put aside to be answered later. We have been and will continue to operate on principles, systems of distribution, and beliefs about rights that implicitly or explicitly provide answers to the ethical questions. But which are the best answers?

T. L. B.

NOTES

1. It might be held that human rights (to health care) require the use of certain distributive principles. On the other hand, it might be held that certain distributive principles confer human rights (to health care). The problem of whether rights *or* principles of distributive justice have priority cannot be considered here.

2. Following the general approach suggested in this paragraph, we need to distinguish two senses of such words as "required," "obligated," etc.: (1) required or obligated by a universal moral duty and (2) required or obligated by some stricture one imposes on oneself, such as a rule of conscience or a commitment to charity.

ROBERT SADE

Is Health Care a Right?

I will briefly consider the meaning of the word "right," then present some of the ways in which the perversion of that concept has been implemented politically around the world.

A "right" defines a freedom of action. For instance, a right to a material object is the uncoerced choice of the use to which that object will be put; a right to a specific action, such as free speech, is the freedom to engage in that activity without forceful repression. The moral foundation of the rights of man begins with the fact that he is a living creature: he has the right to his own life. All other rights are corollaries of this primary one; without the right to life, there can be no others.

The freedom to live does not automatically ensure life. For man, a specific course of action is required in order to sustain his life, a course of action which must be guided by reason and reality, and which has as its goal the creation or acquisition of material values, such as food and clothing, and intellectual values, such as self-esteem and integrity. His moral system is the means by which he is able to select those values which will support his life and achieve his happiness.

The right to life implies three corollaries: first, the right to select those values one deems necessary to sustain one's own life; second, the right to exercise one's own judgment of the best course of action to achieve the chosen values; and third, the right to dispose of those values, once gained, in any way one chooses, without coercion by other men. The denial of any one of these corollaries severely compromises or destroys the right to life itself. A man who is not allowed to choose his own goals, is prevented from setting his own course in achieving those goals, and is not free to dispose of the values he has earned is no less than a slave to those who usurp those rights. The right to private property, therefore, is essential and

indispensable to maintaining free men in a free society.

In a free society, man exercises his right to sustain his own life by producing economic values in the form of goods and services which he is, or should be, free to exchange with other men who are similarly free to trade with him or not. The economic values produced, however, are not given as gifts by nature, but exist only by virtue of the thought and effort of individual men. Goods and services are thus owned as a consequence of the right to sustain life by one's own physical and mental effort.

It is the nature of man as a living, thinking being that determines his natural rights. The concept of human rights, or natural rights, was introduced to the civilized world by Aristotle, who spoke of natural justice and of equal treatment before the law for all men, while noting that unequal merit should result in unequal reward. Thomas Aquinas expanded Aristotle's work by describing the existence of a natural law from which arose natural rights. These rights were recognized as prior to and existing apart from positive law: "Written law indeed contains natural right, but it does not institute it, for its force comes, not from the law, but from nature."

One of the most important defenders of human rights was John Locke, who was quite explicit as to what these rights were:

The law of nature . . . which obliges everyone, and reason which is that law, teaches all mankind who will but consult it, that being all equal and independent, no one ought to harm another in his life, health, liberty, or possessions.

In direct line of intellectual succession to Locke were Thomas Jefferson and the founders of the American Republic. The Declaration of Independence speaks of "inalienable rights," and the Constitution of 1787 made the United States the first major gov-

From *Image* 7 (1974), pp. 11–18.

ernment founded on the explicit proposition that the rights of the people are not granted by the state, but arise from the nature of man, and are beyond the right of the state either to grant or to withhold.

We hold these truths to be self-evident: that all men are created equal; that they are endowed by their Creator with certain inalienable rights; that among these are life, liberty, and the pursuit of happiness.

One of the models for the Declaration of Independence was the Bill of Rights for Virginia, which contained this statement:

. . . all men are born equally free and independent and have certain inherent rights—among which are enjoyment of life, liberty, and pursuing and obtaining happiness and safety.

The only fundamental change in this idea when it was incorporated in the Declaration of Independence was in Jefferson's realization that there is no right to obtain happiness, there is only the right to pursue it.

Since 1787, conceptual clarity in the consideration of rights has been gradually lost. As great a jurist as Justice Oliver Wendell Holmes remarked that "a right is but a prophecy that the state will use its courts and its might to sustain a man's claim." The greatest perversion of the concept of rights occurred during the presidency of Franklin Delano Roosevelt, when "right" was surreptitiously transferred from the freedom to pursue a value to the value itself: now all Americans had the right to a job, the right to a house, the right to a clean this and a decent that. The day of "natural rights" was gone, and the "parasite rights" of the New Deal crept up in the night.

As if dissatisfied with the rape and mutilation of the idea of rights, modern politicians have now reduced it to utter absurdity. The Democrats, in their 1972 platform, promised to secure the right of the American people to health. Not to health care, but to health itself.

Good Health is the least this society should promise its citizens . . . We endorse the principle that good health is a right of all Americans.

If they thought it would make political hay, no doubt they would also promise to secure the inherent right of the people to good looks and superior intelligence.

In fact, there is a limited, specific sense in which health may be thought of as a right. It is that no man

may harm the health of another, under sanction of the same moral force protecting the right to life. To invert the logic of rights and claim that there is an obligation upon society to provide health for its citizens is not only logically absurd and morally indefensible, but it is also medically impossible. Statistics from the Department of Health, Education, and Welfare show that last year 67% of deaths were due to diseases known to be caused or exacerbated by alcohol, tobacco smoking, overeating, or were due to accidents. Each of these factors is either largely or wholly correctable by individual action. Many common illnesses have a relationship like that of mortality to personal habits and excesses. We could, of course, make alcohol and tobacco illegal, prescribe diets for everyone (to be enforced by the FBI and FDA as a joint project), and put an end to airplanes and automobiles. The history of the Eighteenth Amendment in particular, and western civilization in general should not stop us. After all, The Health of the Nation is at stake.

The concept of medical care as the patient's right is immoral because it denies the most fundamental of all rights, that of a man to his own life and the freedom of action to support it. Medical care is neither a right nor a privilege: it is a service that is provided by doctors and others to people who wish to purchase it. It is the provision of the service that a doctor depends upon for his livelihood, and is his means of supporting his own life.

The very question of whether health care is a right or a privilege is an invalid one, because it is based on an erroneous supposition. The word "privilege" is derived from the Latin privus, private, and lex, law, forming the word privilegium, which meant "a law for or against a private person." A privilege is a "right or immunity granted as a peculiar benefit or favor." The fallacy of the right-or-a-privilege question is revealed by rephrasing the question: Should health care be granted to a limited number of people (as a privilege), or should it be granted to everyone (as a right)? This question should properly be answered by two questions: Granted by whom? And at whose expense? The answers are: granted by an arbitrary coercive agency, the government, at the expense of every taxpayer and every health professional. Health care cannot morally be granted to anyone. It is a service that must be treated as any other service: it must be purchased by those who wish to buy it, or given as a gift to the sick by the only human beings who are competent to give that gift—the health professionals themselves.

. . .

There is no such thing as free medical care. Health care is purchasable, meaning that somebody has to pay for it, individually or collectively, at the expense of forgoing the current or future consumption of other things. The question is whether the decision of how to allocate the consumer's dollar should belong to the consumer or to the state. I have already shown that the choice of how a doctor's services should be rendered belongs only to the doctor; in the same way, the choice of whether to buy a health service rather than some other service or commodity belongs to the consumer as a logical consequence of the right to his own life.

. . .

The immorality of all legislative acts that are based on the principle of health care as a right is best illustrated by noting their effects on a group that will be most affected by nationalization of the health care industry—physicians. Remembering that doctors also are citizens, and as such have the same rights as all other citizens, we may note that any doctor who is forced by law to join a group or a hospital he does not choose, or is prevented by law from prescribing a drug he thinks is best for his patient, or is compelled by law to make any decision he would not otherwise have made is being forced to act against his own mind, which means forced to act against his own life. He is also being forced to violate his most fundamental professional commitment, that of using his own best judgment at all times for the maximal benefit of his patient.

These acts of force against physicians are attacks on very basic political principles. If they are allowed to pass unprotested, they can be, and probably will be, used against every other citizen or group of citizens in the country.

. . .

The foundation of excellence in medical care is the doctor-patient relationship. . . . This relationship is attacked and eroded from virtually every side with increasing government control of medicine. Although it is impossible to assign numerical values to as subjective a phenomenon as this, a survey of seven major nations uncovered several mechanisms by which bureaucratization undermines the doctor-patient relationship.

The undermining factors include a decrease in time available to establish rapport due to increase in both patient load and paperwork for physicians. There is an erosion of mutual trust between doctor and patient; the patient recognizes that the records being kept of his illness are not confidential, but available for scrutiny by bureaucrats whose job it is to ensure efficient and frugal operation of the system; the physician, because he is paid by the state, is assigned a central role in protecting the solvency of the system by uncovering malingering and assigning benefits of the system as an agent of the state rather than as servant of the patient.

An eloquent description of the nature of the doctor-patient relationship in a country with a well-developed socialized medical system comes from a Russian physician:

The largest part of the ten minutes allocated as the norm for a patient's visit is consumed in writing.

And the patient? How do you think he feels when he walks into the physician's office with his ailments and sees that the doctor's attention is riveted not to the person but to the papers. Questions are asked abruptly. At times the patient's answers reach the doctor's ears but not his consciousness.

Listening to the complaints with one ear, and with his head bent over his papers, writing, the doctor sometimes does not even look at his patient. . . .

Late at night the doctor returns home, barely dragging his weary limbs, and starts to write what he had not been able to put down during the day while he was with his patients. . . .

As for the patient, he is not so much treated as "officially processed."

Under the present system, consideration and concern for the sick patient sink into the background. The very process of medical thought is bureaucratized. The doctor-thinker is transformed into the doctor-bureaucrat.

To gain the trust of his patient, the physician must project a sense of interest in his patient's illness. The loss of interest in his work was described by a Swedish physician of the effects (upon Swedish physicians) of the nationalization of Swedish medicine:

The details and the complicated working schedule have not yet been determined in all hospitals and districts, but the general feeling of belonging to a free profession, free to decide—at least in principle—how to organize its work, has been lost. Many hospital-based physicians regard their work now with an apathy previously unknown.

The reduction of time available to develop rapport and treat sick patients has occurred virtually everywhere that state medicine has been introduced. In Germany, the average office visit in panel practice was six minutes and the number of patients seen in one day has varied between 50 and 100. The average visit in Britain of 12 minutes includes traveling time for house calls, finding and filing patients' cards, entering clerical details and issuing certificates, history taking, time for the patient to dress and undress, clinical examination, time for thought and advising the patient. In Sweden the situation is just as bad.

·   ·   ·

High-quality medical care requires more than a good doctor-patient relationship and contented physicians. It requires also a sound scientific foundation and an active program of basic medical and biological research. Making available to the population of a country billions of dollars' worth of braces, orthopedic appliances, and reconstructive operations to thousands of victims of polio can be accomplished in the short run by political manipulation of the medical system. A far more significant achievement is the isolation of the polio virus, and the immunization of an entire population against it, completely wiping out the disease. This kind of fundamental advance is possible only through basic research, which thrives only in an atmosphere of scientific freedom of investigation. It takes decades to destroy the research capital and potential of a nation but this is precisely the effect of socialization of medicine.

·   ·   ·

Let us look now at a few vital statistics. Does government control of the health industry actually improve the health statistics of a nation? There is no evidence that it does, but considerable evidence that the health indices are far more closely related to social and economic factors than systems of medical care. The only statistics supporting the notion of superior health care under collectivist systems has been that of infant mortality. The United States, we are told, ranks only 12th to 18th in the world in infant mortality. What we are not told is that infant mortality means different things in different countries; statistical methods vary from country to country, and even within countries (e.g., the United States); there are no standard criteria for determining infant mortality; even if there were standard criteria, countries with a population of small average stature have infants of small size, therefore an artificially lower infant mortality; reporting of births is the responsibility of parents in some countries; reporting of deaths is not rigidly enforced in others; legalized abortions in some countries have an unknown effect on lowering infant mortality; there are known to be racial differences in deaths of infants.

If the U.S. is to be compared to another nation, it should be one of about equal population, spread out over an entire continent, and of multiethnic origin. Such a country is the Soviet Union. In the U.S., with its emphasis on free enterprise in medical care and with a chaotic nonsystem, the infant mortality in 1970 was 19.7 per 1,000 births. In Russia, in the same year, following a 60-year tradition of state-controlled medicine, with a heavy emphasis on public health and preventive medicine, the infant mortality rate was 26.0, an increase of 30% over ours. Whatever benefits we get from nationalization of the health system, improved health will not be one of them.

TOM L. BEAUCHAMP AND RUTH R. FADEN

The Right to Health and the Right to Health Care

Proclamations of general human rights such as those to life, liberty, property, safety, and happiness have been a staple of major political and legal documents in the last 200 years. Declarations of more detailed and specific rights such as the right to health care traditionally played no significant role in such documents. Recently this historical trend has been reversed, and many particular rights have been either declared or proposed for consideration. Biomedical ethics and health policy have increasingly been drawn into these discussions about rights. The following rights, for example, have been demanded, and in some cases given legal status: the right to die, the right to life, the right to commit suicide, the right to health care, the right to treatment, the right to privacy, and the right to have an abortion.

In this paper only issues pertaining to the right to health and the right to health care will be examined. However, our position on the nature and justification of rights applies to virtually all rights mentioned above.

We begin with a brief set of reminders about the history of claims to a right to health or to health care. However, throughout the section we concentrate on a highly questionable use of the distinction between positive and negative rights employed in the documents comprising part of this history.

HISTORICAL LANDMARKS

Chapman and Talmadge[1] have documented an extensive history of discussions about rights to health and health care in the United States—dating at least from the quarantine laws of 1796. As early as 1813, Congress passed laws granting a right to effective cowpox vaccines, which were to be distributed free of charge to any citizen. Subsequently, protective laws

controlling adulterated medicines and drugs, hygiene, sanitation, and water supplies were passed. With the exception of the vaccination laws, these early measures could be plausibly construed as recognitions of *negative* rights, because they were intended to protect individuals from identifiable health hazards that to some extent resulted from the actions of others. However, discussions of *positive* rights were by no means nonexistent.[2] In the early 1910s, for example, attention was focused on European health insurance schemes and in particular on Britain's National Health Insurance Act which was passed in 1911. These European programs were seriously studied by the American Medical Association (AMA), which established its own Committee on Social Insurance in 1916. The AMA's interest in national health insurance programs continued approximately until 1921, when the "liberal" period in AMA history ended and with it any immediate hope of securing national health insurance legislation.

Serious modern concern about a right to health care, together with many discussions concerning other rights on an international level, can probably be traced roughly to the December 10, 1948, "Universal Declaration of Human Rights" of the United Nations General Assembly.[3] Article 25 of this document specifically mentions a right to medical care and a right to a standard of living adequate to provide for one's health and well-being. The UN document, however, does not appear to declare entitlements. Its preamble gives the impression that the document is to be read as a blueprint for future actions and declarations of entitlements rather than as an assertion of rights that persons in their native countries now possess. The UN document has proved difficult to interpret because of its origins in political rhetoric and compromise. It includes rights taken from classic Western declarations of independence, while also including rights to vari-

From *The Journal of Medicine and Philosophy* 4 (June 1979), pp. 118, 122–130.

ous goods and services that were adapted from statements by socialist states regarding minimum standards of living. Still, this document is historically significant because it, perhaps more than any other single source, broadens the scope of rights to include positive rights to be provided with an extensive set of goods and services. The document also asserts positive rights to allocations from collective entities, even though the individual recipient may not be a member of the collective entity.

RECENT PROPOSALS BASED ON NEGATIVE RIGHTS

The distinction between positive and negative rights is only implicit in the aforementioned sources. However, it has recently been employed by a number of writers in order to develop a programmatic position on the issue of rights to health or health care. Unfortunately, the distinction has been abused and misunderstood by many of these writers, especially by those who oppose the claim that there is a positive right to health care. For example, Kuenzi and Sade argue that:

A "right" merely defines a *freedom of action*—free speech, peaceable assembly, press, etc. The only right that a government can guarantee, then, is that of freedom of action in those areas outlined by our constitution. Health Care [by contrast] is a *service* provided by doctors and others functioning in a free society, to people who wish to purchase it.[4]

A "right" [in classical historical writings] defines a freedom of action. . . . The greatest perversion of the concept of rights occurred during the presidency of Franklin Delano Roosevelt, when "right" was surreptitiously transferred from the freedom to pursue a value to the value itself: now all Americans had the right to a job, the right to a house, [etc.]. . . . Modern politicians have [subsequently] reduced [the idea of rights] to utter absurdity.[5]

The negative rights analysis rests in part on a position classically defended by John Stuart Mill: the state may and in some cases ought to intervene to limit the liberty of a person or group if and only if that person or group is producing harm to others. It follows that the state is permitted to and in some cases ought to limit the freedom of action of those who cause harm to others. Insofar as society as a unit ought to limit the liberty of those who cause harm, those who deserve protection have a right to be protected. Such a right is denoted by the expression "a negative right to health," which can be a highly confusing use of the

term because it can incorporate the notion of a protective service tendered by the state. This form of justification, based on liberty-limiting principles, is classically used to defend narrow or conservative social health programs asserting a right to be protected against controllable health hazards that are socially caused. Such public health programs as toxic substance and environmental pollution control, occupational safety regulations, and sanitation are perhaps the most obvious and oft-cited examples of protective measures not provided by the state.

These writers also commonly discuss the implications of their views for proposals regarding a national health program. They maintain that there is no state obligation to provide health goods and services. They contend that at most there exists a right to health (not health care), in the sense of a right to be protected from risks or hazards to health that are the result of the individual or collective actions of others. They propose a noninterference right according to which individuals are born with a specific birthright, namely, a right to some number of healthy units assigned to them in the contingent process Rawls[6] dubs the "natural lottery." Thus, they argue for a state obligation to promulgate and enforce protective and preventive measures when the actions of others threaten the health of individuals. Where the interfering actions of others have compromised the health of innocent individuals, these writers commit themselves to a state obligation to provide therapeutic and palliative services. Even on these conservative arguments, then it is possible that positive obligations to provide benefits may flow from negative rights. The very distinction between negative and positive rights has thus been obscured and abused by this approach.

CONFUSIONS IN THESE PROPOSALS

Unfortunately, these arguments, especially Sade's, are examples of several standard fallacies of irrelevance *(ignoratio elenchi)*. Even if it were true that in early Western philosophical writings and political constitutions the emphasis was exclusively on negative rights, it would follow neither that the concept of rights employed in such documents is limited to negative rights nor that it is a perversion of the concept of rights that positive claims be included. The above arguments also make the mistake of deriving a normative position (that it is a perversion to recognize positive "rights") from purely conceptual and historical (and thus, nonnormative) premises. Furthermore, even were the above arguments not instances of inductive fallacies, the historical claims on which they rest are almost certainly false, as we have seen. The point of our previous discussion of the early history of rights claims was to show that as early as 1813, laws implicitly granting positive rights were passed and that preliminary but serious discussion of positive rights had been initiated long before the Roosevelt period.

Finally, these programmatic proposals rest on an arguable empirical assumption: namely, that the class of risks to health that are socially caused or caused by others is clearly demarcated or at least unambiguously restricted in scope. Yet, the class of socially caused diseases is far from clearly defined and agreed upon. Emphasis is increasingly being placed not on biological factors in the etiology of disease but rather on the social bases of disease and ill health. Certain writers, such as Dan Beauchamp,[7] use the identical conception of a negative right to health here under discussion to justify an extraordinarily broad program of state-supported health services and regulation. Beauchamp construes virtually all major diseases to be largely socially rather than individually caused—two of his controversial and favorite examples being alcoholism and illness caused by smoking. If Beauchamp rather than, for example, Szasz,[8] Kuenzi,[9] Sade,[10] or Kass is correct about the extent to which ill health is rooted in socially induced causes, then a national health program based on a negative right to health would obligate the state to provide preventive and curative goods and services for all manner of controllable and treatable diseases. From this perspective, perhaps the only diseases to which we cannot claim a right to be protected against are those dispersed by a pure form of the natural lottery—that is, the class of purely naturally caused diseases and disorders.

There are further problems in these empirical assumptions about the extent of socially caused disease and ill health. A national health program based exclusively on these negative rights contentions would paradoxically, and without apparent justification, exclude the obligation to control, prevent, or treat certain natural lottery conditions for which we might otherwise feel obligated to provide state benefits. These would include conditions that, from an epidemiological perspective, are not inconsequential public health problems. The bulk of these conditions would probably be genetic: for example, cystic fibrosis, sickle cell, hemophilia, and phenylketonuria (PKU). However, this class would also include certain infectious diseases—for example, pandemics of new strains of influenza—as well as the effects of natural disasters, certain self-inflicted injuries, and perhaps even diseases associated with the aging process. In order to justify the provision of state-supported services for any of the above conditions, we would on these views have to look beyond rights claims—for example, to charity or other humanitarian reasons.

An even more problematic result of the exclusive negative rights theory is that it would create starkly different state obligations within identical disease categories. The identical illness may in some cases be disproportionately caused in some individuals by social factors and in other individuals by biologic or genetic factors. Consider, for example, the role of familial hypercholesterolemia in coronary heart disease. Here it is possible that certain victims of the same disease would be denied state services while others would have a right to treatment merely on grounds of the causal origin of the illness. The same problem would arise if the etiology of a state of ill health were unknown. In cases of unknown etiology there would always be an impossible difficulty in determining which way to turn the presumption of causal responsibility, because the entire issue of whether a condition qualifies for state protection and services turns on causal agency. An exclusively negative conception of the right to health is thus unsatisfactory, on both theoretical and practical grounds.

MORAL ARGUMENTS FOR THE RIGHT TO HEALTH CARE

If our arguments thus far are acceptable, those interested in justifying a positive right to health care will seek a moral principle or set of moral principles sufficient to show that there is a social obligation to provide some level of health care. The immediate problem for moral philosophy, then, may seem to be that of discovering such a principle or set of principles. However, problems stand in the way of any attempt to justify general programs involving massive social allocations by appeal to general moral principles.

Reservations about the power of moral philosophy to handle these problems may be rooted in the all too general character of moral principles when applied to such issues. Policies governing practical matters of great complexity cannot, after all, be directly and consistently derived from highly abstract principles. Such derivations cannot be achieved in law, and even less can they be achieved in philosophy. There also is no single consistent set of material principles of distributive justice that reliably applies when concrete issues of justice arise. There are many such principles in the form of social rules. They sometimes apply and sometimes do not apply when questions of social justice emerge, for different contexts require different orderings of the importance of such principles.

It thus seems to us impossible to apply general principles of justice directly to complex issues of social policy—such as how to construct a national health policy so as to insure maximal fairness. Moreover, just as policymakers stand in danger of arbitrary judgments because of their own moral and evaluative preferences, so do philosophers committed in advance to some single inflexible conception of justice and social order, for example, that society should be egalitarian rather than libertarian. Philosophers interested in public policy would instead do well to start in the midst of policy problems, where financial exigencies and political realities already exist and cannot be eradicated.

COST/BENEFIT ANALYSIS AS AN ALTERNATIVE

In the instance of the right to health care, a framework more appropriate than a general philosophical system for ascertaining our obligations is the mechanism usually referred to as cost/benefit analysis (which has its own more general theoretical roots in utilitarianism). This particular thesis about the appropriateness of cost/benefit procedures has been argued elsewhere and need not be repeated here.[11] However, it is useful to consider how policy decisions might be reached on this basis regarding a social program of health services (to which everyone has an equal claim, as most proponents of a positive right to health care propose). Such a program is a mandatory public insurance scheme in which each of us is both a possible beneficiary and loser in a context of scarce resources. While a small-scale program would not impose a severe burden for those taxpayers who would make it possible, a broad program covering, for example, Medicare, kidney dialysis, cryogenic techniques, psychiatric treatment, the totally implantable heart, basic biomedical research, surgery, dental care, mass screening programs including antenatal diagnosis, and all other envisionable health needs could quickly mount to an intolerable burden, one

unaffordable now and in the future. This context of scarce resources permits the following unrefined, but nonetheless compelling generalization: the broader the health program envisioned, the weaker are our obligations to set it in place.

Thus we find unacceptable the egalitarian theories of health care delivery advanced by Robert Veatch. According to them, justice requires a priority ordering of health goods and services so that they are made available to "the sickest insofar as health care can improve their health."[12] This noble ideal would elicit the approval of all who are generous, but it would chill the enthusiasm of those in the realistic business of macroallocation. For example, Veatch's claim that "the medically worst off have a *complete* claim of justice on health care resources" even in cases of psychiatry, nuclear-powered hearts, and hemodialysis, seems a demand impossible of satisfaction.[13] We wish the option were actualizable. However it is doubtful that society can provide the resources for all these laudable goals, in which case justice would not require it.

IS THERE AN OBLIGATION TO PROVIDE HEALTH CARE?

Two qualifications must be placed on the conclusions thus far reached in this section. First, it does not follow from our arguments that there is no social obligation whatsoever to provide health care goods and services. It follows only that one must restrict, by careful argument, the scope of any claim made to a right to health care. Consider as an example Charles Fried's proposals that as a national policy we ought to provide to all a decent minimum of health care, goods, and services, but no more than a decent minimum.[14] It is hard to imagine that we are not obliged by a string of moral principles such as beneficence, nonmaleficence, and justice to provide a decent minimum of health care. Some critics of a national health policy have occasionally advanced excessive suggestions to the effect that we have no positive obligations to help even the desperately needy. We have not joined forces with those who advance such proposals by the logic of our arguments merely because we appeal to cost/benefit considerations. It is possible, of course, that cost/benefit considerations could in principle lead to the conclusion that it is never cost efficient in financial terms for the state to provide health services. But, as utilitarians have often pointed out, many other social costs that we would probably not be willing to bear would follow from such a narrow focus on financial costs. At any event, we would argue that utility, if nothing else, could support a decent minimum proposal.[15] On the other hand, counterproposals in defense of rights (positive or negative) must not only be principled but carefully restricted in scope when set forth as policy pronouncements. Moreover, the development of such a health program should take place within a carefully delineated, systematic framework of principles for macroallocation, as has been argued elsewhere.[16]

Second, we should (in consistency) ask whether the moral justification underlying valid claims to a negative right to health can be successfully repeated for a positive right to health care. It would seem that there is a significant parallel, as follows: the most obvious and popular argument for a positive right has been that it would be unjust not to provide such care, because if such care were provided only through free-market contracts and insurance schemes, individuals would be harmed because they would be deprived of an adequate level of human welfare. In short, this argument from justice turns on the now familiar distributive principle that we are entitled to health care goods and services if we would be harmed in fundamental ways without them. This position asserts a right to be protected against all diseases and disorders that render a decent level of welfare impossible—whether they are caused naturally or socially. Protection against end-stage diseases such as glomerulonephritis provides one commonly cited example where large social allocations have already been made.

However, the class of diseases preventing a decent functional level of human welfare is perhaps even less clearly agreed upon and defined than is the class of socially caused diseases discussed in the previous section. And even if this class of diseases could be satisfactorily identified, we would be left with the problem of determining exactly which health care services society is obligated to provide, because it is easily possible that the class could be so broad as to exhaust or exceed available resources. Macroallocation problems again emerge as a central issue in analyzing claims on behalf of a positive right to health care. The interesting theoretical question is thus not so much whether there is a right, but what the limits are to the obligation generating the right. What is needed as a practical matter is some principled or procedural way of identifying which or what kinds of health care services we should grant individuals a legal right to obtain.

CONCLUSION

We have argued in this section that some concrete mechanism for determining public policy—such as cost/benefit analysis constrained by a decent minimum criterion—should be the determinative mechanism for deciding allocative questions of national health policy. We see no reason why this method of deciding such policy matters would violate principles of justice, nor do we see reasons to suppose that even from the perspective of a nonutilitarian theory of justice, such as Rawls's, this proposal would be found morally deficient.[17]

The larger objective of this paper has been to counter the common view about the right to health and health care that social allocations for health care goods and assistance must be made because there are preexisting rights to health and health care. We have attempted to stand this contention on its head by arguing that if there is a right to health care goods and assistance it is only because there already exists an obligation to allocate resources for the goods and assistance. We conclude that the major issues about rights to health and to health care turn on the justifiability of social expenditures rather than on some notion of natural, inalienable, or preexisting rights.

NOTES

1. C. B. Chapman and J. M. Talmadge, "The Evolution of the Right to Health Concept in the United States," *Pharos* 34 (January 1971), 30–51.

2. For an analysis of positive and negative rights, see the introduction to this chapter.

3. "Universal Declaration of Human Rights," in *Human Rights: A Compilation of International Instruments of the United Nations* (New York: United Nations, 1973).

4. D. E. Kuenzi, "Health Care, a Right?," *Missouri Medicine* 70 (February 1973), 111.

5. R. Sade, "Is Health Care a Right?," *Image* 7 ((1974), 11–19.

6. John Rawls, *A Theory of Justice* (Cambridge, Mass.: Harvard University Press, 1971).

7. Dan Beauchamp, "Public Health and Social Justice," *Inquiry* 13 (March 1976), 3–14.

8. Thomas Szasz, "The Right to Health," *Georgetown Law Journal* 57 (March 1969), 734–751.

9. D. E. Kuenzi, *op. cit.*

10. R. Sade, *op. cit.*

11. Tom L. Beauchamp, "Morality and the Social Control of Biomedical Technology," in *The Moral Uses of New Knowledge in*

the *Biomedical Sciences,* H. Tristram Engelhardt, Jr., and Stuart F. Spicker, eds. (Boston: Reidel Publishing Co., 1981).

12. Robert M. Veatch, "What Is a 'Just' Health Care Delivery?" in *Ethics and Health Policy,* Robert M. Veatch and Roy Branson, eds. (Cambridge, Mass.: Ballinger Publishing Co., 1976), pp. 134, 137.

13. *Ibid.,* p. 141.

14. Charles Fried, "Equality and Rights in Medical Care," *Hastings Center Report* 6 (February 1976), 29–34.

15. We are inclined to agree with the approach to justification argued for by Michael Bayles, "National Health Insurance and Non-covered Services," *Journal of Health Politics, Policy and*

Law 2 (Fall 1977), 335–348. We would not, however, follow the suggestions for a procedural mechanism proposed in his paper.

16. Tom L. Beauchamp, "Morality and the Social Control of Biomedical Technology," *op. cit.*

17. Rawls acknowledges as much, if what he calls "the basic structure of society" is shaped by his nonutilitarian principles of justice. In addition to *A Theory of Justice* (see note 6 above), see his "The Basic Structure as Subject," *American Philosophical Quarterly* 14 (April 1977), 159–165.

CHARLES FRIED

Equality and Rights in Medical Care

In this article I present arguments intended to support the following conclusions:

1. To say there is a right to health care does not imply a right to equal access, a right that whatever is available to any shall be available to all.
2. The slogan of equal access to the best health care available is just that, a dangerous slogan which could be translated into reality only if we submitted either to intolerable government controls of medical practice or to a thoroughly unreasonable burden of expense.
3. There is sense to the notion of a right to a decent standard of care for all, dynamically defined, but still not dogmatically equated with the best available.
4. We are far from affording such a standard to many of our citizens and that is profoundly wrong.
5. One of the major sources of the exaggerated demands for equality are the pretensions, inflated claims, inefficiencies, and guildlike, monopolistic practices of the health professions.

Reprinted with permission of the author from *Hastings Center Report,* Vol. 6 (February 1976), pp. 29–34.

BACKGROUND

The notion of some kind of a right to health care is not likely to be found in any but the most recent writings, not to mention legislation. After all, even the much more well-established institution of free, universal public education has not achieved the status of a federal constitutional right, is not a constitutional right by the law of many states, and stands as a right more as an inference from the practices and legislation of states, counties, and municipalities. The federal constitutional litigation regarding rights in that area has been restricted to the provision *equally* of whatever public education is in fact provided. So it should not be surprising that the notion of a right to health care is something of a novelty. Moreover, it is only fairly recently that health care could deliver a product which was as unambiguously beneficial as elementary schooling. Nevertheless, if one looks to the laws, practices, and understandings of states, counties, and municipalities, one sees growing up through the last century, and certainly in the twentieth century, an understanding which might be thought of as the inchoate recognition of a right to health care. Indeed, there are those who might say that such an inchoate recognition might be discerned as far back as Elizabethan England.

As one considers this progress, one should not misrepresent history, for in that history lies an important lesson. For the progress may represent not simply a progress in our ideas of social justice, but a progress in what medicine could do. The fact is that the increasingly general provision of medical care may be correlated as well with what medical care could accomplish as with any changing social doctrines. What could medicine accomplish a hundred or even fifty years ago? It is well known that the improvements in health that were wrought in those days were largely the result of improved sanitation, working conditions, diet, and the like. Beyond that, specifically medical ministrations could do very little. They could provide ease, amenities, relief, but rarely a cure. So society may be forgiven if it did not provide elaborate medical care to the poor until recently, since provision of medical care in essence would have meant simply the provision of amenities and placebos. And since society appeared little concerned to assure the amenities to its poor generally, it is no great surprise that it had scant inclination to provide these amenities to the sick poor.

The detailed history of the extension of medical care to the poor, and indeed to those who were not poor but lived in out-of-the-way places, has yet to be written. The emergence of a notion of a right to health care and the embodiment of such a notion in legislation and court decisions must also await difficult historical research. Nevertheless, it is worth noting that, at least in American public discourse, the idea of a right to medical care developed into something which had the appearance of inevitability only recently, in what might be called the intermediate, perhaps golden, age of modern medicine. This was a period when advances in treating acute illness, advances such as the antibiotics, could really make a large difference in prolonging life or restoring health; but the most elaborate technologies which may make only marginal improvements in situations previously thought to be hopeless had not yet been generally developed. In this recent "Golden Age" we could unambiguously afford a notion of a general right to medical care because there were a number of clear successes available to medicine, and these successes were not unduly costly. Having conquered the infectious diseases, medical science has undertaken the degenerative diseases, the malignant neoplasms, and the diseases of unknown etiology; and one must say

that the ratio between expense and benefit has become exponentially more unfavorable. So it is really only now that the notion of a right to health care poses acute analytical and social problems. It is for that reason that neither history nor legal analysis will much illuminate our future course. What we do now will be a matter of our choosing, and for this reason careful analysis of the notion of a right to health care is crucial.

EQUALITY AND RIGHTS:
ANALYTICAL DISTINCTIONS

First, something should be said by way of at least informal definition of this term "right." A right is more than just an interest that an individual might have, a state of affairs or a state of being which an individual might prefer. A claim of right invokes entitlements; and when we speak of entitlements, we mean not those things which it would be nice for people to have, or which they would prefer to have, but which they must have, and which if they do not have they may demand, whether we like it or not. Although I would not want to say that a right is something we must recognize "no matter what," nevertheless a right is something we must accord unless _____ and what we put in to fill in the unless clause should be tightly confined and specific.

This notion of rights has interesting and not altogether obvious relations to the concept of equality, and confusions about those relations are very likely to lead to confused arguments about the very area before us—rights to health care and equality in respect to health care.

First, it should be noted that equality itself may be considered a right. Thus, a person can argue that he is not necessarily entitled to any particular thing—whether it be income, or housing, or education, or health care—but that he is entitled to equality in respect to that thing, so that whatever anyone gets he should get, too. And this is a nice example of my previous proposition about the notion of rights generally. For to recognize a right to equality may very well be—I suppose it often is—contrary to many other policies that we may have, and particularly contrary to attempts to attain some kind of efficiency. Yet, by the very notion of rights, if there is a right to equality, then granting equality cannot depend on whether or not it is efficient to do so.

Second, there is the relation between rights and equality which runs the other way, too: to say that a class of persons, or all persons, have a certain right implies that they all have that right equally. If it is said that all persons within the jurisdiction of the United States have a constitutionally protected right to freedom of speech, whatever that may mean, one thing seems clear: that this right should not depend on what it is one wants to say, who one is, and the like. Indeed, if the government against whom this right is protected were to make such distinctions, for instance, subjecting to constraints the speech of ''irresponsible persons,'' that would be the exact concept of denial of freedom of speech to those persons.

These relations between the notion of right and of equality suggest the great importance of being very clear and precise about how a particular right is conceived: confusions in this regard are rampant in respect to health, and are the source of much pointless controversy. But because the point is quite general, let me first take an example from another area. If we were sloppy in our thinking about what the right of freedom of speech is—and many people are as sloppy about that as they are about their definition of the rights in the area which is our immediate concern—if we were sloppy about that definition, we might, for instance, consider that there has been a denial of right because some people have access to radio or television in getting their ideas across, while others have only the street-corner soapbox to broadcast their views. Indeed, there are those who might find it unjust that even on the soapbox the timid or inarticulate are much less effective than the bold or eloquent. All of these disparities, of course, may or may not be regrettable but they have nothing to do with freedom of speech as a right, given the premise that there is a right to free speech and that this right must be an equal right. It seems clear to me that it is very different from the right to be heard, believed, admired, and applauded. The right to speak freely is just that: a right to be free of constraints and impositions on whatever speaking one might wish to do, should you be able to find someone to listen.

Now this analogy is offered as more than a distant irrelevance. Is it not very similar to many things that are said in the area of health? For analogous to the claim that the right to freedom of speech really implies a right to be heard by the multitude, is the notion that whatever rights might exist in respect to health care are rights to health, rather than to health *care*. And of course the claim is equally absurd in both instances. We may sensibly guarantee that all will be equally free of constraints on the speaking they wish to do, but we should not guarantee that all will be

equally effective in getting their views across. Similarly, we may or may not choose to guarantee all equality of access to health care, but we cannot possibly guarantee to all equality of health.

Consider how these clarifications operate upon the historical development I alluded to at the beginning of this analysis. The right whose recognition might be said to have been implicit in social practices throughout the past hundred years was a right not to health care as such, nor yet a right to health, but rather a right to a certain standard of health care, which was defined in terms of what medicine could reasonably do for people. It is this notion which has become so difficult in our present situation, where the apparatus of medicine has become so much more elaborate, pretentious, and costly than it was in earlier times.

Bringing together the historical and the analytical sides, we might conclude that our present dilemma comes from the fact that there are very many expensive things that medicine can do which might possibly help. And if we commit ourselves to the notion that there is a right to whatever health care might be available, we do indeed get ourselves into a difficult situation where overall national expenditure on health must reach absurd proportions—absurd in the sense that far more is devoted to health at the expense of other important social goals than the population in general wants. Indeed, more is devoted to health than the population wants relative not only to important social goals—for example, education or housing—but relative to all the other things which people would like to have money left over to pay for. And if we recognize that it would be absurd to commit our society to devote more than a certain proportion of our national income to health, while at the same time recognizing a ''right to health care,'' we might then be caught on the other horn of the dilemma. For we might then be required to say that because a right to health care implies a right to equality of health care, then we must limit, we must lower the quality of the health care that might be purchased by some lest our commitment to equality require us to provide such care to all and thus carry us over a reasonable budget limit.

Consider the case of the artificial heart. It seems to me not too fanciful an assumption that such a device is technically feasible within a reasonable time, and likely to be hugely expensive both in terms of its actual implantation and in terms of the subsequent *it may be with the poor that the low cost method (prevention) should be instituted — they are a separate culture.*

care required by those benefiting from the device. Now if the right to health care is taken to mean the right to whatever health care is available to anybody, and if this entails that it is a right to an equal enjoyment of whatever care anyone else enjoys, then what are we to do with respect to the artificial heart? Might we decide not to develop such a device? Though the development and experimental use of it involves an entirely tolerable burden, the general provision of the artificial heart would be an intolerable burden, and since if we provide it to any we must provide it to all, therefore perhaps we should provide it to none.

This solution seems to me both uncomfortable and unstable. For surely there is something odd, if not perverse, about forgoing research on such devices, not because the research might fail, but because it might succeed. Might not this research then go on under some kinds of private auspices if such a governmental decision were made? Would we then go further and forbid even private research, rather than simply refusing to fund it? I can well imagine the next step, where artificial heart research and implantation would become like abortion or sex change operations in the old days: something one went to Sweden or Denmark for. Nor is a lottery device for distributing a limited number of artificial hearts likely to be more stable or satisfactory. For there, too, would we forbid people to go outside the lottery? Would it be a crime to cross national boundaries with the intent of obtaining an artificial heart? The example makes a general point about instituting an all-inclusive "right to health care," with the necessary concomitant of an equal right to whatever health care is available. For if we really instituted such a right and limited the provision of health care to a reasonable level, we would have to institute as well a degree of stringent state control, which it is both unlikely we can achieve and undesirable for us even to try to achieve. There is something that goes very deeply against the grain about any scheme which prohibits scientists from making discoveries which no one claims are harmful as such, but which will cause trouble because we can't give them to everybody. There is something which goes against the grain in a system which might forbid individual doctors to render a service, not because it is harmful, but because its benefits are not available to all.

Or take a much less dramatic case—dental care. It is said that ordinary basic prophylactic care is so lacking for tens of millions of our citizens that quite

No → how does one acquire a right in the event if anyone wanted to or could — at the right time? the place.

unnecessarily they do not have their own teeth while still in their prime. I take it that to provide the kind of elaborate dental care deployed on affluent suburban families to rural populations, and to all even poorer urban dwellers, would be a prodigiously expensive undertaking, one that would cost each of us quite heavily. But if we followed the slogan, "The best available made available to all," that is what is meant. My guess is the American people would not want to bear this burden and that as a form of transfer payment the poor would prefer just to have the money to spend on other things. But this shows the dangerousness of slogans, for perhaps the greatest part of the dental damage could be remedied at far less cost by fluoridation and by relatively routine care provided by a type of modestly trained person who is only now beginning to exist. Care of this sort can be afforded and should be provided. But this would mean abandoning the concept of equality and accepting the fact that the poor would be getting less elaborate care than those who are not poor.

Now it might be said that I am exaggerating. The case put forward is the British National Health Service, which is alleged to provide a model of high level care at reasonable costs with equality for all. But I would caution planners and enthusiasts from drawing too much from this example. The situation in Great Britain is very different in many ways. The country is smaller and more homogeneous. Moreover, even in Great Britain there are disparities between the care available between urban and rural areas; there are long waits for so-called "elective procedures"; and there is a small but significant and distinguished private sector outside of National Health which is the focus of great controversy and rancor. Finally, Great Britain is a country where a substantial portion of the citizenry is committed to the socialist ideal of equalizing incomes and nationalizing the provisions of all vital services. Surely this is a very different situation from that in the United States. Indeed, it may be that the cry for equality of access to health care bears to a general yearning for social equality much the same relation that the opposition to fetal research bears to the opposition to abortion. In each case it is a very large ideological tail wagging a relatively small and confused dog.

My point is analytical. My point is that apart from a rather general commitment to equality and, indeed, to state control of the allocation and distribution of resources, to insist on the right to health care, where that right means a right to equal access, is an anomaly. For as long as our society considers that inequalities of wealth and income are morally acceptable—acceptable in the sense that the system that produces these inequalities is in itself not morally suspect—it is anomalous to carve out a sector like health care and say that *there* equality must reign.

TOWARD A BETTER DEFINITION OF THE RIGHTS INVOLVED

After all, is health care so special? Is it different from education, housing, food, legal assistance? In respect to all of these things, we recognize in our society a right whose enjoyment may not be made wholly dependent upon the ability to pay. But just as surely in respect to all these things, we do not believe that this right entails equality of enjoyment, so that whatever diet one person or class of persons enjoys must be enjoyed by all. The argument, put forward for instance by some members of the Labor Party in Great Britain, that the independent schools in that country should be abolished because they offer a level of education better than that available in state schools, is an argument which would be found strange and repellent in the United States. Rather, in all of these areas — education, housing, food, legal assistance—there obtains a notion of a decent, fair standard, such that when this standard is satisfied all that exists in the way of *rights* has been accorded. And it is necessarily so; were we to insist on equality all the way up, that is, past this minimum, we would have committed ourselves to a political philosophy which I take it is not the dominant one in our society.

Is health care different? Everything that can be said about health care is true of food and is at least by analogy true of education, housing, and legal assistance. The real task before us is not, therefore, I think, to explain why there must be complete equality in medicine, but the more subtle and perilous task of determining the decent minimum in respect to health which accords with sound ethical judgments, while maintaining the virtues of freedom, variety, and flexibility which are thought to flow from a mixed system such as ours. The decent minimum should reflect some conception of what constitutes tolerable life prospects in general. It should speak quite strongly to things like maternal health and child health, which set the terms under which individuals will compete and develop. On the other hand, techniques which will offer some remote relief from conditions that rarely strike in the prime of life, and which strike late in the life because something must,

might be thought of as too esoteric to be part of the concept of minimum decent care.

On the other hand, the notion of a decent minimum should include humane and, I would say, worthy surroundings of care for those whom we know we are not going to be able to treat. Here, it seems to me, the emphasis on technology and the attention of highly trained specialists is seriously mistaken. Not only is it unrealistic to imagine that such fancy services can be provided for everyone "as a right," but there is serious doubt whether these kinds of services are what most people really want or can benefit from.

In the end, I will concede very readily that the notion of minimum health care, which it does make sense for our society to recognize as a right, is itself an unstable and changing notion. As my initial historical remarks must have suggested, the concept of a decent minimum is always relative to what is available over all, and what the best which is available might be. I suppose (to revert to my parable of the artificial heart) that if we allowed an artificial heart to be developed under private auspices and to be available only to those who could pay for it, or who could obtain it from specialized eleemosynary institutions, then the time might well come when it would have been so perfected that it would be a reasonable component of what one would consider minimum decent care. And the process of arriving at this new situation would be a process imbued with struggle and political controversy. But since I do not believe in utopias or final solutions, a resolution of the problem of the right to health care having these kinds of tensions within it neither worries me nor leads me to suspect that I am on the wrong track. To my mind, the right track consists in identifying what it is that health care can and cannot provide, in identifying also the cost of health care, and then in deciding how much of this health care, what level of health care, we are ready to underwrite as a floor for our citizenry.

PRACTICAL PROPOSALS

Although the process of defining the decent minimum is inherently a political process, there is a great deal which analysis and research can do to make the process rational and satisfactory. Much of this is a negative service, clearing away misconceptions and fallacies. For instance, as I have already argued, to state that our objective is to provide the best medical care for all, regardless of the ability to pay, must be shown up for the misleading slogan that it is. But there are more subtle misconceptions as well. The most pervasive of these deal with the situation of the medical profession.

Many observers look at the medical profession, its history of resistance to social change, and the fact that doctors as a profession enjoy the highest incomes of any group in the nation—somewhere around $50,000 a year on the average—and they draw their own conclusions. They draw the conclusion that therefore what is needed is necessarily more regulation. They look at the oversupply of surgeons in this country. They note the obvious fact of over-recourse to surgery which seems to result, and they conclude that what is needed is more government regulation. For instance, the problems of supply would be met by a kind of doctors' draft, requiring service in underserviced rural areas. Now I would, for a moment, suggest that we consider some alternative explanations and alternative reforms. Perhaps, after all, the irrationalities in the supply of medical personnel, together with the high incomes earned, are the result not of market forces run wild, but the result of a guild system as tight and self-protective as any we know. It is, perhaps, an irony that the medical profession, having persuaded the public of the necessity of strictly limiting entry into the profession, having persuaded the public of the indispensability of highly trained specialists, is now faced with the threat of a kind of doctors' draft to make these rare specialists available to all. Perhaps clearer thinking might indicate that many of the things which highly paid and highly trained doctors do might be done by an army of less pretentious persons.

It is well known, of course, that doctors' fees as such represent the smaller portion of the total health care budget, so it might be thought that I am taking aim at an obvious, vulnerable, and somewhat irrelevant target. Yet this is not so. Though the fees of doctors represent the smaller portion of the medical budget, doctors themselves control almost all of the decisions—from the decision about hospitalization, to the decision whether to prescribe drugs by brand or generic name—which do influence the total cost of medical care. And it is in this respect that doctors have resisted most attempts to make their behavior rational and cost-effective. In general, it is said that this is because no doctor would sacrifice the individual interests of his patient, and this may be a sincere claim. But a certain skepticism is in order. What

choice do the patients have to choose more economical systems of delivery? What doctor, for that matter, even gives his patient the choice between a brand and a generic prescription drug?

But it is in the choice of delivery systems themselves that the consumer is most restricted. Most consumers do not have the choice between a variety of delivery systems from prepaid group plans to the present individual fee-for-service system, with each plan costing what it really costs. If the consumer did have this choice, we might soon find out whether the alleged advantages of the fee-for-service system were something the consumer was willing to pay for. But of course we will never find this out if we are committed to underwrite, out of general revenues, the cost of this most expensive possible delivery system. "The best available to all." That is what we tend to do today for those groups whose medical care we do underwrite. The result is that we are trying to drive down the cost of this most expensive delivery system not by changing its organization but by bureaucratic control. What if, instead, each person were assured a certain amount of money to purchase medical services as he chose? If the restrictive practices of the profession itself could be avoided, would this not help a vast variety of delivery systems to grow up, all competing for the consumer's federally assured dollar? And then those who would want what might be considered as fancier or more individualized services could get them, provided only that they were willing to pay more for them.

Finally, there is a feature of our modern situation which is responsible for the present crisis in health care, and for the impossible dilemma posed by the promise of a right to health care. This is a feature of the society and the culture as a whole. I refer to our culture's inability to face and cope with the persistent facts of illness, old age, and death. Because we are little able to come to terms with the hazards which illness proposes, because the old are a burden and an embarrassment, because we pretend that death does not exist, we employ elaborate ruses to put these things out of the ambit of our ordinary lives. The reason why we hospitalize so much more than is rationally required surely goes beyond the vagaries of the health insurance system. Is it not also the result of the fact that the ill are an embarrassment to us, and that we seek to put them away, so we do not have to care for them, while assuaging our consciences that those "best qualified" to care for them are doing so? And in order that the ruse will work, we greatly overstate what it is that these "qualified" people can do for the ill. Needless to say, they are our willing accomplices in this piece of deception. So it is with the mentally retarded, the aged, and the dying. All of these persons are defined as having an abnormal condition not only justifying but requiring their isolation from us and their care in the hands of "specialists." Perhaps it is time that we recognize that this is part of the neurosis of our age. And of course, those whom we hire to perform our proper human role toward the sick, the old, and the dying can get away with charging a very high price for relieving us of our ordinary human obligations. But is this medical care?

Finally, to avoid misunderstanding, a general theoretic point must be made. My argument must sound harsh and callous—unfeelingly, if not unerringly economic. I have elsewhere argued that it is of the essence of the physician's role and of the patient's expectations that the doctor faced with the patient's

need will do everything in his power to alleviate that need.[1] I believe that. I believe that for the individual physician to do less than his best because of some economic calculation of equity or efficiency is a breach of trust. The doctor in his dealings with his patient must not act like a bureaucrat, policy maker, or legislator. But policy makers, voters, and legislators must think in different terms. It is monstrous if an individual doctor thinks like a budget officer when he cares for his patient in need; but it is chaotic and incoherent if budget officers and voters making general policy think like doctors at the bedside.

NOTES

1. In my book, *Medical Experimentation: Personal Integrity and Social Policy* (Amsterdam and New York: Associated Scientific Publishers/Elsevier, 1974).

NORMAN DANIELS

Health Care Needs and Distributive Justice

WHY A THEORY OF HEALTH-CARE NEEDS?

A theory of health-care needs must come to grips with two widely held judgments: that there is something especially important about health care, and that some kinds of health care are more important than others. The philosophical task is to assess, explain, and justify or modify these distinctions we make about the importance of different wants, interests, or needs.

• • •

NEEDS AND PREFERENCES

NOT ALL PREFERENCES ARE CREATED EQUAL

Before turning to health-care needs in particular, it is worth noting that the concept of needs has been in

philosophical disrepute, and with some good reason. The concept seems both too weak and too strong to get us very far toward a theory of distributive justice. Too many things become needs, and too few. And finding a middle ground seems to involve many of the issues of distributive justice one might hope to resolve by appeal to a clear notion of needs.

It is easy to see why too many things appear to be needs. Without abuse of language, we refer to the means necessary to reach any of our goals as needs. To reawaken memories of Miller's, the neighborhood delicatessen of my childhood, I need only the smell of sour pickles in a barrel. To paint my son's swing set, I need a clean brush.[1] The problem of the importance of needs seems to reduce to the problem of the importance or urgency of preferences or wants in general (leaving aside the fact that not all the things we need are expressed as preferences).

But just as not all preferences are on a par—some are more important than others—so too not all the

From *Philosophy & Public Affairs* 10 (Spring 1981), pp. 146–155, 158–161, 163, 165–166, 168, 171–179. Copyright ©1981 by Princeton University Press. Reprinted by permission of the author and Princeton University Press.

things we say we need are. It is possible to pick out various things we say we need, including needs for health care, which play a special role in a variety of moral contexts. Taking a cue from T. M. Scanlon's discussion in "Preference and Urgency," we should distinguish *subjective* and *objective* criteria of well-being.[2] We need *some* such criterion to assess the importance of competing claims on resources in a variety of moral contexts. A *subjective* criterion uses the relevant individual's own assessment of how well-off he is with and without the claimed benefit to determine the importance of his preference or claim. An *objective* criterion invokes a measure of importance independent of the individual's own assessment, for example, independent of the *strength* of his preference.

In contexts of distributive justice and other moral contexts, we do *in fact* appeal to some *objective* criteria of well-being. We refuse to rely solely on subjective ones. If I appeal to my friend's duty of beneficence in requesting $100, I will most likely get a quite different reaction if I tell him I need the money to get a root-canal than if I tell him I need the money to go to the Brooklyn neighborhood of my childhood to smell pickles in a barrel. Indeed, it is not likely to matter in his assessment of *obligations* that I strongly *prefer* to go to Brooklyn. Nor is it likely to matter if I insist I feel a great *need* to reawaken memories of my childhood—I am overcome by nostalgia. (He might give me the money for either purpose, but if he gives it so I can smell pickles, we would probably say he is not doing it out of any duty at all, that he feels no obligation.) Similarly, if my appeal was directed to some (even utopian) social welfare agency rather than my friend, it would adopt objective criteria in assessing the importance of the request independent of my own strength of preference. . . .

The real issue behind Scanlon's insightful discussion is the choice between objective *truncated* or selective scales of well-being and either objective or subjective *full-range* or "satisfaction" scales of well-being. I shall return shortly to consider why the truncated scale *ought to be* (and not just *is*) the measure used in issues of social justice.

One indication that we appeal to an objective, truncated standard is that I might say the root-canal, but not the smell of pickles in a barrel, is something I *really* need (assuming the dentist is right). It is a *need* and not just a desire. The implication is that some of

the things we claim to need fall into special categories which give them a weightier moral claim in contexts involving the distribution of resources (depending, of course, on how well-off we already are within those categories of need).[3] Our task is to characterize the relevant categories of needs in a way that *explains* two central properties these special needs have. First, these needs are *objectively ascribable:* we can ascribe them to a person even if he does not realize he has them and even if he denies he has them because his preferences run contrary to the ascribed needs. Second, and of greater interest to us, these needs are *objectively important:* we attach a special weight to claims based on them in a variety of moral contexts, and we do so independently of the weight attached to these and competing claims by the relevant individuals. So our philosophical task is to characterize the class of things we need which has these properties and to do so in such a way that we explain why such importance is attached to them.

NEEDS AND SPECIES-TYPICAL FUNCTIONING

One plausible suggestion for distinguishing the relevant needs from all the things we can come to need is David Braybrooke's distinction between "course-of-life needs" and "adventitious needs." *Course-of-life needs* are those needs which people "have all through their lives or at certain stages of life through which all must pass." *Adventitious needs* are the things we need because of the particular contingent projects (which may be long-term ones) on which we embark. Human course-of-life needs would include food, shelter, clothing, exercise, rest, companionship, a mate (in one's prime), and so on. Such needs are not themselves deficiencies, for example, when they are anticipated. But a deficiency with respect to them "endangers the normal functioning of the subject of need *considered as a member of a natural species*."[4] A related suggestion can be found in McCloskey's discussion of the human and personal needs we appeal to in political argument. He argues that needs "relate to what it would be detrimental to us to lack, *where the detrimental is explained by reference to our natures as men and specific persons*."[5]

The suggestion here is that the needs which interest us are those things we need in order to achieve or maintain species-typical normal functioning. Do such needs have the two properties noted earlier? Clearly they are objectively ascribable, assuming we can come up with the appropriate notion of species-typical functioning. (So, incidentally, are adventitious needs, assuming we can determine the relevant goals by reference to which the adventitious needs become determinate.) Are these needs objectively important in the appropriate way? In a broad range of contexts we do treat them as such—a claim I shall not trouble to argue. What is of interest is to see *why* being in such a need category gives them their special importance.

A tempting first answer might be this: whatever our specific chosen goals or tasks, our ability to achieve them (and consequently our happiness) will be diminished if we fall short of normal species functioning. So, whatever our specific goals, we need these course-of-life needs, and therein lies their objective importance. We need them whatever else we need. For example, it is sometimes said that whatever our chosen goals or tasks, we need our health, and so appropriate health care. But this claim is not strictly speaking true. For many of us, some of our goals, perhaps even those we feel most important to us, are not necessarily undermined by failing health or disability. Moreover, we can often adjust our goals—and presumably our levels of satisfaction—to fit better with our dysfunction or disability. Coping in this way does not necessarily diminish happiness or satisfaction in life.

Still, there is a clue here to a more plausible account: impairments of normal species functioning reduce the range of opportunity we have within which to construct life-plans and conceptions of the good we have a reasonable expectation of finding satisfying or happiness-producing. Moreover, if persons have a high-order interest in preserving the opportunity to revise their conceptions of the good through time, then they will have a pressing interest in maintaining normal species functioning by establishing institutions—such as health-care systems—which do just that. So the kinds of needs Braybrooke and McCloskey pick out by reference to normal species functioning are objectively important because they meet this high-order interest persons have in maintaining a normal range of opportunities. I shall try to refine this admittedly vague answer, but first I want to characterize health-care needs more specifically and show that they fit within this more general framework.

HEALTH CARE NEEDS

DISEASE AND HEALTH

To specify a notion of health-care needs, we need clear notions of health and disease. I shall begin with a narrow, if not uncontroversial, "biomedical" model of disease and health. The basic idea is that health is the absence of disease, and diseases (I here include deformities and disabilities that result from trauma), are *deviations from the natural functional organization of a typical member of a species.*[6] The task of characterizing this natural functional organization falls to the biomedical sciences, which must include evolutionary theory since claims about the design of the species and its fitness to meeting biological goals underlie at least some of the relevant functional ascriptions. The task is the same for man and beast, with two complications. For humans we require an account of the species-typical functions that permit us to pursue biological goals as social animals. So there must be a way of characterizing the species-typical apparatus underlying such functions as the acquisition of knowledge, linguistic communication, and social cooperation. Moreover, adding mental disease and health into the picture complicates the issue further, most particularly because we have a less well-developed theory of species typical mental functions and functional organization. The "biomedical" model clearly presupposes we can, in theory, supply the missing account and that a reasonable part of what we now take to be psychopathology would show up as diseases.[7]

• • •

Though I have deliberately selected a rather narrow model of disease and health, at least by comparison to some fashionable construals, *health care needs* emerge as a broad and diverse set. Health care needs will be those things we need in order to maintain, restore, or provide functional equivalents (where possible) to normal species functioning. They can be divided into:

1. adequate nutrition, shelter
2. sanitary, safe, unpolluted living and working conditions
3. exercise, rest, and other features of healthy life-styles
4. preventive, curative, and rehabilitative personal medical services
5. non-medical personal (and social) support services

Of course, we do not tend to think of all these things as included among health-care needs, partly because we tend to think narrowly about personal medical services when we think about health care. But the list is not constructed to conform to our ordinary notion of health care but to point out a functional relation between quite diverse goods and services, and the various institutions responsible for delivering them.

DISEASE AND OPPORTUNITY

The *normal opportunity range* for a given society will be the array of "life-plans" reasonable persons in it are likely to construct for themselves. The range is thus relative to key features of the society—its stage of historical development, its level of material wealth and technological development, and even important cultural facts about it. Facts about social organization, including the conception of justice regulating its basic institutions, will of course determine how that total normal range is distributed in the population. Nevertheless, that issue of distribution aside, normal species-typical functioning provides us with one clear parameter relevant to defining the normal opportunity range. Consequently, impairment of normal functioning through disease constitutes a fundamental restriction on individual opportunity relative to the normal opportunity range.

There are two important points to note about the normal opportunity range. Obviously some diseases constitute more serious curtailments of opportunity than others relative to a given range. But because normal ranges are society relative, the same disease in two societies may impair opportunity differently and so have their importance assessed differently. Thus the social importance of particular diseases is a notion we plausibly ought to relativize between societies, assuming for the moment that impairment of opportunity is a relevant consideration. Within a society, however, the normal opportunity range abstracts from important individual differences in what might be called *effective opportunity*. From the perspective of an individual with a particular conception of the good (life plan or utility function), one who has developed certain skills and capacities needed to carry out chosen projects, *effective* opportunity range will be a subspace of the normal range. A college teacher whose career and recreational skills rely little on certain kinds of manual dexterity might find his effective opportunity diminished little compared to what a skilled laborer might find if disease impaired that dexterity. By appealing to the normal range I abstract from these differences in effective range, just as I avoid appeals

directly to a person's conception of the good when I seek a measure for the social importance (for claims of justice) of health care needs.[8]

What emerges here is the suggestion that we use impairment of the normal opportunity range as a fairly crude measure of the relative importance of health-care needs at the macro level. In general, it will be more important to prevent, cure, or compensate for those disease conditions which involve a greater curtailment of normal opportunity range. Of course, impairment of normal species functioning has another distinct effect. It can diminish satisfaction or happiness for an individual, as judged by that individual's conception of the good. Such effects are important at the micro level—for example, to individual decision-making about health-care utilization. But I am here seeking the appropriate framework within which to apply principles of justice to health care at the macro level. So we shall have to look further at considerations that weigh against appeals to satisfaction at the macro level.

TOWARD A DISTRIBUTIVE THEORY

SATISFACTION AND NARROWER MEASURES OF WELL-BEING

. . .We can characterize health-care needs as things we need to maintain, restore, or compensate for the loss of normal species functioning. Since serious impairments of normal functioning diminish our capacities and abilities, they impair individual opportunity range relative to the range normal for our society. If we suppose people have an interest in maintaining a fair and roughly equal opportunity range, we can give at least a plausible *explanation* of why they think health-care needs are special and important (which is not to say we actually do distribute them accordingly).

In what follows, I shall urge a normative claim: we ought to subsume health care under a principle of justice guaranteeing fair equality of opportunity. Actually, since I cannot here defend such a general principle without going too deeply into the general theory of distributive justice, I shall urge a weaker claim: *if* an acceptable theory of justice includes a principle providing for fair equality of opportunity, then health-care institutions should be among those governed by it. Indeed, I shall sketch briefly how one general theory, Rawls' theory of justice as fairness, might be extended in this way to provide a distributive theory for health care. *But my account does not pre-*

suppose the acceptability of Rawls' theory. If a rule or ideal code-utilitarianism, or some other theory, establishes a fair equality of opportunity principle, my account will probably be compatible with it (though some of the argument that follows may not be).

•   •   •

EXTENDING RAWLS' THEORY TO HEALTH CARE

Rawls' *index of primary social goods*—his truncated scale of well-being used in the contract—includes five types of social goods: (a) a set of basic liberties; (b) freedom of movement and choice of occupations against a background of diverse opportunities; (c) powers and prerogatives of office; (d) income and wealth; (e) the social bases of self-respect. Actually, Rawls uses two simplifying assumptions when using the index to assess how well-off (representative) individuals are.

•   •   •

The most promising strategy for extending Rawls' theory without tampering with useful assumptions about the index of primary goods simply includes health-care institutions among the background institutions involved in providing for fair equality of opportunity. Once we note the special connection of normal species functioning to the opportunity range open to an individual, this strategy seems the natural way to extend Rawls' view that *the subject* of theories of social justice are the *basic institutions* which provide a framework of liberties and opportunities within which individuals can use fair income-shares to pursue their own conceptions of the good. Insofar as meeting health-care needs has an important effect on the distribution of health, and more to the point, on the distribution of opportunity, the health-care institutions are plausibly included on the list of basic institutions a fair equality of opportunity principle should regulate.

Including health-care institutions among those which are to protect fair equality of opportunity is compatible with the central intuitions behind wanting to guarantee such opportunity in the first place. Rawls is primarily concerned with *the opportunity to pursue careers*—jobs and offices—that have various benefits attached to them. So equality of opportunity is *strategically* important: a person's well-being will be measured for the most part by the primary goods that accompany placement in such jobs and offices. Rawls argues it is not enough simply to eliminate formal or legal barriers to persons seeking such jobs—for

example, race, class, ethnic, or sex barriers. Rather, positive steps should be taken to enhance the opportunity of those disadvantaged by such social factors as family background. The point is that none of us *deserves* the advantages conferred by accidents of birth—either the genetic or social advantages. These advantages from the "natural lottery" are morally arbitrary, and to let them determine individual opportunity—and reward and success in life—is to confer arbitrariness on the outcomes. So positive steps, for example, through the educational system, are to be taken to provide fair equality of opportunity.

But if it is important to use resources to counter the advantages in opportunity some get in the natural lottery, it is equally important to use resources to counter the natural disadvantages induced by disease (and since class-differentiated social conditions contribute significantly to the etiology of disease, we are reminded disease is not just a product of the natural component of the lottery). But this does not mean we are committed to the futile goal of eliminating all natural differences between persons. Health care has as its goal normal functioning and so concentrates on a specific class of obvious disadvantages and tries to eliminate them. That is its *limited* contribution to guaranteeing fair equality of opportunity.

•   •   •

WORRIES AND QUALIFICATIONS

I would like to address [a worry that arises] in response to the approach to equality of opportunity that I have been sketching, though no doubt there are others.

[This] worry [is] about what commitments the appeal to equal opportunity generates. . . . Certain "hard" cases raise the issue sharply. What does asking for the restoration of normal opportunity range mean for the terminally ill, on whom we lavish exotic life-prolonging technology, or for the severely mentally retarded? We are not required to pour all our resources into the worst cases, for that would undermine our ability to protect the opportunity of many others. But I am not sure what the approach requires here, if it delivers an answer at all. Similarly, the approach provides little help with another sort of hard case, the resource allocation decisions in which we must choose between services which remove serious impairments of opportunity for a few people and those which remove significant but less serious impairments from many. But these shortcomings are not special to the approach I sketch: distributive theories generally founder on such cases. It seems reasonable to test my approach first in the cases where we have a better understanding of what kind of health care is owed. In any case, I do not rule out here the strong response sketched earlier to the worry about exhaustiveness, namely that our problem with at least the first kind of hard case derives from the fact that it takes us beyond the domain of justice into other considerations of right.

The . . . worry also has more fundamental sources. Suppose supplying a car to everyone who cannot afford one would do more to remove individual impairments of normal opportunity range than supplying certain health care services to those who need them. Does the opportunity approach commit us now to supply cars instead of treatments?[9] The example is an instance of a far more general problem, namely, that socioeconomic (and other) inequalities affect opportunity (broadly or narrowly construed), not just the health-care and educational needs we have picked out as strategically important. But my approach does not require me to deny that certain inequalities in wealth and income may conflict with fair equality of opportunity and that guaranteeing fair equality of opportunity may thus constrain acceptable inequalities in these goods. Rather, my approach rests on the calculation that certain institutions meet needs which quite generally have a central impact on opportunity range and which should therefore be governed directly by the opportunity principle.

Finally, the . . . worry can be traced to the fear that health-care needs are so *expansive* (and expensive), given the advance of technology, that they create a bottomless pit. Fried, for example, argues that recognizing individual right claims to the satisfaction of health-care needs would force society to forgo realizing other social goals. He cautions we would end up worshipping the opportunity to pursue our goals but having to forgo the pursuit. Here we have the other form of the social hijacking argument, hijacking by needs rather than by preferences.[10]

Two points can be offered in response to Fried's version of the . . . worry. First, the narrow model I have given of health-care needs excludes some of the kinds of cases Fried uses to demonstrate the threat of the bottomless pit. Thus Fried's example of retarding the effects of normal aging does not emerge as a *need*

on my analysis, since normal aging does not involve a departure from normal species functioning. Such uses of health-care technology may be thought important in a particular society. Then, arguments about the relative merits of this use of scarce resources may be advanced. But such arguments would not rest on claims about basic health-care needs and thus may have different justificatory force. Still, technology does expand the ways (and costs) we have of meeting genuine health care needs. So my account of needs at best reduces but does not eliminate Fried's worry.

Second, there is a difference between Fried's account of individual rights and entitlements and the one I am assuming here (which is quite Rawlsian). Fried is worried that if we posit a fundamental individual right to have needs satisfied, no other social goals will be able to override the right claims to all health care needs.[11] But no such fundamental right is *directly* posited on the view I have sketched. Rather, the particular rights and entitlements of individuals to have certain needs met are specified only *indirectly,* as a result of the basic health-care institutions acting in accord with the general principle governing opportunity. Deciding which needs are to be met and what resources are to be devoted to doing so requires careful moral judgment. The various institutions which affect opportunity must be weighed against each other. Similarly, the resources required to provide for fair equality of opportunity must be weighed against what is needed to provide for other important social institutions. Clearly, health-care institutions capable of protecting opportunity can be maintained only in societies whose productive capacities they do not undermine. The bugaboo of the bottomless pit is less threatening in the context of such a theory. The price paid is that we are less clear—in general and abstracting from the application of the theory to a given society—just what the individual claim comes to. This price is worth paying.

These worries emphasize the sense in which my account is sketchy and programmatic. It is worth a reminder that my account is incomplete in other ways. I have not argued that opportunity-based considerations are the only ones that should bear on the design of health care systems. Other important social goals—some protected by right claims or other claims of need—may require the use of health-care technology. I have not considered when, if ever, these needs or rights take precedence over other wants and preferences or over some health-care needs.[12] Similarly, there is the question whether the demand for equality in health care extends beyond some decent adequate minimum—which we may suppose is defined by reference to fair equality of opportunity. Should those health-care services not considered basic be allowed to operate on a market basis? Should we insist on equality even here? These issues are not addressed by my analysis.[13]

Finally, my account is incomplete because I have concentrated on social obligations to maintain and restore health and have ignored individual responsibility to do so. But there is substantial evidence that individuals can do much to avoid incurring risks to their health—by avoiding smoking, excess alcohol, and certain foods, and by getting adequate exercise and rest. Now, nothing in my approach is incompatible with encouraging people to adopt healthy lifestyles. The harder issue, however, is deciding how to distribute the burdens that result when people "voluntarily" incur extra risks and swell the costs of health care by doing so (by over 10 percent, on some estimates). After all, the consequences of such behavior cannot be easily dismissed as the arbitrary outcome of the natural lottery. Should smokers be forced to pay higher insurance premiums or special health-care taxes? I do not believe my account forces us to ignore the source of health-care risks in assigning such burdens. But at this point little more can be said because much here depends on very specific details of social history. In the United States, government subsidies of the tobacco industry, the legality of cigarette advertising, the legality of smoking in public places, and special subculture pressures on key groups (for example, teenagers) all undermine the view that we have clear-cut cases of informed, individual decision-making for which individuals must be held fully accountable.

APPLICATIONS

The account of health-care needs sketched here has a number of implications of interest to health planners. Here I can only note some of them and set aside the many difficulties that face drawing implications from ideal theory for non-ideal settings.[14]

ACCESS

My account is compatible with (but does not imply) a multi-tiered health-care system. The basic tier would include health-care services that meet important health-care needs, defined by reference to their effects on opportunity. Other tiers would include services that meet less important health-care needs or

other preferences. However the upper tiers are to be financed—through cost-sharing, at full-price, at "zero" price[15]—there should be no obstacles, financial, racial, sexual, or geographical to *initial access to* the system as a whole.

The equality of initial access derives from basic facts about the sociology and epistemology of the determination of health-care needs.[16] The "felt needs" of patients are (unreliable) initial indicators of real health care needs. Financial and geographical barriers to initial access—say to primary care—compel people to make their own determinations of the importance of their symptoms. Of course, every system requires some patient self-assessment, but financial and geographical barriers impose different burdens in such assessment on particular groups. Indeed, where sociological barriers exist to people utilizing services, positive steps are needed (in the schools, at work, in neighborhoods) to make sure unmet needs are detected.

It is sometimes argued that the difficult access problems are ones deriving from geographical barriers and the maldistribution of physicians within specialties. In the United States, it is often argued that achieving more equitable distribution of health care providers would unduly constrain physician liberties. It is important to see that no fundamental liberties need be violated. Suppose that the basic tier of a health-care system is redistributively financed through a national health insurance scheme that eliminates financial barriers, that no alternative insurance for the basic tier is allowed, and that there is central planning of resource allocation to guarantee needs are met. To achieve a more equitable distribution of physicians, planners *license those eligible for reimbursement* in a given health-planning region according to some reasonable formula involving physician-patient ratios.[17] Additional providers might practice in an area, but they would be without benefit of third-party payments for all services in the basic tier (or for other tiers if the national insurance scheme is more comprehensive). Most providers would follow the reimbursement dollar and practice where they are most needed.

Far from violating basic liberties, the scheme merely puts physicians in the same relation to market constraints on job availability that face most other workers and professionals. A college professor cannot simply decide there are people to be taught in Scarsdale or Chevy Chase or Shaker Heights; he must accept what jobs are available within universities, wherever they are. Of course, he is "free" to ignore the market, but then he may not be able to teach. Similarly, managers and many types of workers face the need to locate themselves where there is a need for their skills. So the physician's sacrifice of liberty under the scheme (or variants on it, including a National Health Service) is merely the imposition of a burden already faced by much of the working population. Indeed, the scheme does not change in principle the forces that already motivate physicians; it merely shifts where it is profitable for some physicians to practice. The appearance that there is an enshrined liberty under attack is the legacy of a historical accident, one more visible in the United States than elsewhere, namely, that physicians have been more independent of institutional settings for the delivery of their skills than many other workers, and even than physicians in other countries. But this too shall pass.

RESOURCE ALLOCATION

My account of health-care needs and their connection to fair equality of opportunity has a number of implications for resource-allocation issues. I have already noted that we get an important distinction between the use of health-care services to meet health-care needs and their use to meet other wants and preferences. The tie of health-care needs to opportunity makes the former use special and important in a way not true of the latter. Moreover we get a crude criterion—impact on normal opportunity range—for distinguishing the importance of different health-care needs, though I have also noted how far short this falls of being a solution to many hard allocation questions. Three further implications are worth noting here.

There has been much debate about whether the United States' health-care system overemphasizes acute therapeutic services as opposed to preventive and public health measures. Sometimes the argument focuses on the relative efficacy and cost of preventive, as opposed to acute, services. My account suggests there is also an important issue of distributive justice here. Suppose a system is heavily weighted toward acute interventions, yet it provides equal access to its services. Thus anyone with severe respiratory ailments—black lung, brown lung, asbestosis, emphysema, and so on—is given adequate and com-

prehensive services as needed. Does the system meet the demands of equity? Not if they are determined by the approach of fair equality of opportunity. The point is that people are differentially at risk of contracting such diseases because of work and living conditions. Efficacy aside, preventive measures have distinct distributive implications from acute measures. The opportunity approach requires we attend to both.

My account points to another allocational inequity. One important function of health-care services, here personal medical services, is to restore handicapping dysfunctions, for example, of vision, mobility, and so on. The medical goal is to cure the diseased organ or limb where possible. Where cure is impossible, we try to make function as normal as possible, through corrective lenses or prosthesis and rehabilitative therapy. But where restoration of function is beyond the ability of medicine per se, we begin to enter another area of services, nonmedical social support (we move from (4) to (5) on the list of health-care needs). Such support services provide the blind person with the closest he can get to the functional equivalent of vision—for example, he is taught how to navigate, provided with a seeing-eye dog, taught Braille, and so on. From the point of view of their impact on opportunity, medical services and social support services that meet health-care needs have the same rationale and are equally important. Yet, for various reasons, probably having to do with the profitability and glamor of personal medical service and careers in them as compared to services for the handicapped, our society has taken only slow and halting steps to meet the health-care needs of those with permanent disabilities. These are matters of justice, not charity; we are not facing conditions of scarcity so severe that these steps to provide equality of opportunity must be forgone in favor of more pressing needs. The point also has implications for the problem of long-term care for the frail elderly, but I cannot develop them here.

A final implication of the account raises a different set of issues, namely, how to reconcile the demands of justice with certain traditional views of a physician's obligation to his patients. The traditional view is that the physician's direct responsibility is to the well-being of his patients, that (with their consent) he is to do everything in his power to preserve their lives and well-being. One effect of leaving all resource-allocation decisions in this way to the micro-level decisions of physicians and patients, especially where third-party payment schemes mean little or no rationing by price, is that cost-ineffective utilization results. In the current cost-conscious climate, there is pressure to make physicians see themselves as responsible for introducing economic considerations into their utilization decisions. But the issue raised here goes beyond cost-effectiveness. My account suggests that there are important resource-allocation priorities that derive from considerations of justice. In a context of moderate scarcity, this suggests it is not possible for physicians to see as their ideal the maximization of the quality of care they deliver regardless of cost: pursuing that ideal upsets resource-allocation priorities determined by the opportunity principle. Considerations of justice challenge the traditional (perhaps mythical) view that physicians can act as the unrestrained agents of their patients. The remaining task, which I pursue elsewhere, is to show at what level the constraints should be imposed so as to disturb as little as possible of what is valuable about the traditional view of physician responsibility.[18]

These remarks on applications are frustratingly brief, and fuller development of them is required if we are to assess the practical import of the account I offer. Nevertheless, I think the account offers enough that it is attractive at the theoretical level to warrant further development of its practical implications.

NOTES

1. For emphasis, we often refer to things we simply desire or want as things we need. Sometimes we invoke a distinction between noun and verb uses of "need," so that not everything we say we need counts as *a need*. Any distinction we might draw between noun and verb uses depends on our purposes and the context and would still have to be explained by the kind of analysis I undertake above.

2. T. M. Scanlon, "Preference and Urgency," *Journal of Philosophy* 77, no. 19 (November 1975), 655–669.

3. *Ibid.*, p. 660.

4. David Braybrooke, "Let Needs Diminish That Preferences May Prosper," in *Studies in Moral Philosophy,* American Philosophical Quarterly Monograph Series, No. 1 (Oxford: Blackwell, 1968), p. 90 (my emphasis).

5. McCloskey, unlike Braybrooke, is committed to distinguishing a narrower noun use of "need" from the verb use. See H. J. McCloskey, "Human Needs, Rights, and Political Values," *American Philosophical Quarterly* 13, no. 1 (January 1976), 2f (my emphasis).

6. The account here draws on a fine series of articles by Christopher Boorse; see "On the Distinction Between Disease and Illness," *Philosophy & Public Affairs* 5, no. 1 (Fall 1975); 49–68; "What a Theory of Mental Health Should Be," *Journal of the Theory of Social Behavior* 6, no. 1, 61–84; "Health as a Theoreti-

cal Concept," *Philosophy of Science* 44 (1977), 542–573. See also Ruth Macklin, "Mental Health and Mental Illness: Some Problems of Definition and Concept Formation," *Philosophy of Science* 39, no. 3 (September 1972), 341–365.

7. Boorse, "What a Theory of Mental Health Should Be," p. 77.

8. One issue here is to avoid "hijacking" by past preferences which themselves define the effective range. Of course, effective range may be important in microallocation decisions.

9. Using medical technology to enhance normal capacities or functions—say strength or vision—makes the problem easier: the burden of proof is on proposals that give priority to altering the normal opportunity range rather than protecting individuals whose normal range is compromised.

10. See Charles Fried, *Right and Wrong* (Cambridge, Mass.: Harvard University Press, 1978), chap. 5. The problem also worries Braybrooke, "Let Needs Diminish."

11. It is not clear to me how much Fried's side-constraints resemble Nozick's.

12. My account has the following bearing on the debate about Medicaid-funded abortions. Non-therapeutic abortions do not count as health-care needs, so *if* Medicaid has as its only function the meeting of the health-care needs of the poor, then we cannot argue for funding the abortions just like any other procedure. Their justifications will be different. But if Medicaid should serve other important goals, like ensuring that poor and well-off women can equally well control their bodies, then there is justification for funding abortions. There is also the worry that not funding them will contribute to other health problems induced by illegal abortions.

13. Except where conditions of extensive scarcity leave basic health-care needs unmet and so no room for less important uses of health-care services, or except where the existence of a market-based health-care system threatens the ability of the basic system to deliver its important product.

14. I discuss these difficulties in "Conflicting Objectives and the Priorities Problem," to appear in Peter Brown, Conrad Johnson, and Paul Vernier, eds., *Income Support: Conceptual and Policy Issues* (Rowman and Littlefield, forthcoming). My *Justice and Health Care Delivery* develops some applications in detail.

15. The strongest objections to such mixed systems is that the upper tier competes for resources with the lower tiers. See Claudine McCreadie, "Rawlsian Justice and the Financing of the National Health Service," *Journal of Social Policy* 5, no. 2 (1976), 113–131.

16. See Avedis Donabedian, *Aspects of Medical Care Administration* (Cambridge: Harvard, 1973).

17. I ignore the crudeness of such measures. For fuller discussion of these manpower distribution issues see my "What is the Obligation of the Medical Profession in the Distribution of Health Care?" presented to the Conference on Health Care and Human Rights, University of Cincinnati Medical Center, 6 March 1980.

18. See Avedis Donabedian, "The Quality of Medical Care: A Concept in Search of a Definition," *Journal of Family Practice* 9, no. 2 (1979), 277–284; and Daniels, "Cost-Effectiveness and Patient Welfare," in Marc Basson, ed., *Rights and Responsibilities in Modern Medicine,* Ethics, Humanism, and Medicine Series (New York: Alan R. Liss, 1981).

ROBERT M. VEATCH

What Is a "Just" Health Care Delivery?

MAJOR THEORIES OF DISTRIBUTING HEALTH CARE

. . . Competing bases for distribution can, for purposes of policy analysis, be summarized in three major competing theories of justice. Each has been used to support some health care policy and implicitly some National Health Insurance proposals.

THE UTILITARIAN THEORY OF A JUST HEALTH CARE DELIVERY

At first it seems reasonable to distribute health care so as to maximize the health of the society. The goal should be to improve the major social measures of health—infant mortality, average life expectancy, days of hospitalization, days of morbidity by disease—as much as possible. This is a health application of classical utilitarianism. According to the utilitarian position, the objective is to increase the net good in society to the greatest possible amount without regard to how that good is distributed except insofar as the distribution itself contributes to the total amount of good (through decreasing marginal utility or decreasing social unrest).

While health planning—as seen in the practices of cost-benefit analysis, PPBS, and the social indicators movement—seems based squarely on utilitarian, good-maximizing premises, I am convinced they are mistaken. The argument that utilitarian theory cannot account for our sense of justice is an old one. Suppose that in some hypothetical society the National Health Planning Council was considering ways of improving the health of the nation's citizens. Suppose also that the professional staff for the council had gathered data and made computer projections and had reached the conclusion that one particular plan would most improve the aggregate health indicators for the nation. It was the case in this society that one small group

could be identified as having multiple chronic diseases consuming huge amounts of health resources. These individuals tended to be lower class, of low intelligence, and often brain damaged, so that health instruction had little usefulness. The proposed plan is to identify this group, amounting to 0.1 percent of the population, and ban them from the health care delivery system. The computers indicated that even though this would lower life expectancy for this particular group, it would in aggregate increase not only average life expectancy, but also all the other measures of health.

A second part of the plan would be the identification of the healthiest 10 percent of the population. This group would be encouraged to double their reproduction. Since their contribution to the health statistics would increase, all of the averages would improve.

The utilitarian theory of a just health care delivery would support the plan. In fact, since the sickest in the population would soon die off, morbidity (as opposed to mortality) would be directly improved.

Now utilitarian members of the National Health Planning Council may object. They may point out that the harm of death is critical and must be added to the calculation of goods and harms. Nonhealth harms also might have to be taken into account, such as social malaise or rebellion of the relatives of the sickest ones. It is not logical, however, that the feelings of social guilt would be one such harm, because one would not or should not feel guilty about doing what morality requires. Put more cautiously, the utilitarian should feel even more guilty if he fails to exclude the sickest, because he is consciously choosing to avoid producing the greatest good for the greatest number. One cannot appeal to nonconsequentialist feelings of justice, since those are ruled out by definition in the theory being advocated.

These additional harms would indeed increase the burden of the professional staff of the council—

From Robert M. Veatch and Roy Branson, eds., *Ethics and Health Policy* (Cambridge, Mass.: Ballinger Publishing Company, 1976), pp. 131–142.

provided they conceded that nonhealth harms could be traded off against health goods. (That is a controversial concession to be taken up later.) New computer projections, however, might add in these nonhealth harms.[1] It is conceivable that even after these are added in, the banning of the one in a thousand still turns out to be utility maximizing.

It is the conclusion of nonutilitarians—and I would include myself—that such an outcome would not in itself be sufficient to justify the plan. Furthermore, even if it were the case that adding in enough social harms would always reveal that those policies we find morally objectionable were also not utility maximizing, it does not follow that they are morally wrong because they are not utility maximizing. It could be that they are not utility maximizing because they are wrong (and therefore generate guilt, which is a disutility).

I am convinced the plan of banning the sick is wrong because it is unjust. I am much more convinced that it is wrong than I am convinced of its disutility. In fact, since utility calculations in an area as complex as health care are so intricate, we should always be very uncertain of our judgments—much more uncertain than we actually are—if we based them on the utilitarian theory of a just health care delivery.

THE EGALITARIAN THEORY OF A JUST HEALTH CARE DELIVERY

I propose as an alternative to utilitariansim an egalitarian theory of a just health care delivery. An egalitarian theory of justice is fundamentally opposed to calculating goods—health or otherwise—in the aggregate. It is based on the premise that, at least insofar as health goes, every human being has an equal claim. Since it is health care we are trying to distribute we can formulate the principle as follows: (1) Everyone has a claim to the amount of health care needed to provide a level of health equal to other persons' health.

This sounds much like the first principle (that justice requires that everyone get the resources needed to be healthy). In this form, however, it recognized that healthiness as a goal can generate infinite demands so the egalitarian dimension is made more explicit: those whose health is worst are entitled to enough health care to get them as healthy as others. We would target our efforts on the sickest.

This sounds very similar to the principle articulated by Bernard Williams: "Leaving aside preventative medicine, the proper ground of distribution of medical care is ill health: this is a necessary truth."[2] It is also built on a similar understanding of equality. Williams, in his exposition of the concept of equality, recognized, as we must, that there are obvious physical, intellectual, and genetic differences among humans. There are also differences in ascribed and achieved roles. Beyond this, however, there are fundamental equalities. Common to our humanity is our ability to suffer and feel pain, our desire for affection, and related psychophysiological qualities. Humans may even be unequal in these; however, at least the question is open to empirical testing. Beyond these is what Williams calls "desire for self-respect." Drawing in part on the Kantian maxim that humans are to be treated each as an end and never as a means, Williams argues that each human is "owed the effort of understanding, and that on achieving it, each man is to be (as it were) abstracted from certain conspicuous structures of inequality in which we find him."[3] There is something essential about humans independent of their social, economic, and intellectual condition. This essential quality is sufficient to generate a claim of equality of treatment—at least in certain fundamental ways. This quality (which must be something closely related to Williams's notion of a claim of respect) produces a strong egalitarian claim that cannot be refuted by empirical arguments pointing to the differences among humans in other less essential ways.

The present form of principle (1) also sounds rather similar to Outka's. Beginning with the formal principle that justice requires similar treatment for similar cases, Outka maintains that this leads to the substantive principle that access to health care should be equal for people with similar categories of illness.[4] However, he recognizes a fundamental problem with the formula of this type. To return to our [first] formula, if everyone has a claim to the amount of health care needed to provide a level of health equal to other persons' health, the system will collapse as soon as the person most in need of health care is in need because he has a condition that cannot be treated. If health care is distributed strictly in proportion with ill health, as Williams at least considers "a necessary truth," a group of the incurably sick who are the most ill must end up with *all* the medical resources. This is certainly inefficient. Furthermore, if they do not benefit from the commitment of resources, it is hard to see why it is just that they get those resources. Outka apparently recognized that and thus allows for discrimination according to categories of illness. In doing so, however, his formula of treating similar categories of illness similarly could justify the National Health Planning Council's scheme to ban the 0.1 percent with serious multiple illnesses. Similar cases are treated similarly, but the priority for the neediest can be lost.

A modification might be to recognize that the neediest have a just claim only when something fruitful can come from the resource commitment. Thus: (2) Everyone has a claim to the amount of health care needed to provide a level of health equal, insofar as possible, to other person's health. This principle still will have to be both clarified and modified, but that is the principle in its stark form.

Another qualification is to shift from the duty to actually produce equal health (as far as possible) to a duty to provide an opportunity of equal health. One should not be required to improve his health (if, for instance, he prefers to abjure exercise or proper diet), and justice does not demand that we impose health care or that we provide repeated treatments because an individual does not take advantage of treatments rendered. Thus: (3) Justice requires everyone has a claim to health care needed to provide an opportunity for a level of health equal, as far as possible, to other persons' health.

Two other qualifications may be necessary in the egalitarian principle—one correcting for merit and another correcting for previous social wrong. Both of these qualifications are discussed later. . . .

THE RAWLSIAN MAXIMIN THEORY OF A JUST HEALTH CARE DELIVERY

The third major theory of justice is receiving a great deal of attention in contemporary policy analysis because of the provocative and exciting work of John Rawls.[5] In brief summary Rawls concludes that two distributional principles are required:

1. Each person is to have an equal right to the most extensive total system of equal liberties compatible with a similar system of liberty for all.
2. Social and economic inequalities are to be arranged so that they are both: (a) to the greatest benefit of the least advantaged, consistent with the just savings principle, and (b) attached to

offices and positions open to all under conditions of fair equality of opportunity.[6]

It is often now presumed that this set of distributional principles is the major competitor to the utilitarian societal-good-maximizing principle, and that it properly captures the sense of moral commitment to the least well off that I have attributed to egalitarianism. But that is not the case. The maximin principle is a hybrid principle of moral right in a social distributional context, not a principle of justice that withstands Rawls's own tests.

In order to choose among the three principles of justice there must be a test of justification. There are a number of standard tests—techniques sometimes called "metaethical theories." We might ask what God would approve, what an ideal observer would approve as morally required, what accords with personal or societal feelings or institutions, or what accords with the natural law. Rawls's own method is not precisely the one I would normally support,[7] but it produces conclusions generally consistent with my own ideas.

Rawls asks us to imagine a society of persons formulating rules for social practices. These individuals are self-interested, rational, have access to relevant scientific facts including knowledge of human psychological traits. One clearly counterfactual condition is added, that these individuals have no specific knowledge of their own place in the society, his class, social status, "his fortune in the distribution of natural assets and abilities, his intelligence and strength and the like."[8] They are under a "veil of ignorance." Rawls now asks us to formulate a theory of justice using the original position method as a test. Would such a group indeed accept Rawls's two principles as principles of justice, as Rawls claims?

I am persuaded they would not uniformly adopt them as practices considered most just or fair.[9] Consider a hypothetical test case. Suppose that total amount of primary goods could be quantified for purposes of comparison. Those in the original position are presented with two alternatives (health policies or policies from other areas). One (policy A) would provide every member of the society with 10,000 units of the good, while the second (policy B) would provide everyone with 11,000, except that one percent would receive 100,000. Presumably the incentive to the elite would produce breakthroughs that would trickle down.

Since policy B clearly is more beneficial to the least well off, according to Rawlsian principles it is more just. I am not convinced that people in the original position under the veil of ignorance would find B more just. In fact I do not even find it plausible to conclude that B is always more right. Some (but not necessarily all) reasonable people might choose A. The smaller the marginal increase to the least well off in comparison to the increase in goods to the elite, the less plausible is the Rawlsian formula of justice. The egalitarian theory of justice is one that finds equality of distribution per se a just-making characteristic.

If equality of distribution per se is a just-making characteristic (perhaps one that has to be qualified by consideration of merit or previous social harm), then the maximin formula is not a pure principle of justice at all, but rather a synthesis of both just-making and other right-making characteristics (such as utility maximizing). Rawls specifically acknowledges that he is using the term ''justice''in the narrower sense. Justice ''is not to be confused with the principles defining the other virtues, for the basic structure, and social arrangements generally, may be efficient or inefficient, liberal or illiberal, and many other things, as well as just or unjust.''[10]

Suppose in a health crisis resulting from a hurricane three people are in equal need of health care but the rescue team can treat only one. One of the injured is a physician who, if treated first and well, will be able to treat the others, but only to the point of partial restoration of their health (because of the time that passes). I find it plausible to conclude that it is prudent and right to give the health care to the physician first, and that even the other injured parties would agree to the priority for the physician; but I am not prepared to say that is just or fair. Furthermore, the waiving of the claim to equal treatment by the other injured parties seems to have more weight as a justification than would, say, the maximin argument offered by the physician. In other words, the waiving of the claim to equal distribution in favor of the maximin distribution is more justified if it comes from the least well off themselves rather than other members of the society. This claim that the least well off have more right to waive the equal right to health care than the more well off cannot, I believe, be accounted for by Rawlsian theory.

If that is the case the maximin principle may (under certain partially indeterminant conditions) lead to the most right social policy; it would not, however, be the most just. I would argue that often the maximin would not lead to the most right policy—especially in cases where the least well off would prefer equality.

A health policy that focuses on a distribution that will maximize aggregate health indicators or aggregate economic indicators is most suspect. One that focuses on maximizing the health of the least well off is far superior, but it too is questioned. Justice requires health care sufficient to provide an opportunity for a level of health equal, as far as possible, to the health of others, and requires equality as the ordering principle for funding of health care.

REMAINING SPECIAL PROBLEMS

At several points in the development of the egalitarian principle of health care delivery I have had to postpone consideration of particularly vexing problems. I want now to take up: (1) the conflict between the generally least well off and the medically least well off; (2) claims based on merit; (3) claims of compensatory justice; (4) the question of which diseases have priority; and (5) the conflict between justice and rightness in a health care policy.

THE LEAST WELL OFF: GENERALLY AND MEDICALLY

The principle that justice requires that everyone has a claim to the amount of health care needed to provide an opportunity for a level of health equal, as far as possible, to the health of other persons produces a priority for health care for the sickest insofar as health care can improve their health, qualified by individual freedom to reject that health care if it is not desired. This forces us to deal with the question why the medically least well off ought to be the focus of our distribution principle rather than the generally least well off. This basis of distribution means that the very wealthy, but sick, have a greater claim to a part of the national resources than the very poor person who happens to be healthy. The principles of Pareto optimality would require that the good be given out in as general a form as possible. In this case we might give funds to the generally least well off permitting them to buy housing or food rather than health care if that were their particular need. Since the wealthy but sick individual is not least well off, the funds would, in this example, not be spent for health care at all. According to this approach desire would be one basis on which health care is distributed.[11]

This is a critical challenge to the claim that justice requires that health care be distributed so as to provide an opportunity to equalize the health of the medically least well off. The question is, Why should the wealthy, even the sick wealthy, be included in a health care program at all?

Two answers seem appropriate. First, it could be argued that health is a prior requirement for receipt of any other goods. Rawls has argued that liberty is such a good. One cannot trade off liberty for other goods, because liberty by its very nature is required for enjoyment of the others. Health is, in some ways, like liberty. Certainly death-preventing medical care is like liberty in this respect. However, other forms of health care are not always prior in this way. I think it is meaningful to say that one is generally well off or well off on balance though sick, while it is not meaningful to say that with regard to either death or lack of liberty. Thus it appears that some kinds of health care could receive an absolute priority, taking them out of the general calculation of goods, but by itself is not an altogether convincing argument for separating all health care allocation from the general allocation of goods.

Another argument is a more pragmatic one. While I am not convinced that all with a particular illness, in principle, have an equal claim to health care at government expense without regard to their general financial means, I am convinced that adopting a practice of behaving as if they *did* have an equal claim will serve the interests of the generally least well off as well as the medically least well off, and may promote equality as well. The test case is deciding whether two individuals equally sick, one of whom is poor, the other wealthy, ought to be given equal access to health care under a national health insurance program, or whether their general state ought to be taken as relevant in deciding about health care allocation.

Two arguments support the decision to give the two equal health care independent of how well off they are generally. First, to support the policy of giving funds to the generally least well off one has to be convinced that distribution of a more generalized medium (money) would really be the policy adopted as an alternative. There is strong reason to believe that that is not the case. It is dangerous to assume that if a national health program is not adopted the funds saved will be allocated so as to be more beneficial to the generally least well off. The generally least well off should take what they can get, even if it also benefits those who are not generally least well off. This is, of course, not necessarily an argument from egalitarian justice as we have defined it. If, however, giving equal health care to the poor and the rich added to the welfare of each, it would at least reduce the ratio of their relative welfare and might, if one assumed decreasing marginal utility, decrease the absolute difference. It would not, of course be the policy that would most radically decrease the difference; giving health care only to the poor would decrease it even more. That policy might suffer from the same practical consideration as giving the more generalized medium only to the poor: it might simply never be adopted. This argument for giving equal opportunity for health to the rich and the poor is not a very strong one from the point of view of egalitarian justice.

The second argument for including the medically least well off who generally are better off is stronger. There is reason to believe that having the more wealthy included in the same health system as the poor directly benefits the health care given to the poor. There are at least two ways the poor might benefit from including the wealthy. First, some goods are what might be called social or collective goods. They are not readily divisible. Some practices count as good if, and only if, a critical mass of people participate in the practice. The good of voting or of not walking on the grass accrues only if a critical mass join in the practice. Not everyone need participate, but a large number must. Those who do not will be "free riders." Society can tolerate a certain number of these free riders, but when the critical threshold is crossed, it is not simply the free riders who lose, it is everyone. Some elements of a national health care program may be social or collective goods of this type. Support for health research, for complex equipment, and for highly specialized skilled workers requires a large base of support. If the mass of the middle class were excluded it is quite possible there would not be sufficient support for the social good to result.

This is not the only, or even the primary, way that the poor will benefit by the participation of the relatively wealthy in a national health care program. If those in powerful places must participate in the same health care system as those least well off, the quality of that system may improve not because it adds a critical mass, but because it adds a group with sufficient power to make sure that the care is of high quality and that the patient is treated with respect and dignity. Inclusion of the wealthy might not improve their health at all; it might, in fact, decrease it. An inclusive system, then, might improve the health opportunity of the least well off (improve it even more than if only the poor were included), while it would not improve and might even diminish health opportunity for the better off. The interesting implication of these arguments centering on benefit to the poor if the more wealthy are included is that those well off might have an obligation to participate in the national health care system, whereas if the basis for their inclusion was the general priority of health over other goods, there might be a right to participate, but hardly an obligation.

All arguments considered, a strong case can be made for the general rule of treating the distribution of health care as a phenomenon independent from the more general distribution of goods. The wealthy sick as well as the poor sick should be treated as if they had an equal claim on health care, independent of their general condition. This, of course, may not mean that the burden of paying for the health care would necessarily be the same for the two groups.

MERIT

One historically significant qualifier of the egalitarian principle of distribution is merit. Merit (or some modification of it) can, in principle, be a legitimate qualifier to the egalitarian principle that everyone should have an equal claim to health care sufficient to provide an opportunity to achieve a level of health equal, as far as possible, to other persons'. Consider two individuals (say identical twins) who have had equal genetic and environmental opportunities. Both open small grocery stores, but one works diligently, putting in a sixteen-hour day for twenty years, while the other is slothful, working short days and squandering his resources. It seems to me to be fair (or just) that the first brother has more accumulated goods at the end of the twenty years (even if the memories of experiences may possibly have been richer for the slothful brother).

In principle, justice requires taking into account effort or merit as a consideration of a fair or just distribution of health care. At the same time, I see the gravest danger in including effort or merit as a qualifier of a principle for just distribution of health care. (''Merit'' is a confusing term because it seems to include not only the subjective component of effort, but also native abilities as well. ''Diligence'' or ''ef-

fort'' seems to me to generate the stronger claim.) It seems almost impossible to separate merit or effort from class privilege, inherited wealth and skills, and the social and value biases of those who would be doing the classifying. The error rate in ranking on the basis of effort or merit would seem to be extremely great. Furthermore, the enterprise of ranking individuals on the basis of merit or effort is itself potentially malicious and degrading. Qualifying the egalitarian distribution principle for merit or effort could be justified for some practices in some forms of social organization. However, we are talking about a national policy on the distribution of health care. The dangers appear so great that, with one qualification, any such effort ought to be abandoned.

That one exception is the case of health need resulting from what is seen as a voluntary decision to take a health risk to engage in behavior that is not worthy of public subsidy, such as professional automobile racing, alcohol consumption, smoking, and recreational stunt flying. All are presumed to be voluntary behavior and are thus radically different from health needs as they are normally conceptualized. (If alcoholism were judged a nonvoluntary genetically or psychiatrically determined ''disease,'' it would be excluded from the list.) Furthermore, all are generally not considered activities worthy of public subsidy. This separates them from professional fire fighting, which is voluntary behavior but worthy of subsidy.

Even if these voluntary health-risky behaviors not worthy of public support are thought to generate a lower claim for just health care allocation, humaneness still requires including treatment for such conditions in a national health system. The source of funding for such care, however, might be radically different because of the nature of the medical condition. I have elsewhere supported the view that while all such conditions should be covered by national health insurance, the behaviors should be taxed, where possible, in an amount that would equal the projected costs of the medical treatment.[12]

COMPENSATORY JUSTICE

Another major problem with the general egalitarian principle that everyone has an equal claim to health care sufficient to provide an opportunity for a level of health equal, as far as possible, to the health of others is the claim of those who have suffered previous social wrongs that have previously deprived them of health care opportunities. The question is, Do we have a special obligation of justice to provide health care to those who are sick because of previous social wrongs over and above the obligation to distribute health care on the basis of equality for opportunities for health? Of course, those who have suffered significant social wrongs will often rank high solely on this criterion of need, but is there an additional claim for those whose need derives from previous social harms? In general there is. The duty to provide compensatory justice is a legitimate modifier of the general principle of egalitarian justice. I am not persuaded, however, that the compensatory justice qualifier ought to have significant bearing on the general egalitarian principle for purposes of health care distribution. The question is once again a pragmatic one. If we assume that health need alone will tend to identify those who have suffered previous social wrong, we must compare the justice resulting from the established preference for health care to the wronged group with the risks of singling that group out for an additional priority. I see a great danger in singling out any group for special health care on any basis other than ability to meet medical need. Creating a special class will once again create a two-class health system, with all of the risks involved. While compensatory justice is, in principle, an appropriate qualifier to the egalitarian principle of distribution, I am not convinced that it would add materially to the welfare of those who were previously wronged by society. I remain open for such evidence including expressions of opinions of the wronged groups and would readily incorporate a compensatory justice qualifier if such evidence were found. In this particular case, however, it seems prudent not to create a special health system with special priorities over and above the criteria related to health need.

WHICH DISEASES HAVE PRIORITY?

The thrust of the entire argument has been toward the position that priority go to the diseases or disease combinations that create the most hardship or suffering—to those which make one medically the least well off. The medically worst off have a complete claim of justice on health care resources in order to bring them, as far as possible, up to the level of health of others. This is strikingly different from the usual criteria of distribution in most of the national health insurance proposals, which for the most part focus heavily not on the nature of the diseases or medical conditions but on absolute limits on health care consumption in dollars or days or, in the case of catastrophic illness proposals, the size of the medical bill. . . .

The task of ranking diseases from worst to most benign is rather repulsive as well as gargantuan. Fortunately much of the ranking is unnecessary. We have the capacity to provide available health care necessary to improve the health, insofar as possible of the medically least well off. In fact we can probably work our way up the list of the worst diseases before the question of limits is even raised—if we approach the allocation of health care from this medical egalitarian perspective. Furthermore, we probably can agree on some medical conditions that impose (or ought to impose) so slight a burden that they should not be included in any national health program at this point in history. Alopecia (baldness), most cosmetic surgery, and personal attendance by a physician-traveling companion for general reasons of health safety are examples. The use of certain futuristic biomedical technologies for the satisfaction of medical tastes such as *in vitro* fertilization, prenatal sex selection, or electrical stimulation of the brain's "pleasure centers" might be others.

The real difficulties come in a fairly narrow range. We may not be sure whether patients claiming a need for hemodialysis, semiannual or annual physical examinations, nuclear-powered artificial hearts, dental prostheses, experimental treatments of the aging process, or psychoanalysis have the greatest medical need. If our task is to identify those most in need of health care we need not choose between penicillin for pneumonia and insulin for the diabetic. Certainly both qualify. Only when we get to the borders of our capacity to provide health care does the problem arise. Here the egalitarian claim is that, difficult though it may be, we must include those conditions which constitute the greatest assault on one's health—however that may be defined. The answer will clearly require an understanding of the human norms of healthiness, something requiring arduous philosophical reflection. This, however, is the appropriate task, rather than arbitrarily assigning dollar or day limits to the use of health care resources in a national program. To choose the latter is to distribute health in proportion to the luck of the natural and social lottery and according to our ability to buy health care in the private market.

1. See Chapter Six, "Ethics and Health Care: Computers and Distributive Justice," by Joseph Fletcher, in Robert M. Veatch and Roy Branson, eds., *Ethics and Health Policy* (Cambridge, Mass.: Ballinger, 1976).

2. Bernard Williams, "The Idea of Equality," in *Justice and Equality,* ed. by Hugo Bedau (Englewood Cliffs, N.J.: Prentice-Hall, Inc., 1971), p. 127.

3. *Ibid.*, p. 125.

4. Gene Outka, "Social Justice and Equal Access to Health Care," *Journal of Religious Ethics* 2 (No. 1, 1974), 23–24.

5. John Rawls, *A Theory of Justice* (Cambridge, Mass.: Harvard University Press, 1971).

6. Rawls, p. 302.

7. Robert Veatch, "The Metaethical Foundation for an Ethic of the Life Sciences," *Hastings Center Studies* (No. 1, 1973), 50–65.

8. Rawls, p. 137.

9. Others, some for different reasons, hold that Rawls's principles do not meet his own tests. See Robert Paul Wolff, "A Refutation of Rawls' Theorem on Justice," *Journal of Philosophy* 63 (1966), 179–90; Brian Barry, "On Social Justice," *The Oxford Review* (Trinity Term, 1962), 33–43; Robert Nozick, "Distributive Justice," *Philosophy and Public Affairs* 3 (No. 1, 1973), 45–126; Brian Barry, *The Liberal Theory of Justice* (New York: Oxford University Press, 1973).

10. Rawls, p. 9.

11. Several analysts have advocated market mechanisms and direct money transfers to the poor rather than social service programs. See Vincent Taylor, "How Much Is Good Health Worth?" *Policy Sciences* 1 (1970), 49–72; Martin S. Feldstein, "A New Approach to National Health Insurance," *The Public Interest* 23 (Spring 1971), 93–105.

12. Robert M. Veatch, "Who Should Pay for Smokers' Medical Care?" *Hastings Center Report* 4 (November, 1974), 8–9.

Applications of Health Care Principles

JAMES F. CHILDRESS

Priorities in the Allocation of Health Care Resources

I want to concentrate on [two] major questions in the allocation of resources for and within health care:[1]

1. What resources (time, energy, money, etc.) should be put into health care and into other social goods such as education, defense, eliminating poverty, and improving the environment?

2. Within the area of health care (once we have determined its budget), how much time, energy, money, etc., should we allocate for prevention and how much for rescue or crisis medicine? . . .

The . . . two questions involve "first-order determinations" or macroallocation decisions—how much of a good will be made available? . . .

From *Soundings* 62 (Fall 1979), 258–269.

I. HEALTH CARE VS. OTHER SOCIAL GOODS

Current evidence does not indicate that our great expenditures in health and medical care in, say, the last twenty years have brought us closer to health. In particular, our exotic technologies offer only marginal returns in reducing morbidity and premature death. The advances in health in the last century can be accounted for largely by improvements in living conditions rather than in medical care. Therefore, the pursuit of some other social goods, such as improving the environment and reducing poverty, has beneficial effects on health.

If we accepted the WHO definition of health ("a state of complete physical, mental and social well-being"), all social goods would relate directly or indirectly to health. Practically all allocation decisions would concern the aspects of health to be emphasized and the most effective and efficient means to their realization. But if we assume a narrower and more adequate definition of health (without developing the arguments for it at this point), we have to confront the conflict between health care, especially medical care, and some other social goods, not all of which serve as instruments to better health. For example, should hospitals always have priority over museums and opera houses? One philosopher, Antony Flew, has argued that "morally, so long as hospitals are needed, hospitals must always have priority over amusement parks" on the grounds that pain is not symmetrical with pleasure and that the prior or more fundamental duty is to alleviate pain.[2] But it is not evident (a) that hospitals are primarily to alleviate pain, and (b) that they should always take priority over all other social goods that do not contribute to the aim of hospitals, whether it is the alleviation of pain or some other goal. Health may be a condition for many values for individuals and the community, but it does not have finality or ultimacy. It is not true that when it comes to health, no amount is too much.

Paul Ramsey has said that he does not know how to go about resolving this first priority question—health care in relation to other social goods—because it is "almost, if not altogether incorrigible to moral reasoning" and "to rational determination."[3] Perhaps, as Ramsey suggests, it is basically a *political* question, i.e., one to be resolved through political processes that can reflect the values, preferences and informal priorities of the society. Can one complain of *injustice* if a society puts more money into space programs or defense than health care? "Wrong" priorities may not be unjust unless there are certain basic needs or rights that must be satisfied for justice to be realized.

Suppose we say that just policies give to each according to their needs and that medical care is a basic human need. Medical needs are unpredictable, random, and overwhelming, according to one line of argument, and society ought to be prepared to meet those needs. Such an argument would depend on a vision of human life that we cannot assume in our society—a vision that would rank needs and make health the most important one. Even if we distinguish needs and wants, demands for health care appear to be virtually without limit. And we have to ask how much we are willing to devote to the provision of medical care which, as we have seen, may not be all that important for health.

Another line of argument is that there is what Charles Fried calls a right to a decent minimum of health/medical care,[4] and that society should make sure that there is enough in the budget to meet this need. An argument for equal access to medical care does not necessarily imply a minimum for individuals and thus for the health budget. It may only mean equal access to what is available. And what is available may be meager. But a right to a *decent minimum* establishes a base for individual medical care and, consequently, for the health budget. It would provide a standard for determining the minimum amount for the health care budget. But, again, in the absence of a shared vision of humanity, we may have to resort to the political process to define the decent minimum for individuals.

In short, to determine how to allocate resources for health care in relation to other social goods, we need to resolve several matters: the definition of health, its value, its causes, whether there is a right to a decent minimum of health/medical care, and what that minimum is.

II. PREVENTION VS. RESCUE OR CRISIS MEDICINE

Within the health care budget, how much should we allocate for *prevention* and how much for *rescue* or *crisis medicine*? This question is only one of several that could be raised and profitably discussed about allocative decisions within the health care budget. For example, another very important question concerns *basic research* vs. *applied research*. In response to Ivan Illich, who claims that modern medicine is a major threat to health, Dr. Lewis Thomas replies that we do not really have modern medicine yet.[5] Medicine has "hardly begun as a science." Most diseases cannot be prevented because we do not understand their mechanisms. Until we have more basic research, he contends, we will simply develop more and more "half-way technologies," such as transplanted and artificial organs, that merely compensate for the incapacitating effects of certain diseases whose course we can do little about. A "half-way technology" is designed to "make up for disease, or to postpone death." Usually it is very expensive and requires an expansion of hospital facilities. By contrast, a "high technology" based on an understanding of disease mechanisms is very simple and inexpensive. Compare the treatment of polio by half-way technologies, such as iron lung and support systems, with the simple and inexpensive high technology—the polio vaccine.

I want to concentrate on prevention and crisis or rescue medicine. Although this conflict rarely emerges in a clear and manageable form in debates about public policy, it is present and needs identification and analysis so that we can appreciate the "trade-offs" that we frequently, if unwittingly, make. *Prevention* includes strengthening individuals (e.g., through vaccines), changing the environment, and altering behavioral patterns and lifestyles. As I have indicated, many recent commentators insist that the most effective and efficient way to improve the nation's health is through *prevention* since our current emphasis on rescue medicine now produces only marginal returns. DHEW's *Forward Plan for Health, Fiscal Years 1977-81*, holds: "Only by preventing disease from occurring, rather than treating it later, can we hope to achieve any major improvement in the Nation's health."[6]

This recommendation is at odds with our current macroallocation policies. For example, in 1976 expenditures for health amounted to 11.4% of the federal budget. When that amount (42.4 billion dollars) is assigned to four major determinants of health (human biology, lifestyle, environment, and the health care system), the results are striking: 91% went to the health care system, while 3% went to human biology, 1% to lifestyle, and 5% to environment.[7]

Nevertheless, the evidence for the effectiveness and efficiency of a preventive strategy to reduce morbidity and premature mortality by concentrating on human biology, lifestyle, and environment is by no means conclusive. The appropriate mix of preventive and rescue strategies will depend in part on the state of knowledge of causal links. Despite the dramatic example of polio, some other conditions, such as renal failure, are not the result of a single disease or factor. As a consequence, prevention appears to be only a remote possibility. In some cases prevention (which might involve extensive and expensive screening in order to identify a few persons at risk) may be less cost-effective than therapy after the disease has manifested itself. As Thomas suggests, our uncertainty in these areas is an argument for increased research.

Even if a preventive program (at least in certain areas) would be more effective and efficient, its implementation would not be free of moral, social, and political difficulties. Effectiveness and efficiency, or utility, are not the only relevant standards for

evaluating policies of allocation of resources within health care (which is defined broadly and includes more than medical care). I shall concentrate on (1) the symbolic value of rescue efforts (what is symbolized about both the victim and the rescuer), (2) the duty of compensatory justice generated by the principle of fairness, (3) the principle of equal access, and (4) the principle of liberty.

1. Our society often favors rescue or crisis intervention over prevention because of our putative preference for known, identified lives over statistical lives. The phrase "statistical lives" (Thomas Schelling) refers to unknown persons in possible future peril.[8] They may be alive now, but we do not know which ones of them will be in future peril. Mining companies often are willing to spend vast sums of money to try to rescue trapped miners when they will spend little to develop ways to prevent such disasters even if they could save more lives *statistically* in the long run. At 240 million dollars a year, we could save the lives of 240 workers at coke ovens. We do not know which ones will be saved, and we are not likely as a society to respond enthusiastically to this expenditure. But we cannot ignore statistical lives in a complex, interdependent society, particularly from the standpoint of public policy.

The principle of equality is not violated by including statistical lives in public policy deliberations. It is not merely a matter of sacrificing present persons for future persons, for there are two different distinctions to consider: on the one hand, the distinction between *known* and *unknown* persons; on the other hand, the distinction between *present* and *future* peril.[9] Existing and known persons who may not be in present danger may be in future danger if certain preventive measures are not taken. Thus, preventive measures may aid existing persons who are at risk and not merely future persons.

Following Max Weber, it is possible to distinguish between "goal-rational" (*zweckrational*) and "value-rational" (*wertrational*) conduct.[10] Conduct that is "goal-rational" involves instrumental rationality—reasoning about means in relation to ends. Conduct that is "value-rational" involves matters of value, virtue, character, and identity that are not easily reduced to ends, effects, or even rules of right conduct. There is thus an important distinction between *realizing* a goal and *expressing* a value, attitude or virtue. In the context of debates about prevention and rescue intervention, the "goal-rational" approach concentrates on effectiveness and efficiency in statistical terms, while the "value-rational" approach focuses on the values, attitudes, and virtues that policies express.

This distinction between "value-rational" and "goal-rational" conduct may illuminate the 1972 congressional decision to make funds available for almost everyone who needs renal dialysis or transplantation. This decision followed widespread publicity in the media about particular individuals who were dying of renal failure. One patient was even dialyzed before the House Ways and Means Committee. Now we have a program that costs over a billion dollars each year. Some argue that this decision was an attempt to preserve society's cherished myth that it will not sacrifice individual lives in order to save money. Of course, we make those sacrifices all the time (e.g., when we fail to pass and enforce some safety measures). But society's myth is not as threatened when the sacrificed lives are statistical rather than identified. Hence, decisions to try to rescue identified individuals have symbolic value. It has been said that the Universalists believe that God is too good to damn human beings, and the Unitarians believe that human beings are too good to be damned. Similarly, the symbolic value argument suggests that rescue attempts show that individuals are "priceless" and that society is "too good" to let them die without great efforts to save them. This is society's myth. And, so the argument goes, when Congress acted to cover the costs of renal dialysis, it acted in part to preserve this myth, for the "specific individuals who would have died in the absence of the government program were known.[11] They were identified lives. The policy was "value-rational," if not "goal-rational."

Insofar as this argument focuses on the way rescue interventions symbolize the value of the victims, it encounters difficulties as a basis for allocative decisions. Consider two possibilities. (a) We keep the same total lifesaving budget, but withdraw resources from *preventive* efforts in order to put them in *rescue* efforts so that we can gain the symbolic value of crisis interventions. As Charles Fried argues, "surely it is odd to symbolize our concern for human life by actually doing less than we might to save it," by saving fewer lives than we might in a maximizing strategy. (b) Another possibility is to keep the same prevention

budget, but to take resources from other areas of the larger budget (cf. my discussion of I) so that we can increase crisis interventions. In this case, however, "we symbolize our concern for human life by spending more on human life than in fact it is worth."[12]

The symbolic-value argument focuses not only on the symbolic value of the victims, but also on what is symbolized about the agents: the virtue and character of the society and its members, what is sometimes called "agent-morality." Conduct that is "value-rational," in contrast to "goal-rational," may thus be based on an answer to the questions "Who are we?" or "Who shall we be?" Allocation policies may be thought of as ways for the society to define and to express its sense of itself, its values, and its integrity. From this standpoint, it is possible to argue that rescue efforts should be important, if not dominant, in allocative decisions. As Lawrence Becker notes, "we have (rationally defensible) worries about the sort of moral character represented by people who propose to stand pat and let present victims die for the sake of future possibilities. One who can fail to respond to the call for help is not quite the same sort of character as one who can maximize prevention."[13] Although "agent-morality" has strong appeal, and no doubt influences many of our decisions, it is difficult to determine how much weight it should have in our policy deliberations.

2. In some situations the principle of fairness can generate a duty of *compensatory justice* that assigns priority to identified lives in present danger. In such situations society has an obligation to try to rescue individuals even though it departs from a strategy that would save more lives in the long run. These situations involve some unfairness because of an inequality in the distribution of risks which the society has assigned, encouraged, or tolerated. Suppose that a person who has worked in a coal mine under terrible conditions which should have been corrected is trapped in a cave-in or comes down with a disease related to his working conditions. Fairness requires greater expenditures and efforts for him in order to equalize his risks. Likewise, if society fails to correct certain environmental conditions that may interact with a genetic predisposition to cause some diseases, it may have a duty of compensatory justice. A policy of compensatory justice in health-related matters, of course, faces numerous practical difficulties, such as identifying causation. But it is important to underline the point that the principle of fairness can generate a duty of compensatory justice which sets limits on

utility and efficiency in some situations. Those who argue that individuals voluntarily choose to bear risks and thus waive any claim to compensatory justice need to show that the individuals in question really understand the risks and voluntarily assume them (e.g., do the workers in an asbestos factory have an opportunity to find other employment, to relocate, etc.?). But even the voluntary assumption of risks should not always be construed as a waiver of a claim to compensatory justice when the person is injured (e.g., research-related injuries).[14]

3. If we include statistical lives in a preventive strategy, while allowing for compensatory justice, we still face difficult questions about *distributive justice,* particularly the principle of equality or equal access. It is not enough to maximize aggregate health benefits. Our policies should also meet the test of distributive justice, which is, indeed, presupposed by compensatory or corrective justice. For example, consider a program to reduce hypertension (high blood pressure) which affects approximately 24 million Americans and poses the risk of cardiovascular disease. In order to reduce the morbidity and mortality from cardiovascular disease, Weinstein and Stason propose an anti-hypertensive program on the basis of cost-effectiveness analysis. They recommend the intensive management of known hypertensives instead of public screening efforts. As they recognize, this proposal appears to be disadvantageous to the poor who would probably be unaware of their hypertensive condition because of their limited access to medical care. This inequity might be diminished by Weinstein's and Stason's proposal to give priority to target screening in black communities over community-wide screening, since hypertension is more common among blacks than among whites, and similarly to selective screening in low-income communities.[15]

The formal principle of equality, or justice, is "treat similar cases in a similar way." Of course, such a formulation does not indicate the relevant similarities. When we discuss equal access to medical care, we most often consider medical need, in contrast to geography, finances, etc., as the relevant similarity that justifies similar treatment. Suppose we decide that an effective and efficient strategy to improve the nation's health will not permit us to do all we could do in rescue or crisis medicine. A decision to forgo the development of some technology or therapy may condemn some patients to continued ill health and perhaps to death. Can such a policy be justified?

One possible approach that still respects the formal principle of justice and rules out arbitrary distinctions between patients (e.g., geography and finances) would exclude "entire classes of cases from a priority list." According to Gene Outka, it is more "just to discriminate by virtue of categories of illness, for example, rather than between rich ill and poor ill.[16] Society could decide not to allocate much of its budget for treatment of certain diseases that are rare and noncommunicable, involve high costs, and have little prospect for rehabilitation. The relevant similarity under conditions of scarcity would not be medical need but category of illness. While certain forms of treatment would not be developed and distributed for some categories of illness, care would, nonetheless, be provided. Patients would not be abandoned.

In allocating funds for research into the prevention and treatment of certain diseases, it is important to consider such criteria as the pain and suffering various diseases involve, their costs, and the ages in life when they are likely to occur.[17] By applying criteria such as pain and suffering, we might decide to concentrate less on killer diseases, such as forms of cancer, and more on disabling diseases, such as arthritis. Thus, says Franz Ingelfinger, national health expenditures would reflect the same values that individuals express: "it is more important to live a certain way than to die a certain way."[18]

One danger in establishing priorities among diseases should be noted: a decision about which diseases to treat may in fact conceal a decision about which population groups to treat since some diseases may be more common among some groups.[19] Injustice may result from these priorities.

4. The principle of *liberty* also poses some moral, social, and political difficulties for an effective and efficient preventive strategy. Mounting evidence indicates that a key determinant of an individual's health is his or her *lifestyle.* Leon Kass argues that health care is the individual's duty and responsibility, not a right.[20] And Lester Breslow offers seven rules for good health that are shockingly similar to what our mothers always told us! The rules, based on epidemiological evidence, are: don't smoke, get seven hours sleep each night, eat breakfast, keep your weight down, drink moderately, exercise daily, and don't eat between meals. At age 45, one who has lived by 6 of these rules has a life expectancy eleven years longer than someone who has followed fewer than 4.[21] In his

book, *Who Shall Live?*, Victor Fuchs contrasts the states of Utah and Nevada, which have roughly the same levels of income and medical care, but are at the opposite ends of the spectrum of health. For example, mortality for persons ages 20-59 is approximately 39% higher in Nevada than in Utah. Fuchs asks:

What, then, explains these huge differences in death rates? The answer almost surely lies in the *different lifestyles* of the residents of the two states. Utah is inhabited primarily by Mormons, whose influence is strong throughout the state. Devout Mormons do not use tobacco or alcohol and in general lead stable, quiet lives. Nevada, on the other hand, is a state with high rates of cigarette and alcohol consumption and very high indexes of marital and geographical instability. The contrast with Utah in these respects is extraordinary.[22]

On the one hand, we have increasing evidence that individual behavioral patterns and lifestyles contribute to ill health and premature mortality. On the other hand, we have the liberal tradition that views lifestyles as matters of private choice, not to be interfered with except under certain conditions (e.g., harm to others).

Each person has what Charles Fried calls a *life plan* consisting of aims, ends, values, etc. That life plan also includes a *risk budget,* for we are willing to run certain risks to our health and survival in order to realize some ends.[23] We do not sacrifice all our other ends merely to survive or be healthy. Our willingness to run the risk of death and ill health for success, friendship, and religious convictions discloses the value of those ends for us and gives our lives their style. Within our moral, social, and political tradition, the principle of liberty sets a presumption against governmental interference in matters of lifestyle and voluntary risk-taking. But that presumption may be overridden under some conditions. Let me make a few points about those conditions, which are similar to just war criteria:

1. An important goal is required to override liberty. One such goal might be *paternalism:* to protect a person even when his or her actions do not harm anyone else. This goal is rarely a sufficient justification for interference with liberty. Usually we require that restrictions of liberty be based, at least in part, on the threat of harm to others or to the society (e.g., compulsory vaccinations). We have difficulties with purely paternalistic arguments in requiring seatbelts, helmets, etc. Another goal might be to *protect the financial resources of the community*. If we get national health insurance, we can expect increased pressure to interfere with individual liberty. Why? People simply will not want to have their premiums or taxes increased to pay for the *avoidable afflictions* of others. They will charge that such burdens are unfair.

2. To override the presumption against interfering with liberty, we need strong evidence that the behavior or lifestyle in question really contributes to ill health. This second standard must be underlined because there is a tendency to use a term like "health," which has the ring of objectivity, to impose other values without articulating and defending those values. In Albert Camus' novel, *The Plague,* a doctor and a priest fighting the plague in an Algerian city engage in the following conversation. The priest says to the doctor: "I see that you too are working for the salvation of mankind." "That is not quite correct," the doctor replies, "Salvation is too big a word for me. I am working first of all for man's health." The danger is that "salvation" or "morality" or a certain style of life will be enforced in the name of health although it has little to do with health and more to do with the legislation of morality.

3. Another condition for overriding the presumption against interfering with liberty is that the interference be the *last resort*. Other measures short of interference, such as changing the environment, should be pursued and sometimes continued even when they are less effective and more costly than measures that restrict liberty.

4. A fourth condition is a reasonable assurance that the restriction will have the desired result as well as a net balance of good over evil.

5. Even when we override the principle of liberty, it still has an impact. It requires that we use the least coercive means to reduce risk-taking. For example, information, advice, education, deception, incentives, manipulation, behavior modification, and coercion do not equally infringe liberty. In addition to choosing the least restrictive and the least coercive means, we should evaluate the means on other moral grounds.

These considerations and others come into play when we try to determine whether (and which) incursions into personal liberty are justified. To allocate resources to prevention rather than to rescue is not a simple matter, for successful prevention may infringe autonomy and other moral principles.

NOTES

1. For a similar list of priority questions, see Gene Outka, "Social Justice and Equal Access to Health Care," *Journal of Religious Ethics* 2 (Spring 1974), pp. 11–32.

2. Antony Flew, "Ends and Means," *The Encyclopedia of Philosophy,* edited by Paul Edwards (New York: Macmillan Publishing Co., and The Free Press, 1967), Vol. 2, p. 510.

3. Paul Ramsey, *The Patient as Person* (New Haven: Yale University Press, 1970), pp. 240, 268.

4. Charles Fried, "Equality and Rights in Medical Care," *Implications of Guaranteeing Medical Care,* edited by Joseph G. Perpich (Washington, D.C.: National Academy of Sciences, Institute of Medicine, 1976), pp. 3–14.

5. Lewis Thomas, "Rx for Illich," *The New York Review of Books* (Sept. 16, 1976): 3–4, and *The Lives of a Cell: Notes of a Biology Watcher* (New York: The Viking Press, 1974), pp. 31–36.

6. U.S. Department of Health, Education, and Welfare. Public Health Service. *Forward Plan for Health: FY 1977-81* (DHEW Publication No. [OS] 76-50024), p. 15. Cf. Marc LaLonde, *A New Perspective on the Health of Canadians: A Working Document* (Ottawa, Canada: The Government of Canada, 1974).

7. These categories and figures are presented in Michael S. Koleda, et al., *The Federal Health Dollar: 1969-1976* (Washington, D.C.: National Planning Association, Center for Health Policy Studies, 1977).

8. Thomas Schelling, "The Life You Save May Be Your Own," *Problems in Public Expenditure Analysis,* edited by Samuel B. Chase, Jr. (Washington, D.C.: The Brookings Institution, 1966), pp. 127–66. Cf. Warren Weaver, "Statistical Morality," *Christianity and Crisis,* Vol. XX, No. 24 (Jan. 23, 1961), 210–13.

9. Charles Fried, *An Anatomy of Values: Problems of Personal and Social Choice* (Cambridge, Mass.: Harvard University Press, 1970), pp. 224f. Fried's argument is important for much of this section of the paper.

10. See Max Weber, *Max Weber on Law in Economy and Society,* edited and annotated by Max Rheinstein and translated by Edward Shils and Max Rheinstein (New York: Simon and Schuster, 1967), p. 1. The translators use the term "purpose-rational" for "zweckrational."

11. Richard Zeckhauser, "Procedures for Valuing Lives," *Public Policy,* Vol. 23 (Fall 1975), 447–48. Contrast Richard A. Rettig, "Valuing Lives: The Policy Debate on Patient Care Financing for Victims of End-Stage Renal Disease," *The Rand Paper Series* (Santa Monica, Cal.: The Rand Corporation, 1976).

12. Fried, *An Anatomy of Values,* p. 217.

13. Lawrence C. Becker, "The Neglect of Virtue," *Ethics* 85 (January 1975), 110–22. See also, Lewis H. LaRue, "A Comment on Fried, Summers, and the Value of Life," *Cornell Law Review* 57 (1972), 621–31 and Benjamin Freedman, "The Case for Medical Care, Inefficient or Not," *The Hastings Center Report* 7 (April 1977), 31–39.

14. For a fuller discussion of compensatory justice, see James F. Childress, "Compensating Injured Research Subjects: The Moral Argument," *The Hastings Center Report* 6 (December 1976), 21–27. Cf. also Charles Fried, *An Anatomy of Values,* p. 220.

15. See Milton C. Weinstein and William B. Stason, "Allocating Resources: The Case of Hypertension," *The Hastings Center Report* 7 (October 1977), 24–29; "Allocation of Resources to Manage Hypertension," *The New England Journal of Medicine* 296 (1977), 732–739; and *Hypertension: A Policy Perspective* (Cambridge: Harvard University Press, 1976).

16. Gene Outka, "Social Justice and Equal Access to Health Care," p. 24.

17. Conrad Taeuber. "If Nobody Died of Cancer. . . ." *The Kennedy Institute Quarterly Report,* Vol. 2, No. 2 (Summer 1976), 6–9.

18. Franz Ingelfinger, Editorial, *The New England Journal of Medicine* 287 (December 7, 1972), 1198–99.

19. Jay Katz and Alexander Morgan Capron, *Catastrophic Diseases: Who Decides What?* (New York: Russell Sage Foundation, 1975), p. 178.

20. Leon Kass, "Regarding the End of Medicine and the Pursuit of Health," *The Public Interest,* No. 40 (Summer 1975), 39.

21. See Nedra B. Belloc and Lester Breslow, "Relationship of Physical Status and Health Practices," *Preventive Medicine* 1 (1972), 409–21, and Nedra B. Belloc, "Relationship of Health Practices and Mortality," *Preventive Medicine* 2 (1973), 67–81.

22. Victor R. Fuchs, *Who Shall Live? Health, Economics and Social Choice* (New York: Basic Books, 1974), p. 52. (Italics added.)

23. Fried, *An Anatomy of Values,* part III, chapters 10–12.

MILTON C. WEINSTEIN AND WILLIAM B. STASON

Allocating Resources: The Case of Hypertension

Hypertension, or high blood pressure, is one of America's foremost health problems. It affects about 24 million Americans—11 million men and 13 million women—and is the single most important risk factor for that class of disease—cardiovascular disease—that kills and cripples more people than any other. The higher the blood pressure, the greater the risk of strokes, heart attacks, and other disabling or fatal events.

On the basis of prevalence alone, hypertension is unrivaled among major health problems. Its impact on health and life expectancy are even more striking. A person with a blood pressure of 140/90 (see box) has nearly twice the risk of an untoward cardiovascular event or early death as one with an average blood pressure. At a blood pressure of 160/100 the risk rises to approximately three times the average risk, and at 160/110 to over four times. Half the hypertensives in the United States are under the age of fifty-four, and more than 20 percent are under the age of forty-four. The implications are particularly ominous for blacks, who comprise 18 percent of hypertensives, compared to only 9 percent of the total U.S. population, and for whom access to quality medical care has been limited.

In the vast majority of patients, perhaps as many as 98 percent, the cause is unknown and the diagnosis is "essential" hypertension. For these patients treatment is aimed at the only measurable manifestation of the disease, elevated blood pressure. A wide variety of medications are effective in lowering blood pressure. Moreover, there is strong evidence that reduction in blood pressure by drug treatment reduces the risks associated with hypertension. The Veterans Administration Cooperative Study found this to be the case in middle-aged men, at least for those with initial

From *Hastings Center Report* 7 (October 1977), 24–29. Reprinted with permission of The Hastings Center: Institute of Society, Ethics and the Life Sciences, 360 Broadway, Hastings-on-Hudson, N.Y. 10706.

diastolic pressures of 105 mm Hg or higher. While some doubt remains as to whether these findings can be generalized to lower but still elevated pressures, to women, and to younger persons, this study has been largely responsible for bringing hypertension into the national spotlight.

Unfortunately, antihypertensive treatment is not a free ride. The drugs and associated medical supervision cost from $100 to $500 per patient per year, equivalent to many thousands of dollars over a lifetime. It is estimated that if treatment were provided for all Americans with blood pressures of 160/95 or above, the cost would run over five billion dollars a year, or nearly 4 percent of the total current health expenditures in the United States. Moreover, the medications used to treat hypertension have side effects ranging from minor and transient problems such as lethargy and diarrhea to severe and disabling problems such as impotence, depression, and, possibly, cancer. The pros and cons of treatment must be weighed carefully by the physician and by the policy maker alike in deciding what initiatives are justified.

Despite the importance of hypertension and the presumed efficacy of antihypertensive treatment, 30 to 50 percent of American hypertensives are not even aware that they have high blood pressure; half of those who know they have it are not under treatment; and of those who are being treated, only half have brought their blood pressures under control.

POLICY QUESTIONS ON HYPERTENSION

This evident failure of the medical care system to accomplish effective treatment of as many as 20 million of the 24 million hypertensives raises major public policy questions. On the one hand, it can be argued that a major national effort should be undertaken to provide treatment to as many of the untreated hypertensives as possible. Some advocate mass public screening programs; many such programs have been fostered at the state and local levels, by public and private agencies. On the other hand, treatment is costly, accompanied by side effects, and of uncertain efficacy in the 70 to 80 percent of hypertensives whose diagnostic blood pressures are in the "mild" range of 95 mm Hg to 104 mm Hg. Furthermore, many who are found to be hypertensive will not achieve blood pressure control because they will drop out of treatment, because they will fail to adhere to treatment regimens, or because their providers will fail to prescribe effective treatment. Considerable expenditures beyond pure treatment costs may be required to alter the health care system sufficiently to slow this attrition process.

In these times of escalating health care costs, it is becoming ever more apparent that we shall not be able to undertake every promising health initiative. With the average per capita expenditure on health care in the United States at $600 per year, and more than 8 percent of our gross national product going into health care, we are reaching the limits of our ability to treat health care as if it were a free good. This realization presents new and difficult ethical problems, since the goal of providing each individual with the best possible medical care is now coming directly into conflict with our collective interest in cost containment.

Somehow we must set priorities for health care investments. Hypertension detection and treatment must compete for resources with other programs and activities both within and outside of health care. More hypertension treatment might mean fewer nutrition programs or fewer coronary care units. Moreover, the limited resources available for hypertension must be allocated in the best possible way, consistent with societal goals and principles. How should hypertension treatment resources be allocated—by blood pressure level, age, sex, or other criteria? Considering that many patients do not adhere to medical regimens, is treatment of hypertension nevertheless a wise use of resources? Are public screening programs an appropriate use of resources? Under what conditions? For what target populations? Generally, how should resources be divided among screening for unaware hypertensives, treatment of known hypertensives, and interventions to promote adherence to medical regimens among those under treatment? Our analysis of policy toward hypertension[1] is a systematic effort to clarify the issues that bear most heavily on such questions of resource allocation, and, tentatively, to suggest some answers.

CHOOSING ALLOCATION CRITERIA

Perhaps the most difficult problem of all is to choose criteria by which to judge the merits of the existing allocation of health resources, and by which to set priorities for their prospective allocation. Medical, economic, political, psychological, and ethical considerations all come into play. Both the health and economic outcomes implied by such criteria, and the process by which they are implemented, are of concern.

COST-EFFECTIVENESS

One way to judge the merits of alternative resource allocations is to determine which one results in the greatest aggregate health benefits, as measured by reductions in mortality and morbidity. If the goal is to maximize these benefits across all health care interventions, then we will want to set priorities according to the health benefits produced per dollar spent. By rank-ordering competing investments according to this ratio, and using this as a priority index, the objective of maximizing aggregate health benefits within a given health care budget can be achieved. This is the cost-effectiveness, or efficiency, criterion for allocating health care resources.

One problem in quantifying health benefits in the cost-effectiveness framework is the need to combine several dimensions of health benefit—improved life expectancy, reduced disability, pain and suffering—into a single measure. Different individuals will assign different values to each of these dimensions. Tradeoffs—for example, between length of life and quality of life—must somehow be taken into account. One, albeit imperfect, method for doing this is to construct an index such as "quality-adjusted life years" to summarize the amount of health benefit. Another method is to attempt to value all health benefits in economic terms based on earnings, or some other measure of economic value such as willingness to pay for improved life or health. We tend to favor the former approach, despite its subjectivity, for reasons we will discuss.

EQUITY

The imperative to get the most health from our investments in health care makes the cost-effectiveness criterion for allocating health resources powerful and appealing. But other values and criteria will, and should, also enter into the decision process. One is equity, or the distribution of health benefits among the members of society. As a society we might prefer that a given amount of health benefit (that is, a number of increased years of life expectancy or good health) be spread equitably among different segments of the population. We might be satisfied if a hypertension program erred on the side of devoting more resources to the poor and disadvantaged who lack access to medical care, but we would be less content if the affluent benefited disproportionately at public expense. But equity between socioeconomic groups is only part of the story. Equity is also an issue between sexes, geographical regions, and, possibly, between age groups (although we are nearly all, at one time or another in our lives, both young and old). It is clearly crucial that conclusions based on cost-effectiveness considerations be tested against the yardstick of equity as well.

PSYCHOLOGICAL AND POLITICAL FACTORS

Similarly, other factors may enter into decisions. Psychological factors such as anxiety, guilt, and the satisfaction of saving lives may be important. The widely debated difference between identified and statistical lives is important to many, and may explain our willingness as a nation to underwrite the treatment of end-stage renal failure to save identified lives despite the costs, and our unwillingness to spend much on environmental health to save statistical ones. The criterion of political acceptability is also a significant one, as we determine which diseases and population groups receive the most attention. Perhaps most important of all to many of us is that the process of making the decisions be fair and just, independent of the health and economic consequences of the decisions. The conclusions of any cost-effectiveness analysis must be tempered by all these considerations.

ASSESSING COSTS AND BENEFITS

One premise, which we accept but some may dispute, is that it is best to be explicit about the consequences of alternative actions and allocations of resources; hence, that formal analysis is valuable. We believe that the imperative for explicitness and hardnosed evaluation of evidence on costs and benefits is especially great in the health area, where explicitness has been so rare in the past, and where the failure to be systematic in the evaluation of policy may lead to arbitrary and inappropriate measures to contain health costs. A variety of quantitative and analytical methods have been developed over the last several decades to analyze decision problems in a systematic way. Falling loosely under the headings of decision analysis, systems analysis, operations research and cost-benefit analysis, these methods have been applied repeatedly and successfully in the areas of private business and national defense. Increasingly, under the heading of "policy analysis," and with a sensitivity to political issues as well, they are being adapted to a wide range of public policy issues that had previously escaped systematic, decision-oriented analysis.

Our study of hypertension represents an attempt to combine this analytical perspective with that of clinical medicine in addressing a major categorical health problem. The first step in our analysis was to assess the costs and benefits of treatment of hypertension, ignoring the adherence problem for the time being. To do this, we had to use the existing data on the mortality and morbidity risks associated with various levels of blood pressure for persons of varying age and sex. These data came from the Framingham Heart Study. We also had reasonably good data on the direct costs of treatment and on the savings associated with the treatment of strokes and heart attacks prevented. But where data were inadequate, some assumptions had to be made, and allowance for the uncertainty that surrounded them built into the analysis.

The first assumptions were required to estimate the effect of blood pressure control on mortality and morbidity. We recognized that an individual whose blood pressure is controlled from X to Y at age Z does not necessarily become identical in risk to one whose natural blood pressure is Y at age Z. Instead, we assumed that the risk for such an individual is some weighted average of the risks corresponding to the controlled level and the level in the absence of control. We call this weight the "fraction of benefit." An important consideration is that the fraction of benefit may not remain constant throughout the course of therapy but instead may increase directly with duration of blood pressure control due to prevention or reversal of cardiovascular disease. For similar reasons, the fraction of benefit is likely to depend upon the age at which blood pressure control is initiated, since the duration of blood pressure elevation prior to treatment is indicative of the extent of cumulative cardiovascular damage to that time. In the absence of empirical data, we assessed a set of subjective estimates of fraction of benefit as a function of age at initiation and duration of therapy. To account for uncertainty, we investigated the implications of several alternative fraction-of-benefit assumptions (including full benefit) and used the principles of decision analysis to derive the implications of varying degrees of belief in the assumptions.

The second set of assumptions had to do with the estimation of the effects of the prevention of morbid events and the side effects of drug treatments on the quality of life. We used a measure of "quality-adjusted life years." For a patient dying suddenly, following a life unencumbered by morbidity from heart attacks or strokes, a measure of benefit is simply the number of years of life expectancy conferred by treatment. For the individual who suffers a morbid event such as a stroke, does not die, but is subsequently disabled, it is necessary to calibrate the value of these years of life of impaired quality against healthy years. The tradeoff between life years and disability may be assessed, in principle, by evaluating responses to the question: "Taking into account your pain and suffering, immobility, age, and lost earnings, what fraction of a year of life would you be willing to give up in order to have good health for the remaining fraction of the year instead of your present level of disability for the full year?" An answer near 1.0 implied that the disability is nearly as bad as death; an answer near 0.0 implies a mild or negligible level of disability. To be sure, this tradeoff concept is a difficult one, and different people may hold different values. It is a very real tradeoff, however, and one that is faced daily, either explicitly or implicitly, by both providers and patients. In the absence of empirical answers to the value question, we assigned, subjectively, a quality-adjustment scale to years of life with the disabling effects of strokes and heart attacks and with the side effects of medications. As with the fraction-of-benefit assumption, we conducted several sensitivity studies to test the importance of the particular assumption used. When an assumption is found to be a critical determinant of cost-effectiveness, the importance of further research is highlighted. Such turned out to be the case for the subjective side effects of treatment and for the efficacy of treatment in mild and moderate hypertension, but not for the quality-of-life adjustments for disability from strokes or heart attacks.

The third methodological assumption related to the tradeoff between costs and benefits received immediately and costs and benefits received well in the future. Economists are inclined to "discount" future economic benefits and costs—that is, to value them less than present benefits and costs—to account for the ability of invested resources to yield future returns. Whether the principle of discounting also applies to health benefits is debatable, but we concluded that it is necessary to discount future quality-adjusted life years just as it is necessary to discount future dollars. The reason is, we emphasize, not because future lives are worth less than present lives in any absolute, utilitarian sense (in fact, we find such a concept morally repugnant), but rather because it is in the interest of those future lives to spend the resources on life saving at the point in time where the greatest benefit can be derived. The argument on this point is subtle, and we have described it in more detail elsewhere.[2]

WHAT MEASURES ARE MOST COST-EFFECTIVE?

Given these assumptions and the empirical data available, we derive several conclusions that bear upon the allocation of resources to the treatment of hypertension.

1. The medical costs saved by prevention of strokes and heart attacks in treated hypertensives do not come close to "paying for" the costs of antihypertensive treatment. Only 15 to 25 percent of gross treatment costs can be expected to be recovered. Therefore, treatment must be justified in terms of the prolongation and improved quality of life it provides rather than absolute cost savings.

2. Cost-effectiveness considerations suggest priorities for treatment by blood pressure level, age, and sex. Figure 1 shows, for men and women, our best estimates of the net cost per year of increased quality-adjusted life expectancy as a function of pretreatment diastolic blood pressure and age. Since these estimates assume full adherence to therapy, they are optimistic. In any case, it appears to be more cost-effective to treat higher blood pressures, younger men, and older women. The potential value of initiating treatment early in life for men is particularly impressive. Better data are urgently needed to verify the effectiveness of treatment in young people. (See Figure 1.)

3. Estimates of cost-effectiveness are indeed sensitive to the fraction of benefit, that is, the extent to which treatment eliminates excess risk. More research, based on observational data, if controlled

studies are found not to be feasible or cost-effective would have great value.

4. The dollar cost of antihypertensive drugs is a major determinant of cost-effectiveness, and the use of generic drugs shoud be encouraged to lower these costs.

5. The importance of the mild, chronic, and often subjective side effects of treatment may substantially diminish the net effectiveness of treatment by their adverse effects on the quality of life. Side effects should be carefully monitored in the course of treatment, and research to learn more about their prevalence, and patient attitudes toward them, would be extremely valuable in guiding future policy decisions.

INCOMPLETE ADHERENCE TO THERAPY

The next major extension in the analysis was to introduce the problem of incomplete adherence to therapy. We found a substantial adverse effect on the cost-effectiveness of therapy. Figure 2 shows that if treatment were provided to all persons in the United States with diastolic blood pressures of 105 mm Hg or above, the average cost per year of quality-adjusted life expectancy could be as high as $10,500, compared to $4,850 under full adherence. For treatment of mild hypertension (95-104 mm Hg diastolic), these figures range as high as $20,400, compared to $9,880 under full adherence. The difference between the "maximum cost" and "minimum cost" assumptions has to do with whether nonadherers continue to purchase drugs at the same rate as adherers, or only in proportion to consumption.

Interventions to improve adherence are generally of unproven efficacy, although, in demonstration programs, some are promising, including patient education and counseling, patient contracts with providers, instruction in home blood pressure measurement, and tangible incentives offered to encourage close attention to regimens. Furthermore, the potential of physician education should not be ignored. We found in our analysis that if even moderate effectiveness for an intervention can be established, the cost-effectiveness of treatment can be substantially improved. Therefore, major efforts should be under-

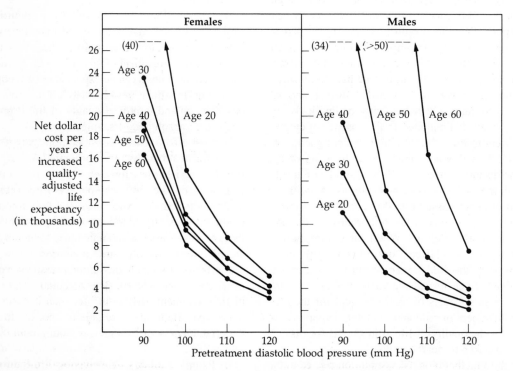

Figure 1. Estimated Cost-Effectiveness of Treating Hypertension, by Sex, Age, and Pretreatment Diastolic Blood Pressure, and Assuming Full Adherence to Therapy.

Source: *Milton C. Weinstein and William B. Stason*, Hypertension: A Policy Perspective (*Cambridge: Harvard University Press, 1976*).

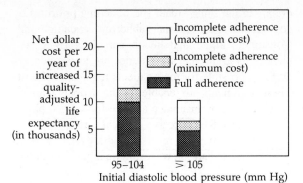

Figure 2. Impact of Incomplete Adherence and Pretreatment Blood Pressure Level on Cost-Effectiveness of Treatment.
Source: William B. Stason and Milton C. Weinstein, *"Allocation of Resources to Manage Hypertension,"* The New England Journal of Medicine 296:732–739, 1977.

taken to develop a portfolio of strategies to improve adherence. Development of such methods should be a goal of every provider and health care institution, and would have obvious implications for the management of many health care problems beyond hypertension.

SCREENING FOR HYPERTENSION

We also examined the cost-effectiveness of screening for hypertension and concluded that large-scale, public mass screening programs are not cost-effective at the present time, largely because of the impact of attrition and poor adherence to therapy. A community with limited resources would probably do better to concentrate its efforts on improving adherence of known hypertensives, even at a sacrifice in terms of the numbers screened. This conclusion holds even if such proadherence interventions are rather expensive and only moderately effective, and even if screening is very inexpensive. Public screening programs in black communities are likely to be substantially more cost-effective than community-wide screening because of the extraordinarily high prevalence and severity of hypertension in blacks. Implementation of such targeted screening programs is recommended, provided that resources for ensuring treatment and follow-up are available. Finally, screening by health care providers in their regular practices is more cost-effective than public screening. This is true, in large part, because the attrition and costs associated with referral are eliminated. Routine screening by providers could be encouraged by the use of financial incentives, through existing and projected fiscal reimbursement mechanisms.

ETHICAL IMPLICATIONS

Some of the ethical implications of our analysis and its conclusions require emphasis. Since our findings are based largely upon efficiency grounds, we should also examine them to see whether they stand up to the test of equity. The recommendation for the intensive management of known hypertensives at a sacrifice of public screening efforts might be troubling since it is the poor who tend to have limited access to health care and who, therefore, are less likely to be aware of their conditions and already under treatment. This dilemma is mitigated, in part, by the conclusion that targeted screening in black communities should have higher priority than community-wide screening. In addition, perhaps selective screening in low-income communities in general should be contemplated on equity grounds. If hypertension screening helps to foster more involvement in primary health care in a disadvantaged community, then this indirect benefit must be recognized; if it becomes a substitute for comprehensive care, however, then it may even be a disservice.

Another dimension of the equity issue relates to the setting of priorities for treatment by age and sex. Is it acceptable, say, to give high priority to treating younger men or older women? This could be difficult to justify, particularly if the population as a whole shares the cost of treatment through taxes and insurance premiums. On the other hand, it can be argued that it is not necessary that each categorical program distribute benefits equally to all demographic groups, provided that the totality of health care does not discriminate against one group or another.

A particularly difficult ethical problem is raised by the conclusion that it is more cost-effective to apply proadherence interventions to known hypertensives (that is, to try to encourage them to change their health behaviors) than to identify those who are unaware. Why should public, or collectively raised, resources be used to cajole people to take care of themselves when others might be denied the basic information about their condition that would even allow them to make a choice? Is there not an obligation, above all, to provide the information to all before we seek to modify the behavior of the informed few whose free will ought to let them decide whether or not they want to take their medicines? We believe that these arguments, while important, can easily be oversimplified. The question of what determines health behavior, and how much free will is involved in personal health-care decisions, is a complex one. Consider the analogy to smoking or weight reduction. People pay to join groups to help motivate their behaviors, because they cannot help themselves. Information and education alone have been shown in several studies to have minimal or no effect on health behavior. Therefore, it is not obvious that the responsibility of the government or health care provider stops with the provision of information, for example, through screening. Is it not an equally valid undertaking to help people realize improved health by developing such needed health practices as faithful adherence to antihypertensive regimens? We believe that it is.

Perhaps the most perplexing ethical problem posed by our analysis is its explicitness about the relation between economic resources, on the one hand, and human lives and health, on the other. By taking the cost-effectiveness approach, we have avoided the need to assign dollar values to human lives (as is required in benefit-cost analyses, in which all benefits and costs are expressed in monetary terms). We have thereby sidestepped one troublesome ethical problem. But we are still making judgments about the relative merits of life-saving or health-improving investments by asserting that an investment with a lower cost per unit of health benefit (that is, per quality-adjusted life year saved) should have higher priority for the use of limited resources than an investment with a higher cost per unit of health benefit.

For some, the idea of mentioning human lives and dollars in the same breath and of setting priorities by cost-effectiveness criteria is abhorrent, even immoral. Consumers argue that health care is a right, and physicians argue that their duties are to provide everything possible for their patients regardless of cost. These arguments are tenable for the patients who are fully covered by insurance and fee-for-service physicians because they perceive medical care as free. For those in society who must bear the ever-increasing costs of health care, however, these arguments do not hold.

We believe that societal interests are best served by using limited health care resources in the most efficacious possible way. One way or another, priorities for health expenditures will have to be set. Health services of marginal value may have to be denied. Better this, however, than to be denied more necessary services because resources to provide them—physicians, hospital beds, or equipment—are not available because they are being fully used for less critical problems. And better to be systematic about determining the alternative ways in which our health care dollars might be spent than to let decisions be made in an inconsistent, often arbitrary way. To be sure, the process of allocating health resources matters. But so, too, do the consequences matter: our lives and the qualities of our lives.

NOTES

1. Milton C. Weinstein and William B. Stason, *Hypertension: A Policy Perspective* (Cambridge: Harvard University Press, 1976).

2. See, for example, Milton C. Weinstein and William B. Stason, "Foundations of Cost-Effectiveness Analysis for Health and Medical Practices," *New England Journal of Medicine,* 296: 716–721, 1977.

RASHI FEIN

High Blood Pressure, Economics, and Equity: A Response to Weinstein and Stason

[Weinstein and Stason] attempt "to determine how resources can be used most efficiently within programs to treat hypertension and to provide a yardstick for comparison with alternative health-related uses of these resources."* It is clear that economists are destined to have an increasingly important role in assisting health-sector decision makers. United States health expenditures now exceed $140 billion per annum and account for almost 9 per cent of America's Gross National Product (the market value of all goods and services produced). Federal health expenditures alone total about $50 billion and 12 per cent of total federal outlays. Given the quantity of resources allocated to and consumed by the health sector as it produces and distributes medical-care services of all kinds, and given the substantial sums accounted for by public expenditures, it is inevitable and desirable that those with a special expertise in analyzing the allocation of resources be called upon to contribute to decision-making processes. Economists will be asked to consider the relation between various possible resource allocations and "the societal objective of deriving the maximum health benefits from dollars spent" to illuminate our understanding of the forces that determine the allocation of resources and the incentives and regulations that might alter the existing allocation. It therefore behooves those in the health sector and other areas in which economists will apply their analytical processes to understand how economists think and what they think about. Weinstein and Stason provide an example of how clinical information and economic analysis can be wedded to illuminate policy issues.

. . .

Because the methods of cost-effectiveness analysis are elegant and powerful, they may be accepted without sufficient caution. Although Weinstein and Stason are in fact both modest and tentative in their conclusions, it seems useful to indicate that there is a "but, on the other hand" side to the story.

In the first place, as is often the case, the outsider may impute a greater certainty and authority to that which is said by practitioners in a discipline unknown to him than he would to things said in his own field. Aware of the disputes within his discipline, he should remember that similar disagreements are likely in other fields as well. Reputable economists may differ and, indeed, do on a number of matters touched upon in the articles. Such differences (e.g., the distinction between benefit-cost and cost-effectiveness analysis, the importance of examining changes at the margin rather than average impacts and the appropriate rate of discount) may be critically important.

Secondly, the analytical techniques may appear coldly neutral—pure science at its best. This impression is misleading. The various steps in the particular approach involve arithmetic exercises. Yet behind the arithmetic lie values. The reader, for example, should recognize the power of arithmetic and the very substantial impact of the discount rate. Years of life that are off in the distant future do not have the same numerical value as years of life in the near present. Thus, the difference between adding 40 or 30 years to life expectancy is not 10 but a smaller number. Does the discount rate (derived from the rate of return on capital) truly capture our social values? Does it assist or hinder us in understanding the advantages and

From *New England Journal of Medicine* 296 (March 31, 1977), pp. 751–753.

*Ed. note: Dr. Fein's article is a response to two articles that appeared in the same issue of Volume 296 (No. 13) of the *New England Journal of Medicine* as his own. Both articles *preceded* the one reprinted here.

disadvantages of treating the young in contrast to the old?

Thirdly, the reader should note the importance of the adjustment made for the quality of life. The authors pose the question, "what fraction, P, of a year of life would you be willing to give up to be completely healthy for the remaining fraction of a year instead of your present level of health status . . . ?" They assume that "The average patient would be willing to give up 3½ days of life per year." No potential patient, however, can be offered the option of living 361½ days each year and being in a "deep freeze" for the other 3½ days. Is the answer that a patient might give to the Weinstein and Stason question really meaningful? Even if it is, does it not pertain only to one year and not to many? One cannot help wondering whether a patient who says that he would be willing to give up one month of life to be completely healthy for the remaining 11 months really means that he would be willing to die one month earlier and whether that, in turn, permits us to say that he would be willing to settle for 11 years of 100 per cent quality life rather than 12 years of 92 per cent quality. Important as the question of side effects is, and interesting as it is to consider the quality of life, it is not at all clear how the concept is made operational. . . .

Fourthly, the reader should remember that the numerical results are derived from a set of relations that summarize the efficacy of various interventions. The numbers have the danger of implying a false precision, and the more so since some of them are subjective. Not only can relations change, but the nature of the various relations—why they are what they are—is not well understood (and is itself subject to change). It is possible, for example, that the publicity campaign designed to increase the number screened may have a favorable (and unrecognized) impact on other parts of the system—e.g., on the proportion of patients who adhere to the regimen prescribed by their physicians. It is imperative that we recognize the complexity of the various relations lest, in ignoring the possible interaction effects, we underestimate or overestimate the impact of a particular course of action.

Fifthly, there is the often recognized and seldom dealt with problem of definition. The analytical tools used require precise quantification of the impact of various interventions. Inevitably, the impact on health is measured by examination of mortality and (on occasion) morbidity. That is an incomplete measure of the impact of the encounter between physician and patient. Patients seek care. Because economists cannot adequately assess the caring function and measure its value, they tend to relegate it to a footnote, reminding the reader that the numbers in the body of the text are incomplete. Yet, over time, the numbers gain currency. More distressingly, a "climate of opinion" is created: that which is measured is important and vice versa. The caring function is left to the soft-hearted idealists, and all of us are encouraged to become hard-headed realists.

Finally, we must be aware that the purpose of the particular analytical exercise is to increase the "efficiency" of the system. It is within the tradition of economics to set efficiency criteria high on the analytical agenda. Economists have done rather better at this type of analysis than they have been able to do on distribution and equity questions. Yet much of the society's agenda deals with equity and distribution. The fact that distributional considerations are neglected by the analysis has important implications. It may be, for example, that screening is justified even if it yields a low rate of return because it reaches persons whom the private sector would otherwise neglect. One cannot, of course, be certain that such a result will occur. It does seem clear, however, that the question of whom various procedures affect and what distributional questions are involved, is most important. Weinstein and Stason refer briefly to the issue of social equity and suggest the possibility that it would affect their conclusions. There is a danger, however, that their conclusions will be remembered while the fact that they derive from a narrow perspective will be forgotten.

These are troubled times for the American medical-care system. Since so many of the problems are economic, the agenda for action is concerned with mechanisms to increase efficiency. In recent years, moreover, physicians have become increasingly interested in whether various interventions do as much good as has often been assumed and, therefore, whether they merit the resources allocated. The importance of efficiency and effectiveness questions cannot be denied, but they are only part of the agenda. It seems to me that in America equity of access still remains the most important, unsolved question for three reasons, the first being that solutions to the equity question will change the very probabilities that enter into the cost-effectiveness analysis. The Weinstein and Stason conclusions, for example, are heavily determined by patient noncompliance, which, in turn, is markedly affected by economic barriers.[1] An increase in equity can therefore alter the efficiency conclusions. The second reason is that the mechanisms designed to increase equity in fact help create the public-policy structures required if the issue of socially optimal resource allocation is to be addressed effectively. It is the socially responsible macro decisions that will ultimately affect individual behavior at the micro level. Finally, until the equity issues are solved, it will be difficult to address efficiency considerations because we will face a hostile public suspicious that our emphasis on efficiency is designed to avoid providing to all what some of us already have.

It should be clear that Weinstein and Stason do not argue that solutions to the moral issues need to be postponed until the economic problems are solved. Nor can they be criticized for being interested in and examining the important problems inherent in a more efficient allocation of resources. Their two articles are useful and important, and we can, and should, learn from them. What can be added, however, is ''but, on the other hand.''

NOTES

1. F. N. Brand, R. T. Smith, and P. A. Brand, ''Effects of Economic Barriers to Medical Care on Patients' Noncompliance,'' *Public Health Reports* 92 (1977), 72–78.

SUGGESTED READINGS FOR CHAPTER 9

Arrow, Kenneth J., *et al*. ''Government Decision Making and the Preciousness of Life.'' In Tancredi, Laurence R., ed. *Ethics of Health Care*. Washington: National Academy of Sciences, 1974, pp. 33–64.

Bayles, Michael D. ''National Health Insurance and Non-Covered Services.'' *Journal of Health Politics, Policy and Law* 2 (Fall 1977), 335–348.

Beauchamp, Tom L., and Childress, James F. *Principles of Biomedical Ethics*. New York: Oxford University Press, 1979. Chap. 6.

Blocker, H. Gene, and Smith, Elizabeth, eds. *John Rawls' Theory of Social Justice: An Introduction*. Athens, Ohio: Ohio University Press, 1980.

Blumstein, James F. ''Constitutional Perspectives on Governmental Decisions Affecting Human Life and Health.'' *Law and Contemporary Problems* 40 (Autumn 1976), 231–305.

Brown, Lawrence D. ''The Scope and Limits of Equality as a Normative Guide to Federal Health Care Policy.'' *Public Policy* 26 (Fall 1978), 481–532.

Callahan, Daniel. ''How Much Is Enough? A National Perspective.'' *Alabama Journal of Medical Sciences* 17 (January 1980), 76–80.

Childress, James F. *Priorities in Biomedical Ethics*. Philadelphia: Westminster Press, 1981. Chap. 4.

Daniels, Norman. ''Cost-Effectiveness and Patient Welfare.'' In Basson, Marc, ed. *Rights and Responsibilities in Medicine*. New York: Alan R. Liss, 1981, pp. 159–170.

———, ed. *Reading Rawls: Critical Studies of a Theory of Justice*. New York: Basic Books, Inc., 1976.

''Due Process in the Allocation of Scarce Life-saving Medical Resources.'' *Yale Law Journal* 84 (July 1975), 1734–1749.

Fein, Rashi. ''On Achieving Access and Equity in Health Care.'' *Milbank Memorial Fund Quarterly* 50 (October 1972), 157–190.

Feldstein, Paul J. ''National Health Insurance: An Approach to the Redistribution of Medical Care.'' *Health Care Economics*. New York: John Wiley & Sons, 1979. Chap. 19.

Freedman, Benjamin. ''The Case for Medical Care: Inefficient or Not.'' *Hastings Center Report* 7 (April 1977), 31–39.

Fried, Charles. ''Rights and Health Care—Beyond Equity and Efficiency.'' *New England Journal of Medicine* 293 (July 31, 1975), 241–245.

Fuchs, Victor. *Who Shall Live?* New York: Basic Books, 1974.

Green, Ronald M. ''Health Care and Justice in Contract Theory Perspective.'' In Veatch, Robert M., and Branson, Roy, eds. *Ethics and Health Policy*. Cambridge Mass.: Ballinger Publishing Co., 1976, pp. 111–126.

Havighurst, Clark C. ''The Ethics of Cost Control in Medical Care.'' *Soundings* 60 (Spring 1977), 22–39.

Hiatt, Howard H. ''Protecting the Medical Commons: Who Is Responsible?'' *New England Journal of Medicine* 293 (July 31, 1975), 235–241.

Jonsen, Albert R. ''Health Care: Right to Health-Care Services.'' In Reich, Warren T., ed. *Encyclopedia of Bioethics*. New York: Free Press, 1978. Vol. 2, pp. 623–630.

Journal of Medicine and Philosophy 4 (1979). Special issue on the Right to Health Care.

Kass, Leon. ''The End of Medicine.'' *The Public Interest* 40 (Summer 1975), 11–42.

Katz, Jay, and Capron, Alexander M. *Catastrophic Diseases: Who Decides What? A Psychological and Legal Analysis*. New York: Russell Sage Foundation, 1975.

Lomasky, Loren E. ''Medical Progress and National Health Care.'' *Philosophy and Public Affairs* 10 (Winter 1981), 65–88.

Outka, Gene. ''Social Justice and Equal Access to Health Care.'' *Journal of Religious Ethics* 2 (Spring 1974), 11–32.

Ramsey, Paul. *The Patient as Person*. New Haven: Yale University Press, 1970. Chap. 7.

Relman, Arnold S. ''The Allocation of Medical Resources by Physicians.'' *Journal of Medical Education* 55 (February 1980), 99–104.

Sade, R. ''Medical Care as a Right: A Refutation.'' *New England Journal of Medicine* 285 (December 2, 1975), 1288–1292.

———. ''Concepts of Rights: Philosophy and Application to Health Care.'' *Linacre Quarterly* 46 (November 1979), 330–344.

''Scarce Medical Resources.'' *Columbia Law Review* (April 1969), 620–692.

Shelp, Earl, ed. *Justice and Health Care*. Boston: D. Reidel, 1981.

Shelton, Robert L. ''Human Rights and Distributive Justice in

Health Care Delivery." *Journal of Medical Ethics* 4 (December 1978), 165–171.

Smith, Harmon L. "Distributive Justice and American Health Care." In Finnin, William M., and Smith, Gerald A., eds. *The Morality of Scarcity: Limited Resources and Social Policy.* Baton Rouge; Louisiana State University Press, 1979, pp. 67–79.

Szasz, Thomas S. "The Right to Health." *Georgetown Law Journal* 57 (March 1969), 734–751.

Veatch, Robert M., and Branson, Roy, eds. *Ethics and Health Policy.* Cambridge, Mass.: Ballinger Publishing Co., 1975.

———. *Case Studies in Medical Ethics.* Cambridge, Mass.: Harvard University Press, 1977. Chap. 9.

Weinstein, Milton C., and Stason, William B. "Foundations of Cost-Effectiveness Analysis for Health and Medical Practices." *New England Journal of Medicine* 296 (March 31, 1977), 716–721.

Goldstein, Doris Mueller. *Bioethics: A Guide to Information Sources.* Detroit: Gale Research Company, 1982. See under "Equality and Rights in Health Care," "Health Care for Particular Groups," and "Allocation of Scarce Medical Resources."

Lineback, Richard H., ed. *Philosopher's Index.* Vols. 1– . Bowling Green, Ohio: Philosophy Documentation Center, Bowling Green State University. Issued quarterly. See under "Allocation," "Cost-Benefit Analysis," "Distributive Justice," "Health Care," "Human Rights," "Medicine," "Resources," and "Rights."

Walters, LeRoy, ed. *Bibliography of Bioethics.* Vols. 1– . New York: Free Press. Issued annually. See under "Health Care," "Resource Allocation," and "Selection for Treatment." (The information contained in the annual *Bibliography of Bioethics* can also be retrieved from BIOETHICSLINE, an online data base of the National Library of Medicine.)

10.
Health Policy

Many health risks are produced in individuals by their own autonomous behaviors, while other risks are environmental or genetic, or are caused by the behaviors of other persons. Cost-effective health policy strategies for dealing with this broad range of health risks are generally considered socially acceptable as long as individuals desire the protection of these policies or at least do not object to active protection. However, some public policies, laws, and regulations are designed specifically to protect and promote the health of individuals opposed to them. Examples of policies that are objectionable to some include: (1) laws requiring motorcyclists to wear safety helmets and motorists to wear seat belts; (2) taxation, allocation, and scaled insurance schemes designed specifically to prevent smoking, obesity, and alcohol abuse; (3) prohibition of dangerous recreational activities, such as hang gliding or stunt flying; and (4) banning the purchase of possible harmful or inefficacious drugs and chemicals. Controversial health policies in these areas (especially 2) are studied in the first section of this chapter.

Public policies that involve tampering with or otherwise controlling individual lifestyles can be contrasted to those that govern, for example, occupational safety and health, environmental pollution, and the shipment of dangerous materials. The latter are attempts to protect workers and citizens from harm inflicted by others, for example, by employers' negligence or by those who pollute the environment. Traditionally, justifications of policies aimed at protecting against harm from all these sources have been either paternalistic or based on a conception of social justice. Paternalistic policies regulate or prohibit risky behaviors against the wishes of those who engage in them, while justifications that protect persons for reasons of social justice contend that society owes such protection to all its members. This chapter begins with arguments for and against these two forms of justification, and the second section considers controversies that surround cost-benefit analysis. In the third section, problems of risks in occupational settings are studied, along with problems of consent or refusal to work in the presence of such risks. Finally, the fourth section focuses on public support of prenatal screening programs.

LIFESTYLE INTERVENTION AND PATERNALISM

Paternalism is here discussed in a rather different context than in other chapters. As mentioned previously, laws governing seat-belt use, smoking, obesity, alcohol, recreation, and drugs are commonly "justified" by appeal to paternalistic arguments. One critical element in the controversy over such justifications concerns the quality of consent or refusal by the persons whose liberty might be restricted by such policies. The case may be argued that those whose health is affected by smoking, alcohol abuse, or obesity are engaging in what may be for them substantially nonvoluntary behavior, even though they knowingly engage in the behavior and might rationally oppose policies that penalized them for such behavior. Laws that prohibit substantially voluntary behaviors require *strong* paternalism, and laws that prohibit substantially nonvoluntary behaviors require *weak* paternalism. (These distinctions are discussed in the last section of Chapter 1.)

The theory of strong paternalism invokes a public's right to override the informed and voluntary actions of individuals in cases of purely self-regarding behavior. As Daniel Wikler, Dan Beauchamp, and Robert Veatch note in this chapter, this theory has been heavily criticized on grounds that it involves an invasion of individual autonomy and gives the state excessive power to enact legislation opposed by the individuals. Weak paternalistic interventions, by contrast, have been thought to be justified in many instances, especially when persons may die or suffer serious injury through decisions that are only partially voluntary. On the other hand, it may only be *because* there is questionable voluntariness or definite nonvoluntariness that the intervention in their lives is justified, not because of the dangerous or unreasonable character of their action. This is one of the major points of dispute about paternalism.

One challenge to paternalism asks whether it helps resolve controversial health policy questions. Paternalism could actually turn out to be irrelevant to policy, because there could always be a more appealing and plausible nonpaternalistic justification for interventions when those interventions are actually justified. For example, policy makers may enact laws to control smoking, alcohol, fluoridated water, insurance rates, and other health-related matters not because they are thereby protecting people against themselves but rather because such practices harm the health of other persons, cost society too much money, potentially can protect the health of many persons, tend to disrupt families, or the like. These arguments are based on a harm principle, not on the paternalistic principle. (Paternalism may turn out to have its most interesting health-connected applications in the case of laws intended to reduce *accidental* injuries that result from intentional but nonetheless hazardous behaviors such as working without a protective mask.)

HEALTH POLICY AND SOCIAL JUSTICE

Health policies to protect people from hazards caused by others or from risks of their own creation have often been promoted on grounds of justice rather than paternalism. According to this approach, problems of public health should be handled as are such other social problems as poverty, poor housing, and racial and sexual discrimination, which require massive social allocations for their alleviation. In each case, society is said to owe the eradication or alleviation of these problems to affected parties as a matter of justice. (See discussions of the terms "justice" and "distributive justice" in Chapter 1.)

Justice-based approaches taken to problems of lifestyle intervention and regulation have proved difficult to bring to bear on practical problems such as those of public health, but Dan Beauchamp outlines in this chapter a theory of distributive justice that he believes would directly and beneficially serve health policy. He argues as follows: Death and disability are more likely to be dramatically reduced through preventive programs than through advances in biomedical technology. Thus, he proposes that we allocate funds to eradicate or at least reduce environmental pollution, automobile hazards that produce injuries and deaths, tobacco use, alcohol use, drugs that induce deaths and disabilities, hazards of the workplace, and the ineffective distribution of medical care. However, broad preventive measures are costly and will place a new burden on the dominant classes in society, who have resisted such allocations and will continue to do so, according to Beauchamp. Their resistance is rooted in a conception of justice that emphasizes individual responsibility and effort—especially responsibility for one's own health. Some of Beauchamp's arguments for the conclusion about individual responsibility are challenged in the essay by Veatch, who offers a needs-based approach that appeals heavily to principles of equal treatment.

Beauchamp's proposals for federal action could also prove to be unrealistic when placed in the framework of present financial resources, since society might not as a *collective* unit be willing to bear such costs. It is problems of precisely this sort that have led to discussions of acceptable risk and cost-benefit analysis as tools for solution.

ACCEPTABLE RISK

The topic of acceptable risk has been lumped together with the subjects of criteria of risk, risk-benefit analysis, the regulation of risk, objective evaluation of risks, and fair decisions about the control of risk. Because risk assessment is now a major factor in decisions about whether or not to permit substances in a workplace or to produce a new technology, the concept of risk and the scope of the risks under consideration should be made clear.

The term "risk" is commonly used to refer to a possible future harm, and statements of risk are usually probabilistic estimates of such harms. However, the *probability* of a harm's occurrence is only one way of expressing a risk and should be distinguished from the *magnitude* of the possible harm—a second way of expressing risk. When such vague expressions as "minimal risk" or "high risk" are used, they commonly refer to an aggregation of the chance of suffering a harm (probability) and the severity of the harm (magnitude) if suffered. Uncertainty may, of course, be present in formal assessments of either the probability or the magnitude of harm, and commonly much uncertainty exists in health policy. For example, in the workplace there is much uncertainty as to dangers, diagnosis, and prognosis. In some cases the probability of exposure to a risk may be known with some precision, while virtually nothing is known about the magnitude of harm; or the magnitude may be precisely expressible, while the probability is too indefinite to be calculated accurately. In other cases a "wild guess" best describes the accuracy with which risks of physical and chemical hazards can be determined—especially for lifelong risks such as the risk of smoking or the risk of a worker who constantly changes locations, who works with multiple substances, and whose physical condition is in part attributable to factors independent of the workplace. (See the essay by Stephen Stich in Chapter 12 for further discussion of the practical difficulties involved in risk assessment.)

There is no general consensus on what level of probability of a serious harm constitutes a risk high enough to demand steps to reduce or eliminate the risk or to require that information be provided to those affected; some speculative (perhaps intuitive) guidelines have been suggested, however. For example, it has been held that risks (expressing probabilities of death per year of an individual's exposure to a given risk) below 1 in 1 million are acts of God too infrequent to merit attempts at control; that risks in the vicinity of 1 in 100,000 may be sufficient to justify issuing warnings; that risks of 1 in 10,000 merit public subsidies in an attempt to eliminate or reduce the risk; and that risks of serious harm greater than 1 in 1,000 are unacceptable.[1] Because the risks of industrial work often fall in the category of 1 in 10,000, some have said that disclosures concerning these risks are morally required.

It is reasonable to ask, however, whether it is adequate that workers, pregnant women, and others affected (such as their families) be protected through health policies that merely expand their information base (and thus perhaps their options). As Ruth Faden and Tom Beauchamp note in this chapter, this question suggests a need to analyze the function or goal of disclosures of risk. The main goal in regulating risks in the workplace has always been and probably always will be to determine an objective level of acceptable risk and then to ban or limit conditions of exposure above that level. It is doubtful that this outcome is the primary goal of mere disclosures of risk, which allow individuals affected to make a subjective determination of what is an acceptable risk to them. At present the government establishes safety standards and controls enforcement, and it may be that workers' safety and health as well as that of pregnant women can be maximally protected (i.e., morbidity and mortality statistics could be kept at their lowest levels) by reasonable government regulations and enforcement. This problem leads to a consideration of issues found in the final two sections of this chapter.

COST-BENEFIT ANALYSIS

Cost-benefit analysis has become widely used in both government and industry as a systematic analytical framework that can serve as the basis for developing health policies. The work of Weinstein and Stason, in Chapter 9, uses this form of analysis, and other applications appear in this chapter—most notably in the Supreme Court decision on the chemical benzene.

Cost-benefit analysis is held out as a device for the clarification of the overt and covert tradeoffs often made in public policy decisions. These are tradeoffs, for example, between lives that will be lost and money expended on new technology that might save them, between environmental quality and factory productivity, and between the quality of gasoline and the quality of the health of those who produce it. The simple idea behind these often complicated procedures is that the cost-benefit analyst should measure or at least carefully describe costs and benefits by some acceptable device, at the same time identifying uncertainties and possible tradeoffs, in order to present policy makers with specific, relevant information on the basis of which a decision can be reached. Although such analysis proceeds by using different quantitative units—for example, number of accidents, statistical deaths, dollars expended, and number of workers fired—cost-benefit analysis often attempts in the end to convert and express these seemingly incommensurable units of measurement into a common one, usually monetary. This monetary conversion is not essential to cost-benefit calculations, however.

Perhaps the main argument favoring use of cost-benefit analysis is that without a systematic evaluative system we may stand condemned to the arbitrary preferences of those who emerge in society as the makers of policy. Their decisions may be based on paternalism, on self-interest, or on an idiosyncratic sense of justice. For example, policy makers need to be able to ascertain in a systematic manner whether the cost of decreasing a risk is worthwhile when the risk is one of death; they must also be able to make that decision when expenditures to combat the risk may dictate that resources must be severely limited in other areas where there are also risks of death. It is this reduction of intuitive weighing and the avoidance of purely political calculations in making decisions that seem of greatest promise in the cost-benefit approach.

The cost-benefit method contains weaknesses, however, as even its proponents agree. There are difficulties in making commensurable all the units it is desirable to compare, and this problem can itself lead to arbitrary decision making. For example, the likelihood of skin cancer is increased by allowing the Concorde to land in the United States. Weighing the former convenience against the likelihood of the latter untoward event is not one that can easily be done in cost-benefit terms. Cost-benefit methods have also proved difficult to implement. Economists have generally discussed how such analyses can be carried out in theory rather than providing practical examples, and those who might wish to structure such an analysis have sometimes been left without any means for reducing all tradeoff variables to a unified form. Another significant objection to cost-benefit analysis is the question of whose values are to count in the weighing and assessment of harms and benefits. The old and the young weigh priorities differently, and some but not all persons place the absence of suffering over the promotion of happiness—to take only two examples. This fact of plurality forces a choice concerning whose voice is to be heard. Also, labeling something a cost (say, environmental damage) or a benefit (say, electric power) itself depends upon an already formed evaluative viewpoint preceding the influence of cost-benefit outcomes. These and other problems are explored in this chapter in the essay by Michael S. Baram.

Despite these deficiencies and the embryonic status of cost-benefit analysis, the cost-benefit approach continues to be viewed in government policy circles as holding out great promise as a rational and ethically justified methodology for public policy analysis. As mentioned, the specific example in this chapter of problems in which cost-benefit analysis can play a role is the issue of standards for occupational exposure to the carcinogen benzene, a problem recently examined by the U.S. Supreme Court and the federal Occupational Safety and Health Administration (OSHA). In this case all parties recognize that benzene is a carcinogen and that we must be cautious about the level allowed in a product or workplace. The question is how to settle for a conservative estimate of health risks as weighed against the substantial benefits of benzene products and the costs of reducing chemical levels. The entire hazard cannot simply be banned, because too many significant benefits not directly related to health would be lost. Gasoline, for example, would be banned. Here it seems appropriate to ask how much society would pay to reduce risks that are continually reducible to lower levels at increasingly greater financial costs. A halt should be called when an acceptable level of risk is reached, where acceptability is determined by what must be given up elsewhere in the way of harms and benefits. Cost-benefit analysis can, *at least in theory,* contribute substantially toward the goal of reaching this level of acceptability.

OCCUPATIONAL RISKS

Information gathered about risks to safety and health does not always determine acceptable occupational risk. Indeed, the information often leaves many regulatory alternatives for policymakers in government. Often a situation of substantial ambiguity prevails, where even the most informed expert is uncertain about the risks—and the dose levels at which there should be concern about health and safety are no clearer. Epidemiology may offer the only method of discovering occupational health risks, and epidemiological studies may deliver conflicting conclusions—for example, about whether there is *any* increased risk of brain cancer from routine work in petrochemical plants. Moreover, the tradeoffs involved—as between control of health hazards and increased production costs or between cessation of production and negative employment effects—are assessed differently by different parties. Worker representatives and management generally disagree about acceptable levels of risk, about appropriate epidemiological evidence, and about acceptable increases in corporate costs to control or eliminate risk. Workers' assessments can also differ markedly from those of government.

This particular feature of the relationship between government and workers is analogous to that between physicians and patients. Physicians, like bureaucrats, have expert technical information and expert skill in evaluating risks and alternatives. It does not follow that physicians should interpret what is best for their patients merely because of their expertise. Such judgments are often nonmedical, even though they require medical information. Just as patients are sometimes unwilling to assume risks that their physicians think eminently reasonable given the alternatives (the psychological risks of having a breast removed being a prime example), so labor may disagree with government and with physicians in occupational medicine. Thus, it will sometimes be problematic to protect workers by health and safety standards alone. These protections may satisfy the moral demands of justice and beneficence without satisfying those of autonomy, for workers may need information in light of which they can decide about levels of risk they are willing to assume as well as about employment in general. Here we obviously confront the problems of informed consent and informed refusal discussed elsewhere in this volume. (See especially Chapters 5 and 11.) These problems of risk, consent, and refusal are discussed in this chapter by Ruth Faden and Tom Beauchamp. Their essay is followed by an article by Tabitha Powledge on occupational risks and genetic screening. Her arguments consider the need for risk information about possible genetic differences among persons in their susceptibility to environmentally caused health problems. Such information might lead to genetic screening to prevent occupational diseases such as emphysema. Screening itself, however, is surrounded by a set of issues.

PRENATAL SCREENING

The capacity to screen for diseases and disease traits on a mass, public-health basis has increased dramatically. There is every reason to suspect that we will continue to enlarge the class of diseases for which screening is possible and that therefore the number and kinds of mass screening programs will continue to increase as well.

A central moral problem for all screening programs is whether participation in the program ought to be compulsory or merely voluntary. "Voluntary" here means that every individual is free to decide whether to participate in the program and also free to refuse participation (even if the program is administered by a public-health agency and even if health care providers are compelled by law to participate in the program). For example, the state of Maryland currently has a law that compels hospitals to offer newborn screening for PKU (phenylketonuria)[2] and other metabolic disorders to all women immediately following childbirth and to obtain the informed consent of all women who decide to participate. Thus, participation in Maryland's newborn screening program is voluntary for patients but not for health care providers, in the sense that health care providers are obligated by law to offer screening. In their article reproduced in this chapter, Harold Green and Alexander Capron pose the question of under what conditions, if any, a compulsory genetic screening program is permissible on constitutional grounds.

Although the problem of whether participation should be compulsory or mandatory applies to all genetic screening programs, other moral issues are encountered in many screening programs. For example, publicly funded screening for Tay-Sachs disease, an affliction that mostly affects Jews of Eastern European descent, raises questions about justice (including racial discrimination) as well as about the allocation of scarce medical resources. Similarly, screening programs for sickle cell trait, which can produce negative consequences if mismanaged, raise questions about the appropriate use of cost-benefit analysis. However, the most morally vexing and controversial of all screening programs are those involving prenatal diagnosis in order to obtain information about fetuses. These programs necessarily entail the problem of abortion, for discovery of defective fetuses commonly leads to abortion. In prenatal diagnosis programs, various medical tests are used to determine whether pregnant women are carrying defective fetuses. Identification of an abnormality is often not possible before the fourth or fifth month of pregnancy. Should the woman or couple choose to terminate the pregnancy, a second trimester abortion is thus required.

In the essay by Ruth Faden on ''Public Policy Implications of Prenatal Diagnosis,'' these issues of prenatal diagnosis are examined. The central question posed is whether the eradication of birth defects ought to be accepted as a public policy goal. The selection by LeRoy Walters that precedes this essay focuses on a new and highly controversial prenatal diagnosis program—MSAFP screening—and examines the moral issues raised by that particular technological advance.

T. L. B.

NOTES

1. *Royal Commission on Environmental Pollution* (1976), 6th Report, Cmnd 6618. HMSO: London.
2. An inborn error of metabolism that, if untreated, can lead to mental retardation.

DAN E. BEAUCHAMP

Public Health and Individual Liberty

INTRODUCTION

The focus of this article is upon the growing tensions between the goals of protecting the public health and individual liberty. This issue is especially acute in the present period, in which the limits of medicine in effecting substantial future improvements of the health of the public are widely discussed. The term "lifestyle" has entered the vocabulary of health policy.

The document that precipitated this shift in attention was undoubtedly Canada's *New Perspectives on the Health of Canadians*.[1] Few policy documents in the field of health have been as influential or as widely quoted. Within the past five years a flood of editorials, articles and books has proclaimed the new gospel. Leon Kass captured the spirit of the time in the title of his widely read article, "Regarding the End of Medicine and the Pursuit of Health."[2]

This new attention to lifestyle risks has contributed to a growing skepticism about the appropriateness and feasibility of a more activist public role in enhancing the public's health. Some feel that, aside from increased health education,[3,4] the government can or should do little to regulate or change the lifestyles of the American public. Because lifestyles are individual problems (so the argument goes), the legitimacy of governmental policy is questionable and its effectiveness weak. Aaron Wildavsky stated the position in this way[4]:

We are not talking about peripheral or infrequent aspects of human behavior. We are talking about some of the most deeply rooted and often experienced aspects of human life—what one eats, how often and how much; . . . whether one smokes or drinks and how much; even the whole question of human personality. . . . To oversee these decisions would require a larger bureaucracy than anyone has yet

From *Annual Review of Public Health*, 1 (1980), 121–136.

conceived and methods of surveillance bigger than big brother.

Tampering with the lifestyles of the public may seem patently paternalistic. As the authors of the *New Perspective on the Health of Canadians* remarked, there is in Canada a widespread sentiment that individuals should be free to "choose their own poison."[1] It is likely that this viewpoint is at least as prevalent in the U.S.

Even the right to health care now seems a potential casualty of the argument that medicine doesn't matter very much.[2,5,6] Can equality be a goal of health care policy if so much depends on individual lifestyles? Perhaps the most articulate spokesman for this point of view is Leon Kass. Kass argues that there really is no way in which we can clearly speak of health as a right because health cannot be given by one to another.[2] Health is a product of living wisely—the reward of individual duty and virtue.[2]

The lifestyle controversy is a serious challenge for public health. If, as a community and a society, we are not justified in accepting reasonable governmental restrictions on lifestyle risks, a future in which early death and serious disability are sharply reduced may be beyond our grasp.

PUBLIC HEALTH AND PATERNALISM: THE DILEMMA OF VOLUNTARY RISKS

Perhaps the clearest recent treatments of paternalism in the philosophical literature are Gerald Dworkin's.[7,8] According to Dworkin, paternalism is "the interference with a person's liberty of action justified by reasons referring exclusively to the welfare, good, happiness, needs, interests or values of the person being coerced."[7] Paternalism is the restriction of the liberty of a class of individuals to confer a benefit on that same class of individuals.[8] Dworkin's definitions strive to capture the essence of paternalism: the provision of benefits for the individuals' own good—benefits that individuals might not prefer.[7,8] A third criterion, which Dworkin discusses obliquely, is that individuals might obtain these benefits if they acted otherwise. Dworkin provides an illustrative list of policies that he defines as paternalistic.[7,8]

Laws requiring motorcyclists to wear safety helmets when operating their machines; laws forbidding persons from swimming at a public beach when lifeguards are not on duty; laws regulating the use of certain drugs which may have harmful consequences to the user but do not lead to anti-social conduct; laws compelling people to spend a specified fraction of their income on the purchase of retirement annuities. . . .

As Feinberg notes, because there is a presumption for liberty in our society, limiting liberty has to be justified.[9] Limiting the liberty of a class of individuals to confer a benefit on that same class is deemed suspect. Presumably, the individuals whose liberty is restricted may not prefer these benefits, as they could act otherwise. We should limit liberty only to prevent harms to others or harms to some important public interest. This distinction has been made unforgettable in a famous quotation from John Stuart Mill's essay, *On Liberty*.[10]

The only purpose for which power can be rightfully exercised over any member of a civilized community, against his will, is to prevent harm to others. His own good, either physical or moral, is not sufficient warrant. He cannot rightfully be compelled to do or forbear because it will be better for him to do so, because it will make him happier, because, in the opinions of others, to do so would be wise or even right. These are good reasons for remonstrating with him, or reasoning with him, or persuading him, or entreating him, but not for compelling him or visiting him with any evil in case he do otherwise. To justify that, the conduct from which it is desired to deter him must be calculated to produce evil to some one else. The only part of the conduct of any one for which he is amenable to society is that which concerns others. In the part which merely concerns himself, his independence is, of right, absolute. Over himself, over his own body and mind, the individual is sovereign.

As Feinberg,[9] Dworkin,[7,8] and others[9] have argued, both tradition and common sense make us unwilling to reject all forms of paternalism.[6] The consensus appears to be that, indeed, we have come to accept at least weak[9] forms of paternalism, although

we seem wary of expanding these specific instances beyond a short and familiar list. John Knowles, for example, listed governmental measures that he deemed acceptable to protect the health of the public: heavy taxation on alcohol and tobacco are at the head of the list.[11] The *1977-1981 Forward Plan* of HEW gave prominent attention to prevention measures, including a number of limits to voluntary risks, such as taxation on alcohol and tobacco, the labeling of alcoholic beverages, restriction on advertising for a wide number of harmful products, etc.[12] White singles out restrictions on drugs, diet, and automobile operation.[13]

Richard Bonnie argues that the measures advocated exemplify the "new paternalism".[14] Bonnie sees many of these policies as justified because they provide substantial aggregate savings in lives and serious disability, yet they involve only minimal restrictions on individual choice.[14] In the case of drugs (including alcohol), he mentions three permissible forms of "weak paternalism": (a) altering the conditions of availability of harmful substances, (b) deterring individual behavior through (mild) punishment (e.g., fines for smoking in public places), (c) symbolizing the posture of the government toward the behavior, and (d) influencing the content of messages in the mass media.[14]

Thus, although there is concern and anxiety in public health about the appropriate scope and role of government regarding limits to voluntary risks, some argue that some forms of "weak paternalism" are justified.[7,9,11,13,14] Typically, these expansions of the government's power are justified on the bases of the desired health consequences, historical precedent, and because they do not involve serious restriction of the public's liberty. These authors do not so much attempt to resolve the dilemma of paternalism as to argue that mild doses will not be so hard to take (but see Etzioni[15] for a discussion of social influences over personal lifestyles).

Nevertheless, objections to paternalism, even in a weak form, remain substantial and widespread. A recent monograph on ethical dilemmas in lifestyle interventions found widespread concern by health professionals and philosophers over the coercion involved in even weak paternalism, including some forms of persuasion and community organization.[3] It seems likely that the controversy and quasi-legitimacy surrounding public limits over self-regarding and voluntary risks will increase rather than diminish.

BURDENS ON SOCIETY

The major alternative for a justifying principle to limit voluntary risks that avoids paternalism is based on the utilitarian tradition. This alternative points out the costs or secondary harms to others of voluntary risk-taking.[14,16] These secondary harms or costs (economic burdens, usually) are largely indirect in effect. Thus, the argument is made that we restrict smokers' rights and privileges by taxation not to prevent harm to them, but rather to prevent the burden or cost to society of excess morbidity or loss of production. In the case of motorcycle helmet legislation, many courts have adopted the *public ward* theory, arguing that the state is justified in adopting these measures in order to reduce the cost of emergency services and hospital costs, as well as the risk that crash victims who were not wearing helmets will become wards of the state.[14,15,16]

Clearly, John Kaplan points out, Mill would not find these arguments very convincing because the notion of indirect or secondary harms is not only vague, it is subject to limitless expansion.[16] (The Hawaii court[14] acknowledged this point in the motorcycle helmet issue.)

An extreme extension of this particular line of reasoning can be found in a recent article in the *American Journal of Public Health* in which the authors point out the cost of obesity to the nation's fuel bills[17]. The overweight, according to the authors, consume a substantial fraction of the nation's fossil fuel because of the excess food they consume. This excess consumption is quite costly to the society because as much as one-fourth of the nation's food bill is based on fuel costs (farm machinery, transportation, processing, etc.).[17]

These economic justifications for saving lives are reminiscent of a slogan attributed by Sartre to Polish public health officials: "Tuberculosis slows down production."[18] To argue that we are not concerned with crippling diseases or early death per se but rather the avoidance of the burdens these misfortunes place on the rest of us would help to create a climate of callousness and disregard for the value of life and health. Michael Halberstam has charged that these economic arguments "blame the sick" for society's medical bills.[19] But others, such as Leon Kass, would

retort that our drive for a "right to health" is based on a "no-fault" principle.[2] Individuals are left free to pursue unhealthy lifestyles and to present society with the bill for increased medical costs, disability benefits, or benefits to dependents.[2]

Tom Beauchamp suggests cost-benefit or utilitarian principles for justifying some limits to voluntary risks.[20] This approach has the virtue of consistently following through on Mill's basic utilitarianism, for as Dworkin[7,8] and Kaplan[16] point out, Mill was rarely "utilitarian" in his thoughts about paternalism. Mill in his essay *On Liberty* almost always defended self-regarding behavior categorically, setting a high boundary around the personal realm.[10] Beauchamp suggests that "cost-benefit analysis can be employed to make explicit the tradeoffs between . . . lives lost and money expended to save them. . . ."[20]

We have reviewed two contrasting sets of justifying principles for limiting—at least minimally—voluntary risks: weak paternalism and the indirect costs or burdens to the larger society. The disadvantage of the first is that it leaves unanswered the charge of paternalism. The second option makes the major justification for intervention not the prevention of illness or early death, but rather economic savings. Either option may fill many public health officials with some unease.

There is a third option, however, that is open—one that disavows paternalism (even weak paternalism) and the economic argument (although the costs of illness and early death can still remain an important secondary argument for legitimating reasonable restrictions to voluntary risks). This third option is based on the tradition of social justice.[21,22]

PUBLIC HEALTH AND SOCIAL JUSTICE

Traditionally, philosophers have paid relatively little attention to the problem of public health when considering the issue of social justice. The reasons are varied but there is one that needs highlighting.

Justice is broadly concerned with the distribution of benefits and burdens in society.[9,23] This distribution is to be accomplished in accordance with some basic principle: rights, needs, and desert are the leading candidates. Historically, the term "social justice" has been used by those who seek to alter or redistribute the burdens and benefits within society according to the principle of need. These benefits are often secured through the protection of rights or legislative entitlements.

The search by philosophers for a fair or just principle of allocation has led to an important distinction—the distinction between the principle of aggregation and that of distribution. Aggregation refers only to the total amount of good enjoyed by a particular group, whereas distribution refers to the share of that good or benefit that different members of the group have for themselves.[23,24] Aggregative principles are usually associated with utilitarianism, which is that political philosophy that seeks to maximize the total amount of happiness or utility for a society.[23,24]

Social justice, on the other hand, is typically concerned with the distribution or shares of a good in society. In fact, the major criticism of the aggregation principle is that it cares "not a whit" for how the aggregate good that is amassed (such as happiness) is distributed in the population.[25]

Public health does not neatly fall into either of these categories. Although public health produces aggregate benefits (reduction of early death and disability), these benefits are not necessarily converted into other, more general benefits (such as happiness or dollars). Instead, the goals of public health (saving lives, reducing disability) are evaluated against an optimal or ideal community or societal standard that other societies have reached or that is otherwise deemed achievable. Public health is not concerned with shares because its policies are "collective goods" that tend to benefit the entire community like other collective goods (defense, fire, and police protection).[26] It is the level of that collective protection (the rates) that is the crucial standard for evaluation, and this level or standard is the measure of justice obtaining in the community.

Further, public health typically distributes benefits in the form of what Fried terms "statistical lives."[27] It is impossible to say who specifically (e.g. named individuals) receives the benefits of lowered infant mortality rates or lowered rates of liver cirrhosis or coronary disease. These are aggregate gains to the entire community.

SELF AND OTHER IN SOCIAL JUSTICE

In both the paternalist and the burden to society options, the fundamental idea that individuals should normally be able to determine their own good is retained. This is the core notion behind the idea of the self and the central objection to paternalistic interventions. In the burden to society argument, this point is never challenged, but rather the claim is made that one man's good has become another man's shackles in higher taxes and insurance premiums.[11]

It is interesting to see that in the social justice perspective this fundamental idea about the self undergoes a slight but crucial modification. Here we are following the contract tradition of social justice, a tradition brilliantly updated by John Rawls,[25] and drawing particularly on his ideas of the "original position" and the "veil of ignorance."[25] The original position is a position outside and prior to society from which persons view the world without knowing whether they will turn out to be male, female, white, black, rich, poor, sick, healthy, etc. Furthermore, those in the original position do not know their own particular good or plan of life. They can only know "primary goods," or goods which are necessary if everyone's plan of life has a reasonable chance of completion. Ignorance of their own particular good or plan of life leads individuals to agree that fairness demands the provision of those primary goods "individuals would want whatever else they would want."[25] Primary goods would likely include maximum liberty, protection against poverty, ignorance, serious disability, racial discrimination, etc.

The interesting point about the original position is what happens to the idea that individuals should remain free to determine their own good, or the basic idea of the self. The original position forces individuals to consider the interests of others and to recognize that there are certain basic protections that are just and fair, i.e., in the interest of everyone taken together.[28] But oddly, the condition in which individuals do not know their own particular good forces a reconsideration of the unqualified claim that individuals should be free to shape their own plans. This freedom would likely be considered a primary good but its protection would be hedged by the provision of those other primary goods that are necessary for the completion of everyone's plans. Thus, the parties would insist that justice and fairness demand the freedom to pursue one's own plans as a primary good, but would, out of justice and fairness, also consent to reasonable restrictions to this freedom when this is required to provide primary goods that are the necessary means to the completion of everyone's plans. Rawls devotes little serious attention to the impact of the original position on the issue of paternalism. The problem is that the original position and the veil of ignorance expose both the self and other to the same disinterested moral gaze, forcing the consideration of serious and fundamental harms to everyone's interest. In that position of disinterest, deaths in airline crashes because of faulty airline safety practices would not be considered a categorically more serious harm than deaths in automotive crashes because of the absence of mandatory seatbelt laws. This point is discussed further below.

The central point is that in the social justice perspective, the categories of self and others cannot serve to automatically define the boundaries of the moral community. (In Rawls' world the moral community consists only of enforceable obligations to others.) The view here is that the moral community is the project of assuring a decent minimum for human welfare. This project would include accepting reasonable limitations to self-regarding risks, as long as these restrictions promised important gains in reducing the risk of early death and yet avoided serious harms to the basic interests of privacy, autonomy, basic political liberties, or the provision of other primary goods. The acceptance of limits to voluntary risks would be justified, however, not in terms of obligations to self or with reference to narrow or specific benefits for the regulated group, but rather in the broader terms of public health and human welfare as a project for building the just society or community. In the just community or society the risk of premature death (and associated serious disability) would be lowered as much as possible in precisely the same way that protections are provided against poverty, old age, unemployment, and racial discrimination. To see how these ideas may be given more substance, let us examine more closely how members in the original position (or persons who take an objective, disinterested moral point of view) would approach the issue of death as a harm.

THE HARM OF EARLY DEATH

Those in the original position would know that death itself, although perhaps the most serious harm confronting human beings, is itself not capable of eradication. What is susceptible to change is premature death. But what constitutes a premature death? How would those in the original position come to an agreement on this crucial issue?

It is not likely that the members would choose the goal of prolonging life (added years at the end of life such as increasing the life expectancy for those who survive to age 70 or 75). Such a goal would demand a technology and a scientific revolution not in hand or in sight. It is far more likely that premature death would be seen as early death, death before some period widely regarded as the defining point of a ripe life. For the American society, such a boundary might well be the ages 65 or 70.[29] Thus, although death after this age would still remain a harm, death before that time would be regarded as an even more serious harm and one from which citizens deserve basic protection.

For the sake of discussion, let us assume that early death would be defined as death before age 65. It seems plausible that those in the original position would see policies to reduce or minimize the risk of early death as a primary good—one enjoying equal status with the other primary goods of the just community and in the interests of everybody taken together. The evidence that other societies do in fact enjoy much lower risks of early death while still retaining the basic political liberties and other key social goods would only strengthen the case. Refusal to secure this protection would be almost unthinkable. Why would the participants be any more eager to live with high rates of early death than high rates of unemployment, poverty, or violation of civil liberties?

To dramatize this situation, let us consider the present American society and the problem of early death as it would appear to members in the original position. We are fortunate to have James Vaupel's definitive analysis of a problem he calls "the American tragedy."[29] As Vaupel points out, the U.S. ranks 26 among all nations in survival rates at age 65, behind the leaders, Sweden and Norway, and "all other major developed countries and behind Bulgaria, Puerto Rico and Hong Kong."[30] The U.S. ranks just above Finland, which has the highest rates of heart disease in the world. Nevertheless, life expectancy at age 65 for Americans is almost exactly the same as for Swedes; the disparity truly lies in early deaths or deaths before age 65.

To the participants in the original position, over one-quarter of all who enter the American society would die before age 65 [given the survival rates used by Vaupel]. One-third of all males woud die before age 65 and one-half of all black males would fail to reach 65. If the participants were to examine Sweden, however, better than 4 out of 5 males would survive to age 65. Females in the U.S. would experience roughly the same survival rates as Swedish males, whereas almost 9 out of 10 Swedish women could expect to live to age 65.

There is little doubt that those in the original position would find this disparity truly alarming, especially if there were evidence that Sweden was prosperous, democratic, and otherwise not paying exorbitantly for its much lower rates of early death. Although the participants may concede that achieving Sweden's rates of early death might be more difficult in the U.S., it is still likely that those in the original position would regard the rates of early death in the U.S. as intolerable. As Vaupel argues,[31] this level of risk would mean that in the U.S. today the risk of early death (25%) is more grave than the risk of poverty (12%).

We now come to a crucial point in the argument. If the participants agree that this primary good ought be provided (early death ought be minimized) and that this goal necessitates some limits over self-regarding behavior, would these limits be paternalistic as Rawls seems to think?[25]

The answer is surely no. The central idea behind paternalism is the state limiting the freedom of individuals to make their own plans. But we have seen how the idea of social justice would result in individuals consenting to reasonable limits to this freedom in order to secure those primary goods that are necessary means for the completion of everyone's plans.

But the objection may still be raised that this protection—at least in the case of policy to avert early death—is paternalistic because it provides benefits that individuals could obtain if they acted otherwise. As Kass argues, if individuals would act more wisely, the harm of early death could be dramatically reduced.[2] But from the viewpoint of the original position, this line of reasoning would seem wrong if not absurd. The participants in the original position would not refuse to consider reducing the very serious harm of early death simply because the individuals involved could have acted otherwise. They would only refuse to eliminate the harm of early death when those restrictions on lifestyle risks incurred a more serious harm, such as a violation of fundamental liberty, privacy, or autonomy.

The virtue of choosing the goal of minimizing the harm of early death is that it moves the justifying principle away from reasons referring exclusively to the interests of the regulated group.[7,8] The focus is upon the broader societal goal of reducing the harm of early death. This shift helps to move the issue away from what individuals might do if they acted more wisely toward a goal that members of society would regard as urgent and justified. By focusing on the harm itself, a future with a high rate of early death would be as unjust as a future without social security or protection against poverty.

The parties probably would develop other criteria governing the selection of policies to minimize early death, choosing to focus on the most serious and widespread threats such as occupational hazards, highway safety, handguns, automobiles, smoking, use of alcohol and drugs rather than risks such as mountain climbing, skiing, skydiving, and hanggliding.

Further, it is likely that the participants would stipulate that priority be given to risks and hazards in which there is an important commercial or industrial interest—an interest that actively promotes and encourages the widespread adoption and acceptance of risk-bearing activities. The participants would do so for two reasons: (1) As Etzioni argues,[15] commercial interests promoting the hazardous activity dilute the purely voluntary aspect of these activities, thus increasing the legitimacy of intervention. (2) The fact that such institutions encourage these activities and risks offers public avenues for regulation and control that avoid the harm of invasion of privacy and the precedent of established tradition. As Kaplan[16] and Bonnie[14] argue, these are important assets for a social policy that seeks to influence self-regarding behavior or lifestyles.

Finally, the participants would attempt to clearly articulate a set of limits for policies to save lives, especially in cases that involve influencing lifestyles. These limits are discussed in more detail below.

SOCIAL JUSTICE IN THE CONTEMPORARY SOCIETY

Using the criteria developed in the last section it is possible to turn to concrete cases and to approach the topic of social justice and the harm of early death in the contemporary society. For purposes of discussion, the case of policy for alcohol and tobacco will be considered.

The attainment of social justice in the contemporary society is a struggle that is conducted amid the swirl of competing and conflicting interests: commercial interests, consumer interests, minority interests, individual interests (privacy, autonomy), and the interest of the health and safety of the public. The conflicts between these interests grow most evident as the goals of social justice (in our case the reduction in rates of early death) are pressed.

The goal of public health in the contemporary society from Rawls' original position would be to dramatize the urgent priority of minimizing early death and to elevate this interest as a primary social goal and central achievement of the just community. This goal cannot be achieved without an adjustment of the benefits and advantages enjoyed by other important interests in society (industry, the consuming public, etc.). As Anthony Downs has observed, many of our most serious problems in American society (racism, unemployment, poverty) are rooted in advantages and benefits enjoyed by the most influential and the most numerous.[32] The essential challenge to public health in its shared struggle for the just community is to work for a future as free as possible from early death.

This perspective on social justice goes beyond the search for the abstract distributive principles, anticipating realistically and without sentimentality the resistance of key groups to the burdens of dramatically reducing early death. Protecting the health and safety of workers, achieving higher levels of highway safety, and effecting even reasonable restrictions on tobacco and alcohol consumption will be accomplished only by altering institutional arrangements and existing distributions of property and power. Those who stand to lose or suffer inconveniences if this realignment is brought about do not remain passive. Because "one man's prize is another man's loss,"[33] attempts to realize social justice lead to wars and skirmishes over distribution.[34] This conflict and involvement of a wide group of interests is yet more evidence that policies to reduce early death (including limits to voluntary risks) involve far more than restrictions on a class of individuals to benefit that same class of individuals.[8]

POLICY FOR ALCOHOL AND TOBACCO

It is clear that the parties in the original position would give high priority to attempts to discourage the use of tobacco and the heavy use of alcohol for the reason that these hazards contribute substantially to early deaths—perhaps 15 to 20% of the approximately 700,000 early deaths[29] each year.[35] The parties would also focus on these two commodities because of the important interests involved in advertising, promoting, and otherwise encouraging the use of

these commodities, a situation that creates a case of voluntary behavior that at the least is clearly influenced. Likewise, these two commodities offer opportunities for public regulation (affecting the conditions of availability, legal prohibitions against certain uses, and taxation) that avoid invasions of privacy; there is compelling if not overwhelming evidence that these restrictions would have an impact, at least for alcohol[36, 37] (although in this paper the effectiveness of specific interventions is not the central issue).

The form of justification in regulating these hazards is crucial. The issue of the harm of early death should be placed again and again before the public. This harm and injustice must constantly be raised so that the entire community can determine for itself whether the current levels of early death are acceptable and fair, and if not, whether a collective response is justified. In other words, a central goal of developing policy for alcohol and tobacco (and related lifestyle risks) is to allow for the formation of consensus. If we defend regulatory policy for these substances only in terms of protecting the interests of the persons being regulated, we run the risk that the fundamental issue of early death will be buried under familiar clichés about individual freedom and individual responsibility. The issues of individual freedom and responsibility must be weighed against the harm of early death, not used to prevent the harm of early death from being recognized.

Shifting the justifying principles behind these policies would help to avoid the charge of moralism: public health officials could no longer be accused of conducting holy wars against tobacco or alcohol, regulating these commodities on moral grounds. Rather, tobacco and alcohol would be singled out because of their significant contribution to what Vaupel terms our national tragedy of early death.[29]

Paradoxically, focusing on early death would also help to avoid the charge that public health officials seek a zero risk society and attack all risk-bearing activity from nuclear power to skateboarding or hang-gliding. Selecting the goal of minimizing early death would clarify the aims and purposes of public health campaigns and establish a goal that, though ambitious, is certainly not reckless or utopian. Centering on early death avoids the charge that policies regulating the hazards of the workplace, the highways, the marketplace, and a few key lifestyle risks promise the "freedom of the zoo,"[38] as prosperous societies exist in which much lower rates of early death obtain without a loss of basic freedoms (Sweden and Norway are the leading examples).[29] There is evidence that major segments of the U.S. population enjoy much higher survival rates than do others:[29] It can hardly be argued that women and whites enjoy the "freedom of the zoo."

The central goal and standard used by public health is a community or societal goal derived from consideration of the issue of justice and fairness when the interests of all are surveyed from a detached, objective standpoint (the original position). Of course, the goal of minimizing early death is a long-term one and no consideration has been given here to the problem of establishing interim objectives that would be fair and acceptable. In establishing such a goal or standard, consideration should be given to historical trends and to the experience of comparable societies whose record is distinctively better, as well as to the testimony of citizens, experts, advocates, and opponents.

LIMITS TO PUBLIC HEALTH

Although the problem of early death is a serious problem for our society, its elimination is not the only goal of the just community. Equality and justice give rise to other values and protections that constitute important limits to public health and collective action. I will list, without elaboration, the most crucial of these limits:

1. the broad injunction against public health measures that unreasonably and coercively interfere with the fundamental rights of privacy of individual citizens
2. the injunction against pursuing the goals of public health at the expense of other primary goods such as basic education, elimination of poverty, and, especially, basic political liberties
3. the injunction against the undue emphasis on controlling some public health hazards to the exclusion of others, especially when the control of others may achieve more dramatic results in terms of minimizing disability or early death
4. the injunction against measures that increase, over the long run, the risks of death and disability
5. the injunction to consider the problems of "redistributive justice," or the special problems of achieving a transition from one model of justice to another. A corollary of this injunction would be that when two or more policy options promise roughly equivalent results, that option

should be chosen that is least disruptive of other social or economic values. This suggests that, whereas the focus of discussion has been on governmental measures to reduce risks, education should occupy an important role in the campaign to eliminate early death. This educational focus would not be simply on encouraging changes in individual behavior but would seek to mobilize support and legitimacy for the project of minimizing early death in American society.

CONCLUSION

This essay, in exploring the current debate about lifestyle risks and the question of paternalism, scrutinizes and finds wanting the options of "weak paternalism" and "burdens on society" (secondary harms) as justifying principles for governmental intervention. A third alternative, drawn from the tradition of social justice, is offered as justifying selected and limited restrictions of lifestyle risks. This alternative casts the issue of paternalism in a new light, suggesting the need to submit our assumptions about paternalism to closer scrutiny instead of searching for increasingly ingenious ways of fitting self-regarding behavior into other-regarding categories.

What has been argued is actually quite simple. From the standpoint of the original position and the perspective of social justice, the central issue is not to first decide whether some harm is a wrong or an injustice by determining whether it is self-inflicted. The central question is one of reducing serious harms outright while at the same time avoiding the creation of greater harms. This mode of thinking turns the traditional philosophical approach upside down, but it follows more closely the way we think about public health problems in everyday life. The crucial debate in society centers on whether some problem or condition is indeed a serious harm. Once this is decided, we then ask if this harm can be minimized while protecting the other vital interests in society, including the interests of privacy, autonomy, and individual liberty. Of course, we do not decide whether a condition is a serious problem or harm without considering the question of self-regarding versus other-regarding behaviors; still, the primary issue is whether the harm itself is so serious as to merit a collective response.

The argument here should help to focus the current debate about lifestyle risks in proper perspective.

Lifestyle risks are not the only culprits in the problem of early death. This country can make dramatic progress in minimizing early death through more stringent protection of the environment, the workplace, and our modes of transportation. Also, eliminating the great disparities of income and other social advantages between the classes and races would help to close the gap for those groups who bear such a heavy burden. The struggle to minimize early death clearly complements and supports the other goals of social justice: economic equality and justice, full employment, a prosperous economy, and a protected environment.

It is often noted that public health is centrally concerned with the community approach.[39] Although the term ''community'' has various meanings, one meaning is important above all else: the strengthening of community through meeting the needs of all its members, i.e., building the community through the doing of justice. If the ideal of community is to have a redemptive meaning, it must be seen as a project in search of justice. There can be no true community when the demands of justice are ignored.

The obvious truth that many, if not most, lifestyle hazards are powerfully influenced by market forces and societal and cultural constraints[15, 21, 22] has been discussed only in passing. It seemed necessary, instead, to face the hard question: Even if there is a substantial voluntary component in most lifestyle risks (and there surely is), do the demands of justice and community require their reasonable restriction? The answer here is in the affirmative.

NOTES

1. Gov. of Canada/Minist. Natl. Health Welfare. 1974. *A New Perspective on the Health of Canadians.* Ottawa: Minist. Natl. Health Welfare. 76 pp.

2. Kass, L. 1975. Regarding the end of medicine and the pursuit of health. *Public Interest* 40:11–42.

3. Meenan, R. F. 1976. Improving the public's health—Some further reflections. *N. Engl. J. Med.* 294:45–47.

4. Faden, R., Faden, A., eds. 1978. Ethical issues in public health policy: Health education and lifestyle interventions. Health Educ. Monogr. 6(2).

5. Wildavsky, A. 1976. Can health be planned? *Davis Lect., Cent. for Health Admin. Stud.* Univ. of Chicago, Chicago, Ill.

6. Brown, L. 1978. The scope and limits of equality as a normative guide to federal health care policy. *Public Policy* 26:481–532.

7. Dworkin, G. 1972. Paternalism. *Monist* 56:64–84.

8. Dworkin, G. 1971. Paternalism. In *Morality and the Law,*
ed. R. A. Wasserstrom, pp. 107–126. Belmont, Calif: Wadsworth, 149 pp.

9. Feinberg, J. 1973. *Social Philosophy,* pp. 45–52. Englewood Cliffs, NJ: Prentice-Hall. 126 pp.

10. Mill, J. S. 1859. *On Liberty,* p. 13, ed. C. V. Shields. Indianapolis: Bobbs-Merrill, 1977 ed. 141 pp.

11. Knowles, J. 1978. The responsibility of the individual. In *Doing Better and Feeling Worse,* ed. J. Knowles, pp. 57–80. New York: Norton. 278 pp.

12. US Dept. Health, Educ., Welfare, Public Health Serv. 1975. *Forward Plan for Health: FY 1977-81,* pp. 100–103. Washington DC: US DHEW. 259 pp.

13. White, L. S. 1975. How to improve the public's health. *N. Engl. J. Med.* 293:773–774.

14. Bonnie, R. 1978. Discouraging unhealthy personal choices: Reflections on new directions in substance abuse policy. *J. Drug Issues* 8:199–219.

15. Etzioni, A. 1978. Individual will and social conditions: Toward an effective health maintenance policy. *Ann. Am. Acad. Polit. Soc. Sci.* 437:62–73.

16. Kaplan, J. 1971. The role of the law in drug control. *Duke Law J.* 1971:1065–1104.

17. Hannon, B. M., Lohman, T. G. 1978. The energy cost of overweight in the United States. *Am. J. Public Health* 68:765–67.

18. Miranda, J. 1977. *Being and the Messiah,* p. 36. Maryknoll, NY: Orbis. 245 pp.

19. *Washington Post.* Dec. 17, 1978.

20. Beauchamp, T. L. 1978. The regulation of hazards and hazardous behavior. *Health Educ. Monogr.* 6:242–257.

21. Beauchamp, D. E. 1976. Public health as social justice. *Inquiry* 13:3–14.

22. Beauchamp, D. E. 1976. Exploring new ethics for public health: Developing a fair alcohol policy. *J. Health Polit. Policy and Law* 1:338–354.

23. Miller, D. 1976. *Social Justice,* pp. 17–153. Oxford: Clarendon. 367 pp.

24. Barry, B. 1963. *Political Argument,* Chap. 3. New York: Humanities. 364 pp.

25. Rawls, J. 1971. *A Theory of Justice,* pp. 3–192, 249. Cambridge: Harvard Univ. Press. 607 pp.

26. Olson, M. 1965. *The Logic of Collective Action,* pp. 14–15. Cambridge: Harvard Univ. Press. 176 pp.

27. Fried, C. 1970. *An Anatomy of Values,* pp. 207–236. Cambridge: Harvard Univ. Press. 265 pp.

28. Baier, K. 1965. *The Moral Point of View.* New York: Random. 165 pp.

29. Vaupel, J. V. 1976. Early death: An American tragedy. *Law Contemp. Probl.* 40:73–121.

30. *Ibid.,* p. 86.

31. *Ibid.,* p. 82.

32. Downs, A. 1972. Up and down with ecology—The issue-attention cycle. *Public Interest* 20:38–50.

33. Klein, R. In Lekachman, R. 1979. Looking for the left. *Harper's* April, pp. 21–23.

34. Lekachman, R. 1979. See Ref. 31, p. 22. Natl. Inst. Alcohol Abuse and Alcoholism/Alcohol, Drug Abuse, and Mental Health Admin./Public Health Serv. 1978. *Third Special Report to the U.S. Congress on Alcohol and Health,* p. 10. Washington DC: GPO, 98 pp. and Public Health Service/Dept. Health, Education, and Welfare 1979. *Smoking and Health: A Report of the Surgeon General,* Chap. 2. Washington DC: GPO.

35. This estimate assumes that roughly 50,000 to 65,000 early deaths are due to cirrhosis, highway crashes, and other causes that are alcohol-related. Statistics on early deaths due to smoking are hard to come by but the assumption that roughly the same magnitude of deaths (50,000 to 65,000), or 15 to 20% of the 325,000 excess deaths attributed to smoking, are early deaths does not seem unreasonable.

36. Bruun, K., Edwards, G. Lumio, M., Mäkelä, K., Pan, L., Popham, R. E., Room, R., Schmidt, W., Skog, O.L., Sulkunen, P., Österberg, E. 1975. *Alcohol Control Policies in Public Health Perspective.* Helsinki: Finnish Found. Alcohol Studies. 106 pp.

37. Popham, R., Schmidt, W., deLint, J. 1976. The effects of legal restraint on drinking. In *The Social Aspects of Alcoholism, The Biology of Alcoholism,* ed. B. Kissin, H. Begleiter, 4:579–625. New York: Plenum. 643 pp.

38. Fuchs, V. 1974. *Who Shall Live?,* p. 26. New York: Basic. 168 pp.

39. McGavran, E. 1953. What is public health? *Can. J. Public Health* 44:441–451

DANIEL WIKLER

Persuasion and Coercion for Health: Ethical Issues in Government Efforts to Change Lifestyles

What should be the government's role in promoting the kinds of personal behavior that lead to long life and good health? Smoking, overeating, and lack of exercise increase one's chances of suffering illness later in life, as do many other habits. The role played by lifestyle is so important that, as stated by Fuchs:[1] "The greatest current potential for improving the health of the American people is to be found in what they do and don't do for themselves." But the public has shown little spontaneous interest in reforming. If the government uses the means at its disposal to remedy the situation, it may be faced with problems of an ethical nature. Education, exhortation, and other relatively mild measures may not prove effective in inducing self-destructive people to change their behavior. Attention might turn instead to other means, which, though possibly more effective, might also be intrusive or otherwise distasteful. In this essay, I seek to identify the moral principles underlying a reasoned judgment on whether stronger methods might justifiably be used, and, if so, what limits ought to be observed.

. . .

GOALS OF HEALTH BEHAVIOR REFORM

I propose to discuss three possible goals of health behavior reform with regard to their appropriateness as goals of government programs and the problems arising in their pursuit. The first goal can be simply stated: health should be valued for its own sake. Americans are likely to be healthier if they can be induced to adopt healthier habits, and this may be reason enough to try to get them to do so. The second goal is the fair distribution of the burdens caused by illness. Those who become ill because of unhealthy lifestyles may require the financial support of the more prudent, as well as the sharing of what may be scarce medical facilities. If this is seen as unfair to those who do not make themselves sick, lifestyle reform measures will also be seen as accomplishing distributive justice. The third goal is the maintenance and improvement of the general welfare, for the nation's health conditions have their effects on the economy, allocation of resources, and even national security.

HEALTH AS A GOAL IN ITSELF: BENEFICENCE AND PATERNALISM

Much of the present concern for the reform of unhealthy lifestyles stems from concern over the health of those who live dangerously. Only a misanthrope would quarrel with this goal. There are several steps that might immediately be justified: the government could make the effects of unhealthy living habits known to those who practice them, and sponsor research to discover more of these facts. The chief concern over such efforts might be that the government

From *Milbank Memorial Fund Quarterly/Health and Society* 56 (Summer 1978), 303, 306–317.

would begin its urgings before the facts in question had been firmly established, thus endorsing living habits that might be useless or detrimental to good health.

Considerably more debate, however, would arise over a decision to use stronger methods. For example, a case in point might be a government "fat tax," which would require citizens to be weighed and taxed if overweight. The surcharges thus derived would be held in trust, to be refunded with interest if and when the taxpayers brought their weight down.[2] This pressure would, under the circumstances, be a bond imposed by the government upon its citizens, and thus can be fairly considered as coercive.

The two signal properties of this policy would be its aim of improving the welfare of obese taxpayers, and its presumed unwelcome imposition on personal freedom. (Certain individual taxpayers, of course, might welcome such an imposition, but this is not the ordinary response to penalties.) The first property might be called "beneficence," and it is generally a virtue. But the second property becomes paternalism;[3] and its status as a virtue is very much in doubt. "Paternalism" is a loaded word, almost automatically a term of reprobation. But many paternalistic policies, especially when more neutrally described, attract support and even admiration. It may be useful to consider what is bad and what is good about paternalistic practices, so that we might decide whether in this case the good outweighs the bad. For detailed discussions of paternalism in the abstract, see Feinberg,[4] Dworkin,[5] Bayles,[6] and Hodson.[7]

What is good about some paternalistic interventions is that people are helped, or saved from harm. Citizens who have to pay a fat tax, for example, may lose weight, become more attractive, and live longer. In the eyes of many, these possible advantages are more than offset by the chief fault of paternalism, its denying persons the chance to make their own choices concerning matters that affect them. Self-direction, in turn, is valued because people usually believe themselves to be the best judges of what is good for them, and because the choosing is considered a good in itself. These beliefs are codified in our ordinary morality in the form of a moral right to noninterference so long as one does not adversely affect the interests of others. This right is supposed to shield an individual's "self-regarding" actions from intervention by others,

even when those acts are not socially approved ones and even when they promise to be unwise.

At the same time, the case for paternalistic intervention on at least some occasions seems compelling. There may be circumstances in which we lose, temporarily or permanently, our capacity for competent self-direction, and thereby inflict harm upon ourselves that serves little purpose. Like Ulysses approaching the Sirens, we may hope that others would then protect us from ourselves. This sort of consideration supports our imposed guardianship of children and of the mentally retarded. Although these persons often resent our paternalistic control, we reason that we are doing what they would want us to do were their autonomy not compromised. Paternalism would be a benefit under the sort of social insurance policy that a reasonable person would opt for if considered in a moment of lucidity and competence.[5]

Does this rationale for paternalism support governmental coercion of competent adults to assure the adoption of healthy habits of living? It might seem to, at first sight. Although these adults may be generally competent, their decision-making abilities can be compromised in specific areas. Individuals may be ignorant of the consequences of their acts; they may be under the sway of social or commercial manipulation and suggestion; they may be afflicted by severe psychological stress or compulsion; or be under external constraint. If any of these conditions hold, the behavior of adults may fail to express their settled will. Those of us who disavow any intention of interfering with free and voluntary risk-taking may see cause to intervene when a person's behavior is not under his or her control.

Paternalism: Theoretical Problems. There are a number of reasons to question the general argument for paternalism in the coercive eradication of unhealthful personal practices. First, the analogy between the cases of children and the retarded, where paternalism is most clearly indicated, and of risk-taking adults is misleading. If the autonomy of adults is compromised in one or more of the ways just mentioned, it might be possible to restore that autonomy by attending to the sources of the involuntariness; the same cannot ordinarily be done with children or the retarded. Thus, adults who are destroying their health because of ignorance may be educated; adults acting under constraint may be freed. If restoration of autonomy is a realistic project, then paternalistic interference is unjustified. The two kinds of interventions are aimed at the same target, i.e., harmful behavior not freely and competently chosen. But they accomplish the result differently. Paternalistic intervention blocks the harm; education and similar measures restore the choice. The state or health planners would seem obligated to use this less restrictive alternative if they can. This holds true even though the individuals might still engage in their harmful practices once autonomy is restored. This would not call for paternalistic intervention, since the risk woud be voluntarily shouldered.

It remains true, however, that autonomy sometimes cannot be restored. It may be impossible to reach a given population with the information they need; or, once reached, the persons in question may prove ineducable. Psychological compulsions and social pressures may be even harder to eradicate. In these situations, the case for paternalistic interference is relatively strong, yet even here there is reason for caution. Persons who prove incapable of absorbing the facts about smoking, for example, or who abuse drugs because of compulsion or addiction, may retain a kind of second-order autonomy. They can be told that they appear unable to accept scientific truth, or that they are addicted; and they can then decide to reconsider the facts or to seek a cure. In some cases these will be decisions that the individuals are fully competent to carry out; paternalistic intervention would unjustly deny them the right to control their destinies. Coercion would be acceptable only if this second-order decision were itself constrained, compelled, or otherwise compromised—which, in the case of health-related behavior, it may often be.

A second reason for doubting the justifiability of paternalistic interference concerns the subjectivity of the notion of harm. The same experience may be seen as harmful by one person and as beneficial by another; or, even more common, the goodness (or badness) of a given eventuality may be rated very differently by different persons. Although we as individuals are often critical of the importance placed on certain events by others, we nevertheless hesitate to claim special authority in such matters. Most of us subscribe to the pluralistic ethic, for better or for worse, which has as a central tenet the proposition that there are multiple distinct, but equally valid, concepts of good and of the good life. It follows that we must use personal preferences and tastes to determine whether our health-related practices are detrimental.

Unfortunately, it is often difficult to defer to the authority of others in defining harm and benefit. It is common to feel that one's own preferences reflect values that reasonable people adopt; one can hardly regard oneself as unreasonable. To the extent that government planners employ their own concepts of good in attempting to change health practices for the public's benefit, the social insurance rationale for paternalism is clearly inapplicable.

A third reason for criticism of paternalism is the vagueness of the notion of decision-making disability. The conscientious paternalist intervenes only when the self-destructive individual's autonomy is compromised. It is probably impossible, however, to specify a compromising condition. To be sure, there are cases in which the lack of autonomy is evident, such as that of a child swallowing dangerous pills in the belief that they are candy. But the sorts of practices that would be the targets of coercive campaigns to reform health-related behavior are less dramatic and their involuntary quality much less certain. Since the free and voluntary conditions of health-related practice cannot be specified in advance, there is obviously considerable potential for unwarranted interference with fully voluntary choices.

Indeed, the dangers involved in disregarding individuals' personal values and in falsely branding their behavior involuntary are closely linked. In the absence of independent criteria for decision-making disability, the paternalist may try to determine disability by seeing whether the individual is rational, i.e., whether he or she competently pursues what is valuable. An absence of rationality may be reason to suspect the presence of involuntariness and hence grounds for paternalism. The problem, however, is that this test for rationality—whether the chosen means are appropriate for the individual's personal ends—is not fully adequate. Factors that deprive an individual of autonomy—such as compulsion or constraint—not only affect a person's ability to calculate means to ends but also induce ends that are in some sense foreign. Advertisements, for example, may instill desires to consume certain substances whose pleasures would ordinarily be considered trifling. Similarly, ignorance may induce people to value a certain experience because they believe it will lead to their attainment of other ends. Alcoholics, for example, may value intoxication because they think it will enhance their social acceptance. The paternalist on the lookout for non-autonomous, self-destructive behavior will be interested not only in irrational means but also uncharacteristic, unreasonable values.

The difficulty for the paternalist at this point is plain. The desire to interfere only with involuntary risk-taking leads to designating individuals for intervention whose behavior proceeds from externally instilled values. Pluralism commits the paternalist to use the person's own values in determining whether a health-related practice is harmful. What is needed is some way of determining individuals' "true" personal values; but if these cannot be read off from their behavior, how can they be known?

In certain individual cases, a person's characteristic preferences can be determined from wishes expressed before losing autonomy, as was Ulysses' desire to be tied to the mast. But this sort of data is hardly likely to be available to government health planners. The problem would be at least partially solved if we could identify a set of goods that is basic and appealing, and that nearly all rational persons value. Such universal valuation would justify a presumption of involuntariness should an individual's behavior put these goods in jeopardy. On what grounds would we include an item on this list? Simple popularity would suffice: if almost everyone likes something, such approval probably stems from a common human nature, shared by even those not professing to like that thing. Hence we may suspect, that, if unconstrained, they would like it also. Alternatively, there may be experiences or qualities that, while not particularly appealing in themselves, are preconditions to attaining a wide variety of goods that people idiosyncratically value. Relief from pain is an example of the first sort of good; normal-or-better intelligence is an instance of the latter.

The crucial question for health planners is whether *health* is one of these primary goods. Considered alone, it certainly is: it is valued for its own sake; and it is a means to almost all ends. Indeed, it is a necessary good. No matter how eccentric a person's values and tastes are, no matter what kinds of activities are pleasurable, it is impossible to engage in them unless alive. Most activities a person is likely to enjoy, in fact, require not only life but good health. Unless one believes in an afterlife, the rational person must rate death as an incomparable calamity, for it means the loss of everything.

But the significance of health as a primary good should not be overestimated. The health planner may attempt to argue for coercive reform of health-destructive behavior with a line of reasoning that recalls Pascal's wager.[8] Since death, which precludes all good experience, must receive an enormously negative valuation, contemplated action that involves risk of death will also receive a substantial negative value after the good and bad consequences have been considered. And this will hold true even if the risk is small, since even low probability multiplied by a very large quantity yields a large quantity. Hence anyone who risks death by living dangerously must, on this view, be acting irrationally. This would be grounds for suspecting that the life-threatening practices were less than wholly voluntary and thus created a need for protection. Further, this case would not require the paternalistic intervenor to turn away from pluralistic ideals, for the unhealthy habits would be faulted not on the basis of deviance from paternalistic values, but on the apparent lapse in the agent's ability to understand the logic of the acts.

This argument, or something like it, may lie behind the willingness of some to endorse paternalistic regulation of the lifestyles of apparently competent adults. It is, however, invalid. Its premises may sometimes be true, and so too may its conclusion, but the one does not follow from the other. Any number of considerations can suffice to show this. For example, time factors are ignored. An act performed at age 25 that risks death at age 50 does not threaten every valued activity. It simply threatens the continuation of those activities past the age of 50. The argument also overlooks an interplay between the possible courses of action: if every action that carries some risk of death or crippling illness is avoided, the enjoyment of life decreases. This makes continued life less likely to be worth the price of giving up favorite unhealthy habits.[9] Indeed, although it may be true that death would deny one of all chances for valued experiences, the experiences that make up some people's lives have little value. The less value a person places on continued life, the more rational it is to engage in activities that may brighten it up, even if they involve the risk of ending it. Craig Claiborne, food editor of *The New York Times,* gives ebullient testimony to this possibility in the conclusion of his "In Defense of Eating Rich Food":[10]

I love hamburgers and chili con carne and hot dogs. And foie gras and sauternes and those small birds known as ortolans. I love banquettes of quail eggs with hollandaise sauce and clambakes with lobsters dipped into so much butter it dribbles down the chin. I like cheesecake and crepes filled with cream sauces and strawberries with creme fraîche . . .

And if I am abbreviating my stay on this earth for an hour or so, I say only that I have no desire to be a Methuselah, a hundred or more years old and still alive, grace be to something that plugs into an electric outlet.

The assumption that one who is endangering one's health must be acting irrationally and involuntarily is not infrequently made by those who advocate forceful intervention in suicide attempts; and perhaps some regard unhealthy lifestyles as a sort of slow suicide. The more reasonable view, even in cases of imminent suicide, seems rather to be that *some* unhealthy or self-destructive acts are less-than-fully voluntary but that others are not. Claiborne's diet certainly seems to be voluntary, and suggests that the case for paternalistic intervention in lifestyle cannot be made on grounds of logic alone. It remains true, however, that much of the behavior that leads to chronic illness and accidental injury is not fully under the control of the persons so acting. My thesis is merely that, first, this involuntariness must be shown (along with much else) if paternalistic intervention is to be justified; and, second, this can only be determined by case-by-case empirical study. Those who advocate coercive measures to reform lifestyles, whose motives are purely beneficent, and who wish to avoid paternalism except where justified, might find such study worth undertaking.

Any such study is likely to reveal that different practitioners of a given self-destructive habit act from different causes. Perhaps one obese person overeats because of an oral fixation over which he has no control, or in a Pavlovian response to enticing television food advertisements. The diminished voluntariness of these actions lends support to paternalistic intervention. Claiborne has clearly thought matters through and decided in favor of a shorter though gastronomically happier life; to pressure him into changing so that he may live longer would be a clear imposition of values and would lack the justification provided in the other person's case.

The trouble for a government policy of lifestyle reform is that a given intervention is more likely to be tailored to practices and habits than to people. Although we may someday have a fat tax to combat obesity, it would be surprising indeed to find one that imposed charges only on those whose obesity was due to involuntary factors. It would be difficult to reach agreement on what constituted diminished voluntariness; harder still to measure it; and perhaps administratively impractical to make the necessary exceptions and adjustments. We may feel, after examining the merits of the cases, that intervention is justified in the compulsive eater's lifestyle but not in the case of Claiborne. If the intervention takes the form of a tax on obesity *per se,* we face a choice: Do we owe it to those like Claiborne *not* to enforce alien values more than we owe it to compulsive overeaters to protect them from self-destruction? The general right of epicures to answer to their own values, a presumptive right conferred by the pluralistic ethic spoken of earlier, might count for more then the need of compulsive overeaters to have health imposed on them, since the first violates a right and the second merely confers a benefit. But the situation is more complex than this. The compulsive overeater's life is at stake, and this may be of greater concern (everything else being equal) than the epicure's pleasures. Then, too, the epicure is receiving a compensating benefit in the form of longer life, even if this is not a welcome exchange. And there may be many more compulsive overeaters than there are people like Claiborne. On the other hand, the positive causal link between tax and health for either is indirect and tenuous, while the negative relation between tax and gastronomic pleasure is relatively more substantial. (For a fuller discussion of this type of tradeoff, see Bayles.[6] Perhaps the firmest conclusion one may draw from all this is that a thoroughly reasoned moral rationale for a given kind of intervention can be very difficult to carry out.

Paternalism: Problems in Practice. Even if we accept the social insurance rationale for paternalism in the abstract, then there are theoretical reasons to question its applicability to the problem of living habits that are injurious to health. It is still possible that in some instances these doubts can be laid to rest. We may have some noncircular way of determining when self-destructive behavior is involuntary; we may have knowledge of what preferences people would have were their behavior not constrained; and there may be no way to restore their autonomy. While at least a *prima facie* case for paternalistic intervention would exist under such circumstances, I think it is important to note several practical problems that could arise in any attempt to design and carry out a policy of coercive lifestyle reform.

First, there is the distinct possibility that the government that takes over decision-making power from partially incompetent individuals may prove even less adept at securing their interests than they would have been if left alone. Paucity of scientific data may lead to misidentification of risk factors. The primitive state of the art in health promotion and mass-scale behavior modification may render interventions ineffective or even counterproductive. And the usual run of political and administrative tempests that affect all public policy may result in the misapplication of such knowledge as is available in these fields. These factors call for recognizing a limitation on the social insurance rationale for paternalism. If rational persons doubt that the authorities who would be guiding their affairs during periods of their incompetence would themselves be particularly competent, they are unlikely to license interventions except when there is a high probability of favorable cost-benefit tradeoff. This yields the strongest support for those interventions that prevent very serious injuries, and in which the danger posed is imminent.[4]

These reflections count against a rationale for government involvement in vigorous health promotion efforts, as recently voiced by the Secretary of Health, Education, and Welfare[11] and found elsewhere.[12] Their statements that smoking and similar habits are "slow suicide" and should be treated as such make a false analogy, precisely because suicide often involves certain imminent dangers of the most serious sort in situations in which there cannot be time to determine whether the act is voluntary. This is just the sort of case that the social insurance policy here described would cover; but this would not extend to the self-destruction that takes 30 years to accomplish.

Second, there is some possibility that what would be advertised as concern for the individual's welfare (as that person defines it) would turn out to be simple legal moralism, i.e., an attempt to impose the society's or authorities' moral prescriptions upon those not following them. In Knowles's call for lifestyle reform[13] the language is suggestive:

The next major advances in the health of the American people will result from the assumption of individual responsibility for one's own health. This will require a change in lifestyle for the majority of Americans. The cost of sloth, gluttony, alcoholic overuse, reckless driving, sexual intemperance, and smoking is now a national, not an individual responsibility.[14]

All save the last of these practices are explicit *vices;* indeed, the first two—sloth and gluttony—use their traditional names. The intrusion of nonmedical values is evidenced by the fact that of all the living habits that affect health adversely, only those that are sins (with smoking excepted) are mentioned as targets for change. Skiing and football produce injuries as surely as sloth produces heart disease; and the decision to postpone childbearing until the thirties increases susceptibility to certain cancers in women.[15] If it is the unhealthiness of "sinful" living habits that motivates the paternalist toward reform, then ought not other acts also be targeted on occasions when persons exhibit lack of self-direction? The fact that other practices are not ordinarily pointed out in this regard provides no *argument* against paternalistic lifestyle reform. But those who favor pressuring the slothful to engage in physical exercise might ask themselves if they also favor pressure on habits which, though unhealthy, are not otherwise despised. If enthusiasm for paternalistic intervention slackens in these latter cases, it may be a signal for reexamination of the motives.

A third problem is that the involuntariness of some self-destructive behavior may make paternalistic reform efforts ineffective. To the extent that the unhealthy behavior is not under the control of the individual, we cannot expect the kind of financial threat involved in a "fat tax" to exert much influence. Paradoxically, the very conditions under which paternalistic intervention seems most justified are those in which many of the methods available are least likely to succeed. The result of intervention under these circumstances may be a failure to change the life-threatening behavior, and a needless (and inexcusable) addition to the individual's woes through the unpleasantness of the intervention itself. A more appropriate target for government intervention might be the commercial and/or social forces that cause or support the life-threatening behavior.

Although the discussion above has focused on the problems attendant to a paternalistic argument for coercive health promotion programs, I have implicitly outlined a positive case for such interventions as well. A campaign to reform unhealthy habits of living will be justified, in my view, so long as it does not run afoul of the problems I have mentioned. It may indeed be possible to design such a program. The relative weight of the case against paternalistic intervention can be lessened, in any case, by making adjustments for the proportion of intervention, benefit, and intrusion. Health-promotion programs that are only very mildly coercive, such as moderate increases in cigarette taxes, require very little justification; noncoercive measures such as health education require none at all. And the case for more intrusive measures would be stronger if greater and more certain benefits could be promised. Moreover, even if the paternalistic rationale for coercive reform of health-related behavior fails completely, there may be other rationales to justify the intrusion.

NOTES

1. Fuchs, V. R. 1974. *Who Shall Live?* New York: Basic Books, Inc.

2. This measure was concocted for the present essay, but it shares its important features with others which have been actually proposed.

3. ''Coercive beneficence'' is not a fully correct definition of paternalism; but I will not attempt to give adequate definition here (see Gert and Culver, 1976). The term itself is unnecessarily sex-linked; ''Parentalism'' carries the same meaning without this feature. However, ''paternalism'' is a standard term in philosophical writing, and a change from it invites confusion.

4. Feinberg, J. 1973. *Social Philosophy*. Englewood Cliffs, N.J.: Prentice-Hall.

5. Dworkin, G. 1971. Paternalism. In Wasserstrom, R., ed., *Morality and the Law*. Belmont, Calif.: Wadsworth Publishing Co.

6. Bayles, M. D. 1974. Criminal Paternalism. In Pennock, J. R. and Chapman, J. W., eds., *The Limits of Law: Nomos XV*. New York: Lieber, Atherton.

7. Hodson, J. 1977. The Principle of Paternalism. *American Philosophical Quarterly* 14(1): 61–69.

8. The agnostic should adopt the habits which would foster his own belief in God. If he does and God exists, he will receive the infinite rewards of paradise; if he does and God does not exist, he was only wasting the efforts of conversion and prayer. If he does not try to believe in God, and religion is true, he suffers the infinitely bad fate of hell; whereas if God does not exist he has merely saved some inconvenience. Conversion is the rational choice even if the agnostic estimates the chances of God's existing as very remote, since even a very small probability yields a large index when multiplied against an infinite quantity.

9. Readers of the previous footnote might note that a similar difficulty attends Pascal's wager. If the agnostic took steps to foster belief in every diety for which the chance of existing was greater than zero, the inconvenience suffered would be considerable, after all. Yet such would be required by the logic of the wager.

10. Claiborne, C. 1976. In Defense of Eating Rich Food. *The New York Times,* December 8.

11. Department of Health, Education and Welfare. 1975. *Forward Plan for Health FY 1977–81*. (June). Washington, D.C.: U.S. Government Printing Office.

12. McKeown, T., and Lowe, C. R. 1974. *An Introduction to Social Medicine*. Second edition. Oxford: Blackwell's.

13. Knowles, J. H. 1976. The Struggle to Stay Healthy. *Time:* August 9.

14. Elsewhere, however, Dr. Knowles emphasizes that ''he who hates sin, hates humanity'' (Knowles, 1977). Knowles's argument in the latter essay is primarily nonpaternalistic.

15. Medawar, T. B. 1977. Signs of Cancer. *New York Review of Books* 24(10): 10–14.

ROBERT M. VEATCH

Voluntary Risks to Health: The Ethical Issues

In an earlier era, one's health was thought to be determined by the gods or by fate. The individual had little responsibility for personal health. In terms of the personal responsibility for health and disease, the modern medical model has required little change in this view. One of the primary elements of the medical model was the belief that people were exempt from

From *Journal of the American Medical Association* 243 (January 4, 1980), 50–55. Copyright ©1980, American Medical Association.

responsibility for their condition.[1] If one had good health in old age, from the vantage point of the belief system of the medical model, one would say he had been blessed with good health. Disease was the result of mysterious, uncontrollable microorganisms or the random process of genetic fate.

A few years ago we developed a case study[2] involving a purely hypothetical proposal that smokers should be required to pay for the costs of their extra health care required over and above that of nonsmokers. The scheme involved taxing tobacco at a rate calculated to add to the nation's budget an amount equal to the marginal health cost of smoking.

Recently a number of proposals have been put forth that imply that individuals are in some sense personally responsible for the state of their health. The town of Alexandria, Va., refuses to hire smokers as fire fighters, in part because smokers increase the cost of health and disability insurance (*The New York Times,* Dec. 18, 1977, p. 28). Oral Roberts University insists that students meet weight requirements to attend school. Claiming that the school was concerned about the whole person, the school dean said that the school was just as concerned about the students' physical growth as their intellectual and spiritual growth (*The New York Times,* Oct 9, 1977, p. 77). Behaviors as highly diverse as smoking, skiing, playing professional football, compulsive eating, omitting exercise, exposing oneself excessively to the sun, skipping needed immunizations, automobile racing, and mountain climbing all can be viewed as having a substantial voluntary component. Health care needed as a result of any voluntary behavior might generate very different claims on a health care system from care conceptualized as growing out of some other causal nexus. Keith Reemtsma, M.D., chairman of the Department of Surgery at Columbia University's College of Physicians and Surgeons, has called for ''a more rational approach to improving national health,'' involving ''a reward/punishment system based on individual choices.'' Persons who smoked cigarettes, drank whiskey, drove cars, and owned guns would be taxed for the medical consequences of their choices (*The New York Times,* Oct 14, 1976, p. 37). That individuals should be personally responsible for their health is a new theme, implying a new model for health care and perhaps for funding of health care.[3-6]

Some data correlating lifestyle to health status are being generated. They seem to support the conceptual shift toward a model that sees the individual as more personally responsible for his health status. The data of Belloc and Breslow[7-9] make those of us who lead the slovenly lifestyle very uncomfortable. As Morison[3] has pointed out, John Wesley and his puritan brothers of the covenant may not have been far from wrong after all. Belloc and Breslow identify seven empirical correlates of good health: eating moder-

ately, eating regularly, eating breakfast, no cigarette smoking, moderate or no use of alcohol, at least moderate exercise, and seven to eight hours of sleep nightly. They all seem to be well within human control, far less mysterious than the viruses and genes that exceed the comprehension of the average citizen. The authors found that the average physical health of persons aged 70 years who reported all of the preceding good health practices was about the same as persons aged 35 to 44 years who reported fewer than three.

We have just begun to realize the policy implications and the ethical impact of the conceptual shift that begins viewing health status as, in part, a result of voluntary risk taking in personal behavior and lifestyle choices. If individuals are responsible to some degree for their health and their need for health resources, why should they not also be responsible for the costs involved? If national health insurance is on the horizon, it will be even more questionable that individuals should have such health care paid for out of the same money pool generated by society to pay for other kinds of health care. Even with existing insurance plans, is it equitable that all persons contributing to the insurance money pool pay the extra costs of those who voluntarily run the risk of increasing their need for medical services?

• • •

There are several ethical principles that could lead us to be concerned about these apparently voluntary behaviors and even lead us to justify decisions to change our social policy about paying for or providing health care needed as a result of such behavior. The most obvious, the most traditional, medical ethical basis for concern is that the welfare of the individual is at stake. The Hippocratic tradition is committed to having the physician do what he thinks will benefit the patient. If one were developing an insurance policy or a mode of approaching the individual patient for private practice, paternalistic concern about the medical welfare of the patient might lead to a conclusion that, for the good of the patient, this behavior ought to be prevented or deferred. The paternalistic Hippocratic ethic, however, is suspect in circles outside the medical profession and is even coming under attack from within the physician community itself.[10] The Hippocratic ethic leaves no room for the principle of self-determination—a principle at the core of liberal Western thought. The freedom of choice to smoke, ski, and even race automobiles may well justify avoiding more coercive policies regarding these behaviors—assuming that it is the individual's own welfare that is at stake. The hyperindividualistic ethics of Hippocratism also leaves no room for concern for the welfare of others or the distribution of burdens within the society. A totally different rationale for concern is being put forward, however. Some, such as Tom Beauchamp,[11] have argued that we have a right to be concerned about such behaviors because of their social costs. He leaves unanswered the question of why it would be considered fair or just to regulate these voluntary behaviors when and only when their total social costs exceed the total social benefits of the behavior. This is a question we must explore.

Clearly, the argument is a complex one requiring many empirical, conceptual, and ethical judgments. Those judgments will have to be made regardless of whether we decide to continue the present policy or adopt one of the proposed alternatives. At this point, we need a thorough statement of the kinds of questions that must be addressed and the types of judgments that must be made.

ARE HEALTH RISKS VOLUNTARY?

The first question, addressed to those advocating policy shifts based on the notion that persons are in some sense responsible for their own health, melds the conceptual and empirical issues. Are health risks voluntary? Several models are competing for the conceptual attention of those working in the field.

THE VOLUNTARY MODEL

The model that considers the individual as personally responsible for his health has a great deal going for it. The empirical correlations of lifestyle choices with health status are impressive. The view of humans as personally responsible for their destiny is attractive to those of us within modern Western society. Its appeal extends beyond the view of the human as subject to the forces of fate and even the medical model, which as late as the 1950s saw disease as an attack on the individual coming from outside the person and outside his control.

THE MEDICAL MODEL

Of course, that it is attractive cannot justify opting for the voluntarist model if it flies in the face of the empirical reality. The theory of external and uncontrollable causation is central to the medical model.[12] It is still probably the case that organic causal chains almost totally outside human control account now and then for a disease. But the medical model has been under such an onslaught of reality testing in the last decade that it can hardly provide a credible alternative to the voluntarist model. Even for those conditions that undeniably have an organic causal component, the luxury of human innocence is no longer a plausible defense against human accountability.

· · ·

THE PSYCHOLOGICAL MODEL

While the medical model seems to offer at best a limited counter to the policy options rooted in the voluntarist model, other theories of determinism may be more plausible. Any policy to control health care services that are viewed as necessitated by voluntary choices to risk one's health is based on the judgment that the behavior is indeed voluntary. The primary argument countering policies to tax or control smoking to be fair in distributing the burdens for treating smokers' health problems is that the smoker is not really responsible for his medical problems. The argument is not normally based on organic or genetic theories of determinism, but on more psychological theories. The smoker's personality and even the initial pattern of smoking are developed at such an early point in life that they could be viewed as beyond voluntary control. If the smoker's behavior is the result of toilet training rather than rational decision making, then to blame the smoker for the toilet training seems odd.

· · ·

If so-called voluntary health risks are really psychologically determined, then the ethical and policy implications collapse. But it must seriously be questioned whether the model of psychological determinism is a much more plausible monocausal explanation of these behaviors than the medical model. Choosing to be a professional football player, or even to continue smoking, simply cannot be viewed as determined and beyond personal choice because of demonstrated irresistible psychological forces. The fact that so many people have stopped smoking or drinking or even playing professional sports reveals that such choices are fundamentally different from monocausally determined behaviors.

. . .

THE SOCIAL STRUCTURAL MODEL

Perhaps the most plausible competition to the voluntarist model comes not from a theory of organic or even psychological determinism, but from a social structural model. The correlations of disease, mortality, and even so-called voluntary health-risk behavior with socioeconomic class are impressive. Recent data from Great Britain and from the Medicaid system in the United States[13] reveal that these correlations persist even with elaborate schemes that attempt to make health care more equitably available to all social classes. In Great Britain, for instance, it has recently been revealed that differences in death rates by social class continue, with inequalities essentially undiminished, since the advent of the National Health Service. Continuing to press the voluntarist model of personal responsibility for health risk in the face of a social structural model of the patterns of health and disease could be nothing more than blaming the victim,[14-17] avoiding the reality of the true causes of disease, and escaping proper social responsibility for changing the underlying social inequalities of the society and its modes of production.

This is a powerful counter to the voluntarist thesis. Even if it is shown that health and disease are governed by behaviors and risk factors subject to human control, it does not follow that the individual should bear the sole or even primary responsibility for bringing about the changes necessary to produce better health.

. . .

A MULTICAUSAL MODEL AND ITS IMPLICATIONS

The only reasonable alternative is to adopt a multicausal model, one that has a place for organic, psychological, and social theories of causation, as well as voluntarist elements, in an account of the cause of a disease or health pattern. One of the great conceptual issues confronting persons working in this area will be whether it is logically or psychologically possible to maintain simultaneously voluntarist and deterministic theories. In other areas of competing causal theories, such as theories of crime, drug addiction, and occupational achievement, we have not been

very successful in maintaining the two types of explanation simultaneously. I am not convinced that it is impossible.

. . .

RESPONSIBILITY AND CULPABILITY

Even in cases where we conclude that the voluntarist model may be relevant—where voluntary choices are at least a minor component of the pattern of health—it is still unclear what to make of the voluntarist conclusion. If we say that a person is responsible for his health, it still does not follow that the person is culpable for the harm that comes from voluntary choices. It may be that society still would want to bear the burden of providing health care needed to patch up a person who has voluntarily taken a health risk.

To take an extreme example, a member of a community may choose to become a professional fire fighter. Certainly this is a health-risking choice. Presumably it could be a relatively voluntary one. Still it does not follow that the person is culpable for the harms done to his health. Responsible, yes, but culpable, no.

To decide in favor of any policy incorporating the so-called presumption that health risks are voluntary, it will be necessary to decide not only that the risk is voluntary, but also that it is not worthy of public subsidy. Fire fighting, an occupation undertaken in the public interest, probably would be worthy of subsidy. It seems that very few such activities, however, are so evaluated. Professional automobile racing, for instance, hardly seems socially ennobling, even if it does provide entertainment and diversion. A more plausible course would be requiring auto racers to purchase a license for a fee equal to their predicted extra health costs.

But what about the health risks of casual automobile driving for business or personal reasons? There are currently marginal health costs that are not built into the insurance system, e.g., risks from automobile exhaust pollution, from stress, and from the discouraging of exercise. It seems as though, in principle, there would be nothing wrong with recovering the economic part of those costs, if it could be done. A health tax on gasoline, for instance, might be sensible as a progressive way of funding a national health service. The evidence for the direct causal links and the exact costs will be hard, probably impossible, to discover. That difficulty, however, may not be decisive, provided there is general agreement that there are some costs, that the behavior is not socially ennobling, and that the funds are obtained more or less equitably in any case. It would certainly be no worse than some other luxury tax.

THE ARGUMENTS FROM JUSTICE

The core of the argument over policies deriving from the voluntary health-risks thesis is the argument over what is fair or just. Regardless of whether individuals have a general right to health care, or whether justice in general requires the social provision of health services, it seems as though what justice requires for a risk voluntarily assumed is quite different from what it might require in the more usual medical need.

Two responses have been offered to the problem of justice in providing health care for medical needs resulting from voluntarily assumed risks. One by Dan Beauchamp[17-21] and others resolves the problem by attacking the category of voluntary risk. He implies that so-called voluntary behaviors are, in reality, the result of social and cultural forces. Since voluntary behavior is a null set, the special implications of meritorious or blameworthy behavior for a theory of justice are of no importance. Beauchamp begins forcefully with a somewhat egalitarian theory of social justice, which leads to a moral right to health for all citizens. There is no need to amend that theory to account for fairness of the claims of citizens who bring on their need for health care through their voluntary choices, because there are no voluntary choices.

It seems reasonable to concede to Dan Beauchamp that the medical model has been overly individualistic, that socioeconomic and cultural forces play a much greater role in the causal nexus of health problems than is normally assumed. Indeed, they probably play the dominant role. But the total elimination of voluntarism from our understanding of human behavior is quite implausible. Injuries to the socioeconomic elite while mountain climbing or waterskiing are not reasonably seen as primarily the result of social structural determinism. If there remains a residuum of the voluntary theory, then one of justice for health care will have to take that into account.

A second approach is that of Tom Beauchamp,[11] who goes further than Dan Beauchamp. He attacks the principle of justice itself. Dan Beauchamp seems to hold that justice or fairness requires us to distribute resources according to need. Since needs are not the result of voluntary choices, a subsidiary consideration of whether the need results from foolish, voluntary behavior is unnecessary. Tom Beauchamp, on the other hand, rejects the idea that needs per se have a claim on us as a society. He seems to accept the idea that at least occasionally behaviors may be voluntary. He questions whether need alone provides a plausible basis for deciding what is fair in cases where the individual has voluntarily risked his health and is subsequently in need of medical services. He offers a utilitarian alternative, claiming that the crucial dimension is the total social costs of the behaviors. He argues:

Hazardous personal behaviors should be restricted if, and only if: (1) the behavior creates risks of harm to persons other than those who engage in such activities, and (2) a cost-benefit analysis reveals that the social investment in controlling such behaviors would produce a net increase in social utility, rather than a net decrease.

The implication is that any social advantage to the society that can come from controlling these behaviors would justify intervention, regardless of how the benefits and burdens of the policy are distributed.

A totally independent, nonpaternalistic argument is based much more in the principle of justice. This approach examines not only the impact of disease, but also questions of fairness. It is asked, is it fair that society as a whole should bear the burden of providing medical care needed only because of voluntarily taken risks to one's health? From this point of view, even if the net benefit of letting the behavior continue exceeded the benefits of prohibiting it, the behavior justifiably might be prohibited, or at least controlled, on nonpaternalistic grounds. Consider the case, for instance, where the benefits accrue overwhelmingly to persons who do engage in the behavior and the costs to those who do not. If the need for medical care is the result of the voluntary choice to engage in the behavior, then those arguing from the standpoint of equity or fairness might conclude that the behavior should still be controlled even though it produces a net benefit in aggregate.

Both Beauchamps downplay a secondary dimension of the argument over the principle of justice. Even those who accept the egalitarian formula ought to concede that all an individual is entitled to is an equal opportunity for a chance to be as healthy, insofar as possible, as other people.[22] Since those who are voluntarily risking their health (assuming for the moment that the behavior really is voluntary) do have an opportunity to be healthy, it is not the egalitarian dimensions of the principle of justice that are relevant to the voluntary health-risks question. It is the question of what is just treatment of those who have had opportunity and have not taken advantage of it. The question is one of what to do with persons who have not made use of their chance. Even the most egalitarian theories of justice—of which I consider myself to be a proponent—must at times deal with the secondary question of what to do in cases where individuals voluntarily have chosen to use their opportunities unequally. Unless there is no such thing as voluntary health-risk behavior, as Dan Beauchamp implies, this must remain a problem for the more egalitarian theories of justice.

In principle I see nothing wrong with the conclusion, which even an egalitarian would hold, that those who have not used fairly their opportunities receive inequalities of outcome. I emphasize that this is an argument in principle. It would not apply to persons who are truly not equal in their opportunity because of their social or psychological conditions. It would not apply to those who are forced into their health-risky behavior because of social oppression or stress in the mode of production.

From this application of a subsidiary component of the principle of justice, I reach the conclusion that it is fair, that it is just, if persons in need of health services resulting from true, voluntary risks are treated differently from those in need of the same services for other reasons. In fact, it would be unfair if the two groups were treated equally.

For most cases this would justify only the funding of the needed health care separately in cases where the need results from voluntary behavior. In extreme circumstances, however, where the resources needed are scarce and cannot be supplemented with more funds (e.g., when it is the skill that is scarce), then actual prohibition of the behavior may be the only plausible option, if one is arguing from this kind of principle of justice.

This essentially egalitarian principle, which says that like cases should be treated alike, leaves us with one final problem under the rubric of justice. If all voluntary risks ought to be treated alike, what do we make of the fact that only certain of the behaviors are monitorable? Is it unfair to place a health tax on smoking, automobile racing, skiing at organized resorts with ski lifts, and other organized activities that one can monitor, while letting slip by failing to exercise, climbing, mountain skiing on the hill on one's farm, and other behaviors that cannot be monitored? In a sense it may be. The problem is perhaps like the unfairness of being able to treat the respiratory problems of pneumonia, but not those of trisomy E syndrome or other incurable diseases. There may be some essential unfairness in life. This may appear in the inequities of policy proposals to control or tax monitorable behavior, but not behavior that cannot be monitored. Actually some ingenuity may generate ways to tax what seems untaxable—taxing gasoline for the health risks of automobiles, taxing mountain climbing equipment (assuming it is not an ennobling activity), or creating special insurance pools for persons who eat a bad diet. The devices probably would be crude and not necessarily in exact proportion to the risks involved. Some people engaged in equally risky behaviors probably would not be treated equally. That may be a necessary implication of the crudeness of any public policy mechanism. Whether the inequities of not being able to treat equally people taking comparable risks constitute such a serious problem that it would be better to abandon entirely the principle of equality of opportunity for health is the policy question that will have to be resolved.

COST-SAVING HEALTH-RISK BEHAVIORS

Another argument is mounted against the application of the principle of equity to voluntarily health-risking behaviors. What ought to be done with behaviors that are health risky, but that end up either not costing society or actually saving society's scarce resources? This question will separate clearly those who argue for intervention on paternalistic grounds from those who argue on utilitarian grounds or on the basis of the principle of justice. What ought to be done about a behavior that would risk a person's health, but risk it in such a way that he would die rapidly and cheaply at about retirement age? If the concern is from the unfair burden that these behaviors generate on the rest of society, and, if the society is required to bear the costs and to use scarce resources, then a health-risk behavior that did not involve such social costs would surely be exempt from any social policy oriented to controlling such unfair behavior. In fact, if social utility were the only concern, then this particular type of risky behavior ought to be encouraged. Since our social policy is one that ought to incorporate many ethical concerns, it seems unlikely that we would want to encourage these behaviors even if such encouragement were cost-effective. This, indeed, shows the weakness of approaches that focus only on aggregate costs and benefits.

REVULSION AGAINST THE RATIONAL, CALCULATING LIFE

There is one final, last-ditch argument against adoption of a health policy that incorporates an equitable handling of voluntary health risks. Some would argue that, although the behavior might be voluntary and supplying health care to meet the resulting needs unfair to the rest of the society, the alternative would be even worse. Such a policy might require the conversion of many decisions in life from spontaneous expressions based on long tradition and life-style patterns to cold, rational, calculating decisions based on health and economic elements.

It is not clear to me that that would be the result. Placing a health fee on a package of cigarettes or on a ski-lift ticket may not make those decisions any more rational calculations than they are now. The current warning on tobacco has not had much of an impact. Even if rational decision making were the outcome, however, I am not sure that it would be wrong to elevate such health-risking decisions to a level of consciousness in which one had to think about what one was doing. At least it seems that as a side effect of a policy that would permit health resources to be paid for and used more equitably, this would not be an overwhelming or decisive counterargument.

CONCLUSION

The health policy decisions that must be made in an era in which a multicausal theory is the only plausible one are going to be much harder than the ones made in the simpler era of the medical model—but then, those were harder than some of the ones that had to be made in the era where health was in the hands of the gods. Several serious questions remain to be answered. These are both empirical and normative. They may constitute a research agenda for pursuing the question of ethics and health policy for an era when some risks to health may be seen, at least by some people, as voluntary.

NOTES

1. Parsons, T.: *The Social System*. New York, The Free Press, 1951, p 437.

2. Steinfels, P., and Veatch, R. M.: Who should pay for smokers' medical care? *Hastings Cent. Rep.* 4:8–10, 1974.

3. Morison, R. S.: Rights and responsibilities: Redressing the uneasy balance. *Hastings Cent. Rep.* 4:1–4, 1974.

4. Vayda, E.: Keeping people well: A new approach to medicine. *Hum. Nature* 1:64–71, 1978.

5. Somers, A. R., and Hayden, M. C.: Rights and responsibilities in prevention. *Health Educ.* 9:37–39, 1978.

6. Kass, L.: Regarding the end of medicine and the pursuit of health. *Public Interest* 40:11–42, 1975.

7. Belloc, N. B., and Breslow, L.: Relationship of physical status health and health practices. *Prev. Med.* 1:409–421, 1972.

8. Belloc, N. B.: Relationship of health practices and mortality. *Prev. Med.* 2:67–81, 1973.

9. Breslow, L.: Prospects for improving health through reducing risk factors. *Prev. Med.* 7:449–458, 1978.

10. Veatch, R. M.: The Hippocratic ethic: Consequentialism, individualism and paternalism, in Smith, D. H., and Bernstein, L. M. (eds.): *No Rush to Judgment: Essays on Medical Ethics.* Bloomington, Ind., The Poynter Center, Indiana University, 1978, pp 238–264.

11. Beauchamp, T.: The regulation of hazards and hazardous behaviors. *Health Educ. Monogr.* 6:242–257, 1978.

12. Veatch, R. M.: The medical model: Its nature and problems. *Hastings Cent. Rep.* 1:59–76, 1973.

13. Morris, J. N.: Social inequalities undiminished. *Lancet* 1:87–90, 1979.

14. Ryan, W.: *Blaming the Victim*. New York, Vintage Books, 1971.

15. Crawford, R.: Sickness as sin. *Health Policy Advisory Center Bull.* 80:10–16, 1978.

16. Crawford, R.: You are dangerous to your health. *Social Policy* 8:11–20, 1978.

17. Beauchamp, D. E.: Public health as social justice. *Inquiry* 13:3–14, 1976.

18. Syme, L., and Berkman, I.: Social class, susceptibility and sickness. *Am. J. Epidemiol.* 104:1–8, 1976.

19. Conover, P. W.: Social class and chronic illness. *Int. J. Health Serv.* 3:357–368, 1973.

20. *Health of the Disadvantaged: Chart Book,* publication (HRA) 77–628. Hyattsville, Md., U.S. Dept. of Health, Education, and Welfare, Public Health Service, Health Resources Administration, 1977.

21. Beauchamp, D. E.: Alcoholism as blaming the alcoholic. *Int. J. Addict.* 11:41–52, 1976.

22. Veatch, R. M.: What is a 'just' health care delivery? in Branson, R., and Veatch, R. M. (eds.): *Ethics and Health Policy.* Cambridge, Mass., Ballinger Publishing Co, 1976, pp 127–153.

SUPREME COURT OF THE UNITED STATES

Industrial Union Department, AFL-CIO, v. American Petroleum Institute

[Mr. Justice Stevens announced the judgment of the Court and delivered an opinion in which The Chief Justice and Mr. Justice Stewart join and in Parts I, II, III-A-C and E of which Mr. Justice Powell joins.]

The Occupational Safety and Health Act of 1970, 29 U. S. C. § 651 *et seq.* (the Act), was enacted for the purpose of ensuring safe and healthful working conditions for every working man and woman in the Nation. This case concerns a standard promulgated by the Secretary of Labor to regulate occupational exposure to benzene, a substance which has been shown to cause cancer at high exposure levels. The principal question is whether such a showing is a sufficient basis for a standard that places the most stringent limitation on exposure to benzene that is technologically and economically possible.

The Act delegates broad authority to the Secretary to promulgate different kinds of standards. The basic definition of an "occupational safety and health standard" is found in § 3 (8), which provides:

The term "occupational safety and health standard" means a standard which requires conditions, or the adoption or use of one or more practices, means, methods, operations, or processes, reasonably necessary or appropriate to provide safe or healthful employment and places of employment. 29 U. S. C. § 652 (8).

Where toxic materials or harmful physical agents are concerned, a standard must also comply with § 6 (b) (5), which provides:

The Secretary, in promulgating standards dealing with toxic materials or harmful physical agents under this subsection, shall set the standard which most adequately assures, to the

extent feasible, on the basis of the best available evidence, that no employee will suffer material impairment of health or functional capacity even if such employee has regular exposure to the hazard dealt with by such standard for the period of his working life. Development of standards under this subsection shall be based upon research, demonstrations, experiments, and such other information as may be appropriate. In addition to the attainment of the highest degree of health and safety protection for the employee, other considerations shall be the latest available scientific data in the field, the feasibility of the standards, and experience gained under this and other health and safety laws. 29 U. S. C. § 655 (b) (5).

Wherever the toxic material to be regulated is a carcinogen, the Secretary has taken the position that no safe exposure level can be determined and that § 6 (b) (5) requires him to set an exposure limit at the lowest technologically feasible level that will not impair the viability of the industries regulated. In this case, after having determined that there is a causal connection between benzene and leukemia (a cancer of the white blood cells), the Secretary set an exposure limit on airborne concentrations of benzene of one part benzene per million parts of air (1 ppm), regulated dermal and eye contact with solutions containing benzene, and imposed complex monitoring and medical testing requirements on employers whose workplaces contain 0.5 ppm or more of benzene. 29 CFR § 1910.1028, 43 Fed. Reg. 5918 (Feb. 10, 1978), as amended, 43 Fed. Reg. 27962 (June 27, 1978).

On pre-enforcement review pursuant to 29 U. S. C. § 655 (f), the United States Court of Appeals for the Fifth Circuit held the regulation invalid. 581 F. 2d 493 (1978). The court concluded that OSHA had exceeded its standard-setting authority because it had not shown that the new benzene exposure limit was "reasonably necessary or appropriate to provide safe

Industrial Union Department, AFL-CIO v. American Petroleum Institute *et al.* and Ray Marshall, Secretary of Labor v. American Petroleum Institute *et al.*, Supreme Court of the United States, Nos. 78-911 and 78-1036 (July 2, 1980).

or healthful employment'' as required by § 3 (8), and because § 6 (b) (5) does ''not give OSHA the unbridled discretion to adopt standards designed to create absolutely risk-free workplaces regardless of costs.'' Reading the two provisions together, the Fifth Circuit held that the Secretary was under a duty to determine whether the benefits expected from the new standard bore a reasonable relationship to the costs that it imposed. *Id.,* at 503. The court noted that OSHA had made an estimate of the costs of compliance, but that the record lacked substantial evidence of any discernible benefits.

We agree with the Fifth Circuit's holding that § 3 (8) requires the Secretary to find, as a threshold matter, that the toxic substance in question poses a significant health risk in the workplace and that a new, lower standard is therefore ''reasonably necessary or appropriate to provide safe or healthful employment and places of employment.'' Unless and until such a finding is made, it is not necessary to address the further question whether the Court of Appeals correctly held that there must be a reasonable correlation between costs and benefits, or whether, as the Government argues, the Secretary is then required by § 6 (b) (5) to promulgate a standard that goes as far as technologically and economically possible to eliminate the risk.

Because this is an unusually important case of first impression, we have reviewed the record with special care. In this opinion, we (1) describe the benzene standard, (2) analyze the Agency's rationale for imposing a 1 ppm exposure limit, [and] (3) discuss the controlling legal issues. . . .

I

Benzene is a familiar and important commodity. It is a colorless, aromatic liquid that evaporates rapidly under ordinary atmospheric conditions. Approximately 11 billion pounds of benzene were produced in the United States in 1976. Ninety-four percent of that total was produced by the petroleum and petrochemical industries, with the remainder produced by the steel industry as a byproduct of coking operations. Benzene is used in manufacturing a variety of products including motor fuels (which may contain as much as 2% benzene), solvents, detergents, pesticides, and other organic chemicals. 43 Fed. Reg., at 5918.

The entire population of the United States is exposed to small quantities of benzene, ranging from a few parts per billion to 0.5 ppm, in the ambient air.

Tr. 1030–1032. Over one million workers are subject to additional low-level exposures as a consequence of their employment. The majority of these employees work in gasoline service stations, benzene production (petroleum refineries and coking operations), chemical processing, benzene transportation, rubber manufacturing and laboratory operations.

Benzene is a toxic substance. Although it could conceivably cause harm to a person who swallowed or touched it, the principal risk of harm comes from inhalation of benzene vapors. When these vapors are inhaled, the benzene diffuses through the lungs and is quickly absorbed into the blood. Exposure to high concentrations produces an almost immediate effect on the central nervous system. Inhalation of concentrations of 20,000 ppm can be fatal within minutes; exposures in the range of 250 to 500 ppm can cause vertigo, nausea, and other symptoms of mild poisoning. 43 Fed. Reg., at 5921. Persistent exposures at levels above 25–40 ppm may lead to blood deficiencies and diseases of the blood-forming organs, including aplastic anemia, which is generally fatal.

Industrial health experts have long been aware that exposure to benzene may lead to various types of nonmalignant diseases. By 1948 the evidence connecting high levels of benzene to serious blood disorders had become so strong that the Commonwealth of Massachusetts imposed a 35 ppm limitation on workplaces within its jurisdiction. In 1969 the American National Standards Institute adopted a national consensus standard of 10 ppm averaged over an eight-hour period with a ceiling concentration of 25 ppm for 10-minute periods or a maximum peak concentration of 50 ppm. 43 Fed. Reg., at 5919. In 1971, after the Occupational Health and Safety Act was passed, the Secretary adopted this consensus standard as the federal standard, pursuant to 29 U. S. C. § 655 (a).

As early as 1928, some health experts theorized that there might also be a connection between benzene in the workplace and leukemia. In the late 1960s and early 1970s a number of epidemiological studies were published indicating that workers exposed to high concentrations of benzene were subject to a significantly increased risk of leukemia. In a 1974 report recommending a permanent standard for benzene, the National Institute of Occupational Health and Safety (NIOSH), OSHA's research arm, noted that these studies raised the ''distinct possibility'' that benzene caused leukemia. But, in light of the fact that all known cases had occurred at very high exposure levels, NIOSH declined to recommend a change in the 10 ppm standard, which it considered sufficient to protect against nonmalignant diseases. NIOSH suggested that further studies were necessary to determine conclusively whether there was a link between benzene and leukemia and, if so, what exposure levels were dangerous.

Between 1974 and 1976 additional studies were published which tended to confirm the view that benzene can cause leukemia, at least when exposure levels are high. In an August 1976 revision of its earlier recommendation, NIOSH stated that these studies provided "conclusive" proof of a causal connection between benzene and leukemia. Vol. I, Ex. 2–5. Although it acknowledged that none of the intervening studies had provided the dose-response data it had found lacking two years earlier, id., at 9, NIOSH nevertheless recommended that the exposure limit be set as low as possible. As a result of this recommendation, OSHA contracted with a consulting firm to do a study on the costs to industry of complying with the 10 ppm standard then in effect or, alternatively, with whatever standard would be the lowest feasible. Tr. 505–506.

In October 1976 NIOSH sent another memorandum to OSHA, seeking acceleration of the rule-making process and "strongly" recommending the issuance of an emergency temporary standard pursuant to 29 U. S. C. § 655 (c) for benzene and two other chemicals believed to be carcinogens. NIOSH recommended that a 1 ppm exposure limit be imposed for benzene. Vol. I, Ex. 2–6. Apparently because of the NIOSH recommendation, OSHA asked its consultant to determine the cost of complying with a 1 ppm standard instead of with the "minimum feasible" standard. Tr. 506–507. It also issued voluntary guidelines for benzene, recommending that exposure levels be limited to 1 ppm on an 8-hour time-weighted average basis wherever possible. Vol. II, Ex. 2–44.

In the spring of 1976 NIOSH had selected two Pliofilm plants in St. Mary's and Akron, Ohio, for an epidemiological study of the link between leukemia and benzene exposure. In April, 1977 NIOSH forwarded an interim report to OSHA indicating at least a five-fold increase in the expected incidence of leukemia for workers who had been exposed to benzene at the two plants from 1940 to 1949. The report submitted to OSHA erroneously suggested that expo-

sures in the two plants had generally been between zero and 15 ppm during the period in question. As a result of this new evidence and the continued prodding of NIOSH, Vol. I, Ex. 2–7, OSHA did issue an emergency standard, effective May 21, 1977, reducing the benzene exposure limit from 10 ppm to 1 ppm, the ceiling for exposures of up to 10 minutes from 25 ppm to 5 ppm, and eliminating the authority for peak concentrations of 50 ppm. 42 Fed. Reg. 22516 (May 3, 1977). In its explanation accompanying the emergency standard, OSHA stated that benzene had been shown to cause leukemia at exposures below 25 ppm and that, in light of its consultant's report, it was feasible to reduce the exposure limit to 1 ppm. 42 Fed. Reg., at 22517, 22521.

On May 19, 1977, the Court of Appeals for the Fifth Circuit entered a temporary restraining order preventing the emergency standard from taking effect. Thereafter, OSHA abandoned its efforts to make the emergency standard effective and instead issued a proposal for a permanent standard patterned almost entirely after the aborted emergency standard. 42 Fed. Reg. 27452 (May 27, 1977).

In its published statement giving notice of the proposed permanent standard, OSHA did not ask for comments as to whether or not benzene presented a significant health risk at exposures of 10 ppm or less. Rather, it asked for comments as to whether 1 ppm was the minimum feasible exposure limit. 42 Fed. Reg., at 27452. As OSHA's Deputy Director of Health Standards, Grover Wrenn, testified at the hearing, this formulation of the issue to be considered by the Agency was consistent with OSHA's general policy with respect to carcinogens. Whenever a carcinogen is involved, OSHA will presume that no safe level of exposure exists in the absence of clear proof establishing such a level and will accordingly set the exposure limit at the lowest level feasible. The proposed 1 ppm exposure limit in this case thus was established not on the basis of a proven hazard at 10 ppm, but rather on the basis of "OSHA's best judgment at the time of the proposal of the feasibility of compliance with the proposed standard by the affected industries." Tr. 30. Given OSHA's cancer policy, it was in fact irrelevant whether there was any evidence at all of a leukemia risk at 10 ppm. The important point was that there was no evidence that there was *not* some risk, however small, at that level. The fact that OSHA did not ask for comments on whether there was a safe level of exposure for benzene was indicative of its further view that a demonstration of such absolute safety simply could not be made.

Public hearings were held on the proposed standard, commencing on July 19, 1977. The final standard was issued on February 10, 1978. 43 Fed. Reg. 5918. In its final form, the benzene standard is designed to protect workers from whatever hazards are associated with low-level benzene exposures by requiring employers to monitor workplaces to determine the level of exposure, to provide medical examinations when the level rises above 0.5 ppm, and to institute whatever engineering or other controls are necessary to keep exposures at or below 1 ppm.

In the standard as originally proposed by OSHA, the employer's duty to monitor, keep records and provide medical examinations arose whenever *any* benzene was present in a workplace covered by the rule. Because benzene is omnipresent in small quantities, NIOSH and the President's Council on Wage and Price Stability recommended the use of an "action level" to trigger monitoring and medical examination requirements. Tr. 1030–1032; Vol. XIV, Ex. 41–28. OSHA accepted this recommendation, providing under the final standard that, if initial monitoring discloses benzene concentrations below 0.5 ppm averaged over an eight-hour work day, no further action is required unless there is a change in the company's practices. If exposures are above the action level, but below the 1 ppm exposure limit, employers are required to monitor exposure levels on a quarterly basis and to provide semiannual medical examinations for their exposed employees. Neither the concept of an action level, nor the specific level selected by OSHA, is challenged in this proceeding.

Whenever initial monitoring indicates that employees are subject to airborne concentrations of benzene above 1 ppm averaged over an eight-hour workday, with a ceiling of 5 ppm for any 15-minute period, employers are required to modify their plants or institute work practice controls to reduce exposures within permissible limits. Consistent with OSHA's general policy, the regulation does not allow respirators to be used if engineering modifications are technologically feasible. Employers in this category are also required to perform monthly monitoring so long as their workplaces remain above 1 ppm, provide semiannual medical examinations to exposed workers, post signs in and restrict access to "regulated areas" where the permissible exposure limit is exceeded, and conduct employee training programs where necessary.

The standard also places strict limits on exposure to liquid benzene. As originally framed, the standard totally prohibited any skin or eye contact with any liquid containing any benzene. Ultimately, after the standard was challenged, OSHA modified this prohibition by excluding liquids containing less than 0.5% benzene. After three years, that exclusion will be narrowed to liquids containing less than 0.1% benzene.

The permanent standard is expressly inapplicable to the storage, transportation, distribution, sale or use of gasoline or other fuels subsequent to discharge from bulk terminals. This exception is particularly significant in light of the fact that over 795,000 gas station employees, who are exposed to an average of 102,700 gallons of gasoline (containing up to 2% benzene) annually, are thus excluded from the protection of the standard.

As presently formulated, the benzene standard is an expensive way of providing some additional protection for a relatively small number of employees. According to OSHA's figures, the standard will require capital investments in engineering controls of approximately $266 million, first-year operating costs (for monitoring, medical testing, employee training and respirators) of $187 million to $205 million and recurring annual costs of approximately $34 million. 43 Fed. Reg., at 5934. The figures outlined in OSHA's explanation of the costs of compliance to various industries indicate that only 35,000 employees would gain any benefit from the regulation in terms of a reduction in their exposure to benzene. Over two-thirds of these workers (24,450) are employed in the rubber manufacturing industry. Compliance costs in that industry are estimated to be rather low, with no capital costs and initial operating expenses estimated at only $34 million ($1390 per employee); recurring annual costs would also be rather low, totalling less than $1 million. By contrast, the segment of the petroleum refining industry that produces benzene would be required to incur $24 million in capital costs and $600,000 in first-year operating expenses to provide additional protection for 300 workers ($82,000 per employee), while the petrochemical industry would be required to incur $20.9 million in capital costs and $1 million in initial operating expenses for the benefit of 552 employees ($39,675 per employee). 43 Fed. Reg., at 5936–5938.

Although OSHA did not quantify the benefits to each category of worker in terms of decreased exposure to benzene, it appears from the economic impact study done at OSHA's direction that those benefits may be relatively small. Thus, although the current exposure limit is 10 ppm, the actual exposures outlined in that study are often considerably lower. For example, for the period 1970–1975 the petrochemical industry reported that, out of a total of 496 employees exposed to benzene, only 53 were exposed to levels between 1 and 5 ppm and only seven (all at the same plant) were exposed to between 5 and 10 ppm. Economic Impact Study, Vol. I, table 4.2. See also tables 4.3–4.8 (indicating sample exposure levels in various industries).

II

The critical issue at this point in the litigation is whether the Court of Appeals was correct in refusing to enforce the 1 ppm exposure limit on the ground that it was not supported by appropriate findings.

Any discussion of the 1 ppm exposure limit must, of course, begin with the Agency's rationale for imposing that limit. The written explanation of the standard fills 184 pages of the printed appendix. Much of it is devoted to a discussion of the voluminous evidence of the adverse effects of exposure to benzene at levels of concentration well above 10 ppm. This discussion demonstrates that there is ample justification for regulating occupational exposure to benzene and that the prior limit of 10 ppm, with a ceiling of 25 ppm (or a peak of 50 ppm) was reasonable. It does not, however, provide direct support for the Agency's conclusion that the limit should be reduced from 10 ppm to 1 ppm.

The evidence in the administrative record of adverse effects of benzene exposure at 10 ppm is sketchy at best. OSHA noted that there was "no dispute" that certain nonmalignant blood disorders, evidenced by a reduction in the level of red or white cells or platelets in the blood, could result from exposures of 25–40 ppm. It then stated that several studies had indicated that relatively slight changes in normal blood values could result from exposures below 25 ppm and perhaps below 10 ppm. OSHA did not attempt to make any estimate based on these studies of how significant the risk of nonmalignant disease would be at exposures of 10 ppm or less. Rather, it stated that because of the lack of data concerning the

linkage between low-level exposures and blood abnormalities, it was impossible to construct a dose-response curve at this time. OSHA did conclude, however, that the studies demonstrated that the current 10 ppm exposure limit was inadequate to ensure that no single worker would suffer a nonmalignant blood disorder as a result of benzene exposure. Noting that it is "customary" to set a permissible exposure limit by applying a safety factor of 10–100 to the lowest level at which adverse effects had been observed, the Agency stated that the evidence supported the conclusion that the limit should be set at a point "substantially less than 10 ppm" even if benzene's leukemic effects were not considered. 43 Fed. Reg., at 5924–5925. OSHA did not state, however, that the nonmalignant effects of benzene exposure justified a reduction in the permissible exposure limit to 1 ppm.

OSHA also noted some studies indicating an increase in chromosomal aberrations in workers chronically exposed to concentrations of benzene "probably less than 25 ppm." However, the Agency took no definitive position as to what these aberrations meant in terms of demonstrable health effects and stated that no quantitative dose-response relationship had yet been established. Under these circumstances, chromosomal effects were categorized by OSHA as an "adverse biological event of serious concern which may pose or reflect a potential health risk and as such, must be considered in the larger purview of adverse health effects associated with benzene." 43 Fed. Reg., at 5932–5934.

With respect to leukemia, evidence of an increased risk (i.e., a risk greater than that borne by the general population) due to benzene exposures at or below 10 ppm was even sketchier. Once OSHA acknowledged that the NIOSH study it had relied upon in promulgating the emergency standard did not support its earlier view that benzene had been shown to cause leukemia at concentrations below 25 ppm, . . . there was only one study that provided any evidence of such an increased risk. That study, conducted by the Dow Chemical Co., uncovered three leukemia deaths, versus 0.2 expected deaths, out of a population of 594 workers; it appeared that the three workers had never been exposed to more than 2 to 9 ppm of benzene. The authors of the study, however, concluded that it could not be viewed as proof of a relationship between low-level benzene exposure and leukemia because all three workers had probably been occupationally exposed to a number of other potentially carcinogenic chemicals at other points in their careers and because no leukemia deaths had been uncovered among workers who had been exposed to much higher levels of benzene. In its explanation of the permanent standard, OSHA stated that the possibility that these three leukemias had been caused by benzene exposure could not be ruled out and that the study, although not evidence of an increased risk of leukemia at 10 ppm, was therefore "consistent with the findings of many studies that there is an excess leukemia risk among benzene exposed employees." 43 Fed. Reg., at 5928. The Agency made no finding that the Dow study, any other empirical evidence or any opinion testimony demonstrated that exposure to benzene at or below the 10 ppm level had ever in fact caused leukemia. See 581 F. 2d, at 503, where the Court of Appeals noted that OSHA was "unable to point to any empirical evidence documenting a leukemia risk at 10 ppm. . . ."

In the end OSHA's rationale for lowering the permissible exposure limit to 1 ppm was based, not on any finding that leukemia has ever been caused by exposure to 10 ppm of benzene and that it will *not* be caused by exposure to 1 ppm, but rather on a series of assumptions indicating that some leukemias might result from exposure to 10 ppm and that the number of cases might be reduced by reducing the exposure level to 1 ppm. In reaching that result, the Agency first unequivocally concluded that benzene is a human carcinogen. Second, it concluded that industry had failed to prove that there is a safe threshold level of exposure to benzene below which no excess leukemia cases would occur. In reaching this conclusion OSHA rejected industry contentions that certain epidemiological studies indicating no excess risk of leukemia among workers exposed at levels below 10 ppm were sufficient to establish that the threshold level of safe exposure was at or above 10 ppm. It also rejected an industry witness' testimony that a dose-response curve could be constructed on the basis of the reported epidemiological studies and that this curve indicated that reducing the permissible exposure limit from 10 to 1 ppm would prevent at most one leukemia and one other cancer death every six years.

Third, the Agency applied its standard policy with respect to carcinogens, concluding that, in the absence of definitive proof of a safe level, it must be assumed that *any* level above zero presents *some* increased risk of cancer. As the Government points out in its brief, there are a number of scientists and public health specialists who subscribe to this view, theorizing that a susceptible person may contract cancer from the absorption of even one molecule of a carcinogen like benzene. Brief for Federal Parties, at 18–19.

Fourth, the Agency reiterated its view of the Act, stating that it was required by § 6 (b) (5) to set the standard either at the level that has been demonstrated to be safe or at the lowest level feasible, whichever is higher. If no safe level is established, as in this case, the Secretary's interpretation of the statute automatically leads to the selection of an exposure limit that is the lowest feasible. Because of benzene's importance to the economy, no one has ever suggested that it would be feasible to eliminate its use entirely, or to try to limit exposures to the small amounts that are omnipresent. Rather, the Agency selected 1 ppm as a workable exposure level . . . and then determined that compliance with that level was technologically feasible and that "the economic impact of . . . [compliance] will not be such as to threaten the financial welfare of the affected firms or the general economy." 43 Fed. Reg., at 5939. It therefore held that 1 ppm was the minimum feasible exposure level within the meaning of § 6 (b) (5) of the Act.

Finally, although the Agency did not refer in its discussion of the pertinent legal authority to any duty to identify the anticipated benefits of the new standard, it did conclude that some benefits were likely to result from reducing the exposure limit from 10 ppm to 1 ppm. This conclusion was based, again, not on evidence but rather on the assumption that the risk of leukemia will decrease as exposure levels decrease. Although the Agency had found it impossible to construct a dose-response curve that would predict with any accuracy the number of leukemias that could be expected to result from exposures at 10 ppm, at 1 ppm, or at any intermediate level, it nevertheless "determined that the benefits of the proposed standard are likely to be appreciable." 43 Fed. Reg., at 5941. In light of the Agency's disavowal of any ability to determine the numbers of employees likely to be adversely affected by exposures of 10 ppm, the Court of Appeals held this finding to be unsupported by the record. 581 F. 2d, at 503.

It is noteworthy that at no point in its lengthy explanation did the Agency quote or even cite § 3 (8) of the Act. It made no finding that any of the provisions of the new standard were "reasonably necessary or appropriate to provide safe or healthful employment and places of employment." Nor did it allude to the possibility that any such finding might have been appropriate.

III

Our resolution of the issues in this case turns, to a large extent, on the meaning of and the relationship between § 3 (8), which defines a health and safety standard as a standard that is "reasonably necessary and appropriate to provide safe or healthful employment," and § 6 (b) (5), which directs the Secretary in promulgating a health and safety standard for toxic materials to "set the standard which most adequately assures, to the extent feasible, on the basis of the best available evidence, that no employee will suffer material impairment of health or functional capacity. . . ."

In the Government's view, § 3 (8)'s definition of the term "standard" has no legal significance or at best merely requires that a standard not be totally irrational. It takes the position that § 6 (b) (5) is controlling and that it requires OSHA to promulgate a standard that either gives an absolute assurance of safety for each and every worker or that reduces exposures to the lowest level feasible. The Government interprets "feasible" as meaning technologically achievable at a cost that would not impair the viability of the industries subject to the regulation. The respondent industry representatives, on the other hand, argue that the Court of Appeals was correct in holding that the "reasonably necessary and appropriate" language of § 3 (8), along with the feasibility requirement of § 6 (b) (5), requires the Agency to quantify both the costs and the benefits of a proposed rule and to conclude that they are roughly commensurate.

In our view, it is not necessary to decide whether either the Government or industry is entirely correct. For we think it is clear that § 3 (8) does apply to all permanent standards promulgated under the Act and that it requires the Secretary, before issuing any standard, to determine that it is reasonably necessary and appropriate to remedy a significant risk of material health impairment. Only after the Secretary has made the threshold determination that such a risk exists with respect to a toxic substance, would it be necessary to decide whether § 6 (b) (5) requires him to select the most protective standard he can consistent with economic and technological feasibility, or whether, as respondents argue, the benefits of the regulation must be commensurate with the costs of its implementation. Because the Secretary did not make the required threshold finding in this case, we have no occasion to determine whether costs must be weighed against benefits in an appropriate case.

M I C H A E L   S .   B A R A M

Cost-Benefit Analysis: An Inadequate Basis for Health, Safety, and Environmental Regulatory Decision Making

INTRODUCTION

The use of cost-benefit analysis in agency decision making has been hailed as the cure for numerous dissatisfactions with governmental regulation. Using this form of economic analysis arguably promotes rational decision making and prevents health, safety, and environmental regulations from having inflationary and other adverse economic impacts. Closer analysis, however, reveals that the cost-benefit approach to regulatory decision making suffers from major methodological limitations and institutional abuses. In practice, regulatory uses of cost-benefit analysis stifle and obstruct the achievement of legislated health, safety, and environmental goals.

From *Ecology Law Quarterly* 8 (1980), 473–475, 477–492. Reprinted with permission of the author.

This article critically reviews the methodological limitations of cost-benefit analysis, current agency uses of cost-benefit analysis under statutory requirements, the impact of recent Executive orders mandating economic balancing analyses for all major regulatory agency decisions, and agency efforts to structure their discretion in the use of cost-benefit analysis. The article concludes that if the health, safety, and environmental regulators continue to use cost-benefit analysis, procedural reforms are needed to promote greater accountability and public participation in the decision-making process. Further, to the extent that economic factors are permissible considerations under enabling statutes, agencies should conduct cost-effectiveness analysis, which aids in determining the least costly means to designated goals, rather than cost-benefit analysis, which improperly determines regulatory ends as well as means.

COST-BENEFIT ANALYSIS AS A MEANS TO STRUCTURE AGENCY DISCRETION

DELEGATION OF AUTHORITY TO ACHIEVE MULTIPLE OBJECTIVES

In response to increasing concerns about risks to health, safety, and environmental quality, Congress has enacted several statutes providing new schemes for agency decision making. These statutes specify the problems to be addressed and the procedures to be followed, but provide little guidance on the analytical processes the federal agency should use in reaching regulatory decisions.

The statutes typically prescribe a variety of general policy objectives, decisional criteria, and legislative findings to guide the agency in dealing with the substantive aspects of its decision making. These factors usually fall into two competing categories: (1) the reduction of certain risks to health, safety, or environmental quality; and (2) the minimization of adverse economic effects on regulated entities, their employees, and consumers. In addition, an agency may be required to consider using the best practicable or available technology to reduce risks, promote energy conservation or national security, protect the small business sector, or encourage innovation.

Agencies must also consider the additional, and often inconsistent, objectives and requirements imposed by other statutes. Operating with limited resources and conflicting objectives, federal agencies must therefore "make policy when Congress could make none" and afford "a fair degree of predictabil-

ity of decision in the great majority of cases and of intelligibility in all."[1]

. . .

USE OF COST-BENEFIT ANALYSIS

Defining Cost-Benefit Analysis. Cost-benefit analysis derives from simple profit and loss accounting traditionally practiced by business organizations.[2] Cost-benefit analysis

involves translating the attribute performances of alternatives into dollar quantities. The favorable attribute performances are added together to become the benefits. The sum of the unfavorable attribute performances is the cost. Thus, the cost-benefit analysis can be viewed as a process of deriving dollar values for each entry in a performance matrix and aggregating all of the performances into one attribute, either net benefits (benefit minus cost) or a benefit to cost ratio.[3]

A decision is justifiable when net benefit is positive or a benefit-to-cost ratio is greater than one.

Policy analysts have broadened the meaning of cost-benefit analysis to encompass virtually any analytical method that organizes information on alternative courses of action or displays possible tradeoff opportunities, thereby structuring decision making. Thus, the cost-benefit rubric encompasses many different types of analyses. Some of these analyses simply adopt a previously determined objective, leaving only the "cost" side of the balance sheet to be developed. For example, in establishing an emission standard for the discharge of ionizing radiation from a nuclear reactor, an analyst may be "given" a pre-existing standard for the ambient level of radiation necessary to protect human health near the reactor. This standard represents a conclusive determination of the degree of societal benefit to be achieved and reduces the analyst's task to finding the most cost-effective method to meet the ambient standard. Hence, the analysis in this truncated format is a simpler task of cost-effectiveness analysis. *Cost-benefit analysis,* then, is used by the decision maker to establish societal goals as well as the means for achieving these goals, whereas *cost-effectiveness analysis* only compares alternative means for achieving "given" goals. This article focuses on cost-benefit analysis.

Adoption of Cost-Benefit Analysis by Federal Agencies. The continuing efforts of regulatory agencies to balance competing considerations, such as public health and economic feasibility, are beset by a number of special problems. The technical problems include an ever-expanding, but limited and generally inconclusive data base, disagreement among experts on methods for using data, lack of consensus as to findings and their applicability to problems at hand, and unquantifiable attributes. Regulators must also value low-probability, high-cost events while taking into consideration the diverse and changing values of our pluralistic society. Moreover, an atmosphere of "crisis management" is promoted by statutory time limitations and pressures from various interests.

Mandated by statutes and recent Executive orders to conduct complex "balancing analyses" to reach decisions, regulatory agencies are under considerable pressure to adopt cost-benefit analysis.[4] The use of cost-benefit analysis in regulatory decision processes has been promoted by economic consultants and advisory committees to the agencies drawn from the scientific and engineering communities, including the National Academy of Sciences. In addition, regulated industries have urged agencies to use cost-benefit analysis in considering the economic impacts of regulations.

•   •   •

METHODOLOGICAL ISSUES IN REGULATORY USES OF COST-BENEFIT ANALYSIS

Many studies have identified the methodological limitations in the use of cost-benefit analysis as a basis for governmental decision making. Nevertheless, regulatory agencies continue to use cost-benefit analysis on many questions that present significant difficulties. The problems discussed in this section are not uniquely attributable to the analytical restraints of cost-benefit analysis, but stem from estimates based on scanty technical facts and the consideration of diverse values. Furthermore, many of the cost-benefit analysis problems are fundamental problems of the regulatory process itself, including good faith objectivity, effective citizen participation, and agency accountability. Other problems arise from unresolved constitutional problems, including the congressional delegation of broad and unguided authority to agencies and presidential intervention to promote consideration of economic factors conflicting with statutory requirements that stress health, safety, or environmental considerations. The following discussion briefly inventories methodological issues raised by

the use of cost-benefit analysis in regulatory agency decision making.

INADEQUATE IDENTIFICATION OF COSTS AND BENEFITS OF PROPOSED ACTION

One of the first steps in cost-benefit analysis is identifying the implications of regulatory options. Forecasting techniques notoriously fail to identify the possible primary, secondary, and tertiary consequences of a proposed action—particularly if that action sets a standard with diffuse health or environmental consequences that extend geographically and temporally. For example, analysts have great difficulty estimating the specific social and economic costs and benefits of regulatory options for controlling carcinogens. Cost-benefit analysis "offers no protection against historically bad assumptions. . . . [F]oolproof techniques for forecasting unforeseen consequences are by definition nonexistent."

The problem of inadequate or impossible measurement of attributes is related to the deficiencies of forecasting techniques. For instance, the "skimpy science" of toxicity is an acknowledged problem for regulatory officials seeking to measure costs and benefits of possible regulatory options for the control of toxic substances. Without the knowledge, techniques, trained personnel, and funds to measure these factors adequately, gross error in estimation may result. Similarly, many environmental effects, such as changes in ecosystems, cannot be estimated with confidence because no acceptable method exists to measure these attributes.

Furthermore, characterization of attributes may be problematic. An attribute deemed a benefit by an agency official may pose the problem of beneficiaries who do not desire the benefit or who do not even consider the attribute to be a benefit. For example, "cheap energy" is normally characterized as a benefit in a proceeding considering the construction of an energy facility. It may, however, be immaterial to those who have enough energy, or may be viewed as a cost to proponents of resource conservation.

Even if costs and benefits are identified, they may not be included in subsequent analysis for pragmatic reasons. Attributes may be too costly or too complex to measure. Exclusion may be based on a tenuous causal connection between the planned action and the possible attribute, as with the predicted probabilities of secondary or tertiary effects of a proposed agency action. Identified attributes also may be excluded for self-serving reasons. For example, if consideration of a possible disastrous consequence of a regulatory decision would tilt the outcome of the analysis against a favored agency action, it might be omitted from the final balancing process.

QUANTIFYING THE VALUE OF HUMAN LIFE AND OTHER TRADITIONALLY UNQUANTIFIABLE ATTRIBUTES

Cost-benefit analysis works best when (1) a socially accepted method, such as market pricing, is available to measure the costs and benefits, and (2) the measurement can be expressed in dollars or some other commensurable unit. Regulatory agencies using cost-benefit analysis face a critical problem when confronted with attributes that defy traditional economic valuation.

Analysts are well aware of these problems. Some refrain from placing their own values on immeasurable attributes and redirect their analyses. More typically, analysts recommend cautious use of cost-benefit analysis. Inconclusive analyses of valuation difficulties in cost-benefit literature reflect the hope that the problem will fade or be forgotten. For instance, although Stokey and Zeckhauser maintain that the complexity and importance of measuring intangible costs and benefits should not be underestimated, they ultimately conclude that perhaps quantification should be consciously postponed.

In some cases, it may be best to avoid quantifying some intangibles as long as possible, carrying them along instead in the form of a written paragraph of description. Maybe we will find that the intangible considerations point toward the same decision as the more easily quantified attributes. Maybe one or a few of them can be adequately handled by a decision-maker without resort to quantification. We will find no escape from the numbers. . . . Ultimately the final decision will implicitly quantify a host of intangibles; there are no incommensurables when decisions are made in the real world.[5]

This use of cost-benefit analysis is morally and intellectually irresponsible.

Today, a number of agencies assign monetary values to human life. The Nuclear Regulatory Commission (NRC) uses a value of $1,000 per whole-body rem in its cost-benefit analysis. This figure, multiplied by the number of rems capable of producing different types of deaths, provides dollar values for human life. The Environmental Protection Agency's Office of Radiation Programs establishes its environmental radiation standards at levels that will not cost more than $500,000 for each life to be saved. The

Consumer Product Safety Commission uses values ranging from $200,000 to $2,000,000 per life in its analyses.

But the fundamental issue is whether cost-benefit analysis is appropriate at all. Without an answer to this question from Congress or the courts, consideration turns to lesser issues: the proper method of valuation, the substantive basis for valuation (possibly relying on insurance statistics, jury awards, or potential lifetime earnings), and the extent agencies should articulate these issues and provide procedures for participation in the valuation process.

To date, agencies have expressed surprisingly little concern about these unresolved problems associated with cost-benefit analysis. Although officials deny valuing unquantifiable factors, these valuations are implicit in any cost-benefit based policy decision involving risks to human life. Responsible decision making demands that implicit valuations be acknowledged and addressed explicitly.

• • •

IMPROPER DISTRIBUTION OF COSTS AND BENEFITS

Every regulatory decision on health, safety, or environmental problems results in costs and benefits that will be distributed in some pattern across different population sectors, and in many cases, over several generations. For example, a decision to allow the commercial distribution of a toxic substance may result in economic benefits to the industrial users, their shareholders and employees, and consumers. It may also result, however, in adverse health effects and property damage to plant employees and those living near the plant. In addition, future generations may suffer mutagenic health effects or the depletion or pollution of natural resources.

Analysts and decision makers using cost-benefit analysis recognize these implications. Nonetheless, in the absence of public policy directives, analysts frequently apply personal assumptions about the allocation of costs and benefits while calling for objective "fairness" in dealing with distributional problems. Thus according to Stokey and Zeckhauser:

1. A program should be adopted when it will yield benefits to one group that are greater than the losses of another group, provided that the two groups are in roughly equivalent circumstances and the changes in welfare are not of great magnitude. . . .

2. If the benefits of a proposed policy are greater for one group than the costs for another group, and if it redresses the discriminatory effects of earlier policy choices, that policy should be undertaken. . . .

3. It is not so clear whether policies should be undertaken if they will benefit some groups only by imposing significant costs on others. It is sometimes proposed that a policy change should be adopted if and only if it passes a two-part test: (a) it yields positive net benefits, and (b) the redistributional effects of the change are beneficial. . . .[6]

Such earnest analytical approaches to determining fair distributions of costs and benefits ignore constitutional precepts underlying public sector decision making. Constitutional guarantees of due process, equal protection, property rights, and representative government should carry greater weight in solving the distributional problem than assumptions about fairness developed by economists and analysts.

Issues of temporal distribution, involving the allocation of costs and benefits for future generations, transcend even these constitutional values. Future generations possess neither present interests nor designated representatives to advance those interests. Our laws and values favor current benefits to those that accrue later. Cost-benefit analysis also reflects a preference for current benefits over future ones. Distribution over time, therefore, like the discount rate, is essentially an ethical issue for the nation. The assumptions that analysts must make about temporal distributions in using cost-benefit analysis are inadequate precisely because analysts, and not society, have made them.

PROMOTING SELF-INTEREST AND OTHER ANALYTICAL TEMPTATIONS

Users of cost-benefit analysis can easily play a "numbers game" to arrive at decisions that promote or justify agency actions reached on other grounds. The purportedly objective framework of cost-benefit analysis can be used to promote rather than to analyze options by manipulating the discount rate, assigning arbitrary values to identified costs and benefits, excluding costs that would tilt the outcome against the preferred option, and using self-serving assumptions about distributional fairness. Indeed, the very use of cost-benefit analysis leads some observers to conclude that the action under consideration is scheduled

for approval. Even self-corrective measures are suspect. For example, the use of safety factors ostensibly chosen to avoid certain effects may prove to be a facile solution that does not alter the preferred analytical result if these factors are determined only *after* completing a preliminary analysis. Furthermore, these factors are usually based on technical estimates and do not properly consider the value-laden aspects of large, irreversible risks.

In addition, the "technology-forcing function" of regulatory programs can be stifled by limited technical and economic information. Governmental officials must often rely on the regulated industry for news of recent technological developments. Industry information is likely to be unduly pessimistic about the costs, reliability, and availability of new techniques. Thus, cost-benefit analysis based upon industrial information may become a mechanism for economically convenient regulation that tends to perpetuate the technological status quo. This result is particularly predictable when regulatory agencies have not defined their objectives. If such objectives were established initially, they would "drive" the regulatory process and more readily force development of new technology.

SPECIAL PROBLEMS OF ACCOUNTABILITY

The use of cost-benefit analysis raises new issues in addition to the usual problems of ensuring agency accountability to the courts, Congress, the President, and the public. Certainly the jargon, presumably objective numbers, and analytical complexities of cost-benefit analysis obscure the subjective assumptions, uncertain data, and arbitrary distributions and valuations of the decision-making process, thereby preventing meaningful review of agency activity. Agency uses of cost-benefit analysis tend to promote the role of experts and diminish the participatory and review roles of nonexperts.

Senator Muskie has voiced his concern about agencies including "questionable benefits" that can make projects appear "economically sound."[7] He has called for evaluating projects at different stages of completion "to find if the validity of benefits claimed at project authorization can be reaffirmed during and after construction."[8] No governmental agency has adopted this approach despite its obvious value in improving subsequent uses of cost-benefit analysis.

In its cost-benefit analysis of nuclear reactor licensing decisions, NRC estimates the population that will live near the reactor site in the future. Yet neither NRC nor any other governmental body attempts to control actual population growth in the areas surrounding nuclear plants. Thus the estimated cost-benefit basis for approving a proposed activity is not used as a planning tool for maintaining predicted costs and benefits once the activity is undertaken. The actual costs and benefits consequently may vary considerably from those projected in the analysis.

Additionally, the combination of fragmented regulatory jurisdiction over pervasive problems and increased agency reliance on cost-benefit analysis ultimately leads to increased societal risk. For example, a trace metal such as mercury constitutes a health and environmental quality hazard. It is regulated by several agencies, including the Environmental Protection Agency (EPA), Occupational Safety and Health Administration (OSHA), Consumer Product Safety Commission (CPSC), and Food and Drug Administration (FDA). Each agency may permit some activity introducing an additional incremental amount of the pollutant into the environment because the minor amount of calculable human exposure or environmental harm in each instance is offset by a broad range of postulated societal benefits. Even though each agency may be making careful and objective decisions, without overall interagency accounting for the increasing risk to the general population and the environment from these many small decisions, the total societal risk will continue to aggregate.

The above taxonomy of methodological problems reveals the need for a "best efforts" approach, fostered by Congress and the President, and administered by the agencies and the courts, to exclude the use of cost-benefit analysis under certain conditions and to resolve rational and humanistic concerns. This best efforts approach should focus on: (1) improving the technical and objective quality of cost-benefit analysis; (2) establishing the limits and societal implications of cost-benefit analysis; (3) improving public participation; and (4) designing more effective measures for congressional and executive oversight of agency practices.

NOTES

1. Friendly, *The Federal Administrative Agencies: The Need for a Better Definition of Standards,* 75 Harv. L. Rev. 873, 874 (1962).

2. See E. J. Mishan, *Cost-Benefit Analysis* 6 (1973).

3. Battelle Pacific Northwest Labs, Review of Decision Methodologies for Evaluating Regulatory Actions Affecting Public Health and Safety (December 1976), p. 53. See also E. Stokey and R. Zeckhauser, *A Primer for Policy Analysis* (N.Y.: Norton, 1978), pp. 136–137.

4. However, the courts have given the regulatory agencies a relatively free hand to establish procedures for conducting cost-benefit analysis. *See* Vermont Yankee Nuclear Power Corp. v. Natural Resources Defense Council, Inc., 435 U.S. 519 (1978). In that case, the NRDC challenged an AEC rulemaking procedure dealing with spent fuel from a reactor and the use of the rule in cost-benefit analysis for licensing Vermont Yankee's light water reactor. The District of Columbia Court of Appeals overturned the rulemaking because of the AEC's failure to employ certain procedural devices beyond the statutory minima. The Supreme Court held that the circuit court had improperly intruded into the AEC's rulemaking authority and remanded the case.

5. Stokey and Zeckhauser, *supra* note 3, p. 153.

6. *Ibid.,* pp. 281–282.

7. Letter from Senator Edmund Muskie to Comptroller General Elmer Staats (August 5, 1977), reprinted in General Accounting Office, *Improved Formulation and Presentation of Water Resources Project Alternatives Provide a Basis for Better Management Decisions* 18 (February 1, 1978), p. 19.

8. *Ibid.*

VICTOR R. FUCHS

What Is Cost-Benefit Analysis?

Many physicians approach cost-benefit and cost-effectiveness analysis (CBA/CEA) with something akin to what Sir James Frazer described as "the awe and dread with which the untutored savage contemplates his mother-in-law."[1] This is unwise and unnecessary. The recently published report of the Office of Technology Assessment[2] makes it clear that CBA/CEA is neither a purgative nor a panacea nor a placebo. This well-written, carefully documented study explains the strengths and weaknesses of CBA/CEA, reviews attempts to apply it in health care, and offers a set of policy options and recommendations for future action. The report deserves the attention of physicians and should do much to dispel mystery and allay concern.

In simplest terms, CBA is an analytic technique designed to help a decision maker consider systematically all the consequences of a possible course of action, arrayed as costs and benefits.[3] One of its strengths (and also one of its problems) is that it forces the analyst-decision maker to attach a value to each identifiable consequence. That this is frequently difficult to do goes without saying. Evaluation of health benefits such as reductions in mortality, disability, or pain is particularly difficult, and that is why CEA is often substituted for CBA. In CEA alternative courses of action that have similar health benefits are compared, thus reducing the problem primarily to a comparison of costs.[4] Such comparisons are not free of problems either, but they are usually not as troublesome as the evaluation of benefits. CBA/CEA has been applied to many fields, including education, transportation, and defense. Within the health-care field, several dozen papers have been published on CBA/CEA in such illnesses as poliomyelitis,[5] rubella,[6] myocardial infarction,[7] hypertension,[8] appendicitis,[9] and pneumococcal pneumonia.[10]

Critics of CBA contend that it is either impossible

to place a value on certain benefits (e.g., saving a human life) or, if not impossible, immoral. Such objections lack merit in a world in which choices must be made; every choice necessarily reflects a set of values. We do not, as the critics imply, have an option between evaluating and not evaluating. The only option is whether to evaluate explicitly, systematically, and openly, as CBA/CEA forces us to do, or whether to evaluate implicitly, haphazardly, and secretly, as has been done so often in the past. Even the decision to allocate a potentially life-saving scarce resource among patients by some random process such as a coin toss or lottery involves evaluation. If the patients have equal prospects of benefiting medically from the resource, giving each an equal chance to receive it implies an equal value of life for each patient. If the patients differ in their prospects of benefiting, giving each an equal chance implies a different set of values.

Although researchers at the Office of Technology Assessment could find only a few examples of CBA/CEA actually being used in health-care decision making, interest in this technique is increasing rapidly. This interest is derived from a growing realization that we live in a world of scarce resources and that the fundamental economic problem of society is to allocate these resources in a way that will best satisfy human wants. Health is a basic human want, perhaps the most basic, but it is only one of many competing wants. Neither this society nor any other can allocate to health all the resources that physicians and other health professionals believe might benefit their patients. What, then, is to be done? Given the wide range of potential choices in the use of health-care facilities, personnel, and technologies, decision makers clearly need a better understanding of the consequences of the alternatives.

Consider some field other than health—say, energy. Few physicians would be upset to learn that CBA/CEA is being applied to evaluate the feasibility

From New England Journal of Medicine 303 (October 16, 1980), 937–938.

of alternative sources of energy; indeed, most would be troubled if the government embarked on a multi-billion-dollar project for shale oil or solar energy without first conducting a systematic analysis. Yet that is precisely what has occurred in the health-care field. Government health-care expenditures have doubled every five or six years for more than two decades, and private expenditures have grown only slightly less rapidly. This growth has proceeded, for the most part, without the systematic appraisal of programs or technologies that CBA/CEA would provide.

The report from the Office of Technology Assessment is skeptical of the idea that CBA/CEA in itself will be effective in controlling health expenditures. To be sure! There must be a will to do so, and there must also be financial and organizational mechanisms to implement that will. Given the will and the mechanisms, however, CBA/CEA offers the most rational, humane basis for cost control. Physicians should hardly fear such efforts but should welcome and cooperate actively in them. Mounting pressure from taxpayers, business firms, and labor unions to control expenditures makes some constraints inevitable. It is in the best interests of patients and physicians for these constraints to be derived from careful study of costs and benefits rather than from capricious budget ceilings and regulatory roulette.

That CBA/CEA has its problems and its limitations is made abundantly clear in the Office of Technology Assessment report. What needs to be spelled out just as clearly is the even greater danger inherent in other strategies for rationing scarce resources. When constraints on medical practice are imposed without regard to costs and benefits, the nation's health suffers more than is necessary. Of course, no technique, whether in medicine or economics, is likely to be valuable unless it is competently employed. Some studies, such as a recent CBA of cardiac surgery,[11] lose much of their value because of such conceptual errors as double counting of benefits and omission of certain categories of costs.

Are there ever situations in which CBA/CEA would not be desirable? Clearly there are. Sometimes the application of systematic analysis would not be worth the costs. After all, CBA/CEA itself involves the use of scarce resources, and their costs may outweigh the benefit of additional information. At other times, society may prefer that certain evaluations not be made explicit. In other words, the costs and benefits of the decision-making process itself must be

considered; in some cases, society may prefer a less explicit, less systematic process. Furthermore, even where CBA/CEA is applied, it will be important to insulate the individual practitioner from explicit involvement on a day-to-day basis because of potential conflict with the commitment to do what is best for each patient. Thus, the best time for evaluations and tradeoffs will usually be when decisions are made about construction of facilities, authorization of new technologies, training of personnel, and setting of standards and procedures. Practicing physicians have a great deal to contribute to those decisions. Although it is not important for every physician to know how to perform CBA/CEA, it will become essential for every physician to understand why these analyses are performed. The report from the Office of Technology Assessment and the many background papers on which it is based are useful contributions toward that end.

NOTES

1. Frazer, J. *The golden bough: a study in magic and religion.* abridged. New York: Macmillan, 1922.

2. Office of Technology Assessment. *The implications of cost-effectiveness: analysis of medical technology.* Washington, D.C.: Government Printing Office, 1980.

3. Zeckhauser, R., Harberger, A., Haveman, R., Lynn, L., Niskanen, W., and Williams, J., eds. Benefit-cost and policy analysis. Chicago: Aldine, 1975.

4. Weinstein, M. C., and Stason, W. B. Foundations of cost-effectiveness analysis for health and medical practices. *N. Engl. J. Med.* 1977; 296:716–21.

5. Weisbrod, B. A. Costs and benefits of medical research: a case study of poliomyelitis. *J. Polit. Econ.* 1971; 79(3):527–44.

6. Farber, M. E., and Finkelstein, S. N. A cost-benefit analysis of a mandatory premarital rubella-antibody screening program. *N. Engl. J. Med.* 1978; 300:856–9.

7. Cretin, S. Cost/benefit analysis of treatment and prevention of myocardial infarction. *Health Serv. Res.* 1977; 12:174–89.

8. McNeil, B. J., Varady, P. D., Burrows, B. A., and Adelstein, S. J. Measures of clinical efficacy: cost-effectiveness calculations in the diagnosis and treatment of hypertensive renovascular disease. *N. Engl. J. Med.* 1975; 293:216–21.

9. Neutra, R. R. Indications for the surgical treatment of suspected acute appendicitis: a cost-effectiveness approach. In: Bunker, J. P., Barnes, B. A., and Mosteller, F., eds. Costs, risks and benefits of surgery. New York: Oxford University Press, 1977:277–307.

10. Willems, J. S., Sanders, C. R., Riddiough, M. A., and Bell, J. C. Cost effectiveness of vaccination against pneumococcal pneumonia. *N. Engl. J. Med.* 1980; 303:553–69.

11. Crosby, I. K., Wellons, H. A., Jr., Martin, R.P., Schuch, D., and Muller, W. H., Jr. Employability—a new indication for aneurysmectomy and coronary revascularization. *Circulation.* 1980; 62: Part 2, no. 2:I-79–83.

RUTH R. FADEN AND TOM L. BEAUCHAMP

The Right to Risk Information and the Right to Refuse Health Hazards in the Workplace

Gaps in information workers have about risks in the workplace prompted the *Wall Street Journal* to run a story in 1977 on the "Workers' Right to Know."[1] As much an editorial as a feature article, this story proposed a congressional investigation of the need for "full disclosure of hazards by companies" whose workplaces present significant risk to workers. The article pointed out that no federal agency has clear authority to disclose risks to workers or to control company disclosures. Since 1977 there have been congressional and agency hearings on this and related issues. Yet in early 1979 the *New York Times*[2] virtually repeated the *Wall Street Journal* appeal, this time in reference to women employees at American Cyanamid. In the early 1980s it was still being argued on the floor of the U.S. House of Representatives that new national legislation is needed, especially in light of persistent failures by various manufacturers to disclose hazards to their workers.[3]

The idea that there is a moral obligation to disclose relevant information to workers has already obtained currency in other quarters as well. The "Code of Ethical Conduct for Physicians Providing Occupational-Medical Services," for example, calls on member physicians to communicate health hazards "to individuals or groups potentially affected."[4] Recently passed bills in the state of New York and the city of Philadelphia support the claim that workers have a right to know. The New York bill declares that employees and their representatives have a right to "*all* information relating to toxic substances"—a right that cannot be "waived as a condition of employment."[5] Such a moral thesis has been defended in a demanding form by both Joseph Fletcher[6] and Chief Counsel Weiner of the California Department of In-

dustrial Relations.[7] This problem of a right to know is addressed in this paper, along with other rights of employees to effect safety standards in the workplace and even to refuse various kinds of hazardous work.

I

First, consider some elementary background history. By the late 1970s it became apparent that a right-to-know movement had taken hold in the United States, especially in matters of consumer protection. The belief that citizens in general—though not workers in particular—have a right to know about significant risks is reflected in an extraordinarily diverse set of laws and federal regulations such as The Freedom of Information Act; The Federal Insecticide, Fungicide, and Rodenticide Amendments and Regulations; The Motor Vehicle and School Bus Safety Amendments; the Truth-in-Lending Act; The Pension Reform Act; the Real Estate Settlement Procedures Act; The Federal Food, Drug, and Cosmetic Act; The Consumer Product Safety Act; and The Toxic Substances Control Act. These acts commonly require explanations of products, guidebooks, and warranties, and the implicit message is that manufacturing companies and other businesses have a moral (and obviously in some cases a legal) obligation to disclose information without which individuals could not adequately decide about matters of participation, usage, employment, or enrollment.[8]

The related idea that there is a corporate or government responsibility to provide adequate information to workers about hazards in the workplace potentially could have a pervasive and revolutionary effect on major American corporations. There are over 30,000 pesticides alone now in use in the United States. There are approximately 1/4 million industrial chemicals. About 25 million largely uninformed American workers are exposed to toxic substances

©1981 Ruth R. Faden and Tom L. Beauchamp. Work on this essay was supported by a grant from the National Library of Medicine.

now regulated by the Occupational Safety and Health Administration (OSHA), and toxic substances present only one dimension of the problem of risks in the workplace. Some representative harms that products, substances, or activities in the workplace may cause are:

Benzene (leukemia)

Asbestos (asbestosis)

Lead (destruction of reproductive capacities)

Microwave radiation (cataractogenic effects)

Petrochemicals (brain tumors, sterility)

Machines (ear damage from noise, etc.)

Construction (injury due to accident)

Cotton textiles (byssinosis)

Coal dust (black lung)

II

The most developed model of disclosure obligations and rights of informed refusal has thus far been found in the body of literature on so-called informed consent. This literature has been developed largely from contexts of fiduciary relationships between physicians and patients or between scientific investigators and subjects, where there are broadly recognized moral and legal obligations to disclose known risks (and benefits) associated with a proposed treatment or research maneuver. No parallel obligation has traditionally been legally recognized in nonfiduciary relationships, such as that between management and workers, and except for special and limited regulations that require warnings or signs about individual substances or conditions, there is currently no general legal requirement that employers warn workers about the above-mentioned hazards in the workplace. There may nonetheless be moral requirements, and the law may need substantial revision.

The recent history of the development of informed consent and refusal requirements in fiduciary relationships provides relevant data for discussions of nonfiduciary contexts and offers one model of disclosure that seems promising for the workplace. This model, however, rather clearly has only limited application in the workplace. There is no reasonable analogy drawn in the law between fiduciary relationships and the employer-employee relationship. Nor is there any parallel in the union-employee relationship, for unions are not fiduciaries in the eyes of the law. Consequently neither employers nor unions have a duty to warn of risk or to disclose relevant information in an informed consent context. Employers can be sued for fraudulent misrepresentation of the risks of a job, but not for failure to disclose risk. Dangers in the workplace have thus far been handled largely by workmen's compensation laws. These laws were originally designed for problems of accident in instances of immediately assessible damage, where the risks of accident are already known by employees. Duties to warn or to disclose are pointless under this no-fault conception of workmen's compensation, and there is no functional equivalent of the concept of formal, voluntary assumption of a risk. To be compensated for an injury a worker must only show that an injury occurred; there is no need to show that someone was responsible, and therefore no reason to show that there should have been a warning or a valid consent. The problem here is one of legal causation: the physician may be sued by causing an injury through nondisclosure or underdisclosure; management may not, unless fraudulent misrepresentation is involved.

Reasons traditionally invoked for establishing such starkly different arrangements of responsibility, causation, and compensation for medicine and for industry may now be crumbling, however. It has been relatively easy in the past to disassociate the disclosure of information from causation of industrial "accidents" and from problems of compensation, but the fact that asbestos or cotton fibers, for example, present serious long-term risks of injury, disease, and death is different from the fact that radial saws and pathways along steel girders lead to similarly serious accidents. Every worker on the job already knows of the existence of the latter dangers (though not of the magnitude of those risks, e.g., plant injury rates), and, as *Canterbury v. Spence* and other cases make clear, there is no duty even in fiduciary contexts to disclose what a reasonable person in the situation would already know. Recently discovered risks to health in the workplace thus *do* carry with them a *need* for information without which the person may suffer harms, and on the basis of which a person may wish to forgo employment completely or to refuse certain work environments within a place of employment. Accordingly, the party capable of providing the information should perhaps be held responsible for *not* providing it.

At the present time it appears that we are unprepared by our legal tradition to deal with these questions about workers' needs for information. We are therefore ripe for a discussion of the responsibility of employers—and perhaps other parties—to make disclosures about risks.

III

It is perhaps more imperative in the case of employee-employer relationships that there be disclosure requirements for risk information *because* no fiduciary relationship or common goal exists between the parties—the employment relationship often being confrontational, with few interests and goals shared in common, and therefore entailing increased risks to workers. The relative powerlessness of employees in the employer-employee relationship may not be sufficient to justify *employer* disclosure obligations, but it does seem to call for relevant disclosures by some party. By what criteria, however, shall such disclosure obligations be determined to begin and end, and how is negligence to be determined? It will clearly not do to argue that there is never any obligation on employers because workmen's compensation relieves them of responsibility and makes the issue moot. This response is appropriate only from a narrow legal perspective, and it is worth remarking again that the law's focus on causation requires a certain blindness to broader moral issues.

Accordingly, let us consider the argument that the withholding of relevant information by a fiduciary unduly deprives individuals of opportunities to know and refuse, thus undermining autonomy. Here we must not press the analogy to medicine very hard, for it is implausible to suppose that employers can be conceived as fiduciaries. As customarily conceived, both the government and unions have a relationship to employees more closely approximating a fiduciary relationship than do employers. This only indicates, however, that in some contexts the government or a union leader is a more likely candidate to be held culpable for not providing information than an employer, and the question still must be faced whether an employer or any other party must be bound to any stringent disclosure requirements. One plausible view is the following: Because large employers, unions, and government agencies must deal with multiple numbers of employees and complicated causal conditions, no standard *more* demanding than the objective reasonable person standard proposed in *Canterbury* is appropriate for general industry disclosures. That is, no party would be held responsible for disclosing information beyond that needed to make an informed choice about the adequacy of safety precautions, industrial hygiene, long-term hazards, etc.—as determined by what the reasonable person would judge to be the worker's need for information that is material to a decision about employment or working conditions. It does not follow, however, that this general standard of disclosure—which would in practice be used for disclosures to unions who represent employees (or to groups of employees)—is adequate for all individual disclosures. At least in the case of extremely serious hazards—such as those involved in short-term but very concentrated doses of radiation—the subjective standard rejected in *Canterbury* may be more appropriate.*

Accordingly, in cases where disclosures to *individual* workers may be expected to have significant subjective impact and variance, the objective reasonable person standard should perhaps be supplemented by a subjective standard that takes account of independent informational needs. An alternative that might be viable would be to include the following as a component of all general disclosures under the reasonable person standard: "If you are concerned about the possible effect of hazards on your individual health, and you seek clarification or personal information, a company physician may be consulted by making an appointment." (Of course, an entirely subjective standard would be inappropriate, because workers will rarely know what information would be relevant for their deliberations, and underdisclosures would regularly occur.)

IV

Despite the direction of the arguments thus far, there are reasons why in practice it will prove far more difficult to honor the "right to know" for workers through disclosure duties than for patients. There are, for example, more complicated questions about the kinds of information to be disclosed, by whom, to whom, under what conditions, and what to do if workers themselves are inhibited from acting on any concerns they might have about such information (as, e.g., in the case of industries where ten persons stand in line for every available position). In the workplace the intractability of these questions is magnified by the massive number of persons directly affected and

---

*Ed. note: *Canterbury v. Spence* and the standards mentioned here are discussed in the introduction to Chapter 5 of this volume.

by the legitimate interests of third parties—in this case the federal government and the public whose cost concerns it represents. However, we must set these considerations aside here in order to consider what is perhaps the single greatest difficulty about the right to know about risks in the workplace: the right to refuse hazardous work assignments and to have effective mechanisms for workers to reduce the risks they face.

Some issues turn on the options available to informed workers to reduce or remove personal risks. In certain limited cases, it may be possible for informed workers to reject employment because health and safety conditions are perceived as unacceptable. This is most likely to occur in a job market where workers have alternative employment opportunities or where a worker is being offered a new assignment with the option of remaining in his or her current job. Usually, however, workers are not in a position to respond to information about health hazards by seeking employment elsewhere. For the information to be useful to the worker, it must be possible for the worker to effect change while staying on the job.

The Occupational Safety and Health Act of 1970 (OSH Act) confers a series of rights on employees which, at least ideally, go a long way toward making meaningful a duty to disclose hazards in the workplace.[9] Specifically, the OSH Act grants workers the right to request an OSHA inspection where they believe an OSHA standard has been violated or an imminent hazard exists. Under the Act, employees also have the right to participate in OSHA inspections of the worksite and to consult freely with the inspection officer. Perhaps most importantly, employees requesting an inspection or otherwise exercising their rights under the OSH Act are explicitly protected in the Act from discharge or any form of discrimination by current or future employers.

While these worker rights under the OSH Act are important, it can be argued that they do not go far enough in ensuring that workers have effective mechanisms for initiating inspections of suspected health hazards. It should be noted that federal, state, and municipal employees are not covered by the OSH Act and that unions are not afforded the same protections against discrimination as individual employees. There are also serious questions about the ability of the Occupational Safety and Health Administration to enforce provisions of the OSH Act. If workers are to make effective use of disclosed information about health hazards, they must have unimpeded access to an effective and efficient regulatory system.

It is also essential that workers have an adequately protected right to refuse unsafe work. It is difficult to determine the extent to which this right is currently legally protected. Although the OSH Act does not grant a general right to refuse unsafe work,[10] provisions to this effect exist in some state occupational safety laws. In addition, the Secretary of Labor has issued a regulation which interprets the OSH Act as including a limited right to refuse unsafe work.[11] A limited right to refuse is also protected explicitly in the Labor-Management Relations Act (LMRA) and implicitly in the National Labor Relations Act (NLRA).[12] Unfortunately, these statutory protections vary significantly in the conditions under which they grant a right to refuse and the consequences which they permit to follow from such refusals. For example, the OSHA regulation allows workers to walk off the job where there is a "real danger of death or serious injury,"[13] while the LMRA permits refusals only under "abnormally dangerous conditions."[14] Thus, under the LMRA, the nature of the occupation determines the extent of danger justifying refusal, while under OSHA it is the character of the threat which is determinative. By contrast, under the NLRA a walkout may be justified for even minimal safety problems, so long as the action can be construed as a concerted activity for mutual aid and protection and there does not exist a no-strike clause in any collective bargaining agreements.[15] However, employees refusing to work under the NLRA may lose the right to be reinstated in their positions if permanent replacements can be found.[16]

The relative merits of the different statutes are further confused by questions of overlapping authorities. It is by no means always clear (1) when a worker is eligible to claim protection under each law, (2) which law affords a worker maximum protection in a particular circumstance, and (3) whether or under what conditions a worker can seek relief through more than one law or directly through the courts.

The overall legal situation concerning the right to refuse hazardous work is far too complicated to be adequately treated here. Any definitive treatment of the problem will need to consider not only narrow legal questions of jurisdiction and remedy but also important policy and moral questions raised by the conflicting interests of employees and employers. Unfortunately, these questions have not received much attention outside particular legal circles. Consider, for example, the issue of whether a meaningful right to refuse hazardous work entails an obligation to continue to pay nonworking employees, or to award the employees back pay, should the issue be resolved in their favor. It could be argued that workers without union strike benefits or other income protections are unable to exercise their right to refuse unsafe work because of undue economic pressures. On the other hand, it could be argued that to permit such workers to draw a paycheck is to legitimize strike with pay, a practice generally considered unacceptable by management and by Congress.

Also unresolved is whether the right to refuse unsafe work should be restricted to cases of obvious, imminent, and serious risks to health or life (the current OSHA and LMRA position) or expanded to include lesser risks and also uncertain risks—e.g., exposure to suspected toxic or carcinogenic substances. Certainly, if "the right to know" is to lead to meaningful worker action, workers must be able to remove themselves from exposure to suspected hazards, as well as obvious hazards. Related to this issue is the question of the *proper standard* for determining whether a safety walkout is justified. At least three different standards have been proposed (and even imposed): a good-faith standard which requires only a determination that the worker honestly (subjectively) *believes* that the health hazard exists; a reasonable person standard which requires that the belief be reasonable under the circumstances as well as honestly held; and an objective standard which requires evidence, generally established by expert witnesses, that the threat actually existed.[17] (The similarities between these three standards and the three standards proposed for the duty to disclose are obvious and pertinent.) Although the possibility of worker abuse of the right to refuse has been a major factor in a current trend to reject the good-faith standard, recent commentary has argued that this trend raises serious equity issues in the proper balancing of this concern with the needs of workers confronted with basic self-preservation issues.[18]

Still another related issue is whether the right to refuse hazardous work should be protected only until review is initiated, at which time the worker must return to the job, or whether the walk-out should be permitted until the alleged hazard is at least temporarily removed. So long as the hazards covered under a right to refuse are restricted to those risks which are obvious in the environment and which are easily established as health hazards, this issue is relatively easy to resolve. However, where the nature of the risk is less apparent—as in the case of the risks treated in this paper—a major role of the right to refuse may be to call attention to an alleged hazard and to compel regulatory action. When this occurs, requiring workers to continue to be exposed while OSHA or the NLRB conduct their investigations may be unacceptable to workers, and certainly will be unacceptable if the magnitude of potential harm is perceived as great. On the other hand, compelling employers to remove suspected hazards during the evaluation period may in some cases result in intolerable economic burdens. What is needed is a delineation of the conditions under which workers may be compelled to return to work while an alleged hazard is being evaluated and the conditions under which employers must be compelled to remove alleged hazards. This problem is only a special case of the larger issue of setting standards for acceptable risks in the workplace.

In conclusion, legal rights, no matter how adequate, are of no practical consequence if workers remain ignorant of their options. To take the right to refuse as an example, it is doubtful that many workers, and particularly non-unionized workers, are even aware that they have a legally protected right to refuse hazardous work, let alone that there are at least three different statutory provisions which apply. Even if workers were generally aware that they had such a right, it is extremely unlikely that they could prudently weave their way through the maze of legal options unaided. If there is to be a meaningful right to know in the workplace, not only will there have to be adequate legal protection of this and related worker rights, there will also have to be an adequate program to educate workers about their rights and how to exercise them.

NOTES

1. Gail Bronson, "The Right to Know," *The Wall Street Journal* (Eastern Edition), July 1, 1977, p. 4.

2. Editorial. January 1, 1979.

3. George Miller, "The Asbestos Coverup," *Congressional Record* (May 17, 1979), pp. E2363–64, and "Asbestos Health Hazards and Company Morality," *Congressional Record* (May 24, 1979), pp. E2523–24.

4. Adopted by the Board of Directors of the American Occupational Medical Association (July 23, 1976), as reprinted in *Bulletin of the New York Academy of Medicine* 54 (September 1978), Appendix, pp. 818–19.

5. State of New York, 1979–1980 Regular Sessions, 7103-D, Article 28, para. 880. This bill passed but has as yet received no appropriation.

6. Joseph Fletcher, "The Right to Know," in Thomas P. Vogl, ed., *Public Information in the Prevention of Occupational Cancer: Proceedings of a Symposium* (December 2–3, 1976) (Washington: National Academy of Sciences, 1977), p. 55.

7. P. Weiner, "Testimony to OSHA on Employee Access to Records," December 5, 1978.

8. On this point, cf. Harold J. Magnuson, "The Right to Know," *Archives of Environmental Health* 32 (1977), pp. 40–44.

9. 29 U.S.C. § 651–678 (1970).

10. Susan Preston, "A Right Under OSHA to Refuse Unsafe Work or A Hobson's Choice of Safety or Job?" *University of Baltimore Law Review* 8(3): Spring 1979, 519–550.

11. This interpretation of the OSH Act was upheld by the Supreme Court on February 26, 1980, see *Law Week,* 48:33, p. 4189–4195, Feb. 26, 1980.

12. Susan Preston, "A Right Under OSHA to Refuse Unsafe Work or A Hobson's Choice of Safety or Job?" *University of Baltimore Law Review* 8(3): Spring 1979, 519–550.

13. 29 U.S.C. § 143 (1976), as cited in Susan Preston, "A

Right Under OSHA to Refuse Unsafe Work or A Hobson's Choice of Safety or Job?" *University of Baltimore Law Review* 8(3): Spring 1979, p. 543.

14. 29 CFR § 1977.12 (1978), as cited in Susan Preston, "A Right Under OSHA to Refuse Unsafe Work or A Hobson's Choice of Safety or Job?" *University of Baltimore Law Review* 8(3): Spring 1979, 525–526.

15. Nicholas Ashford and Judith P. Katz, "Unsafe Working Conditions: Employee Rights Under the Labor Management Relations Act and the Occupational Safety and Health Act," *Notre Dame Lawyer,* 52:802, June 1977, 802–837.

16. Susan Preston, "A Right Under OSHA to Refuse Unsafe Work or A Hobson's Choice of Safety or Job?" *University of Baltimore Law Review* 8(3): Spring 1979, p. 543.

17. Nancy K. Frank, "A Question of Equity: Workers' 'Right to Refuse' Under OSHA Compared to the Criminal Necessity Defense," *Labor Law Journal,* 31:10, October 1980, 617–626.

18. Nancy K. Frank, "A Question of Equity: Workers' 'Right to Refuse' Under OSHA Compared to the Criminal Necessity Defense," *Labor Law Journal,* 31:10, October 1980, 617–626.

TABITHA POWLEDGE

Can Genetic Screening Prevent Occupational Disease?

Occupational health, like nutrition, is one of medicine's neglected children. When the subject crops up, everybody agrees that it is very important. But the subject does not come up unless, as in the recent cases of vinyl chloride and asbestos, we are presented with examples too arresting to be ignored.

A much more glamorous field of investigation, the genetic basis for differences in susceptibility to various environmental insults is, however, being linked to occupational health—and in the process is raising serious social and moral questions about the ways in which workers should be protected against the rapidly proliferating hazards of our industrial economies.

One important example of this trend is the theory that an inherited deficiency of alpha$_1$-antitrypsin (an

inhibitor of protease) is a major factor in predisposition to lung disorders. Much of the literature on alpha$_1$-antitrypsin argues the need for the identification of deficient individuals so they can be warned that they are at unusually high risk and should modify their surroundings accordingly. The pernicious effect of smoking on development of pulmonary disease is most often stressed as the factor that triggers disease in susceptible individuals, but occupational triggers have also been suggested.

There have already been *in vitro* studies by Parimal Chowdhury and Donald Luria of New Jersey Medical School linking cadmium with reduction of alpha$_1$-antitrypsin concentrations, providing a possible explanation for the high rate of emphysema in workers exposed to cadmium and ultimately a possible rationale for excluding alpha$_1$-antitrypsin deficient workers from jobs which involve exposure to cadmium. Alpha$_1$-antitrypsin deficiency has also been investi-

From *New Scientist* 2 (September 2, 1976), 486–488. This first appeared in *New Scientist,* London, the weekly review of science and technology.

gated in Saskatchewan grain handlers, who are occupationally exposed to a lot of dust and have a high incidence of lung problems. In Sweden, 200,000 newborn infants have been screened for alpha$_1$-antitrypsin, and a prospective follow-up on those found to be deficient is in progress. Hundreds of California 13-year-olds have also been screened, and those identified as deficient (plus their families) warned about future risks. Again, the emphasis is on avoiding smoking, but Jack Lieberman of the City of Hope National Medical Centre in California also observes, ''Tests for alpha$_1$-antitrypsin deficiency should eventually become an important part of pre-employment examinations in industry so that susceptible individuals can be kept out of those work areas where the risk would be greatest.''

Another example comes from the histocompatibility antigen system so useful in matching tissues of donor and recipient in organ transplantation. An enormous amount of work has been done on associations between these antigens, which are present on most body cells, and disease, exceeding in energy, enthusiasm and medical respectability the similar flurry of work on associations between blood groups and disease in vogue in the 1960s.

Although several antigens in this complex system appear to have a positive statistical relationship with many disorders, the strongest and most widely-accepted to date is that of the B27 antigen and ankylosing spondylitis, a chronic but non-lethal and treatable arthritis of the lower spine. More than 90 per cent of ankylosing spondylitis patients possess the B27 antigen, compared with less than 8 per cent of controls. On the other hand, even the most generous researchers estimate that no more than 20 per cent of those who possess the B27 antigen will develop the disorder. In fact, a recent major review by Jane Schaller and Gilbert Omenn of Washington University concluded that these antigens, while possibly important in clinical research into disease classifications and mechanisms, had ''little value as diagnostic or prognostic tests.''

Nevertheless, there have been attempts to use these associations in occupational medicine. Histocompatibility antigens have been studied in British asbestos workers, resulting in the conclusion that the B27 antigen ''may provide a useful marker of an enhanced susceptibility to the tissue-damaging effects of as-

bestos dust.'' And William Gough and colleagues from the Cornell Medical Centre of New York Hospital have argued that B27-positive offspring of ankylosing spondylitis patients ''avoid occupations such as driving, dentistry, surgery, and professional athletics, which are likely to place excessive strain on the back.'' Thus some professionals are, on the basis of current data, willing to warn a child against dreams of becoming a surgeon, and even against such an everyday pursuit as driving a car, because he or she might (only might) develop a disease widely conceded to be treatable.

''BLAME THE VICTIM''

Plans ''to identify those workers with a genetic potential to hyper-react to industrial chemicals'' have actually been around since the early 1960s; the first suggestion of industrial screening for alpha$_1$-antitrypsin deficiency, for instance, came almost a decade ago from H. E. Stokinger and L. D. Scheel. There has not been much enthusiasm for such genetic categorizations, particularly among workers, partly because it is feared (not unreasonably) that people will be refused jobs because of them. Some groups (both British and American Science for the People groups, for instance) think of it as just one more example of the ''blame the victim'' mentality. While Stokinger and Scheel argue that ''the tests do not deny employment; they merely orient job placement to the advantage of both the employer and the employed,'' there is reason for workers to suspect that the lion's share of the advantages may accrue to the former.

The most flagrant current example involves what one might call the quintessential genetic category— sex. The protagonist is 34-year-old Norma James of Whitby, Ontario, who opted for permanent sterilization rather than lose her well-paid job in the lead battery plant of General Motors, whose night shift hours left her free during the day to care for her four children.

Because of lead's disastrous fetal effects, GM has a company policy of not employing women of child-bearing age in any operations involving lead exposure in either the US or Canada unless they can prove they are sterile. James was one of seven women the company transferred to shift work; four of the others have filed a complaint of discrimination against GM with the Ontario Human Rights Commission. General Motors spokesman John Crellin said: ''The restrictions on women who might become pregnant are part of the overall programme to protect employees and their children from the harmful effects of lead.''

Feminists, many union activists, and occupational health specialists agree with GM about the necessity for protection of workers and their families; what they do not agree on is that exclusion of possibly fertile women provides that protection. The evidence that lead exposure is damaging to male reproductive capacity as well as women's reproductive system is quite persuasive—and not even new. A review prepared by researchers at the US National Institute for Occupational Safety and Health describes a 1914 study of pregnancy among wives of male house painters, many of whom suffered from lead colic; the stillbirth rate was much increased over that of the rest of the town. More recent research on male workers exposed to lead in a storage battery plant reveals significant alterations in sperm number, morphology and motility. More than 30 years ago, studies of lead-exposed rats of both sexes showed increased mortality, stunted growth, and sterility—in the second generation. In light of these data the NIOSH researchers ask ''must we now transfer male employees from high lead exposure areas, or require proof of their inability to reproduce as has previously been the public health approach for females?''

That approach is not likely to prove popular, since it would leave work with lead and other such toxic substances to be performed—as one commentator has remarked—by 60-year-old eunuchs. And exclusion of women only in the case of lead exposure is all the more remarkable when it is compared with the very similar problem of hazards in the operating room.

The ill effects of long-term exposure to low levels of anesthetic gases in operating theatres include both reproductive and non-reproductive morbidity and mortality. Increased rates of spontaneous abortion and congenital abnormalities among both male and female operating room personnel have been noted by several researchers. The reproductive risks may fall more heavily on women than men but there have been no calls for complete exclusion of women from the operating room.

Feminists explain these differing responses to similar cases by arguing that the operating room has historically been dependent upon the services of women, whereas jobs involving lead exposure are well paid and only recently have been opened to women, who are competing, in hard economic times, against men.

SAFETY ON THE CHEAP

The arguments thus often reduce to economic ones. On the face of it, engineering the workplace to be safe for everyone sounds sensible, but there are powerful forces working against this solution and reinforcing the idea of screening for genetic susceptibility as an alternative. There are arguments for instance about whether it is technically possible to cleanse an area entirely of a particular toxic substance. Monitoring and the institution of controls will almost certainly be more expensive than pre-employment screening to eliminate vulnerable workers. Employers understandably want their safety measures to cost as little as possible.

The idea that hypersusceptibility is responsible for a significant amount of occupation disease, however, is not supported by the evidence, according to a recent thorough and massive report to the Ford Foundation by Nicholas Ashford of the Center for Policy Alternatives at MIT. ''However, continuing adherence to this belief,'' he argues, ''prevents more progressive and innovative measures from being taken.''

On the other hand, there are some respected voices in medicine who argue, albeit regretfully, that attention to individual susceptibilities is the wave of the future as far as occupational health is concerned. Such a position was adopted a few months ago by Barton Childs, Chairman of the Committee for the Study of Inborn Errors of Metabolism of the National Research Council, National Academy of Sciences. Childs concludes that the chief usefulness of medical genetics is its growing ability to identify populations at risk, so that efforts at preventive medicine can be concentrated on those individuals most susceptible to disease.

It would be rational to exert more ''control over indiscriminate manipulation of the environment, partly by more rigorous testing of anything which is health related,'' he said, but as a practical matter, the more probable route will be ''an individual design for living based upon a comprehensive knowledge of the genotype and compensating for specific genetic deficiences.'' The latter is more likely to succeed because it is based on self-interest, whereas environmental improvement, however desirable, he noted wryly, ''requires a degree of public attention to the commonweal not notably evident in modern times.''

LEROY WALTERS

Ethical Perspectives on Maternal Serum Alpha-Fetoprotein Screening

In this essay, I shall discuss ethical issues involved in screening programs designed to detect prenatally two types of NTDs*: anencephaly and open spina bifida. The term "screening" serves as a reminder that we are considering a public health program and a public policy issue rather than simply patient-initiated transactions with providers of health care.

• • •

WHAT ARE THE MAJOR POTENTIAL BENEFITS AND RISKS OF MSAFP SCREENING?

In most of this section, I assume that adequate quality control will be an integral part of any proposed MSAFP screening program. At the end of the section, I shall return to the issue of quality control.

Assuming that a proposed MSAFP screening program will be efficiently administered by competent health professionals and will maintain excellent quality control in diagnostic laboratories, what benefits are to be expected from it? The major potential benefit cited by most advocates of MSAFP screening is a reduction in the incidence of NTDs among newborn infants. Estimates of the number of infants born in the United States each year with anencephaly or spina bifida vary from 5,000 to 8,000,[1] but general agreement exists that the number of such births would decrease as a result of a screening program.

One way of describing the potential benefit of MSAFP screening is in terms of cost-benefit analysis. Peter Layde and his associates at the Center for Disease Control in Atlanta have calculated that screening

From *Maternal Serum Alpha-Fetoprotein: Issues in the Prenatal Screening and Diagnosis of Neural Tube Defects,* Conference Proceedings, Barbara Gastel, *et al.,* eds. (Washington, D.C.: U.S. Government Printing Office, 1980), pp. 64, 66–71. Slightly revised by the author.

Ed. note: neural tube defects.

a theoretical cohort of 100,000 American pregnant women would cost just over $2,000,000. If 87% of anencephalic fetuses and 63% of spina-bifida fetuses were detected and aborted, the program would result in 128 abortions of affected fetuses and in savings to society of more than $4,000,000.[2] The net benefit of such a program would thus be approximately $2,000,000. Similarly favorable cost-benefit ratios have been obtained in two British analyses.[3]

Another way of characterizing the potential benefits is to speak of the suffering that families would be spared. For the family, the unexpected birth of an anencephalic infant is a tragedy. The unexpected birth of a child with open spina bifida will confront the family with either a stillbirth, a neonatal death, or a difficult decision about treatment or nontreatment. If treatment is elected and is successful, the family may need to defray substantial medical expense. Layde and associates estimate the cost of medical care for a child having spina bifida to be $16,807 during the first 20 years of life whereas the average cost of care for an unaffected child is approximately $2,400 in terms of 1977 dollars.[4]

The psychological effects on the family of raising a child with spina bifida also merit brief elaboration. In the late 1960s and early 1970s, Tew and Laurence conducted a survey of 59 Welsh families with a child having spina bifida and 59 matched control families without handicapped children. The divorce rate in the affected families was twice that in control families,[5] and sibling maladjustment in affected families occurred almost four times as often as in control families. The health of mothers in particular was often compromised as they "struggled on" rather than promptly seeking health care.[6] MSAFP screening would help to reduce these financial and psychological burdens.

In addition to the direct economic and familial benefits described above, an MSAFP screening program probably would have an indirect benefit: it would assist obstetricians in the early identification of special conditions of pregnancy. The early detection of twins is one obvious example. Recent studies also suggest that elevated MSAFP levels may be associated with slower-than-average fetal growth and a tendency toward spontaneous abortion or perinatal death.[7]

On the risk side of the ratio, probably the most feared and discussed risk is that of false positives. The magnitude of this risk depends markedly on the stage of the MSAFP screening program. At the initial serum screening stage, approximately 5 percent of women would have elevated values. Of these 5 percent, more than 95 percent are not, in fact, carrying fetuses afflicted with NTDs. Some psychological stress would inevitably accompany the abnormal test results.

At the stage of amniocentesis, false positives would entail both psychological and physical risks. On the average, only 7 percent of the pregnant women undergoing amniocentesis would, in fact, be carrying affected fetuses. In the remaining 93 percent, pregnant women and fetuses not afflicted with NTDs would be exposed to the risks of amniocentesis. Estimates of the potential hazards associated with amniocentesis vary significantly among the three major studies conducted in the United States, Canada, and Great Britain. After surveying the three studies, the British Working Group on Screening for Neural Tube Defects accepted the compromise figure of 2 percent excess fetal loss and infant morbidity as being attributable to amniocentesis.[8] The U.K. Collaborative Study has estimated the excess risk of fetal loss following amniocentesis at between 0.5% and 1.5%.[9]

The ultimate false-positive problem that may arise in MSAFP screening is that in rare cases unaffected fetuses may be mistakenly identified as affected and therefore aborted. In the U.K. Collaborative Study, 68 of 13,490 amniocenteses yielded false-positive results. In 8 of these cases, or 0.06% of the total amniocenteses, unaffected fetuses were aborted. The ratio of unaffected fetuses aborted to affected fetuses detected was 1:43.5.[10] In their cost-benefit analysis of a hypothetical MSAFP screening program, Layde and associates estimate that a program screening 100,000 women would result in the termination of 128 affected and 18 unaffected pregnancies; according to their model, the ratio of unaffected fetuses aborted to affected fetuses aborted would be approximately 1:7.[11]

A second major type of risk in MSAFP screening programs is that false negatives sometimes occur. That is, some pregnant women whose serum AFP values fall within the normal range are, in fact, carrying fetuses with open spina bifida or even anencephaly. In the U.K. Collaborative Study of over 19,000 pregnancies, the false-negative rate during the 16th to 18th gestational weeks was 12% to 16% for anencephaly and 12% to 30% for open spina bifida.[12] More recent results from a Glasgow series of 11,500 pregnancies attained false-negative rates of 0% for anencephaly and 19.8% for open spina bifida.[13]

It may be worth noting that false positives and false negatives constitute a tradeoff in AFP screening. Programs that set relatively low cutoff points for "normal" serum AFP values will have a higher detection rate for true positives (that is, affected fetuses), but at the price of also having a higher false positive rate. Conversely, programs that set relatively high cutoff points for elevated serum AFP values will have both a lower detection efficiency and a lower false-positive rate. Program planners' value judgments concerning the relative acceptability of false-positives and false negatives will significantly influence their choices of cutoff points.

Various commentators have mentioned, but not elaborated on, several other potential psychological risks of screening programs. These risks include the anxiety experienced by parents between the time of amniocentesis and the time when test results are received,[14] the potential effect of selective abortion on children already born into a family,[15] and a possible trend in the society at large toward intolerance of children and adults who have somehow managed to "slip through the screen."[16]

At the beginning of this section, I mentioned the assumption that MSAFP screening would be performed by competent professionals, supported by laboratories with rigorous standards of quality control. The assumption that a sufficient number of such persons and facilities exist for a large-scale screening program in the United States has been questioned by several groups, including representatives of the American College of Obstetricians and Gynecologists, the American Academy of Pediatrics, the American Society of Human Genetics, the Spina

Bifida Association of America, and the Public Citizen Health Research Group.[17] In part because of these publicly expressed reservations, the U.S. Food and Drug Administration is currently preparing proposed rules for the sale, distribution, and use of AFP test kits. The adequacy of the American health care system to provide AFP screening and of the FDA's rules to provide reasonable standards of quality for a large-scale screening program will significantly affect the risk-benefit ratio in any such program.

WHAT RESOURCE ALLOCATION QUESTIONS ARE RAISED BY MSAFP SCREENING PROGRAMS?

MSAFP screening will raise numerous allocation questions. Of them, I will select two for brief discussion. First, who should have access to local or regional screening programs? Second, what priority should be given to a possible national MSAFP screening program in comparison with other health-care needs?

The question of access to local or regional MSAFP screening programs is important because of the patchwork character of health-care financing. Differences among coverage and reimbursement policies are particularly pronounced for preventive health services.

The problem of access to MSAFP screening becomes especially critical at two points: the point of entry into the program and the point where follow-up services may be required. Some pregnant women may be deterred from enrolling in local or regional MSAFP screening programs because of the cost of the initial serum screen. Others may have no difficulty in paying the $12 cost of the initial serum screen or even the additional $27 cost of a repeat screen. They could, however, find the payment of $50 for an ultrasound scan or $62 for amniocentesis a formidable barrier to continued participation in a screening program.

This barrier is formidable because private and public health insurance programs are so unpredictable in their coverage of, and reimbursement for, prenatal diagnostic services, genetic counseling, and selective abortion. The Pregnancy Discrimination Act (Public Law 95-555), enacted in October, 1978, has had a significant impact on private health insurers which, prior to that time, frequently did not cover such pregnancy-related services as amniocentesis. How-

ever, levels of reimbursement for pregnancy-related services vary markedly from plan to plan.[18] Medicaid coverage policies also vary from state to state. There is no legal barrier to the provision of prenatal diagnostic services by the states, but specific information about the coverage and reimbursement of such services is unavailable from the Health Care Financing Administration. Medicaid coverage of abortion has been a highly controversial public issue. Under the terms of the Hyde Amendment, which the U.S. Supreme Court recently upheld as constitutional, no Federal funds may be provided to the states for abortion following a positive prenatal diagnosis. However, nine states and the District of Columbia use their own funds to cover abortion on request, and an additional eleven states are under court order to provide medically necessary abortions.[19]

In light of these differences in coverage, prudence would dictate that every local or regional MSAFP screening program formulate in advance a policy concerning access. Justice—or at least beneficence—would seem to require that every pregnant woman who desires such testing be provided access to serum screening and to necessary follow-up services without regard to her ability to pay or the comprehensiveness of her health insurance coverage. To put the matter bluntly, a woman who is told that her serum AFP value is elevated but who cannot afford genetic counseling, ultrasound, or amniocentesis is probably worse off than a woman who has not been screened at all.

To their credit, the existing MSAFP screening programs in Long Island, N.Y., and Maine and the proposed program in Baltimore County have given careful consideration to access. In Maine, the Foundation for Blood Research provides both the initial serum screen and necessary follow-up services gratis to pregnant women who are not covered by health insurance and are unable to pay.[20] The planners of the screening program in Baltimore County have contacted third-party payers in an effort to secure a commitment by the insurers to cover necessary prenatal diagnostic services.[21]

The second resource allocation question is perhaps the most difficult of all: What priority should be given to a possible MSAFP screening program in comparison with other health-care needs? In the past, we have sometimes assumed that we as a society could provide comprehensive, high-quality health care for all. However, the gradually increasing fraction of the gross national product going to the health-care sector is a constant reminder that some limits must be set. According to one projection from the Health Care Financing Administration, it is conceivable that the annual health-care budget, both public and private, will grow from the 1978 figure of $192.4 billion to $757.9 billion in 1990.[22]

The dollar cost of a national MSAFP screening program would be significant. The British Working Group on Screening for Neural Tube Defects estimated that the establishment of a national screening program for 450,000 pregnancies per year in Great Britain would cost an initial 1,707,800 pounds in capital expenditures and an additional 2,235,100 pounds in operating expenditures per year at November, 1978, prices.[23] Translated into dollars, these figures are $4,087,619 for capital investment and $5,349,712 for annual operating expenses. If costs are proportionate in the United States, which has five times as many births per year, the cost of a national screening program here might be $20,438,095 in initial capital expenditures and $26,748,560 in annual operating expenditures. Layde and his associates estimate that the cost of screening 100,000 women would be $2,047,780.[24] Extrapolated to a national program in which 75% of American pregnant women participate, that estimate would yield an annual cost, including capital and administrative expenditures, of $46,075,050 for screening 2,250,000 pregnancies.

These cost figures are virtually meaningless unless related to the potential risks and benefits of a national MSAFP screening program and to other possible investments in the health-care arena. For example, what priority should this type of national screening program have relative to a national hypertension screening program or a significant new program of research into the causes of NTDs? These are some of the difficult, almost intractable, allocation decisions that must be made in the next several years.

WHAT ISSUES OF FREEDOM AND COERCION DO MSAFP SCREENING PROGRAMS RAISE?

The most obvious question of freedom and coercion raised by MSAFP screening is the following: From an ethical standpoint, should future MSAFP screening programs be voluntary or mandatory? In one sense, the answer to this question is simple. The U.K. Collaborative Study and the few pilot studies in the United States have been totally voluntary. To my knowledge, no one has proposed that MSAFP screening be mandatory. In fact, the most extensive study of public policy on screening for NTDs, the British Working Group report, clearly endorses the view that MSAFP screening programs should be voluntary.[25]

However, some commentators on the ethics of genetic screening have *in general* advocated the adoption of mandatory programs for the prevention of birth defects. Ethicist Joseph Fletcher is perhaps the most unabashed spokesperson for the mandatory option. In his book, *Humanhood,* Fletcher writes:

What means of control would be appropriate to various diseases? How shall we carry out a policy of mutual coercion mutually agreed upon? For example, mandatory screening, if we still leave it up to parents to choose whether to continue an affected pregnancy up to term, would not satisfy the ethical imperative. Would criteria for issuing or refusing marriage licenses do it? Would we have to have mandatory practices such as sterilization, contraception, and abortion, to back up our minimum standards?[26]

Even if our society refuses to adopt Joseph Fletcher's proposed mandatory screening programs —or his radical suggestion about measures within them—more subtle questions of freedom and coercion may nonetheless arise, even in voluntary MSAFP screening programs. For example, a health care system that provides ample coverage for prenatal diagnostic services and induced abortion but only minimal coverage of the services required by handicapped children could strongly influence the decisions of couples about selective abortion.

A final question of freedom and coercion concerns informed consent in MSAFP screening programs. In speaking of informed consent, I am referring not to a signed document but rather to an ongoing process of communication, comprehension, and autonomous decision-making. The information to be conveyed in MSAFP screening programs is complex. In how many other public health programs are potential screenees presented with a series of five probabilities for the multiple stages of the screening process? Several excellent models of informational documents and counseling procedures have already been developed, both in Great Britain and the United States.[27] One hopes that these models will be widely adopted and further refined as MSAFP screening becomes more widely diffused. Indeed, it can be argued that a significant component in the quality of MSAFP screening programs is the quality of the consent process within those programs.

In summary, three of the major ethical issues in MSAFP screening are the potential risks and benefits of screening, the allocation of scarce resources, and freedom and coercion in screening. These issues bear a striking resemblance to three much-discussed principles in contemporary moral philosophy—beneficence, justice, and autonomy.

NOTES

1. Milunsky, A. Prenatal detection of neural tube defects: False positive and negative results. *Pediatrics* 1977; 59:782. Layde, P., Allmen, S., and Oakley, G. P., Jr. Maternal serum alpha-fetoprotein screening: a cost-benefit analysis. *Am. J. Public Health* 1979; 69:567.

2. Layde *et al*. Maternal serum alpha-fetoprotein screening:570. These figures are expressed in 1977 dollars.

3. Hagard, S., *et al*. Screening for spina bifida cystica: a cost-benefit analysis. *Br. J. Prev. Soc. Med*. 1976; 30:40–53. Glass, N. J., and Cove, A. R. Cost effectiveness of screening for neural tube defects. In: Scrimgeour, J. B., ed. *Towards the prevention of fetal malformation*. Edinburgh: Edinburgh University Press, 1978: 217–223.

4. Layde *et al*. Maternal serum alpha-fetoprotein screening:571.

5. Tew, B. J., *et al*. Must a family with a handicapped child be a handicapped family? *Dev. Med. Child Neurol*. 1974; 16(6, Supplement No. 32):96–97.

6. Tew, B., and Laurence, K. M. Mothers, brothers and sisters of patients with spina bifida. *Dev. Med. Child Neurol*. 1973; 15(6, Supplement No. 29):72–74.

7. Brock, D. J. H., *et al*. Significance of elevated mid-trimester maternal plasma-alpha-fetoprotein values. *Lancet* 1979; 1:1281–1282.

8. Working Group on Screening for Neural Tube Defects. Report. London: Department of Health and Social Security, July 1979:27.

9. Wald, N. J., *et al*. Amniotic-fluid alpha-fetoprotein measurement in antenatal diagnosis of anencephaly and open spina bifida in early pregnancy. *Lancet* 1979; 2:656.

10. *Ibid.*: 651, 660.

11. Layde *et al*. Maternal serum alpha-fetoprotein screening:570.

12. Wald, N. J., *et al*. Maternal serum-alpha-fetoprotein measurement in antenatal screening for anencephaly and spina bifida in early pregnancy. *Lancet* 1977; 1:1327.

13. Ferguson-Smith, M. A., *et al*. Avoidance of anencephalic and spina bifida births by maternal serum alpha-fetoprotein screening. *Lancet* 1978; 1:1330.

14. Blumberg, B. D., *et al*. The psychological sequelae of abortion performed for a genetic indication, *Am. J. Obstet. Gynecol*. 1975; 122:799–808.

15. Meyerowitz, S., and Lipkin, M., Jr. Psychosocial aspects. In: Brent, R. L., and Harris, M. I., eds. Prevention of embryonic, fetal, and perinatal disease. DHEW Publication No. (NIH) 76–853 (Washington, D.C.: U.S. Government Printing Office, 1976):281.

16. Callahan, D. The meaning and significance of genetic disease: philosophical perspectives. In: Hilton, B., *et al.,* eds. *Ethical issues in human genetics*. New York: Plenum Press, 1973:86–87.

17. Dickson, D. Alpha-fetoprotein screening: too hot to handle? *Nature* 1979; 280:6–7.

18. U.S. Statutes, Vol. 92, p. 2076. Muller, C. F. Insurance coverage of abortion, contraception, and sterilization. *Fam. Plann. Perspect*. March/April 1978; 10(2):72.

19. Public funding for abortions now in legislative arena. Planned Parenthood-World Population Washington Memo. July 18, 1980:3.

20. Personal communication from Edward M. Kloza, Foundation for Blood Research, Scarborough, Maine.

21. Personal communication from Neil Anton Holtzman, Department of Pediatrics, Johns Hopkins University Medical School.

22. Freelander, M., *et al*. Projections of national health expenditures, 1980, 1985, and 1990. *Health Care Financing Review* 1980; 1:2.

23. Working Group. Report:55.

24. Layde *et al*. Maternal serum alpha-fetoprotein screening:568.

25. Working Group. Report:61.

26. Fletcher, J. Our duty to the unborn. In: Fletcher J. Humanhood:111.

27. Working Group. Report: 37–38. Informational pamphlet in: Haddow, J. E. Informed consent and patient education about neural tube defects. In: Haddow, J. E., and Macri, J. N., eds. Screening for neural tube defects in the United States (Proceedings of the First Scarborough Conference, Scarborough, Maine, September 6–8, 1977). Portland, ME: Pilot Press, 1977:26.

RUTH R. FADEN

Public Policy Implications of Prenatal Diagnosis

It is generally agreed that prenatal diagnosis represents a significant technological advance which at the same time poses dilemmatic questions for public policy. Some policy questions are, of course, not unique to prenatal diagnosis: Questions of whether and to what extent prenatal diagnosis ought to receive public funds and of who ought to have access to the procedure are typical examples. Most important technological advances pose such problems for systems of allocation, as well as problems in the determination of efficacy, safety and overall public benefit. Whether the technology be therapeutic, as in the case of coronary by-pass procedures and heart transplantation, diagnostic, as in the case of positron emission transaxial tomography, or preventive, as in the case of screening for various genetic defects, formidable barriers stand in the way of any attempt to assess and evaluate the ethical, or even the social and economic impacts, of new advances. In the wake of these barriers, public and scientific controversy ensues.

Despite this shared background of controversy, it can be argued that prenatal diagnosis has generated even more controversy and heated public debate than is normally encountered through a technological advance in health care. The purpose of this essay is to catalogue some of the reasons why this unusual degree of controversy has emerged and to evaluate some of the positions that have been expressed on major issues. My thesis is that at least some of the controversy concerning prenatal diagnosis stems from the failure to have straightforwardly addressed the most basic of all moral questions concerning prenatal diag-

nosis: Ought we to accept the eradication of birth defects as a goal of our public policies?

Perhaps one reason why this question has been overlooked is that, at least in its milder form, the answer is obvious to many persons. It could be said that we are living in the (second) Era of Prevention in health policy. As many commentators have noted, we are rapidly recognizing that there are limits to the way therapeutic technologies can be employed to improve morbidity and mortality statistics. Increasingly, we are looking to preventive interventions to repeat the successes of earlier periods in the public health movement: preventing heart disease is a good thing; preventing smallpox is a good thing; preventing tooth decay is a good thing; and, many now say, preventing *birth defects* is a good thing. But does the latter "defect" really belong in the same category with these other diseases?

Let us examine at least two premises almost certainly found in any argument that preventing birth defects is a good thing. The first premise is "Birth defects are not desirable and are not in fact desired by parents." It follows that, all other things being equal, it is preferable not to have birth defects than to have them; and, all other things being equal, parents would prefer not to have children born with defects than to have children born defective. I take it that this first premise is unobjectionable. However, consider further the second premise: "The prevention of birth defects is desirable." This premise holds that, all other things being equal, it is more desirable to reduce the prevalence of birth defects in a community (and in this sense to *prevent* birth defects) than to permit the existing prevalence rates to continue unabated. Until recently, this premise has generally been considered as uncontroversial as the first premise. At the level of health policy, we have had for many years varied national programs devised to prevent birth defects (in the above sense of "prevent"). Consider, for example, efforts to control exposure to teratogens and

This paper is published here for the first time. ©1981 Ruth R. Faden. It is based on two presentations made at the 1980 meetings of the Society for Health and Human Values and a National Center for Health Care Technology and the Food and Drug Administration conference on maternal serum alpha-fetoprotein: *Maternal Serum Alpha-Fetoprotein: Issues in the Prenatal Screening and Diagnosis of Nueral Tube Defects,* Conference Proceedings, Barbara Gastel *et al.,* eds. (Washington, D.C.: Government Printing Office, 1980).

mutagens in the workplace and in medical care; programs to improve the nutritional status of pregnant women; mass use of silver nitrate drops in newborns to prevent blindness; and, finally, large-scale funding of basic biomedical research into the causes of numerous birth defects.

Yet prenatal diagnosis is *morally* different from most of these other programs. In most programs, it has been possible to prevent birth defects without preventing the birth of those who have these defects. This generalization holds, of course, even more clearly for prevention programs outside the birth defect area. Programs to prevent heart disease, for example, do not generally entail preventing the birth of people with this condition. But in prenatal diagnosis situations, it is commonly necessary to prevent the person who has it from existing in order to prevent the disease. There is as yet no alternative. This reality has created a psychological trap for many participants in this controversy—particularly, I would argue, for those who are advocates or parents of the handicapped. To argue for a program to prevent the birth of people with defects seems to some to require taking the position that life as a handicapped person is not worth living, or at least is worth considerably less than other lives. This is patently not the case. It is morally and conceptually possible to hold the positions that (1) many people with birth defects lead productive, worthwhile, and meaningful lives and at the same time that (2) I am grateful not to be one of them and grateful that my child is not one of them. To advocate a program with the primary or secondary goal of preventing birth defects is not in any way to diminish the human worth—the value that ought properly to be placed—on those who suffer the defect. I realize of course that substantial issues in moral philosophy about the nature and grounds of respect for persons surround this claim, but on most influential theories of personhood and respect this generalization can be supported.

This brings me to the central problem contributing to the controversy over prenatal diagnosis. It has been my thesis that, at least as a matter of public health policy, the prevention of birth defects has been considered a relatively noncontroversial issue, *all other things being equal*. However, the reliance on abortion to effect ''prevention'' has seemed to many the ''something'' that has made all other things unequal. So long as it is not possible to prevent certain birth

defects without aborting human fetuses, a program of prenatal diagnosis with the goal of primary prevention will be viewed by many as morally wrong. Because such a significant proportion of the American public holds abortion to be immoral, and because of the deeply held value placed on autonomy in reproductive choices, a program of *compulsory* prenatal diagnosis is currently unthinkable as a public policy option. Also unthinkable is the other extreme—a public policy *prohibiting* prenatal diagnosis. Respect for autonomy and the significant public interest in cost control clearly weigh against any form of prohibition. However, between these two extremes of compulsion are a host of public policy questions yet to be resolved.

The most obvious paradox in our implicit current public policy on birth defects is that while there is public support for prenatal diagnosis research and services, a regulation also prohibits the allocation of federal funds for abortion. One dimension of this paradox is the issue whether we ought as a matter of public policy to promote the use of prenatal diagnosis as part of a program generally leading to the abortion of defective fetuses. Much has been made of cost containment, for example, the figure that up to 400 million dollars could be saved each year through a single prenatal diagnosis program—the screening of all pregnant women over the age of 35.[1] However, this figure of 400 million dollars assumes that in every instance where a defective fetus is identified, the pregnancy will be terminated by abortion. Clearly, the cost-benefit balance of prenatal diagnosis—the primary factor in whether to allocate public funds to prenatal diagnosis—depends critically on the willingness of prospective parents to abort defective fetuses. We have already established that a policy of compulsory abortion is out of the question on grounds of respect for autonomy, but given the compelling public interest in aborting the birth of severely defective persons would it not be appropriate, indeed is it not essential to a sound public policy, to encourage women to abort defective fetuses?

In attempting to answer this question, I shall make the following assumption: There is nothing inherently objectionable about persuasion as a form of social influence. Generally speaking, persuasive communications and public health-education programs are thought to be the least objectionable forms of government intervention—that is, least objectionable from the perspective of the principle of autonomy. Further, it could be argued that many prospective parents are altogether unaware of prenatal diagnosis. Indeed there is evidence that only well-educated persons have adequate access to prenatal diagnosis. Also, it is possible that many who maintain that they would want to raise a defective child have made this choice in ignorance. They have not had an accurate understanding of the consequences involved—of what it would be like to parent and care for an afflicted person; therefore, an educational campaign to promote prenatal diagnosis and the abortion of defective fetuses, if properly conducted, would result in a broadening rather than a narrowing of autonomous reproductive choices.

A country with a policy to limit population growth would be perfectly consistent and, many would agree, politically and morally responsible in mounting a health education campaign to promote the use of contraception. If a country with a policy to prevent disability through the prevention of birth defects mounted a campaign to promote the use of prenatal diagnosis and selective abortion, it too would be acting consistently. However, in this case, many would dispute the morality of the health education program.

What this simple comparison suggests is that there may not be anything inherently objectionable about government attempts to influence reproductive choices. Instead, the issue in this comparison is again abortion or, more specifically, the moral probity of government efforts to encourage abortion in a pluralistic society which is badly divided on the issue. However, from the perspective of public policy, there may be a relevant difference between abortion of healthy fetuses and abortion of at least severely defective fetuses. Generally speaking, the state's interests in the birth of a normal fetus are not impressive when compared with the interests of the fetus and the mother or parents. Because of the controversy and the uncertain public interest, it may be appropriate for the state to remove itself as completely as possible from the issue. However, in the case of a severely defective fetus, the state has a strong positive interest in the child's not being born, and this factor suggests the justification for some state involvement.

I want to make a sharp distinction here between a program to compel prenatal diagnosis and the abortion of defective fetuses and one limited to encouraging these practices. If we leave aside moral issues for a minute, we can all agree that—whatever the public interest arguments are—they could not be compelling enough to override the certain political opposition to any compulsory program. I am, in fact, very skeptical about the political feasibility of even a health education campaign in this area. At present, we are operating under a more or less explicit government policy which prohibits the use of federal funds for any program which can be construed as promoting abortion. Thus, any educational campaign of the sort I am describing would, at present, be an unlikely candidate for federal funding. There are, admittedly, very disturbing moral questions raised by such a health education program—questions of the kind of persuasive appeals to be used and the choice of the defects to be the targets of the appeals. Also, it is likely that those who oppose abortion on moral grounds would find a government program intended to promote the use of prenatal diagnosis and selective abortion more objectionable than a program to fund abortions for those mothers who have, without government influence, chosen the procedure; but this is an issue which has not yet been discussed.

This brings me to one final point about the goal or the proper goals for a national policy on birth defects. If we are to become serious about preventing birth defects through prenatal diagnosis, then we have to address the issue of the proper purposes of prenatal diagnosis. There is already substantial controversy concerning the use of prenatal diagnosis to identify desired physical traits, such as sex. Less examined is the issue of whether we ought, as a matter of public policy, attempt to apply prenatal diagnosis to the identification of any physical defect, no matter how benign. For example, should we work toward a technology for identifying diabetes through prenatal diagnosis? Is the public goal of eradicating diabetes relevantly similar to the goal of eradicating Down's syndrome or anencephaly? For that matter, is the public goal of eradicating Down's syndrome comparable to the goal of eradicating smallpox? Is it to be greeted with uncritical enthusiasm and uniform international support? These questions concerning the severity and nature of the afflictions to be prevented must be directly confronted before a morally satisfactory and stable public health policy on the prevention of birth defects can be said to be in place.

My own position on these questions is as yet only primitively formed, although I am inclined to the view that the eradication of birth defects is a morally laudable goal, provided that proper commitment to a societal obligation to fully respect and assist handicapped persons who do exist can be maintained.[2]

However, I am not unmindful of arguments that the presence of people with handicaps has a salutary effect on the moral fabric of the wider community, arguments that the handicapped serve to foster such virtues as compassion, inspiration, courage and humility. Before we can agree on the moral probity of any technology with the primary or secondary goal of preventing the birth of handicapped persons, its significance for these and other virtues will have to be weighed against the suffering and costs to be avoided, as well as against the preferences of future parents and society.

NOTES

1. See Amitai Etzioni, "Public Policy Issues Raised by a Medical Breakthrough," *Policy Analysis,* 1(1):69–76, Winter 1975. The figures Etzioni and others cite are based on the work of Aubrey Milunsky, *The Prenatal Diagnosis of Hereditary Disorders,* Charles C Thomas, 1973.

2. I believe it is reasonable to fear that programs to prevent the birth of people with birth defects will have a negative effect on society's treatment of those who are actually born with such handicaps. This is a plausible negative consequence of programs to prevent birth defects, but it is itself a preventable consequence. So long as efforts to reform social attitudes toward, and the life opportunities offered to, the handicapped continue apace with programs to reduce the prevalence of birth defects, it should be possible to avoid harming those handicapped persons who survive. I note without further comment the following editorial: "Two other theoretical problems are presented by selective abortion. Its widespread use might reduce the tolerance shown by society to living defectives. A child with hemophilia or muscular dystrophy living in a society in which most of his potential fellow-sufferers had been destroyed prenatally might be seen by the community as one unfit to be alive. It could also be argued that the ethical justifications for destroying a defective fetus might apply just as well to destruction of the newborn defective child. Could we be at the top of a slippery slope?" Editorial, *British Medical Journal* 4:676, December 21, 1974.

HAROLD P. GREEN AND ALEXANDER M. CAPRON

Issues of Public Policy in Compulsory Genetic Screening

Different questions [than those in voluntary programs] are raised by mandatory genetic screening programs pursuant to statutes prescribing the testing of everyone, or of specific classes of individuals, with penalties or deprivation of benefits for those who refuse to submit to screening. For example, most states presently require screening of newborn infants for phenylketonuria (PKU), an inborn error of metabolism which usually causes mental retardation if not treated early in life. At present some states and the District of Columbia require screening for sickle cell anemia and sickle cell trait for all school children and attempts will doubtless be made before long to go beyond sickle cell disease and require screening for certain genetic conditions and carrier states as a prerequisite to obtaining a marriage license.

Questions have been raised as to whether such genetic screening programs may be unlawful on constitutional grounds, a matter which has never been decided by the courts. Two separate issues are thus presented: (1) whether the legislature has the power to enact compulsory screening measures, and (2) whether, if the power exists, its exercise violates any constitutional prohibitions.

THE POWER TO PROMOTE PUBLIC HEALTH THROUGH GENETIC SCREENING

POWER OF THE FEDERAL GOVERNMENT

The powers exercisable by the federal government are limited to those enumerated in the Constitution,[1] which does not give Congress any express power to

From Green, H. P., and Capron, A. M.: Issues of Law and Public Policy in Genetic Screening. In Bergsma, D. (ed.): "Ethical, Social and Legal Dimensions of Screening for Human Genetic Disease." Miami, Florida: Symposium Specialists for the National Foundation–March of Dimes, *Birth Defects: Original Article Series* 10(6): 57–84, 1974.

legislate with respect to the public health and welfare. Congress does, however, have the power to enact legislation dealing with the public health as an incident to its explicit powers, for example, to regulate commerce or to provide for national defense. It is likely that a mandatory genetic screening statute enacted by Congress would be found by the courts to come within the greatly expanded scope of federal authority (primarily under the commerce clause) that has been recognized in the last few decades. This is probably only a hypothetic possibility, since Congress has not been disposed to enact legislation of this kind which would impinge upon an area that traditionally has been regarded as within the power of the states. Congress does, nevertheless, have direct power to enact health legislation to certain limited areas which are within the scope of its authority, such as the District of Columbia, federal employment or the armed services.

POWER OF THE STATES

Under the Constitution of the United States, exercise of police power (i.e., the power to take action to protect and promote the health, welfare and safety of the public) rests in the first instance with the states. "The range of state power is not defined and delimited by an enumeration of legislative subject-matter"[2] in the United States Constitution. Rather, the scope of the police power of any state is defined and limited by the state's own constitution. Since there is great variation in state constitutions, no useful purpose would be served by attempting to analyze them here in order to determine whether genetic screening would be encompassed by the police power of particular states. This would be a matter for decision by the legislators, and if necessary the judges, of each state.

RELATIONSHIP TO A VALID GOVERNMENTAL PURPOSE

This is not to say that the Constitution of the United States has no bearing on whether a public health measure promulgated by a state (or by federal authorities regarding the District of Columbia) is a valid exercise of the police power. The government may prescribe reasonable regulations in order to protect or promote the health, safety, morals and welfare of the community,[3] but under the Fifth and Fourteenth Amendments to the Constitution any such regulations must be reasonably related to a legitimate state purpose.[4] The threshold question, then, is whether compulsory genetic screening programs would be open to challenge for failing to foster a permissible end that may be sought by the government.

Like the numerous public health measures on the books in every state, a genetic screening program might be expected to serve a number of purposes, including: (1) the provision of information about the incidence and severity of the disease; (2) the protection of members of the public from disease; and (3) the conservation of health resources through the prevention and appropriate treatment of disease. As long as plausible justifications for screening such as these can be found, it is unlikely that the judiciary would seriously entertain a challenge to a screening program on the ground that it lacked efficacy in promoting legitimate state purposes.

•   •   •

CONSTITUTIONAL LIMITATIONS ON GOVERNMENT ACTION

Putting aside the question of governmental power, then, the validity of a compulsory genetic screening program will depend primarily on whether it impinges impermissibly upon individual rights protected by the United States Constitution. In recent years, the courts have elaborated a number of areas in which they apply special scrutiny to the actions of the legislative and executive branches. While judges no longer use the due process clause to strike down economic legislation which they believe to be unwise or unnecessary, other kinds of state action that encroach on personal liberty—especially on so-called fundamental rights—are increasingly found to run afoul of the Constitution. Moreover, neither state nor federal authorities may deny citizens the "equal protection of the laws." Both of these constitutional limitations are relevant in analyzing compulsory genetic screening programs.

DUE PROCESS AND FUNDAMENTAL RIGHTS

In recent years the Supreme Court has identified certain rights as "fundamental" ones, interference with which requires greater justification. Although not all constitutionally guaranteed rights are regarded as fundamental, some of the fundamental rights are those specifically protected by the Constitution, such as freedom of religion and of speech. In other cases, the Court has found fundamental rights not explicitly mentioned in the Constitution, such as the right of privacy,[5] which has recently been held to include the right to make certain decisions about health care free of certain restrictions.[6] A law which restricts those liberties that are "so rooted in the traditions and conscience of our people as to be ranked as fundamental,"[7] is subject to specially rigorous examination as to whether it violates the due process clause. Legislation impinging on such a right must be supported by a heavy burden of justification going far beyond the usual "rational basis" test. The state must show at least that the governmental objective or classification is supported by a compelling interest and that no alternative means, with lesser impingement on these rights, are available for accomplishment of that objective. Indeed, in some cases, the Supreme Court has held that certain activities, within the scope of the fundamental rights, are totally beyond the power of government to regulate.[8]

Among the fundamental rights there are two groups associated with the constitutional right of privacy which have particular relevance to genetic screening: those rights relating to marriage and procreation and those concerning a person's control of his or her own body.

For some time the Supreme Court has given explicit recognition to the rights which protect decisions about one's family.[9] Marriage itself has been termed "fundamental to our very existence and survival"[10] and "one of the basic civil rights of man."[11] Free decision making about procreation is also recognized as a fundamental right.[12] Indeed, it was in the context of state regulation of procreation that the "right of privacy" received forceful articulation in the landmark case of *Griswold v. Connecticut*.[13] In that case, the Supreme Court held unconstitutional a statute making the use of, or assistance in the use of, contraceptives a crime. In reaching this conclusion, the Court found a fundamental "right of privacy older than the Bill of Rights,"[14] and though not mentioned therein still established by the "penumbras" surrounding the First, Fourth, Fifth, Sixth, and Ninth Amendments to the Constitution. The Court held that the marital relationship falls within a constitutionally protected zone of privacy and that the law prohibiting *use* of contraceptives has a "maximum destructive impact"[15] on that relationship. Yet it must be remembered that the decision did not go so far as to declare that married couples have an absolute right to use contraceptives, since the Court suggested that a

statute prohibiting manufacture or sale of contraceptives might be constitutional.

The constitutionally protected zone of privacy was extended in *Eisenstadt v. Baird*[16] to decisions about childbearing by unmarried as well as married persons. Baird had been convicted under a Massachusetts statute prohibiting the distribution of contraceptives to unmarried persons, and the Court affirmed a discharge of his conviction on the ground that there was no rational basis for the separate classification of unmarried persons. In so doing, the Court made clear the fundamental nature of the right at issue: "If the right of privacy means anything, it is the right of the *individual*, married or single, to be free from unwarranted governmental intrusion into matters so fundamentally affecting a person as the decision whether to bear or beget a child."[17]

In *Roe v. Wade*[18] the zone of privacy was found to be "broad enough to encompass a woman's decision whether or not to terminate her pregnancy."[19] The Supreme Court ruled, however, that the right to choose an abortion is not unqualified and must be weighed against the state's interests in protecting the health of pregnant women and in safeguarding potential life. "These interests are separate and distinct. Each grows in substantiality as the woman approaches term and, at a point during pregnancy, each becomes 'compelling'."[20] Since abortion during the first trimester is safer for a woman than continuing her pregnancy to term, the Court held that the decision to abort during this period lies with the woman and her physician, "free of interference by the State."[21] During the second trimester the qualifications of persons performing abortions, the places where they are performed, and so forth, may be regulated to promote the safety of the procedure. During the final trimester, once the fetus is "viable," the state "may, if it chooses, regulate, and even proscribe, abortion except where it is necessary, in appropriate medical judgment, for the preservation of the life or health of the mother."[22]

A number of the major purposes which the state might have in mandating genetic screening, such as preventing disease and saving state resources, are obviously based on the expected connection between screening results and decisions about marriage and procreation. In light of the cases, the question must be confronted whether it is permissible for the state to compel genetic screening for these purposes. This is a problem which has not yet been resolved by the courts. If screening were linked by statute with restrictions on marriage and procreation (e.g., mandatory abortion) or were conducted in such a way as to coerce screenees' decisions on these matters, it would probably be found invalid under the *Griswold* line of cases. It is likely, however, that any restrictions placed on marriage and procreation that would result from genetic screening would be only indirect—that is, the result of choices made by individuals in consequence of the information about themselves brought to their attention by the state. Screening results presented in a noncoercive fashion would probably be comparable to such permissible state activities as sex education classes. Moreover, some restrictions on marriage are permissible; for example, most states already prohibit marriage between persons of a stated degree of relationship. To the extent that such legislation can be justified on genetic grounds, it has yet to be judged in light of post-*Griswold* jurisprudence on marriage-related decisions. This also raises the issue of whether, and how, the state may infringe on one person's liberty to protect another person or the community in general.

One is thus brought to the second aspect of "privacy" which may be relevant to compulsory genetic screening—control over one's own body. As was already suggested, this issue was raised in *Roe,* but in a slightly different context. There the question was whether the state could limit potentially risky but voluntary activities, while in genetic screening the question is whether the individual can limit the state's interference with his or her body by asserting, as Justice Brandeis once wrote, a "right to be let alone—the most comprehensive of rights and the right most valued by civilized men."[23] The Supreme Court did not have to decide that issue in *Roe,* and the Justices felt that it was "not clear" whether the absolute right claimed by some "to do with one's body as one pleases bears a close relationship to the right of privacy."[24] Mr. Justice Blackmun cited two cases to illustrate that the Supreme Court has not found such an absolute right.

The first was *Jacobson v. Massachusetts,*[25] which upheld the conviction of a man who had refused to submit to compulsory smallpox vaccination during an epidemic in Cambridge. He offered to prove that he had been made seriously ill when vaccinated as a child and that there was no way to determine "with any degree of certainty"[26] whether one's blood was in such a condition as to render vaccination danger-

ous. This evidence was excluded by the trial court as immaterial, and the Supreme Court affirmed on the ground that the offers of proof invited the court improperly "to go over the whole ground gone over by the legislature when it enacted the statute in question."[27] *Jacobson* would thus seem neither to condemn nor to sanction legislation mandating genetic screening. On the one hand, it appears that the immediate physical risks of the procedure to the screenee would be so slight as not to justify interfering with the legislative judgment. On the other hand, the state's interest in seeing that screening is done seems much less compelling than in the stemming of an epidemic. While the interference with the person is small, it may be resisted if no interference at all is justified, as Justice Harlan stated in *Jacobson:*

There is . . . a sphere within which the individual may assert the supremacy of his own will and rightfully dispute the authority of any human government, especially of any free government existing under a written constitution, to interfere with the exercise of that will. But it is equally true that in every well-ordered society charged with the duty of conserving the safety of its members the rights of the individual in respect of his liberty may at times, under the pressure of great dangers, be subjected to such restraint, to be enforced by reasonable regulations, as the safety of the general public may demand.[28]

Jacobson thus speaks in terms of protecting others from "great dangers," an apt description of the consequences of many genetic diseases. This concern for the health of future generations is a legitimate one which is also exemplified in the laws restricting marriage to those who have passed an examination for venereal disease.[29] Yet it must be read in the context of the more recent cases such as *Griswold* and *Roe* that exhibit a greater concern for privacy and bodily integrity.

Although the interference sanctioned in *Jacobson* not only served a pressing public need but involved a minimal intrusion, a much greater invasion of privacy—and interference with the right to procreate—was upheld in *Buck v. Bell,*[30] the second case cited by Mr. Justice Blackmun in *Roe.* At issue in *Buck* was a Virginia statute authorizing the sterilization of institutionalized "feeble-minded" persons. The Supreme Court upheld the law against a due process challenge, stating that it would be better if society, rather than having to wait for the misdeeds or destitution of feeble-minded persons' feeble-minded offspring, could instead "prevent those who are manifestly unfit from continuing their kind."[31]

In the nearly 50 years since *Buck* was decided there have been great changes in geneticists' confidence in making sweeping characterizations of "manifest unfitness." Indeed, the increased sophistication of genetics and its ability to identify the inheritance of many more disorders makes the medical model underlying the compulsory sterilization of "imbeciles" seem terrifyingly naive. It is doubtful that any court would accept compulsory sterilization for any of a host of genetic diseases for which carrier screening is now possible—many of them far worse conditions than feeble-mindedness—simply on the authority of *Buck v. Bell.*

. . .

Buck, like *Roe,* thus lends some support to genetic screening intended to protect the screenee's own health or welfare—as where, for example, screening could reveal a late-onset disease which could be prevented or ameliorated through early detection and treatment. It is well to keep in mind, however, the factual background of these cases: in *Buck* the alternative to sterilization was a lifetime in the "State Colony for Epileptics and Feeble Minded" with the constant risk of repeated unwanted pregnancies, and in *Roe* the Court spoke approvingly of the state's interest in safeguarding life and health not in terms of state action to promote better health but only to keep people from engaging in life-threatening conduct (unsafe, nonmedical abortions). Unless the genetic disorder were severe and the means were at hand to prevent its manifestation, compulsory screening would not be justified under this branch of the reasoning in Buck.

The second reason for the *Buck* decision flows from the first: Carrie Buck's sterilization and release were predicted to save the state money, both for her maintenance and for that of any offspring in need of institutional care. *Buck* would thus appear to validate screening designed to reduce health expenditures. Yet the Supreme Court has recently made clear that a potential saving in state funds, or even a requirement to expend them, is not sufficient grounds for the abridgement of fundamental constitutional rights or for the drawing of an invidious classification.[32] It re-

mains to be seen how the Court would weigh the state's financial interests against the claim that mandatory genetic screening violates a right of privacy or of bodily integrity.

Accordingly, while the present state of constitutional law does not provide a definite answer about the validity of compulsory genetic screening, no case stands either as a clear bar to, or an unequivocal precedent for, such a government effort. Clearly, a definite gap remains between the Supreme Court's decisions on "fundamental rights" and the burdens that may be imposed by mandatory genetic screening. This gap can probably best be bridged by legislation assuring that any such screening programs will not unduly infringe on the privacy or self-determination of the people screened.

This analysis is limited, however, to the kinds of mandatory genetic screening programs now in existence. Other kinds of genetic screening—for example, mandatory amniocentesis—would raise more difficult constitutional questions because of the greater burdens and risks involved to the subjects—factors which entered into both the *Jacobson* and *Roe* decisions—because mandatory amniocentesis may in fact approach mandatory abortion. Mandatory counseling and abortion or explicit restrictions on marriage resulting from mandatory screening would probably run afoul of the *Griswold* doctrine. In addition, the uses to which information resulting from mandatory genetic screening is put may raise new, substantial constitutional problems. The use of the results of mandatory screening for purposes of subsequently classifying individuals for special treatment—for example, the classification of XYY males for special education or the use of information for insurance or occupational purposes—might infringe constitutional rights.

EQUAL PROTECTION

If a compulsory genetic screening program were to single out a particular class of persons for screening, members of the class might challenge the program on the ground that it imposed a discriminatory burden on them in violation of the equal protection clause. Although the problem of classification does not admit of "doctrinaire definition,"[33] a classification will be upheld if it can be concluded that the classification is reasonably related to a legitimate purpose of the state.[34] For example, a state may single out the class of persons who handle food in restaurants for mandatory chest x-rays or other forms of screening.

In recent years, however, the Supreme Court has announced a new and more stringent test applicable in equal protection cases where statutes involve classifications which are "constitutionally suspect." Where the classification is drawn on racial, religious or ethnic lines, it is regarded as inherently suspect and a more stringent test is applied. This trend is illustrated in two recent Supreme Court decisions involving laws prohibiting miscegenation. In *McLaughlin v. Florida*[35] the Court held that racial classifications are "conditionally suspect" and that such a classification will be upheld "only if it is necessary, and not merely rationally related, to the accomplishment of a permissible state policy."[36] In the second case, *Loving v. Virginia*,[37] the Court explicitly rejected the rational basis test in favor of imposing a "very heavy burden of justification" on the state.

Accordingly, if a statute singles out blacks for mandatory sickle cell screening, Jews for Tay-Sachs screening or persons of Mediterranean descent for Cooley anemia screening, this would, presumably, involve a "suspect" classification imposing a heavy burden of justification, perhaps even a showing of necessity, upon the state. If the program were regarded as essentially beneficial and if the burdens were regarded as minimal, the stringency of the test might be reduced.

NOTES

1. *McCulloch v. Maryland*, 4 Wheat. 316 (1819).
2. *New York v. O'Neill*, 359 U.S. 1, 6 (1959).
3. *West Coast Hotel Co. v. Parrish*, 300 U.S. 379 (1937).
4. *Meyer v. Nebraska*, 262 U.S. 390 (1923).
5. See, e.g., *Stanley v. Georgia*, 394 U.S. 557 (1969); *Griswold v. Connecticut*, 381 U.S. 479 (1965).
6. *Roe v. Wade*, 410 U.S. 113 (1973).
7. *Snyder v. Massachusetts*, 291 U.S. 97, 105 (1934).
8. E.g., *Stanley v. Georgia*, 394 U.S. 557 (1969) (mere private possession of obscene materials may not be made a crime); *Griswold v. Connecticut*, 381 U.S. 479 (1965) (statute penalizing possession or use of contraceptives invalid).
9. See e.g., *Pierce v. Society of Sisters*, 268 U.S. 510 (1925); *Meyer v. Nebraska*, 262 U.S. 390 (1923). See also *Maynard v. Hill*, 125 U.S. 190 (1888).
10. *Loving v. Virginia*, 388 U.S. 1, 12 (1967).
11. *Skinner v. Oklahoma*, 316 U.S. 535, 541 (1942).
12. *Eisenstadt v. Baird*, 405 U.S. 438 (1972); *Griswold v. Connecticut*, 381 U.S. 479 (1965).
13. 381 U.S. 479 (1965).
14. Id. at 486.
15. Id. at 485.
16. 405 U.S. 438 (1972).
17. Id. at 453 (emphasis in original).
18. 410 U.S. 112 (1973).

19. Id. at 153.
20. Id. at 162–63.
21. Id. at 163.
22. Id. at 165.
23. *Olmstead v. United States*, 277 U.S. 438, 478 (1928) (Brandeis, J., dissenting).
24. 410 U.S. at 154.
25. 197 U.S. 11 (1905).
26. Id. at 36.
27. Id.
28. Id. at 29.
29. See *Peterson v. Widule*, 157 Wis. 641, 147 N.W. 966 (1914).
30. 274 U.S. 200 (1927).
31. Id. at 207.
32. See e.g., *Argersinger v. Hamlin*, 407 U.S. 25 (1972); *Shapiro v. Thompson*, 394 U.S. 618 (1969).
33. *Williamson v. Lee Optical Co.*, 348 U.S. 483, 489 (1955).
34. *Railway Express v. New York*, 336 U.S. 106 (1949).
35. 379 U.S. 184 (1964).
36. Id. at 196.
37. 388 U.S. 1 (1967).

SUGGESTED READINGS FOR CHAPTER 10

LIFESTYLE INTERVENTIONS AND BEHAVIOR CHANGE

Beauchamp, Dan E. "Public Health as Social Justice." *Inquiry* 13 (March 1976), 3–14.

———. *Beyond Alcoholism: Alcohol and Public Health Policy*. Philadelphia: Temple University Press, 1978.

Beauchamp, Tom L. "The Regulation of Hazards and Hazardous Behaviors." *Health Education Monographs* 6 (Summer 1980), 242–257.

Faden, Ruth, and Faden, Alan. "The Ethics of Health Education as Public Health Policy." *Health Education Monographs* 6 (Summer 1978), 180–197.

Kelman, Herbert. "Manipulation of Human Behavior: An Ethical Dilemma for the Social Scientist." In Bennis, W. D., *et al.*, eds. *The Planning of Change*. New York: Holt, Rinehart, and Winston, 1969.

Knowles, J. H. "The Responsibility of the Individual." *Daedalus* 106 (Winter 1977), 57–80.

Lalonde, M. *A New Perspective on the Health of Canadians*. Ottawa: Government of Canada, 1974.

Navarro, Vincente. "Justice, Social Policy, and the Public's Health." *Medical Care* 15 (May 1977), 363–370.

Warwick, Donald, and Kelman, Herbert. "Ethical Issues in Social Intervention." In Zaltman, G., ed. *Processes and Phenomena of Social Change*. New York: John Wiley, 1973, pp. 377–417.

Wikler, Daniel I. "Coercive Measures in Health Promotion: Can They be Justified?" *Health Education Monographs* 6 (Summer 1978), 223–241.

COST-BENEFIT ANALYSIS

Beauchamp, Tom L. "Utilitarianism and Cost-Benefit Analysis: A Reply to MacIntyre." In Beauchamp, T., and Bowie, N. E., eds. *Ethical Theory and Business.* Englewood Cliffs, N.J.: Prentice-Hall, 1979, pp. 276–282.

Bunker, John P., Barnes, Benjamin A., and Mosteller, Frederick, eds. *Costs, Risks, and Benefits of Surgery.* New York: Oxford University Press, 1977.

Buxton, M. J., and West, R. R.: "Cost-Benefit Analysis of Long-Term Haemodialysis for Chronic Renal Failure." *British Medical Journal* 2 (May 17, 1975), 376–379.

Inman, Robert P. "On the Benefits and Costs of Genetic Screening." *American Journal of Human Genetics* 30 (March 1978), 219–223.

MacIntyre, Alasdair. "Utilitarianism and Cost-Benefit Analysis." In Beauchamp, T., and Bowie, N. E., eds. *Ethical Theory and Business.* Englewood Cliffs, N.J.: Prentice-Hall, 1979, pp. 266–276.

Mooney, Gavin H. "Cost-Benefit Analysis and Medical Ethics." *Journal of Medical Ethics* 6 (December 1980), 177–179.

Rettig, Richard A. "The Policy Debate on Patient Care Financing for Victims of End-Stage Renal Disease." *Law and Contemporary Problems* 40 (Autumn 1976), 196–230.

Rhoads, Steven E. "How Much Should We Spend to Save a Life?" *Public Interest* 51 (Spring 1978), 74–92.

Schor, Irving M., Bierman, Steven F., and Fuchs, Victor R. "Cost-Benefit and Cost-Effectiveness Analysis." *New England Journal of Medicine* 304 (February 12, 1981), 432.

Taurek, John M. "Should the Numbers Count?" *Philosophy and Public Affairs* 6 (Summer 1977), 293–316.

U.S., Congress, Office of Technology Assessment, *The Implications of Cost-Effectiveness Analysis of Medical Technology.* Washington: Government Printing Office, August 1980. See especially the appendix prepared by the Hastings Center and entitled "Values, Ethics, and CBA in Health Care."

OCCUPATIONAL SAFETY AND HEALTH

Ashford, Nicholas. "Worker Health and Safety: An Area of Conflicts." *Monthly Labor Review* 98 (1975).

———. *Crisis in the Workplace.* Cambridge, Mass.: MIT Press, 1976.

Blackstone, William T. "On Rights and Responsibilities Pertaining to Toxic Substances and Trade Secrecy." *Southern Journal of Philosophy* 16 (Spring 1978), 589–603.

Bloom, Barry. "News about Carcinogens: What's Fit to Print?" *The Hastings Center Report* 9 (August 1979), 5–7, with a response by Arthur C. Upton, "Carcinogen Testing and Public Information," *The Hastings Center Report* 10 (February 1980), 9–10.

Bulletin of the New York Academy of Medicine 54 (September 1978). Special issue devoted to "Ethical Issues in Occupational Medicine."

Fischhoff, Baruch. "Informed Consent for Transient Nuclear Workers." In Kasperson, R., and Kates, R., eds. *Equity Issues in Radioactive Waste Management.* Cambridge, Mass.: Oelgeschlager, Gunn, and Hain, 1981.

Frank, Nancy K. "A Question of Equity: Workers' 'Right to Refuse' Under OSHA Compared to the Criminal Necessity Defense." *Labor Law Journal* 31 (October 1980), 617–626.

Johnson, Deborah G., and Ringen, Knut. "Health Risks and Equal Opportunity." *Hastings Center Report* 10 (December 1980), 25–26.

Magnuson, Harold J. "The Right to Know." *Archives of Environmental Health* 32 (January–February 1977), 40–44.

McGarity, Thomas O., and Shapiro, Sidney A. "The Trade Secrets Status of Health and Safety Testing Information: Reforming Agency Disclosure Policies." *Harvard Law Review* 93 (March 1980), 837–888.

Preston, Susan. "A Right under OSHA to Refuse Unsafe Work or A Hobson's Choice of Safety or Job?" *University of Baltimore Law Review* 8 (Spring 1979), 519–550.

Vogl, Thomas P., ed. *Public Information in the Prevention of Occupational Cancer.* Washington: National Academy of Sciences, 1977.

GENETIC SCREENING

Annas, George, and Coyne, B. "Fitness for Birth and Reproduction: Legal Implications of Genetic Screening." *Family Law Quarterly* 9 (Fall 1975), 463–490.

Baker, Robert. "Protecting the Unconceived." In Davis, John W., Hoffmaster, Barry, and Shorten, Sarah, eds. *Contemporary Issues in Biomedical Ethics.* Clifton, N.J.: Humana Press, 1978, pp. 89–100.

Bayles, Michael D. "Catch-22 Paternalism and Mandatory Genetic Screening." In Robison, Wade L., and Pritchard, Michael S., eds. *Medical Responsibility: Paternalism, Informed Consent, and Euthanasia.* Clifton, N.J.: Humana Press, 1979, pp. 29–42.

Buckley, John J., ed. *Genetics Now: Ethical Issues in Genetic Research.* Washington: University Press of America, 1978.

Capron, Alexander M., *et al. Genetic Counseling: Facts, Values, and Norms.* New York: Alan R. Liss, 1979.

Fletcher, John C. "Prenatal Diagnosis: Ethical Issues." In Reich, Warren T., ed. *Encyclopedia of Bioethics.* New York: Free Press, 1978. Vol. 3, pp. 1336–1346.

Gastel, Barbara, *et al. Maternal Serum Alpha-Fetoprotein: Issues in the Prenatal Screening and Diagnosis of Neural Tube Defects.* Washington: Government Printing Office, 1981.

Kolata, Gina B. "Prenatal Diagnosis of Neural Tube Defects." *Science* 209 (September 12, 1980), 1216–1218.

Kopelman, Loretta. "Genetic Screening in Newborns: Voluntary or Compulsory?" *Perspectives in Biology and Medicine* 22 (Autumn 1978), 83–89.

Lappe, Marc. *Genetic Politics: The Limits of Biological Control.* New York: Simon and Schuster, 1979.

Layde, Peter M., Von Allmen, Stephen D., and Oakley, Godfrey P. "Maternal Serum Alpha-Fetoprotein Screening: A Cost-Benefit Analysis." *American Journal of Public Health* 69 (June 1979), 566–573.

Milunsky, Aubrey. "Prenatal Diagnosis: Clinical Aspects." In Reich, Warren T., ed. *Encyclopedia of Bioethics.* New York: Free Press, 1978. Vol. 3, pp. 1332–1336.

———, ed. *Genetic Disorders and the Fetus.* New York: Plenum Press, 1979.

National Academy of Sciences. *Genetic Screening: Programs, Principles, and Research.* Washington: National Academy of Sciences, 1975.

Omenn, Gilbert S. "Genetics and Epidemiology: Medical Interventions and Public Policy." *Social Biology* 26 (Summer 1979), 117–125.

Powledge, Tabitha M. "Genetic Screening." In Reich, Warren T., ed. *Encyclopedia of Bioethics.* New York: Free Press, 1978. Vol. 2, pp. 567–573.

———, and Fletcher, John. "Guidelines for the Ethical, Social, and Legal Issues in Prenatal Diagnosis." *New England Journal of Medicine* 300 (January 1979), 168–172. [Hastings Center Task Force Report]

Ruse, Michael. "Genetics and the Quality of Life." *Social Indicators Research* 7 (January 1980), 419–441.

Veatch, Robert M. *Case Studies in Medical Ethics*. Cambridge, Mass.: Harvard University Press, 1977. Chap. 8.

Walters, LeRoy. "Genetics, Reproductive Biology, and Bioethics." In Neumann, Marguerite, ed. *The Tricentennial People: Human Applications of the New Genetics*. Ames, Iowa: Iowa State University Press, 1978, pp. 66–80.

BIBLIOGRAPHIES

Goldstein, Doris Mueller. *Bioethics: A Guide to Information Sources*. Detroit: Gale Research Company, 1982. See under "Genetic Counseling and Screening" and "Treatment for Defective Newborns and Infanticide."

Lineback, Richard H., ed. *Philosopher's Index*. Vols. 1– . Bowling Green, Ohio: Philosophy Documentation Center, Bowling Green State University. Issued quarterly. See under "Birth Control," "Birth Defects," "Cost-Benefit Analysis," "Genetic Engineering," "Genetic Screening," "Liberty," "Medicine," "Mentally Retarded," "Public Policy," "Quality of Life," "Risk(s)," and "Social Control."

Walters, LeRoy, ed. *Bibliography of Bioethics*. Vols. 1– . New York: Free Press. Issued annually. See under "Eugenics," "Genetic Screening," and "Occupational Medicine." (The information contained in the annual *Bibliography of Bioethics* can also be retrieved from BIOETHICSLINE, an online data base of the National Library of Medicine.)

Part V

BIOMEDICAL RESEARCH

11.
Research Involving Human Subjects

Chapters 4 and 5 discussed a series of ethical problems that arise in the context of clinical care. In parallel fashion the present chapter explores several ethical issues raised by research involving human subjects, including special problems raised by research involving children.

CONCEPTUAL QUESTIONS

The definition of "research involving human subjects" (or "human research") can perhaps be best approached by way of considering the concepts of "therapy" and "research." In the biomedical and behavioral fields, "therapy" refers to a class of activities designed solely to benefit an individual or the members of a group. Therapy may take several forms: it may be a treatment for a disease, or it may be diagnostic procedures or even preventive measures. In contrast, "research" refers to a class of scientific activities designed to develop or contribute to generalizable knowledge. Examples of research are the comparative study of alternative methods for training pigeons, the search for the best among alternative drug therapies, and the laboratory analysis of a chemical reaction. The term "human research," then, refers to research that involves human subjects.

Two subtypes of human research can be identified. (1) *Therapeutic* research, as the phrase suggests, is closely akin to therapy. However, unlike therapy, which is designed *solely* to benefit patients, therapeutic research has a dual purpose: it is performed *primarily* for the benefit of the patient-subjects; at the same time, the treatments are administered in a systematic and controlled way, so that treatment results can be applied to other contexts or to future subjects and patients. An example of therapeutic research is a study that compares the relative effectiveness of two similarly promising anticancer drugs administered to cancer patients. (2) *Nontherapeutic* research, on the other hand, is performed primarily for the purpose of gaining new knowledge, not for the benefit of the subjects involved in the study. For example, healthy human volunteers who need no drugs for therapeutic purposes frequently participate in the early phases of drug testing, when the safety of new drugs for human use is being evaluated. The essays by Hans Jonas and Charles Fried in this chapter discuss the distinction between therapeutic and nontherapeutic research.

THE MORAL JUSTIFICATION OF RESEARCH INVOLVING HUMAN SUBJECTS

In literature on human research, including codes of research ethics, surprisingly little attention is paid to the general justification for involving human subjects in research. This silence at the most general level of justification is particularly striking when one considers that the traditional ethic of medicine has been exclusively a patient-benefit ethic. The motto *primum non nocere* (do no harm) has generally been interpreted to mean "Do nothing that is not intended for the direct benefit of the patient." We must ask, then, whether good reasons can be given for deviating in any way from therapy, as that term was defined above.

The primary argument in favor of human research appeals to the principle of beneficence (as was briefly noted in Chapter 1). It asserts that the social benefits to be gained from such research are substantial and that the harms resulting from the cessation of such investigations would be exceedingly grave. In their essays in this chapter, Leon Eisenberg and Thomas Chalmers advance such claims. They note that the therapeutic value of many reputed "therapies" is in fact unknown; indeed, these treatments may be no more useful than the bloodletting technique so much in vogue during the eighteenth and early nineteenth centuries. On this view, the only alternative to a perpetual plague of medically induced illness is the vigorous pursuit of biomedical research, particularly research involving human subjects.

A second approach to the justification of human research is based on a joint appeal to the principles of beneficence and justice. According to this view, beneficence requires that each of us make at least a modest positive contribution to the good of our fellow-citizens or the society as a whole. If our participation in research promises significant benefit to others, at little or no risk to ourselves, then such participation may become a duty of beneficence. In addition, if we fail to fulfill this modest duty, while most of our contemporaries perform it, we may be acting unjustly, since we are not performing our fair share of a communal task. Eisenberg and Richard McCormick advance qualified versions of this argument in their essays in this chapter.

The justice argument can be further elaborated by reference to the past. Every person currently alive is the beneficiary of earlier subjects' involvement in research. To be specific, the willingness of past human volunteers to take part in studies of antibiotics (like penicillin) and vaccines (like the polio vaccine) contributes to the health of us all. Accordingly, it seems unfair for us to reap the benefits of already-performed research without making a reciprocal contribution to the alleviation of disability and disease.

Hans Jonas vigorously challenges both of these approaches to the general justification of human research. In answer to the consequential argument advanced by Eisenberg and Chalmers, Jonas asserts that while human research generally contributes to medical progress, most research involving human subjects is not *essential* to the well-being or survival of the human species. According to Jonas, progress, even medical progress, is "an optional goal, not an unconditional commitment." On this view, only a national health emergency or a similar "clear and present danger" would provide a sufficient justification for nontherapeutic human research.

Implicit in Jonas's characterization of most human research as optional is a rejection of the thesis of a general moral duty to participate in such research. Thus, there is no injustice involved in our not volunteering to take part in nontherapeutic studies. In Jonas's view, most volunteers of the past, including investigators involved in self-experimentation, performed acts of altruism and moral heroism. If we of the present owe any debt to the past, it is a debt of gratitude to these bygone heroes, not an obligation to society required by a reciprocity principle of justice.

A presupposition of Jonas's position on the general justification of human research is that autonomy rights—for example, the right to be free from invasions of one's body and the right to consent—are supremely important. Jonas also regards all nontherapeutic research involving human subjects as an infringement of the individual's "primary inviolability"; in Kantian terms, he objects to the use of a person as a means rather than an end. Because of this primary commitment to protecting the rights, dignity, and inviolability of the individual, Jonas is unwilling to accept either ordinary social benefits or the notion of universal duties to society as sufficient justifications for human research.

But the principle of autonomy can be taken in another direction, as well. One additional justification, not explicitly mentioned by either Eisenberg or Jonas, is sometimes advanced in support of research involving human subjects. Investigators, it is asserted, should be free to decide what kinds of research they will perform and how they wish to conduct that research. According to this view, the freedom of scientific inquiry should be protected from outside interference, unless there are strong reasons for overriding the presumption of freedom. Thus, if an investigator can find human subjects who are willing to take part in some proposed research, he or she should generally be allowed to proceed with the research. Critics of this freedom-of-inquiry position reply that there is a significant difference between the freedom to do research and the freedom to involve human subjects in research. For example, there may be a qualitative distinction between analyzing the properties of a chemical compound, on the one hand, and soliciting the participation of human subjects in a research project, on the other. In addition, critics of the freedom-of-inquiry viewpoint argue that the knowledge differential between most investigators and most subjects is so great that some intervention by society is justified, if only to ensure that the consent of prospective subjects is adequately informed. (See the final section of Chapter 12 for a more detailed discussion of these issues.)

RESEARCH DESIGN AND BENEFIT-HARM RATIO

If human research as a practice can be justified in certain circumstances, then one can proceed to consider what rules should be applied to the conduct of research. Many of these rules have been developed in the various codes of research ethics, beginning with the Nuremberg Code. Perhaps the most prominent rule discussed in the codes is the informed consent requirement. However, some codes also devote significant attention to the proper design of research and to the minimization of risks to subjects.

The requirement of adequate research design is end-oriented or utilitarian in character. The central aim of this requirement is to ensure that human research will be conducted efficiently—that is, in a way that maximizes the amount of information gained from exposing human subjects to the minimum amount of risk. From this general rule flow several specific stipulations. First, as David Rutstein notes, studies that are so poorly designed that they cannot possibly produce reliable data should not be performed at all.[1] The codes of research ethics add a second stipulation, that research involving humans should be based upon prior laboratory and animal studies. A third stipulation is perhaps the obverse side of the first: all studies that involve human subjects should be carefully controlled, so that the biases of the investigator do not invalidate research results. Fourth, careful methods of statistical analysis should be employed in interpreting the data derived from human research, so that the greatest possible informational benefit is derived from each study.

Even if the optimal research design is selected for a particular study, questions about the probability and magnitude of anticipated harms and benefits resulting from the study may remain. A maximum level of anticipated harm is suggested in the Nuremberg Code: "No experiment should be conducted where there is *a priori* reason to believe that death or disabling injury will occur." A minimum limit of anticipated benefit is specified by Rutstein, who argues that no experiment which promises only "trivial" results should be performed.[2] As for the benefit-harm ratio, the codes stipulate that the anticipated benefits of a proposed study should be proportionate to the risk of harm to human subjects.

This chapter does not attempt to explore all aspects of research design[3] and risk-benefit analysis. Rather, it focuses on one type of research design that has been the object of rather intense debate—the randomized clinical trial. In this research design, ill patients are assigned on a random basis to one of two or more alternative treatments; the relative efficacy of the treatments is then determined by closely monitoring the progress of patient-subjects assigned to each treatment. The technique of randomization is chosen to avoid investigator bias in selecting subjects for various treatments and also to cancel out unknown variables, for example, variables related to age, sex, or income level. (The essays by Thomas Chalmers and Charles Fried propose several rules for the ethical conduct of randomized clinical trials.)

INFORMED CONSENT

Since the Nuremberg trials, no aspect of human research has received greater attention than the issue of consent. In the Nuremberg Code itself consent was discussed in the first and longest article. Given the context of the Nuremberg judgment, it is not surprising that the emphasis at the time was on subjects' consent being truly voluntary and uncoerced. Subsequently, in judicial decisions dealing with medical care rather than research, the term "informed consent" was coined, to give equal attention to the disclosure of all facts that would be important for a patient's reaching a free and knowledgeable decision. In parallel fashion, several codifications of research ethics, including the Helsinki Declaration (the second selection in this chapter), have gradually developed the concept of informed consent in the context of research.

Each element of the concept raises its own issues. The "information" aspect of informed consent may refer to "reasonable" *disclosures* by investigators about various features of the research, or it may refer to the requirement that the prospective subjects actually *comprehend* what they have been told. The consent component refers to an uncoerced decision to take part in the already disclosed or comprehended procedure or project, but there remains the question whether voluntariness is to be judged by objective standards (of an ideal, reasonable person) or subjective standards that refer solely to a particular individual[4] (as discussed in Chapter 5).

A variety of justifications or rationales for the informed-consent requirement have been advanced. According to Paul Ramsey, the informed-consent rule serves as a deontological check on any effort to justify human research solely on a utilitarian basis: "The principle of informed consent is the cardinal *canon of loyalty* joining men together in medical practice and investigation." A more legally oriented approach is presented by Charles Fried, who views informed consent against the backdrop of legal doctrines concerning liability and medical malpractice, battery and negligence. The law of battery protects patients and subjects against unauthorized interventions ("touching" being the legal term), while the law of negligence holds investigators liable for falling short of the customary standard in informing patients or subjects about the potential risks of a particular intervention.[5] While beneficence-based arguments for the informed-consent requirement can also be developed—for example, that it minimizes harm to subjects and encourages self-scrutiny by investigators[6]—autonomy-based justifications have predominated both in the relevant court decisions and in the general literature that discusses the ethics of research involving human subjects.

In this chapter, Chalmers, Fried, and Ingelfinger discuss several special problems in the application of the informed-consent requirement. Chalmers raises the question: How much information should be disclosed to participants in randomized clinical trials? His answer and Fried's differ. Chalmers argues that patient-subjects should not be informed that their treatment will be allocated on a random basis, on grounds that most informed patient-subjects would refuse randomization, thus rendering completion of the trial and the assembly of data impossible. By contrast, Fried emphasizes the investigator's duty to provide full information to subjects concerning both the fact of randomization and the progress of the trial. Franz Ingelfinger's essay acknowledges the value of informed consent as an ideal but questions whether either adequate comprehension or free choice is ever achieved in practice.

The requirements of adequate research design, favorable benefit-harm ratio, and reasonably free and sufficiently informed consent are generally regarded as *necessary* conditions of ethically acceptable human research. However, it is not clear that these three conditions are *sufficient* to justify proposed research involving human subjects. One might wish to add a justice requirement—that the risks and benefits of research should be fairly allocated among different social classes and other social groups. A few commentators, including Charles Fried,[7] have proposed a fifth requirement, which is also based on considerations of justice: In their view, all subjects who accept the risks of research for the sake of society should also receive equitable compensation for injuries sustained in the course of their participation in that research.

RESEARCH INVOLVING CHILDREN

Ethical guidelines for human research generally presuppose that the subjects who take part in research are adults who have normal mental capacities and who are not pregnant, seriously ill, institutionalized, or in desperate need of money. Special subject groups who differ in one or more respects from this model of the normal adult human subject include the mentally retarded, the dying, the comatose, fetuses, and children. In this chapter we examine the ethical issues raised by research involving one of these special subject groups, namely, children.

The term "child" (or "minor") is frequently applied to humans of widely divergent ages, from newborn infants to adolescents on the verge of attaining legal majority. The documents selected for inclusion in this chapter presuppose that the term refers to biologically immature human beings who either lack completely the capacity to consent (e.g., young infants) or who because of their early stage of intellectual development possess only limited ability to comprehend and give consent (e.g., seven-year-olds). Intellectually speaking, the later stages of childhood gradually shade into adulthood; thus, the ethical issues raised by research involving older groups of children gradually become less similar to those raised by research involving young infants and begin to resemble issues raised by research involving adults.

The general justification for including children in biomedical research is that, physiologically speaking, children are not merely "little adults." For example, many drugs produce totally different effects in adults and children, or even in newborn infants and two-year-olds. Unless carefully controlled studies of pediatric reactions to such drugs are performed, children are likely to receive either ineffective or highly toxic doses of drugs. Proponents of research on children also emphasize the need for additional data concerning the normal development of children—for instance, data concerning resistance to disease, nutritional needs, and body size and weight.

Therapeutic pediatric research, that is, research performed primarily for the benefit of a particular child, is usually thought to raise fewer ethical and legal difficulties than nontherapeutic research. In general, parents are legally empowered to give permission—often termed proxy consent—for pediatric treatment. Since therapeutic research is closely akin to pure therapy, it is frequently assumed that parents are also authorized to permit their children's participation in therapeutic research. This assumption, however, is questioned by some commentators since therapeutic research, in contrast to therapy, is not directed *solely* to the benefit of patients.

Should parents also be permitted to give consent for the participation of their children in *nontherapeutic* research? Answers to this question differ. Paul Ramsey adopts the most stringent position on the moral justifiability of nontherapeutic pediatric research. His argument can be summarized as follows:

1. No nontherapeutic research should be performed without the informed consent of the research subject.
2. Young children are incapable of giving informed consent.
3. Therefore, no nontherapeutic research involving young children should be performed.

A second and somewhat less restrictive position is proposed by Richard McCormick. McCormick suggests that in some cases the risks of nontherapeutic pediatric research may be minimal, while the potential benefits of the research to children as a class may be substantial. To this consideration McCormick adds a second, which is premised on the social nature of human beings. In his view, all members of society are mutually interdependent and therefore owe to each other the performance of certain minimal moral duties. Among these duties is the obligation to take part in minimally risky nontherapeutic research that promises great benefit to the society as a whole. Since children, too, are members of the society, they stand under a similar obligation, although they may be too immature to recognize the fact. Because children, like adults, morally *ought to* want to promote the social good, it is in McCormick's view morally legitimate for their parents to consent for them to do so. By implication, then, it is permissible for parents to provide proxy consent for their children's participation in minimally risky nontherapeutic research.

A hypothetical example may serve to highlight the differences between the positions of Ramsey and McCormick on the moral justifiability of nontherapeutic pediatric research. Suppose that a researcher plans to obtain small blood samples from newborn infants in an effort to understand why such infants are naturally immune to certain diseases. Suppose, further, that the researcher's long-term aim is to develop an anti-pneumonia vaccine for use among infants. Since the research would not be directly beneficial to the newborns from whom the blood samples would be taken, it would not be morally acceptable in Ramsey's view. However, McCormick would probably argue that the proposed research falls within the range of what newborn infants "owe" to society and that the research is therefore appropriate from a moral point of view.

Even if one agrees with McCormick that nontherapeutic pediatric research is morally justifiable in certain circumstances, there remains the problem of formulating appropriate rules for research involving children. These rules would presumably parallel the rules outlined above for research involving adults but with one obvious difference: Some alternative to the informed consent of the research subject must be found, at least in the case of young pediatric subjects. Two attempts to develop rules for the conduct of pediatric research are included in this chapter, the one a set of recommendations proposed by an interdisciplinary advisory commission in the United States, the other a series of guidelines developed by a working party of the British Paediatric Association.

L. W.

NOTES

1. David D. Rutstein, ''The Ethical Design of Human Experiments,'' in Paul A. Freund, ed., *Experimentation with Human Subjects* (New York: George Braziller, 1970), p. 384.

2. Rutstein, *op. cit.,* p. 398.

3. See William G. Cochran, ''Experimental Design: I. The Design of Experiments,'' in David L. Sills, ed., *International Encyclopedia of the Social Sciences* (New York: Macmillan, 1968), Vol. 5, pp. 245–254.

4. Alexander M. Capron, ''Informed Consent in Catastrophic Disease Research and Treatment,'' *University of Pennsylvania Law Review* 123 (December 1974), pp. 404–418.

5. See Charles Fried, *Medical Experimentation: Personal Integrity and Social Policy* (New York: American Elsevier, 1974), pp. 14–25.

6. Capron, *op. cit.,* pp. 371–374.

7. Fried, p. 542 in this chapter.

The Nuremberg Code

The great weight of the evidence before us is to the effect that certain types of medical experiments on human beings, when kept within reasonably well-defined bounds, conform to the ethics of the medical profession generally. The protagonists of the practice of human experimentation justify their views on the basis that such experiments yield results for the good of society that are unprocurable by other methods or means of study. All agree, however, that certain basic principles must be observed in order to satisfy moral, ethical and legal concepts.

1. The voluntary consent of the human subject is absolutely essential.

This means that the person involved should have legal capacity to give consent; should be so situated as to be able to exercise free power of choice, without the intervention of any element of force, fraud, deceit, duress, overreaching, or other ulterior form of constraint or coercion; and should have sufficient knowledge and comprehension of the elements of the subject matter involved as to enable him to make an understanding and enlightened decision. This latter element requires that before the acceptance of an affirmative decision by the experimental subject there should be made known to him the nature, duration, and purpose of the experiment; the method and means by which it is to be conducted; all inconveniences and hazards reasonably to be expected; and the effects upon his health or person which may possibly come from his participation in the experiment.

The duty and responsibility for ascertaining the quality of the consent rests upon each individual who initiates, directs or engages in the experiment. It is a personal duty and responsibility which may not be delegated to another with impunity.

2. The experiment should be such as to yield fruitful results for the good of society, unprocurable by other methods or means of study, and not random and unnecessary in nature.

3. The experiment should be so designed and based on the results of animal experimentation and a knowledge of the natural history of the disease or other problems under study that the anticipated results will justify the performance of the experiment.

4. The experiment should be so conducted as to avoid all unnecessary physical and mental suffering and injury.

5. No experiment should be conducted where there is an *a priori* reason to believe that death or disabling injury will occur; except perhaps, in those experiments where the experimental physicians also serve as subjects.

6. The degree of risk to be taken should never exceed that determined by the humanitarian importance of the problem to be solved by the experiment.

7. Proper preparations should be made and adequate facilities provided to protect the experimental subject against even remote possibilities of injury, disability, or death.

8. The experiment should be conducted only by scientifically qualified persons. The highest degree of skill and care should be required through all stages of the experiment of those who conduct or engage in the experiment.

9. During the course of the experiment the human subject should be at liberty to bring the experiment to an end if he has reached the physical or mental state where continuation of the experiment seems to him to be impossible.

10. During the course of the experiment the scientist in charge must be prepared to terminate the experiment at any stage, if he has probable cause to believe, in the exercise of the good faith, superior skill and careful judgment required of him that a continuation of the experiment is likely to result in injury, disability, or death to the experimental subject.

From *Trials of War Criminals Before the Nuremberg Military Tribunals Under Control Council Law No. 10*. Vol. II, Nuremberg, October 1946–April 1949.

WORLD MEDICAL ASSOCIATION

Declaration of Helsinki*

INTRODUCTION

It is the mission of the medical doctor to safeguard the health of the people. His or her knowledge and conscience are dedicated to the fulfillment of this mission.

The Declaration of Geneva of The World Medical Association binds the doctor with the words "The health of my patient will be my first consideration," and the International Code of Medical Ethics declares that, "Any act or advice which could weaken physical or mental resistance of a human being may be used only in his interest."

The purpose of biomedical research involving human subjects must be to improve diagnostic, therapeutic and prophylactic procedures and the understanding of the aetiology and pathogenesis of disease.

In current medical practice most diagnostic, therapeutic or prophylactic procedures involve hazards. This applies *a fortiori* to biomedical research.

Medical progress is based on research which ultimately must rest in part on experimentation involving human subjects.

In the field of biomedical research a fundamental distinction must be recognized between medical research in which the aim is essentially diagnostic or therapeutic for a patient, and medical research, the essential object of which is purely scientific and without direct diagnostic or therapeutic value to the person subjected to the research.

Special caution must be exercised in the conduct of research which may affect the environment, and the welfare of animals used for research must be respected.

*Recommendations guiding medical doctors in biomedical research involving human subjects.

Adopted by the 18th World Medical Assembly, Helsinki, Finland, 1964, and revised by the 29th World Medical Assembly, Tokyo, Japan, October 1975. Reprinted with permission of the World Medical Association, Inc. from the "Declaration of Helsinki," revised edition.

Because it is essential that the results of laboratory experiments be applied to human beings to further scientific knowledge and to help suffering humanity, The World Medical Association has prepared the following recommendations as a guide to every doctor in biomedical research involving human subjects. They should be kept under review in the future. It must be stressed that the standards as drafted are only a guide to physicians all over the world. Doctors are not relieved from criminal, civil and ethical responsibilities under the laws of their own countries.

I. BASIC PRINCIPLES

1. Biomedical research involving human subjects must conform to generally accepted scientific principles and should be based on adequately performed laboratory and animal experimentation and on a thorough knowledge of the scientific literature.

2. The design and performance of each experimental procedure involving human subjects should be clearly formulated in an experimental protocol which should be transmitted to a specially appointed independent committee for consideration, comment and guidance.

3. Biomedical research involving human subjects should be conducted only by scientifically qualified persons and under the supervision of a clinically competent medical person. The responsibility for the human subject must always rest with a medically qualified person and never rest on the subject of research, even though the subject has given his or her consent.

4. Biomedical research involving human subjects cannot legitimately be carried out unless the importance of the objective is in proportion to the inherent risk to the subject.

5. Every biomedical research project involving human subjects should be preceded by careful assessment of predictable risks in comparison with

foreseeable benefits to the subject or to others. Concern for the interests of the subject must always prevail over the interests of science and society.

6. The right of the research subject to safeguard his or her integrity must always be respected. Every precaution should be taken to respect the privacy of the subject and to minimize the impact of the study on the subject's physical and mental integrity and on the personality of the subject.

7. Doctors should abstain from engaging in research projects involving human subjects unless they are satisfied that the hazards involved are believed to be predictable. Doctors should cease any investigation if the hazards are found to outweigh the potential benefits.

8. In publication of the results of his or her research, the doctor is obliged to preserve the accuracy of the results. Reports of experimentation not in accordance with the principles laid down in this Declaration should not be accepted for publication.

9. In any research on human beings, each potential subject must be adequately informed of the aims, methods, anticipated benefits and potential hazards of the study and the discomfort it may entail. He or she should be informed that he or she is at liberty to abstain from participation in the study and that he or she is free to withdraw his or her consent to participation at any time. The doctor should then obtain the subject's freely given informed consent, preferably in writing.

10. When obtaining informed consent for the research project the doctor should be particularly cautious if the subject is in a dependent relationship to him or her or may consent under duress. In that case the informed consent should be obtained by a doctor who is not engaged in the investigation and who is completely independent of this official relationship.

11. In case of legal incompetence, informed consent should be obtained from the legal guardian in accordance with national legislation. Where physical or mental incapacity makes it impossible to obtain informed consent, or when the subject is a minor, permission from the responsible relative replaces that of the subject in accordance with national legislation.

12. The research protocol should always contain a statement of the ethical considerations involved and

should indicate that the principles enunciated in the present Declaration are complied with.

II. MEDICAL RESEARCH COMBINED WITH PROFESSIONAL CARE (CLINICAL RESEARCH)

1. In the treatment of the sick person, the doctor must be free to use a new diagnostic and therapeutic measure, if in his or her judgment it offers hope of saving life, reestablishing health or alleviating suffering.

2. The potential benefits, hazards and discomfort of a new method should be weighed against the advantages of the best current diagnostic and therapeutic methods.

3. In any medical study, every patient—including those of a control group, if any—should be assured of the best proven diagnostic and therapeutic method.

4. The refusal of the patient to participate in a study must never interfere with the doctor-patient relationship.

5. If the doctor considers it essential not to obtain informed consent, the specific reasons for this proposal should be stated in the experimental protocol for transmission to the independent committee (I, 2).

6. The doctor can combine medical research with professional care, the objective being the acquisition of new medical knowledge, only to the extent that medical research is justified by its potential diagnostic or therapeutic value for the patient.

III. NON-THERAPEUTIC BIOMEDICAL RESEARCH INVOLVING HUMAN SUBJECTS (NON-CLINICAL BIOMEDICAL RESEARCH)

1. In the purely scientific application of medical research carried out on a human being, it is the duty of the doctor to remain the protector of the life and health of that person on whom biomedical research is being carried out.

2. The subjects should be volunteers—either healthy persons or patients for whom the experimental design is not related to the patient's illness.

3. The investigator or the investigating team should discontinue the research if in his/her or their judgment it may, if continued, be harmful to the individual.

4. In research on man, the interest of science and society should never take precedence over considerations related to the well-being of the subject.

ROYAL COLLEGE OF NURSING OF THE UNITED KINGDOM

Ethics Related to Research in Nursing

INTRODUCTION

As a profession committed to the improvement of health services to society nurses are obliged to develop new knowledge and skills as well as to utilize the knowledge and skills already available. Such a commitment to the development of nursing theory and the improvement of nursing practice presupposes a commitment to research.

The ethics of nursing research must be consistent with the ethics of nursing practice. The following statements are intended as guidelines for nurses undertaking or associated with research.

The researcher has obligations to the subjects of study, to sponsors/employers, to colleagues and to the development and promotion of knowledge.

Nurses in authority in places where research is to be undertaken have obligations to the subjects of the study, to the governing body of the institution or place of work, to the sponsors of the study and to the research worker.

Nurses practising in places where research is being carried out have obligations to patients/clients and to the development and promotion of knowledge through research. When assisting in the conduct of research they have obligations to adhere to the ethical code binding upon all research workers.

PART I: NURSES UNDERTAKING RESEARCH

1. RESPONSIBILITY TO SUBJECTS

Subjects here are taken to include individuals, e.g., patients or staff, or collectivities of all kinds, e.g., formal organizations or geographical areas.

a. Before agreeing to undertake any project or piece of research the nurse researcher must be satisfied that the knowledge sought is not already available.

b. The researcher is responsible for obtaining freely given and informed consent from each individual who is to be a subject of study or personally involved in a study. The researcher should explain as fully as possible and in terms meaningful to the subjects what the research is about, who is undertaking and financing it and why it is being undertaken. He/she must make explicit the subject's right to refuse to participate or to withdraw at any stage of the project, and this right must be respected.*

c. If the subject for any reason is unable to appreciate the implications of participation, informed consent must be obtained from relatives or legal guardian.†

d. If the subject is a patient the researcher should discuss the proposed research with the patient's doctor or the appropriate medical officer.

e. If the nature of the research is such that fully informing subjects before the study would invalidate results, then whatever explanation is possible should be given to the subject. There must be provision for appropriate explanation to the subject on completion of the study.

f. Explanation to subjects should include information as to how their names came to the knowl-

---

* "It should be clearly understood that the possibility or probability that a particular investigation will be of benefit to humanity or to posterity would afford no defense in the event of legal proceedings. The individual has rights that the law protects and nobody can infringe those rights for the public good." Report of the Medical Research Council for 1962-63 (Cmnd. 2382), pages 21–25.

† "The situation in respect of minors and mentally subnormal or mentally disordered persons is of particular difficulty. In the strict view of the law parents and guardians of minors cannot give consent on their behalf to any procedures which are of no particular benefit to them, and which may carry some risk of harm." Ibid.

Reprinted with permission of the Royal College of Nursing of the United Kingdom from *Ethics Related to Research in Nursing* (London: Royal College of Nursing of the United Kingdom, 1977), pp. 1–7.

edge of the researcher. He/she should identify him/herself and the organization responsible for the study and leave with the subject a note giving this information together with a brief statement concerning the nature of the study.

g. Research subjects must be assured protection against physical, mental, emotional or social injury. No harm must come to them as a result of being involved in the study insofar as the present state of knowledge allows.

h. The nature of any promise of confidentiality or restriction on the use of information must be made clear to the subjects and adhered to.

i. The researcher should be aware of and seek to avoid the danger of raising false hopes or unnecessary anxieties.

j. The researcher should be aware that the use of records can present particular problems in relation to confidentiality.

k. In most instances the approval of the appropriate ethics committee will be necessary, but in any case the researcher would be wise to seek advice on the ethical aspects of the study.

2. INTEGRITY OF THE RESEARCHER

a. The nurse researcher must possess knowledge and skills compatible with the demands of the investigation to be undertaken and must recognize and not overstep the boundaries of his/her research competence. He/she should not accept work he/she is not qualified to carry out. (Those learning to do research should only work under the guidance of an experienced researcher.)

b. The researcher has responsibility to acknowledge personal limitations and to state limitations on his/her detachment from the area of study and any ways in which his/her presence may have affected the subjects of the study.

c. The researcher has responsibility, within the limits imposed by his/her regard for the interests of the subjects, to publish or to make otherwise available the results of the research, displaying or making available schedules or other research tools and reporting all relevant data, including negative evidence. Limitations on the validity of the conclusions should be stated and the extent to which they can be generalized.

d. As is common practice in any publication, acknowledgements should be made of the con-

tributions of others, but permission must be obtained before names are cited or quotations or acknowledgements made apart from those in already published works which are governed by copyright.

e. The researcher should be aware that he/she has some responsibility for the use made of the research and should not ignore its misuse.

f. He/she has a responsibility for the advancement of the theory and methods of the science in which he/she is working.

g. The researcher is responsible for adherence to the code of ethics by members of his/her team or by any students working under his/her guidance.

3. RELATIONS WITH SPONSORS, EMPLOYERS, AND COLLEAGUES

a. The researchers has the obligation to make clear to his/her employer or sponsor that he/she cannot undertake work outside his/her research competence and to decline work where limitations of his/her competence or of facilities in terms of money, time, personnel or equipment are such as to make the achievement of the research aims improbable.

b. The researcher must make clear to his/her employer and/or sponsor that "solutions" to problems cannot be guaranteed and should make explicit the limitations of the proposed research.

c. The terms under which research is being carried out should be stated in a clear way with as much detail as possible to avoid misunderstanding. A contract should show the mutual obligations of employer and employees or between the sponsors and those undertaking research. The contract should include terms of reference and should be specific about the use of research findings and research material, the right to publish and (where appropriate) trade secrets.

d. The researcher has a responsibility to notify and obtain agreement from employer and/or sponsor for any proposed departure from the terms of reference or proposed change in the nature of the project. He/she has an obligation to strive to complete the project within the agreed time and resources. Whether the aims of the project are achieved or not the researcher has an obligation to provide the sponsor and/or employer with a report on the work making clear any limitations in the validity or generality of the material.

e. When research is undertaken in a formal organization, it is wise to clarify in advance the responsibility of the research worker to the organization, the lines of communication, and the means of settling any problems that may arise. The right of the facilitators to interim reports in certain circumstances and to see the research report before publication should be respected. This in no way sanctions modifications or withholding of results. The responsibility for the published results must rest with the researcher.

f. The researcher has an obligation to make sure that professional colleagues with a responsibility for the subject are informed of the proposed research.

g. (i) a. The nurse as researcher has no responsibility for the service, care/treatment or advice given to patients/clients and should make this clear. Intervention should be confined to occasions when a potentially harmful situation appears imminent.

　　　b. He/she must exercise great care not to interfere in the professional/client or employer/employee relationship.

　(ii) If the nature of the project specifically identifies procedures or practices which are to be the subject for controlled experimental investigation, agreement must be reached in advance with those responsible for the service, care or advice as to the respective responsibilities of the researcher and the employees of the organization.

　(iii) Action research presupposes interaction between the researcher and the subjects and the intervention must be mutually agreed.

PART II: NURSES IN POSITIONS OF AUTHORITY WHERE RESEARCH IS TO BE CARRIED OUT

1. a. Nurses with authority to sanction or commission research within the units or organizations where they work must satisfy themselves that the research is necessary because the knowledge sought is not already available; that the achievement of the project's aims by the means proposed is possible and that the project will not impose unnecessary

hardship or unacceptable increase of work on the subjects of the study or the staff. In reaching these decisions the nurse should take account of other research which may be in progress, and may find helpful the assistance of an experienced researcher or research committee.

b. Consent to participate in a study cannot be given on behalf of another person and the nurse agreeing to allow a study or commissioning a project must satisfy him/herself that the researcher obtains free and informed consent from the subjects of the study. Particular care is necessary when the subjects stand in special relationship to the investigator, e.g., students to their teacher.

c. Any promises of anonymity or confidentiality given by the researcher must be respected also by the nurse commissioning or agreeing to the research being undertaken. Raw data should not be available to anyone outside the immediate research team. No attempt must be made to probe behind the statistical material to identify any person, institution, or place. Research findings must not be used for disciplinary purposes.

d. Any nurse commissioning or taking part in commissioning a project or employing a research worker must respect his/her right to refuse to undertake a project which in his/her opinion is outside his/her research competence or not possible within the resources available.

e. Any nurse commissioning or taking part in commissioning a project should make every effort to use such findings as have implications for the work in hand.

PART III: NURSES PRACTISING IN PLACES WHERE RESEARCH IS BEING CARRIED OUT

1. RESPONSIBILITIES AS A PRACTITIONER

a. Nurses in the course of their normal, non-research duties may be called upon to act as witnesses that free and informed consent has been obtained from patients/clients in relation to research. They should satisfy themselves that the patient/client has understood what he is agreeing to and any risks or discomforts involved and that he is entitled to withdraw at any time.

b. In the event of research seen to be having an adverse effect upon a subject the nurse practitioner has an obligation to intervene by informing the researcher and the appropriate person in authority.

c. Nurses asked to participate in research as data collectors in addition to their duties have an obligation to make it known if these extra activities will be or have become detrimental to their normal work.

2. RESPONSIBILITIES AS DATA COLLECTORS

a. Nurses agreeing to assist with data collection must adhere to the ethical code binding on all research workers. This includes accuracy and integrity in data collecting.

b. Nurses acting as data collectors must recognize that they are now committed to two separate roles. Information which is confidential to them as nurses cannot be made available to the research team unless this has been previously agreed by the nurse in consultation with an ethical committee. Data collected for a research team is confidential to the research team and cannot be used in daily work or for any other purpose without permission of the head of the research team and the subject.

c. Nurses invited to participate in trials of commercial products must exercise special care to avoid being involved in inappropriate methods of data collection and any association with advertising of a product.

Moral Justification

LEON EISENBERG

The Social Imperatives of Medical Research

Peculiar to this time[1] is the need to restate a proposition that, a decade ago, would have been regarded as self-evident, namely, that fostering excellence in medical research is in the public interest. Contemporary news accounts and learned journals alike have announced as exposé what always has been true: that doctors are fallible, that researchers are not all noble, and that what appeared to be true in the light of yesterday's evidence proves false by tomorrow's. The sins committed in the name of medical research are stressed in entire disproportion to the human gains that continue to flow from the enterprise. That a significant amount of funded research will inevitably fail to yield the expected answers is taken as a sign of boondoggling, because the nature of science is not understood. We are asked for guarantees of absolute safety as if this were an attainable goal.

Some of the specific criticism has been just and instructive, some of it merely misinformed, some of it completely irrelevant. A constructive response to the criticism of medical research would have been easier had not distrust been aroused at the same time by the misapplications of technical knowledge (the spread of weapons systems, wire tapping, computerization, nuclear wastes) and the use of technical devices by government against its own people. Those of us who argue for the necessity of scientific research in

[handwritten marginalia: totalities in tonsillectomies but not experimentation gain would not der...]

medicine are too often regarded as if we were indifferent to misuses of it and as though we were apologists for the Establishment. I know of no remedy other than to redouble our effort to explain the nature and the justification of well-designed medical research, the calculus of risk and benefit that is an integral part of it, and the design of methods to maximize its potential for gain. If we permit it to be circumscribed with a bureaucracy of regulation so cumbersome as to impede its progress, we incur a risk to society from the restriction of medical science that will far outweigh the aggregate risk to all the subjects in experimental studies.

[handwritten: don't burden]

MEDICAL PRACTICE AND MEDICAL RESEARCH

One source of misunderstanding is the confusion of what is usual and customary in medical practice with what is safe and useful. The critics of research are often exquisitely aware of the dangers in an experiment (indeed, the responsible investigator is at pains to spell them out as precisely as he or she can). At the same time, these critics, surprisingly naive about the extent to which medical practice rests on custom rather than evidence, fail to appreciate the necessity for controlled trials to determine whether what is traditional does harm rather than good.

Consider, for example, the fact that about 1 million tonsillectomies and adenoidectomies are done each year in the United States; T and A's make up 30 percent of all surgery on children. Set aside budgetary considerations, even though the outlay—about $500 million—represents a significant "opportunity cost" in resources lost to more useful medical care.[2] During the 1950s, T and A's resulted in some 200 to 300 deaths per year.[3] Current mortality has been estimated at one death per 16,000 operations.[4] Yet this procedure (whose origins are lost in antiquity) continues at epidemic rates though there is no evidence that it is effective[5] except for a few uncommon conditions.[6] Doctors disagree so widely about the "indications" for T and A that within one state (Vermont) there is a fivefold variation by area of residence in the probability that a person will have his or her tonsils removed by age 20.[7] Thus, we have a procedure of dubious value employed at high frequency despite significant mortality and dollar costs. Why? It is done because doctors and parents believe in it; having become usual and customary, it is not subject to the systematic scrutiny of an experimental design.

Compare the human cost from this single routine and relatively minor procedure to the risk to human subjects in nontherapeutic and therapeutic research. Cardon and his colleagues[8] surveyed investigators conducting research on 133,000 human subjects over the past 3 years. In nontherapeutic research, which involved some 93,000 subjects, there was not one fatality, there was only one instance of permanent disability (0.001 percent), and there were 37 cases of temporary disability (0.04 percent). In therapeutic research (that is, clinical research carried out on sick people who stood to benefit directly from the knowledge gained), among 39,000 patients, 43 died (0.1 percent) and 13 suffered permanent disability (0.03 percent). (Most of the deaths were of patients on cancer chemotherapy.) The risk to experimental subjects in nontherapeutic research is comparable to the rates for accidental injury in the general population (when one makes appropriate calculation for days of risk per year). Tonsillectomy, a relatively minor surgical procedure, produces more deaths per 100,000 each year than the total from all nontherapeutic research! If we add into our calculation the deaths resulting from major surgical procedures that may be performed more often than is warranted—for example, the current rate of 647 hysterectomies per 100,000 females projects to loss of the uterus for half the female population by age 65[9]—and from excessive and injudicious prescription of powerful drugs, it becomes clear that the gain in public safety from exacting scrutiny of medical practice by means of controlled trials would far outweigh any possible gain from the most restrictive approach to medical research. Let me not be misunderstood: I do not deny the necessity for surveillance of the ethics of the research community; the point I stress is that medical research, applied to medical practice, stands alone in its ability to avert unnecessary human suffering and death.

THE SOURCES OF MEDICAL ERROR

Among the reasons given for the persistence of medical error are venality on the part of physicians, professional incompetence, and lack of commitment to the public weal. There are venal physicians; we need look no further than the exposure of Medicaid mills to find them. But that hardly accounts for the overprescription of surgery when we recognize that surgery is performed on physicians' families even more often than it is on the general public[10]; physicians as consumers follow the advice they proffer as providers. There are incompetent doctors, and we still lack adequate methods for weeding them out; but anesthetic and surgical deaths occur in the best of hands because of the risks inherent in the procedures. Not all doctors are actuated by the public interest, but this hardly explains what concerns us about physician behavior. Although these factors contribute to wrong-headedness in medical practice, a far more important source is simply the doctor's conviction that what he or she does is for the patient's welfare. When good evidence is lacking, the best and most dedicated of us do wrong in the utter conviction of being right.

BLOODLETTING AS PANACEA

Let me offer a historical illustration from the career of a man with many admirable qualities, a leading U.S. physician of the late 18th century. Benjamin Rush was uncommon among his peers in having a university degree in medicine (from Edinburgh); he was appointed professor of chemistry at the College of Philadelphia (soon to become the Medical School of the University of Pennsylvania, the first medical school in America) and later professor of the institute and practices of medicine. He was among the most steadfast of patriots, a signer of the Declaration of Independence, a member of the Pennsylvania delegation that voted to adopt the Constitution of the United States, and a founder of the first antislavery society.[11] His book *Medical Inquiries and Observations upon the Diseases of the Mind* was the first comprehensive American treatise on mental illness.[12] Thus, we have a physician with as good an education as his time could provide, a leading member of the faculty of the premier school of medicine, and a man dedicated to the public interest.

In 1793, a severe epidemic of yellow fever fell upon the city of Philadelphia.[13] It is estimated that more than one-third of its population of 50,000 fled the city and that more than 4,000 lives were lost. Panic beset the medical community, and doctors were among those who took flight to escape the pestilence. From illness and defection at the height of the epidemic, only three physicians were available to treat more than 6,000 patients. Rush dispatched his wife and children to the safety of the countryside and remained behind to fulfill his medical responsibility.

Rush was an adherent of the Brunonian system of medicine, according to which febrile illnesses re-sulted from an excess of stimulation and a corresponding excitement of the blood. In keeping with this theory, he ministered to his patients by vigorous bleeding and purging, the latter to "divert the force of the fever to [the bowels] and thereby save the liver and brains from a fatal and dangerous congestion." Rush went from patient to patient, letting blood copiously and purging with vigor. His desperate remedies, contemporary critics contended, were more dangerous than the disease, a criticism history has borne out.

His beliefs were not something he reserved for others. He himself was taken with a violent fever. He instructed his assistant to bleed him "plentifully" and give him "a dose of the mercurial medicine." From illness and treatment combined, he almost died; his convalescence was prolonged. That he did recover persuaded him that his methods were correct. Thus, when the epidemic subsided, he wrote: "Never before did I experience such sublime joy as I now felt on contemplating the success of my remedies. . . . The conquest of a formidable disease was through the triumph of a principle in medicine."[14] Neither dedication so great that he risked his life to minister to others, nor willingness to treat himself as he treated others, nor yet the best education to be had in his day was sufficient to prevent Rush from committing grievous harm in the name of doing good. Convinced of the correctness of his theory of medicine and lacking a means for the systematic study of treatment outcome, he attributed each new instance of improvement to the efficacy of his treatment and each new death that occurred despite it to the severity of the disease.

INTRODUCTION OF THE NUMERICAL METHOD

Bloodletting continued to be a widely used medical remedy until the middle of the 19th century. Accordint to Osler,[15] it was finally abandoned because of the introduction into American medicine of the "numerical method" of the French physician Pierre Charles Alexandre Louis. Louis had been disenchanted with his medical education and his experience as a practitioner. He withdrew from practice to devote himself to study. As one contemporary commented:[15]

He consecrated the whole of his time and talent to rigorous, impartial observation. All private practice was relinquished and he allowed no considerations of personal emolument to interfere with the resolution he had formed. For some time, his extreme minuteness in inquiry and accuracy of descrip-

Louis's observation led to stopping bloodletting

tion were the subjects of sneering and ridicule, and "to what end?" was not infrequently and tauntingly asked.

One result of his study, an essay on bloodletting, appeared in Paris in 1835.[16] Within a year, it was translated into English by G. C. Putnam.[17] In a preface to the volume James Jackson, physician to the Massachusetts General Hospital, wrote:[18]

If anything may be regarded as settled in the treatment of diseases, it is that bloodletting is useful in the class of diseases called inflammatory; and especially in inflammation of the thoracic viscera. To this general opinion or belief on this subject, M. Louis gives support by his observations; but the result of these observations is that the benefits derived from bleeding in the diseases, which he has here examined, are not so great and striking as they had been represented by many teachers. If the same methods should be obtained by others, after making observations as rigorous as M. Louis, many of us will be forced to modify our former opinions. . . . The author does not pretend that the questions, here discussed, are decided forever. He makes a valuable contribution to the evidence, on which they must be decided; he points out the mode, in which this evidence should be collected, and in which its material should be analyzed; seeking truth only, he calls on others to adduce facts, which, being gathered from various quarters, may show us, with a good degree of exactness, the precise value of the remedy in question.

Louis himself began his monograph with the comment:[19]

The results of my researches on the effects of bloodletting in inflammation are so little in accord with the general opinion, that it is not without a degree of hesitation I have decided to publish them. After having analyzed the facts, which relate to them, for the first time, I thought myself deceived, and began my work anew; but having again from this new analysis, obtained the same results, I could no longer doubt their correctness.

He was led to conclude:

We infer that bloodletting has had very little influence on the progress of pneumonitis . . .; that its influence has not been more evident in the cases bled copiously and repeatedly, than in those bled only once and to a small amount; that we do not at once arrest inflammations, as is too often finally imagined; that, in cases where it appears to be otherwise, it is undoubtedly owing, either to an error in diagnosis, or to the fact that the bloodletting was practiced at an advanced period of the disease, when it had nearly run its course.

Yet, so strong was the power of authority, that he was moved to comment:[20]

I will add that bloodletting, notwithstanding its influence is limited, should not be neglected in inflammations which are severe and are seated in an important organ.

Louis's precise observations, his stress on the importance of studying series of cases, and his insistence on reexamining standard belief were to have an enormous influence. Many American physicians went to Paris to become his pupils and returned to these shores persuaded of the value of his method. Insofar as it can be said that any single contribution led to the abandonment on this continent of bloodletting as a panacea, it was Louis's numerical method. It had its roots in the earlier applications of elementary statistics to public health and became far more powerful as a method when the concepts of probability statistics were applied to its simple tabulations.[21] From these beginnings stems much of the progress in medical science.

IMPORTANCE OF CLINICAL DESCRIPTION AND CLASSIFICATION

I have thus far stressed the contributions of the controlled clinical trial[22] to the provision of more effective remedies and to the elimination of harmful ones. But before physicians can treat, they must be able to discriminate disorders one from another. Here, careful delineation of desease patterns, both immediate and longitudinal, and attention to ways in which patients resemble and differ from each other provide the necessary groundwork for identifying the underlying pathophysiology. The process begins with the report of a puzzling and hitherto undescribed group of cases. Initially attention is directed at differentiating the new syndrome from superficially similar conditions. Some decades pass during which doctors disagree on the diagnosis and include or exclude a penumbra of cases which markedly affect the reported outcome. Next a fundamental pathogenic lesion is discovered, and confirmed by other workers, to be present in "typical" cases. As the mechanism of the disease is clarified, the disease itself is redefined in terms of the underlying pathology. Now new and variant clinical forms can be identified, cases that would not have met the original criteria. Let me illustrate this by an example from hematology.

In 1925 Cooley and Lee separated out from the group of childhood anemias (known as von Jaksch's anemia) five cases with hepatosplenomegaly, skin pigmentation, thick bones, and oddly shaped red cells with decreased osmotic fragility. Cooley's anemia was renamed thalassemia in 1932 by Whipple and Bradford, who noted that the children came from families of Mediterranean origin. The genetic basis of thalassemia was established by Wintrobe in 1940 in a paper which distinguished thalassemia minor (the heterozygous state) from thalassemia major (the homozygous state). Fifteen years later Kunkel discovered the normal minor hemoglobin component hemoglobin A_2 and found it to be elevated in individuals with thalassemia minor.[23] A subsequent explosion of research on the hemoglobin molecule has led to the recognition of some 50 combinations of genetic errors which can produce the clinical picture of thalassemia. . . .

BASIC RESEARCH AND DISEASE PREVENTION

Hand in hand with the controlled clinical trial and with the continuing search for diagnostic precision must go fundamental research in basic biology. Much of our armamentarium for the treatment and prevention of disease is at the level of what Lewis Thomas[24] has called "halfway technology," measures which, though useful, only partly reverse the disease process, are costly, and are toxic. Consider the situation this nation faced not long ago in coping with poliomyelitis. Each year it took 2,000 lives and left 3,000 persons with severe paralysis. The hospital cost for acute and chronic care, the iron lung, the wet pack, and physiotherapy exceeded $1 billion a year. For an investment of $40 million in the basic research which led to Ender's method of cultivating the polio virus in the chick embryo, and not more than several hundred million dollars for applied technology and population trials, an enormous human and financial loss has been averted.[25]

The psychiatrist today is in the position of the pediatrician a generation ago. Chemotherapy aborts acute psychotic episodes, but recurrence is common, permanent disability frequent, and drug toxicity considerable. We have strong evidence for familial predisposition but cannot specify modes of inheritance or what is inherited, or distinguish the potential patient before illness occurs. The hope of prevention must rest upon increased support for fundamental research in neurobiology, genetics, and epidemiology.[26] The problem is not a gap in the application of knowledge but a gap in knowledge itself.

Basic research does not begin and end with molecular biology. Vaccination provides a model for infectious diseases and perhaps even for neoplasms; it is simply irrelevant to behavior-linked health problems: the consequences of smoking, overeating, drinking, drugging, and reckless driving. Belloc and Breslow have shown that seven personal health habits sum to a powerful prediction of morbidity[27] and mortality[28] for middle-aged adults. To recognize that cultural patterns, social forces, and idiosyncratic personal behaviors have major effects on health[29] is not equivalent to knowing how to alter them. It does, however, argue for the urgency of research in the social as well as the biological sciences if physicians are to learn how to intervene effectively.[30]

THE RESTRICTION OF RISK
AND THE RISK OF RESTRICTION

Health will be held hazard to custom until the current preoccupation with the dangers of research is placed in the appropriate context: namely, weighing in the very same scales the dangers of not doing research. Surveillance of research ethics requires simultaneous assessment of the scientific and the ethical soundness of the protocols themselves. "A poorly or improperly designed study involving human subjects—one that could not possibly yield scientific facts (that is, reproducible observations) relevant to the question under study—is by definition unethical.[31] Commendation for a high rate of rejection of research proposals implies that the proper goal for a research review committee is blocking human studies. To the contrary, the systematic imposition of impediments to significant therapeutic research is itself unethical because an important benefit is being denied to the community.

This is not a call for unrestricted rights for medical researchers. If I do not accept the view that medical researchers are worse than lawyers or philosophers, I will not argue that they are better. They are simply human; that is to say, fallible. As in the case of all professional activity, social controls are necessary. But in establishing those controls, it is necessary to weigh fully the possible resultant losses. The decision not to do something poses as many ethical quandaries as the decision to do it. Not to act is to act.[32]

Important ethical issues in medical research have been overlooked in the preoccupation with ethical absolutes. Consider, for example, the clear social class bias in the likelihood of being a subject in a medical experiment. For that there can be no justification. Even if risk in research be inevitable, inequity in exposure because of caste or class need not be. The patients on whom clinical research is most often done are clinic patients, those who by reason of economic circumstance and education are the least able to assert their rights against medical authority.

It was not long ago, to our shame, that this practice was explicitly justified on the ground that the poor paid society back for the "privilege" of receiving charitable care by being suitable clinical material for research and teaching. Few would defend that position in so callous a way today. Yet the practice continues, less by plan than by fallout from our two-track medical care system. Researchers are located in teaching hospitals. Teaching hospitals are a major medical resource for the poor. The poor become the patients on whom studies are done because of their convenience as a study population and our insensitivity to the injustice of the practice. It is not enough to say that we now offer explanation and choice and obtain informed consent. Indeed, we do. But the quality of consent is not the same when the social position of doctor and patient are disparate as it is when they are more nearly equals.

Enhancing the human quality of the community in which we live is the responsibility of every citizen; one way to meet that responsibility is by sharing in the risks of the search to diminish human suffering. Richard Titmuss[33] has pointed to the health benefits to the United Kingdom from a public policy based on a voluntary blood donor system [but see Sapolsky and Finkelstein for a contrary view[34]]. I suggest that there will be moral gain as well as health gain to the United States to the extent that we succeed in creating a community of shared responsibility for health research.

INFORMED CONSENT IN THE ABSENCE OF INFORMATION

What does "informed" consent mean in the real world of medical practice? When risks are specifiable so that it is possible to make a rational decision by weighing alternatives, it is clearly the physician's duty to inform the patient fully. That has long been a hallmark of good medical practice and sound clinical

investigation; it is no contemporary discovery. But what does "informed" mean when what is available to the physician, let alone the patient, is not information but noise? In what sense is there a choice to be made between treatment A and treatment B if there is no proof that either works or that one is superior to the other? What right have I lost if, in a national health scheme, I am assigned to a randomized trial without being asked my preference, when that preference can only be capricious? The very justification for a randomized trial is that there is insufficient information to permit a rational, that is, informed, choice. In a free society we will reserve the right for any citizen to opt out. But when we respect the privilege to be guided by superstition, astrology, or simple orneriness, let us drop the adjective "informed" and speak only of "consent."

DO WE NEED MEDICAL RESEARCH?

A major undercurrent in the criticism of medical research is a growing belief that it is basically irrelevant to contemporary human needs. The argument runs something like this: what doctors do has only marginal effects on health; anyway, what researchers learn, when it does add to knowledge, doesn't get into practice; besides, from a higher moral view, what really matters is learning to live with the existential realities of pain and dying and not to permit technical iatrogenesis to alienate man from his nature.[35] To what extent is this credible?

There is good evidence for the proposition that the increase in longevity over the past century in industrialized nations has been principally the result of social forces: better nutrition, better hygiene, and changed behavior.[36] An instructive example is the striking decline in mortality from tuberculosis over the last 100 years, with only a small additional decrement visible after the introduction of streptomycin. But there is no assurance that further social change will eliminate the residual cases. Moreover, chemotherapy is decisive in the treatment of the tuberculosis that is still with us; the lack of a prominent effect on aggregate mortality statistics reflects the lesser prevalence of the disease as a public health problem, not the ineffectiveness of treatment. But the major defect of the proposition, as a general indictment of medical care, is at a more fundamental level. Doctors, at best, postpone death; death itself is inevitable. Most of what doctors do is to mitigate discomfort and pain and to enhance function in the presence of chronic disease, an effect that is not registered in mortality tables.[37] Sole reliance on longevity and mortality leaves unmeasured the benefits most patients consult doctors for and the major benefits they have always derived from them.[38] Morbidity rates, and the consequent demand for medical resources,[39] cannot be predicted from mortality data.[40]

The second theme, the failure to translate research into practice, . . . is grossly exaggerated. Lag undoubtedly occurs in the transfer of medical skills from highly specialized centers to rural areas; the much more troublesome problem is the indiscriminate introduction into practice of new drugs and surgical innovations well before their indications and limitations are clear, often in such ways as to compromise their usefulness. The major barriers to the treatment of life-threatening disease stem not from failing to use what we know but from not knowing what to use.

Eighty percent of the deaths in this country are caused by cardiovascular, neoplastic, cerebrovascular, and renal disease.[24] For the very great majority of the specific disorders within these categories the treatments we have are only palliatives. Palliatives are important, and certainly they should be distributed fairly; but the most evenhanded and prompt distribution of all available remedies would have only a small effect on death rates. As to resource allocation, the percentage of the health dollar (well under 2 percent) devoted to applied and basic medical research in toto is so small a part of total health costs that complete diversion of those funds would have negligible effects on health care delivery. The one clear result would be to end all prospect for improving the quality of the care delivered.

The idea that pain and dying are integral parts of man's fate, though put forth as a truism, is in fact a theological view of the human condition.[35] To comprehend its meaning, it is necessary to ask: How much pain? Death at what age? Whose pain and whose death? By what standards: today's or a century ago's, white American or black American, Indian or African? Perhaps, with a life expectancy exceeding the Biblical threescore and ten, affluent white Americans can afford the luxury of wondering whether medical research makes much sense in view of the risks and costs it entails. That is, we can if we mistake our fate for man's fate, ourselves for all of humankind.

A THIRD WORLD PERSPECTIVE ON RESEARCH

The armchair view of medical research as fun and games undergoes radical transformation from the standpoint of the third world, where infant mortality may be as high as 20 percent and life expectancy no more than 30 years. "People are sick because they are poor, they become poorer because they are sick and they become sicker because they are poorer."[41] Six infectious diseases that are almost unknown on our shores plague Africa, Asia, and Latin America: Malaria afflicts an estimated quarter billion; the mosquito that spreads it is becoming resistant to the standard pesticides and the plasmodium to chloroquin. Trypanosomiasis afflicts perhaps 20 million; we lack effective weapons against either the vector or the parasite; the treatment in use can be more dangerous than the disease. Leishmaniasis claims some 12 million; there is no known treatment. Filariasis and onchocerciasis infect 300 million; treatment is ineffective. Schistosomiasis afflicts 250 million; as nations attempt to improve their agricultural productivity through irrigation, the snail vector multiplies. Finally, there are 12 to 15 million lepers in the world; the current treatment requires 7 years; drug-resistant lepra bacilli have begun to appear.

In the face of all this, there is a clear moral imperative in developed nations for medical research in tropical diseases, to seek to permit two-thirds of the world's population to share in the freedom from pain and untimely death we have achieved for ourselves. In the forceful words of Barry Bloom:[41]

Discourse about medicine and ethics has focused almost entirely on problems of a wealthy society, and relatively little attention has been given to those affecting the vast majority of people in the world. There is a preponderant concern with individualism and individual rights, most recently reflected in the enormous preoccupation with death and dying. Imagine the impact of the anguished disquisitions about the Karen Quinlan case on the reader in Bangladesh or Upper Volta. The public agitation over "pulling the plug" on a single machine seems almost perverse when juxtaposed against the unmet health needs, the desperate struggle for survival of millions of people around the globe. I do not deny that there are serious problems of individual liberty at stake or that the Quinlan case may serve as a model for delimiting the role of the family, physician, or state in authorizing medical treatment for those unable to speak for themselves. But when the model so fills the horizon as to obscure the reality, then all perspective is lost.

•   •   •

Because science is incomplete, reason imperfect, and both can be put to damaging uses, some would abandon science and reason in favor of mysticism, hermeneutics, and transcendental rapture. It is not knowledge but ignorance that assures misery. It is not science but its employment for inhuman purposes that threatens our survival. The fundamental ethical questions of science are political questions:[42] Who shall control its products? For what purposes shall they be employed?

Four years after the community protests against the dangers of [Louis Pasteur's] research, the citizens of France, by public subscriptions in gratitude for his contribution to human welfare, erected the Pasteur Institute. In the ceremony of dedication, Pasteur, overcome by his feelings, asked his son to read his remarks, which concluded:[43]

Two opposing laws seem to be now in contest. The one, a law of blood and of death, ever imagining new means of destruction, forces nations always to be ready for battle. The other, a law of peace, work and health, ever evolving means of delivering man from the scourges which beset him. The one seeks violent conquests, the other the relief of humanity. The one places a single life above all victories, the other sacrifices hundreds of thousands of lives to the ambition of a single individual. The law of which we are the instruments strives even in the midst of carnage to cure the wounds due to the law of war. Treatment by our antiseptic methods may save the lives of thousands of soldiers. Which of these two laws will ultimately prevail, God alone knows. But this we may assert: that French science will have tried, by obeying the law of Humanity, to extend the frontiers of life.

NOTES

1. A. Etzioni and C. Nunn, *Daedalus* 103, 191 (1974).

2. H. H. Hiatt, *N. Engl. J. Med.* 293, 235 (1975).

3. H. Bakwin, *J. Pediatr.* 52, 339 (1958).

4. L. W. Pratt, *Trans. Am. Acad. Ophthalmol. Otolaryngol.* 74, 1146 (1970).

5. W. Shaikh, E. Vayda, W. Feldman, *Pediatrics* 57, 401 (1976).

6. C. Guilleminault, F. L. Eldridge, F. B. Simons, W. C. Dement, *ibid.* 58, 23 (1976).

7. J. Wennberg and A. Gittelsohn, *Science* 182, 1102 (1973).

8. P. V. Cardon, F. W. Dommel, R. R. Trumble, *N. Engl. J. Med.* 295, 650 (1976).

9. J. Bunker, V. C. Donahue, P. Cole, M. Notman, *ibid.,* p. 264.

10. J. Bunker and B. Brown, *ibid.,* 290, 1051 (1974).

11. G. W. Corner, *The Autobiography of Benjamin Rush* (Princeton Univ. Press, Princeton, N.J., 1948).

12. B. Rush, *Medical Inquiries and Observations Upon the Diseases of the Mind* (Kimber & Richardson, Philadelphia, 1812; reprinted by Hafner, New York, 1962).

13. W. S. Middleton, *Ann. Med. Hist.* 10, 434 (1928).

14. *Ibid.,* p. 442.

15. W. Osler, *Bull. Johns Hopkins Hosp.* 8, 161 (1897).

16. W. J. Gaines and H. G. Langford, *Arch. Intern. Med.* 106, 571 (1960).

17. P. C. A. Louis, *Researches on the Effects of Bloodletting in Some Inflammatory Diseases and on the Influence of Tartarized Antimony and Vesication in Pneumonitis,* translated by C. G. Putnam with preface and appendix by J. Jackson (Hilliard, Gray, Boston, 1836).

18. *Ibid.,* pp. v–vi.

19. *Ibid.,* p. 1.

20. *Ibid.,* p. 22.

21. G. Rosen, *Bull. Hist. Med.* 29, 27 (1955).

22. A. L. Cochrane, *Effectiveness and Efficiency: Random Reflections on Health Services* (Nuffield Provincial Hospitals Trust, London, 1972).

23. D. J. Weatherall, *Johns Hopkins Med. J.* 139, 194 (1976).

24. L. Thomas, *Daedalus* 106, 35 (1977).

25. H. H. Fudenberg, *J. Invest. Dermatol.* 61, 321 (1973).

26. L. Eisenberg, *Bull. N.Y. Acad. Med.* 51, 118 (1975).

27. N. B. Belloc and L. Breslow, *Prev. Med.* 1, 409 (1972).

28. ———, *ibid.* 2, 67 (1973).

29. L. Eisenberg, *N. Engl. J. Med.* 296, 903 (1977).

30. A. Kleinman, L. Eisenberg, B. Good, *Ann. Intern. Med.,* 88, 251 (1978).

31. D. D. Rutstein, *Daedalus* 98, 523 (1969).

32. L. Eisenberg, *J. Child Psychol. Psychiatr.* 16, 93 (1975).

33. R. Titmuss, *The Gift Relationship: From Human Blood to Social Policy* (Pantheon, New York, 1971).

34. H. M. Sapolsky and S. N. Finkelstein, *Public Interest* (Winter, 1977), p. 15.

35. I. Illich, *Medical Nemesis: The Expropriation of Health* (Calder & Boyars, London, 1975).

36. T. McKeown, *The Role of Medicine: Dream, Mirage or Nemesis?* (Nuffield Provincial Hospitals Trust, London, 1976).

37. W. McDermott, *Daedalus* 106, 135 (1977).

38. L. Eisenberg, in *Research and Medical Practice* (Ciba Foundation Symposium 44, Elsevier/Excerpta Medica/North-Holland, Amsterdam, 1976), pp. 3–23.

39. A. Barr and R. F. L. Logan, *Lancet* 1977-I, 994 (1977).

40. D. P. Forster, *ibid.,* p. 997.

41. B. R. Bloom, *Hastings Center Rep.* 6, 9 (1976).

42. L. Eisenberg, *J. Med. Philos.* 1, 318 (1976).

43. R. Vallery-Radot, *The Life of Pasteur* (Doubleday, Page, Garden City, N.Y., 1923), p. 444.

HANS JONAS

Philosophical Reflections on Experimenting with Human Subjects

Experimenting with human subjects is going on in many fields of scientific and technological progress. It is designed to replace the overall instruction by natural, occasional experience with the selective information from artificial, systematic experiment which physical science has found so effective in dealing with inanimate nature. Of the new experimentation with man, medical is surely the most legitimate; psychological, the most dubious; biological (still to come), the most dangerous. I have chosen here to deal with the first only, where the case *for* it is strongest and the task of adjudicating conflicting claims hardest. . . .

THE PECULIARITY OF HUMAN EXPERIMENTATION

Experimentation was originally sanctioned by natural science. There it is performed on inanimate objects, and this raises no moral problems. But as soon as animate, feeling beings become the subjects of experiment, as they do in the life sciences and especially in medical research, this innocence of the search for knowledge is lost and questions of conscience arise. The depth to which moral and religious sensibilities can become aroused over these questions is shown by the vivisection issue. Human experimentation must sharpen the issue as it involves ultimate questions of personal dignity and sacrosanctity. One profound difference between the human experiment and the physical (besides that between animate and inanimate, feeling and unfeeling nature) is this: The physical experiment employs small-scale, artificially devised substitutes for that about which

knowledge is to be obtained, and the experimenter extrapolates from these models and simulated conditions to nature at large. Something deputizes for the "real thing"—balls rolling down an inclined plane for sun and planets, electric discharges from a condenser for real lightning, and so on. For the most part, no such substitution is possible in the biological sphere. We must operate on the original itself, the real thing in the fullest sense, and perhaps affect it irreversibly. No simulacrum can take its place. Especially in the human sphere, experimentation loses entirely the advantage of the clear division between vicarious model and true object. Up to a point, animals may fulfill the proxy role of the classical physical experiment. But in the end man himself must furnish knowledge about himself, and the comfortable separation of noncommittal experiment and definitive action vanishes. An experiment in education affects the lives of its subjects, perhaps a whole generation of schoolchildren. Human experimentation for whatever purpose is always *also* a responsible, nonexperimental, definitive dealing with the subject himself. And not even the noblest purpose abrogates the obligations this involves.

This is the root of the problem with which we are faced: Can both that purpose and this obligation be satisfied? If not, what would be a just compromise? Which side should give way to the other? The question is inherently philosophical as it concerns not merely pragmatic difficulties and their arbitration, but a genuine conflict of values involving principles of a high order. May I put conflict in these terms. On principle, it is felt, human beings *ought* not to be dealt with in that way (the "guinea pig" protest); on the other hand, such dealings are increasingly urged on us by considerations, in turn appealing to principle, that claim to override those objections. Such a claim must be carefully assessed, especially when it is swept

Reprinted with permission of George Braziller, Inc. from *Experimentation with Human Subjects* by Paul A. Freund (ed.). Copyright © 1969, 1970 by the American Academy of Arts and Sciences. This essay is included, on pp. 105–131, in a 1980 reedition of Jonas's *Philosophical Essays: From Current Creed to Technological Man*, published by the University of Chicago Press.

along by a mighty tide. Putting the matter thus, we have already made one important assumption rooted in our "Western" cultural tradition: The prohibitive rule is, to that way of thinking, the primary and axiomatic one; the permissive counter-rule, as qualifying the first, is secondary and stands in need of justification. We must justify the infringement of a primary inviolability, which needs no justification itself; and the justification of its infringement must be by values and needs of a dignity commensurate with those to be sacrificed.

. . .

HEALTH AS A PUBLIC GOOD

The cause invoked [for medical experimentation] is health and, in its more critical aspect, life itself—clearly superlative goods that the physician serves directly by curing and the researcher indirectly by the knowledge gained through his experiments. There is no question about the good served or about the evil fought—disease and premature death. But a good to whom and an evil to whom? Here the issue tends to become somewhat clouded. In the attempt to give experimentation the proper dignity (on the problematic view that a value becomes greater by being "social" instead of merely individual), the health in question or the disease in question is somehow predicated on the social whole, as if it were society that, in the persons of its members, enjoyed the one and suffered the other. For the purposes of our problem, public interest can then be pitted against private interest, the common good against the individual good. Indeed, I have found health called a national resource, which, of course it is, but surely not in the first place.

In trying to resolve some of the complexities and ambiguities lurking in these conceptualizations, I have pondered a particular statement, made in the form of a question, which I found in the *Proceedings* of the earlier *Daedalus* conference: "Can society afford to discard the tissues and organs of the hopelessly unconscious patient when they could be used to restore the otherwise hopelessly ill, but still salvageable individual?" And somewhat later: "A strong case can be made that society can ill afford to discard the tissues and organs of the hopelessly unconscious patient; they are greatly needed for study and experimental trial to help those who can be salvaged."[1] I hasten to add that any suspicion of callousness that the "commodity" language of these statements may suggest is immediately dispelled by the name of the speaker, Dr. Henry K. Beecher, for whose humanity and moral

sensibility there can be nothing but admiration. But the use, in all innocence, of this language gives food for thought. Let me, for a moment, take the question literally. "Discarding" implies proprietary rights—nobody can discard what does not belong to him in the first place. Does society then own my body? "Salvaging" implies the same and, moreover, a use-value to the owner. Is the life-extension of certain individuals then a public interest? "Affording" implies a critically vital level of such an interest—that is, of the loss or gain involved. And "society" itself—what is it? When does a need, an aim, an obligation become social? Let us reflect on some of these terms.

WHAT SOCIETY CAN AFFORD

"Can Society afford . . .?" Afford what? To let people die intact, thereby withholding something from other people who desperately need it, who in consequence will have to die too? These other, unfortunate people indeed cannot afford not to have a kidney, heart, or other organ of the dying patient, on which they depend for an extension of their lease on life; but does that give them a right to it? And does it oblige society to procure it for them? What is it that *society* can or cannot afford—leaving aside for the moment the question of what it has a *right* to? It surely can afford to lose members through death; more than that, it is built on the balance of death and birth decreed by the order of life. This is too general, of course, for our question, but perhaps it is well to remember. The specific question seems to be whether society can afford to let some people die whose death might be deferred by particular means if these were authorized by society. Again, if it is merely a question of what society can or cannot afford, rather than of what it ought or ought not to do, the answer must be: Of course, it can. If cancer, heart disease, and other organic, noncontagious ills, especially those tending to strike the old more than the young, continue to exact their toll at the normal rate of incidence (including the toll of private anguish and misery), society can go on flourishing in every way.

Here, by contrast, are some examples of what, in sober truth, society cannot afford. It cannot afford to let an epidemic rage unchecked; a persistent excess of deaths over births, but neither—we must add—too great an excess of births over deaths; too low an average life expectancy even if demographically balanced by fertility, but neither too great a longevity with the necessitated correlative dearth of youth in the social body; a debilitating state of general health; and things of this kind. These are plain cases where the whole condition of society is critically affected, and the public interest can make its imperative claims. The Black Death of the Middle Ages was a *public* calamity of the acute kind; the life-sapping ravages of endemic malaria or sleeping sickness in certain areas are a public calamity of the chronic kind. Such situations a society as a whole can truly not "afford," and they may call for extraordinary remedies, including, perhaps, the invasion of private sacrosanctities.

This is not entirely a matter of numbers and numerical ratios. Society, in a subtler sense, cannot "afford" a single miscarriage of justice, a single inequity in the dispensation of its laws, the violation of the rights of even the tiniest minority, because these undermine the moral basis on which society's existence rests. Nor can it, for a similar reason, afford the absence or atrophy in its midst of compassion and of the effort to alleviate suffering—be it widespread or rare—one form of which is the effort to conquer disease of any kind, whether "socially" significant (by reason of number) or not. And in short, society cannot afford the absence among its members of *virtue*, with its readiness for sacrifice beyond defined duty. Since its presence—that is to say, that of personal idealism—is a matter of grace and not of decree, we have the paradox that society depends for its existence on intangibles of nothing less than a religious order, for which it can hope, but which it cannot enforce. All the more must it protect this most precious capital from abuse.

For what objectives connected with the medico-biological sphere should this reserve be drawn upon—for example, in the form of accepting, soliciting, perhaps even imposing the submission of human subjects to experimentation? We postulate that this must be not just a worthy cause, as any promotion of the health of anybody doubtlessly is, but a cause qualifying for transcedent social sanction. Here one thinks first of those cases critically affecting the whole condition, present and future, of the community we have illustrated. Something equivalent to what in the political sphere is called "clear and present danger" may be invoked and a state of emergency proclaimed, thereby suspending certain otherwise inviolable prohibitions and taboos. We may observe that averting a disaster always carries greater weight than promoting a good. Extraordinary danger excuses extraordinary means. This covers human experimentation, which we would like to count, as far as possible, among the extraordinary rather than the ordinary means of serving the common good under public auspices. Naturally, since foresight and responsibility for the future are of the essence of institutional society, averting disaster extends into long-term prevention, although the lesser urgency will warrant less sweeping licenses.

SOCIETY AND THE CAUSE OF PROGRESS

Much weaker is the case where it is a matter not of saving but of improving society. Much of medical research falls into this category. As stated before, a permanent death rate from heart failure or cancer does not threaten society. So long as certain statistical ratios are maintained, the incidence of disease and of disease-induced mortality is not (in the strict sense) a "social" misfortune. I hasten to add that it is not therefore less of a human misfortune, and the call for relief issuing with silent eloquence from each victim and all potential victims is of no lesser dignity. But it is misleading to equate the fundamentally human response to it with what is owed to society: it is owed by man to man—and it is thereby owed by society to the individuals as soon as the adequate ministering to these concerns outgrows (as it progressively does) the scope of private spontaneity and is made a public mandate. It is thus that society assumes responsibility for medical care, research, old age, and innumerable other things not originally of the public realm (in the original "social contract"), and they become duties toward "society" (rather than directly toward one's fellow man) by the fact that they are socially operated.

Indeed, we expect from organized society no longer mere protection against harm and the securing of the conditions of our preservation, but active and constant improvement in all the domains of life: the waging of the battle against nature, the enhancement of the human estate—in short, the promotion of progress. This is an expansive goal, one far surpassing the disaster norm of our previous reflections. It lacks the urgency of the latter, but has the nobility of the free, forward thrust. It surely is worth sacrifices. It is not at all a question of what society can afford, but of what it is committed to, beyond all necessity, by our mandate. Its trusteeship has become an established, ongoing, institutionalized business of the body politic. As eager beneficiaries of its gains, we now owe to "society," as its chief agent, our individual contributions toward its *continued pursuit*. I emphasize "continued pursuit." Maintaining the existing level requires no more than the orthodox means of taxation and enforcement of professional standards that raise no problems. The more optional goal of pushing forward is also more exacting. We have this syndrome: Progress is by our choosing an acknowledged interest of society, in which we have a stake in various degrees; science is a necessary instrument of progress; research is a necessary instrument of science; and in medical science experimentation on human subjects is a necessary instrument of research. Therefore, human experimentation has come to be a societal interest.

The destination of research is essentially melioristic. It does not serve the preservation of the existing good from which I profit myself and to which I am obligated. Unless the present state is intolerable, the melioristic goal is in a sense gratuitous, and this not only from the vantage point of the present. Our descendants have a right to be left an unplundered planet; they do not have a right to new miracle cures. We have sinned against them, if by our doing we have destroyed their inheritance—which we are doing at full blast; we have not sinned against them if by the time they come around arthritis has not yet been conquered (unless by sheer neglect). And generally, in the matter of progress, as humanity had no claim on a Newton, a Michelangelo, or a St. Francis to appear, and no right to the blessings of their unscheduled deeds, so progress, with all our methodical labor for it, cannot be budgeted in advance and its fruits received as a due. Its coming-about at all and its turning out for good (of which we can never be sure) must rather be regarded as something akin to grace.

THE MELIORISTIC GOAL, MEDICAL RESEARCH, AND INDIVIDUAL DUTY

Nowhere is the melioristic goal more inherent than in medicine. To the physician, it is not gratuitous. He is committed to curing and thus to improving the power to cure. Gratuitous we called it (outside disaster conditions) as a *social* goal, but noble at the same time. Both the nobility and the gratuitousness must influence the manner in which self-sacrifice for it is elicited, and even its free offer accepted. Freedom is certainly the first condition to be observed here. The surrender of one's body to medical experimentation is entirely outside the enforceable "social contract."

Or can it be construed to fall within its terms—

namely, as repayment for benefits from past experimentation that I have enjoyed myself? But I am indebted for these benefits not to society, but to the past "martyrs," to whom society is indebted itself, and society has no right to call in my personal debt by way of adding new to its own. Moreover, gratitude is not an enforceable social obligation; it anyway does not mean that I must emulate the deed. Most of all, if it was wrong to exact such sacrifice in the first place, it does not become right to exact it again with the plea of the profit it has brought me. If, however, it was not exacted, but entirely free, as it ought to have been, then it should remain so, and its precedence must not be used as a social pressure on others for doing the same under the sign of duty.

. . .

THE "CONSCRIPTION" OF CONSENT

. . . The mere issuing of the appeal, the calling for volunteers, with the moral and social pressures it inevitably generates, amounts even under the most meticulous rules of consent to a sort of *conscripting*. And some soliciting is necessarily involved. . . . And this is why "consent," surely a nonnegotiable minimum requirement, is not the full answer to the problem. Granting then that soliciting and therefore some degree of conscripting are part of the situation, who may conscript and who may be conscripted? Or less harshly expressed: Who should issue appeals and to whom?

The naturally qualified issuer of the appeal is the research scientist himself, collectively the main carrier of the impulse and the only one with the technical competence to judge. But his being very much an interested party (with vested interests, indeed, not purely in the public good, but in the scientific enterprise as such, in "his" project, and even in his career) makes him also suspect. The ineradicable dialectic of this situation—a delicate incompatibility problem— calls for particular controls by the research community and by public authority that we need not discuss. They can mitigate, but not eliminate the problem. We have to live with the ambiguity, the treacherous impurity of everything human.

SELF-RECRUITMENT OF THE COMMUNITY

To whom should the appeal be addressed? The natural issuer of the call is also the first natural addressee: the physician-researcher himself and the scientific confraternity at large. With such a coincidence—indeed, the noble tradition with which the whole business of human experimentation started—almost all of the associated legal, ethical, and metaphysical problems vanish. If it is full, autonomous identification of the subject with the purpose that is required for the dignifying of his serving as a subject—here it is; if strongest motivation—here it is; if fullest understanding—here it is; if freest decision—here it is; if greatest integration with the person's total, chosen pursuit—here it is. With the fact of self-solicitation the issue of consent in all its insoluble equivocality is bypassed per se. Not even the condition that the particular purpose be truly important and the project reasonably promising, which must hold in any solicitation of others, need be satisfied here. By himself, the scientist is free to obey his obsession, to play his hunch, to wager on chance, to follow the lure of ambition. It is all part of the "divine madness" that somehow animates the ceaseless pressing against frontiers. For the rest of society, which has a deep-seated disposition to look with reverence and awe upon the guardians of the mysteries of life, the profession assumes with this proof of its devotion the role of a self-chosen, consecrated fraternity, not unlike the monastic orders of the past, and this would come nearest to the actual, religious origins of the art of healing.

. . . .

"IDENTIFICATION" AS THE PRINCIPLE OF RECRUITMENT IN GENERAL

If the properties we adduced as the particular qualifications of the members of the scientific fraternity itself are taken as general criteria of selection, then one should look for additional subjects where a maximum of identification, understanding, and spontaneity can be expected—that is, among the most highly motivated, the most highly educated, and the least "captive" members of the community. From this naturally scarce resource, a descending order of permissibility leads to greater abundance and ease of supply, whose use should become proportionately more hesitant as the exculpating criteria are relaxed. An inversion of normal "market" behavior is demanded here—namely, to accept the lowest quotation last (and excused only by the greatest pressure of need); to pay the highest price first.

The ruling principle in our considerations is that the "wrong" of reification can only be made "right"

by such authentic identification with the cause that it is the subject's as well as the researcher's cause—whereby his role in its service is not just permitted by him, but *willed*. That sovereign will of his which embraces the end as his own restores his personhood to the otherwise depersonalizing context. To be valid it must be autonomous and informed. The latter condition can, outside the research community, only be fulfilled by degrees; but the higher the degree of the understanding regarding the purpose and the technique, the more valid becomes the endorsement of the will. A margin of mere trust inevitably remains. Ultimately, the appeal for volunteers should seek this free and generous endorsement, the appropriation of the research purpose into the person's own scheme of ends. Thus, the appeal is in truth addressed to the one, mysterious, and sacred source of any such generosity of the will—"devotion," whose forms and objects of commitment are various and may invest different motivations in different individuals. The following, for instance, may be responsive to the "call" we are discussing: compassion with human suffering, zeal for humanity, reverence for the Golden Rule, enthusiasm for progress, homage to the cause of knowledge, even longing for sacrificial justification (do not call that "masochism," please). On all these, I say, it is defensible and right to draw when the research objective is worthy enough; and it is a prime duty of the research community (especially in view of what we called the "margin of trust") to see that this sacred source is never abused for frivolous ends. For a less than adequate cause, not even the freest, unsolicited offer should be accepted.

THE RULE OF THE "DESCENDING ORDER" AND ITS COUNTERUTILITY SENSE

We have laid down what must seem to be a forbidding rule to the number-hungry research industry. Having faith in the transcendent potential of man, I do not fear that the "source" will ever fail a society that does not destroy it—and only such a one is worthy of the blessings of progress. But "elitistic" the rule is (as is the enterprise of progress itself), and elites are by nature small. The combined attribute of motivation and information, plus the absence of external pressures, tends to be socially so circumscribed that strict adherence to the rule might numerically starve the research process. This is why I spoke of a descending order of permissibility, which is itself permissive, but where the realization that it is a *descending* order is not without pragmatic import. Departing from the august norm, the appeal must needs shift from idealism to docility, from high-mindedness to compliance, from judgment to trust. Consent spreads over the whole spectrum. I will not go into the casuistics of this penumbral area. I merely indicate the principle of the order of preference: The poorer in knowledge, motivation, and freedom of decision (and that, alas, means the more readily available in terms of numbers and possible manipulation), the more sparingly and indeed reluctantly should the reservoir be used, and the more compelling must therefore become the countervailing justification.

Let us note that this is the opposite of a social utility standard, the reverse of the order by "availability and expendability": The most valuable and scarcest, the least expendable elements of the social organism, are to be the first candidates for risk and sacrifice. It is the standard of *noblesse oblige;* and with all its counterutility and seeming "wastefulness," we feel a rightness about it and perhaps even a higher "utility," for the soul of the community lives by this spirit.[2] It is also the opposite of what the day-to-day interests of research clamor for, and for the scientific community to honor it will mean that it will have to fight a strong temptation to go by routine to the readiest sources of supply—the suggestible, the ignorant, the dependent, the "captive" in various senses.[3] I do not believe that heightened resistance here must cripple research, which cannot be permitted; but it may indeed slow it down by the smaller numbers fed into experimentation in consequence. This price—a possibly slower rate of progress—may have to be paid for the preservation of the most precious capital of higher communal life.

EXPERIMENTATION ON PATIENTS

So far we have been speaking on the tacit assumption that the subjects of experimentation are recruited from among the healthy. To the question "Who is conscriptable?" the spontaneous answer is: Least and last of all the sick—the most available of all as they are under treatment and observation anyway. That the afflicted should not be called upon to bear additional burden and risk, that they are society's special trust and the physician's trust in particular—these are elementary responses of our moral sense. Yet the very destination of medical research, the conquest of disease, requires at the crucial stage trial and verification on precisely the sufferers from the disease, and their total exemption would defeat the purpose itself. In acknowledging this inescapable necessity, we enter the most sensitive area of the whole complex, the one most keenly felt and most searchingly discussed by the practitioners themselves. No wonder, it touches the heart of the doctor-patient relation, putting its most solemn obligations to the test. There is nothing new in what I have to say about the ethics of the doctor-patient relation, but for the purpose of confronting it with the issue of experimentation some of the oldest verities must be recalled.

THE FUNDAMENTAL PRIVILEGE OF THE SICK

In the course of treatment, the physician is obligated to the patient and to no one else. He is not the agent of society, nor of the interests of medical science, nor of the patient's family, nor of his co-sufferers, nor of future sufferers from the same disease. The patient alone counts when he is under the physician's care. By the simple law of bilateral contract (analogous, for example, to the relation of lawyer to client and its "conflict of interest" rule), the physician is bound not to let any other interest interfere with that of the patient in being cured. But manifestly more sublime norms than contractual ones are involved. We may speak of a sacred trust; strictly by its terms, the doctor is, as it were, alone with his patient and God.

There is one normal exception to this—that is, to the doctor's not being the agent of society vis-à-vis the patient, but the trustee of his interests alone: the quarantining of the contagious sick. This is plainly not for the patient's interest, but for that of others threatened by him. (In vaccination, we have a combination of both: protection of the individual and others.) But preventing the patient from causing harm to others is not the same as exploiting him for the advantage of others. And there is, of course, the abnormal exception of collective catastrophe, the analogue to a state of war. The physician who desperately battles a raging epidemic is under a unique dispensation that suspends in a nonspecifiable way some of the structures of normal practice, including possibly those against experimental liberties with his patients. No rules can be devised for the waiving of rules in extremities. And as with the famous shipwreck examples of ethical theory, the less said about it the better. But what is allowable there and may later be passed over in forgiving silence cannot serve as a precedent. We are concerned with non-extreme, non-emergency conditions where the voice of principle can be heard and claims can be adjudicated free from duress. We have conceded that there are such claims, and that if there is to be medical advance at all, not even the superlative privilege of the suffering and the sick can be kept wholly intact from the intrusion of its needs. About this least palatable, most disquieting part of our subject, I have to offer only groping, inconclusive remarks.

THE PRINCIPLE OF "IDENTIFICATION" APPLIED TO PATIENTS

On the whole, the same principles would seem to hold here as are found to hold with "normal subjects": motivation, identification, understanding on the part of the subject. But it is clear that these conditions are peculiarly difficult to satisfy with regard to a patient. His physical state, psychic preoccupation, dependent relation to the doctor, the submissive attitude induced by treatment—everything connected with his condition and situation makes the sick person inherently less of a sovereign person than the healthy one. Spontaneity of self-offering has almost to be ruled out; consent is marred by lower resistance or captive circumstance, and so on. In fact, all the factors that make the patient, as a category, particularly accessible and welcome for experimentation at the same time compromise the quality of the responding affirmation that must morally redeem the making use of them. This, in addition to the primacy of the physician's duty, puts a heightened onus on the physician-researcher to limit his undue power to the most important and defensible research objectives and, of course, to keep persuasion at a minimum.

Still, with all the disabilities noted, there is scope among patients for observing the rule of the "descending order of permissibility" that we have laid down for normal subjects, in vexing inversion of the utility order of quantitative abundance and qualitative "expendability." By the principle of this order, those patients who most identify with and are cognizant of the cause of research—members of the medical profession (who after all are sometimes patients themselves)—come first; the highly motivated and educated, also least dependent, among the lay patients come next; and so on down the line. An added consideration here is seriousness of condition, which again operates in inverse proportion. Here the profession must fight the tempting sophistry that the hopeless case is expendable (because in prospect already expended) and therefore especially usable; and gener-

ally the attitude that the poorer the chances of the patient, the more justifiable his recruitment for experimentation (other than for his own benefit). The opposite is true.

NONDISCLOSURE AS A BORDERLINE CASE

Then there is the case where ignorance of the subject, sometimes even of the experimenter, is of the essence of the experiment (the "double blind"-control group-placebo syndrome). It is said to be a necessary element of the scientific process. Whatever may be said about its ethics in regard to normal subjects, especially volunteers, it is an outright betrayal of trust in regard to the patient who believes that he is receiving treatment. Only supreme importance of the objective can exonerate it, without making it less of a transgression. The patient is definitely wronged even when not harmed. And ethics apart, the practice of such deception holds the danger of undermining the faith in the *bona fides* of treatment, the beneficial intent of the physician—the very basis of the doctor-patient relationship. In every respect, it follows that concealed experiment on patients—that is, experiment under the guise of treatment—should be the rarest exception, at best, if it cannot be wholly avoided.

This has still the merit of a borderline problem. The same is not true of the other case of necessary ignorance of the subject—that of the unconscious patient. Drafting him for nontherapeutic experiments is simply and unqualifiedly impermissible; progress or not, he must never be used, on the inflexible principle that utter helplessness demands utter protection.

When preparing this paper, I filled pages with a casuistics of this harrowing field, but then scrapped most of it, realizing my dilettante status. The shadings are endless, and only the physician-researcher can discern them properly as the cases arise. Into his lap the decision is thrown. The philosophical rule, once it has admitted into itself the idea of a sliding scale, cannot really specify its own application. It can only impress on the practitioner a general maxim or attitude for the exercise of his judgment and conscience in the concrete occasions of his work. In our case, I am afraid, it means making life more difficult for him.

It will also be noted that, somewhat at variance with the emphasis in the literature, I have not dwelt on the element of "risk" and very little on that of "consent." Discussion of the first is beyond the layman's competence; the emphasis on the second has been lessened because of its equivocal character. It is a truism to say that one should strive to minimize the risk and to maximize the consent. The more demanding concept of "identification," which I have used, includes "consent" in its maximal or authentic form, and the assumption of risk is its privilege.

NO EXPERIMENTS ON PATIENTS UNRELATED TO THEIR OWN DISEASE

Although my ponderings have, on the whole, yielded points of view rather than definite prescriptions, premises rather than conclusions, they have led me to a few unequivocal yeses and noes. The first is the emphatic rule that patients should be experimented upon, if at all, *only* with reference to *their disease*. Never should there be added to the gratuitousness of the experiment as such the gratuitousness of service to an unrelated cause. This follows simply from what we have found to be the *only* excuse for infracting the special exemption of the sick at all—namely, that the scientific war on disease cannot accomplish its goal without drawing the sufferers from disease into the investigative process. If under this excuse they become subjects of experiment, they do so *because,* and only because, of *their* disease.

This is the fundamental and self-sufficient consideration. That the patient cannot possibly benefit from the unrelated experiment therapeutically, while he might from experiment related to his condition, is also true, but lies beyond the problem area of pure experiment. I am in any case discussing nontherapeutic experimentation only, where *ex hypothesi* the patient does not benefit. Experiment as part of therapy—that is, directed toward helping the subject himself—is a different matter altogether and raises its own problems but hardly philosophical ones. As long as a doctor can say, even if only in his own thought: "There is no known cure for your condition (or: You have responded to none); but there is promise in a new treatment still under investigation, not quite tested yet as to effectiveness and safety; you will be taking a chance, but all things considered, I judge it in your best interest to let me try it on you"—as long as he can speak thus, he speaks as the patient's physician and may err, but does not transform the patient into a subject of experimentation. Introduction of an untried therapy into the treatment where the tried ones have failed is not "experimentation on the patient."

Generally, and almost needless to say, with all the rules of the book, there is something "experimental" (because tentative) about every individual treatment, beginning with the diagnosis itself; and he would be a poor doctor who would not learn from every case for the benefit of future cases, and a poor member of the profession who would not make any new insights gained from his treatments available to the profession at large. Thus, knowledge may be advanced in the treatment of any patient, and the interest of the medical art and all sufferers from the same affliction as well as the patient himself may be served if something happens to be learned from his case. But his gain to knowledge and future therapy is incidental to the *bona fide* service to the present patient. He has the right to expect that the doctor does nothing to him just in order to learn.

In that case, the doctor's imaginary speech would run, for instance, like this: "There is nothing more I can do for you. But you can do something for me. Speaking no longer as your physician but on behalf of medical science, we could learn a great deal about future cases of this kind if you would permit me to perform certain experiments on you. It is understood that you yourself would not benefit from any knowledge we might gain; but future patients would." This statement would express the purely experimental situation, assumedly here with the subject's concurrence and with all cards on the table. In Alexander Bickel's words: "It is a different situation when the doctor is no longer trying to make [the patient] well, but is trying to find out how to make others well in the future."[4]

But even in the second case, that of the nontherapeutic experiment where the patient does not benefit, at least the patient's own disease is enlisted in the cause of fighting that disease, even if only in others. It is yet another thing to say or think: "Since you are here—in the hospital with its facilities—anyway, under our care and observation anyway, away from your job (or, perhaps, doomed) anyway, we wish to profit from your being available for some other research of great interest we are presently engaged in." From the standpoint of merely medical ethics, which has only to consider risk, consent, and the worth of the objective, there may be no cardinal difference between this case and the last one. I hope that the medical reader will not think I am making too fine a point when I say that from the standpoint of the subject and his dignity there is a cardinal difference that crosses the line between the permissible and the impermissible, and this by the same principle of "identification" I have been invoking all along. Whatever the rights and wrongs of any experimentation on any patient—in the one case, at least that residue of identification is left him that it is his own affliction by which he can contribute to the conquest of that affliction, his own kind of suffering which he helps to alleviate in others; and so in a sense it is his own cause. It is totally indefensible to rob the unfortunate of this intimacy with the purpose and make his misfortune a convenience for the furtherance of alien concerns.

• • •

CONCLUSION

. . . I wish only to say in conclusion that if some of the practical implications of my reasonings are felt to work out toward a slower rate of progress, this should not cause too great dismay. Let us not forget that progress is an optional goal, not an unconditional commitment, and that its tempo in particular, compulsive as it may become, has nothing sacred about it. Let us also remember that a slower progress in the conquest of disease would not threaten society, grievous as it is to those who have to deplore that their particular disease be not yet conquered, but that society would indeed be threatened by the erosion of those moral values whose loss, possibly caused by too ruthless a pursuit of scientific progress, would make its most dazzling triumphs not worth having. Let us finally remember that it cannot be the aim of progress to abolish the lot of mortality. Of some ill or other, each of us will die. Our mortal condition is upon us with its harshness but also its wisdom—because without it there would not be the eternally renewed promise of the freshness, immediacy, and eagerness of youth; nor would there be for any of us the incentive to number our days and make them count. With all our striving to wrest from our mortality what we can, we should bear its burden with patience and dignity.

NOTES

1. *Proceedings of the Conference on the Ethical Aspects of Experimentation on Human Subjects,* November 3–4, 1967 (Boston, Massachusetts; hereafter called *Proceedings*), pp. 50–51.

2. Socially, everyone is expendable relatively—that is, in different degrees; religiously, no one is expendable absolutely: The "image of God" is in all. If it can be enhanced, then it is not by anyone being expended, but by someone expending himself.

3. This refers to captives of circumstance, not of justice. Prison inmates are, with respect to our problem, in a special class. If we hold to some idea of guilt, and to the supposition that our judicial system is not entirely at fault, they may be held to stand in a special debt to society, and their offer to serve—from whatever motive—may be accepted with a minimum of qualms as a means of reparation.

4. *Proceedings,* p. 33.

Informed Consent

PAUL RAMSEY

Consent as a Canon of Loyalty

One need not read very far in medical ethics—and especially not in the literature concerning medical experimentation or the ethical "codes" that have been formulated since the medical cases at the Nuremberg

Reprinted with permission of the publisher from *The Patient as Person* (New Haven, Conn.: Yale University Press, 1970), pp. 2, 5, 6, 8–11.

trials—without realizing that medical ethics has not its sole basis in the overall benefits to be produced. It is not a consequence-ethics alone. It is not solely a teleological ethics, to use the language of philosophy. It is not even an ethics of the "greatest possible medical benefits for the greatest possible number" of people. That calculus too easily comes to mean the "greatest possible medical benefits regardless of the number" of patients who without their proper consent may be made the subjects of promising medical investigations. Medical ethics is not solely a benefit-producing ethics even in regard to the individual patient, since he should not always be helped without his will.

As stated in the *Ethical Guidelines for Organ Transplantation* of the American Medical Association,[1] so also of medical experimentation involving human subjects: "Man participates in these procedures: he is the patient in them; or he performs them. All mankind is the ultimate beneficiary of them." Observe that the respect in which man is the patient and man the performer of medical care or medical investigation (the relation between doctor and patient/subject) places an independent moral limit upon the fashion in which the rest of mankind can be made the ultimate beneficiary of these procedures. In the language of philosophy, a deontological dimension or test holds chief place in medical ethics, beside teleological considerations. That is to say, there must be a determination of the rightness or wrongness of the action and not only of the good to be obtained in medical care or from medical investigation.

A crucial element in answer to the question, What constitutes right action in medical practice? is the requirement of a reasonably free and adequately informed consent. In current medical ethics, this is a chief *canon of loyalty* (as I shall call it) between the man who is patient/subject and the man who performs medical investigational procedures. Physicians discuss the consent-requirement just as ethicists discuss fairness- or justice-claims: these tests must be satisfied along with the benefits (the "good") obtained.

. . .

THE ETHICS OF CONSENT

Hopefully while not exceeding an ethicist's putative competence or trespassing upon the competence of medical men, I wish to undertake an analysis of the consent-requirement itself. The principle of an informed consent is a statement of the fidelity between the man who performs medical procedures and the man on whom they are performed. Other aspects of medical ethics—for example, the requirement of a good experimental design and of professional skill at least as good as is customary in ordinary medical practice—treat the man as a purely passive subject or patient. These are also the requirements that hold for

an ethical experiment upon animals. But any human being is more than a patient or experimental subject; he is a *personal* subject—every bit as much a man as the physician-investigator. Fidelity is between man and man in these procedures. Consent expresses or establishes this relationship, and the requirement of consent sustains it. Fidelity is the bond between consenting man and consenting man in these procedures. The principle of an informed consent is the cardinal *canon of loyalty* joining men together in medical practice and investigation. In this requirement, faithfulness among men—the faithfulness that is normative for all the covenants or moral bonds of life with life—gains specification for the primary relations peculiar to medical practice.

Consent as a canon of loyalty can best be exhibited by a paraphrase of Reinhold Niebuhr's celebrated defense of democracy on both positive and negative grounds: "Man's capacity for justice makes democracy possible; man's propensity to injustice makes democracy necessary."[2] Man's capacity to become joint adventurers in a common cause makes the consensual relation possible; man's propensity to overreach his joint adventurer even in a good cause makes consent necessary. In medical experimentation the common cause of the consensual relation is the advancement of medicine and benefit to others. In therapy and in diagnostic or therapeutic investigations, the common cause is some benefit to the patient himself; but this is still a joint venture in which patient and physician can say and ideally should both say, "I cure."

Therefore, I suggest that men's capacity to become joint adventurers in a common cause makes possible a consent to enter the relation of patient to physician or of subject to investigator. This means that *partnership* is a better term than *contract* in conceptualizing the relation between patient and physician or between subject and investigator. The fact that these pairs of people are joint adventurers is evident from the fact that consent is a continuing and a repeatable requirement. We can legitimately appeal to permissions presumably granted by or implied in the original contract only to the extent that these are not incompatible with the demands of an ongoing partnership sustained by an actual or implied *present* consent and terminable by any present or future dissent from it. For this to be at all a human enterprise—a covenantal relation between the man who performs these procedures and the man who is patient in them—the latter must make a reasonably free and an adequately informed consent. Ideally, he must be constantly engaged in doing so. This is basic to the cooperative enterprise in which he is one partner.

. . .

The foregoing paragraphs describe the basis of the requirement that experimentation involving human subjects should be undertaken only when an informed consent has been secured. There are enormous problems, of course, in knowing how to subsume cases under this moral regulation expressive of respect for the man who is the subject in medical investigations no less than in applying this same moral regulation expressive of the meaning of medical care. What is and what is not a mature and informed consent is a preciously subtle thing to determine. Then there are questions about how to apply this rule that arise from those sorts of medical research in which the patient's knowing enough to give an informed consent may alter the findings sought; and there is debate about whether the use of prisoners or medical students in medical experimentation, or paying the participants, would not put them under too much duress for them to be said to consent freely even if fully informed. Despite these ambiguities, however, to obtain an understanding consent is a minimum obligation of a common enterprise and in a practice in which men are committed to men in definable respects. The *faithfulness*-claims which every man, simply by being a man, places upon the researcher are the morally relevant considerations. This is the ground of the consent-rule in medical practice, though obviously medical practice has also its consequence-features.

Indeed, precisely because there are unknown future benefits and precisely because the results of the experimentation may be believed to be so important as to be overriding, this rule governing medical experimentation upon human beings is needed to ensure that for the sake of those consequences no man shall be degraded and treated as a thing or as an animal in order that good may come of it. In this age of research medicine it is not only that medical benefits are attained by research but also that a man rises to the top in medicine by the success and significance of his research. The likelihood that a researcher would make a mistake in departing from a generally valuable rule of medical practice because he is biased toward the research benefits of permitting an "exception" is exceedingly great. In such a seriously important moral matter, this should be enough to rebut a policy of being open to future possible exceptions to this canon of medical ethics. On grounds of the faithfulness-claims alone, we must surely say that future experience will provide no morally significant exception to the requirement of an informed consent—although doubtless we may learn a great deal more about the meaning of this particular canon of loyalty, and how to apply it in new situations with greater sensitivity and refinement—or we may learn more and more how to practice violations of it.

Doubtless medical men will always be learning more and more about the specific meaning which the requirement of an informed consent has in practice. Or they could learn more and more how to violate or avoid this requirement. But they are not likely to learn that it more and more does not govern the ethical practice of medicine. It is, of course, impossible to demonstrate that there could be *no* exceptions to this requirement. But with regard to unforeseeable future possibilities or apparently unique situations that medicine may face, there is this rule-assuring, principle-strengthening, and practice-upholding rule to be added to the requirement of an informed consent. *In the grave moral matters of life and death, of maiming or curing, of the violation of persons or their bodily integrity, a physician or experimenter is more liable to make an error in moral judgment if he adopts a policy of holding himself open to the possibility that there may be significant, future permissions to ignore the principle of the consent than he is if he holds this requirement of an informed consent always relevant and applicable.* If so, he ought as a practical matter to regard the consent-principle as closed to further morally significant alteration or exception. In this way he braces himself to respect the personal subject while he treats him as patient or tries procedures on him as an experimental subject for the good of mankind.

The researcher knows that his judgment will generally be biased by the fact that he strongly desires one of the consequences (the rapid completion of his research for the good of mankind) which he could hope to attain by breaking or avoiding the requirement of an informed consent. This, too, should strengthen adherence in practice to the principle of consent. If every doer loves his deed more than it ought to be loved, so every researcher his research—and, of course, its promise of future benefits for mankind. The investigator should strive, as Aristotle suggested, to hit the mean of moral virtue or excellence by "leaning against" the excess or the defect to which he knows himself, individually or professionally, and mankind generally in a scientific age, to be especially inclined. To assume otherwise would be to assume an equally serene rationality on the part of men in all moral matters. It would be to assume that a man is as able to sustain good moral judgment and to make a proper choice with a strong interest in results obtainable by violating the requirement of an informed consent as he would be if he had no such interest.

Thus the principle of consent is a canon of loyalty expressive of the faithfulness-claims of persons in medical care and investigation. Let us grant that we cannot theoretically rule out the possibility that there can be exceptions to this requirement in the future. This, at least, is conceivable in extreme examples. It is not logically impossible. Still this is a rule of the highest human loyalty that ought not in practice to be held open to significant future revision. To say this concerning the there and then of some future moral judgment would mean here and now to weaken the protection of coadventurers from violation and self-violation in the common cause of medical care and the advancement of medical science. The material and spiritual pressures upon investigators in this age of research medicine, the collective bias in the direction of successful research, the propensities of the scientific mind toward the consequences alone are all good reasons—even if they are not all good moral reasons—for strengthening the requirement of an informed consent. This helps to protect coadventurers in the cause of medicine from harm and from harmfulness. This is the edification to be found in the thought that man's propensity to overreach a joint adventurer even in a good cause makes consent necessary.

This negative aspect of the ethics of medical research is essential even if only because the constraints of the consent-requirement serve constantly to drive our minds back to the positive meaning or warrant for this principle in the man who is the patient and the man who performs these procedures. An informed consent alone exhibits and establishes medical practice and investigation as a voluntary association of free men in a common cause. The negative constraint of the consent-requirement serves its positive meaning. It directs our attention always upon the man who is the patient in all medical procedures and a partner in all investigations, and away from that celebrated "nonpatient," the future of medical science. Thus consent lies at the heart of medical care as a joint adventure between patient and doctor. It lies at the heart of man's continuing search for cures to all man's diseases as a great human adventure that is carried forward jointly by the investigator and his subjects. Stripped of the requirement of a reasonably free and an adequately informed consent, experimentation and medicine itself would speedily become inhumane.

No one today would propose to eliminate the consent-requirement directly, but this can be done more subtly, or by indirection. Even while retaining it, the consent-requirement can be effectively annulled, or transformed into a disappearing, powerless guideline, simply by writing into it a "quantity-of-benefits-to-come"-exception clause. Thus we could make ourselves ready to override or avoid the consent-requirement in view of future good to be achieved. To do this is to make ourselves conditionally willing to use a subject in medical investigations as a mere means.

NOTES

1. Report of the Judicial Council, E. G. Shelley, M.D., Chairman, and approved by the House of Delegates of the American Medical Association, June 1968.

2. *The Children of Light and the Children of Darkness* (New York: Scribner's, 1949), p. xi.

FRANZ J. INGELFINGER

Informed (but Uneducated) Consent

The trouble with informed consent is that it is not educated consent. Let us assume that the experimental subject, whether a patient, a volunteer, or otherwise enlisted, is exposed to a completely honest array of factual detail. He is told of the medical uncertainty that exists and that must be resolved by research endeavors, of the time and discomfort involved, and of the tiny percentage risk of some serious consequences of the test procedure. He is also reassured of his rights and given a formal, quasilegal statement to read. No exculpatory language is used. With his written signature, the subject then caps the transaction, and whether he sees himself as a heroic martyr for the sake of mankind, or as a reluctant guinea pig dragooned for the benefit of science, or whether, perhaps, he is merely bewildered, he obviously has given his "informed consent." Because established routines have been scrupulously observed, the doctor, the lawyer, and the ethicist are content.

But the chances are remote that the subject really understands what he has consented to—in the sense that the responsible medical investigator understands the goals, nature, and hazards of his study. How can the layman comprehend the importance of his perhaps not receiving, as determined by the luck of the draw, the highly touted new treatment that his roommate will get? How can he appreciate the sensation of living for days with a multi-lumen intestinal tube passing through his mouth and pharynx? How can he interpret the information that an intravascular catheter and radiopaque dye injection have an 0.01 per cent probability of leading to a dangerous thrombosis or cardiac arrhythmia? It is moreover quite unlikely that any patient-subject can see himself accurately within the broad context of the situation, to weigh the inconveniences and hazards that he will have to undergo against the improvements that the research project

may bring to the management of his disease in general and to his own case in particular. The difficulty that the public has in understanding information that is both medical and stressful is exemplified by [a] report [in the *New England Journal Of Medicine,* August 31, 1972, page 433]—that only half the families given genetic counseling grasped its impact.

Nor can the information given to the experimental subject be in any sense totally complete. It would be impractical and probably unethical for the investigator to present the nearly endless list of all possible contingencies; in fact, he may not himself be aware of every untoward thing that might happen. Extensive detail, moreover, usually enhances the subject's confusion. Epstein and Lasagna showed that comprehension of medical information given to untutored subjects is inversely correlated with the elaborateness of the material presented.[1] The inconsiderate investigator, indeed, conceivably could exploit his authority and knowledge and extract "informed consent" by overwhelming the candidate-subject with information.

Ideally, the subject should give his consent freely, under no duress whatsoever. The facts are that some element of coercion is instrumental in any investigator-subject transaction. Volunteers for experiments will usually be influenced by hopes of obtaining better grades, earlier parole, more substantial egos, or just mundane cash. These pressures, however, are but fractional shadows of those enclosing the patient-subject. Incapacitated and hospitalized because of illness, frightened by strange and impersonal routines, and fearful for his health and perhaps life, he is far from exercising a free power of choice when the person to whom he anchors all his hopes asks, "Say, you wouldn't mind, would you, if you joined some of the other patients on this floor and helped us to carry out some very important research we are doing?" When "informed consent" is obtained, it is not the student,

Reprinted with permission from *The New England Journal of Medicine,* Vol. 287, No. 9, pp. 465–466, Aug. 31, 1972.

the destitute bum, or the prisoner to whom, by virtue of his condition, the thumb screws of coercion are most relentlessly applied; it is the most used and useful of all experimental subjects, the patient with disease.

When a man or woman agrees to act as an experimental subject, therefore, his or her consent is marked by neither adequate understanding nor total freedom of choice. The conditions of agreement are a far cry from those visualized as ideal. Jonas would have the subject identify with the investigative endeavor so that he and the researcher would be seeking a common cause: "Ultimately, the appeal for volunteers should seek . . . free and generous endorsement, the appropriation of the research purpose into the person's [i.e., the subject's] own scheme of ends."[2] For Ramsey, "informed consent" should represent a "covenantal bond between consenting man and consenting man [that] makes them . . . joint adventurers in medical care and progress."[3] Clearly, to achieve motivations and attitudes of this lofty type, an educated and understanding, rather than merely informed, consent is necessary.

Although it is unlikely that the goals of Jonas and of Ramsey will ever be achieved, and that human research subjects will spontaneously volunteer rather than be "conscripted,"[2] efforts to promote educated consent are in order. In view of the current emphasis on involving "the community" in such activities as regional planning, operation of clinics, and assignment of priorities, the general public and its political leaders are showing an increased awareness and understanding of medical affairs. But the orientation of this public interest in medicine is chiefly socioeconomic. Little has been done to give the public a basic understanding of medical research and its requirements not only for the people's money but also

for their participation. The public, to be sure, is being subjected to a bombardment of sensation-mongering news stories and books that feature "breakthroughs," or that reveal real or alleged exploitations—horror stories of Nazi-type experimentation on abused human minds and bodies. Muckraking is essential to expose malpractices, but unless accompanied by efforts to promote a broader appreciation of medical research and its methods, it merely compounds the difficulties for both the investigator and the subject when "informed consent" is solicited.

The procedure currently approved in the United States for enlisting human experimental subjects has one great virtue: patient-subjects are put on notice that their management is in part at least an experiment. The deceptions of the past are no longer tolerated. Beyond this accomplishment, however, the process of obtaining "informed consent," with all its regulations and conditions, is no more than elaborate ritual, a device that, when the subject is uneducated and uncomprehending, confers no more than the semblance of propriety on human experimentation. The subject's only real protection, the public as well as the medical profession must recognize, depends on the conscience and compassion of the investigator and his peers.

NOTES

1. Epstein, L. C., and Lasagna, L.: "Obtaining informed consent: form or substance." *Arch. Intern. Med.* 123:682–688, 1969.

2. Jonas, H.: "Philosophical reflections on experimenting with human subjects." *Daedalus* 98:219–247, Spring 1969.

3. Ramsey, P.: "The ethics of a cottage industry in an age of community and research medicine." *N. Engl. J. Med.* 284:700–706, 1971.

THOMAS C. CHALMERS

The Ethics of Randomization as a Decision-Making Technique, and the Problem of Informed Consent

"Do no harm while nature heals" was the motto of my father, who practiced medicine at the end of the nineteenth and early part of the twentieth century. This was a relatively easy course for him to follow in those days when the only effective medicines were digitalis and morphine, and life-threatening treatments such as major surgery were just beginning to be used. Nowadays the busy physician makes several decisions a week which are critical to the life and health of his patient. Whether alone or with consultations, he makes these decisions by means of so-called clinical judgment, a subtle distillation of his personal experience and the knowledge that he has been able to glean from the medical literature.

The major danger in basing action on personal experience is the unavoidable excess influence of the most recent experience. The last case or two, especially if dramatically successful, or unsuccessful, cannot help but have more influence on the next decision than those cases encountered in the more distant past. As an aside I should like to suggest that the older clinician is the more able decision maker not only because he has had more experience, but also because a growing defect in memory for recent events allows him to give a more equal weight to his experiences, no matter when they occurred.

The second important component of clinical judgment is a knowledge of the medical literature, both basic and clinical. Unfortunately, basic research has, almost by definition, little immediate application to the treatment of patients. The practicing physician must be able to evaluate and rely on the clinical medicine literature when he treats patients, and he must be ready to defend his decisions by referring to the articles written by his peers or to his own research experience. When the treatment is symptomatic, it probably makes little difference what the physician does. The potent factor is his interest in his patient. However, when the treatment is life-threatening, as with major surgery or other drastic regimens, then the physician and his patient are in trouble because the clinical literature is so notoriously unscientific. By this I mean that the conclusions of the authors are seldom borne out by the data. Less than 20 percent of the clinical trials reported in the medical literature are controlled, and unfortunately the more drastic and dangerous the therapy the less are controls employed. The major defect in most reports of new therapies is the complete inability of the author or the reader to separate out the effects of the treatment under study from the effects of selection of patients for that treatment. In addition, the physician attempting to decide about life-threatening therapies rarely considers another important selection factor, the multiple variables that determine whether a series of patients is written up or not, and whether a paper is accepted for publication or not. So the final reported series may represent a very small and unidentifiable sub-group of the total number of patients presenting with the disorder under study, and it is next to impossible to apply that information correctly in making decisions about individual members of the total population with that disease.

It is clear by now that I am trying to develop a case for the controlled clinical trial in the initial investigation of a life-threatening therapy. A carefully constructed protocol will contain a randomization procedure by which clearly defined patients are assigned to the new or conventional therapy. In that case the relative efficacy of the new treatment and the population

From *Report of the Fourteenth Conference of Cardiovascular Training Grant Program Directors, National Heart and Lung Institute* (Washington, D.C.: U.S. Department of Health, Education, and Welfare, 1967).

to which it can be applied can be clearly determined. If the new treatment turns out to be best, the patients assigned to that will have been the lucky ones. If the new treatment is comparatively bad, the controls will be the lucky ones. In either case, the patients will be carefully treated and may thus do better than those who are not studied at all.

• • •

From the scientific standpoint, there is no doubt about the need for controlled trials of all new procedures which may on the average be more harmful than helpful. Yet in the last 30 years any number of new procedures have been introduced, only to be discarded or modified many years later when the slow process of individual clinical experience suggested that they were actually dangerous, or at least not as effective as the original proponents had thought. It is unlikely that total ignorance of scientific methodology is the reason for the great scarcity of well-controlled trials of new therapies in clinical medicine. It is more likely that those who introduced and publicized the new methods felt that it was unethical to withhold the possibility of benefit from any available patients, and that they certainly had to decide who was suitable for the operation according to their best clinical judgment rather than according to some very un-doctorlike randomization procedure. To me it seems clear that to randomize patients into a group receiving a new therapy being evaluated, and a group receiving the standard therapy, whether it be a similar treatment or no treatment, depending on what is currently accepted for the disease, is much more ethical and is much more in the interest of the individual patients than is treatment of consecutive selected patients as if the new therapy had already been established; or conversely, the withholding of a new therapy from a group of patients as if it had already been proven to be ineffective.

Three problems remain to be discussed with regard to this discussion of randomization: when to start, what to tell the patients, and when to stop.

One often hears experienced clinical investigators insist that a randomized controlled trial should never be started until the techniques of a new therapy have been worked out in a preliminary group of patients. I am convinced that from the ethical standpoint this is very dangerous reasoning. New therapeutic procedures are always changed and are usually improved by experience with the first few patients. However, it

is extremely difficult for the investigators not to acquire enthusiasm, or the opposite emotional response, when they have tried out the new therapy in a consecutive series of patients. If they have worked out a good dosage regimen or what they consider an effective operative procedure, they are almost by definition convinced that the new treatment has enough merit so that they cannot ethically deprive a control group from receiving it. Or they might prematurely discard a new treatment because of poor results, when in fact a randomized control group might have done much worse. So I believe that it is important to randomize from the very first patient not only to protect future patients but also to protect the first patients, who should have a chance to fall into the control group when the new treatment may well be ineffective because of the inexperience of the person who is applying it. The control patient can always be removed from that group and placed in the experimental group if and when the new treatment seems to be superior to the old.

The second problem has to do with the obtaining of informed consent in therapeutic trials in life-threatening procedures. There can be no argument against the requirement that the investigating physician must obtain completely informed consent from patients taking part in trials which are done for the sake of research and from which they do not necessarily have more to gain than to lose. But I believe that the situation is somewhat different when randomization is carried out because the physician does not know which therapy is better for the individual patients. There are two potent arguments against informing patients with a life-threatening disease that the decision about whether or not they should have a life-threatening operation will be made by chance rather than by clinical judgment. (1) It is not in the best interest of the patients because it seems likely that 9 out of 10 would refuse these studies, and therefore the operation, if so informed. If they were in their right senses, they would find a doctor who thought he knew which was the better treatment, or they would conclude that if the differences were so slight that such a trial had to be carried out, they would prefer to take their chances on no operation. Assuming that there is a 50 percent chance that the operation will prove to be effective, then half the patients who were scared out of the operation by having been asked for their informed consent, would have been mistreated. Furthermore, it is probable that a very sick patient needs to have complete confidence in the fact that his doctor has the knowledge to make the right decisions with regard to his care. In the course of a traumatic illness the loss of that confidence may do great harm to the patient. It is a rare patient who could be expected to be objective enough about his own serious illness to welcome the fact that his physician has enough knowledge to avoid decisions based on ignorance.

The second argument against informing patients that the decision to operate or not will be based on randomization lies in the fact that it is not customary in the ordinary practice of medicine to inform patients of all the details with regard to how decisions are made in their treatment. Few patients would be saved by established surgical procedures if the physician and surgeon had to recount in every detail the complications of the operation. The most vigorous advocates of portacaval shunt surgery would be able to do no more operations if they were required to explain to each patient that of the 50 reports in the literature the only controlled studies showed no effects, and all of the enthusiastic reports were totally uncontrolled. The physician must assume some responsibility for making decisions in the best interest of his patients.

Although in my opinion the physician may withhold information from the patient about the exact details of how decisions are made in a randomized study, he must inform the patient of the pros and cons of each therapeutic maneuver under consideration, and he must assure the patient that he will not carry out any therapy that he knows to be wrong. He must inform the patient that he is taking part in a study of a procedure that has not yet been established as efficacious. In other words, the patient should know that he is taking part in a research project and should be free to refuse to take part. And it should go without saying that all physicians concerned in a randomized study must be convinced that the knowledge necessary to make a decision [about] that patient is not available.

This brings me to the third problem, and to me the most serious one, that must be faced by the physician concerned with the ethics of controlled trials, namely how one makes the decision about when to stop the trial, when a decision should be made to treat all patients according to the apparent results of the trial. The biostatistician tells us that we must determine

from the variability before we start the trial what a reasonable number of experiences would be, and that usually we should not stop until there is less than a 10 or 15 percent chance that we are missing a real difference, or less than a 5 percent chance that the difference we might have demonstrated is a true one and not one due to chance. This is entirely reasonable from the standpoint of the application of the conclusion to future patients. The conclusion can be reached either by the fixed sample technique with occasional peeking by a disinterested person, or by the sequential analysis technique. Either way one should be reasonably sure before stopping a study that the conclusions would be valid and not reversed by further experience. One owes this to the patients who were randomized into the less favorable treatment, if there is a difference.

But what about the rights of the patient who enters a study at a time when one treatment is leading the other, but when the study is being continued because the difference is not significant? One can easily argue that since the difference is not significant, the result can be reversed by further experience. But one can also argue that the welfare of that one patient is more assured if he receives the treatment that is ahead rather than the one that is currently behind in the evaluation. In other words, randomization could be unfair to him because he might be assigned to a treatment that has a less than 50 percent chance of being shown to be the correct one. This argument can then be reduced to the ridiculous by pointing out that the first patient in a study makes it more or less likely that one treatment will come out ahead. The situation is not analogous to the oft-quoted coin flipping rule that the results of previous flips do not influence the next one. In the case of the controlled trial the result of each comparison adds to the evidence for or against the superiority of one or the other treatment. To this problem I can see no solution, and I would appreciate consideration by this group of the argument that if one considers solely the welfare of the individual patient one can never do a controlled trial.

The fact that the investigator is also the patient's physician requires that he tell the subject of the investigation which treatment is ahead. In situations in which both the disease and the treatment are life-threatening, it is unlikely that the patient would consent to be assigned to the treatment that is less likely to prove effective.

In summary, I should like to present you for discussion three conclusions: (1) In the gradual evolution of our knowledge with regard to the prevention and treatment of disease the controlled clinical trial is by far the most effective way of saving people from the misapplication of dangerous and ineffective treatments. (2) We now know how to design scientifically precise and reliable trials of all preventive and therapeutic maneuvers. (3) Currently there are serious ethical and legal barriers to the conduct of any but the most insignificant trials.

CHARLES FRIED

Informed Consent and Medical Experimentation

GENERAL LEGAL PRINCIPLES APPLIED TO MEDICAL EXPERIMENTATION[1]

At the outset we must distinguish between therapeutic and nontherapeutic experimentation.[2] Experimentation is clearly nontherapeutic when it is carried out on a person solely to obtain information of use to others, and in no way to treat some illness that the experimental subject might have. Experimentation is therapeutic when a therapy is tried with the sole view of determining the best way of treating that patient. There is a sense, as a number of commentators have observed, in which so far as there is more or less uncertainty about the best way to proceed in the patient's case, treatment is often experimental.[3] Also, what is learned in treating one patient will be of use in treating others. This may be so, but it in no way obscures the distinction between therapeutic and nontherapeutic research, since therapeutic research is carried out only and only so far as that subject's interests require. Any benefits to others are incidental to this dominant goal. These are clear cases at the extreme.

There are in practice large numbers of gradations in between. Much research is mainly therapeutic, in the sense that the patients' interests are foremost, but nevertheless things may be done which are not dictated solely by the need to treat that patient: tests may be continued even after all the information needed to determine the best treatment of the particular patient has already been completed; or substances may be injected for a period or in doses not strictly necessary for the cure of that patient, but with the motive of developing information of use to others.[4] Moving in from the clear case at the other extreme, that of nontherapeutic research, it must be recognized that persons who become research subjects in nontherapeutic experimentation may often be the beneficiaries of a degree of medical attention which they might not otherwise enjoy, and which thus redounds to their benefit.[5] And there are all possible degrees and gradations in between.

NONTHERAPEUTIC EXPERIMENTATION[6]

No special doctrines apply to nontherapeutic experimentation. Indeed, to the extent that the experimentation is nontherapeutic, the fact that it is being carried out by doctors should be entirely irrelevant. The usual privileges under which doctors work, and the usual special doctrines according to which the liabilities of doctors are judged should not be applicable, since they proceed from the premise that the doctor must be given considerable latitude as he works in the presumed interests of his patient. But that is not the case in nontherapeutic research. The doctor confronts his subject simply as a scientist.

In general, the law imposes a strict duty of disclosure, wherever an individual with a great deal to lose is exposed to a risk or is asked to relinquish rights by someone with considerably greater knowledge.[7] And

Reprinted with permission of the publisher from *Medical Experimentation: Personal Integrity and Social Policy* (New York: American Elsevier Publishing Co., Inc., 1974), pp. 25–36.

this is true, whether the relation is one of buyer and seller or involves some public interest. Persons selling cosmetics,[8] automobiles[9] or pharmaceuticals[10] are required to make full disclosures of all the hazards involved in the products they sell. But policemen seeking damaging admissions from suspects are also required to issue a warning of constitutional rights and to offer legal assistance before those rights are waived.[11] There is no reason why the case should be any different where a researcher asks an experimental subject to risk his health.

Indeed the case might be made that the developing doctrines of strict liability would argue for the imposition of liability without fault, and regardless of disclosures for harm occasioned in the course of nontherapeutic experimentation.[12] In general, it is coming to be believed that those who are in a better position to appreciate the risks of a course of conduct, who are in a better position to insure against those risks or otherwise spread their cost to the broadest group of beneficiaries, and finally whose responsible decisions in evaluating the propriety of the risks we can influence by imposing upon them the costs of those decisions, should be strictly liable (that is liable without fault) for the risks that their conduct imposes.[13] These conditions are amply met in the case of nontherapeutic experimentation. Finally, if the financial pressures of caring for and compensating subjects injured in nontherapeutic experiments meant that experimenters exercised greater caution and carefully evaluated the benefits to be expected from the research, this would be a highly desirable consequence. It is for this reason that a number of commentators have suggested either strict liability for nontherapeutic experimentation or some form of compulsory medical experimentation insurance. In either case the experimental subject would be assured of proper medical care as well as compensatory payments for any injuries he suffers in the experiment. Since most subjects of nontherapeutic experimentation are either idealistic persons for whom the small amounts of compensation are not a significant inducement, or disadvantaged persons for whom the small compensation acts as an all too significant inducement, this added responsibility would seem fair and appropriate.

THERAPEUTIC EXPERIMENTATION

Legal decisions and commentators have always stated that a practitioner is only justified in using "ac-cepted remedies" unless his patient specifically consents to the use of an "experimental" remedy.[14] This statement has seemed reactionary and unreasonable to doctors, but if one puts it in the context of general doctrine one might say that its teeth are quite effectively drawn. General principles require the consent of the patient to any therapy, usual or unusual. It is just that as the therapy moves away from the standard and the accepted, the need for explicit consent, full disclosure of risks and alternatives, becomes more acute, and more likely to pose an issue. The doctor who prescribes an accepted remedy, under the principles set forth so far, might have a good defense to the claim that he should have told his client about alternative, untried or experimental remedies.[15]

The obligation to advise the patient of alternative therapies does not extend to all the hypothetical, untried or experimental remedies that various researchers are in the process of developing. Where, however, the therapy used is itself experimental, then this fact and the existence of either alternatives or professional doubts become material facts, which like all material facts should be disclosed. Beyond this, where the experimentation is truly and exclusively therapeutic, there are no particular legal constraints that do not apply to the practice of medicine generally.[16] It is simply that the implication of those general doctrines may take on a special coloring in this context.

MIXED THERAPEUTIC AND NONTHERAPEUTIC RESEARCH: THE PROBLEM OF THE RANDOMIZED CLINICAL TRIAL

The kind of medical experimentation which causes the greatest legal and ethical perplexities is what might be called mixed therapeutic and nontherapeutic experimentation: The patient is indeed being treated for a particular illness, and a serious effort is being made to cure him. The systems of treatment, however, are not chosen solely with the view to curing the particular patient of his particular ills. Rather, the treatment takes place in the context of an experiment or a research program to test new procedures, or to compare the efficacy of various established procedures.[17] Nor is it the case that this research purpose is limited to carefully reporting the results of treatments in particular cases. Rather, therapies are tried, continued or varied, and patients are assigned to treatment categories partially in response to the needs of the research design, i.e., not exclusively by considering the particular patient's needs at the particular time. Usually it will be the case that there is genuine doubt about which is the best treatment, or the best treatment modality, so that the doctors participating in the experiment do not believe they are compromising the interests of their patients.[18] Or where this is not completely true, it is often the case that no serious or irreversible harms or risk are imposed in pursuing the research design rather than pursuing singlemindedly the interests of the particular patient. The clearest case, and the one which is the focus of our concern in this essay, is the randomized clinical trial (RCT), in which patients are assigned to treatment categories by some randomizing device, with the thought that in this way any bias of the experimenter and any unsuspected interfering factor can be eliminated by the statistical method used.[19] And generally it is said that the alternative therapies between which patients are randomized both have a great deal to recommend them, so that there is no real sense in which one or the other group is being deliberately disadvantaged—at least until the results of the experiments are in.[20]

What is the legal status of experimentation having both therapeutic and nontherapeutic aspects? Since there is a general obligation to obtain consent to a therapy, and since that obligation becomes more exigent as the treatment to be used departs from the ordinary and the accepted, there is at least the legal obligation to obtain consent for the use of the treatment contemplated, with full disclosure of the expected benefits and hazards. This much is straightforward, and not peculiar to the area of mixed therapeutic and nontherapeutic experimentation and RCTs. Moreover, as we have seen, a number of courts have insisted that the disclosure made in obtaining consent include a disclosure of the existence and characteristics of alternative therapies.[21] Certainly if the therapy proposed is experimental in the sense of innovative, this fact along with some description of more traditional alternatives should be part of the disclosure.

The crucial question, and one as to which there is no decided case, asks whether it is also necessary to disclose first that an experiment is being conducted, and second and more delicately the nature of the experiment and the experimental design.

Specifically, in the case of the RCT must the doctor disclose the fact that the patient's therapy will be determined by a randomizing procedure rather than by an individualized judgment on the part of the physician? Some physicians active in mixed therapeutic and nontherapeutic experimentation have argued that it is both unnecessary and undesirable to make this last disclosure.[22] It is undesirable because some patients might be scared off, withdraw from the experiment and seek help elsewhere. It is also undesirable because of those patients who, while remaining in the experiment, might be caused such a degree of distress and anxiety that it would interfere with their cure. The disclosure of randomization is argued to be unnecessary since the medical evidence regarding the alternative treatments will often be evenly balanced (that is why the experiment is being conducted—to help resolve the doubts) so that it is in no way inaccurate to tell the patient that medical opinion is divided on the best therapy, and that the patient will receive the best available therapy according to current medical judgments. To tell the patient that he is being randomized, on this view, would add nothing of relevance regarding the expected outcome of his treatment, and thus nothing of relevance to his choice whether or not to consent to the treatment.

There are no authoritative decisions holding that consent in the absence of a disclosure that the patient is being randomized or that his treatment is being determined by reference to factors other than his individual concerns is invalid consent because of incomplete disclosure. The general principle holds that a person must be given all material information relating to the proposed therapy. But is the fact of randomization or of the existence of an experiment such material information? The information would seem to deal rather with the way in which the therapy is chosen than with the characteristics of the therapy itself. Nevertheless, it would seem that most patients would consider the information regarding the choice mechanism as highly relevant,[23] and would feel that they had been "had" upon discovering that they had received or not received surgery because of a number in a random number table. But does this sentiment create a duty; does it mean, for instance, that consent to the treatment was ineffective and the participating doctors are guilty of a battery?

Though there is no authoritative decision to point to, there are analogies from other areas of law which would suggest that full candid disclosure should include disclosure of randomization. The very fact that the doctor acts in the dual capacity of therapist and researcher, and that his role as researcher to some degree does or may influence his decisions as a therapist, would argue that the fullest disclosure of all the circumstances relating to that dual role, and to the basis on which functions are exercised and decisions made would be required.[24] If the relation were not that of doctor and patient, but of lawyer and client,[25] or of trustee and beneficiary of a trust fund,[26] or of a director or officer of a corporation and the corporation,[27] there would be a strict duty to disclose the existence of any interest which the fiduciary has that may conflict with or influence the exercise of his functions in his fiduciary capacity. The fiduciary owes a duty of strict and unreserved loyalty to his client.[28]

Imagine the case of a lawyer for a public defender organization who has agreed to participate in a foundation-sponsored research project on sentencing. As part of the research protocol his decision as to whether to plead certain categories of offenders guilty or to go to trial is determined at random. This is intended to discover how that decision affects the eventual outcome of the case at the time of sentencing and parole. His clients are not told that this is how the lawyer's "advice" as to plea is determined.[29]

The law of conflict of interests and of fiduciary relations clearly provides that the fiduciary may not pursue activities that either do in fact conflict with the exercise of his judgments as a fiduciary, or might conflict with or influence the exercise of his judgment, or might appear to do so, without the explicit consent of his client.[30] And if the consent is obtained other than on the basis of the fullest disclosure of all facts not only which the fiduciary deems relevant but which he knows his client might consider relevant, the disclosure is incomplete, the consent is fraudulently obtained, and the fiduciary is in breach of his fiduciary relationship.[31] There is no reason why the doctor should not be held to be in a fiduciary relationship to his patient, and therefore why the same fiduciary obligations that obtain for a lawyer, a money manager, a corporation executive or director should not obtain for a doctor.[32]

However the issue of informing patients of the fact of randomization might be resolved, it would seem that there is a continuing duty on the part of the patient's physician to inform himself about the progress of the experiment and to inform his patient about any significant new information coming out of the experiment that might bear on the patient's choice to remain in the study or to seek other types of therapy.[33] This is an important issue in RCTs involving long-term courses of treatment. If patients abandon one alternative on the basis of early, inconclusive results,

no definitive conclusion can be drawn from the trial. Failure to make continuing disclosures and to offer continuing options to the patient in the light of developing information may not constitute the tort of battery, however, since there may be no physical contact requiring a new consent. The wrong which is done to the patient would be in the nature of negligent practice, and as to that the determinative standard is the standard of practice of a respected segment of the profession. The physician who does not keep his patient continuously informed may argue that to do so would interfere with the experiment, and he might find experts to testify that such continuing disclosure in the course of an experiment is not thought to be good practice.[34] The argument should not be accepted uncritically since the practice which the doctor in the case of an RCT would refer to would not be traditional therapeutic practice, but rather the practice of experimentation itself. Indeed it would seem that the doctrine of the case, holding that a physician had a duty to inform his patient that his broken leg was not healing properly and that there was another method of treatment available in a nearby city which was more likely to result in cure,[35] is equally applicable to the case of a participant in an RCT who has been assigned to a treatment category which, as the experiment progresses and the data comes in, appears to be the less successful treatment. Nor would the device, by which only a supervising committee and not the patient's physician has access to the results of the experiment for a determined period of time,[36] insulate the physician from the consequences of this doctrine.[37]

NOTES

1. See generally, J. Katz, *Experimentation with Human Beings* (1972); Berger, "Reflections on Law and Experimental Medicine," 15 *U.C.L.A. L. Rev.* 436 (1968); Freund, "Ethical Problems in Human Experimentation," 273 *N. Engl. J. Med.* 687 (1965), Hirsh, "The Medico-Legal Framework for Medical Research" in *New Dimensions in Legal and Ethical Concepts for Human Research,* 169 Annals N.Y. Acad. Sci. (1970) [herinafter cited as *Annals*]; Jaffe, "Law as a System of Control," in 98 *Daedalus, Ethical Aspects of Experimentation with Human Subjects* (1969) [issue cited hereinafter as *Daedalus*]; Kaplan, "Experimentation—An Articulation of a New Myth," 46 *Neb. L. Rev.* 87 (1967); Note, 75 *Harv. L. Rev.* 1445 (1962); Note, 20 *Stan. L. Rev.* 99 (1967); Note, *Syr. L. Rev.* 1067 (1973).

2. See Halushka v. University of Saskatchewan, 53 D.L.R. 2d 436 (1965);Hyman v. Jewish Chronic Disease Hosp., 42 Misc. 2d 427, 248 N.Y.S. 2d 245 (Sup. Ct. 1964), rev'd per curiam, 21 App. Div. 2d 495, 251 N.Y.S. 2d 818, rev'd 15 N.Y. 2d 317, 206 N.E. 2d 338, 258 N.Y.S. 2d 397 (1965); USDHEW, *NIH, Institutional Guide to DHEW Policy on Protection of Human Subjects*

(1971) [hereinafter cited as *NIH*]; Capron, "The Law of Genetic Therapy," in Katz, *supra* note 1, at 574; Grad, "Regulation of Clinical Research by the State," in *Annals;* "Symposium," 36 *Fordham L. Rev.* 673 (1968).

3. See Fortner v. Koch, 272 Mich. 273, 261 N.W. 762 (1835); Freund, "Legal Frameworks for Human Experimentation," in *Daedalus;* Grad, *supra;* Katz, *supra.*

4. See *NIH,* at 6.

5. This was argued in defense of the experiments in Hyman v. Jewish Chronic Disease Hospital discussed in Katz, *supra,* Chapter 1.

6. See authorities cited *supra* note 1.

7. See generally, W. Prosser, *Torts* §99 (4th ed., 1971); Calabresi, "Toward A Test for Strict Liability in Torts," 81 *Yale L.J.,* 1055 (1972).

8. Larsen v. General Motors Corp., 391 F. 2d 495 (8th Cir. 1968); Witt v. Chrysler Corp., 15 Mich. App. 576, 167 N.W. 2d 100 (1969), Blitzstein v. Ford Motor Co., 288 F. 2d 738 (5th Cir. 1961).

9. Crotty v. Shartenberg's-New Haven, Inc., 147 Conn. 460, 162 A. 2d 513 (1960)(hair remover); Reynolds v. Sun Ray Drug Company, 135 N.J.L. 475, 52 A. 2d 666 (Ct. Err. & App. 1947) (lipstick); Esborg v. Bailey Drug Co., 61 Wash. 2d 347, 378 P. 2d 298 (1963) (hair tint).

10. Martin v. Bengue, Inc., 25 N.J. 359, 136 A. 2d 626 (1957); Marcus v. Specific Pharmaceuticals, 82 N.Y.S. 2d 194 (N.Y. Sup. Ct. 1948); Halloran v. Parke, Davis & Co., 245 App. Div. 727, 280 N.Y.S. 58 (1935).

11. Miranda v. Arizona, 384 U.S. 436 (1966).

12. See Calabresi, "Reflections on Medical Experimentation" in *Daedalus;* Freund, in *Daedalus;* Havighurst, "Compensating Persons Injured in Human Experimentation" 169 *Science* 153 (1970); Note, "Medical Experimentation Insurance" 70 *Colum. L. Rev.* 965 (1970); cf. Ehrenzweig "Compulsory Hospital-Accident Insurance: A Needed First Step Toward the Displacement of Liability for Medical Malpractice" 31 *U. Chi. L. Rev.* 279 (1964); R. Keeton, "Compensation for Medical Accidents" 121 *U. Pa. L. Rev.* 590 (1973); Note, "Medical Malpractice Litigation: Some Suggested Improvements and a Possible Alternative" 18 *U. Fla. L. Rev.* 623 (1966).

13. Calabresi, *The Cost of Accidents: An Economic and Legal Analysis* (1970).

14. Slater v. Baker, 2 Wils. K.B. 359, 95 Eng. Rep. 860 (1767); Carpenter v. Blake, 60 Barb. N.Y. 488 (1871); Langford v. Kosterlitz, 107 Cal. App. 175, 290 P. 80 (1930); Comment, "Non-Therapeutic Research Involving Human Subjects," 24 *Syr. L. Rev.* 1067 (1973), at 1069–1071.

15. Fortner v. Koch, *supra* note 3; Curran, "Governmental Regulation of the Use of Human Subjects in Medical Research"in *Daedalus.*

16. There may come a point, of course, where the procedure is so risky, the benefits so uncertain, and the basis of the treatment so speculative that to use it even with consent is tantamount to unprofessional conduct and quackery. The vagueness of the boundary is, of course, a cause for disquiet for practitioners working with new therapies.

17. See authorities collected at Katz, *supra* note 1, at 376–79; A. L. Cochrane, *Effectiveness and Efficiency* (1972); Chalmers, "Controlled Studies in Clinical Cancer Research," 287 *N. Engl. J. Med.* 75 (July 13, 1972); Shaw and Chalmers, "Ethics in Cooperative Trials" in *Annals;* Veterans Administration Cooperative Study Group, "Effects of Treatment on Morbidity in Hypertension" 213 *J.A.M.A.* 1143 (1970); also reported in Freis *et al., Anti-*

Hypertensive Therapy—Principles and Practice (F. Gross, ed. 1966).

18. Chalmers, "The Ethics of Randomization as a Decision Making Technique and the Problem of Informed Consent," in *US-DHEW Report of the 14th Annual Conference of Cardiovascular Training Grant Program Directors, National Heart Inst.* (1967); Chalmers, *supra;* Shaw and Chalmers, *supra;* Cochrane, *supra;* Chalmers, "When Should Randomization Begin?" *Lancet* 858 (April 20, 1968); Moore, "Ethical Boundaries in Initial Clinical Trials" in *Daedalus;* Mather *et al.,* "Acute Myocardial Infarction, Home and Hospital Treatment" *Br. Med. J.* 334 (August 7, 1971): Rutstein, "The Ethical Design of Human Experimentation" in *Daedalus.*

19. See Chalmers and Cochrane, *supra;* and see generally *The Quantitative Analysis of Social Problems* (Tufte, ed. 1970); Campbell and Erlebacher, "Regression Artifacts in Quasi-Experimental Design" in *The Disadvantaged Child–Compensatory Education,* vol. 3 (1970).

20. Thus, for instance, in a major RCT of the efficacy of simple as compared to radical mastectomy for cancer of the breast, Sir John Bruce writes: "one of the important ethical necessities before a random clinical trial is undertaken is a near certainty that none of the treatment options is likely to be so much inferior that harm could accrue to those allocated to it. In the present instance . . . it looked as if the mode of primary treatment made no significant difference, at least in terms of survival." "Operable Cancer of the Breast—A Controlled Clinical Trial," 28 *Cancer* 1443 (1971).

21. See *supra* note 25 [in original text].

22. See Chalmers, "The Ethics of Randomization as a Decision Making Technique and the Problem of Informed Consent," *supra* note 18; Chalmers, discussion in *Annals,* at 513–16; Lasagna, "Drug Evaluation Problems in Academia and Other Contexts" in *Annals.*

23. Cf. Alexander, "Psychiatry—Methods and Processes for Investigation of Drugs," in *Annals;* Park *et al.,* "Effects of Informed Consent in Research Patients and Study Results" 145 *J. Nerv. Ment. Dis.* 349 (1967), quoted in Katz, *supra* note 1, at 690.

24. Freund, *supra* note 3.

25. See American Bar Association, *Canons of Professional Ethics,* Canon 6, at 11 (1963). Canon 6 states clearly that the lawyer's duty, within the law is "solely" to his client, and should not be influenced by other interests or loyalties.

26. See *Scott on Trusts, §*2.5, 39–43 (3d. ed. 1967).

27. See Geddes v. Anaconda Copper Co., 254 U.S. 590 (1920) (director); Bingham v. Ditzler, 309 Ill. App. 581, 33 N.E. 939 (1941) (officer).

28. See, e.g., Guth v. Loft, 23 D. Ch. 255, 5 A. 2d 503 (1939); In re Westhall's Estate, 125 N.J. Eq. 340, 5 A. 2d 757 (1939); People v. People's Trust Co., 180 App. Div. 494, 167 N.Y.S. 767 (1917).

29. Professor Paul Freund has suggested that it would be improper for a judge to randomize in sentencing. 273 *N. Engl. J. Med.* 657 (1965). Whatever the objection to this may be, it is quite different from the objections I raise in my hypothetical cases or in medical practice. The convicted criminal is not the client of the judge and the judge does not owe him an undivided duty of loyalty. Indeed it is his job to consider social interests in sentencing the individual, and the randomized experiment may be a way of doing this.

30. See, e.g., In re Schummer's Will, 206 N.Y.S. 113, 210 App. Div. 296 (1924); affirmed In re Schummer's Estate, 154 N.E.

600, 243 N.Y. 548 (1926); In re Westhall's Estate, 5 A. 2d 757, 125 N.J. Eq. 551 (1939); Bearse v. Styler, 34 N.E. 2d 672, 309 Mass. 288 (1941).

31. See, e.g., Goodwin v. Agassiz, 186 N.E. 659, 283 Mass. 358 (1933); Daily v. Superior Court, 4 Cal. App. 2d 127, 40 P. 2d 936 (1935); Christensen v. Christensen, 327 Ill. 448, 158 N.E. 706 (1927).

32. Hammonds v. Aetna Cas. & Sur. Co., 237 F. Supp. 96 (N.D. Ohio 1965); motion denied, 243 F. Supp. 79 (1965); Stafford v. Schultz, 42 Cal. 2d 767, 270 P. 2d 1 (1954); Lockett v. Goodill, 71 Wash. 2d 654, 430 P. 2d 589 (1967).

33. See *supra* notes 45 and 46 [in original text] and accompanying text.

34. E.g., Chalmers, "Controlled Studies in Clinical Cancer Research," 287 *N. Engl. J. Med.* 75 (July 13, 1972); Shaw and Chalmers, "Ethics in Cooperative Trials," in *Annals;* cf. V.A. Cooperative Study Group, *supra* note 17.

35. Tvedt v. Haugen, 70 N.D. 338, 294 N.W. 183 (1940).

36. Chalmers, "Controlled Studies in Clinical Cancer Research" *supra* note 17.

37. The position I propose here is supported by Zeisel, "Reducing the Hazards of Human Experimentation through Modifications in Research Design," in *Annals.* See also Rutstein, "The Ethical Design of Human Experimentation" in *Daedalus.*

Research Involving Children

PAUL RAMSEY

Children in Medical Investigation

From consent as a canon of loyalty in medical practice it follows that children, who cannot give a mature and informed consent, or adult incompetents, should not be made the subjects of medical experimentation unless, other remedies having failed to relieve their grave illness, it is reasonable to believe that the administration of a drug as yet untested or insufficiently tested on human beings, or the performance of an untried operation, may further *the patient's own recovery.*

Now that is not a very elaborate moral rule governing medical practice in the matter of experiments involving children or incompetents as human subjects. It is a good example of the general claims of childhood specified for application in medical care and research. It is also a qualification immediately entailed by the meaning of consent in medical investigations as a joint undertaking between men. Again, one has to be prudent (which does not mean overcautious or scrupulous) in order to know how to care

for child-patients in this way. One must know the possible relation of a proposed procedure to the child's own recovery, and also its likely effectiveness compared with other methods that have been or could be tried. These considerations may provide the doctor with necessary and sufficient reason for investigations upon children, perhaps even very hazardous ones. One has to proportion the peril to the diagnostic or therapeutic needs of the child.

Practical medical judgment has undeniable and ominous room for its determinations, since a "benefit" is whatever is *believed* to be of help to the child. Still the limits this rule imposes on practice are essentially clear; where there is no possible relation to the child's recovery, a child is not to be made a mere object in medical experimentation for the sake of good to come. The likelihood of benefits that could flow from the experiment for many other children is an equally insufficient warrant for child experimentation. The individual child is to be tended in illness or in dying, since he himself is not able to donate his illness or his dying to be studied and worked upon solely for the advancement of medicine. Again, future

Reprinted with permission of the publisher from *The Patient a Person* (New Haven, Conn.: Yale University Press, 1970), pp. 11–17.

experience may tell us more about the meaning of this particular rule expressive of loyalty to a human child, and we may learn a great deal more about how to apply it in new situations with greater sensitivity and refinement—or we may learn more and more how to practice violations of it. But we are committed to refraining from morally significant exceptions to this rule defining impermissible medical experimentation upon children.

To experiment on children in ways that are not related to them as patients is already a sanitized form of barbarism; it already removes them from view and pays no attention to the faithfulness-claims which a child, simply by being a normal or a sick or dying child, places upon us and upon medical care. We should expect no morally significant exceptions to this canon of faithfulness to the child. To expect future justifiable exceptions is, in some sense, already to have forgotten the child.

To the layman, the most startling chapters in Dr. M. H. Pappworth's rather too sensational volume *Human Guinea Pigs*[1] are those in which he catalogues case after case of catheterization, percutaneous biopsy, and other hazardous experiments performed upon children, or upon women and their unborn children, *having no relation to their treatment*. Experts have estimated that catheterization of the right heart causes about one death per one thousand cases; of the left heart, five deaths per one thousand cases; and that the death rate in liver biopsy is from one to three per one thousand.[2] Moreover, a study of 55 deaths from heart catheterization has shown that there is "a close relation between the mortality rate and the patient's age." Deaths from this procedure result with greatest frequency in the first two months of life.[3] A parent is competent to consent for his child, and morally may venture to consent for his child to be subjected to these hazards, if the child is afflicted by a malady that is equally or more dangerous to him and to which the investigational procedure is definitely related. The diagnostic procedure may in fact prove to be of no benefit in the child's own treatment. But no parent is morally competent to consent that his child shall be submitted to hazardous or other experiments having no diagnostic or therapeutic significance for the child himself.

Pappworth's book has been criticized for, among other things, drawing the worst conclusion from the fact that articles in medical journals reporting an experiment often fail to state that consent was obtained or how it was obtained. This may be a valid objection,

especially since an indication that a piece of research was funded by the National Institutes of Health now means that a "peer" research committee in the medical center where the experimentation was conducted certified that consent would be obtained. But mention or failure to mention that consent was obtained is surely not the point. Nor is the point merely that, upon reading some of these cases of experiments, even hazardous ones, brought upon children with no relation to their own possible treatment, one has great difficulty understanding how any parent psychologically *could* consent to the procedure. The point is rather that morally no parent *should* consent—or be asked to consent to any such thing even if he is quite capable of doing so, and even if in fact his informed consent was obtained in all cases where this fact is not mentioned in the reports.

To attempt to consent for a child to be made an experimental subject is to treat a child as not a child. It is to treat him as if he were an adult person who has consented to become a joint adventurer in the common cause of medical research. If the grounds for this are alleged to be the presumptive or implied consent of the child, that must simply be characterized as a violent and a false presumption. Nontherapeutic, nondiagnostic experimentation involving human subjects must be based on true consent if it is to proceed as a human enterprise. No child or adult incompetent can choose to become a participating member of medical undertakings, and no one else on earth should decide to subject these people to investigations having no relation to their own treatment. That is a canon of loyalty to them. This they claim of us simply by being a human child or incompetent. When he is grown, the child may put away childish things and become a true volunteer. This is the meaning of being a volunteer: that a man enter and establish a consensual relation in some joint venture for medical progress—where before he could not, nor could anyone else, "volunteer" him for submission to unknown possible hazards for the sake of good to come.

If the requirement of parents, investigators, and state authorities in regard to their wards is "Never subject children to the unknown possible hazards of medical investigations having no relation to their own treatment," we must understand that the maladies for which the individual needs treatment and protection need not already be resident within the compass of the child's own skin. He can properly be regarded as one of a population, and we can add to the foregoing words: "except in epidemic conditions." Dr. Salk tried his polio vaccine on himself and his own children first. Then it was tested on selected children within a normal population. This involved some risk for the children vaccinated, and for other children as well, that the disease *might* be contracted from the vaccine itself, or that there might be unexpected injurious results. But the normal population of children was already subjected to waves of crippling epidemics summer after summer. A parent consenting for his child to be used in this trial was balancing the risks from the trial against the hazards from polio itself for that same child.

Physician-investigators are often in a quandary in which they are torn between the warrants for giving an experimental drug, and the warrants for withholding it from anyone in order to test it. Neither act seems justified, or both acts are equally warranted, when there is no available remedy and the indications are that a new drug may succeed. This situation also justifies a parent or guardian in consenting for a child, since we are supposing the hazard of the proposed treatment to be less or no greater than the hazard of the disease itself when treated by the established procedures. That would be a medical trial having clear relation to the treatment or protection of the child himself. He is not made, without his consent, the subject of medical investigations of possible benefit only to other children, other patients, or for the future advancement of medical science.

These may have been the circumstances surrounding the field trial of the vaccine for rubella (German measles) made in Taiwan, if this was in epidemic conditions, or in expectation of epidemic conditions, early in 1968 by a medical team from the University of Washington, headed by Dr. Thomas Grayston.[4] The vaccine was given to 3,269 young grade-school boys in the cities of Taipei and Taichung, while roughly an equal number were left unvaccinated for comparison purposes. The latter group were given Salk polio vaccine so that they would derive some benefit from the experience to which they were subjected. This generous "payment" does not alter the moral dilemma of withholding the rubella vaccine from a selected group. Yet there may have been an equipoise between the hazards of contracting rubella or other damage from the vaccine and the hazards of

contracting it if not vaccinated. There could have been a likelihood favoring the vaccinated of the two comparison groups.

These considerations, we may suppose, produced the quandary in the conscience of the investigators that was partially relieved by giving the unrelated Salk vaccine to the control group. Such equipoise alone would warrant—and it would sufficiently warrant—a parent or guardian in consenting that his child or ward be used for these research purposes. In the face of actual or predictable epidemic conditions, this would be medical investigation having some measurable or immeasurable relation to a child's own treatment or protection, as surely as the catheterization of the heart of a child with congenital heart trouble may be needed in his own diagnosis and treatment; and to this type of treatment a parent may venture to consent in his child's behalf. If no gulf is to be fixed between maladies beneath the skin and diseases afflicting children as members of a population, then the consent-requirement means: "Never submit children to medical investigation not related to their own treatment, except in face of epidemic conditions, endangering also each individual child." This is simply the meaning of the consent-requirement in application, not a "quantity-of-benefit-to-come" exception clause or a violation of this canon of loyalty to child-patients.

Indeed, a stricter construction of the necessary connection between proxy consent and the foreseeable needs of the child would permit the use of only girl children in field trials of rubella vaccine. Rubella is not the most contagious type of measles. The benefit to the subjects used in these trials (which plus the consent of parents legitimated subjecting them to experiment) was mainly to prevent their giving birth to children with congenital malformations should they later contract rubella during pregnancy. Therefore, there was stronger argument for considering only girl children as part of a population in establishing the necessary connection between experiment and "treatment."

More questionable were the earlier trials of the rubella vaccine performed upon the inmates of a retarded children's home in Conway, Arkansas. These subjects were not specially endangered by an epidemic of rubella. Few of the girls among them will ever be able to become part of the population of child-bearing women, or be in danger of pregnancy while in institutions. Using them simply had the advantage that they were segregated from the rest of the population, and any degree of risk to them would not spread to other people, including women of child-bearing age.

If children are incapable of truly consenting to experiments having unknown hazards for the sake of good to come, and if no one else should consent for them in cases unrelated to their own treatment, then medical research and society in general must choose a perhaps more difficult course of action to gain the benefits we seek from medical investigations. Surely it was possible to secure normal adult volunteers to consent to segregate themselves from the rest of the population for the duration of a rubella trial.[5] That method was simply more costly and inconvenient. At the same time, this illustrates the general fact that if we as a society are to proceed to the conquest of diseases, indeed, if we are to teach medical skills with fairness and justice to the poor and the ward patients, and with no violation of the basic claims of child-hood, then there must be far greater encouragement

generally in our society of a willingness to engage as joint adventurers for medical progress than has been achieved, or believed morally required by the principle of consent, in the past.

NOTES

1. Boston: Beacon, 1968.

2. Henry K. Beecher, "Medical Research and the Individual," in Daniel H. Labby (ed.), *Life or Death: Ethics and Options* (Seattle: University of Washington Press, 1968), p. 148.

3. Eugene Braunwald, "Deaths Related to Cardiac Catheterization," *Circulation,* Supplement III to vols. 27 and 28 (May 1968), pp. 17–26.

4. *New York Times,* October 17, 1968.

5. *New York Times,* April 5, 1969, reported that a hundred monks and nuns, from both Anglican and Roman Catholic orders, living in enclosed communities, were the voluntary subjects in testing American, British, and Belgian vaccines against German measles. This project was organized and directed by Dr. J. A. Dudgeon of London's Great Ormond Street Hospital for Sick Children.

RICHARD A. McCORMICK

Proxy Consent in the Experimentation Situation

It is widely admitted within the research community that if there is to be continuing and proportionate progress in pediatric medicine, experimentation is utterly essential. This conviction rests on two closely interrelated facts. First, as Alexander Capron has pointed out,[1] "Children cannot be regarded simply as 'little people' pharmacologically. Their metabolism, enzymatic and excretory systems, skeletal development and so forth differ so markedly from adults' that drug tests for the latter provide inadequate information about dosage, efficacy, toxicity, side effects, and contraindications for children." Second, and consequently, there is a limit to the usefulness of prior

Reprinted with permission of the author and the publisher from *Perspectives in Biology and Medicine,* Vol. 18, No. 1 (Autumn 1974), pp. 2–20. Copyright 1974 by The University of Chicago Press.

experimentation with animals and adults. At some point or other experimentation with children becomes necessary.

LEGAL CONSIDERATION

At this point, however, a severe problem arises. The legal and moral legitimacy of experimentation (understood here as procedures involving no direct benefit to the person participating in the experiment) is founded above all on the informed consent of the subject. But in many instances, the young subject is either legally or factually incapable of consent. Furthermore, it is argued, the parents are neither legally nor morally capable of supplying this consent for the child. As Dr. Donald T. Chalkley of the National Institutes of Health puts it: "A parent has no legal right to give consent for the involvement of his child in an activity not for the benefit of that child. No legal guardian, no person standing *in loco parentis,* has that right.''[2] It would seem to follow that infants and some minors are simply out of bounds where clinical research is concerned. Indeed, this conclusion has been explicitly drawn by the well-known ethician Paul Ramsey. He notes: ''If children are incapable of truly consenting to experiments having unknown hazards for the sake of good to come, and if no one else should consent for them in cases unrelated to their own treatment, then medical research and society in general must choose a perhaps more difficult course of action to gain the benefits we seek from medical investigations.''[3]

Does the consent requirement taken seriously exclude all experiments on children? If it does, then children themselves will be the ultimate sufferers. If it does not, what is the moral justification for the experimental procedures? The problem is serious, for, as Ramsey notes, an investigation involving children as subjects is ''a prismatic case in which to tell whether we mean to take seriously the consent-requirement.''[4]

Before concluding with Shirkey that those incompetent of consent are ''therapeutic orphans,''[5] I should like to explore the notion and validity of proxy consent. More specifically, the interest here is in the question, Can and may parents consent, and to what extent, to experiments on their children where the procedures are nonbeneficial for the child involved? Before approaching this question, it is necessary to point out the genuine if restricted input of the ethician in such matters. Ramsey has rightly pointed up the difference between the ethics of consent and ethics in the consent situation. This latter refers to the meaning and practical applications of the requirement of an informed consent. It is the work of prudence and pertains to the competence and responsibility of physicians and investigators. The former, on the other hand, refers to the principle requiring an informed consent, the ethics of consent itself. Such moral principles are elaborated out of competences broader than those associated with the medical community.

A brief review of the literature will reveal that the question raised above remains in something of a legal and moral limbo. The *Nuremberg Code* states only that ''the voluntary consent of the human subject is absolutely essential. This means that the person involved should have legal capacity to give consent.''[6]

Nothing specific is said about infants or those who are mentally incompetent. Dr. Leo Alexander, who aided in drafting the first version of the *Nuremberg Code,* explained subsequently that his provision for valid consent from next of kin where mentally ill patients are concerned was dropped by the Nuremberg judges, ''probably because [it] did not apply in the specific cases under trial.''[7, 8] Be that as it may, it has been pointed out by Beecher[9] that a strict observance of Nuremberg's rule 1 would effectively cripple study of mental disease and would simply prohibit all experimentation on children.

The *International Code of Medical Ethics* (General Assembly of the World Medical Association, 1949) states simply: ''Under no circumstances is a doctor permitted to do anything that would weaken the physical or mental resistance of a human being except from strictly therapeutic or prophylactic indications imposed in the interest of his patient.''[10] This statement is categorical and if taken literally means that ''young children and the mentally incompetent are categorically excluded from all investigations except those that directly may benefit the subjects.''[11] However, in 1954 the General Assembly of the World Medical Association (in *Principles for Those in Research and Experimentation*) stated: ''It should be required that each person who submits to experimentation be informed of the nature, the reason for, and the risk of the proposed experiment. If the patient is irresponsible, consent should be obtained from the individual who is legally responsible for the individual.''[12] In the context it is somewhat ambiguous whether this statement is meant to apply beyond experimental procedures that are performed for the patient's good.

The *Declaration of Helsinki* (1964) is much clearer on the point. After distinguishing ''clinical research combined with professional care'' and ''nontherapeutic clinical research,'' it states of this latter: ''Clinical research on a human being cannot be undertaken without his free consent, after he has been fully informed; if he is legally incompetent the consent of the legal guardian should be procured.''[13] In 1966 the American Medical Association, in its *Principles of Medical Ethics,* endorsed the Helsinki statement. It distinguished clinical investigation ''primarily for treatment'' and clinical investigation ''primarily for the accumulation of scientific knowledge.'' With regard to this latter, it noted that ''consent, in writing, should be obtained from the subject, or from his legally authorized representative if the subject lacks the capacity to consent.'' More specifically, with regard to minors or mentally incompetent persons, the AMA statement reads: ''Consent, in writing, is given by a legally authorized representative of the subject under circumstances in which an informed and prudent adult would reasonably be expected to volunteer himself or his child as a subject.''[14]

In 1963, the Medical Research Council of Great Britain issued its *Responsibility in Investigations on Human Subjects*.[15] Under title of ''Procedures Not of Direct Benefit to the Individual'' the Council stated: ''The situation in respect of minors and mentally subnormal or mentally disordered persons is of particular difficulty. In the strict view of the law parents and guardians of minors cannot give consent on their behalf to any procedures which are of no particular benefit to them and which may carry some risk of harm.'' Then, after discussing consent as involving a full understanding of ''the implications to himself of the procedures to which he was consenting,'' the Council concluded: ''When true consent in this sense cannot be obtained, procedures which are of no direct benefit and which might carry a risk of harm to the subject should not be undertaken.'' If it is granted that every experiment involves some risk, then the MRC statement would exclude any experiment on children. Curran and Beecher[16] have pointed out that this strict reading of English law is based on the advice of Sir Harvey Druitt, though there is no statute or case law to support it. Nevertheless, it has gone relatively unchallenged.

Statements of the validity of proxy consent similar to those of the *Declaration of Helsinki* and the American Medical Association have been issued by the American Psychological Association[17] and the Food and Drug Administration.[18] The most recent formulation touching on proxy consent is that of the Department of Health, Education, and Welfare in its *Protection of Human Subjects: Policies and Procedures*.[19] In situations where the subject cannot himself give consent, the document refers to ''supplementary judgment.'' It states: ''For the purposes of this document, supplementary judgment will refer to judgments made by local committees in addition to the subject's consent (when possible) and that of the parents or legal guardian (where applicable), as to whether or not a subject may participate in clinical research.'' The DHEW proposed guidelines admit that the law on parental consent is not clear in all respects. Proxy consent is valid with regard to established and gener-

ally accepted therapeutic procedures; it is, in practice, valid for therapeutic research. However, the guidelines state that ''when research might expose a subject to risk without defined therapeutic benefit or other positive effect on that subject's well-being, parental or guardian consent appears to be insufficient.'' These statements about validity concern law, in the sense (I would judge) of what would happen should a case determination be provoked on the basis of existing precedent.

MEDICAL ETHICS

After this review of the legal validity of proxy consent and its limitations, the DHEW guidelines go on to draw two ethical conclusions. First, ''When the risk of a proposed study is generally considered not significant, and the potential benefit is explicit, the ethical issues need not preclude the participation of children in biomedical research.'' Presumably, this means that where there is risk, ethical issues do preclude the use of children. However, the DHEW document did not draw this conclusion. Rather, its second ethical conclusion states: ''An investigator proposing research activities which expose children to risk must document, as part of the application for support, that the information to be gained can be obtained in no other way. The investigator must also stipulate either that the risk to the subjects will be insignificant or that, although some risk exists, the potential benefit is significant and far outweighs that risk. In no case will research activities be approved which entail substantial risk except in the cases of clearly therapeutic procedures.'' These proposed guidelines admit, therefore, three levels of risk within the ethical calculus: insignificant risk, some risk, and substantial risk. Proxy consent is, by inference, ethically acceptable for the first two levels but not for the third.

The documents cited move almost imperceptibly back and forth between legal and moral considerations, so that it is often difficult to know whether the major concern is one or the other, or even how the relationship of the legal and ethical is conceived. Nevertheless, it can be said that there has been a gradual move away from the absolutism represented in the *Nuremberg Code* to the acceptance of proxy consent, possibly because the *Nuremberg Code* is viewed as containing, to some extent, elements of a reaction to the Nazi experiments.

Medical literature of the noncodal variety has revealed this same pattern or ambiguity. For instance, writing in the *Lancet,* Dr. R. E. W. Fisher reacted to the reports of the use of children in research procedures as follows: "No medical procedure involving the slightest risk or accompanied by the slightest physical or mental pain may be inflicted on a child for experimental purposes unless there is a reasonable chance, or at least a hope, that the child may benefit thereby."[20] On the other hand, Franz J. Ingelfinger, editor of the *New England Journal of Medicine,* contends that the World Medical Association's statement ("Under no circumstances. . ." [above]) is an extremist position that must be modified.[11] His suggested modification reads: "Only when the risks are small and justifiable is a doctor permitted. . . ." It is difficult to know from Ingelfinger's wording whether he means small and therefore justifiable or whether "justifiable" refers to the hoped-for benefit. Responses to this editorial were contradictory. N. Baumslag and R. E. Yodaiken state: "In our opinion there are no conditions under which any children may be used for experimentation not primarily designed for their benefit."[21] Ian Shine, John Howieson, and Ward Griffen, Jr., came to the opposite conclusion: "We strongly support his [Ingelfinger's] proposals provided that one criterion of 'small and justifiable risks' is the willingness of the experimentor to be an experimentee, or to offer a spouse or child when appropriate."[22]

Curran and Beecher had earlier disagreed strongly with the rigid interpretation given the statement of the Medical Research Council through Druitt's influence. Their own conclusion was that "children under 14 may participate in clinical investigation which is not for their benefit where the studies are sound, promise important new knowledge for mankind, and there is no discernible risk."[23] The editors of *Archives of Disease in Childhood* recently endorsed this same conclusion, adding only "necessity of informed parental consent."[24] Discussing relatively minor procedures such as weighing a baby, skin pricks, venipunctures, etc., they contend that "whether or not these procedures are acceptable must depend, it seems to us, on whether the potential gain to others is commensurate with the discomfort to the individual." They see the Medical Research Council's statement as an understandable but exaggerated reaction to the shocking disclosures of the Nazi era. A new value judgment is required in our time, one based on the low risk-benefit ratio.

This same attitude is proposed by Alan M. W. Porter.[25] He argues that there are grounds "for believing that it may be permissible and reasonable to undertake minor procedures on children for experimental purposes with the permission of the parents." The low risk-benefit ratio is the ultimate justification. Interestingly, Porter reports the reactions of colleagues and the public to a research protocol he had drawn up. He desired to study the siblings of children who had succumbed to "cot death." The research involved venipuncture. A pediatric authority told Porter that venipuncture was inadmissible under the Medical Research Council code. Astonished, Porter showed the protocol to the first 10 colleagues he met. The instinctive reaction of nine out of 10 was "Of course you may." Similarly, a professional market researcher asked (for Porter) 10 laymen about the procedure, and all responded that he could proceed. In other words, Porter argues that public opinion (and therefore, presumably, moral common sense) stands behind the low risk-benefit ratio approach to experimentation on children.

This sampling is sufficient indication of the variety of reactions likely to be encountered when research on children is discussed.

THE VIEWS OF ETHICIANS

The professional ethicians who have written on this subject have also drawn rather different conclusions. John Fletcher argues that a middle path between autonomy (of the physician) and heteronomy (external control) must be discovered.[26] The Nuremberg rule "does not take account of exceptions which can be controlled and makes no allowance whatsoever for the exercise of professional judgment." It is clear that Fletcher would accept proxy consent in some instances, though he has not fully specified what these would be.

Thomas J. O'Donnell, S. J., notes that, besides informed consent, we also speak of three other modalities of consent.[27] First, there is presumed consent. Life-saving measures that are done on an unconscious patient in an emergency room are done with presumed consent. Second, there is implied consent. The various tests done on a person who undergoes a general checkup are done with implied consent, the consent being contained and implied in the very fact of his coming for a checkup. Finally, there is vicarious consent. This is the case of the parent who consents for therapy on an infant. O'Donnell wonders whether these modalities of consent, already accepted in the therapeutic context, can be extended to the context of clinical investigation (and by this he means research not to the direct benefit of the child). It is his conclusion that vicarious consent can be ethically operative "provided it is contained within the strict limits of a presumed consent (on the part of the subject) proper to clinical research and much narrower than the presumptions that might be valid in a therapeutic context." Practically, this means that O'Donnell would accept the validity of vicarious consent only where "danger is so remote and discomfort so minimal that a normal and informed individual would be presupposed to give ready consent." O'Donnell discusses neither the criteria nor the analysis that would set the "strict limits of a presumed consent."

Princeton's Paul Ramsey is the ethician who has discussed this problem at greatest length.[3] He is in clear disagreement with the positions of Fletcher and O'Donnell. Ramsey denies the validity of proxy consent in nonbeneficial (to the child) experiments simply and without qualification. Why? We may not, he argues, submit a child either to procedures that involve any measure of risk of harm or to procedures that involve no harm but simply "offensive touching." "A subject can be wronged without being harmed," he writes. This occurs whenever he is used as an object, or as a means only rather than also as an end in himself. Parents cannot consent to this type of thing, regardless of the significance of the experiment. Ramsey sees the morality of experimentation on children to be exactly what Paul Freund has described as the law on the matter: "The law here is that parents may consent for the child if the invasion of the child's body is for the child's welfare or benefit.[28, 29]

In pursuit of his point, Ramsey argues as follows: "To attempt to consent for a child to be made an experimental subject is to treat a child as not a child. It is to treat him as if he were an adult person who has consented to become a joint adventurer in the common cause of medical research. If the grounds for this are alleged to be the presumptive or implied consent of the child, that must simply be characterized as a violent and a false presumption." Thus, he concludes simply that "no parent is morally competent to consent that his child shall be submitted to hazardous *or other experiments* having no diagnostic or therapeutic significance for the child himself" (emphasis added). Though he does not say so, Ramsey would certainly conclude that a law that tolerates proxy consent to any

purely experimental procedure is one without moral warrants, indeed, is immoral because it legitimates (or tries to) treating a human being as a means only.

A careful study, then, of the legal, medical, and ethical literature on proxy consent for nontherapeutic research on children reveals profoundly diverging views. Generally, the pros and cons are spelled out in terms of two important values: individual integrity and societal good through medical benefits. Furthermore, in attempting to balance these two values, this literature by and large either affirms or denies the moral legitimacy of a risk-benefit ratio, what ethicians refer to as a teleological calculus. It seems to me that in doing this, current literature has not faced this tremendously important and paradigmatic issue at its most fundamental level. For instance, Ramsey bases his prohibitive position on the contention that nonbeneficial experimental procedures make an "object" of an individual. In these cases, he contends, parents cannot consent for the individual. Consent is the heart of the matter. If the parents could legitimately consent for the child, then presumably experimental procedures would not make an object of the infant and would be permissible. Therefore, the basic question seems to be, Why cannot the parents provide consent for the child? Why is their consent considered null here while it is accepted when procedures are therapeutic? To say that the child would be treated as an object does not answer this question; it seems that it presupposes the answer and announces it under this formulation.

TRADITIONAL MORAL THEOLOGY

There is in traditional moral theology a handle that may allow us to take hold of this problem at a deeper root and arrive at a principled and consistent position, one that takes account of all the values without arbitrarily softening or suppressing any of them. That handle is the notion of parental consent, particularly the theoretical implications underlying it. If this can be unpacked a bit, perhaps a more satisfying analysis will emerge. Parental consent is required and sufficient for therapy directed at the child's own good. We refer to this as vicarious consent. It is closely related to presumed consent. That is, it is morally valid precisely insofar as it is a reasonable presumption of the child's wishes, a construction of what the child would wish could he consent for himself. But here the notion of "what the child would wish" must be pushed further if we are to avoid a simple imposition of the adult world on the child. Why *would* the child so wish? The answer seems to be that he would choose this if he were capable of choice because he *ought* to do so. This statement roots in a traditional natural-law understanding of human moral obligations.

. . .

The natural-law tradition argues that there are certain identifiable values that we *ought* to support, attempt to realize, and never directly suppress because they are definitive of our flourishing and well-being. It further argues that knowledge of these values and of the prescriptions and proscriptions associated with them is, in principle, available to human reason. That is, they require for their discovery no divine revelation.

MORAL LEGITIMACY OF PROXY CONSENT

What does all this have to do with the moral legitimacy of proxy consent? It was noted that parental (proxy, vicarious) consent is required and sufficient for therapy directed to the child's own good. It was further noted that it is morally valid precisely insofar as it is a reasonable presumption of the child's wishes, a construction of what the child would wish could he do so. Finally, it was suggested that the child *would* wish this therapy because he *ought* to do so. In other words, a construction of what the child *would* wish (presumed consent) is not an exercise in adult capriciousness and arbitrariness, subject to an equally capricious denial or challenge when the child comes of age. It is based, rather, on two assertions: *(a)* that there are certain values (in this case life itself) definitive of our good and flourishing, hence values that we *ought* to choose and support if we want to become and stay human, and that therefore these are good also for the child; and *(b)* that these "ought" judgments, at least in their more general formulations, are a common patronage available to all men, and hence form the basis on which policies can be built.

Specifically, then, I would argue that parental consent is morally legitimate where therapy on the child is involved precisely because we know that life and health are goods for the child, that he *would* choose them because he *ought* to choose the good of life, his own self-preservation as long as this life remains, all things considered, a human good. To see whether and to what extent this type of moral analysis applies to experimentation, we must ask, Are there other things that the child *ought,* as a human being, to choose precisely because and insofar as they are goods definitive of his growth and flourishing? Concretely, *ought* he to choose his own involvement in nontherapeutic experimentation, and to what extent? Certainly there are goods or benefits, at least potential, involved. But are they goods that the child *ought* to choose? Or again, if we can argue that a certain level of involvement in nontherapeutic experimentation is good for the child and therefore that he *ought* to choose it, then there are grounds for saying that parental consent for this is morally legitimate and should be recognized as such.

Perhaps a beginning can be made as follows. To pursue the good that is human life means not only to choose and support this value in one's own case, but also in the case of others when the opportunity arises. In other words, the individual *ought* also to take into account, realize, make efforts in behalf of the lives of others, for we are social beings and the goods that define our growth and invite to it are goods that reside also in others. It can be good for one to pursue and support this good in others. Therefore, when it factually is good, we may say that one *ought* to do so (as opposed to not doing so). If this is true of all of us up to a point and within limits, it is no less true of the infant. He would choose to do so because he *ought* to do so. Now, to support and realize the value that is life means to support and realize health, the cure of disease, and so on. Therefore, up to a point, this support and realization is good for all of us individually. To share in the general effort and burden of health maintenance and disease control is part of our flourishing and growth as humans. To the extent that it is good for all of us to share this burden, we all *ought* to do so. And to the extent that we *ought* to do so, it is a reasonable construction or presumption of our wishes to say that we would do so. The reasonableness of this presumption validates vicarious consent.

It was just noted that sharing in the common burden of progress in medicine constitutes an individual good for all of us *up to a point*. That qualification is crucially important. It suggests that there are limits beyond which sharing is not or might not be a good. What might be the limits of this sharing? When might it no longer be a good for all individuals and therefore something that all need not choose to do? I would develop the matter as follows.

Adults may donate (*inter vivos*) an organ precisely because their personal good is not to be conceived individualistically but socially, that is, there is a natural order to other human persons which is in the very notion of the human personality itself. The personal being and good of an individual do have a relationship to the being and good of others, difficult as it may be to keep this in a balanced perspective. For this reason, an individual can become (in carefully delimited circumstances) more fully a person by donation of an organ, for by communicating to another of his very being he has more fully integrated himself into the mysterious unity between person and person.

Something similar can be said of participation in nontherapeutic experimentation. It can be affirmation of one's solidarity and Christian concern for others (through advancement of medicine). Becoming an experimental subject can involve any or all of three things: some degree of risk (at least of complications), pain, and associated inconvenience (e.g., prolonging hospital stay, delaying recovery, etc.). To accept these for the good of others could be an act of charitable concern.

There are two qualifications to these general statements that must immediately be made, and these qualifications explain the phrase "up to a point." First, whether it is personally good for an individual to donate an organ or participate in experimentation is a very circumstantial and therefore highly individual affair. For some individuals, these undertakings could be or prove to be humanly destructive. Much depends on their personalities, past family life, maturity, future position in life, etc. The second and more important qualification is that these procedures become human goods for the donor or subject precisely because and therefore only when they are voluntary, for the personal good under discussion is the good of expressed charity. For these two reasons I would conclude that no one else can make such decisions for an individual, that is, reasonably presume his consent. He has a right to make them for himself. In other words, whether a person *ought* to do such things is a highly individual affair and cannot be generalized in the way the good of self-preservation can be. And if we cannot say of an individual that he ought to do these things, proxy consent has no reasonable presumptive basis.

But are there situations where such considerations are not involved and where the presumption of consent is reasonable, because we may continue to say of all individuals that (other things being equal) they *ought* to be willing? I believe so. For instance, where organ donation is involved, if the only way a young child could be saved were by a blood transfusion from another child, I suspect that few would find such blood donation an unreasonable presumption on the child's wishes. The reason for the presumption is, I believe, that a great good is provided for another at almost no cost to the child. As the scholastics put it, *parum pro nihilo reputatur* ("very little counts for nothing"). For this reason we may say, lacking countervailing individual evidence, that the individual *ought* to do this.

Could the same reasoning apply to experimentation? Concretely, when a particular experiment would involve no discernible risks, no notable pain, no notable inconvenience, and yet hold promise of considerable benefit, should not the child be constructed to wish this in the same way we presume he chooses his own life, because he *ought* to? I believe so. He *ought* to want this not because it is in any way for his own medical good, but because it is not in any realistic way to his harm, and represents a potentially great benefit for others. He *ought* to want these benefits for others.

WHAT THEY OUGHT TO WANT

If this is a defensible account of the meaning and limits of presumed consent where those incompetent to consent are concerned, it means that proxy consent can be morally legitimate in some experimentations. Which? Those that are scientifically well designed (and therefore offer hope of genuine benefit), that cannot succeed unless children are used (because there are dangers involved in interpreting terms such as "discernible" and "negligible," the child should not unnecessarily be exposed to these even minimal risks), that contain no discernible risk or undue discomfort for the child. Here it must be granted that the notions of "discernible risk" and "undue discomfort" are themselves slippery and difficult, and probably somewhat relative. They certainly involve a value judgment and one that is the heavy responsibility of the medical profession (not the moral theologian) to make. For example, perhaps it can be debated whether venipuncture involves "discernible risks" or "undue discomfort" or not. But if it can be concluded that, in human terms, the risk involved or the discomfort is negligible or insignificant, then I believe there are sound reasons in moral analysis for saying that parental consent to this type of invasion can be justified.

Practically, then, I think there are good moral warrants for adopting the position espoused by Curran, Beecher, Ingelfinger, the *Helsinki Declaration,* the *Archives of Disease in Childhood,* and others. Some who have adopted this position have argued it in terms of a low risk-benefit ratio. This is acceptable if properly understood, that is, if "low risk" means for all practical purposes and in human judgment "no realistic risk." If it is interpreted in any other way, it opens the door wide to a utilitarian subordination of the individual to the collectivity. It goes beyond what individuals would want because they *ought* to. For instance, in light of the above analysis, I find totally unacceptable the DHEW statement that "the investigator must also stipulate either that the risk to the subjects will be insignificant, or that *although some risk exists, the potential benefit is significant and far outweighs that risk.*" This goes beyond what all of us, as members of the community, necessarily *ought* to do. Therefore, it is an invalid basis for proxy consent. For analogous reasons, in light of the foregoing analysis I would conclude that parental consent for a kidney transplant from one noncompetent 3-year-old to another is without moral justification.

•   •   •

These considerations do not mean that all non-competents (where consent is concerned) may be treated in the same way, that the same presumptions are morally legitimate in all cases. For if the circumstances of the infant or child differ markedly, then it is possible that there are appropriate modifications in our construction of what he *ought* to choose. For instance, I believe that institutionalized infants demand special consideration. They are in a situation of peculiar danger for several reasons. First, they are often in a disadvantaged condition physically or mentally so that there is a temptation to regard them as "lesser human beings." Medical history shows our vulnerability to this type of judgment. Second, as institutionalized, they are a controlled group, making them particularly tempting as research subjects. Third, experimentation in such infants is less exposed to public scrutiny. These and other considerations suggest that there is a real danger of overstepping the line between what we all ought to want and what only the individual might want out of heroic, self-sacrificial charity. If such a real danger exists, then what the infant is construed as wanting because he *ought* must be modified. He need not *ought to want* if this involves him in real dangers of going beyond this point.

•   •   •

The editor of the *Journal of the American Medical Association,* Robert H. Moser, in the course of an editorial touching on, among other things, the problem of experimentation, asks whether we are ever justified in the use of children. His answer: "It is an insoluble dilemma. All one can ask is that each situation be studied with consummate circumspection and be approached rationally and compassionately."[30] If circumspection in each situation is to be truly consummate, and if the approach is to be rational and compassionate, then the situation alone cannot be the decisional guide. If the situation alone is the guide, if everything else is a "dilemma," then the qualities Moser seeks in the situation are in jeopardy, and along with them human rights. One can indeed, to paraphrase Moser, ask more than that each situation be studied. He can ask that a genuine ethics of consent be brought to the situation so that ethics in the consent situation will have some chance of surviving human enthusiasms. And an ethics of consent finds its roots in a solid natural-law tradition which maintains that there are basic values that define our potential as human beings; that we ought (within limits and with qualifications) to choose, support, and never directly suppress these values in our conduct; that we can know, therefore, what others would choose (up to a point) because they ought; and that this knowledge is the basis for a soundly grounded and rather precisely limited proxy consent.

NOTES

1. A. Capron. *Clin. Res.,* 21:141, 1973.

2. *Med. World News,* June 8, 1973, p. 41.

3. P. Ramsey. *The Patient as Person.* New Haven, Conn.: Yale Univ. Press, 1970, p. 17.

4. *Ibid.,* p. 28.

5. H. Shirkey. *J. Pediatr.,* 72:119, 1968.

6. H. K. Beecher. *Research and the Individual.* Boston: Little, Brown, 1970.

7. Ramsey, *op. cit.,* p. 26.

8. L. Alexander. *Dis. Nerv. Syst.,* 27:62, 1966.

9. *Op. cit.,* p. 231.

10. Beecher, *op. cit.,* p. 236.

11. F. J. Ingelfinger. *N. Engl. J. Med.,* 288:791, 1973.

12. Beecher, *op. cit.,* p. 240.

13. *Ibid.,* p. 278.

14. *Ibid.,* p. 223.

15. *Ibid.,* pp. 262ff.

16. W. J. Curran and H. K. Beecher. *J. Am. Med. Ass.*, 210:77, 1969.

17. Beecher, *op. cit.*, pp. 256ff.

18. *Ibid.*, pp. 299ff.

19. Department of Health, Education, and Welfare. *Federal Register,* 38:31738, 1973.

20. R. E. W. Fisher. *Lancet* (Letters), November 7, 1953, p. 993.

21. N. Baumslag and R. W. Yodaiken. *N. Engl. J. Med.* (Letters), 288:1247, 1973.

22. I. Shine, J. Howieson, and W. Griffen. Jr. *N. Engl. J. Med.* (Letters), 288:1248, 1973.

23. Curran and Beecher, *op. cit.*, p. 81.

24. Editorial. *Arch. Dis. Child.*, 48:751, 1973.

25. A. W. Franklin, A. M. Porter, and D. N. Raine. *Br. Med. J.,* May 19, 1973, p. 402.

26. J. Fletcher. *Law Contemp. Probl.,* 32:620, 1967.

27. T. J. O'Donnell. *J. Am. Med. Ass.*, 227:73, 1974.

28. P. Freund. *N. Engl. J. Med.*, 273:691, 1965.

29. ———. *Trial,* 2:48, 1966.

30. R. H. Moser. *J. Am. Med. Ass.*, 277:432, 1974.

NATIONAL COMMISSION FOR THE PROTECTION OF HUMAN SUBJECTS

Recommendations on Research Involving Children

Definitions. For the purpose of this report:

1. *Children* are persons who have not attained the legal age of consent to general medical care as determined under the applicable law of the jurisdiction in which the research will be conducted.

· · ·

2. *Research* is a formal investigation designed to develop or contribute to generalizable knowledge.

Comment: A research project generally is described in a protocol that sets forth explicit objectives and formal procedures designed to reach those objectives. The protocol may include therapeutic and other activities intended to benefit the subjects, as well as procedures to evaluate such activities. Research objectives range from understanding normal and abnormal physiological or psychological functions or social phenomena, to evaluating diagnostic, therapeutic or preventive interventions and variations in services or practices. The activities or procedures involved in research may be invasive or noninvasive and include surgical interventions; removal of body tissues or fluids; administration of chemical substances or forms of energy; modification of diet, daily routine or service delivery; alteration of environment; observation; administration of questionnaires or tests; randomization; review of records, etc.

3. *Minimal risk* is the probability and magnitude of physical or psychological harm that is normally encountered in the daily lives, or in the routine medical or psychological examination, of healthy children.

Comment: In any assessment of the degree of risk to children that is presented by proposed research activities, the age of the prospective research subjects should be taken into account. The possible effects of disruption of normal routine, separation from parents, or unusual discomfort should be considered, as well as more obvious physical or psychological harms. Examples of medical procedures presenting no more than minimal risk would include routine immunization, modest changes in diet or schedule, physical examination, obtaining blood and urine specimens, and developmental assessments. Similarly, many

From U.S., National Commission for the Protection of Human Subjects of Biomedical and Behavioral Research, *Research Involving Children: Report and Recommendations* (Washington, D.C.: U.S. Department of Health, Education, and Welfare, 1977), pp. xix–xxi, 1–20.

routine tools of behavioral research, such as most questionnaires, observational techniques, noninvasive physiological monitoring, psychological tests and puzzles, may be considered to present no more than minimal risk. Questions about some topics, however, may generate such anxiety or stress as to involve more than minimal risk. Research in which information is gathered that could be harmful if disclosed should not be considered of minimal risk unless adequate provisions are made to preserve confidentiality. Research in which information will be shared with persons or institutions that may use such information against the subjects should be considered to present more than minimal risk.

4. *Institutional Review Board* (IRB) is (1) a committee required under P.L. 93-348 and approved by the Department of Health, Education, and Welfare to review research involving human subjects at an institution receiving support for such research under the Public Health Service Act, or (2) any substantially similar committee which reviews research involving human subjects that is conducted, supported or regulated by a federal agency or department. . . .

Recommendation 1. Since the Commission finds that research involving children is important for the health and well-being of all children and can be conducted in an ethical manner, the Commission recommends that such research be conducted and supported, subject to the conditions set forth in the following recommendations.

Comment: The Commission recognizes the importance of safeguarding and improving the health and well-being of children, because they deserve the best care that society can reasonably provide. It is necessary to learn more about normal development as well as disease states in order to develop methods of diagnosis, treatment and prevention of conditions that jeopardize the health of children, interfere with optimal development, or adversely affect well-being in later years. Accepted practices must be studied as well, for although infants cannot survive without continual support, the effects of many routine practices are unknown and some have been shown to be harmful.

Much research on childhood disorders or conditions necessarily involves children as subjects. The benefits of this research may accrue to the subjects

directly or to children as a class. The Commission considers, therefore, that the participation of children in research related to their conditions should receive the encouragement and support of the federal government.

The Commission recognizes, however, that the vulnerability of children, which arises out of their dependence and immaturity, raises questions about the ethical acceptability of involving them in research. Such ethical problems can be offset, the Commission believes, by establishing conditions that research must satisfy to be appropriate for the involvement of children. Such conditions are set forth in the following recommendations.

Recommendation 2. Research involving children may be conducted or supported provided an Institutional Review Board has determined that: (a) the research is scientifically sound and significant; (b) where appropriate, studies have been conducted first on animals and adult humans, then on older children, prior to involving infants; (c) risks are minimized by using the safest procedures consistent with sound research design and by using procedures performed for diagnostic or treatment purposes whenever feasibile; (d) adequate provisions are made to protect the privacy of children and their parents, and to maintain confidentiality of data; (e) subjects will be selected in an equitable manner; and (f) the conditions of all applicable subsequent recommendations are met.

Comment: This recommendation sets forth general conditions that should apply to all research involving children. Such research must also satisfy the conditions of one *or more* of Recommendations (3) through (6), as applicable; Recommendation (7); Recommendation (8), if permission of parents or guardians is not a reasonable requirement; Recommendation (9), if the subjects are wards of the state; and Recommendation (10), if the subjects are institutionalized.

Respect for human subjects requires the use of sound methodology appropriate to the discipline. The time and inconvenience requested of subjects should be justified by the soundness of the research and its design, even if no more than minimal risk is involved. In addition, research involving children should satisfy a standard of scientific significance, since these subjects are less capable than adults of determining for themselves whether to participate. If necessary, the IRB [Institutional Review Board] should obtain the advice of consultants to assist in determining scientific soundness and significance. . . .

Whenever possible, research involving risk should be conducted first on animals and adult humans in order to ascertain the degree of risk and the likelihood of generating useful knowledge. Sometimes this is not relevant or possible, as when the research is designed to study disorders or functions that have no parallel in animals or adults. In such cases, studies involving risk should be initiated on older children to the extent feasible prior to including infants, because older children are less vulnerable and they are better able to understand and to assent to participation. In addition, they are more able to communicate about any physical or psychological effects of such participation.

In order to minimize risk, investigators should use the safest procedures consistent with good research design and should make use of information or materials obtained for diagnostic or treatment purposes whenever feasible. For example, if a blood sample is needed, it should be obtained from samples drawn for diagnostic purposes whenever it is consistent with research requirements to do so.

Adequate measures should be taken to protect the privacy of children and their families, and to maintain the confidentiality of data. The adequacy of procedures for protecting confidentiality should be considered in light of the sensitivity of the data to be collected (i.e., the extent to which disclosure could reasonably be expected to be harmful or embarrassing).

Subjects should be selected in an equitable manner, avoiding overutilization of any one group of children based solely upon administrative convenience or availability of a population living in conditions of social or economic deprivation. The burdens of participation in research should be equitably distributed among the segments of our society, no matter how large or small those burdens may be.

In addition to the foregoing requirements, research must satisfy the conditions of the following recommendations, as applicable.

Recommendation 3. Research that does not involve greater than minimal risk to children may be conducted or supported provided an Institutional Review Board has determined that: (a) the conditions of Recommendation (2) are met; and (b) adequate provisions are made for assent of the children and permission of their parents or guardians, as set forth in Recommendations (7) and (8).

Comment: If the IRB determines that proposed research will present no more than minimal risk to children, the research may be conducted or supported

provided the conditions of Recommendation (2) are met and appropriate provisions are made for parental permission and the children's assent, as described in Recommendations (7) and (8) below. If the IRB is unable to determine that the proposed research will present no more than minimal risk to children, the research should be reviewed under Recommendations (4), (5) and (6), as applicable.

Recommendation 4. Research in which more than minimal risk to children is presented by an intervention that holds out the prospect of direct benefit for the individual subjects, or by a monitoring procedure required for the well-being of the subjects, may be conducted or supported provided an Institutional Review Board has determined that: (a) such risk is justified by the anticipated benefit to the subjects; (b) the relation of anticipated benefit to such risk is at least as favorable to the subjects as that presented by available alternative approaches; (c) the conditions of Recommendation (2) are met; and (d) adequate provisions are made for assent of the children and permission of their parents or guardians, as set forth in Recommendations (7) and (8).

Comment: The Commission emphasizes that the purely investigative procedures in research encompassed by Recommendation (4) should entail no more than minimal risk to children. Greater risk is permissible under this recommendation only if it is presented by an intervention that holds out the prospect of direct benefit to the individual subjects or by a procedure necessary to monitor the effects of such intervention in order to maintain the well-being of these subjects (e.g., obtaining samples of blood or spinal fluid in order to determine drug levels that are safe and effective for the subjects). Such risk is acceptable, for example, when all available treatments for a serious illness or disability have been tried without success, and the remaining option is a new intervention under investigation. The expectation of success should be scientifically sound to justify undertaking whatever risk is involved. It is also appropriate to involve children in research when accepted therapeutic, diagnostic or preventive methods involve risk or are not entirely successful, and new biomedical or behavioral procedures under investigation present at least an equally favorable risk-benefit ratio. The IRB should evaluate research protocols of this sort in the same way that comparable decisions are made in clinical practice. It should compare the risk and anticipated benefit of the intervention under investigation (including the monitoring procedures necessary for care of the child) with those of available alternative methods of achieving the same goal, and should also consider the risk and possible benefit of attempting no intervention whatsoever.

To determine the overall acceptability of the research, the risk and anticipated benefit of activities described in a protocol must be evaluated individually as well as collectively, as is done in clinical practice. Research protocols meeting the criteria regarding risk and benefit may be conducted or supported provided the conditions of Recommendation (2) are fulfilled and the requirements for assent of the children and for permission and participation of their parents or guardians, as set forth in Recommendations (7) and (8), will be met. If the research also includes a purely investigative procedure presenting more than minimal risk, the research should be reviewed under Recommendation (5) with respect to such procedure.

Recommendation 5. Research in which more than minimal risk to children is presented by an intervention that does not hold out the prospect of direct benefit for the individual subjects, or by a monitoring procedure not required for the well-being of the subjects, may be conducted or supported provided an Institutional Review Board has determined that: (a) such risk represents a minor increase over minimal risk; (b) such intervention or procedure presents experiences to subjects that are reasonably commensurate with those inherent in their actual or expected medical, psychological or social situations, and is likely to yield generalizable knowledge about the subjects' disorder or condition; (c) the anticipated knowledge is of vital importance for understanding or amelioration of the subjects' disorder or condition; (d) the conditions of Recommendation (2) are met; and (e) adequate provisions are made for assent of the children and permission of their parents or guardians, as set forth in Recommendations (7) and (8).

Comment: An IRB must determine that three special criteria are met in order to approve research presenting more than minimal risk but no direct benefit to the individual subjects. First, the increment in risk must be no more than a minor increase over minimal risk. The IRB should consider the degree of risk presented by the research from at least the following four perspectives: a common-sense estimation of the risk; an estimation based upon investigators' experience

with similar interventions or procedures; any statistical information that is available regarding such interventions or procedures; and the situation of the proposed subjects. Second, the research activity must be commensurate with (i.e., reasonably similar to) procedures that the prospective subjects and others with the specific disorder or condition ordinarily experience (by virtue of having or being treated for that disorder or condition). Finally, the research must hold out the promise of significant benefit in the future to children suffering from or at risk for the disorder or condition (including, possibly, the subjects themselves). If necessary, the advice of scientific consultants should be obtained to assist in determining whether the research is likely to provide knowledge of vital importance to understanding the etiology or pathogenesis, or developing methods for the prevention, diagnosis or treatment, of the disorder or condition affecting the subjects.

The requirement of commensurability of experience should assist children who can assent to make a knowledgeable decision about their participation in research, based on some familiarity with the intervention or procedure and its effects. More generally, commensurability is intended to assure that participation in research will be closer to the ordinary experience of the subjects. The use of procedures that are familiar or similar to those used in treatment of the subjects should not, however, be used as a major justification for their participation in research, but rather as one of several criteria regarding the acceptability of such participation.

In addition to these special criteria, the IRB should assure that the conditions of Recommendation (2) are fulfilled and the requirements for assent of the children and permission and participation of their parents or guardians, as set forth in Recommendations (7) and (8), will be met. If the proposed research includes an intervention or procedure from which the subjects may derive direct benefit, it should also be reviewed under Recommendation (4) with respect to that intervention or procedure.

Recommendation 6. Research that cannot be approved by an Institutional Review Board under Recommendations (3), (4) and (5), as applicable, may be conducted or supported provided an Institutional Review Board has determined that the research presents an opportunity to understand, prevent or alleviate a serious problem affecting the health or welfare of children and, in addition, a national ethical advisory board and, following opportunity for public review and comment, the secretary of the responsible federal department (or highest official of the responsible federal agency) has determined either (a) that the research satisfies the conditions of Recommendations (3), (4) and (5), as applicable, or (b) the following: (i) the research presents an opportunity to understand, prevent or alleviate a serious problem affecting the health or welfare of children; (ii) the conduct of the research would not violate the principles of respect for persons, beneficence and justice; (iii) the conditions of Recommendation (2) are met; and (iv) adequate provisions are made for assent of the children and permission of their parents or guardians, as set forth in Recommendations (7) and (8).

Comment: If an IRB is unable for any reason to determine that proposed research satisfies the conditions of Recommendations (3), (4) and (5), as applicable, the IRB may nevertheless certify the research for review and possible approval by a national ethical advisory board and the secretary of the responsible department. Such review is contingent upon an IRB's determination that the research presents an opportunity to understand, prevent or alleviate a serious problem affecting the health or welfare of children. Thereafter, the research should be reviewed by the national board and secretary, with opportunity for public comment, to determine whether the conditions of Recommendations (3), (4) and (5), as applicable, are satisfied, or, alternatively, the research is justified by the importance of the knowledge sought and would not contravene principles of respect for persons, beneficence and justice that underlie these recommendations. In the latter instance, commencement of the research should be delayed pending Congressional notification and a reasonable opportunity for Congress to take action regarding the proposed research.

The provision for national review and approval under Recommendations (3), (4) and (5) is intended to fit the situation where an IRB has difficulty in applying those recommendations but considers the research of sufficient importance to warrant national review. Such difficulty may be resolved by a determination on the national level pursuant to Recommendation (6a) that the research does satisfy the conditions of the applicable earlier recommendations. Alternatively, the national review may determine either that the research satisfies the conditions of Recommendation (6b) or that it should not be conducted.

The Commission believes that only research of major significance, in the presence of a serious health problem, would justify the approval of research under Recommendation (6b). The problem addressed must be a grave one, the expected benefit should be significant, the hypothesis regarding the expected benefit must be scientifically sound, and an equitable method should be used for selecting subjects who will be invited to participate. Finally, appropriate provisions should be made for assent of the subjects and permission and participation of parents or guardians.

Recommendation 7. In addition to the determinations required under the foregoing recommendations, as applicable, the Institutional Review Board should determine that adequate provisions are made for: (a) soliciting the assent of the children (when capable) and the permission of their parents or guardians; and, when appropriate, (b) monitoring the solicitation of assent and permission, and involving at least one parent or guardian in the conduct of the research. A child's objection to participation in research should be binding unless the intervention holds out a prospect of direct benefit that is important to the health or wellbeing of the child and is available only in the context of the research.

Comment: The Commission uses the term parental or guardian "permission," rather than "consent," in order to distinguish what a person may do autonomously (consent) from what one may do on behalf of another (grant permission). Parental permission normally will be required for the participation of children in research. In addition, assent of the children should be required when they are seven years of age or older. The Commission uses the term "assent" rather than "consent" in this context, to distinguish a child's agreement from a legally valid consent.

Parental or guardian permission, as used in this recommendation, refers to the permission of parents, legally appointed guardians, and others who care for a child in a reasonably normal family setting. The last category might include, for example, step-parents or relatives such as aunts, uncles or grandparents who have established a continuing, close relationship with the child. Recommendation (8) describes circumstances in which the IRB may determine that the permission of parents or guardians is not appropriate because of the nature of the subject under investigation (e.g., contraception, drug abuse) or because of a failure in the relationship with the child (e.g., child abuse, neglect).

Parental or guardian permission should reflect the collective judgment of the family that an infant or child may participate in research. There are some research projects for which documented permission of one parent or guardian should be sufficient, such as research involving no more than minimal risk (as described in Recommendation 3), or research in which risks or discomforts are related to a therapeutic, diagnostic or preventive intervention (as described in Recommendation 4). In such cases, it may be assumed that the person giving formal permission is reflecting a family consensus. For research that is described in Recommendations (5) and (6), the permission of both parents should be documented unless one parent is deceased, unknown, incompetent or not reasonably available, or the child has a guardian or belongs to a single-parent family (i.e., when only one person has legal responsibility for the care, custody and financial support of the child). The IRB should determine for each project whether permission of one or both parents should be required, a substitute mechanism may be used, or the provision may be waived. In making such determination, the IRB should consider the nature of the activities described in the research protocol and the age, status and condition of the subjects.

The IRB should assure that children who will be asked to participate in research described in Recommendation (5) are those with good relationships with their parents or guardians and their physician, and who are receiving care in supportive surroundings. Projects approved under Recommendations (4) and (6) may also require scrutiny of this sort. The IRB may wish to appoint someone to assist in the selection of subjects and to review the quality of interaction between parents or guardian and child. A member of the board or a consultant such as the child's pediatrician, a psychologist, a social worker, a pediatric nurse, or other experienced and perceptive person would be appropriate. The IRB should be particularly sensitive to the difficulties surrounding permission when the investigator is the treating physician to whom the parents or guardian may feel an obligation.

Because of the dependence of infants, the traditional role of parents as protectors, and the general authority of parents to determine the care and upbringing of their children, the IRB may determine that small children should participate in certain research only if the parents or guardians participate themselves by being present during some or all of the conduct of the research. This role will vary according to the nature of the research, the risk involved, the extent to which the research entails possibly disturbing deviations from normal routine, and the age and condition of the children. As a general rule, when infants participate in research that may cause physical discomfort or emotional stress and involves a significant departure from normal routine, a parent or guardian should be present. However, if discomfort arises only as a result of therapeutic interventions that must continue over a considerable period of time, the continual presence of parents need not be required. Parental presence during the conduct of much behavioral research may not be feasible or warranted, especially with older children. Generally, parents or guardians should be sufficiently involved in the research to understand its effects on their children and be able to intervene, if necessary.

The Commission believes that children who are seven years of age or older are generally capable of understanding the procedures and general purpose of research and of indicating their wishes regarding participation. Their assent should be required in addition to parental permission. However, if any child over six years of age is incapacitated so that he or she cannot reasonably be consulted, then parental permission should be sufficient, as it is for infants. The objection of a child of any age to participation in research should be binding except as noted below.

If the research protocol includes an intervention from which the subjects might derive significant benefit to their health or welfare, and that intervention is available only in a research context, the objection of a small child may be overridden. Such would be the case, for example, with a new drug that is not approved by the Food and Drug Administration for general distribution until safety and efficacy have been demonstrated in controlled clinical trials. Access to a drug under investigation generally requires participation in the research. Similar restrictions may be placed on other innovative therapies as a precaution. As children mature, their ability to perceive and act in their own best interest increases; thus, their wishes with respect to such research should carry increasingly more weight. When school-age children disagree with their parents regarding participation in such research, the IRB may wish to have a third party discuss the matter with all concerned and be present during the consent process. Although parents may legally override the objections of school-age children in such cases, the burden of that decision becomes heavier in relation to the maturity of the particular child.

Disclosure requirements for assent and permission are the same as those for informed consent. Similarly, children and parents or guardians should be free from duress. In order to assure understanding and freedom of choice, the IRB may determine that there is a need for an advocate to be present during the decision-making process. The need for third-party involvement in this process will vary according to the risk presented by the research and the autonomy of the subjects. The advocate should be an individual who has the experience and perceptiveness to fulfill such a role and who is not related in any way (except in the role as advocate or member of the IRB) to the research or the investigators.

Finally, the IRB should pay particular attention to the explanation and consent form, if any, to assure that appropriate language is used.

Recommendation 8. If the Institutional Review Board determines that a research protocol is designed for conditions or a subject population for which parental or guardian permission is not a reasonable requirement to protect the subjects, it may waive such requirement provided an appropriate mechanism for protecting the children who will participate as subjects in the research is substituted. The choice of an appropriate mechanism should depend upon the nature and purpose of the activities described in the protocol, the risk and anticipated benefit to the research subjects, and their age, status and condition.

Comment: Circumstances that would justify modification or waiver of the requirement for parental or guardian permission include: (1) research designed to identify factors related to the incidence or treatment of certain conditions in adolescents for which, in certain jurisdictions, they legally may receive treatment without parental consent; (2) research in which the subjects are ''mature minors'' and the procedures involved entail essentially no more than minimal risk that such individuals might reasonably assume on their own; (3) research designed to understand and meet the needs of neglected or abused children, or children designated by their parents as ''in need of supervision''; and (4) research involving children whose parents are legally or functionally incompetent.

There is no single mechanism that can be substituted for parental permission in every instance. In some cases the consent of mature minors should be sufficient. In other cases court approval may be required. The mechanism invoked will vary with the research and the age, status and condition of the prospective subjects.

A number of states have specific legislation permitting minors to consent to treatment for certain conditions (e.g., pregnancy, drug addiction, venereal diseases) without the permission (or knowledge) of their parents. If parental permission were required for research about such conditions, it would be difficult to develop improved methods of prevention and therapy that meet the special needs of adolescents. Therefore, assent of such mature minors should be considered sufficient with respect to research about conditions for which they have legal authority to consent on their own to treatment. An appropriate mechanism for protecting such subjects might be to require that a clinic nurse or physician, unrelated to the research, explain the nature and the purpose of the research to prospective subjects, emphasizing that participation is unrelated to provision of care.

Another alternative might be to appoint a social worker, pediatric nurse, or physician to act as surrogate parent when the research is designed, for example, to study neglected or battered children. Such surrogate parents would be expected to participate not only in the process of soliciting the children's cooperation but also in the conduct of the research, in order to provide reassurance for the subjects and to intervene or support their desires to withdraw if participation becomes too stressful.

Recommendation 9. Children who are wards of the state should not be included in research approved under Recommendations (5) or (6) unless such research is: (a) related to their status as orphans, abandoned children, and the like; or (b) conducted in a school or similar group setting in which the majority of children involved as subjects are not wards of the state. If such research is approved, the Institutional Review Board should require that an advocate for each child be appointed, with an opportunity to intercede that would normally be provided by parents.

Comment: It is important to learn more about the effects of various settings in which children who are wards of the state may be placed, as well as about the circumstances surrounding child abuse and neglect, in order to improve the care that is provided for such children by the community. Also, it is important to avoid embarrassment or psychological harm that might result from excluding wards of the state from research projects in which their peers in a school, camp or other group setting will be participating. Provision must be made to permit the conduct of such studies in ways that will protect the children involved, even though no parents or guardians are available to act in their behalf.

To this end, the IRB reviewing such research should evaluate the reasons for including wards of the state as research subjects and assure that such children

are not the sole participants in a research project unless the research is related to their status as orphans, abandoned children, and the like. The IRB should require, as a minimum, that an advocate for each child be appointed to intercede, when appropriate, on the child's behalf. The IRB may also require additional protections, such as prior court approval.

Recommendation 10. Children who reside in institutions for the mentally infirm or who are confined in correctional facilities should participate in research only if the conditions regarding research on the institutionalized mentally infirm or on prisoners (as applicable) are fulfilled in addition to the conditions set forth herein.

BRITISH PAEDIATRIC ASSOCIATION

Guidelines to Aid Ethical Committees Considering Research Involving Children

These guidelines presume that four premises are accepted.

That research involving children is important for the benefit of all children and should be supported and encouraged and conducted in an ethical manner.

That research should never be done on children if the same investigation could be done on adults.

That research which involves a child and is of no benefit to that child (nontherapeutic research) is not necessarily either unethical or illegal.[1,2]

That the degree of benefit resulting from a research should be assessed in relation to the risk of disturbance, discomfort, or pain—the risk-benefit ratio.

DEFINING "RISK"

Risk, in this context, means the risk of causing physical disturbance, discomfort or pain, or psycho-

logical disturbance to the child or his parents, rather than the risk of serious harm, which no ethical committee would countenance in any case.

Negligible risk—Risk less than that run in everyday life.

Minimal risk—Risk questionably greater than negligible risk.

More than minimal risk.

DEFINING "BENEFIT"

Nontherapeutic research: (a) The procedure is of no benefit to the subject but may benefit the health and welfare of other children or adults. A special case, but an important one, is if the subject suffers from a disorder and the research aims to benefit others suffering from a similar disorder. *(b)* The procedure is of no benefit to the subject but may add to basic biological knowledge—for example, normal values; aging.

Therapeutic research: The procedure is of potential benefit to the subject.

From *Archives of Disease in Childhood* 55 (January, 1980), 75–77. Reprinted with permission of the publisher.

Procedures requiring ethical judgments are usually those which are without benefit to the subject—nontherapeutic research. Most such procedures will fall into one of the following three categories.

(1) The procedure is either *(a)* part of the ordinary care of the infant or child (weighing, measuring, feeding), or *(b)* involves the non-invasive collection of samples—for example, urine, faeces, saliva, hair, or nail clippings, or, at birth, cord blood or placental tissue.

Risk is here likely to be negligible—for example, test weighing a breast-fed baby as part of a study aimed to promote breast feeding.

(2) The procedure involves invasive collection of samples—for example, blood, cerebrospinal fluid, or biopsy tissue—taken from a child who is undergoing treatment. The sample used for research may be *(a)* an additional amount to that required on clinical grounds; or *(b)* not an ordinary part of the child's treatment—for example, collection of biopsy material during a surgical operation.

Risk in *(a)* might be either negligible or minimal; *(b)* might be negligible, minimal, or more than minimal.

Examples—In cystic fibrosis, a research might be considered reasonable which involved an affected child having a sweat test that needed twice as much sweat as required for purely diagnostic purposes. The added discomfort to the child might be assessed as negligible. If in addition a venipuncture was required, this might be judged to put the risk of discomfort and pain into the minimal risk category. But the potential benefit to other child sufferers from this common and serious disease might be deemed such as to make the risk-benefit ratio acceptable.

During the course of an operation for hernia, a fragment of skin from the incision might be required for a research involving tissue culture. The risk could be judged negligible, so that even if the research was not expected to have any direct clinical benefit but only to add to basic biological knowledge, it might be acceptable.

During the course of an abdominal operation, a renal biopsy might be taken for research purposes. The risk here would be judged more than minimal and the benefit would have to be very large to justify it. But suppose the research aimed to resolve the problem of rejection of transplanted kidneys, with result-ing lifesaving consequences both for children and adults with renal failure; this might be considered a benefit of sufficient magnitude to justify the risk.

(3) The procedure is quite apart from the necessary care or treatment of the child. For example, blood sampling; passage of oesophageal tube for pressure recording; application of face mask for respiration studies; placement of infant in plethysmograph chamber for thermal or respiratory studies; needle biopsy of skin or fat; or *x*-ray or isotope studies (see below).

The risk might be negligible, minimal, or more than minimal. The benefit, as defined above in relation to nontherapeutic research, may fall within either the definition *(a)* or *(b)*. If it comes under definition *(a)*, the risk should, to be acceptable, probably be either negligible or minimal. If the benefit comes under definition *(b)*, the risk should be negligible.

Examples—In thalassaemia, a common and lethal disease, progress might depend on taking blood specimens from both affected and unaffected children. The benefit could be assessed as great, so justifying the risk of causing more than minimal discomfort or pain to the children.

Many diabetic children will develop blindness or other severe eye complications in adult life. A research aimed at eventually learning how to prevent this might require several glucose tolerance tests to be done on a diabetic child, not for his own benefit but for the benefit of other diabetic children. The risk of discomfort or pain to that child would be assessed as more than minimal, but might nevertheless be justified by the potential benefit.

The physiology of the initiation of breathing by the baby at birth is poorly understood, and is of clinical importance because some babies fail to breathe. A study of normal newborn babies' first breath, using a face mask, may be judged to cause minimal risk with a justifiable risk-benefit ratio.

APPLYING THE RISK-BENEFIT PRINCIPLE IN THERAPEUTIC RESEARCH

Therapeutic research offers potential benefit to the subject. It includes not only trials of new drugs or procedures but also trials of therapies which, though perhaps widely applied, are yet of unproved value. The risk-benefit principle may still be applicable, the potential benefit as well as the risk relating to the individual subject.

In general, ethical principles in therapeutic research involving children do not usually differ from those applying to adults, except that the age of the subject will often mean that parental understanding and agreement will be required.

In the common type of experiment where two therapies are compared in a controlled trial, two ethical questions are likely to arise.

(1) Is the research necessary? For instance, conventional treatment of a febrile convulsion in a child includes drastic cooling. A research project might question this form of management and entail a controlled trial. An ethical committee might consider it probable that data already existed enabling the question to be answered. The committee might therefore require the researcher first to provide evidence that the world literature had been effectively searched.

(2) Is the design of the trial such that a statistically significant result will emerge with the use of a minimal number of subjects and in a minimum period? Since one set of children will receive what may eventually turn out to be an inferior therapy, it is ethically imperative that this question be answered in the affirmative.

Examples—Current research in treating leukaemia in children often means comparing two different drug regimens. Since both sets of children receive therapies currently considered acceptable, ethical considerations are mainly confined to ensuring that the design of the trial is statistically sound.

A controlled trial of hyposensitising injections of allergens in asthmatic children differs from the foregoing example in that some children (the controls) receive injections of inactive material. This might at first sight seem ethically questionable. However, the following consideration may lead to such a trial being judged acceptable. Until the result of the trial is known the children in either the treatment or the control group have a chance of gaining an advantage. The active therapy may prove superior and those in the treatment group gain an advantage. If, however, there are unpleasant or harmful side effects from the active therapy, the control group will have gained some advantage by not being exposed to those side effects.

X-RAYS AND ISOTOPES

An authoritative pronouncement on the ethical propriety of irradiating children—that is, the use of *x*-rays or isotopes—for research purposes has recently been given by the International Commission on Radiological Protection.[3] It states that "the irradiation, for the purposes of such studies (that is, of no direct benefit to the subject) of children and other persons regarded as being incapable of giving their true consent should only be undertaken if the expected radiation is low (for example, of the order of one-10th of the dose-equivalent limits applicable to individual members of the public) and if valid approval has been given by those legally responsible for such persons."

This means, in common parlance, that exposure to *x*-rays could be justifiable where the dosage was comparable to the normal variation in natural irradiation received by, say, individuals living in two different parts of the British Isles. In fact, using modern equipment, a single radiograph might fall well within such dosage limits, and thus be classifiable as a negligible risk.

PARENTAL PERMISSION AND CO-OPERATION; AGREEMENT BY THE CHILD

Parental (or guardian's) permission should normally be obtained—with rare exceptions such as the comparison of two treatments for some emergency condition—after explaining as fully as possible the nature of the procedure. Whether or not this should be a signed, witnessed declaration remains debatable. It is an advantage if the parents can be present during the procedure. Although the law in Britain does not recognise an age of consent, children much younger than 16 often have enough understanding to collaborate altruistically in a project.

NEW DRUGS; NEW IMMUNISATION PROCEDURES

In general these should be first tested on animals, then on adult volunteers, then on older children able to take part voluntarily in the research, and only then on younger children. However, there are instances where this sequence might be inappropriate; for instance in the development of a vaccine against respiratory syncytial virus, where few uninfected subjects may be available above the age of infancy.

NOTES

1. Dworkin, G. Legality of consent to nontherapeutic medical research on infants and young children. *Arch. Dis. Child.* 1978; 53:443–446.

2. Skegg PDG. English law relating to experimentation on children. *Lancet* 1977; ii:754–755.

3. International Commission on Radiological Protection. *Ann. Int. Commis. Radiol. Protect.* 1977; 1:No 3, 37.

SUGGESTED READINGS FOR CHAPTER 11

GENERAL ISSUES

Annas, George J., *et al. Informed Consent to Human Experimentation: The Subject's Dilemma.* Cambridge, Mass.: Ballinger Publishing Co., 1977.

Barber, Bernard. *Informed Consent in Medical Therapy and Research.* New Brunswick, N.J.: Rutgers University Press, 1980.

Barber, Bernard, *et al. Research on Human Subjects: Problems of Social Control in Medical Experimentation.* New York: Russell Sage Foundation, 1973. New Brunswick, N.J.: Transaction Books, 1978.

Beauchamp, Tom L., *et al.*, eds. *Ethical Issues in Social Science Research.* Baltimore: Johns Hopkins University Press, 1982.

Beecher, Henry K. *Research and the Individual: Human Studies.* Boston: Little, Brown, 1970.

Brieger, Gert H. "Human Experimentation: History." In Reich, Warren T., ed. *Encyclopedia of Bioethics.* New York: Free Press, 1978. Vol. 2, pp. 684–692.

Byar, David P. "Randomized Clinical Trials: Perspectives on Some Recent Ideas." *New England Journal of Medicine* 295 (July 8, 1976), 74–80.

Canada, Medical Research Council. *Ethical Consideration in Research Involving Human Subjects.* Ottawa: Medical Research Council, 1978.

Capron, Alexander M. "Human Experimentation: Basic Issues." In Reich, Warren T., ed. *Encyclopedia of Bioethics.* New York: Free Press, 1978. Vol. 2, pp. 642–699.

———. "Informed Consent in Catastrophic Disease Research and Treatment." *University of Pennsylvania Law Review* 123 (December 1974), 340–438.

Childress, James F. "Compensating Injured Research Subjects: The Moral Argument." *Hastings Center Report* 6 (December 1976), 21–27.

Freund, Paul, ed. *Experimentation with Human Subjects.* New York: George Braziller, 1970.

Fried, Charles. "Human Experimentation: Philosophical Aspects." In Reich, Warren T., ed. *Encyclopedia of Bioethics.* New York: Free Press, 1978. Vol. 2, pp. 699–702.

———. *Medical Experimentation: Personal Integrity and Social Policy.* New York: American Elsevier, 1974.

Gray, Bradford H. *Human Subjects in Medical Experimentation.* New York: John Wiley, 1975.

———, *et al.* "Research Involving Human Subjects." *Science* 201 (September 22, 1978), 1094–1101.

Jones, James H. *Bad Blood: The Tuskegee Syphilis Experiment.* New York: Free Press, 1981.

Katz, Jay, with Capron, Alexander Morgan, and Glass, Eleanor Swift. *Experimentation with Human Beings.* New York: Russell Sage Foundation, 1972.

Robertson, John A. "Compensating Injured Research Subjects: The Law." *Hastings Center Report* 6 (December 1976), 29–31.

———. "The Law of Institutional Review Boards." *UCLA Law Review* 26 (February 1980), 484–549.

U.S., National Commission for the Protection of Human Subjects. *The Belmont Report: Ethical Principles and Guidelines for the Protection of Human Subjects of Research* and *Appendix.* 3 vols. Washington, D.C.: U.S. Government Printing Office, 1978. [Excerpts published in *Federal Register* 44 (April 18, 1979), 23192–23197.]

———. *Institutional Review Boards: Report and Recommendations* and *Appendix.* 2 vols. Washington, D.C.: U.S. Government Printing Office, 1978. [Excerpts published in *Federal Register* 43 (November 30, 1978), 56174–56198.]

Veatch, Robert M. *Case Studies in Medical Ethics.* Cambridge, Mass.: Harvard University Press, 1977. Chapter 11.

———. "Three Theories of Informed Consent." In U.S., National Commission for the Protection of Human Subjects. *The Belmont Report: . . . Appendix:* Volume II. Washington, D.C.: U.S. Government Printing Office, 1978, pp. 26–1 to 26–66.

RESEARCH INVOLVING CHILDREN

Capron, Alexander M. "Legal Considerations Affecting Clinical Pharmacological Studies in Children." *Clinical Research* 12 (February 1973), 141–150.

Curran, William J. "Research on Children." *New England Journal of Medicine* 299 (November 2, 1978), 1001–1002.

Dworkin, Gerald. "Legality of Consent to Nontherapeutic Medical Research on Infants and Young Children." *Archives of Disease in Childhood* 53 (June 1978), 443–446.

Fost, Norman C. "Children and Biomedicine." In Reich, Warren T., ed. *Encyclopedia of Bioethics.* New York: Free Press, 1978. Vol. 1, pp. 150–156.

Holder, Angela R., and Veatch, Robert M. "Can Teenagers Participate in Research without Parental Consent?" *IRB* 3 (February 1981), 5–8.

McCormick, Richard A. "Experimental Subjects: Who Should They Be?" *Journal of the American Medical Association* 235 (May 17, 1976), 297.

———. "Experimentation in Children: Sharing in Sociality." *Hastings Center Report* 6 (December 1976), 41–46.

Pence, Gregory E. "Children's Dissent to Research—A Minor Matter? *IRB* 2 (December 1980), 1–4.

Ramsey, Paul. "The Enforcement of Morals: Nontherapeutic Research on Children." *Hastings Center Report* 6 (August 1976), 21–30.

———. "Children as Research Subjects: A Reply." *Hastings Center Report* (April 1977), 40–41.

Skegg, P.D.G. "English Law Relating to Experimentation on Children." *Lancet* 2 (October 8, 1977), 754–755.

U.S., Department of Health, Education, and Welfare. "Protection of Human Subjects: Proposed Regulations on Research Involving Children." *Federal Register* 43 (July 21, 1978), 31786–31794.

U.S., National Commission for the Protection of Human Subjects. *Research Involving Children: Report and Recommendations* and *Appendix.* 2 vols. Washington, D.C.: U.S. Government Printing Office, 1977. [Excerpts published in *Federal Register* 43 (January 13, 1978), 2084–2114.]

Van Eys, Jan. *Research on Children: Medical Imperatives, Ethical Quandaries, and Legal Constraints.* Baltimore: University Park Press, 1978.

BIBLIOGRAPHIES

Goldstein, Doris Mueller. *Bioethics: A Guide to Information Sources*. Detroit: Gale Research Company, 1982. See under "Research Involving Human Subjects."

Lineback, Richard H., ed. *Philosopher's Index*. Vols. 1– . Bowling Green, Ohio: Bowling Green State University. Issued Quarterly. See under "Children," "Experimentation," and "Research."

Walters, LeRoy. *Bibliography of Bioethics*. Vols. 1– . New York: Free Press. Issued annually. See under "Human Experimentation" and "Human Experimentation/Minors." (The information contained in the annual *Bibliography of Bioethics* can also be retrieved from BIOETHICSLINE, an online data base of the National Library of Medicine.)

12.
Scientific Freedom and Its Limits

The preceding chapter discussed research involving human subjects. In this final chapter we shall explore several additional facets of biomedical research and technology.

RESEARCH INVOLVING ANIMALS

Perhaps the first question to be clarified in any discussion of animal research is: Which animals are to be included within the scope of consideration? The books and articles on the ethics of animal research have devoted surprisingly little attention to this question. One can usually infer from these writings that nonhuman mammals—such as monkeys, dogs, and rats—are to be included in the protected group. Indeed, Christina Hoff explicitly refers to "mammals and other highly organized creatures." A somewhat broader class would be all vertebrates, that is, mammals plus birds, reptiles, amphibians, and fish. Peter Singer's essay cites statistics on the extent of research involving vertebrates. Not included in these statistics, of course, are numerous other categories of animals such as protozoa (for example, paramecia), flatworms, shellfish, or insects. In the discussion which follows, it is assumed that the term "animals" refers to nonhuman vertebrates, although the question of research involving invertebrates may also deserve ethical analysis in its own right.

Two primary issues can be identified in the animal research debate: (1) the consequences of the research and (2) the moral status of animals. Proponents of animal research usually advance arguments that appeal rather straightforwardly to the principle of beneficence. The weak form of the argument can be formulated as follows: Good consequences are achieved through the use of animals in research. A somewhat stronger claim is that at least some of these good consequences can be achieved *only* by means of animal research; that is, no alternative (nonhuman) means to the desired end exists.

The empirical background for the strong claim by proponents of animal research is that intact, live animals respond to research interventions in complex ways that cannot be simulated through any other research technique involving nonanimal systems. For example, administering a drug to a dog or presenting a learning stimulus to a rat may produce a complex reaction that affects multiple physiological systems. At present, such a response simply cannot be duplicated through the manipulation of cells in tissue culture or even through the use of sophisticated computer simulations. In theory at least, human subjects could be substituted for animal subjects and would be capable of producing the same kinds of complex response. However, given the painful, invasive, and even lethal character of much animal research, the use of humans in such research would itself pose serious ethical problems. (See Chapter 11.)

Critics of animal research can also appeal to the principle of beneficence. In response to the weak form of the proponents' argument, the critics urge that alternatives to animal research be more vigorously explored and more actively employed. Both Peter Singer and Alan Bowd advocate such exploration. The strong form of the proponents' argument presents a more formidable challenge, however. If animal research is the only means for achieving a desirable consequence, then the critic can respond by insisting on a conscientious weighing of research benefits against harms to animals. Indeed, reformers like Singer and Hoff recommend the use of precisely this kind of calculus.

A complicating factor in any such effort to assess consequences is the problem of animal sentience, or sensitivity to pain. The notion of sentience raises both conceptual and empirical issues. A broad construal of the concept of sentience might conceivably include primitive ''avoidance'' reactions to aversive stimuli, for example, a paramecium's response to a toxic chemical or a rabbit's reflex reaction to cold. However, a narrower construal of sentience might require the presence of anticipatory or retrospective psychological states, such as fear or regret. Even if one were able to agree on a definition of sentience, there would remain the formidable empirical problem of measuring exactly how much pain is being inflicted upon, or in some sense being experienced by, animal subjects. Hoff comments at some length on the problem of animal sentience.

The second major issue in the animal research debate is the moral status of animals. This issue closely parallels the problem of personhood (Chapter 3) and the question of fetal status (Chapter 6). In an influential essay not reprinted in this book, Joel Feinberg has argued that animals can have rights because they have, or can have, interests. Among the rights ascribed to animals by Feinberg is the right to be treated humanely. In his view, such treatment is owed to animals as their due and therefore involves the principle of justice.[1] In the present chapter, Hoff adopts a similar position, ascribing some rights to animals but assigning a fuller complement of rights to human beings. Singer prefers to avoid the language of rights in discussing animals but nonetheless asserts that humans have an obligation not to inflict suffering on animals. Other philosophers—including Thomas Aquinas, Descartes, and Immanuel Kant—have ascribed no moral status whatever to animals. Descartes regarded animals as mere machines, while Kant argued that because animals lack rationality they need not be treated as ends in themselves.

Kant's position points to the difficult problem of relating the descriptive properties of animals, such as consciousness, to their moral status. (See the introduction to Chapter 3 for a fuller discussion of this problem as it pertains to personhood.) For example, Hoff considers whether humans with extremely limited intellectual capacities—for example, severely retarded individuals—should be involved in painful or fatal research, as animals often are. Her negative answer is based on the premise that we cannot ''safely permit anyone to decide which human beings fall short of worthiness.'' To Singer, positions such as Hoff's are discriminatory. In his words, ''Our respect for the interests of [infants and mentally retarded humans], and our neglect of the members of other species with equal or superior capacities, is mere 'speciesism'—a prejudice in favor of 'our own kind' that is analogous to, and no more justifiable than, racism.''[2]

RESEARCH AT THE MOLECULAR LEVEL

When we move from the world of vertebrate animals to that of bacteria, viruses, and DNA, our ethical problems concerning the research subjects are immediately simplified. Here there is unlikely to be a problem of sentience, and little philosophical ink has been spilled on the moral status of *E. coli* bacteria.

As Robert Sinsheimer explains in his essay, recombinant DNA research involves the joining of segments of DNA—the basic genetic material in all living things. This technique is important for many kinds of laboratory research, but in addition it has potential technological applications in such diverse fields as medicine, agriculture, and industry. Indeed, recombinant DNA methods are already being employed to produce medically important hormones, such as insulin and human growth hormone.

Recombinant DNA research is of philosophical interest primarily as another instance in which risk-benefit analysis seems appropriate. (See Chapter 10 for additional discussion of risk- and cost-benefit analysis.) Robert Sinsheimer depicts the potential benefits of recombinant DNA research and technology but cautions that the enthusiastic use of new technological capabilities in large-scale programs of genetic engineering could introduce "a sudden major discontinuity in the human gene pool" and thus could destroy the delicate balance between biological evolution and human culture. Stephen Stich writes in a more theoretical vein, exploring the difficulties of making predictions in a novel research field as well as analyzing the complexities involved in quantifying and comparing risks and benefits. Stich's prescription for a reasonable public policy on recombinant DNA research in effect combines the principles of autonomy and beneficence: the freedom of scientific inquiry should be protected unless the negative consequences of research significantly outweigh its positive consequences.

SCIENTIFIC INQUIRY AND PUBLIC POLICY

The essays in this chapter by Hans Jonas and Loren Graham raise several conceptual, empirical, and normative issues about science policy. Perhaps the clearest point of disagreement between the two authors concerns the relationship between "science" and "technology." Jonas contends that while traditional science may have been a purely theoretical enterprise—similar in many respects to philosophy—modern science *in practice* is inextricably linked to technology. Because of this linkage, scientists can and should be held morally accountable for the technological applications of their research. Note that Jonas does not deny that a conceptual distinction between science and technology may exist; rather, he claims that the distinction is in practice irrelevant. In contrast, Graham argues that "The division between fundamental studies of physical and biological nature, on the one hand, and technological studies directed toward social or economic goals, on the other, is still a useful one."

The major normative question addressed by Jonas and Graham is the extent to which the freedom of scientific research should be protected. For Jonas, research (with the exception of mathematical research) is a type of action rather than a kind of thought or speech. As such, it is "always subject to legal and moral restraints." Jonas does not expressly deny that there is a presumption in favor of scientific freedom; however, he argues that no special or overriding reasons need be advanced to justify limitations on that freedom. Graham's general strategy is to distinguish numerous varieties of scientific research. In the cases of "Human Subjects Research," "Expensive Science," and "Accidents in Science" Graham is entirely in accord with Jonas's thesis that public controls on research are both necessary and reasonable. However, Graham also identifies several types of research that, in his view, should virtually always be free, and a single category of fundamental knowledge, "Subversive Knowledge," which should remain forever inviolate.

L. W.

NOTES

1. Joel Feinberg, "The Rights of Animals and Unborn Generations," in William T. Blackstone, ed., *Philosophy and the Environmental Crisis* (Athens, Ga.: University of Georgia Press, 1974), pp. 43–68, esp. p. 50.

2. Peter Singer, "Animal Experimentation: Philosophical Perspectives," reproduced in this chapter. I am deeply indebted to Mr. Ray Moseley for his assistance in analyzing the ethical issues raised by animal research.

PETER SINGER

Animal Experimentation: Philosophical Perspectives

Although the practice of conducting scientific experiments on living animals, vivisection, goes back at least to Galen (A.D. 130?–200?), the modern period of experimentation stems from the seventeenth century, when scientific inquiries were beginning to be made in many fields. This was the period of the philosopher and scientist René Descartes (1596–1650). For Descartes and the physiologists who declared themselves his followers, cutting open a fully conscious animal posed no ethical problem, since, Descartes said, animals are mere machines, more complex than clocks but no more capable of feeling pain.

If this convenient view of the nature of nonhuman animals is rejected, however, a serious ethical problem about experimenting on animals does arise, because the infliction of suffering and death on an animal seems, in itself, to be an evil. On the other hand, supporters of vivisection argue that such experiments provide great benefits for humans. Animal experimentation, therefore, raises the issue of whether the end justifies the means (an issue also raised by experiments on humans) and in addition forces us to consider what place nonhuman animals have in our ethical deliberations.

THE NATURE AND EXTENT OF EXPERIMENTS ON ANIMALS

The number of experiments performed on animals has increased remarkably in the last hundred years. The present extent of experimentation, worldwide, is impossible to ascertain with accuracy, since few countries compile the necessary statistics. In the United Kingdom, according to an annual statement published by the Home Office, more than five million

experiments "calculated to cause pain" are performed on live vertebrate animals every year.[1] This figure is low compared to that of the United States, where the number of animals used yearly has been reliably estimated as being in excess of sixty million.[2] Other countries using large numbers of animals include Russia, Japan, West Germany, and France. The worldwide tendency of smaller nations to follow Western scientific techniques has meant that there are now very few nations in which animal experiments are not being performed.

The animals most often used are mice and rats, but dogs, cats, and monkeys are also used in large numbers. It is commonly assumed that animals are experimented upon only for important medical research, but closer scrutiny reveals that only a minority of experiments can be classified as "medical" at all.[3] Many of the most painful experiments are carried out by psychologists and are intended to test theories about learning, punishment, maternal deprivation, and so on. Millions of animals are used to test foodstuffs, pesticides, industrial products, weapons, and even nonessential items like cosmetics, shampoos, and food-coloring agents.

Many of these experiments involve severe and lasting pain for the animals. To test the safety of a foodstuff or cosmetic, the substance is fed in concentrated doses to a group of animals, until a level is found at which half of the sample dies. This means that most of the animals become very sick before some die and others pull through. The dose at which half of the sample dies is supposed to give an indication of the toxicity of the substance, but, since different species have different tolerances, it is at best a very rough guide to the safety of the product for humans (thalidomide, for instance, was tested on several species of animals before being released to humans, and no deformities were found).[3]

Psychologists' experiments about punishment or learning may involve hundreds of severe and inescapable electric shocks. Some psychologists have made monkeys permanently neurotic by rearing them in total isolation (these experiments have been repeated, with minor variations, over and over again). In experiments on stress, monkeys have been locked into iron chairs for more than a year and made to perform tasks in order to avoid electric shock. To study the effects of heatstroke, medical researchers have slowly heated fully conscious dogs to death. Further examples, drawn from recent scientific journals, may be found in Ryder and in Singer.

On the other hand, it is true that many experiments involve little or no suffering for the animals involved. This may be because the experiment is of a harmless nature (such as running a rat through a maze) or because the animal is totally anesthetized during the operation and killed painlessly afterward.

Moreover, some animal experimentation has been of considerable benefit to humans. In such areas as the identification of necessary vitamins and minerals and the development of new surgical techniques and new drugs, discoveries have been made through animal experimentation that could not have been made, or would have been much more difficult to make, had animals not been used. Diabetes is often cited as an example of a disease that has lost its terror through a cure first developed on animals.[4]

LEGISLATION

Laws governing experiments on animals vary from country to country, but in no country does the law prohibit outright painful experiments or require that the experiment be of sufficient importance to outweigh the pain inflicted.

The first law specifically regulating experiments was the British Cruelty to Animals Act of 1876. This law, which has never been amended, requires the use of an anesthetic, except where "insensibility cannot be produced without necessarily frustrating the object of such experiments"; but neither the statute itself nor the officials who administer it make any attempt to assess whether the object of the experiment is itself worth the pain caused. Clearly, a psychologist wishing to test the effects of electric shock on the behavior of dogs cannot anesthetize the animals without frustrating the object of his experiment. Even in toxicity tests of cosmetics anesthetics are not used, because it is thought that they might distort the result of the test.

Therefore such experiments are permitted in Britain.

In the United States, the Animal Welfare Act of 1970 sets standards for the housing, transportation, and handling of animals; but the Act does not control the nature of the experiments performed, except to the extent of requiring research facilities to lodge a report stating that, when painful experiments were performed without the use of pain-relieving drugs, this was necessary to achieve the objectives of the research project. Again, no attempt is made to assess the importance of these objectives, and in fact one section of the law specifically disavows any intention of interfering with the design or performance of research or experimentation. Moreover, since the law is a federal one, facilities not receiving federal funds and not involved in interstate commerce do not have to comply.

A 1972 West German law requires the use of alternatives to experiments on animals whenever possible. Amendments to the same effect have been proposed in Britain, Denmark, and Holland, but it remains to be seen how effective the West German provision will be. Much depends on what is deemed to be a "possible alternative." Many countries, including France, Spain, Brazil, and Japan still have no legislation regulating experiments on animals.

THE CASE FOR EXPERIMENTING ON ANIMALS

The simplest argument for the permissibility of experiments on animals is the Cartesian one: animals do not suffer, and so there is nothing wrong with experimenting upon them. But both common sense and the great majority of experts agree that mammals and probably other vertebrate animals, at least, are capable of suffering both physical pain and some kinds of emotional distress, such as fear.

If animals do suffer, how is their suffering to be justified? The usual justification offered is that the suffering of animals is outweighed by the benefits, for humans, of the discoveries made by the use of animals. Sometimes, however, it is said that the goal of increasing our understanding of the universe is sufficient justification.

Behind these justifications may lie one of a variety of philosophical positions. For instance, it may be said that, as related in Genesis, God has given man "dominion" over the other animals to use as man pleases. Combined with other theological notions, such as the idea that man, alone of all animals, has an immortal soul, this idea has been influential throughout the Christian world. But it can also be turned the other way: as long ago as 1713, Alexander Pope argued against cruel experiments on the grounds that man's dominion requires him to play the role of the good shepherd, caring for his flock.[5]

It has also been said, by writers as diverse as St. Thomas Aquinas, Immanuel Kant, and D. G. Ritchie, that animals are not ''ends in themselves'' or that they have no rights.[6,7] In support of this it is alleged that the status of a being that is an ''end in itself,'' or has rights, belongs only to a being that is rational, capable of autonomous action, or a moral agent. Whereas humans satisfy this requirement, animals, it is alleged, do not. A difficulty with this argument is that *some* humans come no closer to satisfying the requirement than the animals experimented upon. Mentally retarded human beings, for instance, may be no more rational than a dog; yet we do not consider that they are entirely devoid of rights. Other writers have denied that rationality, autonomy, or moral agency is required before we can grant that a being has rights.[8] Still others have taken the approach that we have obligations not to inflict suffering, irrespective of whether we can meaningfully attribute rights to the being in question.[2]

A utilitarian case for animal experimentation is based on the idea that more suffering is alleviated by it than is caused by it. The classical utilitarian writers, however, all accepted that a utilitarian must take *all* suffering—human and animal—into consideration, and this makes the factual claim that animal experimentation relieves more suffering than it causes more difficult to defend. Nevertheless, there are probably some experiments—those that do not involve much suffering for the animals and promise major benefits for humans or animals—that can be defended on this ground.

Finally, defenders of experimentation often accuse their opponents of inconsistency in objecting to the deaths of animals in laboratories while continuing to participate in the practice of rearing and killing animals for food. This argument holds no validity for antivivisectionists who are also vegetarians. Even when directed against someone who does eat meat, it hardly amounts to a positive defense of experimentation.

THE CASE AGAINST EXPERIMENTING ON ANIMALS

Opponents of experiments on animals tend to divide into two groups: absolute abolitionists and reformers. Absolute abolitionists usually rely on the principle that the end does not justify the means. To inflict pain and death on an innocent being is, they maintain, always wrong. They point out that we do not think the possibility of advancing scientific knowledge justifies us in taking healthy human beings and inflicting painful deaths upon them; similarly, they say, the infliction of suffering on animals cannot be justified by reference to future benefits for human or other animals.

The weakness of the absolutist position is that, when the end is sufficiently important, we do sometimes think otherwise unacceptable means are justifiable if there is no other way of achieving the end. We do not like invasions of privacy, but we countenance telephone taps on suspected criminals. Similarly, if the prospects of finding a cure for cancer depended upon a single experiment, should we have any doubt about its justification?

Reformers usually take a more utilitarian line. They concede that some experiments may be justifiable but contend that most are not, because the experiments bring certain suffering and death to animals with no likelihood of significant benefits. In reply to the general argument that experiments on animals benefit humans, the reformers demand that any such benefits be sufficient to offset the costs to the animal subjects; they urge that every experiment come under close prior scrutiny to determine if the benefits are likely to outweigh the costs. Were this done, they maintain, only a small fraction of the experiments now performed would be seen to be justifiable.

Reformers claim[2,3] that alternative methods, not involving animals, could replace many of the experiments now being carried out on animals. Techniques using tissue cultures, for instance, have already replaced animals in the production of certain vaccines, and opponents of animal experimentation suggest that other alternative methods would be developed more rapidly if they were to receive government support.[9]

Although the absolutists and reformers disagree in important respects, they are united in seeking to narrow the ethical gulf that now separates humans from other animals in our conventional morality. This may be the most philosophically interesting question raised by the vivisection controversy, and it has implications that go beyond experimentation to our treatment of animals in general.

THE MORAL STATUS OF ANIMALS

Is there any ethical justification for the sharp distinction we now make between our treatment of members of our own species and members of the other species? Although it is commonly said that humans are superior to other animals in various respects, or that humans are "persons," while animals are not, both Ryder and Singer have pointed out that certain categories of human beings—infants and mentally retarded humans—actually fall below some adult dogs, cats, pigs, or chimpanzees on any test of intelligence, awareness, self-consciousness, moral personality, capacity to communicate, or any other capacity that might be thought to mark humans as superior to other animals. Yet we do not think it legitimate to experiment on these less fortunate humans in the ways in which we experiment on animals. Ryder and Singer claim that our respect for the interests of these humans, and our neglect of the interests of members of other species with equal or superior capacities, is mere "speciesism"—a prejudice in favor of "our own kind" that is analogous to, and no more justifiable than, racism.[2,3]

Certainly it does seem that those supporters of experimentation who have cited the benefits the experiments may bring to humans would need to explain whether this argument also justifies experiments on mentally retarded humans, and, if not, why not. The fact that a being is not a member of our own species does not, in itself, seem to be a sufficient reason for experimenting upon it, if we would refuse to perform a similar experiment upon a member of our own species with similar potentialities.

Defenders of vivisection have had surprisingly little to say about their reasons for disregarding or discounting the interests of nonhuman animals. R. J. White, who has himself carried out experiments in which the heads of monkeys are kept alive and conscious after being severed from their bodies, is perhaps representative of many experimenters when he writes that "the inclusion of lower animals in our ethical system is philosophically meaningless."[10] But White does not explain why the clear proposal of utilitarian writers from Jeremy Bentham onward that pain, as such, is an evil, whatever the species of the being that suffers it, is devoid of meaning. It may sometimes be difficult to compare the suffering of a human and, say, a dog; but if rough comparisons can be made, surely the mere fact that the dog is a "lower animal" is no reason to give less weight to its suffering.

Seen in this light, the argument that restricting experiments on animals interferes with scientific freedom and medical progress also appears less conclusive. We do not grant scientists the freedom to experiment at will on humans, although such experiments might advance medical knowledge. It would seem, therefore, to be incumbent upon the defenders of experiments on animals to show that there is a relevant difference between humans and other animals that justifies experiments on the latter, but not the former; but this is a question to which the experimenters have not addressed themselves.

CONCLUSION

While there has been considerable controversy over the ethics of experiments on humans, there has been little serious discussion of the morality of the far more numerous experiments on animals in recent years. Antivivisectionists have, by and large, been regarded as oversentimental animal lovers or as eccentrics. In the first half of the 1970s, however, three books have appeared containing criticisms of animal experimentation based on carefully reasoned ethical considerations.[2,3,7] It would not be surprising if these books provoke a more serious consideration of the entire issue.

NOTES

1. *Report of the Departmental Committee on Experiments on Animals.* Sir Sydney Littlewood, Chairman. London: Home Office, Her Majesty's Stationery Office, 1965. The result of an official inquiry into animal experiments in Britain; popularly known as the "Littlewood Report," after the committee chairman.

2. Singer, Peter. *Animal Liberation.* New York: Random House, New York Review of Books, 1975. Argues for a radical revision of our attitudes to animals; contains a long chapter discussing experiments, including descriptions of experiments in America and Britain.

3. Ryder, Richard Dudley. *Victims of Science: The Use of Animals in Research.* London: Davis-Poynter, 1975. The most comprehensive account yet published of experiments on animals, the legislation governing experiments, and the case for reform, with principal focus on Britain.

4. "Vivisection–Vivistudy: The Facts and the Benefits to Animal and Human Health." *American Journal of Public Health* 57 (1967): 1597–1626. In four separate papers presented at a symposium, medical and veterinary specialists discuss some of the benefits of animal experimentation for human and animal health.

5. Turner, Ernest S. *All Heaven in a Rage.* London: Michael Joseph, 1964. A historical account of the growth of compassion for

animals, with sections on the beginning of vivisection and the antivivisection movement; p. 48.

6. Passmore, John. "The Treatment of Animals." *Journal of the History of Ideas* 36 (1975): 195–218. Treats the historical ethical issues in cruelty to animals.

7. Regan, Thomas, and Singer, Peter, eds. *Animal Rights and Human Obligations*. Englewood Cliffs, N.J.: Prentice-Hall, 1976.

An anthology of writings, ancient and modern, on ethical aspects of our relations with animals.

8. Feinberg, Joel. "The Rights of Animals and Unborn Generations." *Philosophy and Environmental Crisis*. Edited by William T. Blackstone. Athens: University of Georgia Press, 1974. Argues that animals can possess rights.

9. Ryder, *op. cit.,* Chap. 12.

10. White, Robert J. "Anti-Vivisection: The Reluctant Hydra." *American Scholar* 40 (1971): 503–512. One of the few articles in which an experimenter defends his right to use animals; p. 507.

CHRISTINA HOFF

Immoral and Moral Uses of Animals

One can do something wrong to a tree, but it makes no sense to speak of wronging it. Can one wrong an animal? Many philosophers think not, and many research scientists adopt the attitude that the use of laboratory animals raises no serious moral questions. It is understandable that they should do so. Moral neutrality toward the objects of one's research is conducive to scientific practice. Scientists naturally wish to concentrate on their research and thus tend not to confront the problems that may arise in the choice of techniques. In support of this attitude of indifference, they could cite philosophers who point to features peculiar to human life, by virtue of which painful experimentation on unwilling human beings is rightly to be judged morally reprehensible and that on animals not. What are these features?

Rationality and the ability to communicate meaningfully with others are the most commonly mentioned differentiating characteristics. Philosophers as diverse as Aristotle, Aquinas, Descartes, and Kant point to man's deliberative capacities as the source of his moral preeminence. Animals, because they are irrational, have been denied standing. The trouble is that not all human beings are rational. Mentally retarded or severely brain-damaged human beings are sometimes much less intelligent than lower primates

Reprinted with permission from *The New England Journal of Medicine,* Vol. 302, No. 2, pp. 115–118, January 10, 1980.

that have been successfully taught to employ primitive languages and make simple, logical inferences beyond the capacity of the normal three-year-old child. The view that rationality is the qualifying condition for moral status has the awkward consequence of leaving unexplained our perceived obligations to nonrational humanity.

Some philosophers have therefore argued that man's privileged moral status is owed to his capacity for suffering. To be plausible, this way of explaining man's position as the only being who can be wronged must discount the apparent suffering of mammals and other highly organized creatures. It is sometimes assumed that the subjective experience of pain is quite different for animals and human beings. Descartes, for example, maintains that animals are machines: he speaks of tropisms of avoidance and desire rather than pleasure and pain.[1] Although it is true that human beings can suffer in ways that animals cannot, the idea that animals and human beings experience physical pain differently is physiologically incoherent. We know that animals feel pain because of their behavioral reactions (including writhing, screaming, facial contortions, and desperate efforts to escape the source of pain), the evidence of their nervous systems, and the evolutionary value of pain. (By "animals" I mean mammals, birds, and other organisms of comparable evolutionary complexity.)

There are other sources of human suffering besides pain, but they too are not peculiarly human. One has only to consult the reports of naturalists or go to the zoo or own a pet to learn that the higher animals, at least, can suffer from loneliness, jealousy, boredom, frustration, rage, and terror. If, indeed, the capacity to suffer is the morally relevant characteristic, then the facts determine that animals, along with all human beings, are the proper subjects of moral consideration.

There is, however, another common way of defending human privilege. It is sometimes asserted that "just being human" is a sufficient basis for a protected moral status, that sheer membership in the species confers exclusive moral rights. Each human life, no matter how impoverished, has a depth and meaning that transcends that of even the most gifted dolphin or chimpanzee. One may speak of this as the humanistic principle. Cicero was one of its earliest exponents: "Honor every human being because he is a human being."[2] Kant called it the Principle of Personality and placed it at the foundation of his moral theory.[3] The principle appears evident to us because it is embodied in the attitudes and institutions of most civilized communities. Although this accounts for its intuitive appeal, it is hardly an adequate reason to accept it. Without further argument the humanistic principle is arbitrary. What must be adduced is an acceptable criterion for awarding special rights. But when we proffer a criterion based, say, on the capacity to reason or to suffer, it is clearly inadequate either because it is satisfied by some but not all members of the species *Homo sapiens,* or because it is satisfied by them all—and many other animals as well.

Another type of argument for denying equal consideration to animals goes back at least to Aristotle. I refer to the view that man's tyranny over animals is natural because his superiority as an animal determines for him the dominant position in the natural scale of things. To suggest that man give up his dominance over animals is to suggest that he deny his nature. The argument assumes that "denial of nature" is ethically incoherent. But conformity with nature is not an adequate condition for ethical standards. Being moral does not appear to be a question of abiding by the so-called laws of nature; just as often it seems to require us to disregard what is "natural" in favor of what is compassionate. We avoid slavery and child labor, not because we have discovered that they are unnatural, but because we have discovered that

slaves and children have their own desires and interests and they engage our sympathy. Social Darwinism was an ethical theory that sought to deduce moral rules from the "facts" of nature. Wealthy 19th-century industrialists welcomed a theory that seemed to justify inhumane labor practices by reference to the "natural order of things." It has become clear that these so-called "laws" of nature cannot provide an adequate basis for a moral theory, if only because they may be cited to support almost any conceivable theory.

It is fair to say that no one has yet given good reasons to accept a moral perspective that grants a privileged moral status to all and only human beings. A crucial moral judgment is made when one decides that a given course of action with respect to a certain class of beings does not fall within the range of moral consideration. Historically, mistakes at this level have proved dangerous: they leave the agent free to perpetrate heinous acts that are not regarded as either moral or immoral and are therefore unchecked by normal inhibition. The exclusion of animals from the moral domain may well be a similar and equally benighted error. It is, in any case, arbitrary and unfounded in good moral argument.

Whatever belongs to the moral domain can be wronged. But if one rejects the doctrine that membership in the moral domain necessarily coincides with membership in the human species, then one must state a satisfactory condition for moral recognition. Bentham offers an intuitively acceptable starting point. "The question is not, Can they *reason?,* nor, Can they *talk*? but Can they *suffer*?"[4] The capacity to suffer confers a minimal prima facie moral status on any creature, for it seems reasonable that one who is wantonly cruel to a sentient creature wrongs that creature. Animals too can be wronged; the practical consequences of such a moral position are, however, not as clear as they may seem. We must consider what we may and may not do to them.

I begin with a word about the comparative worthiness of human and animal life. Although animals are entitled to moral consideration, it does not follow that animals and human beings are always equal before the moral law. Distinctions must still be made. One may acknowledge that animals have rights without committing oneself to a radical egalitarianism that awards to animals complete parity with human beings. If hunting animals for sport is wrong, hunting human beings for the same purpose is worse, and such a distinction is not inconsistent with recognizing that animals have moral status. Although some proponents of animal rights would deny it, there are morally critical differences between animals and human beings. Animals share with human beings a common interest in avoiding pain, but the complexities of normal human life clearly provide a relevant basis for assigning to human beings a far more serious right to life itself. When we kill a human being, we take away his physical existence (eating, sleeping, and feeling pleasure and pain), but we deprive him of other things as well. His projects, his friendships, and his sense of himself as a human being are also terminated. To kill a human being is not only to take away his life, but to impugn the special meaning of his life. In contrast, an animal's needs and desires are restricted to his place in time and space. He lives ''the life of the moment.'' Human lives develop and unfold; they have a direction. Animal lives do not. Accordingly, I suggest the following differential principle of life worthiness: Human lives are generally worthier than animal lives, and the right to life of a human being generally supersedes the right to life of an animal.

This differential principle rejects the Cartesian thesis, which totally dismisses animals from moral consideration, and it is consistent with two other principles that I have been tacitly defending: animals are moral subjects with claims to considerations that should not be ignored; and an animal's experience of pain is similar to a human being's experience of pain.

In the light of these principles I shall try to determine what general policies we ought to adopt in regulating the use of animals in experimental science. I am limiting myself to the moral questions arising in the specific area of painful or fatal animal experimentation, but some of the discussion will apply to other areas of human interaction with animals. Space does not allow discussion of killing animals for educational purposes.

Scientists who perform experiments on animals rarely see the need to justify them, but when they do they almost always stress the seriousness of the research. Although it may be regrettable that animals are harmed, their suffering is seen as an unavoidable casualty of scientific progress. The moral philosopher must still ask: is the price in animal misery worth it?

That the ends do not always justify the means is a truism, and when the means involve the painful treatment of unwilling innocents, serious questions arise. Although it is notoriously difficult to formulate the conditions that justify the consequences, it is plausible that desired ends are not likely to justify onerous means in the following situations: when those who suffer the means are not identical with those who are expected to enjoy the ends; when there is grave doubt that the justifying ends will be brought about by the onerous means; and when the ends can be achieved by less onerous means.

When a competent surgeon causes pain he does not run afoul of these conditions. On the other hand, social policies that entail mass misery on the basis of tenuous sociopolitical assumptions of great future benefits do run afoul of the last two conditions and often of the first as well. The use of laboratory animals often fails to satisfy these conditions of consequential justification; the first is ignored most frequently (I shall argue that this can often be justified), but scientists often violate the others as well when they carry out painful or fatal experiments with animals that are poorly designed or could have been just as well executed without intact living animals.

We can be somewhat more specific in formulating guidelines for animal experimentation if we consider the equality of animals and human beings with respect to pain. Because there are no sound biologic reasons for the idea that human pain is intrinsically more intense than animal pain, animals and men may be said to be equals with respect to pain. Equality in this case is a measure of their shared interest in avoiding harm and discomfort. The evil of pain, unlike the value of life, is unaffected by the identity of the individual sufferer.

Animals and human beings, however, do differ in their experience of the aftereffects of pain. When an injury leaves the subject cosmetically disfigured, for example, a human being may suffer from a continuing sense of shame and bitterness, but for the animal the trauma is confined to the momentary pain. Even the permanent impairment of faculties has more serious and lasting aftereffects on human beings than on animals. It can be argued that a person who is stricken by blindness suffers his loss more keenly than an animal similarly stricken.

More important than the subjective experience of privation is the objective diminishment of a valuable being whose scope of activity and future experience have been severely curtailed. In terms of physical privation animals and human beings do not differ, but the measure of loss must be counted far greater in human beings. To sum up: human beings and animals have a parity with respect to the trauma of a painful episode but not with respect to the consequences of the trauma. Yet when an experiment involves permanent impairment or death for the subject and thus considerations of differential life worthiness make it wrong to use most human beings, the pain imposed on the animals should still be counted as intrinsically bad, as if human beings had been made to suffer it, regardless of the aftereffects.

Although I believe that the general inferiority of animal lives to human life is relevant to the formation of public policy, I cannot accept the view that their relative inferiority licenses harming animals except for very serious purposes in rather special circumstances. However, the special circumstances are not necessarily extraordinary. Many experiments, although not as many as is generally supposed, are medically important and needed. The researcher who is working to control cancer and other fatal and crippling diseases may be able to satisfy the conditions that justify the use of laboratory animals. Because I believe that normal human lives are of far greater worth than animal lives, I accept a policy in which those who suffer the means are not those who may enjoy the ends, which violates the first of the conditions of consequential justification mentioned above, by permitting the infliction of pain on animals to save human lives or to contribute substantially to their welfare. However, when researchers intend to harm an animal, they need more than a quick appeal to the worthiness of human life. They ought to be able to show that the resulting benefits are outstandingly compensatory; if the scientist cannot make a good case for the experiment, it should be proscribed. (On the other hand, if suffering is the main consideration in judging the admissibility of experiments with animals, then nonpainful experiments, even fatal ones, may be under fewer constraints than painful, nonfatal experiments. Although this idea may seem paradoxical, it is in accord with the common moral intuition that condones those who put a kitten "to sleep" while condemning those who torment one.) The implementation of this policy raises questions that cannot be dealt with here. Yet one might expect that research proposals involving painful animal experimentation should be reviewed by a panel of experts, perhaps composed of two scientists in the field of the experiment and a scientifically knowledgeable philosopher versed in medical ethics.

In closing, I wish to indicate how I would deal with a possible objection. It may appear that my criteria of life worthiness place human idiots on a par with animals. On what grounds could I prohibit the painful or fatal experimental use of human subjects whose capacity does not differ from that of many animals? I would be prepared to rethink or even abandon a position that could not distinguish between animal and human experimentation. Fortunately, this distinction can be made.

I oppose painful or fatal experimentation on defective, nonconsenting human beings not because I believe that any person, just because he is human, has a privileged moral status, but because I do not believe that we can safely permit anyone to decide which human beings fall short of worthiness. Judgments of this kind and the creation of institutions for making them are fraught with danger and open to grave abuse. It is never necessary to show that an animal's life is not as valuable as that of a normal human being, but just such an initial judgment of exclusion would have to be made for idiots. Because there is no way to circumvent this problem, experiments on human beings are precluded and practically wrong. There are other arguments against experimenting on mentally feeble human beings, but this one seems to me to be the strongest and to be sufficient to support the view that whereas animal experimentation is justifiable, no dangerous or harmful experiments involving unwilling human subjects could be.

Accordingly, I have reached the following conclusions concerning the painful exploitation of animals for human rewards. Animals should not be used in painful experiments when substantial benefits are not expected to result. Even when the objective is important, there is a presumption against the use of animals in painful and dangerous experiments that are expected to yield tenuous results of doubtful value. Animals but not human beings may be used in painful and dangerous experiments that are to yield vital benefits for human beings (or other animals).

Vast numbers of animals are currently being used in all kinds of scientific experiments, many of which entail animal misery. Some of these studies, unfortunately, do not contribute to medical science, and some do not even require the use of intact animals. Even the most conservative corrective measures in the implementation of a reasonable and morally responsible policy would have dramatic practical consequences.

NOTES

1. Descartes, R. Letter to the Marquess of Newcastle. In: Kenny A., ed. *Philosophical letters*. Oxford: Oxford University Press, 1970.

2. Cicero. *De Finibus*.

3. Kant, I. In: Paton HJ, ed. *Groundwork for a metaphysic of morals*.

4. Bentham, J. *The principles of morals and legislation*. New York: Hafner Publishing, 1948:311n.

A L A N   D .   B O W D

Ethical Reservations about Psychological Research with Animals

Behavioral scientists who have concerned themselves with ethical principles in research have dwelt almost exclusively upon issues relating to human subjects.[1] An examination of the literature for the past decade reveals that the questions which have apparently been uppermost in psychologists' minds are the use of deception, inadequate feedback to participants, matters relating to informed consent, subject privacy, and the employment of behavior modification in the schools. Among the reasons that have been cited for the increased sensitivity to the rights of human subjects is "the fact that during the last decade a series of painful and mortifying examples of the abuse of human subjects by scientific investigators has come to light."[2]

Ethical questions relating to research with animals have received only scant or passing consideration by most writers whose stated objectives have been the analysis of issues relating to human subjects. In view of the predominant role of nonhuman experimentation in psychology, and especially in consideration of the nature of much of that experimentation this is a serious omission. The objective of this paper is to examine critically the ethical defense offered for certain prevalent research practices and the institutional factors which help determine and maintain the kinds

Reprinted with permission from *The Psychological Record* 30 (Spring 1980), 201–210.

of attitudes and beliefs psychologists hold toward the animals in their laboratories.

• • •

. . . The ethics involved in animal experimentation have been questioned recently from outside of psychology. An ethologist, Fraser,[3] has argued that since animal behaviorists recognize a broad range of emotions and feelings in animals, in particular aspects of pain and stress, a logically consistent ethical code would not permit the induction of the latter states in experimental subjects. The recently published report of the working party on animal experimentation of the British Psychological Society[4] recommended measures to reduce unnecessary painful animal experimentation; however, it has been criticized for its failure to consider the ethical questions fundamental to traditional practices.[5,6] To consider adequately the philosophical assumptions underlying such practices it is necessary to examine the prevalent contemporary estimation of animals within psychology together with its origins.

ANIMALS: THE PREVALENT VIEW

Contemporary psychology has inherited a view of animals whose origins are an intrinsic part of the Judaeo-Christian tradition. Animals are inherently *less* than mankind. In medieval Christian thought, Aquinas following Socrates attributed to man an immortal soul and the ability to reason, placing humanity apart from the rest of creation. This dogma, reinforced during the enlightenment by Descartes, has survived revolutionary changes in the scientific assessment of the nature of *Homo sapiens* wrought by Darwin and Freud. Today human beings stand apart from other animals by virtue of their apparent dignity. The views of man as the tool-maker or the unique user of language have given way to advances in knowledge about other species. Human intelligence does not define the species' uniqueness, for few would argue that the degree of our humanity is reflected in an IQ score, that the severely retarded are less than human. Indeed, many would argue that the concept of intelligence has little meaning when used for cross-cultural comparisons let alone comparisons across species. In fact many tasks which call upon the human capacity for reason have been shown to be within the capability of animals, particularly certain primates. Donald Hebb in his respected *Textbook* argues that mankind's acquisition of language and the development of intelligence can only be seen in proper perspective when compared with the behavior of nonhuman animals. The argument is difficult to sustain in consideration of the range of human intellectual functioning and current knowledge concerning language acquisition in other primates. Hebb concludes by appealing to the intangible dignity of man, stating that comparative psychological research "does not degrade man but on the contrary dignifies him."[7]

The contemporary view of animals does, of course, recognize humanity's similarity to other living things. As Hebb further points out,

it is quite clear that the anatomical organization of the brains of all mammals is essentially the same; and it seems clear that the principles of behavior, or of brain function, are the same . . . Psychology in the twentieth century is not the study of the human mind, but the study of the *mind*.[7]

There is a contradiction between the accepted physiological identity of human beings and other animals on the one hand, and the notion of humanity's qualitative superiority to animals which is implicit in the writings of most psychologists. Psychologists write about animals, and treat them as if their experience is qualitatively different from that of *Homo sapiens*. Animals in psychological experiments are simply complex research tools. Thus a significant work on research methods in psychology can refer to the deaths of several hundred monkeys from perforated ulcers after many days of exposure to a shock-avoidance schedule as "*an annoying feature* of these experiments"[8] (my emphasis).

The value of animals in research stems from their physiological similarity to mankind; however, certain psychological and philosophical implications are ignored. Animal subjects are generally assumed to function as if they were devoid of conscious experience, although the objective evidence is entirely to the contrary. Indeed it is the similarity of animal responsiveness to stimulation to our own that permits generalization from the behavior of other species to human beings. Psychologists, however, refrain from admitting that animals feel pain (although most would readily recognize the validity of this statement for humans). Rather, animals react to noxious stimuli in a way similar to man: "Physiologically the rat is remarkably similar to man . . . his *reaction to sensations* such as pain, cold or heat is similar"[9] (my emphasis). In this way animals are denied conscious experience. The consequence, of course, is clear. A creature which "reacts to pain" rather than experiencing it, or which "shows fear responses" rather than feeling terror is really no more than a sophisticated measuring instrument and may therefore be treated as if it were no more than a machine. In discussing the advantages of the rat as an experimental subject Lefrancois, for example, writes at length about its physiological, neurological and behavioral similarities to man, concluding without the benefit of logical justification that despite these things "even the most devout humanitarian is unlikely to be too upset if procedures unpleasant to the rat are employed without the rat's consent."[10] As the philosopher Singer maintains,

the researcher's central dilemma exists in an especially acute form in psychology: either the animal is not like us, in which case there is no reason for performing the experiment; or else the animal is like us, in which case we ought not to perform an experiment on the animal which would be considered outrageous if performed on one of us.[11]

THE MAINTENANCE OF ATTITUDES TOWARD ANIMALS

The specialized vocabulary of experimental psychology is an important factor in creating and maintaining attitudes toward laboratory animals. Heim[12] has referred to "hygienic sounding terminology" functioning so as to indoctrinate students in the callousness of much experimental work carried out on lower animals. Terms like "negative reinforcement," "aversive stimulus," and "deprivation" are obvious euphemisms. It is true they have more precise definitions than the words they replace, but the implicit distance they place between the researcher and the unpleasant consequences of his or her actions is also important. There is no semantic reason why starvation should be called deprivation, nor is it reasonable to suppose that the former term could not as easily be defined operationally. The connotations which the word arouses, however, are dispelled if a more neutral one is employed. Thus the animal becomes the "organism" (for no particularly scientific reason), and its reactions indicative of pain at best are called "emotional responses" or lose their relationship to suffering by being subdivided and described as urination, defecation, and rapid ambulatory movement. Finally, the subjects of experiments are "sacrificed" rather than killed.

Because psychologists come to think of laboratory animals as no more than instruments, to attribute emotional states to them because the conditions to which they have been subjected and their consequent behavior suggest they exist, is considered unscientific. However, since it is difficult, even for the most scientific, to describe such behavior without reference to subjective experience, inverted commas are invariably placed around the operative words. Thus animals may give indications of "pain" or "fear" in addition to "insight" or "intelligence." In psychology, as elsewhere, language is able to disguise an unpleasant reality. Thus a photograph of "littermate Scotties," one of which was reared in isolation in a small cage, is captioned "The normal dog is at the left, rather bored with the photographic process; the restricted dog *did not have enough brains* to be bored but kept on being interested in the most trivial events"[13] (my emphasis). In this example a somewhat flippant colloquial expression serves to imply that the severe treatment and its consequences are actually mildly amusing, since only a dog is involved.

The overall effect of customary linguistic practices in the scientific literature is to maintain a *nonscientific* distinction between the human species and others. When combined with the prevailing philosophical assumptions about animals, experiments involving severe pain to nonhumans may be carried out and discussed dispassionately in the almost complete absence of reasoned consideration of the ethical issues involved.

In addition to language practices, psychology students are persuaded to accept prevailing attitudes toward animal research by a variety of social forces. Peer pressure and the attitudes of professors categorize squeamishness and sentimentality as unscientific, it being implied that such natural emotional reactions are irrational while the ability to suppress them is not. The graduate student who for ethical reasons may choose not to subject animals to painful experimental procedures, may find fewer doctoral programs available. Finally, there are subtle prejudices within university psychology departments such that experimental animal research is frequently considered more basic and is invested with a prestige that is denied more applied study.

Contemporary behaviorism has been cited as providing important philosophical rationalizations for current psychological attitudes toward animal experimentation.[14] However, inasmuch as the mechanistic and deterministic features of behaviorism are equally applicable to human and animal behavior, and the denial of mental states makes no distinction between species, the behaviorist philosophy is neutral. In practice, however, it is not uncommon for a behavioral psychologist to reserve purposive constructs for a description of his or her own behavior, while describing that of animals as if they were complex machines. Behaviorism draws no distinctions between human beings and other species, but neither does it presuppose an ethical position. It addresses the methodology of science but not the values of scientists.

ETHICAL JUSTIFICATION FOR PAINFUL EXPERIMENTATION

The use of sentient creatures in experiments involving pain and their subsequent death when no longer useful to the researcher is taken for granted within the scientific community. Psychologists, like other scientists, justify their treatment of animal subjects by two basic arguments. The first is that it is reasonable to sacrifice the interests of animals in order to satisfy the interests of human beings. The benefits of research on animals for the development of life-saving medical techniques are frequently cited as an example. Bachrach[15] like many before him points to the example of the discovery of insulin; however by the same logic one might oppose testing of drugs on animals by reason of the fact that thalidomide was so tested, but proved to have devastating effects on the human fetus. The second argument is that animal interests may be disregarded for the advancement of knowledge, or in the interests of science. This position is frequently cited in psychology texts presumably because it is sometimes difficult to point specifically to immediate benefits accruing to humanity from much psychological research with animals.

$\bullet \quad \bullet \quad \bullet$

The subjecting of animals to severe pain, stress, and deprivation has been and remains a routine procedure in experimental psychology. The starving of rats to 70% or 80% body weight has been considered normal practice for countless experiments in learning and motivation. The vast literature on punishment predominantly involves the effects of electric shock on the behavior of rats, although many species have in fact been exposed to a variety of painful experimental treatments.

The general acceptance of the ethical validity of such procedures is no doubt facilitated by the essentially superstitious attitudes toward the rat which are predominant in Western culture over and above the "scientific" view of animals as research tools. Experiments involving domestic animals, such as dogs or cats, or primate species occasionally excite some controversy but usually for reasons of sentiment alone and not logic. Research on social isolation and maternal deprivation in monkeys,[16] for example, has been the subject of unfavorable press publicity although the related ethical questions have received little attention from the scientific community.[17] Although examples of deprivation, rejection, and relative social isolation among human infants are numerous, psychologists too readily accept the value of experimental animal studies over post hoc analysis of human subjects even when the former involve extreme distress to the animals concerned.

A description of specific studies involving extreme unjustifiable pain to animal subjects is not within the objectives of this paper. All psychologists have some familiarity with research in which animals have been traumatized, mutilated, punished, or subjected to the most severe distress. Few psychologists have considered the ethical implications of such research; they have not done so because they do not consider that for the most part animals should be the subject of ethical concern. However, the hypothetical example of a specific experiment saving human lives or even mar-

ginally affecting the human condition remains hypothetical. An indifferent examination of the literature involving painful animal experimentation reveals that a significant proportion of published research is repetitive or deals with problems to which the answers are self-evident. The argument that their work showed self-evident or trivial results would naturally be denied by the researchers involved. Whether a study's findings are trivial is a relative issue. Clearly, when the interests of the animals involved are considered irrelevant the results may be judged to have some significance. It should also be noted that research which remains unpublished has in all likelihood been judged insignificant by the experimenter's peers (as represented by journal editors and reviewers). In this connection, a British government committee that investigated experiments on animals found that only about one-fourth of the experiments performed ever found their way into print.[18]

It is a generally accepted ethical principle in psychology that

A particular study is ethically unacceptable to the extent that its theoretical or practical values are too limited to justify the impositions it makes on the participants or that scientifically acceptable alternative procedures have not been carefully considered.[19]

ALTERNATIVES

AN ALTERNATIVE ETHIC

It has been argued throughout this paper that the traditional justification for subjecting sentient animals to painful experimentation rests upon unscientific, illogical reasoning. *Homo sapiens* is one species among many. There is no one characteristic peculiar to members of the human species which might distinguish them from other animals in a qualitative sense. Painful experimentation is not permitted upon human beings who are incapable of granting consent for the simple reason that susceptibility to pain is considered evidence enough of the right to be spared it. Similar rights are withheld from nonhumans, it being claimed that human interests supersede those of animals. Thus the traditional ethical position speaks of the researcher's obligation to avoid causing "unnecessary" pain, but provides no detailed terms of reference for the determination of when pain might be considered unnecessary.[20] In practice this judgment is left to the researcher so that the code is, in fact, providing experimenters with a carte blanche. Logic demands that the criterion for sparing a creature pain should be the ability of that creature to suffer. The following basic principle is therefore endorsed:

It is a realistic humanitarian goal to insist that animals, if experimented on by the human species, should not be forced to accept suffering greater than man himself would accept.[21]

ALTERNATIVE RESEARCH METHODS

Although the numbers of animals used in research is constantly increasing there has at the same time been a growth of experimental techniques which replace the whole animal or reduce its use.[17] Some of these alternatives have most immediate application in areas other than psychology, but may replace animal research in areas of physiological psychology, learning, perception, and motivation. Among such techniques are tissue and organ cultures (both animal and human); lower forms such as embryonated eggs, bacteria and simple nonsentient animals; chemical analysis and, particularly, the use of computer models. The employment of film and videotape for teaching purposes is both more humane and educationally efficient than repetitive demonstrations on living animals.

Donald Hebb has written that "animals are fascinating and may be studied for their own sakes. Their behavior presents some of the most engaging puzzles to be found anywhere, which is quite enough reason for trying to solve them."[22] The statement seems best to fit the behavior of animals under natural conditions, and certainly not when subjected to noxious stimulation in the laboratory. As ethologists have proposed, animal behavior may be best understood when observed as it naturally occurs:

The natural laboratory can be profitably used to study questions about imprinting that have been raised but not answered by traditional laboratory experiments. We must move away from the *in vitro,* or test tube approach to the study of behavior and move toward the *in vivo* method that allows interaction with normal environmental factors.[23]

The post hoc observational study of human subjects represents a viable alternative to certain stressful animal experimentation. Unfortunate human examples of maternal rejection, sensory deprivation, or stress are not rare. The argument that it is only by the experimental study of such factors, of necessity on animal subjects, that prediction and explanation are possible must be weighed against the record of actual applied results from such studies, and in the final analysis within the context of the ethical questions involved.

The restrictions placed on psychological research by the ethical position advocated in this paper will be regarded as too severe by some psychologists. No doubt if painful experimentation on sentient animals were to cease, certain research questions would remain for which alternative methods would not necessarily be available. However, the consideration of the necessity of an ethical position should be quite independent of whether certain kinds of research issues would be precluded by its adoption. The acceptance of any ethic implies restrictions upon research activity for logical and moral reasons. The present issue is whether certain types of research are justifiable, particularly when dispassionate consideration is given to the logical implications of traditional distinctions between human beings and animals.

The time has come for psychologists to reevaluate their beliefs regarding the treatment of laboratory animals. It is no longer acceptable for serious writers about psychological research tritely to dismiss opponents of animal experimentation as animal lovers whose ethical views, rather than being based upon reasoned argument, are no more than "an expression of a sincere love of animals and a wish to avoid seeing them injured or hurt."[24] As this paper has attempted to show, there are contradictions inherent in the traditional arguments provided by psychologists in justification of their treatment of animal subjects. The fact that the assumptions underlying these arguments have received so little critical attention is evidence, not so much of their foundation in logic, but of the power of traditional attitudes toward animals within the Western cultural tradition.

NOTES

1. Diener, E., and Crandall, R. 1978. *Ethics in social and behavioral research.* Chicago: University of Chicago Press.

2. Reiss, D. 1977. Freedom of inquiry and subjects' rights: An introduction. *American Journal of Psychiatry,* 134, 891–892, esp. p. 891.

3. Fraser, A. 1975. Ethology and ethics. *Applied Animal Ethology,* 1, 211–212.

4. British Psychological Society, Scientific Affairs Board. 1979. Report of the working party on animal experimentation. *Bulletin of the B.P.S.,* 32, 44–52.

5. Heim, A. 1979. Report of the working party on animal experimentation. *Bulletin of the B.P.S.,* 32, 113–114.

6. Sperlinger, D. 1979. Working party on animal experimentation. *Bulletin of the B.P.S.*, 32, 291–292.

7. Hebb, D. 1964. *A textbook of psychology*. Philadelphia: Saunders.

8. Sidman, M. 1960. *Tactics of scientific research*. New York: Basic Books, p. 11.

9. LeFrancois, G. 1975. *Psychology for teaching* (2nd ed.). Belmont, CA: Wadsworth, p. 41.

10. *Ibid.*, p. 44.

11. Singer, P. 1975. *Animal liberation*. New York: New York Review of Books, p. 49.

12. Heim, A. 1970. *Intelligence and personality*. Harmondsworth, England: Pelican.

13. Hebb, *op. cit.*, p. 127.

14. Ryder, R. 1975. *Victims of science: The use of animals in research*. London: Davis-Poynter.

15. Bachrach, A. J. 1962. *Psychological research: An introduction*. New York: Random House.

16. Harlow, H., and Harlow, M. 1962. Social deprivation in monkeys. *Scientific American*, 207, 5, 136–146.

17. Pratt, D. 1976. *Painful experiments on animals*. New York: Argus Archives.

18. Ryder, R. 1971. Experiments on animals. In S. Godlovitch, R. Godlovitch, and J. Harris (eds.), *Animals, men and morals*, London: Gollancz.

19. American Psychological Association, 1973. *Ethical principles in the conduct of research with human subjects*. Washington, D.C.: A.P.A.

20. American Psychological Association, Committee on Precautions and Standards in Animal Experimentation. 1971. *Principles for the care and use of animals*. Washington, D.C.: A.P.A.

21. Pratt, *op. cit.*, p. 181.

22. Hebb, *op. cit.*, p. 5.

23. Hess, E. H. 1972. "Imprinting" in a natural laboratory. *Scientific American*, 227, 2, 24–31.

24. Bachrach, *op. cit.*, p. 103.

Research at the Molecular Level

ROBERT SINSHEIMER

Troubled Dawn for Genetic Engineering

The essence of engineering is design and, thus, the essence of genetic engineering, as distinct from applied genetics, is the introduction of human design into the formulation of new genes and new genetic combinations. These methods thus supplement the older methods which rely upon the intelligent selection and perpetuation of those chance genetic combinations which arise in the natural breeding process.

The possibility of genetic engineering derives from major advances in DNA technology—in the means of synthesizing, analyzing, transposing and generally manipulating the basic genetic substance of life. Three major advances have all neatly combined to permit this striking accomplishment: these are (1) the

This article first appeared in *New Scientist, London, The Weekly Review of Science and Technology,* Vol. 68 (October 16, 1975). Reprinted with permission.

discovery of means for the cleavage of DNA at highly specific sites; (2) the development of simple and generally applicable methods for the joining of DNA molecules; and (3) the discovery of effective techniques for the introduction of DNA into previously refractory organisms.

The art of DNA cleavage and degradation languished in a crude and unsatisfactory state until the discovery and more recent application of enzymes known as restriction endonucleases. These enzymes protect the host cells against invasion by foreign genomes by specifically severing the intruding DNA strands. For the purposes of genetic engineering, restriction enzymes provide a reservoir of means to cleave DNA molecules reproducibly at a limited number of sites by recognizing specific tracts of DNA ranging from four to eight nucleotides in length.

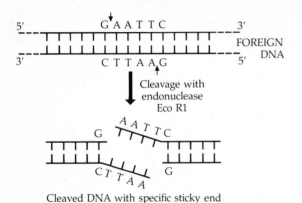

Figure 1.   Endonucleases can cleave double-stranded DNA at one point, or staggered as shown in the diagram. The staggered cut produces sticky ends which can join with sections of DNA severed by the same enzyme.

These sites may be deliberately varied by the choice of the restriction enzyme.

The enzymes cut both strands of the DNA double helix, and the break may be at the same base pair or staggered by several bases (Figure 1). In the latter case the two fragments of DNA are each left with a terminal unpaired strand—a so-called cohesive or "sticky" end. This is particularly valuable in joining together two pieces of DNA end to end.

The number of susceptible tracts in a DNA obviously depends on the particular DNA and the particular enzyme. In some important instances there is only one such tract. For instance, the restriction enzyme coded by the *E. coli* drug resistance transfer factor I—Eco R1—cleaves the DNA of the simian virus 40 at only one site. Similarly it cleaves the circular DNA of the plasmid* PSC 101 at only one site. The DNA of bacteriophage* lambda is, however, severed at five sites. It is possible to produce mutants of lambda with progressively fewer sites, until lambda strains are now available with just one or two sites.

For some purposes more numerous cleavage sites are useful. In a number of laboratories, including my own, the ϕX virus RF can be cut at up to 13 sites using selected restriction enzymes. Because these enzymes yield overlapping fragments, a physical map of the DNA can be formed and correlated with the viral genetic map.

Restriction enzymes thus permit us to obtain specific fragments of DNA. For genetic engineering

Ed. note: Plasmid—A small circle of DNA in a bacterium. Plasmids are capable of autonomous self-replication.

Bacteriophage—A virus that attacks bacteria.

one would like to be able to rejoin such fragments in arbitrary ways. Two general methods have been developed to achieve this, both of which depend on the "sticky end" principle in which complementary single strand ends combine (Figures 1 and 2). Restriction enzymes which inflict staggered cuts automatically produce "sticky ends" in the DNA chain severed. Alternatively, a combination of enzymic and chemical manipulation can create a "sticky end."

MODIFIED PLASMIDS IN *E. COLI*

By these means, then, any arbitrarily selected piece of DNA from any source can be inserted into the DNA of an appropriately chosen plasmid or virus. The new combination must then, for most purposes, be reintroduced into an appropriate host cell. This was achieved just a few years ago when Stanley Cohen, at Stanford, discovered that plasmid DNA could be reintroduced, albeit with low efficiency, into appropriately treated *E. coli* * cells and that these could then subsequently grow and propagate the plasmid. Foreign genes can therefore be introduced into *E. coli* plasmids which can be propagated indefinitely in ordinary bacterial cultures. As one instance, the ribosomal* RNA genes of *Xenopus laevis* (the African clawed toad) have been introduced into an *E. coli* plasmid and propagated for over 100 cell generations. And these genes are transcribed in their new host (Figure 2).

A similar result can, in principle, be achieved with the bacteriophage lambda. A foreign gene can be inserted into lambda DNA; spheroplasts* or treated cells infected with this DNA will yield virus which can then be used to infect normal cells. By clever manipulation a recombinant DNA can be obtained which can subsequently be integrated into the host chromosome and propagated thereafter with the host.

To what purposes may these novel genetic combinations be put? One can conceive of a variety of benign purposes. Unfortunately one can also conceive of malign purposes, and of major, if unintended, hazards.

The first purposes that come to mind are of a purely scientific character. The structure and organization of the eukaryotic (higher organism) genome is

Ed. note: E. coli—A bacterium that inhabits the gastrointestinal tract of most mammals, including humans.

Ribosomes—Complex particles that are the sites of protein synthesis in living cells.

Spheroblasts—Self-reproducing structures that exist in the cytoplasm, outside the nucleus of a cell.

currently being studied intensively. This research has been grossly impeded by the complexity of these genomes and the lack of means to isolate particular portions in adequate quantities for experimental analysis. The insertion of fragments of eukaryotic DNA into plasmids, followed by cloning (cellular multiplication), permits one to grow cultures of any size containing just one particular fragment. At present the choice of fragments to be inserted cannot in general be precisely defined, although some prior selection can be introduced. However, ingenious methods are being devised to permit subsequent selection of those bacterial clones carrying fragments of particular interest.

Clones of bacteria bearing, say, histone* genes, ribosomal RNA genes, genes from individual bands of *Drosophila** DNA, DNA of a certain degree of repetition in the sea urchin genome, and so forth, are currently being investigated. There are numerous questions to ask and numerous matters of interest concerning the transcription and translation of such genes in the bacterial host: for instance, the rates at which they may mutate, and the use of such cloned genes as probes of the eukaryotic genome.

Ed. note: Histone—Protein produced in the nuclei of cells. Drosophila—Fruit fly.

It is very probable that in time the appropriate genes can be introduced into bacteria to convert them into biochemical factories for producing complex substances of medical importance: for example, insulin (for which a shortage seems imminent), growth hormone, specific antibodies, and clotting factor VIII, which is defective in hemophiliacs. Even if these specific genes cannot be isolated from the appropriate organisms, the chances of synthesizing them from scratch are now significant.

Other more grandiose applications of microbial genetic engineering can be envisaged. The transfer of genes for nitrogen fixation into presently inept species might have very significant agricultural applications. Appropriate design might permit appreciable modifications of the normal bacterial flora of the human mouth with a significant impact upon the incidence of dental caries. Even major industrial processes might be carried out by appropriately planned micro-organisms.

However, we must remember that we are creating here novel, self-propagating organisms. And with that reminder, another darker side appears on this scene of brilliant scientific enterprise. For instance, for scien-

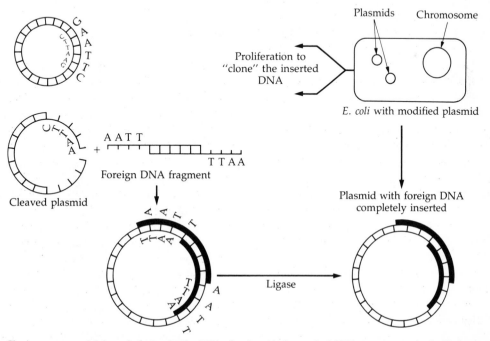

Figure 2.   Cloning a gene: a nick is made in the circular DNA of a plasmid; the required DNA sequence, excised with the same restriction enzyme, is inserted into the gap; the DNA chains are repaired by a ligase enzyme; the plasmids are reintroduced into *E. coli;* when the coli culture multiplies, the plasmids, and the foreign genes with them, are multiplied (cloned) too.

tific purposes there is great interest in the insertion of particular regions of viral DNA into plasmids—particularly, portions of oncogenic (cancer-inducing) viral DNA—so as to be able to obtain such portions and their gene products in quantity and subsequently to study the effects of these substances on their normal host cells. Abruptly we come to the potential hazard of research in this field, in fact the specific hazard which inspired the widely known "moratorium" proposed last year by a committee of the U.S. National Academy, chaired by Paul Berg.

This moratorium and its related issues deserve very considerable discussion. Briefly, it became apparent to the scientists involved—at almost the last hour when all of the techniques were really at hand—that they were about to create novel forms of self-propagating organisms—derivatives of strains known to be normal components of the human intestinal flora—with almost completely unknown potential for biological havoc. Could an *Escherichia coli* strain carrying all or part of an oncogenic virus become resident in the human intestine? Could it thereby become a possible source of malignancy? Could such a strain spread throughout a human population? What would be the consequence if even an insulin-secreting strain became an intestinal resident? Not to mention the more malign or just plain stupid scenarios such as those which depict the insertion of the gene for botulinus toxin* into *Escherichia coli*.

UNKNOWN PROBABILITIES

Unfortunately the answers to these questions in terms of probabilities that some of these strains could persist in the intestines, the probabilities that the modified plasmids might be transferred to other strains, better adapted to intestinal life, the probabilities that the genome of an oncogenic virus could escape, could be taken up, could transform* a host cell, are all largely unknown.

Following the call for a moratorium a conference was held at Asilomar at the end of last February to assess these problems. While it proved possible to rank various types of proposed experiments with respect to potential hazard, for the reasons already

Ed. note: Toxin—A potent poison sometimes produced by bacteria during the decay of food. Botulism is the name given to this type of food poisoning.

In animal cells, transformation is the conversion of normal cells to cancerous cells.

stated it proved impossible to establish, on any secure basis, the absolute magnitude of hazard. Various distinguished scientists differed very widely, but sincerely, in their estimates. Historical experience indicated that simple reliance upon the physical containment of these new organisms could not be completely effective.

In the end a broad, but not universal, consensus was reached which recommended that the seemingly more dangerous experiments be deferred until means of "biological containment" could be developed to supplement physical containment. By biological containment is meant the crippling of all vehicles—cells or viruses—intended to carry the recombinant genomes through the insertion of a variety of genetic defects so as to reduce very greatly the likelihood that the organisms could survive outside of a protective, carefully supplemented laboratory culture.

This seems a sensible and responsible compromise. However, several of the less prominent aspects of the Asilomar conference also deserve much thought. The lens of Asilomar was focused sharply upon the potential biological and medical hazard of this new research, but other issues drifted in and out of the field of discussion. There was, for instance, no specific consideration of the wisdom of diverting appreciable research funds and talent to this field, in lieu of others. An indirect discussion of this question was perhaps implicit in the description of the significance and scientific potential of research in this field presented by those who were impatient of any delay.

Indeed the eagerness of the researchers to get on with the work in this field was most evident. To a scientist this was exhilarating. Obviously these new techniques open many previously closed doorways leading to the potential resolution of long-standing and important problems. I think also there is a certain romance in this joining together of DNA molecules that diverged billions of years ago and have pursued separate paths through all of these millenia. Personally I feel confident one could easily justify this new research direction. But a sociologist of science might see other undercurrents in this impetuous eagerness, and the bright scientific promise should not blind us to the realities of other concerns.

Nor was there any sustained discussion at Asilomar of ancillary issues such as the absolute right of free inquiry claimed quite vigorously by some of the participants. Here, I think, we have come to recognize that there are limits to the practice of any human activity. To impose any limit upon freedom of inquiry is especially bitter for the scientist whose life is one of inquiry; but science has become too potent. It is no longer enough to wave the flag of Galileo.

Rights are not found in nature. Rights are conferred within a human society and for each there is expected a corresponding responsibility. Inevitably at some boundaries different rights come into conflict, and the exercise of a right should not destroy the society that conferred it. We recognize this in other fields. Freedom of the press is a right but it is subject to restraints, such as libel and obscenity and, perhaps more dubiously, national security. The right to experiment on human beings is obviously constrained. Similarly, would we wish to claim the right of individual scientists to be free to create novel self-perpetuating organisms likely to spread about the planet in an uncontrollable manner for better or worse? I think not.

This does not mean we cannot advance our science or that we must doubt its ultimate beneficence. It simply means that we must be able to look at what we do in a mature way.

There was, at Asilomar, no explicit consideration of the potential broader social or ethical implications of initiating this line of research—of its role, as a possible prelude to longer-range, broader-scale genetic engineering of the flora and fauna of the planet, including, ultimately, man. It is not yet clear how these techniques may be applied to higher organisms but we should not underestimate scientific ingenuity. Indeed the oncogenic viruses may provide a key; and mitochondria may serve as analogues for plasmids.

CONTROLLED EVOLUTION?

How far will we want to develop genetic engineering? Do we want to assume the basic responsibility for life on this planet—to develop new living forms for our own purpose? Shall we take into our own hands our own future evolution? These are profound issues which involve science but also transcend science. They deserve our most serious and continuing thought. I can here mention only a very few of the more salient considerations.

Clearly the advent of genetic engineering, even merely in the microbial world, brings new responsibilities to accompany the new potentials. It is always thus when we introduce the element of human design. The distant yet much discussed application of genetic engineering to mankind would place this equation at the center of all future human history. It would in the end make human design responsible for

human nature. It is a responsibility to give pause, especially if one recognizes that the prerequisite for responsibility is the ability to forecast, to make reliable estimates of the consequence.

Can we really forecast the consequence for mankind, for human society, of any major change in the human gene pool? The more I have reflected on this, the more I have come to doubt it. I do not refer here to the alleviation of individual genetic defects—or, if you will, to the occasional introduction of a genetic clone—but more broadly to the genetic redefinition of man. Our social structures have evolved so as to be more or less well adapted to the array of talents and personalities emergent by chance from the existing gene pool and developed through our cultural agencies. In our social endeavours we have, biologically, remained cradled in that web of evolutionary nature which bore us and which has undoubtedly provided a most valuable safety net as we have in our fumbling way created and tried our varied cultural forms.

To introduce a sudden major discontinuity in the human gene pool might well create a major mismatch between our social order and our individual capacities. Even a minor perturbation such as a marked change in the sex ratio from its present near equality could shake our social structures—or consider the impact of a major change in the human life span. Can we really predict the results of such a perturbation? And if we cannot foresee the consequence, do we go ahead?

It is difficult for a scientist to conceive that there are certain matters best left unknown, at least for a time. But science is the major organ of inquiry for a society—and perhaps a society, like an organism, must follow a developmental program in which the genetic information is revealed in an orderly sequence.

The dawn of genetic engineering is troubled. In part this is the spirit of the time—the very idea of progress through science is in question. People seriously wonder if through our cleverness we may not blunder into worse dilemmas than we seek to solve. They are concerned not only for the vagrant lethal virus or the escaped mutant deadly microbe, but also for the awful potential that we might inadvertently so arm the anarchic in our society as to shatter its bonds or conversely so arm the tyrannical in our society as to forever imprison liberty.

It is grievous that the elan of science must be tempered, that the glowing conviction that knowledge is good and that man can with knowledge lift himself out of hapless impotence must now be shaded with doubt and caution. But in this we join a long tradition. The fetters that are part of the human condition are not so easily struck.

We confront again, the enduring paradox of emergence. We are each a unit, each alone. Yet, bonded together, we are so much more. As individuals men will have always to accept their genetic constraints, but as a species we can transcend our inheritance and mould it to our purpose—if we can trust ourselves with such powers. As geneticists we can continue to evolve possibilities and take the long view.

STEPHEN P. STICH

The Recombinant DNA Debate

The debate over recombinant DNA research is a unique event, perhaps a turning point, in the history of science. For the first time in modern history there has been widespread public discussion about whether and how a promising though potentially dangerous line of research shall be pursued. At root the debate is a moral debate and, like most such debates, requires proper assessment of the facts at crucial stages in the argument. . . .

In order to help sharpen our perception of the moral issues underlying the controversy over recombinant DNA research, I shall start by clearing away some frivolous arguments that have deflected attention from more serious issues. We may then examine the problems involved in deciding whether the potential benefits of recombinant DNA research justify pursuing it despite the risks that it poses.

I. THREE BAD ARGUMENTS

My focus in this section will be on three untenable arguments, each of which has surfaced with considerable frequency in the public debate over recombinant DNA research.

The first argument on my list concludes that recombinant DNA research should not be controlled or restricted. The central premise of the argument is that scientists should have full and unqualified freedom to pursue whatever inquiries they may choose to pursue. This claim was stated repeatedly in petitions and letters to the editor during the height of the public debate over recombinant DNA research in the University of Michigan community. The general moral principle which is the central premise of the argument plainly does entail that investigators using recombinant DNA technology should be allowed to pursue their research as they see fit. However, we need only consider a few examples to see that the principle invoked in this "freedom of inquiry" argument is utterly indefensible. No matter how sincere a researcher's interest may be in investigating the conjugal behavior of American university professors, few would be willing to grant him the right to pursue his research in my bedroom without my consent. No matter how interested a researcher may be in investigating the effects of massive doses of bomb-grade plutonium on preschool children, it is hard to imagine that anyone thinks he should be allowed to do so. Yet the "free inquiry" principle, if accepted, would allow both of these projects and countless other Dr. Strangelove projects as well. So plainly the simplistic "free inquiry" principle is indefensible. It would, however, be a mistake to conclude that freedom of inquiry ought not to be protected. A better conclusion is that the right of free inquiry is a qualified right and must sometimes yield to conflicting rights and to the demands of conflicting moral principles. Articulating an explicit and properly qualified principle of free inquiry is a task of no small

From *Philosophy and Public Affairs* 7 (Spring 1978), 187–205. Copyright ©1978 by the Princeton University Press. Reprinted with permission of the publisher.

difficulty. We will touch on this topic again toward the end of Section II.

The second argument I want to examine aims at establishing just the opposite conclusion from the first. The particular moral judgment being defended is that there should be a total ban on recombinant DNA research. The argument begins with the observation that even in so-called low-risk recombinant DNA experiments there is at least a possibility of catastrophic consequences. We are, after all, dealing with a relatively new and unexplored technology. Thus it is at least possible that a bacterial culture whose genetic makeup has been altered in the course of a recombinant DNA experiment may exhibit completely unexpected pathogenic characteristics. Indeed, it is not impossible that we could find ourselves confronted with a killer strain of, say, *E. coli* and, worse, a strain against which humans can marshal no natural defense. Now if this is possible—if we cannot say with assurance that the probability of it happening is zero—then, the argument continues, all recombinant DNA research should be halted. For the negative utility of the imagined catastrophe is so enormous, resulting as it would in the destruction of our society and perhaps even of our species, that no work which could possibly lead to this result would be worth the risk.

The argument just sketched, which might be called the "doomsday scenario" argument, begins with a premise which no informed person would be inclined to deny. It is indeed *possible* that even a low-risk recombinant DNA experiment might lead to totally catastrophic results. No ironclad guarantee can be offered that this will not happen. And while the probability of such an unanticipated catastrophe is surely not large, there is no serious argument that the probability is zero. Still, I think the argument is a sophistry. To go from the undeniable premise that recombinant DNA research might possibly result in unthinkable catastrophe to the conclusion that such research should be banned requires a moral principle stating that *all* endeavors that might possibly result in such a catastrophe should be prohibited. Once the principle has been stated, it is hard to believe that anyone would take it at all seriously. For the principle entails that, along with recombinant DNA research, almost all scientific research and many other commonplace activities having little to do with science should be prohibited. It is, after all, at least logically possible that the next new compound synthesized in an ongoing chemical research program will turn out to be an uncontainable carcinogen many orders of magnitude more dangerous than aerosol plutonium. And, to vary the example, there is a non-zero probability that experiments in artificial pollination will produce a weed that will, a decade from now, ruin the world's food grain harvest.[1]

•   •   •

The third argument I want to consider provides a striking illustration of how important it is, in normative thinking, to make clear the moral *principles* being invoked. The argument I have in mind begins with a factual claim about recombinant DNA research and concludes that stringent restrictions, perhaps even a moratorium, should be imposed. However, advocates of the argument are generally silent on the normative principle(s) linking premise and conclusion. The gap thus created can be filled in a variety of ways, resulting in very different arguments. The empirical observation that begins the argument is that recombinant DNA methods enable scientists to move genes back and forth across natural barriers, "particularly the most fundamental such barrier, that which divides prokaryotes from eukaryotes.* The results will be essentially new organisms, self-perpetuating and hence permanent.[2] Because of this, it is concluded that severe restrictions are in order. Plainly this argument is an enthymeme; a central premise has been left unstated. What sort of moral principle is being tacitly assumed?

The principle that comes first to mind is simply that natural barriers should not be breached, or perhaps that "essentially new organisms" should not be created. The principle has an almost theological ring to it, and perhaps there are some people who would be prepared to defend it on theological grounds. But short of a theological argument, it is hard to see why anyone would hold the view that breaching natural barriers or creating new organisms is *intrinsically* wrong. For if a person were to advocate such a principle, he would have to condemn the creation of new bacterial strains capable of, say, synthesizing human clotting factor or insulin, *even if* creating the new organism generated *no unwelcome side effects*.

There is quite a different way of unraveling the

Ed. note: Prokaryotes are simple organisms, like bacteria, which lack a defined nucleus. Eukaryotes are more complex organisms, which have cells containing defined nuclei. Examples of eukaryotes are plants and animals.

"natural barriers" argument which avoids appeal to the dubious principles just discussed. As an alternative, this second reading of the argument ties premise to conclusion with a second factual claim and a quite different normative premise. The added factual claim is that at present our knowledge of the consequences of creating new forms of life is severely limited; thus we cannot know with any assurance that the probability of disastrous consequences is very low. The moral principle needed to mesh with the two factual premises would be something such as the following:

If we do not know with considerable assurance that the probability of an activity leading to disastrous consequences is very low, then we should not allow the activity to continue.

Now this principle, unlike those marshaled in the first interpretation of the natural barriers argument, is not lightly dismissed. It is, to be sure, a conservative principle, and it has the odd feature of focusing entirely on the dangers an activity poses while ignoring its potential benefits.[3] Still, the principle may have a certain attraction in light of recent history, which has increasingly been marked by catastrophes attributable to technology's unanticipated side effects. I will not attempt a full-scale evaluation of this principle just now. For the principle raises, albeit in a rather extreme way, the question of how risks and benefits are to be weighed against each other. In my opinion, that is the really crucial moral question raised by recombinant DNA research. It is a question which bristles with problems. In Section II I shall take a look at some of these problems and make a few tentative steps toward some solutions. While picking our way through the problems we will have another opportunity to examine the principle just cited.

II. RISKS AND BENEFITS

At first glance it might be thought that the issue of risks and benefits is quite straightforward, at least in principle. What we want to know is whether the potential benefits of recombinant DNA research justify the risks involved. To find out we need only determine the probabilities of the various dangers and benefits. And while some of the empirical facts— the probabilities—may require considerable ingenuity and effort to uncover, the assessment poses no particularly difficult normative or conceptual problems.

Unfortunately, this sanguine view does not survive much more than a first glance. A closer look at the task of balancing the risks and benefits of recombinant DNA research reveals a quagmire of sticky conceptual problems and simmering moral disputes. In the next few pages I will try to catalogue and comment on some of these moral disputes. I wish I could also promise solutions to all of them, but to do so would be false advertising.

PROBLEMS ABOUT PROBABILITIES

In trying to assess costs and benefits, a familiar first step is to set down a list of possible actions and possible outcomes. Next, we assign some measure of desirability to each possible outcome, and for each action we estimate the conditional probability of each outcome given that the action is performed. In attempting to apply this decision-making strategy to the case of recombinant DNA research, the assignment of probabilities poses some perplexing problems. Some of the outcomes whose probabilities we want to know can be approached using standard empirical techniques. Thus, for example, we may want to know what the probability is of a specific enfeebled host *E. coli* strain surviving passage through the human intestinal system, should it be accidentally ingested. Or we may want to know what the probability is that a host organism will escape from a P-4 laboratory. In such cases, while there may be technical difficulties to be overcome, we have a reasonably clear idea of the sort of data needed to estimate the required probabilities. But there are other possible outcomes whose probabilities cannot be determined by experiment. It is important, for example, to know what the probability is of recombinant DNA research leading to a method for developing nitrogen-fixing strains of corn and wheat. And it is important to know how likely it is that recombinant DNA research will lead to techniques for effectively treating or preventing various types of cancer. Yet there is no experiment we can perform or any data we can gather that will enable us to *empirically* estimate these probabilities. Nor are these the most problematic probabilities we may want to know. A possibility that weighs heavily on the minds of many who are worried about recombinant DNA research is that this research may lead to negative consequences for human health or for the environment *which have not yet even been thought of*. The history of technology during the last half-century surely demonstrates that this is not a quixotic concern. Yet here again there would appear to be no data we can gather that would help much in estimating the probability of such potential outcomes.

It should be stressed that the problems just sketched are not to be traced simply to a paucity of data. Rather, they are conceptual problems; it is doubtful whether there is *any clear empirical sense* to be made of objective probability assignments to contingencies like those we are considering.

Theorists in the Bayesian tradition may be unmoved by the difficulties we have noted. On their view all probability claims are reports of subjective probabilities.[4] And, a Bayesian might quite properly note, there is no special problem about assigning *subjective* probabilities to outcomes such as those that worried us. But even for the radical Bayesian, there remains the problem of *whose* subjective probabilities ought to be employed in making a *social* or *political* decision. The problem is a pressing one since the subjective probabilities assigned to potential dangers and benefits of recombinant DNA research would appear to vary considerably even among reasonably well informed members of the scientific community.

The difficulties we have been surveying are serious ones. Some might feel they are so serious that they render rational assessment of the risks and benefits of recombinant DNA research all but impossible. I am inclined to be rather more optimistic, however. Almost all of the perils posed by recombinant DNA research require the occurrence of a sequence of separate events. For a chimerical bacterial strain created in a recombinant DNA experiment to cause a serious epidemic, for example, at least the following events must occur:

1. A pathogenic bacterium must be synthesized.
2. The chimerical bacteria must escape from the laboratory.
3. The strain must be viable in nature.
4. The strain must compete successfully with other microorganisms which are themselves the product of intense natural selection.[5]

Since *all* of these must occur, the probability of the potential epidemic is the product of the probabilities of each individual contingency. And there are at least two items on the list, namely (2) and (3), whose probabilities are amenable to reasonably straightforward empirical assessment. Thus the product of these two individual probabilities places an upper limit on the probability of the epidemic. For the remaining two probabilities, we must rely on subjective probability assessments of informed scientists. No doubt there

will be considerable variability. Yet even here the variability will be limited. In the case of (4), as an example, the available knowledge about microbial natural selection provides no precise way of estimating the probability that a chimerical strain of enfeebled *E. coli* will compete successfully outside the laboratory. But no serious scientist would urge that the probability is *high*. We can then use the highest responsible subjective estimate of the probabilities of (1) and (4) in calculating the "worst case" estimate of the risk of epidemic. If in using this highest "worst case" estimate, our assessment yields the result that benefits outweigh risks, then lower estimates of the same probabilities will, of course, yield the same conclusion. Thus it may well be the case that the problems about probabilities we have reviewed will not pose insuperable obstacles to a rational assessment of risks and benefits.

WEIGHING HARMS AND BENEFITS

A second cluster of problems that confronts us in assessing the risks and benefits of recombinant DNA research turns on the assignment of a measure of desirability to the various possible outcomes. Suppose that we have a list of the various harms and benefits that might possibly result from pursuing recombinant DNA research. The list will include such "benefits" as development of an inexpensive way to synthesize human clotting factor and development of a strain of nitrogen-fixing wheat; and such "harms" as release of a new antibiotic-resistant strain of pathogenic bacteria and release of a strain of *E. coli* carrying tumor viruses capable of causing cancer in man.

Plainly, it is possible that pursuing a given policy will result in more than one benefit and in more than one harm. Now if we are to assess the potential impact of various policies or courses of action, we must assign some index of desirability to the possible *total outcomes* of each policy, outcomes which may well include a mix of benefits and harms. To do this we must confront a tangle of normative problems that are as vexing and difficult as any we are likely to face. We must *compare* the moral desirabilities of various harms and benefits. The task is particularly troublesome when the harms and benefits to be compared are of different kinds. Thus, for example, some of the attractive potential benefits of recombinant DNA research are economic: we may learn to recover small amounts of valuable metals in an economically feasible way, or we may be able to synthesize insulin and other drugs inexpensively. By contrast, many of the risks of recombinant DNA research are risks to human life or health. So if we are to take the idea of cost-benefit analysis seriously, we must at some point decide how human lives are to be weighed against economic benefits.

There are those who contend that the need to make such decisions indicates the moral bankruptcy of attempting to employ risk-benefit analyses when human lives are at stake. On the critics' view, we cannot reckon the possible loss of a human life as just another negative outcome, albeit a grave and heavily weighted one. To do so, it is urged, is morally repugnant and reflects a callous lack of respect for the sacredness of human life.

On my view, this sort of critique of the very idea of using risk-benefit analyses is ultimately untenable. It is simply a fact about the human condition, lamentable as it is inescapable, that in many human activities we run the risk of inadvertently causing the death of a human being. We run such a risk each time we drive a car, allow a dam to be built, or allow a plane to take off. Moreover, in making social and individual decisions, we cannot escape weighing economic consequences against the risk to human life. A building code in the Midwest will typically mandate fewer precautions against earthquakes than a building code in certain parts of California. Yet earthquakes are not impossible in the Midwest. If we elect not to require precautions, then surely a major reason must be that it would simply be too expensive. In this judgment, as in countless others, there is no escaping the need to balance economic costs against possible loss of life. To deny that we must and do balance economic costs against risks to human life is to assume the posture of a moral ostrich.

I have been urging the point that it is not *morally objectionable* to try to balance economic concerns against risks to human life. But if such judgments are unobjectionable, indeed necessary, they also surely are among the most difficult any of us has to face. It is hard to imagine a morally sensitive person not feeling extremely uncomfortable when confronted with the need to put a dollar value on human lives. It might be thought that the moral dilemmas engendered by the need to balance such radically different costs and benefits pose insuperable practical obstacles for a rational resolution of the recombinant DNA debate. But

here, as in the case of problems with probabilities, I am more sanguine. For while some of the risks and potential benefits of recombinant DNA research are all but morally incommensurable, the most salient risks and benefits are easier to compare. The major risks, as we have noted, are to human life and health. However, the major potential benefits are *also* to human life and health. The potential economic benefits of recombinant DNA research pale in significance when set against the potential for major breakthroughs in our understanding and ability to treat a broad range of conditions, from birth defects to cancer. Those of us, and I confess I am among them, who despair of deciding how lives and economic benefits are to be compared can nonetheless hope to settle our views about recombinant DNA research by comparing the potential risks to life and health with the potential benefits to life and health. Here we are comparing plainly commensurable outcomes. If the balance turns out to be favorable, then we need not worry about factoring in potential economic benefits.

· · ·

PROBLEMS ABOUT PRINCIPLES

The third problem I want to consider focuses on the following question. Once we have assessed the potential harms and benefits of recombinant DNA research, how should we use this information in coming to a decision? It might be thought that the answer is trivially obvious. To assess the harms and benefits is, after all, just to compute, for each of the various policies that we are considering, what might be called its *expected utility*. The expected utility of a given policy is found by first multiplying the desirability of each possible total outcome by the probability that the policy in question will lead to that total outcome, and then adding the numbers obtained. As we have seen, finding the needed probabilities and assigning the required desirabilities will not be easy. But once we know the expected utility of each policy, is it not obvious that we should choose the policy with the highest expected utility? The answer, unfortunately, is no, it is not at all obvious.

Let us call the principle that we should adopt the policy with the highest expected utility the *utilitarian principle*. The following example should make it clear that, far from being trivial or tautological, the utilitarian principle is a substantive and controversial moral principle. Suppose that the decision which confronts us is whether or not to adopt policy *A*. What is more, suppose we know there is a probability close to 1 that 100,000 lives will be saved if we adopt *A*. However, we also know that there is a probability close to 1 that 1,000 will die as a direct result of our adopting policy *A,* and these people would survive if we did not adopt *A*. Finally, suppose that the other possible consequences of adopting *A* are relatively inconsequential and can be ignored. (For concreteness, we might take *A* to be the establishment of a mass vaccination program, using a relatively risky vaccine.) Now plainly if we take the moral desirability of saving a life to be exactly offset by the moral undesirability of causing a death, then the utilitarian principle dictates that we adopt policy *A*. But many people feel uncomfortable with this result, the discomfort increasing with the number of deaths that would result from *A*. If, to change the example, the choice that confronts us is saving 100,000 lives while causing the deaths of 50,000 others, a significant number of people are inclined to think that the morally right thing to do is to refrain from doing *A,* and "let nature take its course."

If we reject policy *A*, the likely reason is that we also reject the utilitarian principle. Perhaps the most plausible reason for rejecting the utilitarian principle is the view that our obligation to *avoid doing harm* is stronger than our obligation to do good. There are many examples, some considerably more compelling than the one we have been discussing, which seem to illustrate that in a broad range of cases we do feel that our obligation to avoid doing harm is greater than our obligation to do good.[6] Suppose, to take but one example, that my neighbor requests my help in paying off his gambling debts. He owes $5,000 to a certain bookmaker with underworld connections. Unless the neighbor pays the debt immediately, he will be shot. Here, I think we are all inclined to say, I have no strong obligation to give my neighbor the money he needs, and if I were to do so it would be a supererogatory gesture. By contrast, suppose a representative of my neighbor's bookmaker approaches me and requests that I shoot my neighbor. If I refuse, he will see to it that my new car, which cost $5,000, will be destroyed by a bomb while it sits unattended at the curb. In this case, surely, I have a strong obligation not to harm my neighbor, although not shooting him will cost me $5,000.

Suppose that this example and others convince us that we cannot adopt the utilitarian principle, at least not in its most general form, where it purports to be applicable to all moral decisions. What are the alternatives? One cluster of alternative principles would urge that in some or all cases we weigh the harm a contemplated action will cause more heavily than we weigh the good it will do. The extreme form of such a principle would dictate that we ignore the benefits entirely and opt for the action or policy that produces the *least* expected harm. (It is this principle, or a close relation, which emerged in the second reading of the "natural barriers" argument discussed in the third part of Section I above.) A more plausible variant would allow us to count both benefits and harms in our deliberations, but would specify how much more heavily harms were to count.

On my view, some moderate version of a "harm-weighted" principle is preferable to the utilitarian principle in a considerable range of cases. *However, the recombinant DNA issue is not one of these cases.* Indeed, when we try to apply a harm-weighted principle to the recombinant DNA case we run head on into a conceptual problem of considerable difficulty. The distinction between doing good and doing harm presupposes a notion of the normal or expectable course of events. Roughly, if my action causes you to be worse off than you would have been in the normal course of events, then I have harmed you; if my action causes you to be better off than in the normal course of events, then I have done you some good; and if my action leaves you just as you would be in the normal course of events, then I have done neither. In many cases, the normal course of events is intuitively quite obvious. Thus in the case of the neighbor and the bookmaker, in the expected course of events I would neither shoot my neighbor nor give him $5,000 to pay off his debts. Thus I am doing good if I give him the money and I am doing harm if I shoot him. But in other cases, including the recombinant DNA case, it is not at all obvious what constitutes the "expected course of events," and thus it is not at all obvious what to count as a harm. To see this, suppose that as a matter of fact many more deaths and illnesses will be prevented as a result of pursuing recombinant DNA research than will be caused by pursuing it. But suppose that there *will* be at least some people who become ill or die as a result of recombinant DNA research being pursued. If these are the facts, then who would be harmed by imposing a ban on recombinant DNA research? That depends on what we take to be the "normal course of events." Presumably, if we do not impose a ban, then the research will continue and the lives will be saved. If this is the normal course of events, then if we impose a ban we have *harmed* those people who would be saved. But it is equally natural to take as the normal course of events the situation in which recombinant DNA research is not pursued. And if *that* is the normal course of events, then those who would have been saved are not harmed by a ban, for they are no worse off than they would be in the normal course of events. However, on this reading of "normal course of events," if we *fail* to impose a ban, then we have harmed those people who will ultimately become ill or die as a result of recombinant DNA research, since as a result of not imposing a ban they are worse off than they would have been in the normal course of events. I conclude that, in the absence of a theory detailing how we are to recognize the normal course of events, harm-weighted principles have no clear application to the case of recombinant DNA research.

Harm-weighted principles are not the only alternatives to the utilitarian principle. There is another cluster of alternatives that take off in quite a different direction. These principles urge that in deciding which policy to pursue there is a strong presumption in favor of policies that adhere to certain formal moral principles (that is, principles which do not deal with the *consequences* of our policies). Thus, to take the example most directly relevant to the recombinant DNA case, it might be urged that there is a strong presumption in favor of a policy which preserves freedom of scientific inquiry. In its extreme form, this principle would protect freedom of inquiry *no matter what the consequences;* and as we saw in the first part of Section I, this extreme position is exceptionally implausible. A much more plausible principle would urge that freedom of inquiry be protected until the balance of negative over positive consequences reaches a certain specified amount, at which point we would revert to the utilitarian principle. On such a view, if the expected utility of banning recombinant DNA research is a bit higher than the expected utility of allowing it to continue, then we would nonetheless allow it to continue. But if the expected utility of a ban is enormously higher than the expected utility of continuation, banning is the policy to be preferred.[7]

III. LONG-TERM RISKS

Thus far in our discussion of risks and benefits, the risks that have occupied us have been what might be

termed "short-term" risks, such as the release of a new pathogen. The negative effects of these events, though they might be long-lasting indeed, would be upon us relatively quickly. However, some of those who are concerned about recombinant DNA research think there are longer-term dangers that are at least as worrisome. The dangers they have in mind stem not from the accidental release of harmful substances in the course of recombinant DNA research, but rather from the unwise use of the *knowledge* we will likely gain in pursuing the research. The scenarios most often proposed are nightmarish variations on the theme of human genetic engineering. With the knowledge we acquire, it is conjectured, some future tyrant may have people built to order, perhaps creating a whole class of people who willingly and cheaply do the society's dirty or dangerous work, as in Huxley's *Brave New World*. Though the proposed scenarios clearly are science fiction, they are not to be lightly dismissed. For if the technology they conjure is not demonstrably achievable, neither is it demonstrably impossible. And if only a bit of the science fiction turns to fact, the dangers could be beyond reckoning.

Granting that potential misuse of the knowledge gained in recombinant DNA research is a legitimate topic of concern, how ought we to guard ourselves against this misuse? One common proposal is to try to prevent the acquisition of such knowledge by banning or curtailing recombinant DNA research now. Let us cast this proposal in the form of an explicit moral argument. The conclusion is that recombinant DNA research should be curtailed, and the reason given for the conclusion is that such research could possibly produce knowledge which might be misused with disastrous consequences. To complete the argument we need a moral principle, and the one which seems to be needed is something such as this:

If a line of research can lead to the discovery of knowledge which might be disastrously misused, then that line of research should be curtailed.

Once it has been made explicit, I think relatively few people would be willing to endorse this principle. For recombinant DNA research is hardly alone in potentially leading to knowledge that might be disastrously abused. Indeed, it is hard to think of an area of scientific research that could *not* lead to the discovery of potentially dangerous knowledge. So if the principle is accepted it would entail that almost all scientific research should be curtailed or abandoned.

It might be thought that we could avoid the extreme consequences just cited by retreating to a more moderate moral principle. The moderate principle would urge only that we should curtail those areas of research where the probability of producing dangerous knowledge is comparatively high. Unfortunately, this more moderate principle is of little help in avoiding the unwelcome consequences of the stronger principle. The problem is that the history of science is simply too unpredictable to enable us to say with any assurance which lines of research will produce which sorts of knowledge or technology. There is a convenient illustration of the point in the recent history of molecular genetics. The idea of recombining DNA molecules is one which has been around for some time. However, early efforts proved unsuccessful. As it happened, the crucial step in making recombinant DNA technology possible was provided by research on restriction enzymes, research that was undertaken with no thought of recombinant DNA technology. Indeed, until it was realized that restriction enzymes provided the key to recombining DNA molecules, the research on restriction enzymes was regarded as a rather unexciting (and certainly uncontroversial) scientific backwater.[8] In an entirely analogous way, crucial pieces of information that may one day enable us to manipulate the human genome may come from just about any branch of molecular biology. To guard against the discovery of that knowledge we should have to curtail not only recombinant DNA research but all of molecular biology.

Before concluding, we would do well to note that there is a profound pessimism reflected in the attitude of those who would stop recombinant DNA research because it might lead to knowledge that could be abused. It is, after all, granted on all sides that the knowledge resulting from recombinant DNA research will have both good and evil potential uses. So it would seem the sensible strategy would be to try to prevent the improper uses of this knowledge rather than trying to prevent the knowledge from ever being uncovered. Those who would take the more extreme step of trying to stop the knowledge from being uncovered presumably feel that its improper use is all but inevitable, that our political and social institutions are incapable of preventing morally abhorrent applications of the knowledge while encouraging beneficial applications. On my view, this pessimism is unwarranted; indeed, it is all but inconsistent. The historical record gives us no reason to believe that what is technologically possible will be done, no matter what the moral price. Indeed, in the area of human genetic manipulation, the record points in quite the *opposite* direction. We have long known that the same techniques that work so successfully in animal breeding can be applied to humans as well. Yet there is no evidence of a "technological imperative" impelling our society to breed people as we breed dairy cattle, simply because we know that it can be done. Finally, it is odd that those who express no confidence in the ability of our institutions to forestall such monstrous applications of technology are not equally pessimistic about the ability of the same institutions to impose an effective ban on the uncovering of dangerous knowledge. If our institutions are incapable of restraining the application of technology when those applications would be plainly morally abhorrent, one would think they would be even more impotent in attempting to restrain a line of research which promises major gains in human welfare.[9]

NOTES

1. Unfortunately, the doomsday scenario argument is *not* a straw man conjured only by those who would refute it. Consider, for example, the remarks of Anthony Mazzocchi, spokesman for the Oil, Chemical and Atomic Workers International Union, reported in *Science News,* 19 March 1977, p. 181: "When scientists argue over safe or unsafe, we ought to be very prudent. . . . If critics are correct and the Andromeda scenario has *even the smallest possibility* of occurring, we must assume it will occur on the basis of our experience" (emphasis added).

2. The quotation is from George Wald, "The Case Against Genetic Engineering," *The Sciences,* September/October 1976; reprinted in David A. Jackson and Stephen P. Stich, eds., *The Recombinant DNA Debate* (Englewood Cliffs, N.J.: Prentice-Hall, 1979), pp. 127–133.

3. It is important to note, however, that the principle is considerably less conservative, and correspondingly more plausible, than the principle invoked in the doomsday scenario argument. That latter principle would have us enjoin an activity if the probability of the activity leading to catastrophe is anything other than zero.

4. For an elaboration of the Bayesian position, see Leonard J. Savage, *The Foundations of Statistics* (New York: John Wiley & Sons, 1954); also cf. Leonard J. Savage, "The Shifting Foundations of Statistics," in Robert G. Colodny, ed., *Logic, Laws and Life* (Pittsburgh: University of Pittsburgh Press, 1977).

5. For an elaboration of this point, see Bernard D. Davis, "Evolution, Epidemiology, and Recombinant DNA," *The Recombinant DNA Debate,* pp. 137–154.

6. For an interesting discussion of these cases, see J. O. Urmson, "Saints and Heroes," in A. I. Melden, ed., *Essays In Moral Philosophy* (Seattle: University of Washington Press, 1958). Also see the discussion of positive and negative duties in Philippa Foot, "The Problem of Abortion and the Doctrine of Double Effect," *Oxford Review* 5 (1967). Reprinted in James Rachels, ed., *Moral Problems* (New York: Harper & Row) 1971.

7. Carl Cohen defends this sort of limited protection of the formal free inquiry principle over a straight application of the

utilitarian principle in his interesting essay, "When May Research Be Stopped?" *New England Journal of Medicine* 296 (1977). Reprinted in *The Recombinant DNA Debate*, pp. 203–218.

8. I am indebted to Prof. Ethel Jackson for both the argument and the illustration.

9. This essay is an abridged and somewhat modified version of my essay, "The Recombinant DNA Debate: Some Philosophical Considerations," in *The Recombinant DNA Debate*, pp. 183–202. I am grateful to the editors of *Philosophy & Public Affairs* for their detailed and useful suggestions on modifying the essay to make it appropriate for use in this journal.

Scientific Inquiry and Public Policy

HANS JONAS

Freedom of Scientific Inquiry and the Public Interest

Freedom of inquiry and the idea of it are precious to the Western world as part of its general regard for freedom. Freedom of inquiry is claimed, granted, and cherished as unqualified on the premise that inquiry as such raises no moral problems. Let us take a look at this all-important premise, bearing in mind that "inquiry" today means preeminently *scientific* inquiry in the technical sense.

What are the points of contact between science and morals? At first glance there seem to be none, beyond the internal morality of keeping faith with the standards of science itself. Its sole value is truth, its sole aim the knowledge of truth, its sole business the pursuit of knowledge. This, to be sure, imposes its own code of conduct which can be called the territorial morals of the scientific realm: abiding by the rules of evidence and method, not cheating oneself and others, for example, by sloppy reasoning or experiment, let alone falsifying the latter's outcome—in short, being rigorous and intellectually honest. Ethically this amounts to no more than the command to be a good rather than a bad scientist (that is, when a scientist, be a scientist!) and implies no extrascientific commitment. The same is true for the personal virtues

From *Hastings Center Report* 6 (August 1976), 15–17. Reprinted with permission of the Hastings Center: © Institute of Society, Ethics, and the Life Services, 360 Broadway, Hastings-on-Hudson, N.Y. 10706.

of dedication, persistence, discipline, and the strength to resist one's own prejudices—again simply conditions of success within the vocation, if also praiseworthy qualities in general. Finally, the duty of sharing one's results and evidence with the scientific community seems to lend a social and public dimension to intrascientific morals; but in fact, given the increasingly collective nature of the scientific enterprise, intercommunication belongs—even for the individual investigator—to the technical conditions of doing science well: it still leaves the scientific morality strictly "territorial" and as yet stipulates no obligation of the scientific fraternity beyond itself.

We feel, of course, that this cannot be the whole truth. It may have been true as long as the contemplative sphere and the active sphere were cleanly separate (as they were in premodern times), and pure theory did not intervene in the practical affairs of men. Knowledge could then be considered a private good to the knower, which—being merely a state of mind—could do no harm to the good of others, as it sought only to comprehend but not to change the state of things. Its dissemination, indeed, was sometimes regarded by public powers (such as the Church, but sometimes also the state) as dangerous to the good of the many, for example, by undermining their faith; but a quasi-automatic protection against this lay already in the esoteric character of higher learning as such, which confined its reception to the few; and those few had mainly to defend the right to their own thought against custodial claims on their souls, seeing that it did not trespass on things in the outer world. And, after all, even broadcast widely among the untutored, ideas have at most persuasive and not coercive force.

MERGING THEORY AND PRACTICE IN MODERN SCIENCE

All this lapsed with the rise of natural science at the beginning of the modern age, which entirely altered the traditional relation of theory and practice, making them merge ever more intimately. Even so, the fiction of "pure theory" and its essential "innocence" persisted: under the banner of the general freedom of thought and speech, as distinct from deeds, scientific inquiry too claimed untrammeled freedom for itself on the same distinction—in curious concurrence with the promise of eventual usefulness, which contradicts the plea of theoretical insularity. It took the Industrial Revolution to fulfill the promise of usefulness on a large scale. Until then, the social charter of science still rested on the inherited dignity of "knowledge for its own sake," now joined with the principle of toleration for all thought and belief (including the right to err). So deeply is this twofold respect ingrained in the modern mind that even in today's vastly changed situation, few things sound more odious to Western ears than "interference with the freedom of inquiry."

Sincere as this homage to disinterested knowledge may often be, it would be hypocritical to deny that in fact the emphasis in the case for science has heavily shifted to its practical benefits. From some time in the nineteenth century onward, and accelerating in ours, there was an increasingly irresistible spill-over from theory, however pure, into the vulgar field of practice in the shape of scientific technology. Belatedly and almost suddenly, Francis Bacon's (1561–1626) precocious directive to science to aim at power over nature for the sake of raising man's material estate had become working truth beyond all expectations.

Though the "esotericism" of the proliferating branches of knowledge has even heightened and keeps heightening to the point of virtual inaccessibility to all but the insiders on each twig, yet the public impact of their recondite cerebrations is enormous: an impact not, as it was at most before, on opinions but on conditions and ways of life. And therewith the subject of "science and morals" begins in earnest. For whatever of human doing impinges on the real world and thus on the welfare of others is subject to moral assessment. As soon as there is power and its use, morality is involved. The very praise of the benefits of science exposes science to the question of whether *all* of its works are beneficial. It is then no longer a question of good or bad science, but of good or ill effects of science (and only "good science" can be effectual at all). Is it responsible for either? Clearly, taking credit for the benefits means also taking blame for the damages; it would be better for science to do neither, but this option may be closed. Apportioning praise and blame can be an idle exercise, but it is not when a social privilege—and the freedom of inquiry is nothing else—is implicated in it. Thus it is not idle to ask: if technology, the offspring, has its dark sides, is science, the progenitor, to blame?

The simplistic answer is that the scientist, having no control over the application of his theoretical findings, is not responsible for their misuse. His product is knowledge and nothing else: its use-potential is there for others to take or leave, to exploit for good or for evil, for serious or for frivolous ends. Science by itself is innocent and somehow beyond good and evil. Plausible, but too easy: witness the soul-searching of atomic scientists after Hiroshima. We must take a closer look at the interlocking of theory and practice in the actual way science is nowadays "done" and essentially must be done. We shall then see that not only have the boundaries between theory and practice become blurred, but that the two are now fused in the very heart of science itself, so that the ancient alibi of pure theory and with it the moral immunity it provided no longer hold.

DENYING THE MORAL IMMUNITY OF SCIENCE

The first patent observation is that no branch of science remains whose discoveries are devoid of some technological applicability. The only exception I can think of is cosmology: the expanding universe, the evolution of galaxies, big bang and black holes—these are matters for knowing only and for no possible doing on our part. It is worth our reflection, and surely no accident, that the first science of all, astronomy, the contemplation of the heavens, is also the last to be purely science. Every other unraveling of nature by science now invites some translation of itself into some technological possibility or other, often even starts off a whole technology not conceived of before. If this were all, the theoretician might still argue his sanctuary this side of the step into action: "That threshold is crossed after my work is done and as far as I am concerned, could as well be left uncrossed." But we must remind him that he could not have done the first, "pure" part without massive arrangements from outside under whose broader roof his role becomes part of a contractual division of labor. What is the true relationship? *theory & practice*

First, much of science now lives on the intellectual feedback from precisely its technological application. Second, it receives its assignments from there: in what direction to search, what problems to solve. Third, for solving them, and generally for its own advance, it uses advanced technology itself: its physical tools become ever more demanding. In this sense, even purest science has now a stake in technology, as technology has in science. Fourth, the cost of those physical tools and their staffing must be underwritten from outside: the mere economics of the case calls on the public purse or other sponsorship; and this, in funding the scientist's project (even with "no strings attached") naturally does so in the expectation of some future return in the practical sphere. Here there is mutual understanding. With nothing shamefaced about it, the anticipated payoff is put forward as the recommending rationale in seeking grants or is specified outright as the purpose in offering them. In sum, it has come to be that the tasks of science are increasingly defined by extraneous interests rather than its own internal logic or the free curiosity of the investigator. This is not to disparage those extraneous interests nor the fact that science has become their servant, that is, part of the social enterprise. But it is to say that the acceptance of this functional role (without which there would be no science of the advanced type we have, but also not the type of society living by its fruits) has destroyed the alibi of pure, disinterested theory and put science squarely in the realm of social action where every agent is accountable for his deeds. Add to this the pervasive experience that the pragmatic implications of scientific discoveries prove irresistible to the marketplace—that what they show *can* be done *will* be done, with or without a prior compact—and it is abundantly clear that no insularity of the theoretical realm still saves the scientist from being the generator of enormous consequences. While technically it is still true that

one can be a good scientist without being a good person, it is no longer true that being a good person begins for him outside his professional work: the very doing of it entails moral questions already inside the sacred precinct.

How much "inside" becomes clear when we reflect on the third point in our list, the employment of physical tools—that is, on *how* the scientist *gets* his knowledge. It is then borne in on us that doing science already includes physical action; that thinking and doing interpenetrate in the very procedures of inquiry, and thus the division of "theory and practice" breaks down within theory itself. This has an important bearing on the hallowed "freedom of inquiry," after inquiry has become essentially "research." There was a time when the seekers after knowledge did not need to dirty their hands; of this noble breed the mathematician is the sole survivor. Modern natural science arose with the decision to wrest knowledge from nature by actively operating on it, that is, by intervening in the objects of knowledge. The name for this intervention is "experiment," vital to all modern science. Observation here involves manipulation. But the granting of freedom to thought and speech, from which that of inquiry derives, does not cover *action,* even if subsidiary to thought. Action is always subject to legal and moral restraints. However, two properties of classic experimentation still ensured the "innocence" of this kind of action internal to scientific inquiry: that it dealt with inanimate matter, and on a small scale. Not real thunderstorms but discharges from condensers are generated to learn about lightning. Simulating models, containable within the laboratory, substitute for the real thing. In that respect, the insulation of the cognitive arena from the real world still holds.

Both these guarantees of harmlessness and therefore of freedom in experimentation have lapsed with certain more recent developments in science. As to scale, an atomic explosion, be it merely done for the sake of theory, affects the whole atmosphere and possibly many lives now or later. The world itself has become the laboratory. One finds out by doing in earnest what, having found out, one might wish not to have done. And as to experimentation on animate objects, which came with the younger biological sciences, no surrogate will do, no vicarious model, but the original itself must serve, and ethical neutrality ceases at the latest when it comes to human subjects. What is done to them is a real deed, for whose morality the interest of knowledge is no blanket warrant. In either case of experimentation, that of excessive magnitude and that performed on persons, to which others could be added, the protective line between vicarious and genuine action is obliterated in the execution of research itself—rendering somehow obsolete the conventional distinction of "pure" and "applied" science. Not only the "what," already the "how" of cognition straddles the line. Application takes place in the inquiry itself. (Where it does not directly, as in theoretical physics, the experimental base is vitally drawn upon.) It follows that the "freedom of inquiry" cannot be unqualified.

QUALIFYING FREEDOM OF INQUIRY

We are with reason touchy about interference with this freedom, not only because it had once painfully to be wrested from earlier thought control and is thus a precious and vulnerable possession, but also because we have before our eyes its shameful repression in the East. Yet we must remember that the high privilege of theory had its own theoretical foundation in the distinction of thought and action and is really conditional on it. Never has absolute freedom been claimed for action, and surely never has it been accorded to action. Thus to the extent that the operation of science becomes shot through with action, it comes under the same rule of law, social censorship, moral approval or disapproval, to which any outward acting is exposed in civil society. And, of course, its own internal morals cease to be purely "territorial": the very means of getting to know can raise moral questions before the "extraterritorial" question of how to use the knowledge so obtained poses itself.

It would weaken the case to illustrate it only with notorious atrocities. It is easy to elicit unanimity on such examples: that one must not, in order to find out how people behave under torture (which may be of interest to a theory of man) try out torture on a subject; or kill in order to determine the limit of tolerance to a poison, and the like. We are referring, of course, to the deeds of physicians (some of them prominent ones!) in Nazi concentration camps. Here was "freedom" of inquiry as shameful as its worst suppression. But we know too well, or believe we know, that the perpetrators of such scientific experiments (yes, scientific they could have been) were despicable and their motives base, and we can wash our hands of them. We may go further and question whether in these cases the knowledge sought after is a legitimate scientific aim in the first place; and if we conclude that it is not (for which there would be good reasons) then we could say that we are not really dealing with a case of science, but with one of human depravity. But our problem is not with crooked or perverted science but with bona fide, regular science. Keeping, then, to indubitably legitimate and even praiseworthy goals, we ask whether in *their* pursuit one may, for example, inject cancer cells into noncancerous subjects, or (for control purposes) withhold treatment from syphilitic patients—both actual occurrences in this country and both presumably helpful to a desirable end. I do not rush into an answer, but I do say that here moral and legal issues arise in the inner workings of science long before the question of application arises—issues that crash through the territorial barriers of science and present themselves before the general court of ethics and law. To the public authority of that court even the vaunted freedom of inquiry must bow.

LOREN R. GRAHAM

Concerns about Science and Attempts to Regulate Inquiry[1]

It will be the thesis of this article that discussions of proposals to regulate science do not have general value until a number of basic distinctions have been made among types of concern about science and types of proposal for its regulation. What we need as a first step toward a discussion of possible limits to inquiry is a typology or taxonomy of concerns about science. We can then assess the validity of each concern and address the problem of limits or regulation in a more specific and informed fashion.

• • •

The subsequent discussion will be based on a number of broad categories of concerns about science and technology, some of which have subcategories:

I. Concerns about Technology
  A. Concerns about the physical results of technology—"Destructive Technology"
  B. Concerns about the ethical results of technology—"Slippery Slope Technology"
    1. Biomedical ethics
  C. Concerns about the economic results of technology—"Economically Exploitative Technology"
II. Concerns about Science
  A. Concerns about research on human subjects—"Human Subjects Research"
  B. Concerns about distortions in allocations of resources for science—"Expensive Science"
  C. Concerns about certain kinds of fundamental knowledge
    1. Knowledge itself—"Subversive Knowledge"
    2. Knowledge "inevitably" leading to technology—"Inevitable Technology"

  D. Concerns about accidents in the research itself—"Accidents in Science"
  E. Concerns about the use of science to excite racial, sexual, or class prejudices—"Prejudicial Science"
  F. Concerns about certain modes of knowing—"Ways of Knowing"

The list given above sorts the concerns into the two broad divisions, technology and science. Some critics will respond that this division is no longer tenable. In an eloquent article Hans Jonas maintained "not only have the boundaries between theory and practice become blurred, but . . . the two are now fused in the very heart of science itself, so that the ancient alibi of pure theory and with it the moral immunity it provided no longer holds."[2]

Although I appreciate the argument which Professor Jonas has advanced, for the following reasons I do not consider it a serious challenge to the classification I am presenting here. First, I do not maintain, as Jonas's comment seems to imply, that problems of "science" enjoy a "moral immunity." I will consider ethical and moral issues under the headings both of technology and of science. (Note, for example, "human subjects research.") Second, although I agree that there are some problems which cannot easily be classified as either science or technology, it is my opinion that the great majority of current issues can be so classified without much difficulty, including most of the ones which have recently attracted so much attention in the press. The division between fundamental studies of physical and biological nature, on the one hand, and technological studies directed toward social or economic goals, on the other, is still a useful one. Third, I will consider issues under "Inevitable Technology" where the boundary between theory and practice has become blurred in the way in which Jonas emphasizes.

Concern about the physical results of technology is one of the most familiar and easily identified categories of concern. A prime example is the damage to the environment caused by industrial civilization. A specific case would be damage to the ozone layer alleged to result from the escape to the upper atmosphere of fluorocarbons used in aerosols. Others would be the polluting effects of DDT, supersonic transports, and various energy sources. The large array of issues under this category also include many that are not best described as environmental, such as regulation of the distribution and use of pharmaceutical drugs, food additives and chemicals (like saccharin), explosives, and radioactive materials. All are examples of society's need to prevent the products of technology from spreading in an unmonitored or unregulated way.

This category is the one where the observation "if we can regulate the railroads, so can we regulate science" is most apt, although we should remind ourselves that we are speaking here of technology, not science. The imposition of controls on the use of destructive technology is clearly within the rights and traditional practices of government regulatory agencies. Important questions about the wisdom of the regulations, economic and otherwise, can be raised, but the principle of government regulation is well established.

. . .

SLIPPERY SLOPE TECHNOLOGY

Whereas the previous category dealt with the physical effects of certain technologies, the present one centers upon the ethical effects. Obviously, every act of physical damage contains an ethical dimension, and no clean separation of the two can ever be made. Nonetheless, there exists a significant difference between, on the one hand, a concern whether the physically damaging effects of a certain technology can be excused within existing ethical systems, and, on the other hand, whether a certain technology may be destroying the ethical system itself. The present category deals with the latter concern.

The use of new technology in the biomedical area has recently raised many difficult ethical issues. New possibilities for prenatal diagnosis by amniocentesis, prolongation of life through the use of dialysis and respiratory machines, psychosurgery, and DNA therapy (or "genetic engineering") are only a few

examples of issues which by now have been widely discussed in the press. A whole new field of discussion, biomedical ethics, has developed as a result of the advent of these new technologies. The Institute for the Study of Society, Ethics and the Life Sciences in Hastings-on-Hudson and the Kennedy Institute Center for Bioethics in Washington, D.C., are two of the more active centers among the many where issues of medical ethics are now under close study.

One of the major concerns expressed by observers of technological developments in the biomedical field has been that by blurring or erasing ethical boundaries that were earlier considered absolute, we will go out onto a "slippery slope" of relativistic ethics on which we may lose our balance and tumble to the bottom. Critics often raise the specter of eugenics and medical experimentation under national socialism as the ultimate point of descent. They ask, if we sanction the disconnection of life-support machines in terminal cases, or we perform abortions on genetically defective fetuses in the last months of pregnancy, what ethical limitations exist preventing us from taking a more active role in ending the lives of terminal patients suffering pain, killing a deformed child immediately after birth, or even several months after birth? The possibility of becoming callous to moral values through adoption of the radical proposals or repetition of the less radical ones is worrisome, and properly demands our attention. On the other hand, if we simply prohibit abortions or termination of extraordinary care, we will encourage worse ethical abuses (illegal abortions under frightful conditions, economic injustice, even infanticide by parents). The slippery slope slants in more than one direction.

. . .

Controversial as these issues are, they do not, in themselves, directly involve the question of limits to inquiry. They are immensely difficult questions of the wise use of medical technology. Guidelines are developing which help to prevent abuses while still taking advantage of the benefits of the new technologies, benefits which in many instances are significant and deeply humane.

ECONOMICALLY EXPLOITATIVE TECHNOLOGY

Enormous costs are involved in research and development in certain high technology areas. Should large public sums be spent for the development of an American supersonic transport when only a small portion of the population would ever utilize such transportation? Should large amounts be invested in developing exotic and cosmetic medical treatments if these sums detract from public health programs? How does one decide how much money should be given research on diseases such as cancer and heart disease which afflict highly industrialized societies to a greater degree than underdeveloped societies (where, for example, kwashiorkor and schistosomiasis may be more serious threats)? From a health standpoint, how does one decide the relative importance of research on curative medical technologies as opposed to improvement of environmental conditions, which are increasingly seen as the source of many illnesses?

* * *

A [second] example of economic results of technology is the distortion in the use of natural resources which certain technologies entail. The present effort to slow the exhaustion of fossil fuels by automobiles and home-heating is an example of control of expensive or wasteful technology.

In each of the examples discussed above, the principle of control for economic reasons is already established in the United States, although great controversies about the best means of control remain. In contrast to the centrally planned economies, where direct limitation on outputs of certain technologies is often imposed, in the United States the emphasis has frequently been on economic penalties or rewards (taxes, deductions) on the technology, and on controlling research and development through modulation of federal research grants. This approach seems quite proper. Still, the possibility of controls of a variety of types, particularly in response to crisis situations, is apparent. If these controls are carefully executed within a democratic framework, they are visualizable without damage to political or academic freedom.

As we move now from the subject of concerns about technology to that of concerns about science itself, we come much closer to questions of principle that are essential to our concept of free inquiry.

HUMAN SUBJECTS RESEARCH

The methods of procedure in certain types of research may do damage to human subjects of the re-

search, or be suspected of doing such damage. The adoption of guidelines on research on human subjects by the National Institutes of Health is an example of efforts to avoid damaging effects of this type.

Surely we all admit that limits to inquiry *do* exist within this category. One cannot, for example, morally justify injecting human subjects with pathogenic organisms or toxic chemicals to determine their lethality. Nor can we determine the outer limits of human toleration of physical or psychological deprivation, or of physical pain, by direct experimentation, even if subjects would volunteer for such experiments. The history of medical experiments in Nazi Germany, such as the ones designed to help the Luftwaffe decide how long a downed pilot could survive in icy waters, is still a recent memory warning us against such immoral and crude experiments.

* * *

Most of us would probably agree that greater ethical awareness about [human] research is a laudable development. Research scientists have not only a moral responsibility to avoid damage through individual and corporate examination of the possible effects of their research procedures on human subjects, but also an interest in avoiding such controversies by self-regulation, since the alternative is increasing regulation by bodies outside the scientific community. The fact that the law already provides some avenues for redress to individuals actually harmed is not a sufficient answer to the problem. The responsibility of scientists themselves for the alleviation of public concerns is heavier in this category of research than any other so far discussed.

EXPENSIVE SCIENCE

This is a category of concern about distortions in the allocations of resources for science. One of the most frequent observations made about contemporary science is that research in many areas is no longer possible on individual budgets, or even small institutional budgets, and that large external support is now necessary. Although external support of scientific research is centuries old in several countries, the degree to which such support is obligatory if high-level research is to be continued has changed markedly in this century. Robert Boyle, Antoine Lavoisier, Charles Lyell, and Charles Darwin were all outstanding scientists who were able to support themselves entirely or partly on the basis of their own funds. Now even a Nelson Rockefeller who was a radio astronomer would probably not be eager to undertake the building of a very large array radiotelescope.

• • •

The concerns of fund administrators about scientific research impinge on freedom of inquiry in several indirect ways. . . . If a line of research has no visible practical value, the scientist in the field will probably have fewer possible sources for funds than if he or she can point to a potential valuable technology issuing from that research. If the research is highly unorthodox, it may not receive support even if potential applications are visualizable. Fund administrators traditionally fear controversy, and they fear even more the possibility that the work which they support will bring discredit to the funder (as did the Carnegie Foundation's support in the early decades of this century of the eugenics movement). An administrator of another large private foundation recently offered to show its early archives to an historian, but he said he did not have records on unsuccessful applicants, only on those who received grants. The records of the unsuccessful petitioners might be more interesting.

At the level of decision-making about the construction of the most expensive research installations, such as mammoth high-energy accelerators like the one at Fermi Lab, a worry about distortions in the allocation of resources is a serious one. The important discussions of societal priorities necessary for making such decisions do not present a fundamental limitation on individual freedom, even though in such areas work cannot be done without outside funds. Society obviously does not have an obligation to build a facility costing millions of dollars for every good scientist who wants one. On the other hand, a prosperous society which decided to stop building such facilities would be doing damage of a double nature: it would be inflicting harm on its scientific community and it would be limiting its own curiosity and creativity.

SUBVERSIVE KNOWLEDGE

All the categories of concern about science and technology discussed so far involved side effects; they were based on the physical, ethical, or economic results of individual technologies, the effects of the design of fundamental research in projects involving human beings as subjects, and the economic costs of large fundamental research projects. The concern to be discussed now rests on fundamental knowledge itself.

Some of the best-known cases of interference with science in past centuries have been the results of resistance to fundamental knowledge. In the classic instances the anxiety has had two sources: the new fundamental knowledge was seen as conflicting with the theories of ruling authorities, and it appeared to demote the place of man in nature. The affair of Galileo's censure by the Church is one which can be interpreted in terms of these concerns. The Catholic Church had, undoubtedly without logical necessity, incorporated the basic features of the Ptolemaic system into its body of theological teachings. Furthermore, the rival Copernican theory seemed to demote the place of man by situating his abode outside the center of the Universe.

Historians of science will be quick to point out that the situation was far from being as simple as the foregoing description might seem to indicate. Copernicus dedicated his treatise to a Pope, and his work was not criticized by Rome until many years after his death; Protestant leaders such as Melanchthon and Calvin protested at first more vociferously than the Catholic leaders; the Copernican system was actually not heliocentric but heliostatic; the Catholic Church might not have taken the position it did were it not under the pressures of the Reformation and Counterreformation.

All these qualifications are valuable, but the fact still remains that on a general but nonetheless very significant level the Copernican system as espoused by Galileo was perceived as both contrary to theological teachings and demeaning to the place of man. It was a form of pure knowledge that was seen as a threat in itself. Debates over Darwinism in the last part of the nineteenth century also contained these two elements: conflict with at least some interpretations of religions, and an apparent denigration of the uniqueness of man.

We often assume that such conflicts are now elements of the past, that a mature world which attributes such an important place to science has surely outgrown adolescent anxieties of this type about science. And, indeed, we have improved very much in this regard. The concerns are still there, however, and they have appeared in several new forms. Furthermore, some of these concerns are not trivial.

Some of the popular resistance to studies in the field of ethology and primatology can be related to concerns about the diminution of the uniqueness of man, the narrowing of the distance between humans and the rest of the animal world. The possibility of increasingly successful explanations of human behavior in terms of animal behavior often evokes resistance among intellectuals who would usually consider themselves far from being antiscience. One does not have to accept the vulgarized interpretations of ethology of the type of Robert Ardrey or Desmond Morris to agree that at least part of the resistance here is the ancient one of concern for man's place in nature.

Another example of current concern about the uniqueness of humans is that expressed by the biophysicist Robert Sinsheimer. . . .

Should we attempt to contact presumed "extraterrestrial intelligences"? I wonder if the authors of such experiments have ever considered the impact upon the human spirit if it should develop that there are other forms of life, to whom we are, for instance, as the chimpanzee is to us. Once it were realized someone already knew the answers to our questions, it seems to me, the impact upon science itself would be especially devastating. We know from our own history the shattering impact more advanced civilizations have upon the less advanced. In my view the human race has to make it on its own, for our own self-respect.[3]

This objection to possible research cannot be described, it seems to me, as anything else than another variation of anxiety about man's place in nature of the type often seen in past centuries, though not in a religious context.

On this topic of resistance to fundamental knowledge in itself my position is a simple one, and, I would maintain, of great importance to our intellectual freedom. That position is: "Critical discussion, yes! Regulation, no!"

In fairness to contemporary commentators such as Sinsheimer, who are responsible and helpful critics, I should add that many of them are not suggesting censorship or a ban on research in these areas, but a deep questioning of the amount of national resources that should be invested in certain research. But to ask whether millions of dollars should be directed toward possible contact with another civilization is to transform the question from one of limits to fundamental inquiry to one of allocation of resources, which is the separate category "expensive science."

Another form of concern about fundamental science is the one that states "anything that *can* be done, *will* be done," and therefore, the critics say, it is not justifiable to draw a line between science and technology when one is attempting to discuss the question of limits to inquiry. These commentators continue that since some sorts of knowledge will "inevitably" lead to technology which will "inevitably" be used (even though we all might agree that the specified use is not desirable) we ought to impose limits on the original inquiry. Holders of this viewpoint might even classify certain types of knowledge as "forbidden" in principle.

Although I believe that this form of argument is incorrect as a general position, unnecessarily condemning our civilization to technological determinism, I would like to present it in the strongest form before criticizing it. We will all agree, I think, that fundamental physical research in the first four decades of this century provided the knowledge necessary for the construction of nuclear weapons; most of us would agree that the major political powers in the world now possess these weapons in sufficient numbers that if all were exploded in the atmosphere either our civilization would be destroyed or it would be so altered that many of us would not be eager to survive in whatever remained. If that holocaust should occur, the following argument would ring hollow in the ears of anyone able to hear it: "Science itself has no moral responsibility for what happened, since it was not necessary that nuclear weapons be constructed or used, even though the knowledge necessary for these events was produced by science."

Logically correct though the argument may be, we are all familiar with the failure of logic to handle adequately the most extreme human dilemmas. The simple fact would be that without the development of nuclear physics this ultimate disaster would not have occurred.

But on the basis of this realization should we try to regulate fundamental research in the future in order to avoid such events? I believe that we would not know how to do so even if we wished, and that in the effort we would cause immense damage to our existing values as well as deprive ourselves of many benefits, both material and intellectual. Frightening as our present situation is, it may just force us to be more responsible than we have ever before been.

•   •   •

Taken literally, the "inevitable technology" argument is clearly false. Examples can be given of available technologies which have never been employed on a wide scale. As Harvey Brooks has reminded us, "Artificial insemination among humans is a good example of a technology which, though still in limited use, has never 'taken off.' People prefer the conventional method, and probably always will, when it works."[4]

The alternative of controlling fundamental research instead of technology is illusory, because it assumes the impossible: the foreseeing of the results of fundamental inquiry. Controlling technology is extremely difficult, but it is not impossible.

ACCIDENTS IN SCIENCE

The controversy over recombinant DNA is one which needs to be analyzed on several different levels. The first level is the one which addresses the explicit and most common concern expressed by people who have objected to this research, namely that as a result of an accident in fundamental research the public safety will be threatened. This concern is the one which I have classified as a separate category, "accident in science." The second level is one which concerns those largely unspoken, but nonetheless real concerns which relate to other categories. I will treat them separately.

On the first level, it is important to notice that the opponents of recombinant DNA research in Cambridge, Massachusetts, were not (at least originally) objecting principally to what could be intentionally produced by a successful recombinant DNA technology, but to the possibility during fundamental research of the accidental production of a pathogenic organism immune to normal antibiotics. It is true that one *could* express concerns of the type of category I ("technology") about recombinant DNA work (e.g., its possible use for biological warfare, or an objection to what might intentionally be done to alter the life of plants, animals, or people) but this type of resistance has so far not been the major one. The Cambridge City Council, for example, explicitly excluded these latter concerns from its considerations.

The topic of accidents in research is not a new one; indeed, accidents of various types, ranging enormously in the scale of potential damage, have long been evident. Explosions occur even in undergraduate chemistry laboratories, and electrocution is often a possibility. Even some common chemical elements,

such as mercury or sodium, must be handled with care, and the dangers increase with volatile and explosive chemical compounds, radioactive materials and high-energy experiments. The transportation, distribution, and use of the most hazardous of these materials are already under controls of various types. In biology, unwanted organisms may escape to cause subsequent damage; the release of the gypsy moth in New England many decades ago continues to disturb us today.

•   •   •

The second level of analysis which needs to be applied to recombinant DNA research goes far beyond the issue of public safety. As the controversy has progressed, the objections to this type of research have broadened beyond the original issue to a whole series of concerns that belong outside the category "accidents in science." Jeremy Rifkin has said, "The central issue is the mystery of life itself. It is now only a matter of time until scientists will be able to create new strains of plants, even alter human life." Rifkin's concern is a combination of several types: "destructive technology," "slippery slope technology," and probably a deep fear of science itself, one with non-rational roots. Ethan Singer has commented that DNA research "will eventually tinker with the gene pool of humanity. So the public, like the subject of any experiment, must give its informed consent—but willingly, not by coercion." This statement is a mixture of concerns about "inevitable technology" and "human subjects research." Roger Noll has added his view that since the federal government sponsors much of the research, "I suppose the question, 'Is this worth buying?' is going to be the real issue." This opinion represents a concern for "expensive research," but it is not clear whether Mr. Noll considered it science or technology, and it is furthermore not clear whether the financial concern is a cover for other worries.[5]

It is this mixture of concerns of various categories that made the recombinant DNA case so inflammatory. Any one of the concerns, by itself, could probably be resolved. Some of the anxieties are legitimate, although still not defined (e.g., public safety, which falls under my category "accidents in science"), while others are highly dubious or unacceptable to the scientific community (e.g., concern for the "mystery of life,'' which falls under my category ''subversive knowledge'').

An important step in trying to deal with the concerns expressed about recombinant DNA is the attempt to sort out and evaluate them one by one. This step cannot be accomplished without first dividing ''concerns about science'' from ''concerns about technology,'' the two most general categories. Part of the difficulty of discussing recombinant DNA research is the interweaving of these concerns, which in large part results from the fact that fundamental research in recombinant DNA is based on a novel ''technique''—the introduction into a bacterial cell of a segment of foreign DNA by means of a now familiar multistep procedure—and therefore seems to be technology. Yet the development and use of novel techniques for conducting fundamental research is an old feature in the history of science (e.g., mass spectrometry in chemistry), and in no way defines the work as technology. It is true that the distinction is more complex with recombinant DNA than is usually the case, because the technique which is important to the fundamental research is also, apparently, the main method by which technology will probably proceed; nonetheless, the difference between exploring the nature of living organisms and intentionally trying to produce ones with specific socially useful characteristics is still important.

The separation of recombinant DNA fundamental research from recombinant DNA technology may be somewhat difficult to perform, but it is my opinion that the distinction should be made wherever possible. The policy implications are considerable. In the case of science, the emphasis should be upon keeping the work as free from controls as is consonant with public safety; in the case of technology, the emphasis should be upon the question of whether the application of the science serves a social need. The greater the risk of possible damage, the greater the social need should be before the application is developed and employed in society.

If one concentrates on fundamental research itself, the only concern about recombinant DNA which commands our attention persuasively is that of accidents which might endanger the public. Adequate protection against such accidents now seems feasible, but whatever the outcome of decisions in this area, it seems rather clear that the recombinant DNA case is not typical of many other areas of fundamental research. It would be a great mistake if recombinant DNA were taken as a paradigm case for regulating fundamental research. There have been relatively few actual cases in the recent history of science in which the primary concern expressed by knowledgeable critics was not about an application of science, nor financial, nor an ethical issue in biomedical research, but instead a worry that during the process of fundamental research an accident would result in social damage. The closest parallel to the recombinant DNA case is probably concern about accidents in nuclear research (e.g., the controversy over the Triga reactor at Columbia University), not to be confused with accidents in nuclear power installations (a ''destructive technology'' fear). The category ''accidents in science'' will probably broaden in coming years, but it is difficult to conceive that it would include more than a small portion of all fundamental research.

The recombinant DNA controversy is significant in two other senses: (1) the authentic issues it raises about who should bear the responsibility of devising and enforcing regulations on research, and (2) the possibility that underneath the specific concerns expressed by the public on recombinant DNA lurk much more significant and deeper irrational fears of science. These two issues are extremely difficult ones to resolve (more will be said on the first in the Conclusions), but little progress can be made in handling them unless distinctions have been made about various types of concerns about research, as I have been attempting to do here.

PREJUDICIAL SCIENCE

A type of concern which is separable from those discussed so far is that scientists will present evidence or arguments that exacerbate racial, ethnic, sexual or class prejudices and which might be used in the service of a particular ideology. The old controversies over eugenics and the newer ones over intelligence tests and race can be related to this category, as can, to a certain extent, the current one over sociobiology.

There are governments today which ban such research on principle. The current edition of the East German encyclopedia *Meyers Neues Lexikon* contains in its article on ''Race theory'' *(Rassentheorie)* a condemnation of the subject and then the following statement:

Race theory is still today openly propagandized in the imperialistic countries and especially in West Germany. In the German Democratic Republic the spreading of this doctrine is constitutionally prohibited.[6]

Research on intelligence and race would not be supported in East Germany. Neither is freedom of speech.

So far as formal regulation is concerned, my position on this category of concern is the same as on "knowledge itself": Critical discussion, yes! Regulation, no! I would not be candid, however, if I did not admit that I consider this category of concern to be one in which a pure separation of facts and values will probably never be possible, and may not even be desirable. If I were at present an executive of a research foundation and I were asked to vote on funding a program for projects on race and intelligence, I would vote negatively. I would refer to the fact that current definitions of "intelligence" and "race" are inadequate for the task, that the problem is not one that seems currently solvable, and that money could be used to greater advantage in other areas. And yet I know, and would acknowledge, that my negative opinion on the matter was influenced by my own values, my belief that the more potentially dangerous to society the results of research might be, the more rigorous one should insist that the methodology for that research must be.

· · ·

WAYS OF KNOWING

A final type of concern about science stems not so much from any piece of information that science might produce, nor from any technology that might result from it, but from a critique of its mode of cognition. There are many people who maintain that science is only one of several avenues to knowledge, and these people often resist the tendency of science to expand its claims. The critique of science which these people advance attacks the epistemological bases of science on the ground that it is, at best, so specialized that it misses the most significant modes of reality, and, at worst, fundamentally alienating to the human spirit. The supporters of this view, who vary greatly in their sophistication, often call for supplementing the scientific approach with "other ways of knowing."

A contemporary example of such a critic is Theodore Roszak, who observed in his popular *Where the Wasteland Ends* that "Science is not, in my view, merely *another* subject for discussion, it is *the* subject." He spoke of the "intimate link between the search for epistemological objectivity and the psychology of alienation: that is, to idolatrous consciousness." "It is no mere coincidence," he continued,

"that this devouring sense of alienation from nature and one's fellow man—and from one's own essential self—becomes the endemic anguish of advanced industrial societies."[7]

One should not assume that all proponents of "other ways of knowing" come from outside the scientific community. The distinguished astrophysicist and mathematician Arthur Eddington surprised and irritated some of his scientific colleagues by writing in the late nineteen-twenties and early thirties popular books about science (which were adopted in many universities) in which he spoke of a world of "intimate knowledge" not accessible by scientific methods. Eddington wrote that when we make use of the "eye of the soul" as an avenue of cognition we should dispel the feeling that "we are doing something irrational and disobeying the leading of truth which as scientists we are pledged to serve."[8]

Such viewpoints have always existed in our history and undoubtedly always will. Whether one finds them valuable or not is a deeply personal characteristic. The views, fears, and premonitions of Goethe and Blake are only prominent examples of the many that could be associated with this category.

There is at least one area where this category of concern about science has current practical significance and where the term "regulation" may arise in at least some people's minds. In California and elsewhere, proponents of "creationism" criticizing Darwinian evolution have had some political success in their efforts to revise school textbooks by making the argument that since religious interpretations of the universe and scientific interpretations are based on strikingly different and even incommensurable ways of knowing, the contrasting interpretations should be given equal time. The creationists say that since neither they nor the evolutionists can disprove the views of the other side, both sides should be represented in high school and elementary science textbooks. This specious argument has an appeal to some listeners because of its superficial resemblance to the principle of giving all sides in a true debate opportunity for expressing their opinions.[9]

It is conceivable that this threat to science could become a serious one; the controversies over the MACOS (Man: A Course of Study) project and the resulting attempts to restrict [the National Science Foundation's] autonomy are recent events in which this type of concern played an important role.[10] At the present moment, however, the strength of "alternative modes of cognition" may be receding with the passing of the peak of interest in mysticism and the occult in the late sixties or early seventies. At any rate, a form of special regulation that goes beyond the well-established separation of church and state does not seem appropriate. On the whole, school boards are more sophisticated than they were in the days of the Scopes trial, and one can only hope that the efforts to oppose religious, romantic, or mystical viewpoints to those of science will not receive significant official support.

· · ·

CONCLUSIONS

The first major conclusion which issues from the analysis presented in this article is that there exists a core of categories of concerns about research where regulation should still not be permitted at all. All of them fall under the heading science, and not technology, but not all categories under science are in the core. This core consists of concerns I have labeled "subversive knowledge," "inevitable technology," "prejudicial science," and "ways of knowing." The most inviolable category of all is "subversive knowledge," for this is the area where the truly fundamental threats to science have emerged in past centuries, and where there is always the possibility of new dangers.

In the other core categories a democratic and healthy society should be able to avoid controls, but I will admit that I can imagine extreme and unlikely situations in which a temporary control of "inevitable technology" might be conceivable (a bit of fundamental knowledge which led easily to a serious and uncontrollable destructive application), and perhaps even "prejudicial science" (a bit of fundamental knowledge that would exacerbate social conflict in a temporary and extremely destructive fashion), but our society is presently far from being in such situations. (The circumstances would have to be roughly equivalent to the crying of "fire" in a crowded theater; for a hypothetical example, see reference 11). And in the category "ways of knowing" we might possibly need additional regulation in extremis to *protect* science, not limit it (which is what the principle of separation of church and state already does).

I am not willing, however, to admit that controls of any kind are justified on "subversive knowledge" under circumstances not covered by one of the other categories. It is my opinion, furthermore, that in the three other categories just mentioned ("inevitable technology," "prejudicial science," and "ways of knowing") there is no justification at the present time for regulation of research, and also that the likelihood of the emergence of circumstances which would make such regulation advisable is remote. These four categories ([including] "subversive knowledge") form the inner core where regulation should be stoutly resisted.

The second major conclusion proceeding from this classification and analysis is that outside the inner core we have a group of categories ("destructive technology," "slipper slope technology," "economically exploitative technology," "human subjects research," "expensive science," "accidents in science") in which controls are not only conceivable and justified, but where regulations of one sort or another are already in effect. The most important debate within these categories of concerns is not about academic freedom in principle, but about a compromise between the effort to avoid destructive social effects, on the one hand, and the effort to promote scientific and technical creativity and new advances in human welfare, on the other.

The third conclusion which I would draw from this analysis is that even within those categories of concerns where controls are clearly justified, there exists a danger that creativity will be regulated to death by bureaucracies with momentums of their own. Just as we are wary of the "slippery slope" in biomedical ethics, so also should we resist slipping inadvertently into increasing controls over fundamental science, since such controls can easily lead to abuses. Tremendous damage can be caused by the regulators, while the lack of regulation over some types of research would be quite dangerous to society.

NOTES

1. I would like to express my appreciation to the Rockefeller Foundation for a Humanities Fellowship for 1976–1977, during which time I did research on the relationship of science and sociopolitical values, including research for this article. I would also like to thank colleagues at the Program on Science and International Affairs, Harvard University, the members of the MIT seminar on "Limits to Inquiry," and, especially, Harvey Brooks and David Z. Robinson.

2. Hans Jonas, "Freedom of Scientific Inquiry and the Public Interest," *Hastings Center Report* (August 1976): 16.

3. Robert Sinsheimer, "Comments," *Hastings Center Report* (August 1976): 18.

4. Letter to the author from Harvey Brooks (April 12, 1977).

5. All quotations in this paragraph are from Cheryl M. Fields, "Who Should Control Recombinant DNA?" *The Chronicle of Higher Education*, XIV, No. 4 (March 21, 1977): 1, 4–5.

6. "Rassentheorie," *Meyers Neues Lexikon,* VI (Leipzig, 1963), pp. 817–818.

7. Theodore Roszak, *Where the Wasteland Ends: Politics and Transcendence in Postindustrial Society* (Garden City, N.Y.: Doubleday, 1972), pp. *xxiv,* 168.

8. A. S. Eddington, *Science and the Unseen World* (New York: Macmillan, 1929), p. 49.

9. Dorothy Nelkin, "The Science-Textbook Controversies," *Scientific American,* 234 (April 1976): 33–39. Also see her *Science Textbook Controversies* (Cambridge, Mass.: MIT Press, 1977).

10. "NSF: Congress Takes Hard Look at Behavioral Science Course," *Science,* 188 (May 2, 1977): 426–428.

11. For people who discount the possibility of such a situation, let me portray the following hypothetical scenario. Imagine that you are a scientist in Nazi Germany and that you have just discovered Tay-Sachs disease, an abnormality based on a genetic defect which is more common among Jews than other population groups. Is it not possible that you would try to keep this bit of knowledge away from the eyes of Hitler and National Socialist bureaucrats, and that you might suggest to your trusted colleagues that they do the same?

SUGGESTED READINGS FOR CHAPTER 12

RESEARCH INVOLVING ANIMALS

Clark, Stephen R. L. *The Moral Status of Animals.* New York: Oxford University Press, 1977.

Feinberg, Joel. "The Rights of Animals and Unborn Generations." In Blackstone, William T., ed. *Philosophy and the Environmental Crisis.* Athens: University of Georgia Press, 1974, p. 43.

French, Richard D. "Animal Experimentation: Historical Aspects." In Reich, Warren T., ed. *Encyclopedia of Bioethics.* New York: Free Press, 1978. Vol. 1, pp. 75–79.

———. *Antivivisection and Medical Science in Victorian Society.* Princeton: Princeton University Press, 1975.

Frey, R. G. *Interests and Rights: The Case Against Animals.* Oxford: Clarendon Press, 1980.

Lane-Petter, W. "The Ethics of Animal Experimentation." *Journal of Medical Ethics* 2 (September 1976), 118–126.

Morris, Richard Knowles, and Fox, Michael W. *On the Fifth Day: Animal Rights and Human Ethics.* Washington, D.C.: Acropolis Press, 1978.

Regan, Tom, and Singer, Peter, eds. *Animal Rights and Human Obligations.* Englewood Cliffs, N.J.: Prentice-Hall, 1976.

Rowan, Andrew N. "Laboratory Animals and Alternatives in the 80's." *International Journal for the Study of Animal Problems* 1 (May/June 1980), 162–169.

Ryder, Richard D. "Experiments on Animals." In Godlovitch, Stanley, *et al.,* eds. *Animals, Men, and Morals.* New York: Taplinger, 1972.

———. *Victims of Science: The Use of Animals in Research.* London: Davis-Poynter, 1975.

Singer, Peter. *Animal Liberation.* New York: Random House, New York Review of Books, 1975.

———. "Animals and the Value of Life." In Regan, Tom, ed. *Matters of Life and Death: New Introductory Essays in Moral Philosophy.* New York: Random House, 1980, pp. 218–259.

RESEARCH AT THE MOLECULAR LEVEL

"Biotechnology and the Law: Recombinant DNA and the Control of Scientific Research." *Southern California Law Review* 51 (September 1978), 969–1573. Special issue.

Grobstein, Clifford. *A Double Image of the Double Helix: The*

Recombinant-DNA Debate. San Francisco: W. H. Freeman, 1979.

Jackson, David A., and Stich, Stephen P., eds. *The Recombinant DNA Debate.* Englewood Cliffs, N.J.: Prentice-Hall, 1979.

Lappé, Marc, and Morrison, Robert S., eds. "Ethical and Scientific Issues Posed by Human Uses of Molecular Genetics." *Annals of the New York Academy of Sciences* 265 (1976), 1–208.

"Recombinant DNA and Technology Assessment." *Georgia Law Review* 11 (Summer 1977), 785–878. Special issue.

Research with Recombinant DNA: An Academy Forum, March 7–9, 1977. Washington, D.C.: National Academy of Sciences, 1977.

Richards, John, ed. *Recombinant DNA: Science, Ethics, and Politics.* New York: Academic Press, 1978.

U.S., National Institutes of Health. *Recombinant DNA Research: Documents Relating to "NIH Guidelines for Research Involving Recombinant DNA Molecules."* Multiple volumes. Washington, D.C.: U.S. Government Printing Office, August 1976–

SCIENTIFIC INQUIRY AND PUBLIC POLICY

Davidson, Michael D. "First Amendment Protection for Biomedical Research." *Arizona Law Review* 19 (1977), 893–918.

Ferguson, James R. "Scientific Inquiry and the First Amendment." *Cornell Law Review* 64 (April 1979), 639–665.

Fudenberg, H. Hugh, and Melnick, Vijaya, eds. *Biomedical Scientists and Public Policy.* New York: Plenum Press, 1978.

Gibson, William C. "The Costs of *Not* Doing Medical Research." *Journal of the American Medical Association* 244 (October 17, 1980), 1817–1819.

Green, Harold P. "The Boundaries of Scientific Freedom." *Newsletter on Science, Technology, and Human Values* 20 (June 1977), 17–21.

Holton, Gerald, ed. "Limits of Scientific Inquiry." *Daedalus* 107 (Spring 1978), 1–234. Special issue.

Lakoff, Sanford A. "Moral Responsibility and the 'Galilean Imperative.' " *Ethics* 91 (October 1980), 100–116.

Robertson, John A. "The Scientist's Right to Research: A Constitutional Analysis." *Southern California Law Review* 51 (September 1978), 1203–1279.

Stetten, DeWitt. "Freedom of Enquiry." *Genetics* 81 (November 1975), 415–425.

Thomas, Lewis. "The Hazards of Science." *New England Journal of Medicine* 296 (February 10, 1977), 324–328.

BIBLIOGRAPHY

Goldstein, Doris Mueller. *Bioethics: A Guide to Information Sources.* Detroit: Gale Research Company, 1982. See under "Genetic Intervention."

Lineback, Richard H., ed. *Philosopher's Index.* Vols. 1– . Bowling Green, Ohio: Bowling Green State University, Philosophy Documentation Center. Issued quarterly. See under "Animals," "Genetic Engineering," "Pain," "Research," and "Science."

Walters, LeRoy, ed. *Bibliography of Bioethics.* Vols. 1– . New York: Free Press. Issued annually. See under "Biomedical Research," "Biomedical Technologies," "Genetic Intervention," and "Recombinant DNA Research." (The information contained in the annual *Bibliography of Bioethics* can also be retrieved from BIOETHICSLINE, an online data base of the National Library of Medicine.)

About the Authors

GEORGE J. ANNAS teaches law and medicine in the Department of Socio-Medical Sciences and Community Medicine at the Boston University School of Medicine. He is author of *The Rights of Hospital Patients,* coauthor of *Informed Consent to Human Experimentation,* and coeditor of *Genetics and the Law.* He also writes a regular column on ''Law and the Life Sciences'' for the *Hastings Center Report.*

MICHAEL S. BARAM directs the Program in Law and Technology at Boston University Law School and practices law with the firm of Bracker and Baram. He has published *Alternatives to Regulation for Managing Risks to Health, Safety, and the Environment* and *Environmental Law and the Siting of Facilities.* His articles have focused on regulatory reform, risk management, and other issues related to health, safety, and the environment.

DAN E. BEAUCHAMP teaches in the Department of Health Administration, School of Public Health, and in the Department of Community Medicine and Hospital Administration, School of Medicine, both at the University of North Carolina. He has written numerous articles on public health policy.

TOM L. BEAUCHAMP teaches in the Department of Philosophy and at the Kennedy Institute of Ethics, Georgetown University. He is author of *Philosophical Ethics* and coauthor of *Hume and the Problem of Causation* and *Principles of Biomedical Ethics.* He previously served as consulting philosopher in ethics for the National Commission for the Protection of Human Subjects of Biomedical and Behavioral Research.

SISSELA BOK teaches ethics at Harvard Medical School. She is author of *Lying: Moral Choice in Public and Private Life* and coauthor of *The Teaching of Ethics in Higher Education.* From 1978 to 1980 she was a member of the Ethics Advisory Board to the Secretary of Health, Education and Welfare. She has written many articles on biomedical ethics.

CHRISTOPHER BOORSE teaches in the Department of Philosophy at the University of Delaware. He publishes primarily in the philosophy of language and the philosophy of science. His article in this volume is one of a series he has written on the concepts of health and disease.

ALAN BOWD teaches in the School of Education at the Riverina College of Advanced Education, Wagga Wagga, New South Wales, Australia. He has written several articles concerning the ethical implications of psychological research with animals.

DAN W. BROCK teaches in the Department of Philosophy at Brown University. He has written several articles in both general ethics and biomedical ethics. From 1981 to 1982 he served as staff philosopher to the President's Commission for the Study of Ethical Problems in Medicine and Biomedical and Behavioral Research.

BARUCH BRODY teaches in the Department of Philosophy at Rice University in Houston, Texas. He is author of *Abortion and the Sanctity of Human Life: A Philosophical View, A Beginning Philosophy,* and *Identity and Essence.* He is also coeditor of *Mental Illness: Law and Public Policy.*

DANIEL CALLAHAN is a philosopher and the Director of the Hastings Center, Hastings-on-Hudson, New York. He is author of *Abortion: Law, Choice and Morality, Ethics and Population Limitation,* and *The Tyranny of Survival: On a Science of Technological Limits.*

ALEXANDER M. CAPRON teaches at the University of Pennsylvania Law School. He is coauthor of *Catastrophic Disease: Who Decides What?* and *Experimentation with Human Beings* and author of numerous articles on law and the life sciences. He has served as Executive Director of the President's Commission for the Study of Ethical Problems in Medicine and Biomedical and Behavioral Research.

THOMAS C. CHALMERS is President of Mount Sinai Medical Center and Dean and Professor of Medicine at the City University of New York. He has written several articles on ethical and statistical problems posed by clinical trials. He has also served on review committees and advisory boards for the National Cancer Institute, the National Heart, Lung, and Blood Institute, and other governmental and professional bodies.

JAMES F. CHILDRESS teaches in the Department of Religious Studies at the University of Virginia. He is author of *Civil Disobedience and Political Obligation* and *Priorities in Biomedical Ethics.* He is coauthor of *Principles of Biomedical Ethics.*

PAUL CHODOFF is a physician who teaches in the Department of Psychiatry at George Washington University School of Medicine. He is consultant to several Federal psychiatric hospitals in the District of Columbia.

CHARLES M. CULVER is a physician and clinical psychologist who teaches in the Department of Psychiatry at Dartmouth Medical School. He is coauthor of *Philosophy in Medicine* and has published extensively on problems in biomedical ethics, with special reference to the problem of paternalism.

WILLIAM J. CURRAN is the Francis Glessner Lee Professor of Legal Medicine at the Harvard University School of Public Health. He is coauthor of *Law, Medicine and Forensic Science* and coeditor of *Ethics in Medicine: Historical Perspectives and Contemporary Concerns.* He also writes regular columns on law and health affairs for the *New England Journal of Medicine* and the *American Journal of Public Health.* Professor Curran is a member of the Kennedy Interfaculty Program on Medical Ethics at Harvard.

NORMAN DANIELS teaches in the Department of Philosophy at Tufts University in Boston. He has written several essays on problems of justice and medical ethics. He is author of *Thomas Reid's Inquiry: The Geometry of Visibles and the Case for Realism* and editor of *Reading Rawls.*

PHILIP E. DEVINE teaches in the Department of Philosophy at Rensselaer Polytechnic Institute in Troy, New York. He is author of *The Ethics of Homicide.*

RONALD J. DIAMOND teaches in the Department of Psychiatry at the University of Wisconsin, Madison. He is Medical Director of the Mobile Community Treatment Program of Dane County Mental Health Center.

LEON EISENBERG is the Maude and Lillian Presley Professor of Psychiatry at Harvard Medical School and holds a clinical appointment at the Children's Hospital Medical Center in Boston. He has written many articles on the ethics of both psychiatry and biomedical research.

H. TRISTRAM ENGLEHARDT, JR. is Rosemary Kennedy Professor of the Philosophy of Medicine at the Kennedy Institute of Ethics, Georgetown University. He is a physician and philosopher who teaches in the Department of Philosophy and the Department of Community and Family Medicine at Georgetown. He is author of *Mind-Body: A Categorical Relation,* coeditor of the Philosophy and Medicine monograph series, and associate editor of the *Journal of Medicine and Philosophy.*

RUTH R. FADEN teaches health services administration, behavioral sciences, and population dynamics in the School of Hygiene and Public Health, and psychology in the Graduate School at The Johns Hopkins University. She is also a Senior Research Scholar at the Kennedy Institute of Ethics, Georgetown University. She is coeditor of *Ethical Issues in Social Science Research.* Professor Faden has published numerous articles on biomedical ethics and has served as consultant to several federal agencies on problems in health care.

RASHI FEIN is Professor of the Economics of Medicine and teaches in the Department of Social Medicine and Health Policy at the Harvard Medical School. He is author of several books, including *The Economics of Mental Illness.* He has published essays on national health insurance, the cost of health care, and equity in the allocation of health-care services.

JOEL FEINBERG teaches in the Department of Philosophy at the University of Arizona. He is author of *Doing and Deserving: Essays in the Theory of Responsibility, Social Philosophy,* and *Rights, Justice, and the Bounds of Liberty.* He is editor of *The Problem of Abortion,* as well as several other volumes in applied philosophy.

JOSEPH FLETCHER is Visiting Professor of Medical Ethics at the University of Virginia School of Medicine. He is author of *Morals and Medicine, Situation Ethics, The Ethics of Genetic Control,* and *Humanhood: Essays in Biomedical Ethics.*

CHARLES FRIED teaches at Harvard Law School. He is author of *An Anatomy of Values: Problems of Personal and Social Choice, Medical Experimentation: Personal Integrity and Social Policy,* and *Right and Wrong.*

VICTOR R. FUCHS teaches economics at Stanford University and is Research Associate at the National Bureau of Economic Research in Stanford, California. He is author of several books, including *Who Shall Live? Health, Economics and Social Choice,* and has also edited several works on the economic aspects of health care.

WILLARD GAYLIN is President of the Hastings Center and a practicing psychiatrist. He is author of *Caring* and *Feelings: Our Vital Signs* and is coauthor of *Doing Good: The Limits of Benevolence.*

BERNARD GERT teaches in the Department of Philosophy at Dartmouth College. He is author of *The Moral Rules,* coauthor of *Philosophy in Medicine,* and editor of Thomas Hobbes' *Man and Citizen.*

LOREN R. GRAHAM teaches the history of science at Massachusetts Institute of Technology in Cambridge, Massachusetts. He is the author of *The Soviet Academy of Sciences and the Communist Party, 1927–1932.* He has also published several articles on the history of science and ethics.

HAROLD P. GREEN teaches at the National Law Center, George Washington University. He is also a partner in the law firm of

Fried, Frank, Harris, Shriver and Kampelman in Washington. He has written a number of essays on the legal and public-policy aspects of science and technology.

ALEXANDER Z. GUIORA is a psychiatrist who teaches in the Department of Psychiatry and Psychology at the University of Michigan. He is coauthor of *Perspectives in Clinical Psychology.*

SALLY GUTTMACHER teaches in the Division of Sociomedical Sciences at the Columbia University School of Public Health. She has published several articles on ethics and health policy.

ANDRÉ E. HELLEGERS (d. 1979) was founder and first Director of the Kennedy Institute of Ethics at Georgetown University. His medical specialty was obstetrics and gynecology, and his primary research interest was fetal physiology. Dr. Hellegers wrote numerous essays on ethical problems raised by advances in biology and medicine.

CHRISTINA HOFF teaches in the Department of Philosophy at Clark University in Massachusetts. Her article in this volume is one of several she has written on ethical considerations in the use of animals for research.

TIMOTHY HOWELL is a resident in psychiatry at the University of Wisconsin Hospital and Clinics in Madison. His primary research interests are ethical and philosophical issues in psychiatry and depression and the biochemistry of depression in patients with spinal-cord injuries.

FRANZ J. INGELFINGER (d. 1980) was editor of the *New England Journal of Medicine* from 1967 to 1977. He also taught in the Department of Medicine at Boston University Medical School. In his capacity as editor, Dr. Ingelfinger frequently wrote editorials on issues in biomedical ethics.

HANS JONAS is Professor Emeritus of Philosophy at the New School for Social Research in New York City. He publishes on topics in ancient philosophy, metaphysics, and ethics. He is author of *Gnostic Religion, The Phenomenon of Life: Toward a Philosophical Biology,* and *Philosophical Essays: From Ancient Creed to Technological Man.*

YALE KAMISAR teaches at the University of Michigan Law School. He is author of *Police Interrogation and Confessions: Essays in Law and Policy* and coauthor of *Criminal Justice in Our Time, Constitutional Law: Cases, Comments, and Questions,* and *Modern Criminal Procedure: Cases and Commentaries.*

LEON KASS, a physician and biochemist, is Henry R. Luce Professor in the College at the University of Chicago. He has published essays on concepts of health and disease, the role of the physician, and the social impact of new biomedical technologies.

JAY KATZ is a psychiatrist and teaches law and psychiatry at Yale University Law School. He is coauthor of *Experimentation with Human Beings, Catastrophic Diseases: Who Decides What?,* and *Psychoanalysis, Psychiatry and Law.*

JOHN LORBER is a physician who teaches in the Department of Pediatrics at Sheffield University in England. He has written several articles concerning medical and ethical issues in the treatment of handicapped newborn infants

RICHARD A. McCORMICK is Rose F. Kennedy Professor of Christian Ethics at the Kennedy Institute of Ethics, Georgetown

University. He is author of *How Brave a New World?* and *Notes on Moral Theology: 1965–1980* and coeditor of *Doing Evil to Achieve Good.*

JOSEPH MARGOLIS teaches in the Department of Philosophy at Temple University in Philadelphia. He is author of *Art and Philosophy, Negativities: The Limits of Life,* and *Persons and Minds: The Prospects of Nonreductive Materialism.*

HERBERT MORRIS teaches law and philosophy in the Law School of the University of California at Los Angeles. He is author of *On Guilt and Innocence: Essays in Legal Philosophy and Moral Psychology* and editor of *Freedom and Responsibility: Readings in Philosophy and Law.*

ROLAND PUCCETTI teaches in the Department of Philosophy at Dalhousie University in Halifax, Nova Scotia. He is author of a philosophical work entitled *Persons: A Study of Possible Moral Agents in the Universe.* He has also written two novels, *The Trial of John and Henry Norton* and *The Death of the Führer.*

JAMES RACHELS teaches in the Department of Philosophy at the University of Alabama in Birmingham. He is editor of *Moral Problems and Understanding Moral Philosophy* and coeditor of *Philosophical Issues: A Contemporary Introduction.* He is author of numerous essays in applied ethics.

PAUL RAMSEY is Harrington Spear Paine Professor of Religion at Princeton University. His books on bioethics are *Fabricated Man: The Ethics of Genetic Control, Ethics at the Edges of Life: Medical and Legal Intersections, The Ethics of Fetal Research,* and *The Patient as Person.* He has also written extensively on ethics and the problem of war.

PETER SINGER teaches in the Department of Philosophy at Monash University in Clayton, Victoria, Australia. He is author of *Democracy and Disobedience, Animal Liberation,* and *Practical Ethics.*

ROBERT L. SINSHEIMER is Professor of Biology and Chancellor at the University of California at Santa Cruz. He has been a prominent figure in the public discussion of recombinant DNA research. He has published several articles on the prospects for human genetic engineering.

WILLIAM B. STASON is a physician who is a member of the Center for the Analysis of Health Practices, Harvard School of Public Health. He is coauthor of *Hypertension: A Policy Perspective* and of several essays on the role of cost-effectiveness analysis in the formulation of health policy.

STEPHEN P. STICH teaches in the Department of Philosophy at the University of Maryland in College Park. He is editor of *Innate Ideas* and coeditor of *The Recombinant DNA Debate.*

THOMAS S. SZASZ is a physician and Professor of Psychiatry at the Upstate Medical Center in Syracuse, New York. He is the author of a number of books that examine contemporary psychiatric practice, including *The Myth of Mental Illness, The Ethics of Psychoanalysis, Ideology and Insanity, The Manufacture of Madness,* and *Law, Liberty, and Psychiatry.*

JUDITH JARVIS THOMSON teaches in the Department of Philosophy at the Massachusetts Institute of Technology. She is author of the book *Acts and Events* and has published several articles on bioethics, including "Killing, Letting Die, and the Trolley Problem," and "Rights and Deaths."

ROBERT M. VEATCH is Professor Medical Ethics at the Kennedy Institute of Ethics, Georgetown University. He is author of *Case Studies in Medical Ethics, Death, Dying and the Biological Revolution, A Theory of Medical Ethics,* and *Value-Freedom in Science and Technology.* He has also contributed numerous articles to the literature of bioethics.

LEROY WALTERS is Director of the Center for Bioethics at the Kennedy Institute of Ethics and teaches in the Philosophy Department at Georgetown University. He is editor of the annual *Bibliography of Bioethics* and has published several essays on biomedical ethics and on war and morality.

MILTON C. WEINSTEIN teaches public policy at the John F. Kennedy School of Government, Harvard University, and is a member of the Center for the Analysis of Health Practices at the Harvard School of Public Health. He is coauthor of *Hypertension: A Policy Perspective* and *Clinical Decision Analysis,* as well as of several essays on the role of cost-effectiveness analysis in health policy.

DANIEL WIKLER is a member of the Program in Medical Ethics, Center for Health Sciences, and teaches in the Department of Philosophy at the University of Wisconsin, Madison. He has also served as staff philosopher for the President's Commission for the Study of Ethical Problems in Medicine and Biomedical and Behavioral Research. He has published several articles on bioethics, with special reference to the problems of paternalism and personal identity.

GLANVILLE WILLIAMS is a fellow of Jesus College and Rouse Ball Professor of the Laws of England at Cambridge University. He is a member of the Standing Committee on Criminal Law Revision and a prominent spokesperson for the movement to legalize voluntary euthanasia. He is author of *The Sanctity of Life and the Criminal Law, The Proof of Guilt,* and *The Mental Element in Crime.*